FLIGHT NURSING

Principles and Practice

FLIGHT NURSING

Principles and Practice

Second Edition

EDITED BY

Reneé Semonin Holleran

RN, PhD, CEN, CCRN, CFRN

Chief Flight Nurse
University Air Care
University of Cincinnati
Cincinnati, Ohio

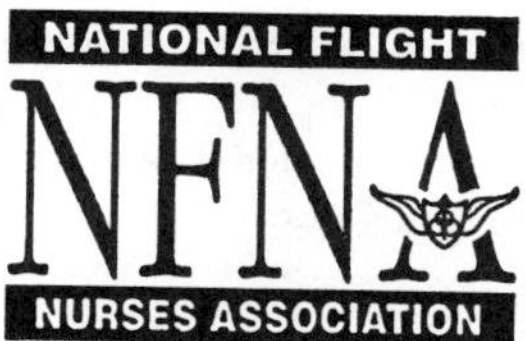

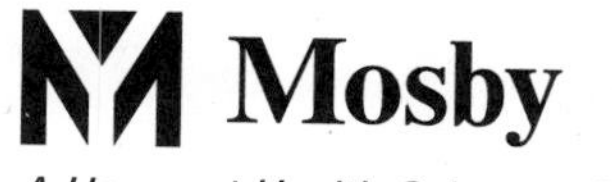

A Harcourt Health Sciences Company

St. Louis London Philadelphia Sydney Toronto

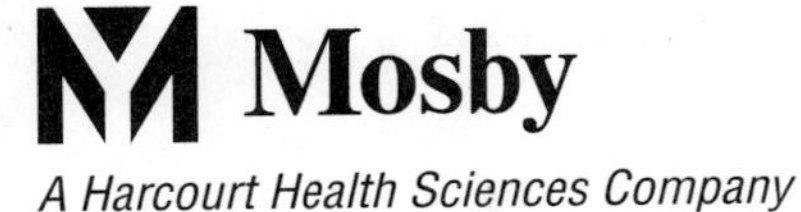

Publisher Nancy Coon
Senior Acquisitions Editor Sally Schrefer
Associate Developmental Editor Rae L. Robertson
Project Manager Linda McKinley
Production Editor Julie Zipfel
Designer Elizabeth Fett
Cover Design Sandy Cicotte

SECOND EDITION

The authors and publisher have exerted every effort to ensure that drug selection and dosage set forth in this text are in accord with current recommendations and practice at the time of publication. The reader is urged to check the package insert for each drug for any change in indications, dosage, warnings and precautions. This is particularly important when the drug is new or infrequently used.

Printed in the United States of America

Mosby, Inc.
11830 Westline Industrial Drive, St. Louis, Mo 63146

ISBN 0-8151-7471-3

00/9 8 7 6 5 4

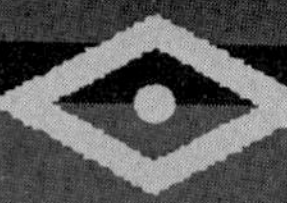

Contributors to the First Edition

WILLA ADELSTEIN, RN, MSN
Clinical Nurse Specialist, Neurosurgery
University Hospital & Clinics
Columbia, Missouri

LORRAINE ASTON-LINQUIST, RN, BS, CCRN
Flight Nurse, Staff for Life
St. Anthony Hospital Systems
Denver, Colorado

ALLISON L. BOLIN, RN, CEN, CCRN
Charge Nurse, Emergency Department
Community Hospital-Santa Cruz
Santa Cruz, California

DEBBIE BOWMAN, RN, BSN
Flight Nurse
State of Oklahoma Teaching Hospitals
Oklahoma City, Oklahoma

CYNTHIA SALE BRISTOL, RN, BSN, CEN
Flight Nurse, LifeSaver
Carraway Methodist Medical Center
Birmingham, Alabama

JEFFREY H. BROADY
Pilot, Mayo Aeromed
Denver, Colorado

CAPTAIN JAMES T. CANTRELL, R-EMT-P
Little Rock Fire Department
Little Rock, Arkansas

DEBORAH A. CHARLSON, RN, BSN
Trauma Coordinator
Washoe Medical Center
Reno, Nevada

TOM CHURCH, RN
Senior Division Director
Care Team, Health Care Service
Fort Worth, Texas

EDDI COHEN, RN, BS, MICN, CCRN, CFRN
Chief Flight Nurse
AIRescue International
Van Nuys, California;
Consultant
EMS Network International
Santa Monica, California

ROSE CORDER, RN, BSN, EMT-P
Assistant Nurse Manager
Hermann Hospital Life Flight
Houston, Texas

NANCY COWLES, RN, BSN
Former Flight Nurse, Flight for Life
Penrose-St. Francis Healthcare Systems
Colorado Springs, Colorado

JANET C. CUNNINGHAM, RN, MS
Pediatric Transport Nurse
Children's Emergency Transport Service
The Children's Hospital
Denver, Colorado

Rhys V. Dapar, MD
Resident, Emergency Medicine
Harbor-UCLA Medical Center
Torrance, California
NAUI #7617

ANNE F. DARGA, RN, MS, CCRN
Former Flight Nurse Specialist
University of Michigan Hospitals, Ann Arbor;
Clinical Nurse Specialist
Cardiology Division, Northern Michigan Hospital
Petoskey, Michigan

TOM DAVIS III
Pilot, Flight for Life
St. Anthony Hospital Systems
Denver, Colorado

CLYDE DeBELL
Mechanic, Flight for Life
St. Anthony Hospital Systems
Denver, Colorado

SUSAN DOUGLAS, RN, TNS, EMT
Life Flight
Georgia Baptist Medical Center
Atlanta, Georgia

J. SUSAN DOUGLASS, RN, CERTIFIED NEPHROLOGY NURSE
Educational Coordinator, Dialysis Unit
University of Michigan Medical Center
Ann Arbor, Michigan

GARY DROTAR
Pilot, Mayo Aeromed
Denver, Colorado

LYNN E. EASTES, RN, MS
Trauma Coordinator/Case Manager
Oregon Health Sciences University
Portland, Oregon

NANCY GRABOWSKI ELLIOTT, RN, BSN, MBA
National Board Member
Board of Directors, National Flight Nurses Association
Seattle, Washington

KIM EVERT, RN, BS, CCRN
Former Flight Nurse, Flight for Life
Penrose-St. Francis Healthcare Systems
Colorado Springs, Colorado

REBECCA J. YORI FEAGAN, RN, MS, CCRN
Unit Administrator, Surgical ICU
University of Colorado Health Sciences Center
Denver, Colorado

VANCE FEREBEE, RN, BSN, CEN, TNS, ADVANCED EMT
Life Flight
Georgia Baptist Medical Center
Atlanta, Georgia

MARY M. FREITAG-HAGNEY, RN, MSN
Nursing Manager, CVICU
St. Anthony Hospital Systems
Denver, Colorado

SANDRA GATES, RN, BSN
Nurse Manager
Hermann Hospital Life Flight
Houston, Texas

MARY BUSER GILLS, MS, RNC, NNP
Clinical Director
Children's Transport Service
The Children's Hospital
Denver, Colorado

MAGGIE GRIMES, RN, BSN, EMT-P
Clinical Specialist
Hermann Hospital Life Flight
Houston, Texas

WALT HINTON, RN, MS
Deputy Commander, Sheriff Air Medics
San Bernandino Sheriff's Department
Rialto, California

FORREST HOLDEN, MD
Emergency Medicine Consultants
Phoenix, Arizona

RENEÉ SEMONIN HOLLERAN, RN PhD, CEN, CCRN, CFRN
Chief Flight Nurse/Emergency Clinical Nurse Specialist
University Air Care
University of Cincinnati Medical Center
Cincinnati, Ohio

BUTCH IGNACIO, RN, BSN, TNS, CEN, EMT
Life Flight
Georgia Baptist Medical Center
Atlanta, Georgia

JOHN JORDAN, RN, BSN
Chief Flight Nurse
Mayo One, Mayo Foundation
St. Mary's Hospital
Rochester, Minnesota

EVA M. KLINE, RN, BSN
Cardiovascular Research Coordinator
Division of Cardiology
University of Michigan Hospitals
Ann Arbor, Michigan

HEATHER LIGHTFOOT, RN, CEN
Flight Nurse, UTMB Life Flight
University of Texas Medical Branch
Galveston, Texas

LESLEY LOOS, RN, CEN, CFRN, TNS
Flight Nurse, Staff for Life
University Hospital & Clinics
Columbia, Missouri

KATHLEEN MAYER, RN, BSN
Flight Nurse, Flight for Life
St. Anthony Hospital Systems
Denver, Colorado

TERRY McCRARY, RN, CCRN, TNS, EMT
Life Flight
Georgia Baptist Medical Center
Atlanta, Georgia

KEVIN MERIGIAN, MD
Medical Toxicology Consultants
Cincinnati, Ohio

MARY E. MITCHELL, RN, BSN, TNS, NREMT
Life Flight
Georgia Baptist Medical Center
Atlanta, Georgia

PAMELA C. MOORE, RN
Director, Pediatric Life Flight
Primary Children's Medical Center
Salt Lake City, Utah

BETTYE MORRIS, RN, TNS, EMT
Chief Flight Nurse, Life Flight
Georgia Baptist Medical Center
Atlanta, Georgia

DAVE NATHAN, BS, EMT-P
Firefighter-Paramedic
Birmingham Fire and Rescue Service
Assistant Chief Communications Technician
LifeSaver, Carraway Methodist Medical Center
Birmingham, Alabama

SHIRLEY NEVILLE, RN, BHS, CCRN, CFRN, CEN, TNS
Flight Nurse, Staff for Life
University Hospital & Clinics
Columbia, Missouri

CYNTHIA NEWTON, RN, TNS, EMT
Life Flight
Georgia Baptist Medical Center
Atlanta, Georgia

MARY ANN NIEHAUS, RN, MSN, CEN, REMT-P
Flight Nurse, University Air Care
University of Cincinnati Medical Center
Cincinnati, Ohio

EDWARD OTTEN, MD
Associate Professor
Director, Prehospital Care
University of Cincinnati Medical Center
Cincinnati, Ohio

PATRICIA A. RAILSBACK, RN, BSN, CCRN, CEN
Nursing Manager
Boston MedFlight
Boston, Massachusetts

BOB RUELL
Flight for Life
St. Anthony Hospital Systems
Denver, Colorado

SUSAN RUELL, BA, EMT
Dispatcher, Communications Center
St. Anthony Hospital Systems
Denver, Colorado

PATRICIA M. SCOTT, EMT
Formerly Mayo AeroMed
Denver, Colorado

GAIL D. SKINNER, RN, BSN
Perinatal Flight Nurse
Samaritan AirEvac
Phoenix, Arizona

DANIEL STORER, MD
Associate Professor
Medical Director, University Air Care
University of Cincinnati Medical Center
Cincinnati, Ohio

MARK SWICORD, RN, RNS, CEN, EMT
Life Flight
Georgia Baptist Medical Center
Atlanta, Georgia

KENDRA TJELMELAND, RN, BSN, CCRN
Research/QA Coordinator
Samaritan AirEvac
Phoenix, Arizona

NANCY TUNE, RN-C, BSN
Reengineering Specialist
Critical Care Educator
Boone Hospital Center
Columbia, Missouri

LORRAINE M. VUKICH, RN, MS, ARNP
Director, Trauma & Flight Services
University Medical Center
Jacksonville, Florida

RUSSELL R. WAGGONER, RN, BSN, CEN, EMT-P, IC
Flight Nurse Specialist
University of Michigan Medical Center
Ann Arbor, Michigan

CHRISTINE M. ZALAR, MA
Partner
Fitch & Associates, Inc.
Platte City, Missouri

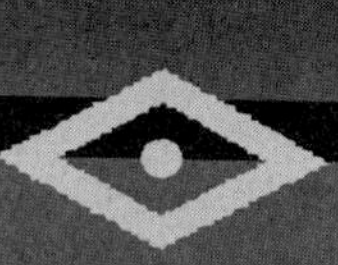

Contributors to the Second Edition

WILLA ADELSTEIN, RN, MSN
Clinical Nurse Specialist, Neurosurgery
University Hospital & Clinics
Columbia, Missouri

TONY BRIGHT, BS
Communications Supervisor
Administrative Assistant
University Air Care
University of Cincinnati Medical Center
Cincinnati, Ohio

KEVIN BROFORD
Line Pilot/Safety Committee Member
PHI Aeromedical Services
University Air Care
Cincinnati, Ohio

SALLY BRUSH, RN, CCRN
Chief Flight Nurse
IHC Life Flight
Intermountain Health Care
Salt Lake City, Utah

EDDI COHEN, RN, BS, MICN, CCRN, CFRN
Chief Flight Nurse
AIRescue International
Van Nuys, California;
Consultant
EMS Network International
Santa Monica, California

TOM CULWELL, RN, BSN, CEN, CCRN, CFRN, EMT-P
Regional Chief Flight Nurse
Critical Air Medicine
San Antonio, Texas

JANET C. CUNNINGHAM, RN, MS
Pediatric Transport Nurse
Children's Emergency Transport Service
The Children's Hospital
Denver, Colorado

LYNN E. EASTES, RN, MS
Trauma Coordinator/Case Manager
Oregon Health Sciences University
Portland, Oregon

MIKE ENGLEBERT
Lead Pilot
PHI Aeromedical Services
University Air Care
Cincinnati, Ohio

CHERYL J. ERLER, RN, MS
Associate Professor
Purdue University
School of Nursing
West Lafayette, Indiana

ILONA FRANCIS, MS, RNC, NNP
Neonatal Nurse Practitioner
Children's Transport Service
The Children's Hospital
Denver, Colorado

MARY BUSER GILLS, MS, RNC, NNP
Clinical Director
Children's Transport Service
The Children's Hospital
Denver, Colorado

JEANETTE GOLTERMANN, RN, MBA, CFRN
Flight Nurse
Loyola Life Star
Maywood, Illinois

SUE HAGER, RN
Flight Nurse
Survival Flight
University of Michigan Medical Center
Ann Arbor, Michigan

KAREN JOHNSON, RN
Flight Nurse
Samaritan Air Evac
Phoenix, Arizona

LESLEY LOOS, RN, CEN, CFRN, TNS
Flight Nurse, Staff for Life
University Hospital & Clinics
Columbia, Missouri

LAURA LOWE, RN, CCRN, EMT
Flight Nurse, Staff for Life
University Hospital & Clinics
Columbia, Missouri

NEMA McELVEEN, RN, CCRN
Flight Nurse
Lifestar Inc.
Savannah, Georgia

HEATHER McLELLAN, RN, BN, CFRN
Medical Operations Manager
STARS
Calgary, Alberta

SHIRLEY NEVILLE, RN, BHS, CCRN, CFRN, CEN, TNS
Flight Nurse, Staff for Life
University Hospital & Clinics
Columbia, Missouri

MICHELLE NORTH
Director of Safety
Rocky Mountain Helicopters
Sacramento, California

EILEEN PATTON, RN, BHS, CCRN, CEN, TNS, EMT-P
Assistant Manager, Staff for Life
University Hospital & Clinics
Columbia, Missouri

NANCY P. VON ROTZ, RN, MSN
Flight Nurse
University Air Care
University of Cincinnati Medical Center
Cincinnati, Ohio

NANCY PROSSER, RN, BSN, CEN
Flight Nurse
University Air Care
University of Cincinnati Medical Center
Cincinnati, Ohio

MICHAEL ROUSE, RN, BSN, CFRN
Flight Nurse
University Air Care
University of Cincinnati Medical Center
Cincinnati, Ohio

LEEANN RUNYAN, RN, CCRN
Flight Nurse, Staff for Life
University Hospital & Clinics
Columbia, Missouri

MICHAEL SNYDER
Flight Nurse
Survival Flight
University of Michigan Medical Center
Ann Arbor, Michigan

MICHAEL SPADAFORA, MD
Assistant Professor of Emergency Medicine
Director, Hyperbaric Medicine
University of Cincinnati
Center for Emergency Care
Cincinnati, Ohio

FRANK THOMAS, MD
Medical Director
IHC Life Flight
Intermountain Health Care
Salt Lake City, Utah

RICHARD S. TOBIASZ, RN, BS, CEN, CCRN, CFRN, EMT-P
Chief Flight Nurse
Flight for Life
Northern Illinois Medical Center
McHenry, Illinois

NANCY TUNE, RN-C, BSN
Reengineering Specialist
Critical Care Educator
Boone Hospital Center
Columbia, Missouri

RUSSELL R. WAGGONER, RN, BSN, CEN, EMT-P, IC
Flight Nurse Specialist
University of Michigan Medical Center
Ann Arbor, Michigan

CHRISTOPHER WAGNER, RN, CEN, CCRN, EMT-P
Flight Nurse
Survival Flight
University of Michigan Medical Center
Ann Arbor, Michigan

JANET WILLIAMS, RN, MSN, CCRN
Flight Nurse
University Air Care
University of Cincinnati Medical Center
Cincinnati, Ohio

JUDY WILSON, RNC, BSN
Maternal Transport Coordinator
Barnes Hospital
BJC Health Systems
St. Louis, Missouri

CHERYL WRAA, RN, BSN, CFRN
Flight Nurse, Clinical Resource Nurse
Life Flight
University of California, Davis Medical Center
Sacramento, California

DONNA YORK, RN, MS, CFRN
Chief Flight Nurse/Nurse Manager
Stanford Life Flight/Medical Transport Program
Stanford Health Services
San Francisco, California

LINDA YOUNG, RN, MNA
Manager CQI/Research
Samaritan AirEvac
Phoenix, Arizona

CHRISTINE M. ZALAR, MA
Partner
Fitch & Associates, Inc.
Platte City, Missouri

Dedication

The second edition of *Flight Nursing: Principles and Practice* is dedicated first to my family, Micke, Erin, and Sara, who despite all the time that nursing takes in my life, still love me. I also have to mention someone who has been the backbone of our program, Jane Swaim. Know that because of you, we are all better nurses today.

Finally, this book is dedicated to the flight nurses of the past, present, and future . . . and to those who have paid the ultimate price for their dedication to patient care by losing their lives trying to save others, as our friend Sandy Sigman did in July 1994.

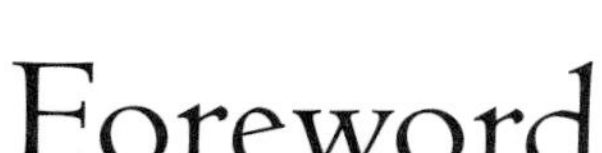

Foreword

This year, 1996, is the National Flight Nurses Association's 15-year anniversary. Flight nursing is a unique specialty performed in a unique environment, with the flight nurse being an integral part of the out-of-hospital transport team. Our role has developed and changed throughout the years, with transport teams expected to care for all ages of critically ill and injured patients. Due to our uniqueness, NFNA recognized the need and developed this comprehensive textbook for flight nurses. In this revision we have once again asked many flight nurses to contribute their expertise to this text. I would personally like to thank everyone for their time, effort, and commitment to this project.

Special thanks to my dear friend and mentor, Reneé Semonin Holleran, for her time, energy, and tenacity exhibited as editor. I would also like to acknowledge NFNA's founders Jean Mason, Marcia Katz, Sally Nielson, and Pat Noonan. Last but not least, I would like to recognize all the flight nurses around the world for their dedication to excellence in the care and safe transport of patients.

CHERYL WRAA
1996-1997
President
National Flight Nurses Association

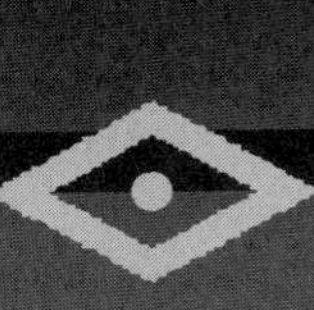

Preface

The National Flight Nurses Association recognized the need for a comprehensive textbook for flight nurses and in 1991 published the first edition of *Flight Nursing: Principles and Practice.* During the years since its publication, the practice of flight nursing has continued to grow and evolve, just as the knowledge that is required to provide patient care before, during, and after transport has increased.

The second edition of *Flight Nursing: Principles and Practice* has been written to carry on the tradition of the first. However, some new chapters and the clinical information and case studies have been updated. Once again, this book was written by practicing flight nurses. Included in this edition are the roles of others who are also an integral part of our flight programs.

The first six chapters of *Flight Nursing: Principles and Practice* include chapters on the role of the flight nurse, flight physiology, extrication and scene management, disaster management, communications, and safety. A portion also contains detailed information about fixed wing transport. Patient care is covered in Chapters 7 through 10. This includes new chapters on patient assessment, preparation of the patient for transport, and patient care issues such as needs of the family and death and dying. The airway and shock chapters have been rewritten and expanded.

Chapters 11 through 18 include chapters related to trauma, and Chapters 19 through 26 address medical emergencies. Chapter 25, which addresses infectious disease, includes information about universal precautions during transport, reporting of infectious exposures, and current treatments. Chapters 27 through 31 incorporate environmental emergencies. Gynecologic, obstetric, and neonatal care are discussed in Chapters 32 through 34.

Finally, Chapters 35 through 37 deal with issues related to air medical management such as risk management, continuous quality management, and marketing. Chapter 38 describes the sources of stress and its management in the air medical environment.

Each clinical chapter ends with a case study. The majority of these are new challenges that have been faced by practicing flight nurses. The contributors have drawn on their own clinical expertise in flight nursing to illustrate pertinent issues related to each clinical situation. The format for each case study varies to allow the individual style of the author.

The writing of the second edition of *Flight Nursing* was achieved through the efforts of the original authors and new authors who are experts with a deep commitment to flight nursing. Just as in the first edition, this second edition represents their contribution and commitment to flight nursing and the National Flight Nurses Association.

ACKNOWLEDGMENTS

The second edition of this book would not have been possible without the work of those who wrote and edited the first edition—particularly Genell Lee. The people who assisted in the work of this second edition include Cheryl Wraa, Jeanette Goltermann, and Mike Rouse.

I would personally like to thank Sally Schrefer for her help in identifying what would make this book better and Rae Robertson, who coordinated all the material, which has come in from all over the United States.

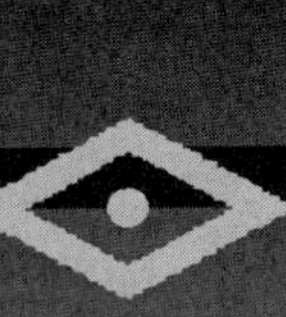

Introduction to the First Edition

In 1980 a steering committee of four flight nurses met to consider the development of a national organization for flight nurses. The members of the steering committee were Jean Mason, R.N., of LifeFlight, Hermann Hospital, Houston, Texas; Marcia Katz, R.N. of LifeFlight, St. Joseph's Hospital, Omaha, Nebraska; Sally Nielson, R.N., of Aircare, University of Iowa Hospital, Iowa City, Iowa; and Pat Noonan, R.N. of Aircare, West Jefferson General Hospital, Marerro, Louisiana. After a year of developing bylaws, the organization was founded in 1981. Jean Mason was elected the first President of the National Flight Nurses Association.

The initial goals established by the organization were:

1. To promote the delivery of quality care to patients.
2. To develop minimum training standards for flight nurses.
3. To develop minimum standards of care for flight nurses.
4. To share flight nursing knowledge.
5. To provide hospitals considering emergency air service programs with assistance in developing appropriate programs.
6. To promote continuing education for all flight crews.
7. To promote quality assurance.
8. To develop and promote optimum working conditions for all flight nurses.

During the first year, the *Flight Nurse Newsletter,* edited by John Jordan, was started. Rose Corder developed the NFNA philosophy (see p. XIX) and Bill Swanson designed the NFNA Logo (see p. XX).

The NFNA will celebrate its 10-year anniversary in 1991. The textbook *Flight Nursing: Principles and Practice* is a culmination of five years of effort on the part of members of NFNA. Its intent is to advance the goals and objectives of the National Flight Nurses Association. This book is dedicated to the efforts and accomplishments of flight nurses past, present, and future.

GENELL LEE, R.N., M.S.N., CEN
Editor-In-Chief

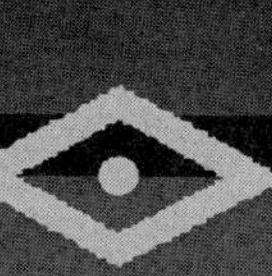

Introduction to the Second Edition

Since the publication of the first edition of *Flight Nursing: Principles and Practice* more than 5 years ago, flight nursing has seen many changes. In 1994 the first flight nursing certification examination was offered. With the creation of the CFRN (Certified Flight Registered Nurse), a core curriculum has been developed and the need for a textbook that specifically contains information about the practice of flight nursing has emerged.

Even though flight nursing continues to evolve, we are not immune to the changes that face the health care system today. We need to continue to demonstrate the need for nursing to be a member of the transport team. We need to be aware of the roles of those we work with and how to foster the collegiality that will see us through difficult times.

Flight nursing is both an art and a science. This text encompasses the unique role of the flight nurse in patient care.

RENEÉ SEMONIN HOLLERAN,
RN, PhD, CEN, CCRN, CFRN

National Flight Nurses Association Organization Philosophy

The National Flight Nurses Association (NFNA) is defined by its bylaws and mission as a volunteer membership organization of professional nurses who practice flight nursing. Flight nursing is a unique and expanded role for a professional nurse that encompasses the air medical transport of critically ill and injured patients. This role is characterized by expanded nursing practice based on the ever-growing body of flight nursing knowledge and the NFNA standards.

The NFNA is the dominant and leading body representing flight nurses as the voice of clinical care in the air medical field with regard to patient and provider advocacy. Its leadership shall be representative of those professional nurses meeting membership criteria.

The NFNA's activities are performed in a manner exemplifying a service ethic and orientation toward the membership these activities are focused on supporting, serving, and facilitating communication among professional nurses who practice or are actively involved in the support, education, and/or management of flight nurses.

MISSION STATEMENT

The National Flight Nurses Association is a nonprofit member organization whose mission is to represent, promote, and provide guidance to professional nurses who practice the unique and distinct specialty of flight nursing.

GOALS

I. Provide leadership for the unique and distinct specialty of flight nursing.
II. Facilitate and provide opportunities for communication and collaboration among flight nurses.
III. Provide representation and networking through forums that support or relate to the practice of flight nursing.
IV. Support and promote scientific research that expands and enhances flight nursing knowledge and/or medical patient care.
V. Promote continuing education related to flight nursing practice.
VI. Serve as an information resource about flight nursing and air medical care delivery systems.

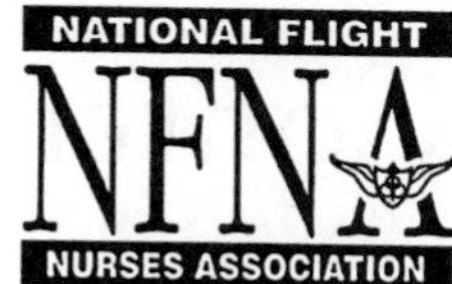

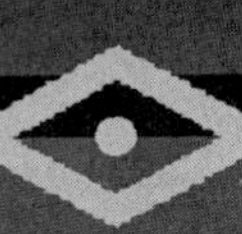

Contents

CHAPTER 1

The Role of the Flight Nurse

Flight nursing provides the opportunity to practice nursing outside the hospital. Historically, nursing outside of the hospital has taken place through the administration of public health and social services. In addition, nurses have played an important role in the care of war casualties, dating from the days of Florence Nightingale to the recent Gulf War.[7]

Flight nursing requires a broad clinical experience with emergency and critical care nursing. Flight nurses work collaboratively with a number of other health care providers, including other nurses, physicians, and prehospital care providers. Depending on the type of flight program, flight nurses' partners may be paramedics, other registered nurses, physicians, or respiratory therapists.[1] The air medical team includes the flight nurse and his or her partner and a medical director, program management, pilots, mechanics, and communication specialists.

The role of the flight nurse is multifaceted and often depends on where the flight nurse works. The responsibilities of the flight nurse include clinical practice, patient advocacy and education, research, and management. Because of these varied functions, the practice requires that flight nurses continue their education, practice skill competencies, and be active in their professional organizations.

The purpose of this chapter is to discuss the history of flight nursing, describe the preparation for flight nursing practice, and address flight nursing interactions with those who provide collaborative patient care before, during, and after transport.

HISTORICAL PERSPECTIVE

The word *nursing* is derived from the Latin word *nutrire,* to nourish.[1] Florence Nightingale is considered the founder of modern nursing practice and was one of the original nurses practicing in the "field."[1] In 1854, Florence Nightingale was put in charge of the Female Nursing Establishment of the English General Hospitals in Turkey during the Crimean War. Within 6 months, the death rate in the military hospitals went from 47% to 2.2% under her leadership. She went to the front lines and visited and cared for the ill and injured until she became ill with Crimean Fever and was sent back to England. Her work during the Crimean War laid the foundation of prehospital nursing practice.

The Civil War in the United States furnished nurses with an opportunity to demonstrate their skills and administer care to ill and injured soldiers. Nurses served in volunteer corps during the Civil War, offering care to both the Union and Confederate Armies.

Clara Barton emerged as the symbol of nursing's philosophy to meet the health needs of all humans, regardless of race, creed, or color. She was an outspoken opponent of slavery and she gave care on the battlefield to Northerners, Southerners, blacks, and whites.[7] She went on to establish the American Red Cross in 1882. Many flight nurses today are MAT (Mobile Assist Teams) nurses, who play an integral role in delivering care to victims of disasters.

In the twentieth century, nurses have been active participants in World War I, World War II, the Korean and Vietnam Wars, and more recently the Gulf War. Hospitals known as Mobile Army Surgical Hospitals (MASH) and Medical Unit Self-contained Transportable (MUST) have been staffed by nurses, physicians, and corpsman only miles from the battle front. The war experiences of the twentieth century have shown that field stabilization and rapid transport can decrease mortality and morbidity rates. Nurses have played a significant role in the delivery of care in the field, particularly through flight nursing.

The origin of flight nursing can be traced to Laureate M. Schimmoler, who formed the Emergency Flight Corps in 1933. The name of the group was later changed to the Aerial Nurse Corps of America.[11] The first public appearance of the Aerial Nurse Corps was at the National Air Races in 1936 in Los Angeles. During this event, these flight nurses provided field hospitals.[11]

Through the influence of Ms. Schimmoler, the military opened its first flight nurse training program in 1942 at the 349th Air Evacuation Group, Bowman Field, Kentucky. This program, which was moved to Texas in 1944, required that the nurse take 6 weeks of training including flight physiology.

During World War II, more than 1.5 million patients were transported by fixed-wing aircraft with educated flight nurses in attendance.[11] After WW II, flight nurse training was conducted by the Air Force. Flight nurses were activated for service during both the Korean and Vietnam Wars.

During the Korean and Vietnam Wars, the value of helicopter transport of the injured was recognized. Many of the physicians, nurses, and corpsmen who spent time in these wars felt that there was a role for helicopter transport in the civilian care of those who were injured or needed to be transported to another care facility.[8]

In 1972, St. Anthony's Hospital in Denver established a civilian-based flight program staffed by nurses with critical care experience. Herman Hospital in Houston, Texas established a flight program in 1976 and added the physician to the flight team.

During the 1980s, there was a boom in the development of hospital-based programs. At one point, there were more than 220 programs. The primary crew member is a registered nurse with either emergency or critical care nursing experience. Other members of the flight team include paramedics, other registered nurses, physicians, and respiratory therapists (Fig. 1-1). Some flight programs continue to offer specialized flight teams such as maternal or neonatal.

The practice of flight nursing evolved from the role of nursing care in the field and continues to develop based on the type of patients who require transport today. Because of the variety of health needs encountered, flight nurses must be prepared to

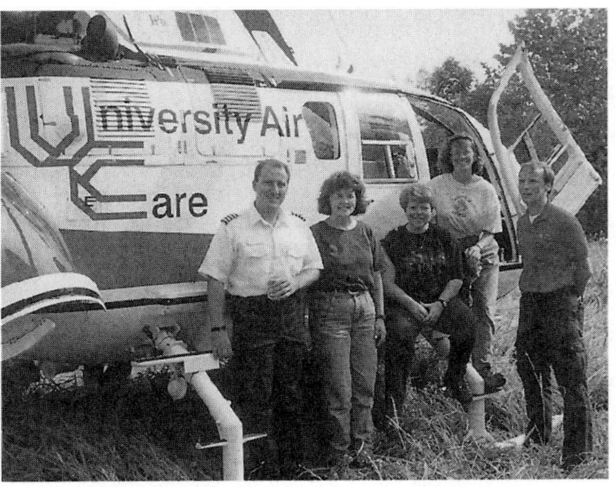

Fig. 1-1 An example of a flight crew. (Courtesy University Air Care, Cincinnati, Ohio.)

provide care in diverse situations. The following section discusses preparation for flight nursing practice.

PREPARATION FOR PRACTICE

The goals of patient transport[6] are to maintain adequate tissue oxygenation; replace lost fluids and/or blood and blood products; immobilize injured body parts; and to deliver early, definitive care such as the administration of thrombolytic therapy, mehthylprednisone for spinal cord injury, or administration of cerebral resuscitative drugs. The education, skills, and experience needed to provide this care before and during transport must be diverse and comprehensive.

The Emergency Nurses Association (ENA) and the National Flight Nurses Association (NFNA) released a joint position paper in 1987 that described the role of nursing in the prehospital environment. This paper was updated in 1995. Essentially, both organizations believe that nurses who practice in the prehospital care environment need to be appropriately educated to function successfully in that role, and that practice should be regulated by state boards of nursing in the state where the flight nurse practices. A summary of this position paper is contained in the box.

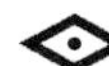

SUMMARY OF THE ENA/NFNA POSITION STATEMENT: THE ROLE OF THE NURSE IN THE PREHOSPITAL CARE ENVIRONMENT

1. ENA and NFNA endorse a collaborative role for specially prepared nurses in the delivery of prehospital care.
2. ENA and NFNA believe that a registered nurse who has received the appropriate knowledge and demonstrated skill proficiency related to prehospital care activities need not become certified as an EMT.
3. ENA and NFNA *do* endorse the need for special educational requirements for nurses practicing in the prehospital care environment.
4. ENA and NFNA believe that the practice of the prehospital care nurse should be based on the use of the nursing process, which includes assessment; formulation of nursing diagnoses, expected outcomes, and a plan of care; evaluation of interventions rendered; collaboration and coordination with others involved with the patient's care; and communication to the receiving facility.
5. ENA and NFNA believe the role of the nurse in prehospital care includes practice, research, education, management, consultation, advocacy, and administrative responsibilities.
6. ENA and NFNA believe that the practice of prehospital nursing should be regulated by state boards of nursing in the state in which each individual nurse practices.

From ENA and NFNA: Role of the registered nurse in the prehospital environment, *Emergency Nurses Association Position Statement*, 1995, Park Ridge, Ill.

Brader et al[1] conducted a national survey to discover the characteristics of flight nursing practice. Their study found that one third of the flight nurses who participated in the flight programs were prepared at the baccalaureate level (BSN) and had 10 to 15 years of nursing experience. Most flight nurses had either emergency or critical care experience, had completed a trauma course, and were certified in PALS, PHTLS/BTLS, and in emergency nursing (CEN). If the flight nurses were members of a professional organization, they belonged to the NFNA or NFNA and ENA.[1]

Currently, there are three curriculums that outline the recommended education and skills needed to practice flight nursing. These are the *Flight Nurse Advanced Trauma Course* from the NFNA; the *Air Medical Crew National Curriculum* from the U.S. Department of Transportation, and the *National Standard Guidelines for Prehospital Nursing* from the ENA. The NFNA has published standards of practice that provide the flight nurse with a framework for flight nursing practice.[9] The box on p. 4 contains a description of the professionalism standards for flight nurses. The performance standards are summarized in Chapter 35.

In 1994, the first flight nursing certification examination was administered. The certified flight reg-

PROFESSIONALISM STANDARDS

1. The flight nurse practices autonomously within the scope of practice defined by each institution.
2. The flight nurse practices in accordance with their state Nurse Practice Acts, state regulations governing prehospital care, NFNA standards, and policies and procedures set forth by medical direction and their institution.
3. The flight nurse assumes responsibility and accountability for their actions.
4. The flight nurse identifies self to patients, significant others, and health care providers.
5. The flight nurse participates in the education of the health care team, clients and their significant others, and the community.

From Hepp H: *National flight nurses standards of flight nursing practice,* St Louis, 1995, Mosby.

istered nurse (CFRN) examination now provides flight nurses with a mechanism of verifying their body of knowledge related to the practice of flight nursing. The advent of the CFRN produced the flight nursing core curriculum, published in 1996, and the initiation of a role delineation study to describe the practice of flight nursing. This study is to be completed in 1997.

The lack of a uniform curriculum and the fact that a flight nurse's job description varies from program to program has led to some controversy as to what kind of preparation is requisite for a flight nurse. A study conducted by Johnson et al[10] found that 44 out of the 50 states had no certification for nurses practicing in the prehospital care environment. In some states, nurses need both an RN and EMT license to practice outside of the hospital. Nurses are required to take the entire EMT course in 61% of the states. The remaining states allow for some type of challenge examination and educational courses to meet the EMT requirements. The researchers found that only 6 states actually had a certification for prehospital nursing.

Some states have prehospital care courses that act as bridge courses for nurses to meet the requirements for EMT and paramedic certification. An example of this is the Prehospital Nursing Course (PNC) that has been proposed in Maryland.[13] The PNC contains various modules related to prehospital care and all but four of these modules could be challenged by nurses. The modules that each nurse is required to complete are disaster/triage, rescue/extrication, vehicle operation, and orientation/role socialization.

There is no question that flight nurses should be prepared to function in the prehospital care environment, particularly if they are first responders. Even if flight nurses are not first responders, they still must be familiar with both the potential hazards of scene work and how to keep themselves and their patients safe.

Bader et al[1] found that flight nursing practice consists of both critical care and emergency nursing skills. The procedures that flight nurses performed included intubation, thoracentesis, cricothyroidotomy, escharotomy, intraosseous insertion, cutdowns, chest tube insertion, central line insertion, birthing delivery, and transport of patients with intraaortic balloon pumps in place. The ability to perform the skills necessary to carry out these procedures depends on the flight team, medical direction, and state boards of nursing.

Learning technical skills and remaining competent in these skills can be accomplished through laboratory practice and supervision of patient care. Many flight programs require that a specific number of procedures be completed in a designated period of time. The box contains a summary of some of the procedures performed by flight nurses.

Critical thinking skills constitute one of the most important interventions flight nurses bring to air medical transport. Flight nurses constantly question, analyze, and evaluate the whole transport process. Critical thinking involves the use of knowledge and skills to explore practice situations.[12] Critical thinking skills include the ability of the flight nurse to be

SUMMARY OF SKILLS FOR FLIGHT NURSING PRACTICE

Airway Management

1. Intubation
   - Oral
   - Nasotracheal
   - Digital/manual
2. Cricothyroidotomy
   - Needle
   - Surgical
3. End-tidal CO_2 monitoring
4. Pulse oximetry

Ventilation Management

1. Needle decompression
2. Chest tube insertion
3. Open thoracotomy—assisting
4. Pericardiocentesis
5. Ventilator management

Circulation Management

1. Vascular access
   - Central line placement
   - Venous cannulation
   - Arterial cannulation
   - Intraosseous line placement
   - Seldinger technique
2. Medication administration
   - Fluids
   - Blood
   - Blood products
   - Vasoactive drugs
   - Experimental drugs
3. Intraaortic balloon pump management
4. Pacing devices
   - Internal
   - External
5. Vital sign monitors
6. Invasive line monitors
   - Blood pressure
   - Pulmonary catheters
   - Intracranial monitors
7. Urinary catheters
8. Nasogastric catheters
9. ECG monitors
10. 12-lead ECG monitors
11. Temperature management
12. Wound care
    - Control of hemorrhage
    - Protection from contamination

Additional Skills

1. Pain management during transport
   - Movement
   - Motion sickness
2. Emotional care
3. Family care

autonomous and organized, and to view practice situations in an in-depth, comprehensive way to better understand what is happening to the air medical patient.[12] This unique competence was identified in Bader et al,[1] who stated that flight nurses were held accountable for these complex skills. "These complex skills included decisions regarding the administration and titration of medications, initiating therapeutic treatment based on physical assessment findings, communicating and documenting significant findings and performing follow-up activities."[1]

Flight nursing requires experience, education, and continuous evaluation of competence. Flight nurses must be physically and mentally fit to meet the demands of patient care during transport.[17] Although there are some general characteristics of flight nursing, overall, the responsibilities of a flight nurse depend on the type of service provided, the crew partner, the type of aircraft in which the crew functions, and state regulations including state boards of nursing. The following box summarizes educational preparation for flight nursing practice.[16]

SUMMARY OF EDUCATIONAL REQUIREMENTS FOR THE FLIGHT NURSE

Registered nurse (some programs require multiple licensure when providing care across the state line)
Advanced cardiac life support (ACLS)
Pediatric advanced life support (PALS)
Emergency nursing pediatric course (ENPC)
Prehospital care orientation course (determined by state EMS agency)
or
Prehospital registered nurse course
or
EMT/EMT-P certification
Certification in a nursing specialty
- Certified emergency nurse (CEN)
- Certified critical care nurse (CCRN)
- Certified flight registered nurse (CFRN)

Trauma course
- Basic trauma life support (BTLS)
- Prehospital trauma life support (PHTLS)
- Advanced trauma life support (ATLS)
- Flight nurse advanced trauma course (FNATC)
- Trauma nursing core course (TNCC)

MEMBERS OF THE FLIGHT TEAM

To reemphasize the earlier discussion, flight nursing practice is collaborative. The flight nurse is a part of a team, with the nurse's most common partner being a paramedic.[1] Other members of the team include the medical director, pilots, mechanics, program management, and communications specialists. The following discussion deals with the role of some of these other team members.

Air Medical Physician Roles

Traditionally, the training of a physician differs from that of a nurse. Physician training includes 4 years of premedical school, 4 years of medical school, a residency program that varies from 3 to 5 years, and a possible fellowship, which also varies in length from 2 to 3 years. Much of a physician's training centers around an understanding of basic science and differential diagnosis of disease processes. The physician team member can make a significant contribution to the care of the air medical patient. Because of their training, physicians can be of great assistance in delineating the causes and therefore the required treatment of a medical condition.

A physician involved in an air medical transport program can function in one of three roles: (1) as a physician flight crew member, (2) for control of medical direction, or (3) as the physician medical director.

The Flight Physician

Six percent of the flight programs in existence today routinely use a physician as a crew member.[5] Only 18% of these physicians are full-time employees of the hospital or flight program. Forty-three percent of these physicians are in a residency program.

The need for or benefit of having a physician as a flight team member has been and continues to be a highly debated subject.[2,15] The level of expertise of flight physicians varies from that of an intern, who is in training, to that of a well-experienced, well-seasoned, board-certified physician specialist.[3] The selection of physician experience depends on the specific program. Unlike the flight nurse certification examination (CFRN), flight physicians have no available certification test.

As a flight crew member, the physician is often, but not necessarily, delegated as the final medical authority. Further, because a physician is routinely on board an aircraft, it may be less necessary to have medical protocols, or standing orders, in existence.

Medical Direction

In programs where flight physicians are not used, control of medical direction of the flight team is often provided by assigning a physician on-line responsibility for the actions of the flight team. This **medical direction physician** has the responsibility of overseeing that appropriate medical backup is available for the non-physician flight team.[14]

Proper medical direction occurs when the physician does one of the following: (1) makes inquiry to the patient's medical condition from the referring institution and relays that information to the flight team, or (2) provides on-line advice to the flight team.

The overall goal of medical direction is to ensure that the appropriate mode of transport (i.e., helicopter vs. fixed wing vs. ground), proper team (i.e., adult vs. neonatal vs. pediatric), and equipment (i.e., ALS, BLS, specialized) are provided to meet the patient's medical requirements.

The Physician Medical Director

The physician medical director has several roles as a team member of the medical flight crew. Specifically, these roles include the following: (1) establishing medical protocols, (2) ensuring adequate training, and (3) providing medical support and advice for problems that may arise during the delivery of medical care by flight crew personnel.

Establishing Medical Protocols For the transport service that does not routinely use physicians as flight team members, the medical director is responsible for establishing medical protocols that enable flight nurses to initiate care and treatment outside their hospital-based nursing practice. These protocols enable the flight nurse to engage in the diagnosis, treatment, and initiation of special procedures which, in the past, have been designated as the responsibility of a physician. This is not to say that the air medical physician director is not responsible for writing these protocols, but rather that the air medical physician is ultimately responsible for the content and accuracy of these protocols. When confusion in treatment results, the team members in conjunction with the medical director should develop new policies and protocols that govern future medical care.

Ensuring Adequate Training The medical director must develop training that ensures that the flight nurses meet an expected level of medical care. This training can occur prospectively, such as in the introduction courses to flight nursing which include training on altitude physiology, medical protocols, and medical procedures. In addition to the initial training, the medical director must provide continuous training and updating of the flight nurses regarding new innovations in patient care. Often this education occurs during flight nursing meetings where new information can be presented.

Finally, a retrospective analysis of patient care should occur in the weekly or monthly flight meetings. At this time, patient charts are reviewed and reinforcement of current policies and procedures is made. In addition, particular problems that may have arisen from these policies and procedures are presented. The discussion that ensues allows all flight team members an opportunity to develop the best possible method for patient care in the future.

Medical Support The physician must serve as the sounding board and provide medical support to the flight crew members. This may be done pretransport so the physician can provide the flight crew member with valuable information regarding the patient's status and with possible diagnostic or therapeutic suggestions. This support can also be provided during the transport, when the flight nurse recognizes that additional medical input may be beneficial in diagnosing or providing care to the patient.

Most counsel is done posttransport. In these situations, the flight crew may wish to discuss the possible diagnostic and therapeutic options related to the patient's condition. Such interactions are beneficial because the flight crew member gains additional insight and the medical director recognizes any need for additional flight team training.

Conflict with the Physician

Conflict can arise among flight crew members, particularly when a flight nurse and a physician disagree about patient treatment. Most often, such conflict is a result of a difference in perspectives. When such conflicts occur, the flight nurse and the physician should work together to resolve the issue. Physicians must attempt to understand flight nurses' concerns as they relate to the delivery of patient care. Likewise, the flight nurse must recognize that the physician may have a different perspective of the issue as it relates to patient treatment. The best patient care results from a collaborative effort between the flight nurse and the physician.

Physicians may participate in the transport process in a number of ways. They may be crew members, provide on-line medical direction, or serve as a medical director. Flight nurses and physicians in collaboration provide patients with the highest quality of care.

The Flight Paramedic

More than 50% of flight services operate with a nurse and paramedic crew.[1] Most flight nurses and flight paramedics receive the same training and many perform the same skills; however, flight nurses are accountable for more complex skills, including administration and titration of certain medications, therapeutic interventions such as the management of an intraaortic balloon pump, and documentation and follow-up activities.[1] However, flight nurses and flight paramedics generally function well as a team.

The use of a flight nurse/paramedic team integrates experience from the hospital setting and the prehospital environment. The flight nurse has experience providing patient care in the context of the emergency or critical care unit and prioritizes patient needs based on this clinical background. When transporting patients from the ER or critical care unit, the flight nurse is typically more familiar with the patient's needs before and during transport, and therefore usually leads the nurse/paramedic team.[1,20]

Conversely, flight paramedics usually lead the prehospital transport because of their expertise in this environment. This is not to say that flight nurses and flight paramedics cannot learn or become accustomed to the unique features of each profession's area of practice, but rather that their experiences and respective areas of expertise enhance patient care during transport.

Nurse/paramedic flight teams have been found to be more cost effective than other flight teams. These flight teams have demonstrated that they can be taught skills such as neuromuscular blocking and chest tube insertion without undue complications.[4,18]

The major concern that has been voiced about the nurse/paramedic flight team is related to medical judgment. However, medical judgment can be acquired with experience,[1] use of medical protocols, and contacting medical control by radio or cellular telephone.

Flight nurse/paramedic teams are the most common kind of transport teams. These teams demonstrate that nurses and paramedics can work together and provide excellent patient care before and during patient transport.

Communication Specialists

As discussed in Chapter 7, communication is the first step in the transport process. The communication specialist is responsible for obtaining patient information, initiating the flight, flight following, and notification of appropriate personnel before, during, and after the transport process. In addition, many communication centers serve as contact areas for flight team members and their friends and family.

Chapter 5 and Chapter 7 discuss communication operations and the communication process. However, the flight nurse must always remember that the communication specialist is the "voice" of the flight team. The communication specialist must be treated as a flight team member and included in decision making and stress management.

Communication specialists play a major role in the transport process. They are integral members of the flight team (Fig. 1-2).

Flight Nurse and Pilot Interaction

Flight nurse and pilot interactions play a critical role in the performance of air medical teams. Team and organization level factors may enhance or impede the ability of well-trained individuals to work together effectively and efficiently. Each crew member's position must be clearly stated and defined. This es-

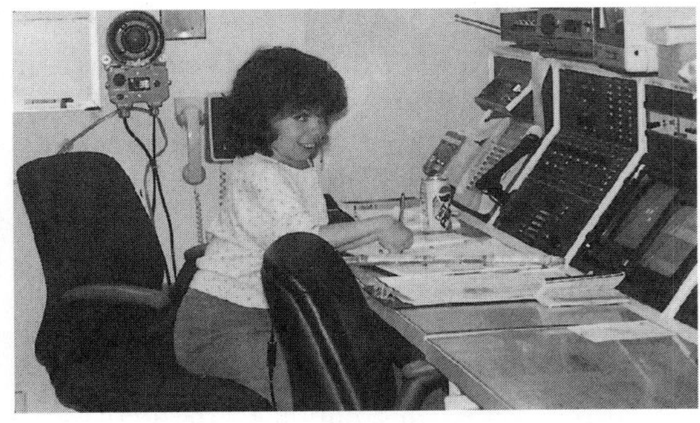

Fig. 1-2 The communication specialist is an integral part of the flight team. (Courtesy University Air Care, Cincinnati, Ohio.)

tablishes structure and determines the flow of communication.

The pilot-in-command (PIC) is the person responsible for the safety of the aircraft, crew, and passengers. The pilot is accountable for nonmedical aspects of the flight, and has final authority in all flight-related issues. Flight crew members assist in flight-related duties as outlined by the PIC. Flight nurses offer assistance in a variety of flight duties. Some of their contributions include air or ground traffic sightings; hazard and obstacle sightings; obstacle avoidance procedures (landing zones); securing cargo (medical equipment); briefing passengers; monitoring radios; and computation of weight and balance requirements.

It is the responsibility of the PIC to create an atmosphere in which crew participation can flourish. The PIC must help maintain a balanced, predictable environment, while responding to changing situations. This implies that shifts of balance will occur and that each crew member should understand that they have the responsibility to participate fully and professionally in every flight.

If the PIC has not succeeded in establishing a comfortable atmosphere of open participation, the flight nurse will not verbally communicate any concerns or discomforts. It is imperative that the PIC must establish clear leadership and command authority, and appropriately apply the use of authority based on the current situation. The pilot must command respect while at the same time create an atmosphere conducive to crew participation.

When time permits, the pilot may also assist the flight nurse by helping to load and unload patients. In addition, the pilot can transport needed medical equipment to the flight team and relay medical information to the receiving hospital.

The flight nurse and the pilot's association can have a positive or negative effect on risk management. Flight nurses are in a valuable position to observe the pilot and assist in making safe decisions. For example, if a pilot expresses concern about the weather, this may be an indication that the pilot does not feel entirely comfortable with all aspects of the flight. An appropriate response from the flight nurse would be to open an objective discussion of alternatives. An inappropriate response would be to indicate displeasure. Accidents have occurred when the pilot, after exhibiting concerns, was met with a negative response or just silence, signifying the desire of the flight crew to continue the flight.

The bond between established crew members and the air medical staff can become quite strong. There are eight goals for a successful relationship between the pilot and flight nurse. These are as follows:

1. Communicate positively
2. Direct assistance as needed
3. Announce decisions clearly
4. Offer assistance
5. Acknowledge the actions of others
6. Be specific
7. Know and understand the teams' aviation roles and responsibilities
8. Be vigilant in understanding the interaction between the crew members, the machine, and the environment

Program Director

In most flight programs, the program director is responsible for coordinating the activities of all systems that are a part of the flight service. The program director may be a flight nurse, physician, pilot, paramedic, or hospital administrator.[19]

The major responsibilities of the program director include[14] formulating administrative policies, directing continuous quality improvement activities, managing vehicle contracts and vendors, maintaining the communications system, preparing and monitoring components of the budget, participating in strategic planning and marketing, serving as a resource for problem solving, and serving as community liaison.

Each flight program dictates the role of the program director. It is important for the flight nurse to know and understand the director's role in the program and the organizational chart and how the flight team functions in the program.[19]

SUMMARY

Flight nursing originated through the work of nursing pioneers like Florence Nightingale and Clara

Barton, who became integral to patient care during the battles fought in the nineteenth century. As principles of flight nursing were incorporated into civilian care, hospital-based flight programs were started and staffed by nurses.

Flight nursing preparation requires experience, advanced skills, and additional education so that the nurse is able to function autonomously and in collaboration with all others who may be involved in the transport process. Flight nursing involves the ability to work with others in a variety of clinical situations. It involves dedication to the profession of nursing and an ability to care for others in diverse and sometimes difficult situations.

REFERENCES

1. Bader G et al: Characteristics of flight nursing practice, *Air Med J* 14(4):214, 1995.
2. Baxt W, Moody P: The impact of a physician as part of the aeromedical pre-hospital team in patients with blunt trauma, *JAMA* 257(23):3246-3250, 1987.
3. Baxt W, Moody P, Ireland HC: Hospital-based rotorcraft aeromedical emergency care services and transport: a multicenter study, *Ann Emerg Med* 14(9):859, 1985.
4. Campbell P: Flight nurse practice: what is the governing body? *J Emerg Nurs* 13(4):198, 1987.
5. Cody G: 1994 air medical program survey, *Air Med J* 13: 9, 1994.
6. Colardyn F: Delivering critical care: a challenge, *J Emerg Med* 11(1):37, 1993.
7. Donahue P: *Nursing: the finest art,* ed 2, St Louis, 1996, Mosby.
8. Hackel A: *History of medical transport systems.* In McClosky K, Orr R, editors: *Pediatric transport medicine,* St Louis, 1995, Mosby.
9. Hepp H: *National Flight Nurses Association standards of flight nursing practice,* St Louis, 1995, Mosby.
10. Johnson R et al: Regulation of prehospital nursing practice: a national survey, *J Emerg Nurs* 19(5):437, 1993.
11. Lee G: History of flight nursing, *J Emerg Nurs* 13(4):212, 1987.
12. Miller M, Babcock D: *Critical thinking applied to nursing,* St Louis, 1996, Mosby.
13. Miller P, Epifanio P: Development of a prehospital nursing curriculum in Maryland, *J Emerg Nurs* 19(3):206, 1993.
14. Pon S and Notterman DA: *Roles of the medical and program directors.* In McClosky K, Orr R, editors: *Pediatric transport medicine,* St Louis, 1995, Mosby.
15. Rhee K, Strozeskim Burney RE: Is a flight physician needed for helicopter emergency services? *Ann Emerg Med* 15(2):174, 1986.
16. Semonin-Holleran R: *Prehospital nursing: a collaborative approach,* St Louis, 1994, Mosby.
17. Shaner S et al: Flight crew physical fitness: a baseline analysis, *Air Med J* 14(1):30, 1995.
18. Smale, J: Endotracheal intubation by paramedics during in-hospital CPR, *Chest* 107(6):1655, 1995.
19. Tellez D, Balazs K, Young L: *Prehospital transport-air medical.* In McClosky K, Orr R, editors: *Pediatric transport medicine,* St Louis, 1995, Mosby.
20. York D: A comparison study of chest tube thoracostomy, *J Air Med Transport* 14(7):255, 1993.

CHAPTER 2

Flight Physiology

COMPETENCIES

1. Provide a simple example of each gas law.
2. Identify appropriate interventions for correcting hypoxia.
3. Provide interventions to prevent the adverse effects of barometric pressure in the air medical patient.
4. Identify the appropriate method of patient transport based on altitude physiology.
5. Perform specific patient care interventions in the event of a slow or rapid decompression.

Air medical transports must be effected safely and expeditiously, and to ensure safe transport, flight nurses must know the effects of flight on patients. Understanding the concepts of flight physiology is crucial because they are the basis for the special skills used by flight nurses in transporting air medical patients. Such concepts include the gas laws and the way they relate to the stresses of flight.

THE GAS LAWS

To provide optimal patient care in the air medical environment, personnel must possess in-depth knowledge of altitude physiology. Altitude physiology exemplifies the concepts of the gas laws, the primary concern of which is to describe the relationships among the interdependent variables of temperature, pressure, volume, and mass of gases. Before the gas laws are addressed, those factors influencing the behavior of gases need to be considered. The four basic variables that affect gas volumetric relationships are temperature, pressure, volume, and the relative mass of a gas or the number of molecules. These variables—T, P, V, and n—are defined as follows[3]:

1. Temperature (T), when expressed as degrees Kelvin (K), indicates the level of energy of a gas sample and is referred to as *absolute temperature,* converted from temperature centigrade, or Celsius (C), or Fahrenheit (F).
2. Pressure (P), defined as absolute or total exerted pressure, is conventionally expressed in atmospheres (torr) or as a given column of mercury in millimeters (mm Hg) or of water balancing the pressure in centimeters (cm of H_2O).
3. Volume (V), is expressed in cubic units, such as cubic meters (m^3) or cubic centimeters (cc), or in liters (L).
4. Relative mass of gas or number of molecules (n) or ions is expressed in gram molecules (the molecular weight of the substance in grams).

Gas laws govern the body's physiologic response to barometric pressure changes by these four variables. When flight nurses are taking care of the air medical patient, these changes become particularly important on ascent and descent.

Boyle's Law

Boyle's Law, which originated from experiments conducted by Robert Boyle in the 1660s, states: "When the temperature remains constant, the volume of a given mass of gas varies inversely as its pressure . . .". This law applies to all gases and may be expressed as follows[28]:

$$\frac{V_1}{V_2} = \frac{P_2}{P_1} \text{ or } P_1V_1 = P_2V_2$$

where

V_1 = The initial volume
V_2 = The final volume
P_1 = The initial pressure
P_2 = the final pressure

Thus at a constant temperature the volume of a gas is inversely proportional to the pressure. The volume of gas in a balloon, for example, expands as the balloon ascends.

Dalton's Law (Law of Partial Pressure)

Dalton's Law relates to the pressure of a mixture of gases and states "The total pressure of a gas mixture is the sum of the individual or partial pressures of all the gases in the mixture. . . .":

$$P = P_1 + P_2 + P_3 + P_4 \text{ (and so on)}$$

P is the total pressure of the gas mixture and P_1, P_2, and P_3 are partial pressures of each gas in the mixture.

The partial pressure of each gas in the mixture is derived by the following equation[28]:

$$P_1 = F_1 \times P$$

where

P_1 = The partial pressure of gas 1
F_1 = The fractional concentration of gas 1 in the mixture
P = The total pressure of the gas mixture[26]

Stated another way, gases in a mixture exert pressure equivalent to the pressure each would exert if present alone in the volume of the total mixture. This means that each gas present in a mixture exerts a partial pressure equal to the fractional concentration (by volume) multiplied by the total pressure.[3]

A mathematical illustration of Dalton's Law is shown in the following example of calculating the partial pressure of oxygen (PO_2) at sea level:

$$PO_2 = 20.95\ (21\%) \times 760 \text{ mm Hg} - 159.6$$

Barometric, or atmospheric, pressure is the pressure exerted against an object or a person by the atmosphere (Table 2-1). At sea level this pressure is 15 psi (pounds per square inch). Increasing altitude results in decreased barometric pressure. Barometric pressure multiplied by the concentration of a gas is equal to the partial pressure of the gas[19]:

TABLE 2-1

Dry atmospheric composition

Gas	Pressure (torr)	Percent
Nitrogen	593.408	78.08
Oxygen	159.22	20.95
Argon	7.144	0.94
Carbon dioxide	0.288	0.03
Hydrogen	0.076	0.01
Neon	0.013	0.0018
Helium	0.003	0.00015

Barometric pressure × Gas concentration = Gas partial pressure

$$760 \text{ mm Hg} \times 21\% \ O_2 = 159.6 \text{ mm Hg } PO_2$$

NOTE: Oxygen concentration remains at 21%, regardless of altitude. However, oxygen availability decreases with altitude because the oxygen molecules are farther apart, thus potentially resulting in hypoxia.

Charles' Law

An additional development in the early formulation of the laws of ideal gases came from the French physicist Charles, who concluded that "When pressure is constant, the volume of a gas is very nearly proportional to its absolute temperature." This is expressed as follows[28]:

$$\frac{V_1}{V_2} = \frac{T_1}{T_2}$$

where

V_1 = The initial volume
V_2 = The final volume
T_1 = The initial absolute temperature
T_2 = The final absolute temperature

Thus the volume is directly proportional to temperature when it is expressed on an absolute scale where all other factors remain constant (where P and n are constant).[3] Consequently, if a mass of gas is kept under a constant pressure, as the absolute temperature of the gas is increased or decreased, the volume will increase or decrease accordingly.[7]

The motion of the molecules in a gas is directly related to temperature. A decrease in the temperature of a gas causes the molecules to move more slowly, whereas an increase in the temperature causes a faster motion. The relationship demonstrates that when a greater force is exerted, the volume expands. An example of this would be to put a shaving cream can into a fire and then watch the effects of Charles' Law take place, but carrying out this experiment is not recommended.

Gay-Lussac's Law

Many times Gay-Lussac's Law is combined with Charles' Law because it too deals with a directly proportional relationship between pressure and temperature. Gay-Lussac's Law expresses the same relationship but is stated as follows:

$$\frac{P_1}{T_1} = \frac{P_2}{T_2}$$

where [V] and [n] are constant. Thus the pressure of gases when volume is maintained constant is directly proportional to the absolute temperature for a constant amount of gas.[3] For example, the pressure in an oxygen tank shows a decrease in the pressure reading as the temperature decreases.

Henry's Law

Henry's Law deals with the solubility of gases in liquids and states, "The quantity of gas dissolved in 1 cm^3 (1 ml) of a liquid is proportional to the partial pressure of the gas in contact with the liquid. . . ." The absolute amount of any gas dissolved in liquid under conditions of equilibrium is dependent on the solubility of the gas in the liquid and the temperature, in addition to the partial pressure of the gas.[28] A simpler interpretation is that the weight of a gas dissolved in a liquid is directly proportional to the weight of the gas above the liquid.[7] An ideal example would be when a can of soda (i.e., a carbonated soft drink) is opened immediately after it has been dropped. The soda was bottled with an equilibrium established between the soda and the gas in the can. When the can is opened, the equilibrium of the gas above the soda is drastically altered, thus releasing the bubbles of gas within the soda. A further example of this law is decompression sickness. When a scuba diver ascends too rapidly from a deep dive, nitrogen bubbles can form in the blood, causing one form of decompression sickness.

Graham's Law (Law of Gaseous Diffusion)

Graham's Law states that the rate of diffusion of a gas through a liquid medium is directly related to the solubility of the gas and inversely proportional to the square root of its density or gram molecular weight.[7] This means that gases will go from a higher pressure or concentration to the region of lower pressure or concentration. Examples would be simple diffusion, or gas exchange at the cellular level. NOTE: Carbon dioxide is 19 times as diffusible as oxygen. Hence uptake of carbon dioxide occurs 19 times faster than uptake of oxygen.

STRESSES OF FLIGHT

The literature on the stresses of flight defines many different stresses. According to the U.S. Air Force,[26] which has done the most research on the subject, eight classical stresses of flight exist:

- Decreased partial pressure of oxygen
- Barometric pressure
- Thermal changes
- Decreased humidity
- Noise
- Vibration
- Fatigue
- G forces

Decreased Partial Pressure of Oxygen

An understanding of the terms *hypoxia, hypoxemia,* and *hypercapnia* is essential for establishing a foundation on which to build a knowledge base.

Hypoxia is a general term that describes the state of oxygen deficiency in the tissues. It refers to a decrease in tissue oxygen or an oxygen supply inadequate to meet tissue needs.[1] It is a general term that describes the state of oxygen deficiency in the tissues. Hypoxia disrupts the intracellular oxidative process and impairs cellular function.[20]

Hypoxemia refers to a decrease in arterial blood oxygen tension. A normal PaO_2 does not guarantee adequate tissue oxygenation; conversely, a low PaO_2 may not mean tissue hypoxia and may be clinically acceptable.[1]

Hypercapnia refers to an increased amount of carbon dioxide in the blood.[24]

Hypoxia

Four stages of hypoxia need to be considered when examining hypoxia and its effects on human pathophysiology. The four stages are divided by altitude. The first stage is the **indifferent stage.** This physiologic zone starts at sea level and extends to 10,000 feet. In this stage the body reacts with a slight increase in heart rate and ventilation. Night vision loss occurs at 5000 feet. The second stage is the **compensatory stage,** which extends from 10,000 to 15,000 feet. This is the stage in which the body attempts to protect itself against hypoxia. An increase in blood pressure, heart rate, and depth and rate of respiration occurs. This stage is when efficiency and performance of tasks requiring mental alertness become impaired. The third stage is the **disturbance stage,** which is from 15,000 to 20,000 feet. This stage is characterized by dizziness, sleepiness, tunnel vision, and cyanosis. Thinking becomes slowed, and muscle coordination decreases. The **critical stage** is the fourth stage of hypoxia. This stage is from 20,000 to 30,000 feet and features marked mental confusion and incapacitation, followed by unconsciousness, usually within a few minutes.[20,23]

Types. Based on the physiologic effects elicited on the body, hypoxia can be divided into four different types: hypoxic hypoxia, hypemic hypoxia, stagnant hypoxia, and histotoxic hypoxia.

Hypoxic hypoxia is a deficiency in alveolar oxygen exchange. Oxygen deficiency may be caused by a reduction in PO_2 in inspired air or the effective gas exchange area of the lung. The result is an inadequate oxygen supply to the arterial blood, which in turn decreases the amount of oxygen available to the tissues.[20] Decreased barometric pressure at altitude causes a reduction in the alveolar partial pressure of oxygen (PAO_2). The blood oxygen saturation, which is 98% at sea level, is reduced to 87% at 10,000 feet and 60% at 22,000 feet. This reduction in the amount of oxygen in the blood decreases the availability of the oxygen to the tissues, causing an impairment of body functions.[5] Hypoxic hypoxia is also referred to as *altitude hypoxia,* because its primary cause is exposure to low barometric pressure. Hypoxic hypoxia interferes with gas exchange in two phases of respiration: ventilation and diffusion. During the ventilation phase, a reduction in PAO_2 may occur. Specific causes include breathing air at reduced barometric pressure, strangulation/respiratory arrest/laryngospasm, severe asthma, breath holding, hypoventilation, breathing gas mixtures with insufficient PO_2, and malfunctioning oxygen equipment at altitude. Causes of reduction in the gas exchange area include pneumonia, drowning, atelectasis, emphysema (chronic obstructive pulmonary disease), pneumothorax, pulmonary embolism, congenital heart defects, and physiologic shunting. Some causes of diffusion barriers are hyaline membrane disease, pneumonia, and drowning.[20]

Hypemic hypoxia is a reduction in the oxygen-carrying capacity of the blood. If the number of red blood cells per unit volume of blood is reduced, as with various types of anemia or with a loss of blood, the oxygen-carrying capacity and thus the oxygen content of the blood are reduced.[5] Even with normal ventilation and diffusion, cellular hypoxia can occur if the rate of delivery of oxygen does not satisfy metabolic requirements.[20] Hypemic hypoxia interferes with the transportation phase of respiration with a reduction in oxygen-carrying capacity. Specific causes of hypemic hypoxia include anemias, hemorrhage, hemoglobin abnormalities, use of drugs (sulfanilamides, nitrites), and intake of chemicals (cyanide, carbon monoxide).[20] Carbon monoxide is significant to air medical crews because it is present in the exhaust fumes of both conventional and jet engine aircraft. It is also present in cigarette smoke. Carbon monoxide binds with hemoglobin 200 times more readily than does oxygen, and it displaces oxygen to form carboxyhemoglobin.[20]

Stagnant hypoxia occurs when conditions exist that result in reduced total cardiac output, pooling of the blood within certain regions of the body, a decreased blood flow to the tissues, or restriction of blood flow.[5,20] Stagnant hypoxia interferes with the transportation phase of respiration by reducing systemic blood flow. Specific causes include heart failure, shock, continuous positive-pressure breathing, acceleration (G forces), and pulmonary embolism. A reduction in regional or local blood flow may be caused by extremes of environmental temperatures, postural changes (prolonged sitting, bed rest, or weightlessness), tourniquets (restrictive clothing, straps), hyperventilation, embolism by clots or gas bubbles, and cerebral vascular accidents.[20]

Histotoxic hypoxia (tissue poisoning) occurs when metabolic disorders or poisoning of the cytochrome oxidase enzyme system results in a cell's inability to use molecular oxygen.[20] Histotoxic hypoxia interferes with the utilization phase of respiration because of metabolic poisoning or dysfunction. Specific causes include respiratory enzyme poisoning or degradation and the intake of carbon monoxide, cyanide, or alcohol.[20] Carbon monoxide can cause both hypemic and histotoxic hypoxia.

Effective Performance Time and Time of Useful Consciousness. Two terms are frequently used synonymously but are not interchangeable: *Effective performance time (EPT)* denotes the amount of time an individual is able to perform useful flying duties in an environment of inadequate oxygen[20]; *time of useful consciousness (TUC)* refers to the elapsed time from the point of exposure to an oxygen-deficient environment to the point where deliberate function is lost.[5,26] EPT more accurately refers to critical (functional) performance than does TUC. With the loss of effective performance in flight, the individual is no longer capable of taking the proper corrective or protective action.[20] Thus for air medical personnel the emphasis is on prevention. Table 2-2 illustrates the average TUC.

In addition to altitude, factors that influence TUC are the rate of ascent, physical fitness, physical activity, temperature, individual tolerance, and self-imposed stresses such as smoking, intake of alcohol and medication, and fatigue.[5] Another factor that dramat-

TABLE 2-2

Average TUC for nonpressurized aircraft

Altitude (in feet)	Time
18,000 and below	30 min
25,000	3-5 min
30,000	90 sec
35,000	30-60 sec
40,000 and above	15 sec or less

ically reduces both EPT and TUC is rapid decompression, which occurs when a quick loss of cabin altitude occurs in a pressurized aircraft. On decompression to altitudes above 10,058 meters (33,000 feet), an immediate reversal of oxygen flow in the alveoli takes place, caused by a higher Po_2 within the pulmonary capillaries. This depletes the blood's oxygen reserve and reduces the EPT at rest by up to 50%. Exercise reduces the EPT considerably.[20]

Causes. Hypoxia has three causes:

1. High altitude
2. Hypoventilation
3. Pathologic condition of the lung

Characteristics. Onset of hypoxia may be gradual or insidious. Intellectual impairment occurs, demonstrated by slowed thinking, faulty memory of events and lessened immediate recall, delayed reaction time, and a tendency to fixate.

Early Signs and Symptoms. The individual symptoms of hypoxia can be identified in subjects under safe and controlled conditions in an altitude chamber. Once recognized, these symptoms do not vary dramatically in similar time exposures or among subjects. Hypoxia can be classified by objective signs (those perceived by an observer) or subjective symptoms (those perceived by the subject).[20] Signs and symptoms that appear on both lists in the box on p. 17 may be seen by observers and recognized when occurring by the hypoxic subject.[5,9,19]

NOTE: Cyanosis has been concluded to be an unreliable sign of hypoxia because the oxygen saturation must be below 75% in persons with normal hemoglobin before it is detectable.[29]

Treatment. The treatment for hypoxia is to administer 100% oxygen. The type of hypoxia needs to be determined so that treatment can be administered accordingly. The following are required steps for air medical crew members:

1. **Administer supplemental oxygen under pressure.** Providing adequate supplemental oxygen is the prime consideration in the treatment of hypoxia. Depending on the severity of the condition, 100% oxygen delivered under positive pressure may be required. Consideration must be given to the altitude and cause of the oxygen deficiency. Equipment malfunction or altitude exposure above 12,192 meters (40,000 feet) cannot be corrected without the addition of positive pressure.
   NOTE: Positive-pressure breathing is the opposite of normal breathing. The physiologic requirements for breathing are as follows:

NORMAL	POSITIVE PRESSURE
Inspiration—active	Inspiration—passive
Expiration—passive	Expiration—active

   The proper method of positive pressure breathing is as follows:

   Inhale slowly → Pause → Exhale forcibly → Pause
2. **Monitor breathing.** After a hypoxic episode, the resulting hyperventilation must be controlled to achieve complete recovery. Maintaining a breathing rate of 12 to 16 breaths per minute or slightly lower will aid recovery.
3. **Monitor equipment.** The most frequently reported causes of hypoxia are lack of oxygen discipline and equipment malfunction. A conscientious preflight check of equipment and frequent in-flight monitoring will reduce this hazard. Inspection of oxygen equipment when hypoxia is suspected may detect its cause. Correction of the malfunction helps bring immediate relief of the hypoxic condition. If treatment for hypoxia does not

SIGNS AND SYMPTOMS OF HYPOXIA

Objective Signs	Subjective Symptoms
Confusion	Confusion
Tachycardia	Headache
Tachypnea	Stupor
Seizures	Insomnia
Dyspnea	Change in judgment or personality
Hypertension	Dizziness
Bradycardia	Blurred vision
Arrhythmias	Tunnel vision
Restlessness	Hot and cold flashes
Slouching	Tingling
Unconsciousness	Numbness
Hypotension (late)	Nausea
Cyanosis (late)	Euphoria
Euphoria	Anger
Belligerence	

remedy the situation, oxygen contamination should be suspected. Use of an alternative oxygen source, such as the emergency oxygen cylinder or portable assembly, should be considered. Descent should be initiated as soon as possible and the contents of the oxygen system analyzed.

4. **Descend.** Increasing the ambient oxygen pressures by descent to lower altitudes, particularly below 3048 meters (10,000 feet), is also beneficial. Descent to lower altitude compensates for malfunctioning oxygen equipment that may have caused the hypoxia.[20]

The treatment of hypoxia of the air medical patient centers around prevention. The air medical crew must accurately anticipate the oxygen needs of the patient to prevent difficulties during flight. If the patient begins to exhibit signs and symptoms of hypoxia, the treatment is administration of 100% oxygen and following the steps described previously. NOTE: The air medical patient is already in a compromised state and will usually experience the effects of hypoxia before air medical crew members do.

Hyperventilation

Hyperventilation at altitude is an important consideration for air medical personnel and also for the air medical patient. Hyperventilation is of concern because it produces changes in cellular respiration. Although unrelated in cause, the symptoms of hyperventilation and hypoxia are similar and often result in confusion and inappropriate corrective procedures. Despite increased knowledge, training, and improved life-support equipment, both hypoxia and hyperventilation are hazards in flying and diving operations.[20] Hyperventilation, an abnormal increase in the rate and depth of breathing that upsets the chemical balance of the blood,[24] is commonly caused by psychologic stress (e.g., fear, anxiety, apprehensiveness, and anger) and environmental stress (e.g., hypoxia, pressure breathing, vibration, and heat). Certain drugs such as salicylates and female sex hormones also cause or enhance hyperventilation, and any condition that creates metabolic acidosis results in hyperventilation at altitude.[5,20] Table 2-3 compares signs and symptoms of hyperventilation to those of hypoxia.

TABLE 2-3

Comparison of signs and symptoms of hyperventilation and hypoxia

Signs/symptoms	Hyperventilation	Hypoxia
Onset of symptoms	Gradual	Rapid (altitude dependent, may also be gradual)
Muscle activity	Spasmodic	Flaccid
Appearance	Pale	Cyanotic
Tetany	Present	Absent
Breathlessness	X*	X
Dizziness	X	X
Dullness and drowsiness	X	X
Euphoria	X	X
Fatigue	X	X
Headache	X	X
Poor judgment	X	X
Lightheadedness	X	X
Faulty memory	X	X
Muscle incoordination	X	X
Numbness	X	X
Deteriorated performance	X	X
Increased respiratory rate	X	X
Delayed reaction time	X	X
Tingling	X	X
Unconsciousness	X	X
Blurred vision	X	X

From Sheffield PJ, Heimbach RD: Respiratory physiology. In DeHart RI, editor *Fundamentals of aerospace medicine,* Philadelphia, 1985, Lea & Febiger.
*X means that the sign or symptom can occur in either condition.

Treatment. At altitude, hyperventilation and hypoxia are treated the same way because of similarities in the signs and symptoms. The following steps describe the treatment:

1. Administer 100% oxygen.
2. Begin positive pressure breathing, which is the same as supplemental oxygen under pressure.
3. Regulate breathing and watch for hyperventilation.
4. Check equipment.
5. Descend.

The treatment for hyperventilation in the air medical patient is administration of oxygen. If this is successfully accomplished, the amount of oxygen in the blood will increase. Oxygen transfers from air to blood 20 times slower than carbon dioxide, and carbon dioxide transfers 20 times faster from blood to air than oxygen, which explains why the amount of carbon dioxide in the blood is directly associated with ventilation. When a patient is hyperventilating from anxiety, the act of putting a mask on his or her face to administer oxygen will probably heighten the anxiety and increase tidal volume. Tidal volume must be reduced.[5] More favorable responses can be obtained by talking to patients to distract them, identifying causes of hyperventilation, and suggesting specific exercises to reduce respiratory rate. Following are several helpful exercises:

1. The patient should count to 10 slowly while exhaling.
2. The patient should inhale and exhale only 10 times per minute.
3. Using a watch with a second hand, the patient should set a respiratory rate between 10 and 12 breaths per minute.
4. The air medical crew member can provide counter pressure by suggesting isometric or active-passive exercises[5] that cause the patient to hold his or her breath, thus reducing the respiratory rate.

Barometric Pressure

Boyle's Law states that at a constant temperature, the volume of a gas is inversely proportional to the pressure. On ascent gas expands, and on descent gas contracts. Therefore trapped or partially trapped gases within certain body cavities (e.g., the gastrointestinal [GI] tract, lungs, skull, middle ear, sinuses, and teeth) expand in direct proportion to the decrease in pressure.[5]

Middle Ear

The middle ear cavity is an air-filled space connected to the nasopharynx by the eustachian tube. The eustachian tube has a slitlike orifice at the throat end that allows air to vent outward more easily than inward. During ascent, air in the middle ear cavity expands but will normally vent into the throat via the eustachian tube when a pressure differential of approximately 15 mm Hg has been reached. A mild fullness is usually detected but disappears as equalization occurs. This constitutes the passive process.[5] On descent, however, a different situation exists. The eustachian tube remains closed unless actively opened by muscle action or high positive pressure in the nasopharynx. If the eustachian tube opens, any existing pressure differential is immediately equalized. If the tube does not open regularly during descent, a pressure differential may develop. If this pressure differential reaches 80 to 90 mm Hg, the small muscles of the soft palate cannot overcome it, and either reascent or a maneuver that is not physiologic is necessary to open the tube.[10] On descent, equalization of pressure in the middle ear can be accomplished by performing the Valsalva maneuver, yawning, swallowing, moving the lower jaw, controlling administration of vasoconstrictors, or using a Politzer bag or bag-valve mask (BVM). These procedures are examples of the active process.

NOTE: It is not recommended that gum chewing be used as a method of pressure equalization because it causes swallowing of air, thereby causing gastric distention.

Barotitis Media. Barotitis media, frequently referred to as an *ear block,* results from failure of the middle ear space to ventilate when going from low to high atmospheric pressure (i.e., on descent).[10] Pressure in the middle ear becomes increasingly negative, and a partial vacuum is created. As the pressure differential increases, the tympanic membrane is depressed inward and becomes inflamed, and petechial hemorrhages develop. Blood and tissue fluids can be drawn into the middle ear cavity, and if equalization with ambient pressure does not take place, perforation of the tympanic membrane occurs. Severe pain, tinnitus, and possibly vertigo and nausea can accompany acute barotitis.[5] Priority is placed on patient briefing before flight and adequate instructions for air medical crews. The ears should be cleared on descent by using the methods previously described. Patients who are sleeping should be awakened before descent so they can clear their ears in the normal manner.

Patients suffering from colds or upper respiratory tract infections must be closely monitored during both ascent and descent for swollen eustachian tubes, a condition that interferes with normal equalization procedures.[5] Air medical crew members with upper respiratory tract infections should not fly.

Mild vasoconstrictors should be administered

early, and the plane should reascend to a higher altitude until symptoms lessen, or the patient's ear block clears. If patients experience ear pain during ascent, which rarely occurs, air medical personnel should not have them execute a Valsalva maneuver, because that would only aggravate the problem; instead, personnel should have them swallow or move their jaw muscles, or administer to them a mild vasoconstrictor.[5] Either the Politzer bag or a source of compressed air may be used. A patient's nose should be sprayed well with a decongestant solution to attain maximum shrinkage of the mucosa. For the Politzer bag method, the olive tip is placed in one nostril, the nose is compressed between the air medical crew member's fingers, and the patient is then instructed to say "kick, kick, kick" while the bag is squeezed, thereby increasing the pressure in the nasopharyngeal cavity to the point at which the eustachian tube will be opened and the middle ear space ventilated.[10] In review, the treatment is as follows:

1. Patient performs Valsalva maneuver
2. Crew member administers vasoconstrictor spray
3. Crew member administers Politzer bag or BVM
4. Aircraft reascends

Delayed Ear Block. A delayed ear block occurs after the flight is terminated and results from breathing 100% oxygen during flight. As the ears clear during descent, 100% oxygen is forced into the middle ear cavity.[5] In addition, the absorption of oxygen by the middle ear and mastoid mucosa also contributes to the relatively negative pressure in those cavities. The patient may be asymptomatic immediately after flight, but if the oxygen in the middle ear is not replaced with air, it is absorbed by the surrounding tissues, and a negative pressure is created within the cavity. **Delayed barotitis media** occurs when oxygen absorption is the primary factor in the development of a pressure differential.[10] This causes a tightness or "stopped-up" sensation in the ears and slight to possibly severe pain. To prevent delayed ear problems, the patient should perform the Valsalva maneuver periodically after the flight.[5] However, if a flight is completed in the late evening hours or during the night, and the individual retires a short time later, a significant pressure differential may develop during sleep because of combined factors of oxygen absorption and infrequent swallowing.[10] Patients who are maintained on 100% oxygen during flight are especially susceptible to this problem.[5]

Barosinusitis (Sinus Block)

The sinuses usually present little problem when subjected to changes in barometric pressure. Because there is a free flow of air between the sinus cavities and the exterior, the sinuses automatically equalize with ambient pressure when the air in them expands or contracts.[5]

Barosinusitis is an acute or chronic inflammation of one or more of the paranasal sinuses produced by the development of a pressure difference, usually negative, between the air in the sinus cavity and that of the surrounding atmosphere.[10] Common causes of barosinusitis are colds and upper respiratory tract infections. Patients suffering from such problems should be closely monitored during ascent and descent.[5] The symptoms of barosinusitis are usually proportional to its severity and may vary from a mild feeling of fullness in or around the involved sinus to excruciating pain. Pain can develop suddenly and be incapacitating.[10] Another symptom is possible persistent local tenderness. The immediate treatment for barosinusitis is to reascend until the pressure within the sinus equals the cabin pressure, administer vasoconstrictors to reduce swelling, and descend as gradually as possible to afford every opportunity for pressure equalization.[5]

Barodontalgia

Barodontalgia, or aerodontalgia, is a toothache that is caused by exposure to changing barometric pressures during actual or simulated flight.[10] The precise cause of barodontalgia has not been determined; however, exposure to reduced atmospheric pressure is obviously a significant factor. This exposure is evidently a precipitating factor, with disease of the pulp the primary cause. Pressure changes do not elicit pain in teeth with normal pulps, regardless of whether a tooth is intact, carious, or restored.[10] Some pathologic conditions may cause no symptoms at ground level but be adversely affected by a change in barometric pressure. It is common for barodontalgia to occur during ascent, with descent bringing relief.[5] Direct barodontalgia is generally manifested by moderate to severe pain, which usually develops during ascent and is well localized. The patient is frequently able to identify the involved tooth. This condition can usually be prevented by high quality dental care, with an emphasis on slow, careful treatment of cavities and the routine use of a cavity varnish. Indirect barodontalgia is a dull, poorly defined pain that involves the posterior maxillary teeth and develops during descent.[10] If patients complain of tooth pain during descent, especially that involving the upper posterior teeth, they may be suffering from barosinusitis and should be treated accordingly.[5]

A crew member who undergoes dental treatment involving deep restorations should be restricted from flying for 48 to 72 hours after treatment to allow time for the dental pulp to stabilize.[10]

Gastrointestinal Changes

Gas contained within body cavities is saturated with water vapor, the partial pressure of which is related to body temperature. In determining the mechanical effect of gas expansion, one must account for the noncompressibility of water vapor, which causes wet gases to expand to a greater extent than do dry gases.[12] The stomach and intestines normally contain a variable amount of gas at a pressure that is equivalent to the surrounding barometric pressure. On ascending to altitude, however, the gases in the GI tract expand. Unless the gases are passed by belching or the passing of flatus, they may produce pain and discomfort, make breathing more difficult, and possibly lead to hyperventilation or syncope.[5] Severe pain may cause a vasovagal reaction consisting of hypotension, tachycardia, and fainting. Abdominal massage and physical activity may promote the passage of gas. If this is unsuccessful, a descent should be initiated to an altitude at which comfort is achieved.[12] Fortunately, severe gas expansion problems generally do not occur below flight level 250. (*Flight level* is defined as true altitude, or the actual height above sea level in feet divided by 100, and can be expressed as FL. For example, 25,000 ft = FL 250.) Because the possibility of decompression does exist, however, certain precautionary measures should be taken to reduce the chances of GI gas expansion difficulties. Such measures include avoiding hasty and heavy meals before flight, which include gas-forming foods, carbonated beverages, and foods that are not easily digested.[5] Normally, the average GI tract has approximately 1 L of gas present at any one time. Wet gas expands to approximately 1½ times its original volume at 9000 feet. Table 2-4 illustrates gas expansion in the GI tract at various altitudes.

One useful example is a pediatric patient with abdominal distention. Gas expansion in the abdominal cavity, if untreated, can increase to such a volume as to raise the diaphragm. With diaphragmatic crowding, lung volume and expansion are decreased. If this distention is large enough, the great blood vessels in the area will be compressed, thus altering the blood supply to vital organs.[5]

Patients with ileus (bowel obstruction) or recent abdominal surgery should have a nasogastric (NG) tube placed before transport. The NG tube should not be clamped but should be vented for ambient air or low intermittent suction during transport. Following abdominal surgery, pockets of air may remain in the abdominal cavity. For this reason, it is generally recommended that patients not be transported by air until 24 to 48 hours after the surgery. Colostomy patients should be advised to carry extra bags because

TABLE 2-4

Gas expansion of 1 L in volume in GI tract at various altitudes

Altitude (in feet)	Amount (times) increased
Sea level	No increase
9,000	1.5
16,500	2
25,000	3
34,000	5
39,000	7
43,000	9

of more frequent bowel movements resulting from gas expansion.[22] Colostomy bags should be empty and properly vented before air medical transport. Penetrating wounds allow for ambient air to travel along the wound tract. According to Boyle's Law, penetrating wounds to the eyes, neck, thorax, abdomen, and lower extremities can cause the introduction of emboli in addition to irreparable damage to nerves and surrounding tissues.

Thermal Changes

An increase in altitude results in a decrease in ambient temperature. As a consequence, cabin temperature fluctuates considerably depending on the temperature outside the aircraft.[5] The ratio of altitude to temperature is fairly constant from sea level to about 35,000 feet. Temperature decreases by 1° C for every 100 m (330 feet) increase in altitude. From FL 350 to FL 990 the temperature fluctuates plus or minus 3° to 5° C. The temperature remains relatively isothermic at approximately −550° C from FL 350 to FL 990.[26] Vibration and thermal change, depending on whether the change is to greater heat or more cold, can have either an antagonistic or a synergistic effect. The body's primary response to heat exposure is vasodilation and activation of cooling mechanisms. Exposure to cold and vibration stimulate vasoconstriction and decreased perspiration.[2] Exposure to whole body vibration appears to interfere with humans' normal cooling responses in a hot environment by reducing blood flow and decreasing perspiration.[21] Turbulence can be produced by high and low temperature changes in the air. Turbulence increases stress during flight by promoting fatigue and increasing susceptibility to motion sickness and disorientation.[21] Both hyperthermia and hypothermia increase the body's oxygen requirement. Hyperthermia increases the metabolic rate, and hypothermia increases energy needs as a result of shivering and thereby increases the body's oxygen consumption.[5] Air medical crews can facilitate maintenance of adequate body temperature by having access to blankets, warm clothing, and warm liquids.[5] An additional way to facilitate thermoregulatory control for the air medical patient is use of a first-aid thermal blanket, which is sometimes called a *space blanket.*

Decreased Humidity

Humidity is the concentration of water vapor in the air; as air cools it loses its ability to hold moisture. Because temperature is inversely proportional to altitude, an increase in altitude produces a decrease in temperature and, therefore, a decrease in the amount of humidity. The fresh air supply is drawn into the aircraft cabin from a very dry atmosphere.[5] Before takeoff, small amounts of moisture are present in the cabin air from clothing and other items on board that retain moisture, in addition to expired air from crew members, patients, and other passengers. As the aircraft altitude increases, trapped moisture is carried away by the air exhausted overboard. Eventually, all the original moisture is lost. The only moisture that remains is supplied by crew members, patients, and other passengers on board and from the fresh air system.[5] For example, on a typical flight of the military jet aircraft known as a C-141 Starlifter, which is a high-speed, high-altitude, long-range aircraft used for troops, cargo, and air medical transport, less than 5% relative humidity remains after 2 hours of flying time. Relative humidity decreases to less than 1% after 4 hours.[5] Propeller-type aircraft are not as dry inside because they do not fly as high; the lowest relative humidities reached on typical propeller aircraft flights range from 10% to 25%.[5] Patients and air crew members may become significantly dehydrated because of the decreased humidity at altitude. The ventilation systems on aircraft draw off what little moisture there is and contribute further to the decrease in the percentage of humidity. For a healthy person, low humidity results in nothing more than chapped lips, scratchy or slightly sore throat, and hoarseness. Steps that the medical crew member can take to minimize problems caused by decreased humidity include mouth care, lip balm, and adequate fluid intake.[5] Patients who receive in-flight oxygen therapy are twice as susceptible to dehydration because oxygen itself is a drying agent. Moisture must be provided by commercial humidification devices for all patients who receive oxygen. Tracheostomy patients in particular require warmed humidification with or without oxygen during air medical transport.[5] Patients who are unconscious or are unable to close their eyelids must be provided with eye care. Administering artificial tears and taping the lids shut prevents corneal drying. Compromised patients predisposed by age, diet, or preexisting medical or surgical complications need special consideration in relation to decreased humidity before air medical transport. Crew members must also protect themselves from dehydration during flight.

Noise

Sound is any undulatory motion in an elastic medium (gaseous, liquid, or solid) capable of producing the sensation of hearing. Normally, the medium is air.[18] Sound waves are variations in air pressure above and below the ambient pressure.[18,27] Sound is described in terms of its intensity, spectrum, and time history. The intensity of a sound wave is the magnitude by which the pressure varies above and below the ambient level. It is measured by a logarithmic scale that expresses the ratio of sound pressure to a reference pressure in decibels (dB), which are units used to describe levels of acoustic pressure, power, and intensity.[26,27] The spectrum of a sound represents the qualities present distributed across frequency. The frequency of periodic motion (e.g., sound and vibrations) is the number of complete cycles of motion taking place in a unit of time, usually 1 second. The international standard unit of frequency is the hertz (Hz), which is 1 cycle per second.[27] Pressure-time histories describe variations in the sound pressure of a signal as a function of time. The frequency content is not quantified in pressure-time histories of signals, so analytic techniques must be applied to the signal to obtain frequency or spectrum characteristics.[27]

Theoretically, sound waves in open air spread spherically in all directions from an ideal source. As a result of this spherical dispersion, the sound pressure is reduced to one half of its original value as the distance is doubled, which is a 6-dB reduction in sound pressure level.[27] Hence a number of factors are involved in the creation of sound. In relation to the definition of sound, it is usually easier to think of sound as comprising intensity, which is commonly thought of as merely loudness, in decibels; frequency, in cycles per second and pitch; and duration, in length of time.

Thus noise, which is dependent on sound, can more easily be defined. Noise may be defined subjectively as a sound that is unpleasant, distracting, unwarranted, or in some other way undesirable.[18] The human hearing mechanism has a wide range and is fairly tolerant, but at times in an aircraft this tolerance is exceeded with the following potential effects:

1. Communications in the form of speech and other auditory signals inside the aircraft or air-to-air or air-to-ground may be degraded.
2. The sense of hearing may be temporarily or permanently damaged.
3. Noise, acting as a stress, may interfere with the flying task.
4. Noise may induce varying levels of fatigue.[18]

The A-level of a decibel (dBA) is a unit of noise measurement that correlates most closely with the way a human ear accommodates sound or noise. The dBA is a single measurement that incorporates both amplitude and selective frequency response features that most closely parallel the human ear. When ambient noise levels exceed 80 to 85 dBA, a person must usually shout to be heard.[5] Essentially, unprotected exposure to noise can produce one or more of the following three undesirable auditory effects: interference with effective communication, temporary threshold shifts (auditory fatigue), or permanent threshold shifts (sensorineural hearing loss).[5] Auditory fatigue incurred by noise is frequently accompanied by a feeling of "fullness," high-pitched ringing, buzzing, or a roaring sound in the ears (tinnitus). Tinnitus usually subsides within a few minutes after cessation of the noise exposure; however, for some individuals the tinnitus may continue for several hours.[5] Most of the truly significant forms of undesirable response to acoustic noise, such as nausea, disorientation, and excessive general fatigue, are associated only with very intense noise, which air medical personnel rarely encounter during normal airlift operations.[5] Other hazards of exposure are loss of appetite and interest, diaphoresis, salivation, nausea or vomiting, headache, fatigue, and general discomfort. Table 2-5 provides an example of the number of decibels resulting from certain sources. Whenever

TABLE 2-5

Number of decibels in relation to source

Decibels	Source
60	Normal conversation at 1 meter
80	Garbage disposal
88	Propeller aircraft flyover at 1000 feet
90	Noisy factory Cockpit of light aircraft
103	Jet flyover at 1000 feet
117	Jet on runway in preparation for takeoff
110-130	Construction site during pile driving

From Glaister DH: The effects of long-duration acceleration. In Ernsting J, King P, editors: *Aviation medicine,* ed 2, London, 1988, Butterworths.

it is not feasible to control the noise at a desirable level, ear protection devices that attenuate the noise on its way from the surrounding air to the tympanic membrane must be worn. Such devices include a helmet, earplugs, and earmuffs. Because effectiveness can vary considerably, depending on a device's basic performance and personal fit, all air medical personnel should be carefully instructed regarding quality and size selection and in techniques for use.[27] Earplugs are inert devices, and headsets and earmuffs are occluding devices. Earplugs must fit tightly to offer the maximum allowable attenuation; the only requirement for using airtight earplugs during flight operations is that the plugs be removed before descent. Pressure changes resulting from decreased altitude tend to pull the plugs inward toward the tympanic membrane.[5]

Vibration

Vibration is the motion of objects relative to a reference position (usually the object at rest) and is described relative to its effect on humans in terms of frequency, intensity (amplitude), direction (with regard to anatomic axes of the human body), and duration of exposure.[27] Most vehicles contain two principal sources of vibration: The first originates within the vehicle; specifically, the power source, and the second comes from the environment, which comprises the terrain over which the land vehicle travels, the turbulence of the air through which the aircraft flies, or the status of the sea in which the ship sails.[24]

Helicopter vibration occurs with broadly similar intensity in all three axes of motion. There may be large differences in the amplitudes of specific harmonics in different modes of light, but the overall amplitude of vibration tends to increase with airspeed and with the loading of the aircraft. Vibration is usually worse during transition to the hover position.[24]

In fixed-wing aircraft, any vibration coming from the power source is usually at a higher frequency than it is in helicopters. The main source of vibration encountered in fixed-wing aircraft originates from the atmospheric turbulence through which the aircraft flies. In consequence, the most severe vibration usually occurs during storm cloud penetration or during high-speed, low-level flight. The response of the aircraft as a whole to atmospheric turbulence is determined by the aerodynamic loading on the wings. An aircraft with a large wing area relative to its weight undergoes greater amplitude, low-frequency excursions from level flight as a result of turbulence.[24]

Resonance frequencies of body structures produce a more pronounced effect than nonresonant frequencies.[4] It has been firmly established that vibration between 1 and 12 Hz causes performance decrement in the cockpit. For example, low-frequency vibration can induce motion sickness, fatigue, shortness of breath, and abdominal and chest pain.[17] Research has established that a human's sensitivity to external vibration is highest between 0.5 and 20 Hz because the human system absorbs most of the vibratory energy applied within this range, with maximal amplification between 5 and 11 Hz. Posture can greatly affect tolerance in test subjects, and wide variability occurs among and in individuals, depending on other factors such as fatigue, physical conditioning, and perceived risk.[6]

When the human body is in direct contact with a source of vibration, mechanical energy is transferred, some of which is degraded into heat within those tissues that have dampening properties. The response to whole body vibration is an increase in muscle activity to maintain posture and possibly to reduce the resonant amplification of body structures. This is reflected in an increase in metabolic rate under vibration and a redistribution of blood flow with peripheral vasoconstriction. The increase in metabolic rate during vibrations is comparable to that seen in gentle exercise. Respiration is increased to achieve the necessary increase in elimination of carbon dioxide (CO_2).[24] Disturbances in dynamic visual acuity, speech, and fine-muscle coordination result from vibration exposure.[4]

The effects of vibration on the body can be reduced by attention to the source of vibration, by modification of the transmission pathway, or by alteration of the dynamic properties of the body.[24] Aircraft manufacturers have eliminated severe vibrations by improving designs and materials; however, some vibrations still occur as a result of engine operation, flap and landing gear extension and retraction, and general aircraft movement. To minimize these reactions, medical crew members should properly secure patients, encourage and assist them with position changes, and provide adequate padding and skin care.[5]

Fatigue

All of the many operational stresses of flight induce fatigue to some degree. Fatigue is an inherent stress of aviation duties. Erratic schedules, hypoxic environments, noise and vibration, and imperfect environmental systems eventually take their toll, and therefore, in aviation, fatigue is always a potential threat to safety.[17] Fatigue is the end product of all the physiologic and psychologic stresses of flight associated with exposure to altitude.[5,26] Factors involved also include self-imposed stresses. The following box shows self-imposed stresses that can have disastrous results.

FACTORS AFFECTING TOLERANCE: DEATH

Factors affecting tolerance to the stresses of flight can be summarized by the acronym *death.*

D = drugs. Use of over-the-counter (OTC) drugs and antihistamines, misuse of prescription drugs, and use of stimulants such as caffeine can cause insomnia, tremors, indigestion, and nervousness.

E = exhaustion (fatigue). Exhaustion can lead to judgment errors, limited response, falling asleep on the job, narrowed attention, and change in circadian rhythm.

A = alcohol. Use of alcohol can cause histotoxic hypoxia, affect efficiency of cells to use oxygen, interfere with metabolic activity, and can result in a hangover with ⅓ oz/hr elimination.

T = tobacco. Besides exposing the body to nicotine, tar, and carcinogens, smoking 2 packs of cigarettes per day results in 8% to 10% of the body's hemoglobin being saturated with carbon monoxide.

H = hypoglycemia (diet). Poor dietary intake can cause nausea, judgment errors, headache, and dizziness.

G Force

To examine force as a stress of flight, an understanding of mass, speed, velocity, and acceleration can help clarify the concepts of exerted forces.

Speed is the rate of movement of a body without specifying the direction of travel.

Velocity is the rate (magnitude) of change of distance and direction of travel of an object and is therefore a vector quantity. The velocity of a body changes if its speed or its direction of travel changes. Velocity is expressed as the rate of change of distance in a specified direction.

Acceleration is the rate of change of velocity of an object, and like velocity, is a vector quantity.[9]

Weight is the force exerted by the mass of an accelerating body.[9]

Mass is a measure of the inertia of an object, e.g., its resistance to being accelerated.[8]

Newton's three laws of motion define the relationship between motion and force.[9]

Newton's First Law of Motion. Unless it is acted on by a force, a body at rest will remain at rest, and a body in motion will move at constant speed in a straight line.

Newton's Second Law of Motion. When a force is applied to a body, the body accelerates, and the acceleration is directly proportional to the force applied and inversely proportional to the mass of the body.

Newton's Third Law of Motion. For every action there is an equal and opposite reaction.

Two types of acceleration must be considered—linear and radial acceleration. Linear acceleration is produced by a change of speed without a change in direction. In conventional aviation, prolonged linear accelerations seldom reach a magnitude that could produce significant changes in human performance, because most aircraft do not exert sufficient thrust to produce extended changes in linear velocity. However, significant linear accelerations that last 2 to 4 seconds are produced during catapult-assisted takeoffs, arrested landings, and when reheat is engaged in certain high-performance aircraft. Large prolonged linear accelerations occur during the launching of spacecraft and when they are slowed on reentering the Earth's atmosphere. Radial acceleration is produced by a change of direction without a change of speed. Such accelerations occur when the line of flight is changed. Aircraft maneuvers are by far the most common source of prolonged acceleration in flight. Accelerations of the order of 6 to 9 G or more can be maintained for many seconds by circular flight in agile military aircraft.[9]

When the main interest is the effect of acceleration on humans, the direction in which an acceleration or inertial force acts is described by the use of a three-axis coordinate system (X, Y, and Z), in which the vertical (Z) axis is parallel to the long axis of the body. Considerable confusion can result if a clear distinction is not made between the applied acceleration and the resultant inertial force because these, by definition, always act in diametrically opposite directions.[9]

Aircraft Motion

Because space is three-dimensional, linear motions in space are described by reference to three linear axes, and angular motions by three angular axes. In aviation it is customary to speak of the longitudinal (fore-aft), lateral (right-left), and vertical (up-down) linear axes and the roll, pitch, and yaw angular axes.[8]

LINEAR AXES	ANGULAR AXES
Longitudinal axis (fore-aft)	Axis of roll
Lateral axis (right-left)	Axis of pitch
Vertical axis (up-down)	Axis of yaw

The relationship of this three-axis system to its action on man is illustrated in Table 2-6.

Long-Duration Positive Acceleration ($+G_z$). The crews of agile aircraft are frequently exposed to sustained positive accelerations by changes in the direction of flight either in turns or recovery from dives. Exposure to positive acceleration usually causes deterioration of vision before causing any disturbance of consciousness. Thus exposure to $+4.5\ G_z$ typically produces complete loss of vision, or "blackout," while hearing and mental activity remain unaffected. Exposure to a positive acceleration stress somewhat greater than that required to produce blackout results in unconsciousness. At moderate levels of acceleration (5 to 6 G), blackout precedes loss of consciousness, but at higher accelerations, unconsciousness occurs before any visual symptoms occur.[9]

Long-Duration Negative Acceleration ($-G_z$). Flight conditions that cause negative accelerations are outside loops and spins and simple inverted flight and recovery from such maneuvers. Tolerance for negative acceleration is much lower than that for positive acceleration, and the symptoms produced by even $-2\ G_z$ are unpleasant and alarming. Furthermore, low levels of negative acceleration produce serious decrements in performance.[9]

Long-Duration Transverse Acceleration ($+G_x$). Accelerations of long duration acting at right angles to the long axis of the body occur rarely in present-day conventional flight. They are usually confined to catapult launches, rocket- and jet-assisted takeoffs, and carrier landings, although forces in excess of $-2\ G_x$ may build up during flat spins. However, the forces in these maneuvers are small relative to man's tolerance and do not cause problems.[9]

The above definitions of the effects of G forces are applicable for high-performance aircraft, mostly fighter-type, and in the event of emergency situations. The longitudinal axis is the most important in air medical transports. However, the effects of G forces are usually encountered only with forces

TABLE 2-6

Three-axis coordinate system for describing action on humans of direction of acceleration and inertial forces

Direction of acceleration	Direction of resultant inertial forces	Physiologic and vernacular descriptors	Standard terminology
Headward	Head-to-foot	Positive G Eyeballs down	$+G_z$
Footward	Foot-to-head	Negative G Eyeballs up	$-G_z$
Forward	Chest-to-back	Transverse A-P-G Supine G Eyeballs in	$+G_x$
Backward	Back-to-chest	Transverse P-A-G Prone G Eyeballs out	$-G_x$
To the right	Right-to-left side	Left lateral G Eyeballs left	$+G_y$
To the left	Left-to-right side	Right lateral G Eyeballs right	$-G_y$

greater than 1.5 G. In terms of practical application for civilian air medical transports, the effects of G force are limited and in most cases negligible.

CABIN PRESSURIZATION

The pressure environment surrounding the earth can be divided into the following four zones that are based on the following physiologic effects: the physiologic zone, the physiologically deficient zone, the space-equivalent zone, and space.

Physiologic zone: from sea level to altitudes up to 10,000 feet

Physiologically deficient zone: altitudes from 10,000 to 50,000 feet

Space-equivalent zone: altitudes from 50,000 to 250,000 feet

Space: altitudes beyond 250,000 feet

In the physiologic zone, humans are well adapted. Although middle ear or sinus problems may be experienced during ascent or descent in this zone, most physiologic problems occur outside this zone and when proper protective equipment is not used. In the physiologically deficient zone, protective oxygen equipment is mandatory, because the decrease in barometric pressure results in oxygen deficiency, causing altitude hypoxia.[13] Additional problems may result from trapped and evolved gases. Travel in the space-equivalent and space zones requires either a sealed cabin or a full-pressure suit.

In general, the most effective way to prevent physiologic problems is to provide an aircraft pressurization system so the occupants of the aircraft are never exposed to pressures outside the physiologic zone. In those cases when ascent above the physiologic zone is required, protective oxygen equipment must be provided.[13] Aircraft pressurization consists of increased barometric pressure within crew and passenger compartments. This reduces the cabin altitude, creating near-the-earth atmospheric conditions within the aircraft.[5] Commercial passenger aircraft normally pressurize to the equivalent of 5000 to 8000 feet, with the aircraft ascending a bit over 40,000 feet (FL 400).[11] The conventional method, used in virtually all current aircraft, is to draw air from outside the aircraft, compress it, and deliver it into the cabin. The desired pressure is maintained within the cabin by controlling the flow of compressed gas out of the cabin and to the atmosphere. The continuous flow of air ventilates the compartment, and in most aircraft, this flow of air also controls the thermal environment within the cabin.[15]

The difference between the absolute pressure within an aircraft and that of the atmosphere immediately outside an aircraft is called the *cabin differential pressure.* Differential pressure is frequently controlled so that it varies with aircraft altitude.[15] The two principal aircraft pressurization systems—isobaric and isobaric-differential—are described as follows[13]:

Isobaric system. Isobaric control maintains a constant cabin pressure while the ambient barometric pressure decreases. Many military and civilian aircraft are equipped with isobaric pressurization systems. This pressurization increases the comfort and mobility of the passengers, negates the requirement for the routine use of oxygen equipment, and minimizes fatigue.

Isobaric-differential system. Tactical military aircraft are not equipped with isobaric pressurization systems, because the added weight would severely limit the range of the aircraft, and the large pressure differential would increase the danger of a rapid decompression during combat situations. Instead, these aircraft are equipped with an isobaric-differential cabin pressurization system. The isobaric function controls cabin altitude until a preset pressure differential is reached. With continued ascent, the preset differential is maintained. Thus cabin altitude progressively increases as the aircraft ascends.

In air medical transports, cabin pressurization is especially important. Not only does it protect the occupants from the physiologic hazards of altitude, but it provides more effective control of cabin temperature and ventilation, promotes greater mobility and comfort, and reduces fatigue. Cabin pressurization does not eliminate all problems, however. Cabin pressure can be lost as a result of structural failure, such as a window or a door blowing out, or through a mechanical malfunction of pressurization equipment.[5]

Decompression

A loss of cabin pressure is referred to as a *decompression.* Aircraft decompression can be slow and gradual, taking place over a period of several minutes, or it can be sudden, occurring within a matter of seconds.[5,26] The risk of injury resulting from decompression increases in proportion to the ratio of the area of the defect in the wall to the volume of the cabin and to the ratio of cabin pressures before and immediately after the decompression.[15] The following factors determine the rate of decompression[13,15]:

1. Volume of the pressurized cabin—the larger the cabin, the slower the rate of decompression if all other factors are constant.
2. Size of the opening—the larger the opening, the faster the rate of decompression. The most important factor is the ratio between the volume of the cabin and a cross-sectional area of the opening.
3. Pressure differential—the initial pressure gradient between the initial cabin pressure and the initial ambient pressure directly influences the rate and severity of decompression. The greater the differential, the more severe the decompression.
4. Pressure ratio—time is directly related to the pressure ratio between the cabin and ambient pressures. The greater the ratio, the longer the decompression.
5. Flight pressure altitude—the altitude at which decompression occurs relates directly to the physiologic problems that occur after the incident.

The box illustrates the physical characteristics of decompression.

Physiologic effects of rapid decompression are hypothermia, gas expansion, hypoxia, and decompression sickness. Hypoxia is by far the most important hazard of cabin decompression of an aircraft flying at high altitudes.[15] The rapid reduction of ambient pressure produces a corresponding drop in the PO_2 and reduces the alveolar oxygen tension. A two- to

PHYSICAL CHARACTERISTICS OF DECOMPRESSION[5,13]

Slow Decompression

Onset is insidious and gradual and can occur without detection. Signs and symptoms are the same as for hypoxia. Decompression can be determined by checking cabin altimeter.

Rapid Decompression

Onset is immediate, in 1 to 3 seconds, and is accompanied by noise, flying debris, and fog.

Noise

When two different air masses collide, a sound is heard that ranges from a "swish" to an explosion.

Flying debris

On decompression, rapidly rushing air from a pressurized cabin causes the velocity of airflow through the cabin to increase rapidly as the air approaches the opening. Loose objects, such as maps, charts, and unsecured medical equipment, can be extracted through the orifice. Dust and dirt hamper vision for a short period of time.

Fog

During rapid decompression, both temperature and pressure suddenly decrease. This decrease reduces the capacity of air to contain water vapor, and fog occurs. The dissipation rate of fog is fairly rapid in fighter aircraft but considerably slower in larger, multiplace aircraft.

threefold performance decrement occurs, regardless of altitude. The reduced tolerance for hypoxia after decompression is caused by (1) a reversal in the direction of oxygen flow in the lungs, (2) diminished respiratory activity at the time of decompression, and (3) decreased cardiac activity at the time of decompression.[13,15]

Following a loss of cabin pressure, the crew members and passengers must take measures to protect themselves from potential physiologic hazards. Because hypoxia is the most immediate hazard, all occupants must breathe 100% oxygen. Air medical personnel must first ensure that they are breathing 100% oxygen before attempting to assist their patients. Patients already suffering from oxygen deficiencies, such as those with coronary disease, anemia, or pneumonia, must be closely monitored after decompression. After preventing or correcting hypoxia, descent is made to an altitude below 10,000 feet if possible.[5]

Decompression Sickness

The first human case of decompression sickness was reported in 1841 by M. Triger, a French mining engineer who noticed symptoms of pain and muscle cramps in coal miners who had been working in an air-pressurized mine shaft.[12] Because tunnel workers were first to suffer from the syndrome now known as decompression sickness, early terminology describing this disorder was related to that occupation; hence the names *caisson disease* and *compressed-air illness.*[12]

There is a distinct difference between compressed-air illness and subatmospheric decompression sickness, although they share the same colloquial nomenclature for the common manifestations. Classically, the main manifestations are limb pain ("the bends"), respiratory disturbances ("the chokes"), skin irritation ("the creeps"), various disturbances of the central nervous system ("the staggers"), and cardiovascular collapse (syncope). These symptoms of subatmospheric decompression sickness virtually always subside or disappear during descent to ground level. Rarely, however, does recovery occur after recompression to ground level, and in some cases the severity of the symptoms may increase, accompanied by a generalized deterioration in the individual's condition, which is known as *postdescent collapse.*[14] Although the finer points of the pathologic processes underlying some of the manifestations of altitude decompression sickness remain unknown, the basic mechanism is supersaturation of the tissues with nitrogen.[12,14] Because the partial pressure of nitrogen in the inspired air falls with ascent to altitude, nitrogen is carried by the blood from the tissues to the lungs, where it exits the body in the expired gas. In addition, because the solubility of nitrogen in the blood is relatively low and some tissues contain large amounts of nitrogen, the rate of fall of the absolute pressure of the body tissues associated with the ascent of altitude is greater than the rate of fall of the partial pressure of nitrogen in the tissues. These tissues, therefore, become supersaturated with nitrogen. Under certain circumstances, supersaturation gives rise to the formation of bubbles of gas, the main constituent of which is initially nitrogen, in specific tissues of the body. Gas exchange is the governing mechanism in the formation of the bubbles, and these bubbles subsequently grow in size through the diffusion of nitrogen and other gases such as oxygen and carbon dioxide from surrounding tissues. The driving pressure for bubble formation in a fluid is the difference between the partial pressure of the gas dissolved in the fluid and the absolute hydrostatic pressure.[14] Henry's Law can be applied as follows: the amount of a gas that will dissolve in a solution and remain in solution is directly proportional to the pressure of the gas over the solution. Nitrogen is metabolically inert. At sea level, the amount of nitrogen dissolved in the body tissues and fluid is in equilibrium with the ambient pressure. At a higher altitude, nitrogen evolves in a manner similar to the formation of bubbles in a carbonated beverage when the bottle cap is removed. Decompression sickness is not usually encountered below a pressure altitude of FL 250.[5] The clinical manifestations of decompression sickness are shown in the box.

In a small number of cases, circulatory collapse or postdecompression collapse may occur. The clinical symptoms vary. Typically, the patient becomes anxious, develops a frontal headache, and feels sick. Facial pallor, coldness, sweaty extremities may occur, and peripheral cyanosis almost always occurs. General or focal signs of neurologic involvement such as weakness of the limbs, apraxia, scotomata, and convulsions may occur. Arterial blood pressure is generally well maintained until late in the development of the illness. Finally, in the worst cases, coma supervenes. Recovery can occur at any stage, although in the past it has been very rare once coma has developed.[14,16,30]

In addition to supersaturation of the tissues with nitrogen, other factors that influence susceptibility are rate of ascent, altitude, time of exposure, reexposure to altitude, body fat, age (if greater than 40 years), exercise before and after flight, presence of infection, and the effects of alcohol ingestion.[12,14,30]

CLINICAL MANIFESTATIONS OF DECOMPRESSION SICKNESS

Skin

Paresthesia (numbness or tingling sensation)
Mottled or diffuse rash of short duration
Itching
Cold or warm sensations

Joints

"Bends" pain (mild to severe) in muscles and joints, caused by nitrogen bubbles in the joint space
Pain is mild at onset, becomes deep and penetrating, and eventually becomes severe
Pain usually affects (in order) knee, shoulder, elbow, wrist or hand, ankle or foot
Pain increases with motion

Lungs

"Chokes" (rare in both diving and aviation)
Deep, sharp pain under sternum
Dry cough
Inability to take a normal breath
Attempted deep breath causes coughing (frequently paroxysmal)
Condition progresses to collapse if exposure to altitude is maintained
"False chokes" (caused by breathing cold, dry oxygen, which dries the throat and causes irritation and a nonproductive cough)

Brain

Visual disturbances
Headache
Spotty motor and/or sensory loss
Unilateral paresthesia
Confusion
Paresis
Seizures

The primary treatment of decompression sickness arising at altitude is recompression to ground level as rapidly as possible. Breathing 100% oxygen also relieves the tissue hypoxia produced by the reduction of local blood flow. The actual management of a case of serious decompression sickness depends on geographic location and availability of a suitable hyperbaric chamber. Therefore, the order of preference of available treatment is as follows[14]:

1. Immediate hyperbaric compression with or without intermittent oxygen breathing should be administered.
2. Where no chamber facility exists, air medical personnel should treat circulatory collapse and arrange for early transfer to a hyperbaric chamber where this facility is available at a reasonable time or distance (less than 6 hours travel time). Surface transport is preferable; flight to a suitable chamber should be at an altitude below 1000 feet, if possible, and not higher than 3000 feet.
3. Air medical crew members should administer full supportive treatment for circulatory collapse where there is no possibility of transfer within a reasonable time to a hyperbaric chamber.

To become an effective health care provider in the airborne environment, each air medical crew member must be thoroughly familiar with the effects of altitude on the human body. Implementation of correct nursing principles is an essential responsibility of each team member to minimize the effects of the stresses of flight.

FLIGHT PHYSIOLOGY CASE STUDY #1

An industrial hydraulic press trapped a 29-year-old man at the substernal level and compressed him to an anterior posterior diameter of approximately 10 inches with positive loss of consciousness for approximately 2 minutes. On his arrival at the local ED his BP was 80 systolic, and he remained awake and oriented. He was taken emergently to the OR for exploratory laparotomy. He had a minor splenic laceration, a grade V laceration to the right lobe of the liver, and a hematoma of the transverse colon. During the operation, he received 22 units of PRBCs. He was transferred by fixed wing to a level I trauma center 310 nautical miles away. He was transferred directly from the referring OR to the receiving OR. In flight he continued to be hemodynamically unstable and hypothermic. Before departure he had received 5 L of IV fluid, 22 units PRBCs, 4 units FFP, 10 units platelets, and 800 ml Hespan. IV access was triple lumen L subclavian, L antecubital, and R antecubital IVs; L radial arterial line. Before departure, the patient was given Norcuron 10 mg and fentanyl 150 μg and orally intubated with an 8.5 ETT. NG and Foley were placed before arrival at the initial OR. Weight was 220 lbs. Vital signs on arrival of the flight team (RN/RN) were BP 80/P, HR 80, on vent 100% oxygen, O_2 saturation 92%.

En route, the patient's abdominal distention continued, in addition to the serosanguineous drainage from his abdominal dressing. The fixed-wing flight time was 1 hour. Because of his continuing hemodynamic instability, rotor-wing transport was accomplished from the airport to the receiving hospital. His IV total during transport was 8 units PRBCs, 1 unit FFP, 6 units platelets, and 1500 ml crystalloid. His total urine output during transport was 1200 ml. He was maintained on Norcuron, Pavulon, and fentanyl IV for transport.

The rotor wing transport time was 10 minutes. He was placed on the vent TV 850, control of 22, FiO_2 100%, and PEEP of 5 cm. He was taken directly to the OR at the trauma center. On repeat exploratory laparotomy, his splenic laceration was managed conservatively. His gallbladder appeared necrotic and was removed, a G tube with a J extension was placed, and multiple drains and packing were placed around the liver. The CTLS spine was negative, and CXR showed pulmonary edema, no pneumothorax. He was transferred to the trauma-burn intensive care unit, hemodynamically stable.

The second postoperative day, he was trached because of pulmonary edema and failure to wean. A large pleural effusion was noted on CXR and 1500 ml were evacuated after a right chest tube insertion. He remained in the intensive care unit for 14 days before being transferred to a general surgery floor. He developed sepsis, and the infection persisted despite treatment with multiple antibiotics.

He was discharged 33 days later with a PICC line for home IV antibiotics, one drain in place for irrigation with antibiotics, and wet-to-dry packing of the abdominal wound.

DISCUSSION

Assessment: On arrival of the flight team to the referring OR, the man was orally intubated 8.5 ETT, 27 cm at the lip line, on vent 75% oxygen, TV 650, rate 12. Patient weight was 220 lbs/100 kg. He had the following lines: L radial art line, L triple lumen subclavian, NS with blood tubing all ports, 16 ga. angiocath R & L antecubital (also NS with blood tubing). His abdomen was distended, continuously oozing serosanguineous drainage, petechiae seen from the nipple line up, bilateral upper and lower extremities mottled, cool to touch, femoral pulses diminished, pedal pulses absent, refill capacity longer than 5 sec, and HR 100 to 110 without ectopy. Positive fogging of ETT and bilateral chest rise symmetrical with ventilation. R base diminished, breath sounds R > L, rhonchi bilateral throughout, and end-tidal CO_2 detector "C" category. Neurologically, previously on neuromuscular blockade (NMB), bilateral pupils 3 mm, ERL, was awake, talking, oriented before arrival at initial OR at referring hospital. Foley intact, draining clear amber urine, NG placed L naris on flight team arrival, positive placement.

Intervention: EET pulled back to 24 cm at lip, ETT cuff inflated with 8 ml NS, increased oxygen to 100%, TV to 850 ml, PEEP 7, and rate to 20. Trialed on transport ventilator for 20 minutes while patient being packaged for transport. C-collar applied, long boarded (padded board), secured (body first, head second), and wrapped in a survival blanket on top of spread and bath blankets. Warmed saline IVs and port-a-warm mattress (neonatal) to axilla, groin, and upper torso. PRBCs continued for transport.

Inflight: During flight, NG was open to ambient air, abdominal dressing continued to be reinforced as a result of increasing drainage and distention. Abdomen was packed and temporarily closed without drains. O_2 saturation increased to 90% to 100%. HR continued to increase 110 to 120, BP stabilized before takeoff 110/P to 138/P; at altitude became unstable, decreasing to 70/P, but responded well to continued fluid resuscitation. His IV total during transport was 8 units PRBCs, 1 unit FFP, 6 units platelets, and 1500 ml crystalloid. His total urine output during transport was 1200 ml. He was maintained on Norcuron, Pavulon, and fentanyl IV during transport. Because of his condition, rotor wing transport was arranged before landing at airport 15 nautical miles from receiving facility. He was flown directly to receiving facility and taken directly to the OR where the trauma team was already scrubbed and awaiting his arrival. Patient outcome as mentioned above.

ALTITUDE CONSIDERATIONS

Prevent hypoxia by administering 100% oxygen, adequate TV, and PEEP if required. Prevent hypemic and stagnant hypoxia, and observe signs and symptoms (subjective). O_2 saturations only give part of the picture regarding oxygenation.

Keep the NG tube open to ambient air. Barosinusitis and barotitis media are difficult to assess in the paralyzed and comatose patient. All air-filled cuffs and balloons should be replaced with normal saline. Watch for increasing distention in the GI tract or along penetrating wound tracts, including incision lines. Remember to apply Boyle's Law.

The man was initially hypothermic, with increased metabolic needs and acidosis. Decreased perfusion from hypotension and hypothermia causes further decompensation of his health state.

The air medical crew should provide oxygen humidified or an in-line humidifier. Crew members should administer sterile lubrication for eyes if NMB or comatose. Ensure that he has adequate fluid intake. Strict I & O and best evidence of fluid resuscitation.

Noise contributes to fatigue and discomfort. A possible option is to make use of hearing protection (even for a patient who is sedated, paralyzed, or comatose) and crew, both rotor wing and fixed wing.

Air medical crew members must ensure proper securing of patient for safety and to decrease vibration. With CTLS precautions, use a pad board if possible before transport. Boarded patients pick up all vibrations. Vibration leads to increased fatigue, skin breakdown, and patient discomfort.

Fatigue is the result of all other stresses. Consider factors affecting tolerance and self-imposed stresses.

FLIGHT PHYSIOLOGY CASE STUDY #2

This case study addresses the issues of stresses of flight and their relationship to an optimum level of care in the air medical environment. In a city in the Dominican Republic, a 10-year-old girl stepped on a downed power line (60,000 volts) and sustained approximately 60% to 70% total body surface area, full-thickness burns to part of the face, thorax, abdomen, arms, and legs, with the right arm requiring amputation. She was spared instant death by a stray dog that pulled her away from the downed power line. Forty-one days postburn she was transferred by air in a twin-engine pressurized plane from Puerto Plata, Dominican Republic, to a tertiary care burn unit in Miami, Florida. Air travel time was 2 hours, 45 minutes at an altitude of 25,000 to 29,000 feet. The girl was then flown by the U.S. Coast Guard via Lear jet from Miami to the end destination airport. Travel time on this leg of the trip was 2 hours, 30 minutes at an altitude of 37,000 to 41,000 feet.

The girl was transferred from the end destination airport to the tertiary care burn unit by ambulance. She was accompanied by her primary care physician and an interpreter. En route, the girl became increasingly dyspneic and hypotensive. The EMS personnel radioed the receiving hospital that they were unable to obtain a blood pressure or pulse, and the girl was in great respiratory distress. They were informed to proceed directly to the ED instead of the burn unit as had previously been arranged.

On arrival at the ED (April 7, 1987, at 1730 hours), the patient assessment yielded the following facts:

Skin: burn areas as previously described; loose, wet dressings in place

Neurologic: patient awake, responsive; bilateral pupils equally round, midline, 4 mm equally reactive to light; able to nod appropriately yes and no (despite low BP) to questions per interpreter; slight to no movement of left arm, leg, and right leg (right arm amputated while in Dominican Republic)

Cardiovascular: burn areas as previously described; no palpable pulses; BP on arrival was 40/Doppler (double-checked by two separate individuals); HR 120, RR 36; color pale; capillary refill delayed > 2 seconds; skin cold, clammy; rectal temperature was 91.6° F; IV of D_5W at KVO to right side scalp vein, patent, intact; bilateral pedal pulses by Doppler only

Respiratory: on nasal oxygen at 2 L/min; bilateral chest rise symmetrical, bilateral breath sounds diminished bilateral bases, rhonchi throughout; respiratory rate 32 to 36 beats/min, irregular in depth; slight suprasternal and supraclavicular retractions

Gastrointestinal: initially unable to auscultate bowel sounds because of dressings; abdomen slightly distended, firm on palpation

Genitourinary: Foley to bedside drainage; scant amount of urine, 10 to 20 ml dark tea-colored urine

The girl's initial treatment consisted of the following procedures: (1) placement on 100% O_2 via non-rebreather mask; (2) patient prepared for intubation; (3) wet dressings removed, and dry, sterile dressings applied; (4) warmer placed over resuscitation table, and warm blankets applied; (5) IV solution changed to warmed, lactated Ringer's, initially run wide open; (6) central venous catheter placed; D_5LR hung, also initially run at wide-open rate; (7) 25 g albumin IV administered; and (8) initial blood work drawn and sent to the lab. The girl was intubated with a 6.0 cuffed endotracheal tube, placed on a ventilator, and ventilated with warmed, humidified 100% O_2.

The following are the initial lab values from April 7, at 1750 hours. L = low and H = high.

BLOOD SURVEY

Test	Level	Reference	Units
WBC	4.4 L	4.5–13.5	k/mm^3
RBC	3.06 L	5.20–6.20	m/mm^3
Hgb	9.2 L	11.0–18.0	g
Hct	27.2 L	34.0–52.0	%
MCV	89.0		
MCH	30.1		
MCHC	33.8		g/dl
PLT	2.0 L	150–400	×1000

Prothrombin time

Seconds	16.3 h	10.7–12.8 sec	
Ratio	1.4		

Activated Partial Thromboplastin Time

Seconds	44.2 h	23.0–28.0 sec	

SERIES A AND B

Test	Level	Reference	Units
Sodium	136	132–145	mEq/L
Potassium	<2.0	3.3–5.0	mEq/L
Chloride	105	99–111	mEq/L
Bicarb	12 L	20–30	mEq/L
Urea NIT	16	5–20	mg/dl
Creatinine	1.0	0.5–0.9	mg/dl
Glucose	196 H	50–135	mg/dl

SERIES D AND E

Test	Level	Reference	Units
Calcium	7.0 L	8.0–10.4	mg/dl
Phosphor	2.2 L	3.2–5.4	mg/dl
Protein	<3.0	5.8–8.0	g/dl
Albumin	1.2 L	3.2–5.2	IU/L
SGOT	21	2–40	IU/L
SGPT	16	2–35	IU/L
LDH	260	140–280	IU/L
ALK	56 L	80–350	IU/L
TOT BILI	0.9	0.1–1.0	mg/dl

URINALYSIS

Specific gravity	1.03 H	1.003–1.030
Bacteria	Mod	
Yeast	Many	

BLOOD CULTURE

Positive culture for:

Pseudomonas aeruginosa
Enterobacter cloacae

BLOOD PRODUCTS

Red blood cells	500 ml
Platelets	550 ml
Single-donor plasma liquid	600 ml
Fresh frozen plasma	150 ml

MEDICATIONS AND IV DRIPS

Tetanus toxoid
Hypertet
Gamma globulin
Magnesium sulfate
Potassium sulfate
Phenobarbital
Phenytoin (Dilantin)
Ketamine hydrochloride
Hydrocortisone sodium succinate (Solu-Cortef)
Tobramycin
Ceftazadime
Vancomycin hydrochloride
Dopamine drip
Lidocaine drip
Isoproterenol (Isuprel) drip

Initial arterial blood gases were apparently venous, with a Po_2 of 21 and a Pco_2 of 60. (The normal venous Po_2 is usually 40 to 50, and the normal venous Pco_2 is usually 40 to 45.) The next set of gases was drawn in the burn unit after the girl was ventilated for 2 hours. During the interim, pulse oximetry was used and showed a steady increase in oxygen saturation. The next set of arterial gases reflected adequate oxygenation. The girl was transferred from the ED to the burn unit for continued care. During the next 2 hours her condition started to deteriorate. She became increasingly difficult to ventilate, started to exhibit signs of disseminated intravascular coagulation (DIC), and her level of consciousness decreased. Two hours later she had the first of two cardiac arrests. She was unable to be resuscitated from the second arrest and died on April 8, less than 20 hours after admission. Her autopsy report follows:

POST CLINICOPATHOLOGIC DIAGNOSIS: ELECTRICAL BURNS

Sixty-five percent TBSA burns with granulation tissue and purulence
Status postamputation of right arm
Bacteremia
Septic shock
Bilateral necrotizing pneumonia
Intravascular coagulation
Focal bacterial pituitaritis
Chronic passive hepatic congestion
Microvesicular fatty change in liver
Hypocellular bone marrow
Pleural effusions (right 200 ml, left 100 ml)
Ascites (300 ml)

ANALYSIS

The purpose of this case study is to examine the aspects of patient care that must be considered when preparing a patient for air medical transport, and the relationship those aspects of care have in terms of altitude physiology. The elements of altitude physiology involving the stresses of flight have been covered in-depth; therefore this case study will identify those aspects that directly correlate to this particular transport.

The largest single factor affecting this patient was hypoxia. Rapid death was the result of a combination of factors with a cumulative effect. Looking at Dalton's Law, it is easy to understand the reason for ensuing hypoxia, hypemic hypoxia, and stagnant hypoxia. Hypoxic hypoxia was a result of the disruption of the ventilatory phase of respiration by two conditions: First, the reduction in PAO_2 (caused by breathing air at reduced barometric pressure and hypoventilation); and second, a reduction in the gas exchange area (caused by pneumonia, atelectasis, and pleural effusions). The girl also experienced a change in the diffusion phase of respiration. She had diffusion barriers caused by pneumonia that contributed to hypoxic hypoxia. Hypemic hypoxia, caused by a change in the transportation phase of respiration, occurred because of the decrease in her hemoglobin, which resulted in a reduction of its oxygen-carrying capacity. Stagnant hypoxia also occurred because of a disruption in the transportation phase of respiration caused by a reduction in systemic blood flow (extremes of environmental temperatures, which result in a decrease in core temperature and postural changes as a result of prolonged inactivity or bed rest).

Barometric pressure adds another stress that adversely affected the pathophysiology of this patient. The gas law involved is Boyle's Law, which in this case also contributed to hypoxia. Because the girl did not have an NG tube in place and vented to the ambient air or to low suction, gastric distention occurred. This adversely affected respirations by partial physical impedance of the chest and lung expansion, thus increasing not only respiratory effort but also metabolic expenditure in a patient who was already in a negative metabolic state.

With regard to reviewing the thermal stress of flight, the temperature within a fixed-wing aircraft can fluctuate considerably, depending on the temperature outside the aircraft. Burn patients are predisposed to ambient temperature changes even without going to altitude because of the difficulty in maintaining adequate body temperature. Wet dressings covered most of the girl's body (from altered tissue permeability and because urine was leaking from around her Foley catheter), thereby allowing heat dissipation and producing a gradual and cumulative increase in hypothermia. Further, a decrease in temperature that leads to shivering causes an increase in metabolic requirements of the body, thereby increasing overall oxygen consumption.

Humidity becomes a factor at altitude. Cooler air is drier, thus contributing to insensible loss from the respiratory tract and increasing dehydration of the patient. The aircraft ventilation system contributes by removing what little moisture is present in the aircraft's ambient air. Humidity also plays an important part in oxygen administration. The patient was on oxygen at 2 L per minute via nasal cannula without humidification. The dry oxygen also dries mucous membranes, thereby increasing the loss of moisture from the entire respiratory system.

Noise can affect the air medical patient in many covert ways. Noise can lead to anorexia, diaphoresis, nausea and vomiting, headache, fatigue, and overall general malaise. This can accentuate the effects of the other stresses of flight, thus further decreasing the patient's compensatory abilities.

Prolonged exposure to vibration can lead to an increase in fatigue, discomfort, or pain. Leaving a patient in the same position for the entirety of a flight can potentiate the effects of vibration. In this case, the total air travel time alone was over 5 hours. Added to that are refueling time, enplaning, deplaning, and surface transport time.

Fatigue is the end product of all physiologic and psychologic stresses of flight associated with altitude exposure. In this case, even if there were not already enough stresses, fatigue could have been all that was needed to shift the delicate balance in the wrong direction.

REFERENCES

1. Borg N, editor: *Core curriculum for critical care nursing,* ed 2, Philadelphia, 1981, WB Saunders.
2. Browne L et al: The nine stresses of flight, *J Emerg Nurs* 13(4):232, 1987.
3. Burton GG, Helmholz HF: Gas laws and certain indispensable conversions. In Burton GG, Hodgkin JE, editors: *Respiratory care: a guide to clinical practice,* ed 2, Philadelphia, 1984, JB Lippincott.

4. Chase NB, Kreutzman RJ: Army aviation medicine. In DeHart RL, editor: *Fundamentals of aerospace medicine,* Philadelphia, 1985, Lea & Febiger.
5. Department of the Air Force: Aeromedical evacuation, U.S. Air Force Pamphlet No 164-2, 1983.
6. deTreville RT: Occupational medical support to the aviation industry. In DeHart RI, editor: *Fundamentals of aerospace medicine,* Philadelphia, 1985, Lea & Febiger.
7. Egan DF, Spearman CB, Sheldon RL: Gases, the atmosphere and the gas laws. In *Egan's fundamentals of respiratory therapy,* ed 4, St Louis, 1982, Mosby.
8. Gillingham KK, Wolfe JW: Spatial orientation in flight. In DeHart RL, editor: *Fundamentals of aerospace medicine,* Philadelphia, 1985, Lea & Febiger.
9. Glaister DH: The effects of long-duration acceleration. In Ernsting J, King P, editors: *Aviation medicine,* ed 2, London, 1988, Butterworths.
10. Hanna HH, Yarington CT: Otolaryngology in aerospace medicine. In DeHart RL, editor: *Fundamentals of aerospace medicine,* Philadelphia, 1985, Lea & Febiger.
11. Hawkins FH: The aircraft cabin and its human payload. In Orlady HW, editor: *Human factors in aviation,* ed 2, England, 1993, Aveberry Technical.
12. Heimbach RD, Sheffield PJ: Decompression sickness and pulmonary overpressure accidents. In DeHart RL, editor: *Fundamentals of aerospace medicine,* Philadelphia, 1985, Lea & Febiger.
13. Heimbach RD, Sheffield PJ: Protection in the pressure environment: cabin pressurization and oxygen equipment. In DeHart RL, editor: *Fundamentals of aerospace medicine,* Philadelphia, 1985, Lea & Febiger.
14. Macmillan AJ: Decompression sickness. In Ernsting J, King P, editors: *Aviation medicine,* ed 2, London, 1988, Butterworths.
15. Macmillan AJ: The pressure cabin. In Ernsting J, King P, editors: *Aviation medicine,* ed 2, London, 1988, Butterworths.
16. Neubauer JC, Dixon JP, Herndon CM: Fatal pulmonary decompression sickness: a case report, *Aviat Space Environ Med* 59(12):1181, 1988.
17. Raymann RB: Air crew health care maintenance. In DeHart RL, editor: *Fundamentals of aerospace medicine,* Philadelphia, 1985, Lea & Febiger.
18. Rood GM: Noise and communication. In Ernsting J, King P, editors: *Aviation medicine,* ed 2, London, 1988, Butterworths.
19. Sharp GR: The earth's atmosphere. In *Aviation medicine,* London, 1978, Trimed Books.
20. Sheffield PJ, Heimbach RD: Respiratory physiology. In DeHart RL, editor: *Fundamentals of aerospace medicine,* Philadelphia, 1985, Lea & Febiger.
21. Spaul WA, Spear RC, Greenleaf JE: Thermoregulatory response to heat and vibration in men, *Aviat Space Environ Med* 57(11):1082, 1986.
22. Spoor DH: The passenger and the patient in flight. In DeHart RL, editor: *Fundamentals of aerospace medicine,* Philadelphia, 1985, Lea & Febiger.
23. Sredl D: *Airborne patient care management: a multidisciplinary approach,* St Louis, 1983, Medical Research Associated Publications.
24. Stoot JR: Vibration. In Ersting J, King P, editors: *Aviation medicine,* ed 2, London, 1988, Butterworths.
25. Thomas CL, editor: *Taber's cyclopedic medical dictionary,* ed 15, Philadelphia, 1985, FA Davis.
26. United States Air Force School of Aerospace Medicine: Flight nurse handouts, June 1995.
27. von Gierke HE, Nixon CW: Vibration, noise and communication. In DeHart RL, editor: *Fundamentals of aerospace medicine,* Philadelphia, 1985, Lea & Febiger.
28. Welch BE: The biosphere. In DeHart RL, editor: *Fundamentals of aerospace medicine,* Philadelphia, 1985, Lea & Febiger.
29. Wilson LM, Price SA: Respiratory pathophysiology. In *Pathophysiology: clinical concepts of disease processes,* ed 2, New York, 1986, McGraw-Hill.
30. Wirjosemito SA, Touhey JE, Workman WT: Type II altitude decompression sickness (DCS): U.S. Air Force experience with 133 cases, *Avia Space Environ Med* 60(3): 256, 1989.

CHAPTER 3

Extrication and Scene Management

COMPETENCIES

1. Perform an initial scene evaluation and identify potential safety hazards.
2. Dress appropriately for exposure to hazardous material spills.
3. Decontaminate a patient who has been exposed to a toxic substance.
4. Identify whom to call when hazardous materials have been spilled.
5. Preserve evidence from a police scene.

Air medical operations are becoming more common in prehospital settings. Often the rescue helicopter has been preceded by rescue personnel who have already freed trapped victims and secured them to backboards. However, when extrication is prolonged or if the helicopter is a first responder, air medical crews need to use their scene management and extrication skills.

Extrication exercises should be included in annual training for air medical personnel who respond directly to traffic collisions. The training officer of the local fire department or rescue team is an excellent resource for either joint agency training exercises or training that is exclusively applicable to air medical personnel.

Most citizens and unskilled rescuers immediately rush to the victims. However, doing so can result in direct injury to both rescuers and victims, and it may delay the extrication process.

RESCUE MANAGEMENT

Following are rescue management guidelines:

1. Evaluate the situation for potential safety hazards.

2. Secure the accident scene.
3. Wear protective clothing appropriate to the hazards on the scene (i.e., gloves, goggles, or self-contained breathing apparatus [SCBA]).[8]
4. Gain access to the victim.
5. Provide life-sustaining care to the victim.
6. Disentangle the victim from the vehicle.
7. Prepare victim for removal from the accident scene (i.e., place cervical collar).
8. Remove victim.
9. Prepare the victim for transport to the hospital.
10. Provide victim with treatment en route.

Scene evaluation begins with the communications center obtaining information about possible problems and circumstances the rescuers will confront. The dispatcher should continue to seek information that might aid the rescuers throughout the incident, such as time of day, weather conditions, location, terrain, and number of victims. Information about fire, spilled fuel, toxic chemicals, overturned or entangled vehicles, and downed electrical lines should also be related to the dispatcher.

The general rule is never to compromise the rescuers to aid victims. The utility company should secure downed electrical lines; the fire department will hose down spilled fuel and contain hazardous materials. The extricator should read placards on heavy trucks or read the manifest in the truck cab to determine the presence of any toxic or radioactive materials.

Scene security is usually provided by law enforcement personnel. Onlookers and the media should be kept well back from the operation. The rescue team should enlist the assistance of responsible adults to walk 100 yards in opposite directions from the scene and divert traffic.[5]

Proper placement of the helicopter is essential so that it does not create a second accident or hazard to personnel on the scene. The pilot retains ultimate responsibility for landing the helicopter safely. Chapter 6 discusses scene landing recommendations.

The rescue team should enter vehicles through the car doors or by breaking out the glass and crawling through. Although one side of a vehicle may be crushed beyond recognition, the opposite-side car door may be operable. If the vehicle is lying on its side and access is gained by opening the top side car door, the rescue crew should be prepared for the car to shift. In the most serious crashes, the roof of the vehicle may need to be cut open.

Once inside the vehicle, the rescue team must perform a rapid triage of the occupants. Initial emergency treatment before extrication is extremely limited. Usually the initial-entry rescuer brings in a rigid cervical collar, a pocket face mask, and trauma dressings. The objectives are to (1) establish and maintain an airway with cervical spine precautions using either the chin-lift maneuver or jaw-thrust maneuver, (2) provide artificial ventilation (but not oxygenation, because the presence of an inadvertent spark can ignite fuel-saturated clothing), (3) control external hemorrhage, and (4) provide CPR. CPR is not effective unless the patient is supine and on a firm surface.

The basic principle of extrication is that the rescuers should remove the vehicle from the victim rather than the other way around. If the vehicle is on its side, the extrication is performed through the roof. If the vehicle is on its wheels or roof, extrication is conducted through the doors. Rescue personnel inside an upright vehicle first unlock the doors and use interior handles while their partners use exterior handles to open the doors.

Once the doors are open, victims can be secured to short backboards that will provide spinal-column immobilization. There may be further obstacles to extrication. Typically a victim's thorax becomes wedged between the forward-displaced seat and the rearward-displaced steering wheel/column, or a victim's feet and legs become trapped under the downward-displaced dashboard and the accelerator or brake pedal.

The victim must be completely immobilized if the seat has been torn from the mechanical track. When the seat tracks snap, there are usually a series of physically jarring pops that could substantially compromise an injured victim.

Pulling the steering wheel usually disentangles the victim's legs and feet because it concurrently lifts the dashboard up and forward.

If the vehicle is resting on its side, extrication can be achieved by cutting an upside down U in the roof. The vehicle should be stabilized in the side position, the occupants should be warned of the very loud noise about to begin, and a heavy aluminized blanket should cover the occupants for their safety. After the three-sided U-shaped cut of the roof is made, the metal flap should be folded down to provide a smooth edge to move the victims across on their way out.

Extrication and Scene Management

Another hazard that rescuers must be aware of is air bags. New cars are now usually equipped with these safety devices. Studies have documented the effectiveness of air bags in decreasing serious injuries to drivers and passengers.[1,6] However, air bags can cause injuries such as facial abrasions and lacerations and contusions to the chest and upper extremities.[1,6]

Undeployed air bags may be a potential hazard to the rescuer and can cause injuries similar to those reported in accidents where the air bag has deployed. If the air bag has not been deployed the rescuer should observe the following precaution[1,6,8]:

1. Disconnect or cut both battery cables.
2. Avoid placing personnel or objects in front of the air bag deployment path.
3. Do not mechanically displace or cut through the steering column until the system has been deactivated.
4. Do not cut or drill into the air bag module.
5. Do not apply heat in the area of the steering wheel hub.

AIRCRAFT CRASH

The crash of even a light aircraft requires the response of a variety of emergency service units including fire, rescue, EMS, and law enforcement. For the response to be quick and effective, it is vital that the person reporting a crash provide as much information about the incident as possible.

The following information should be obtained by communication center personnel and relayed to responders:

1. The time of the crash
2. The type of aircraft (small passenger plane, commuter aircraft, large commercial jet, military transport plane, military fighter aircraft, helicopter)
3. The number of engines, if known
4. Whether or not the wreckage is on fire
5. Whether or not a parachute was observed
6. The number of occupants of the aircraft, if known
7. Identification numbers and markings of the aircraft; military aircraft are marked "U.S. Air Force," "U.S. Navy," or whatever. Commercial aircraft show the name of the carrier. Private aircraft may have a combination of letters and numbers that constitute the identification number
8. The status of any structures struck by the aircraft or its components (on fire, damaged, collapsed)
9. The status of people in those structures, if known
10. Vehicles that were struck by the aircraft or parts of it and the status of any persons inside the vehicles, if known
11. Structures that appear to be endangered by encroaching fire, spilled fuel, military ordnance, and so on

If the air medical team arrives at the crash site before emergency service units, flight crew members must proceed with caution. Survivors of the crash or persons who have been ejected or who have parachuted from the aircraft may be lying on the roadway leading to the crash site. If the aircraft is military, crew members must avoid both the front and rear ends of any externally mounted tanks or pods; they may be containers for missiles or rockets. The crew must be careful not to disturb any armament thrown clear of the aircraft; it may explode if improperly handled. No one should move body parts or components of the aircraft unless it must be done to care for injured persons. When emergency service units arrive on the scene, the air medical crew reports to the officer-in-charge, telling him or her everything known about the incident and the locations of any injured persons who have been assisted.

BUS ACCIDENT

Stopping the Engine

Buses equipped with diesel engines do not need electrical power to keep running once they have been started. If possible, the rescuers should stop the engine using the emergency stop button located on the driver's left-hand switch panel. If the engine does not stop by operating this button, a crew member should discharge CO_2 into the engine air intake located at the left rear corner of the coach, discharging the agent inward and toward the front of the coach. Dry chemical should not be used.

Entering the Coach

The rescuers should enter the coach through the front door if possible. Door unlocking and unlatching mechanisms can be found under the right side wheel well, behind the front medallion, or to the left of the driver's seat, depending on the make and model of the bus. If the rescuers cannot enter through the front door, they can enter the bus through the windshield by removing the rubber locking strip from around the pane and then removing the pane. To enter the restroom (if the bus is equipped with one), the rescuers should open the small flap at the right rear window and lift the latch bar to open the window. Once inside the coach, the air medical team should plan to remove victims confined to stretchers through the side windows.

The Air Suspension System

The flight crew must remember the warning not to place their heads or extremities under any portion of the coach until it is securely blocked. The air suspension system bellows may deflate without warning, in which case the body of the coach may drop suddenly to within 3½ inches of the roadway.

ELECTRICAL EMERGENCIES

High voltages are common on roadside utility poles. Wood poles are sometimes used to support conductors of as much as 500,000 volts. Energized downed lines may or may not arc and burn. There is no assurance that a dead line at the scene of a vehicle accident will not become energized again unless it is cut or otherwise disconnected from the system by a representative of the power company. When an interruption of current flow is sensed in most power distribution systems, automatic devices restore the flow two or three times over a period of minutes.

The dispatcher should advise the power company of the exact location of the accident and the number of the power pole. The rescue team member designated to control bystanders should order spectators and nonessential personnel to leave the danger zone. Depending on the distances between poles, the danger zone may be as large as 600 feet by 1500 feet. Any rescuer should stop the approach immediately if a tingling sensation is felt in the legs and lower torso. This sensation signals energized ground, and that current is entering through one foot, passing through the lower body, and leaving through the other foot. This current flow is possible because of the condition known as **ground gradient.** This means the voltage is greatest at the point of contact with the ground and then diminishes as the distance from the point of contact increases.

If a tingling sensation is felt, the proper procedure is to bend one leg at the knee and grasp the foot of that leg with one hand, turn around, and hop to a safe place on one foot. By moving in this manner the body will not be completing a circuit between sections of ground energized with different voltages. The rescuer should then stand by in a safe place until a representative of the power company can cut the lines or otherwise disconnect them from the power distribution system. The crew member controlling access to the scene must discourage ambulatory accident victims from leaving their vehicles until conductors that are either touching or surrounding the wreckage can be deenergized.

Energized Chain-Link Fence

A lethal current can be conducted through chain-link fence for some distance. If required to work near or climb a chain-link fence that may be energized by a downed conductor, a crew member should not approach the fence with arms extended and fingers pointing forward. If contact is made with an energized fence, the current will cause the person's fingers to curl around the fence mesh and hold the person in place.

The proper approach to the fence is with arms extended and the backs of hands facing forward. If the fence is energized, the current will cause the person to be repelled backward.

HAZARDOUS MATERIALS EMERGENCIES

Emergencies involving hazardous materials occur in all areas of the United States, and flight crews are likely to be involved in the care of those who have been injured. Hall et al.[3] reported that not enough information is being collected to determine the public health consequences of emergencies that involve hazardous materials. They found that 23% of the emergencies involving hazardous materials were transportation related. Respiratory and eye irritation were the most frequently reported health consequences of a toxic spill.

When a hazardous material can be identified from a number or by name, emergency service personnel may obtain advice about managing the emergency from agencies that assist in the management of hazardous materials (box). Agencies such as CHEMTREC and the U.S. Department of Transportation can offer specific information.

However, not every transport vehicle is marked with a placard that identifies the specific materials on board. Many have placards that identify only the category of material being carried. CHEMTREC should be called for advice if a placard with a four-digit number that identifies the material is noted (Fig. 3-1).

Suggested procedures for air medical personnel responding to the scene of a hazardous material transport emergency are as follows:

1. Land the aircraft upwind of the scene.
2. Keep out of low areas where heavier-than-air vapors can accumulate. Wear full protective clothing and a self-contained breathing apparatus if working in the hazard area. The use of special protective clothing (such as an acid suit) and a positive-pressure breathing apparatus is recommended.
3. If the vehicle is on fire, be aware that some corrosive materials react violently with water. Attempt to extinguish a small fire with dry chemical or CO_2. Extinguish a large fire with water spray, fog, or foam. Fight the fire from the maximum distance that hose streams will allow. Stay away from the ends of tank vehi-

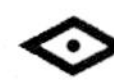

AGENCIES THAT ASSIST IN HAZARDOUS MATERIALS INCIDENTS

Federal Agencies

Environmental Protection Agency (EPA)
Department of Transportation (DOT)
National Response Center (NRC)
United States Coast Guard (USCG)
Centers for Disease Control (CDC)
Federal Aviation Administration (FAA)
United States Armed Forces (Army, Navy, Air Force, Marines)
U.S. Department of Energy (DOE)

Regional and State Agencies

State EPA
State health departments
National Guard
State police
State emergency management agencies

Local Agencies

Emergency management
Fire service (HAZMAT units)
Poison control center
Law enforcement agencies
Public utilities
Sewage and treatment facilities

Commercial Agencies

American Petroleum Institute
Association of American Railroads (AAR) and Hazardous Materials Systems
Chemical Manufacturers Association
HELP (Union Carbide's emergency response system for company shipments)
Chevron (provides assistance with Chevron products)
Railway industry
Local industry
Local contractors
Local carriers and transporters

From Sanders MJ: *Mosby's paramedic textbook,* St Louis, 1994, Mosby.

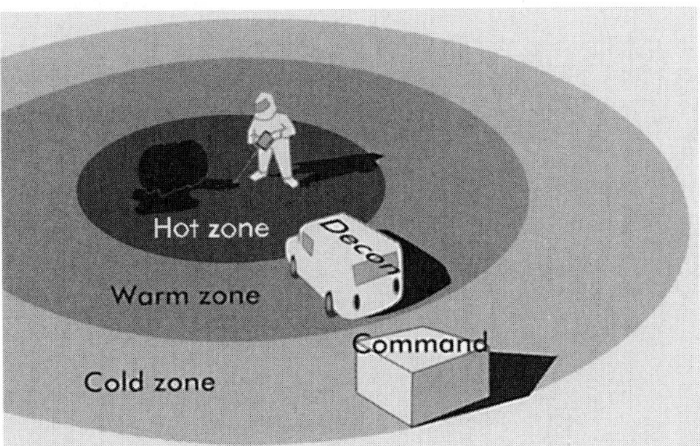

Fig. 3-1 Safety zones for hazardous materials incident. (From Sanders MJ: *Mosby's paramedic textbook,* St Louis, 1994, Mosby.)

cles. Cool down uninvolved containers exposed to heat. Contain large amounts of spilled materials with dikes for later pick-up by personnel qualified in decontamination procedures.

In the event someone has had contact with a dangerous substance, these procedures should be followed:

1. Move the person to a safe place in fresh air.
2. Support respirations if the person is breathing with difficulty. Administer oxygen if it is available.
3. Initiate pulmonary resuscitation efforts if the person is not breathing.
4. Initiate CPR efforts if the person's breathing or heartbeat has stopped.
5. If skin surfaces (or eyes) have been in contact with a dangerous substance, begin flushing immediately with plenty of running water. The person may also be washed with water and a mild detergent.[8]
6. Strip away contaminated clothing and shoes while flushing with water.
7. Continue to flush the exposed skin surfaces (or eyes) until reasonably certain all traces of the dangerous substance have been removed.
8. Isolate contaminated clothing and shoes.

Decontamination

The following steps have been recommended when a person needs to be decontaminated after exposure to a hazardous material[8]:

1. There should be an entry point established for the "dirty" victims and rescuers to remove their clothing.
2. Surface decontamination should be performed using plenty of water unless the contaminant requires another decontaminant.
3. Protective clothing should be removed and stored.
4. Other clothing may have to be removed depending on the level of contamination.
5. Contaminated personnel and victims should be washed at least twice. Water with or without a mild detergent may be used.
6. The victims and personnel should be medically evaluated.
7. Injured individuals should be transported for definitive care.
8. The decontamination site should be cleaned up and contaminated materials disposed of.
9. All equipment that has been used should be decontaminated and cleaned.
10. Contaminated clothing should never be taken home and cleaned.

EXPLOSIVE MATERIALS EMERGENCIES

There has been an increase in the number of injuries and deaths caused by explosives. Between 1980 and 1990 there were 12,261 bombings in the United States. Pipe bombs caused the majority of injuries. The injuries that resulted include both blast and thermal injuries.[4,7] Three classes of explosives are discussed in the following paragraphs.

Class A explosives are the most hazardous types of explosives. They include dynamite, desensitized nitroglycerine, lead azide, mercury, fulminate, black powder, blasting caps, detonators, detonating primers, and certain smokeless propellants.

Class B explosives have a high flammability hazard and include most propellant materials.

Class C explosives include manufactured materials that contain limited quantities of Class A or Class

B explosives as one of their components, such as detonating cord, explosive rivets, and fireworks. Class C explosives will not normally detonate under fire conditions.

A vehicle involved in an accident or fire with a placard indicating the presence of Class A or Class B explosives or blasting agents is a potential danger. It is important to stop traffic in all directions, clear the area of nonessential personnel for 2500 feet in all directions, and deny access to all persons not essential to firefighting or the rescue operation.

RADIOACTIVE MATERIAL EMERGENCIES

The degree of hazard will vary greatly depending on the type and quantity of the radioactive material. External radiation can result from exposure to unshielded radioactive material. Internal radiation can result from inhalation, ingestion, or skin absorption. Runoff from fire control or dilution activities can cause water pollution and thus spread the probability of contamination. Although some radioactive materials may burn normally they do not ignite rapidly.

If only the yellow, black, and white RADIOACTIVE MATERIAL placard is visible, and the material being carried cannot otherwise be identified, people not essential to the firefighting or rescue operation should be kept at least 150 feet upwind of the area; greater distances may be advised by the radiation authority. A rescuer must enter the spill area only to save a life and, when entry is necessary, should stay only the shortest possible time. The rescuer must wear full protective clothing and a positive-pressure breathing apparatus. Persons and equipment exposed to the radioactive material must then be detained until the radiation authority arrives or other instructions are received.

If the vehicle is on fire, damaged containers should not be moved; undamaged containers may be moved if it is possible to do so safely. The crew should attempt to extinguish any small fire with dry chemical, CO_2, water fog, or foam.

It is important to be sure that the victim has been appropriately decontaminated before being placed in the helicopter. If the victim is not appropriately decontaminated, he or she can contaminate both the flight team and the helicopter if they are not protected. If the helicopter is contaminated, it will need to be taken out of service and decontaminated according to decontamination codes and guidelines.[8]

LP-GAS LEAK—NO FIRE

Quick action is necessary when a leak develops in an LP-gas transport vehicle or a large LP-gas storage vessel. A large leak can produce a significant vapor cloud, and the heavier-than-air gas can easily ignite. Vapor releases are usually invisible, and not all LP-gas is odorized.

As emergency service units arrive, firefighters will set up large-diameter hose lines and take positions from which they can apply water to the sides of the tank. The officer in charge will establish a danger zone around the leaking container that should extend for at least 2000 feet from each end of the vessel and for at least 1000 feet from each side. Police officers will evacuate the danger zone and deny access to all nonessential personnel until the emergency is over. If an air medical crew is first to arrive, a member should first request that police close access roads and then alert the gas company, electric company, and telephone company.

When hose lines are in position, the firefighters will disperse the gas by directing water spray across the vapor path. The crew should remain behind the protective spray so that they will be protected if the vapors ignite unexpectedly. No one should enter the vapor cloud. The gas company or plant operating personnel will stop the flow of gas, if possible.

As utility company personnel arrive, the gas company representative will shut off the gas supply. The power company representative will shut off electricity to the surrounding buildings. The telephone company representative should disconnect the telephone service to buildings. A ringing telephone can trigger an explosion of flammable vapors.

REACTION VESSEL EMERGENCIES

Reaction vessels are steel kettles in which chemicals and other products are combined during a manufacturing process. Essentially "mixing bowls," these vessels can range in capacity from a few hundred to several thousand gallons. Some are simple, open, stainless steel vats with hinged lids; others are thick-walled vessels that can be sealed, pressurized, and heated. Large reaction vessels have manholes several feet in diameter, and others have elliptical openings as small as 12 × 16 inches. Mixing vessels have agitators or "beaters" similar to those provided with a kitchen mixer. The edges of the beaters usually come to within a few inches of the vessel wall, and the rescue of a worker behind the beaters (in relation to the manhole) can be a difficult task.

A worker may be injured when he or she fails to follow the established shutdown procedure, enters the vessel, and comes into contact with a hazardous material or a moving beater. A worker may fall and be injured while working inside the vessel. If there is any doubt about the quality of the air within the structure, rescuers will wear self-contained breathing units and a full set of protective clothing.

The rescuer should consult with the plant safety engineer or manager at the vessel location. If a knowledgeable person is not present (as in a multiple-injury situation), look for the **Confined Space Entry Permit** that should be displayed near the entrance to the vessel. From the permit the rescuer should be able to determine the following:

1. Any requirement for special protective clothing.
2. The frequency with which the atmosphere should be analyzed for oxygen concentration.
3. The frequency with which the atmosphere should be checked for explosive vapors.
4. The threshold limit value of any toxic material present.
5. The explosive limits of any flammable materials.
6. What chemicals were in the vessel before shutdown.
7. Any requirement for using nonsparking tools.
8. The frequency with which radiation levels should be checked.
9. Any requirement to use safety harnesses.
10. Any requirement for standby personnel.
11. The type of respiratory protection required.
12. Any requirement for lifelines.

Plant personnel should close feed valves and charging chutes. A rescuer or other responsible person should be assigned to guard the valves and chutes to ensure that they are not inadvertently opened during the rescue operation.

Plant personnel will deenergize the agitator power drive by opening the main disconnect switch and installing a lockout device. The padlock key should be secured until the rescue operation is over.

A rescuer should never be satisfied with someone's assertion that the agitator is "shut off." If there is any doubt that the agitator is inoperative, the rescuer should have plant personnel remove drive belts or chain (or otherwise immobilize) pulleys or flywheels.

CONSTRUCTION SITE EMERGENCIES

If a flight nurse is near a piece of construction equipment when aiding a sick or injured operator, and the engine of the machine is still running, the nurse should not touch any of the operating levers, pedals, or other controls but should ask another operator to shut the engine down. If the injured operator can communicate, he or she should be asked how to shut the machine down.

If another operator is not available and the sick or injured operator cannot provide instructions in the shutdown procedure and, if the equipment is gasoline-powered, the air medical team member should turn the key or master switch to the "off" position. If this does not stop the engine, the cable can be disconnected from the negative terminal of the battery. If the equipment is diesel-powered and has a level-type throttle control, pushing the lever all the way forward past the idle position and then turning the key or throwing the master switch to the "off" position will disrupt the electrical circuit to the engine.

RAILROAD EMERGENCIES

Grade Crossing Accident

In the event an accident occurs at a railroad crossing, the dispatcher should contact the railroad dispatcher with a request to stop all trains that are headed for the crossing.

Stopping the Train

The engineer of a train that is traveling at 60 mph has about 1 second to determine that a collision is imminent and activate the emergency braking system. The train will travel a distance of 7920 feet (1½ miles). Even when traveling at only 30 mph, after the engineer applies the emergency brake a train will travel for ⅔ mile before stopping.

To stop a train before it reaches a grade crossing, a person should be designated to go down the tracks to a point 1½ to 2 miles from the grade crossing and swing a lighted flare slowly back and forth horizontally at right angles to the track. This is the stop signal that is used by all railroads. The locomotive engineer should acknowledge the signal with two whistle blasts and then stop the train. The engineer might either misinterpret or disregard other signs and not stop the train. A flare can be waved day or night; if a flare is not available, a flashlight, battery-powered hand light, or lantern can be waved at night and a flag or other brightly colored object during daylight.

When responding to a derailment, the flight team should quickly assess the situation, report initial observations to the dispatcher, and request that he or she notify the railroad dispatcher of the incident. The railroad dispatcher will arrange to halt rail traffic, to dispatch railroad police, rescue, and clean-up crews, and to notify railroad officials.

If the derailed train can be approached safely, the train conductor should be in or near the caboose. The conductor is in charge of the train and he or she will have documents to show whether the train is carrying hazardous materials.

To reach the caboose when passing close to the wreckage, the rescuers should not go under any derailed cars that are piled high. A precariously perched car can come plunging down without warning.

If the conductor and other train members are incapacitated, the flight crew member can look in the documentation drawer in the caboose for information about the train cargo. There should be car movement waybills and a "consist." Waybills are documents that describe the cargo and identify the shipper and receiver. The consist is a car-by-car listing of the contents of each rail car.

When searching for injured crew members in the locomotive, the flight crew will observe that there are forward and rear cabin doors. If access cannot be achieved by opening these doors inward, a rescuer can come in through the sliding cabin windows. The entire cabin area including nose section, boiler room, and electrical power transmission areas should be searched for injured persons.

Electric locomotives operate from an overhead electricity system that carries 11,000 volts AC. It is important to disconnect that overhead power by pressing the **Pantograph Down** button in the locomotive control cab.

Steam generators are powered by diesel fuel. Fuel shutoff controls are located on each side of the car body under a cover plate marked **Fuel Shut Off.** The rescuer should lift the plate and pull the ring straight out 2 inches; the generator will stop running within 1 to 2 minutes.

Searching the train for injured passengers requires sliding open the side or end car doors, or entering through an emergency window. The flight crew should check the entire car including toilet and baggage areas.

Side entry doors on passenger cars may be locked and will require tools to open. Side doors that slide in the car body panels have electric locks. The conductor and crew members have a skeleton key necessary to open this type of door latch. Access through dual-paned emergency exit windows is accomplished by shattering the outer tempered glass with a heavy, sharp, pointed tool, then removing the inner window's rubber molding and using a pry bar to remove the inner Lexan window.

UNDERGROUND EMERGENCIES

Mine Emergency

In the event of a response to a mine emergency, the air medical team should report directly to the mine office for instructions and follow those instructions explicitly.

Cave Emergency

Preemergency Activities

The air medical team should identify cave rescue specialists, speleologists, and local cavers in the area, catalog their qualifications, and establish procedures for contacting them at the time of a cave emergency.

Rescue equipment and medical supplies should be streamlined. Suggested equipment for cave rescue includes the following[2]:

1. 24 hours of light for a helmet-mounted light.
2. Helmet with a chin strap and headlight attachment.
3. Warm clothes and gloves that are waterproof and allow for mobility.
4. Lug-soled boots that are light and drain water.
5. Specialized caving rope.
6. A litter that can fit through tight spaces.
7. Wet suits when water is expected in the cave.
8. Harnesses and rings resistant to chemicals and water.
9. Equipment to divert water from the victim and rescue crew.
10. Warm food and drink.

The flight crew should participate in cross-training programs so agency rescue personnel can become familiar with cave rescue techniques, and the administrator should develop a continuing education program so rescue personnel can practice rescue techniques in real cave settings.

Care for an Injured Person During Cave Rescue

Caring for victims in a cave presents the flight crew with difficult challenges. Care must be provided in the dark and in muddy conditions. The flight team must be properly trained and experienced before they attempt any cave rescue.

The rescuer should carefully remove the victim from water or water spray, conduct a primary survey for life-threatening problems, and provide basic life support as necessary. The rescuer should remove the victim from drafts, if possible, and if not, should shield the victim using equipment or personnel. Heat loss to the ground can be prevented by placing a ground cover, blanket, articles of clothing, or rope under the victim. Heat loss to the surrounding air can be prevented by replacing the victim's wet clothes with dry clothing that is brought in or worn by the rescuers.

Trench Collapse

Workers and emergency service personnel can be buried under tons of earth when unsupported trench walls collapse. Sheeting and shoring a trench is labor-intensive but it is absolutely necessary if a rescue operation is to be carried out safely. The steps to be followed in case of a trench collapse are as follows:

1. Determine who is in charge.
2. Assess the immediate injury problem.
3. Determine how many people are buried.
4. Determine where people are buried.
5. Assess on-the-scene capabilities of emergency medical services.
6. Request additional resources, if needed.

Hazard control measures that can be taken include the following:

1. See that rescuers are protected.
2. Control traffic movement.
3. Control spectator movement.
4. Make the trench lip safe.
5. Ventilate the trench.
6. Position a safety observer.
7. Make the trench safe.
8. If the trench cannot be made safe, dig to the angle of repose.

Once access to the trapped victims has been achieved, the rescuers can dig them out by hand and remove the mechanisms of entrapment. First, a rescuer should uncover each victim's head and chest and initiate emergency care measures. When all the victims have been assessed and ABCs have been treated, the flight crew member can work to free them completely.

As each victim is freed, he or she should be secured to a backboard before being removed from the trench.

Well Emergencies

Deep wells have shafts that may penetrate the earth for several hundred feet. Depending on the diameter of the shaft, a person who falls into a deep well may become wedged only a few feet from the surface or may go all the way to the bottom. In most cases, rescue (or recovery) is possible only when a parallel shaft is drilled and a horizontal tunnel dug, through which rescuers can pass from the shaft to the well.

Many conditions add to the danger of well emergencies. In shallow wells, the atmosphere in the well may be oxygen deficient. Heavier-than-air toxic gases may be present at the bottom of the well. Methane gas may present the threat of an explosion. Water in the well may cause the victim to drown. Unstable shaft walls may collapse during a rescue operation.

All of these conditions warrant special precautions. To guard against possible shaft-wall collapse, the rescuer should place ground pads (sheets of 4 × 8-foot plywood) around the shaft opening. The pads will distribute the weight of the rescuers and equipment and minimize the possibility of a cave-in. The possibility of an oxygen-deficient atmosphere must be suspected if the victim at the bottom of the shaft is unconscious or incoherent. The rescuer should ventilate the well by having fresh air blown down the shaft. To reach the victim, the rescuer should put on a safety harness that is secured to a lifeline or a harness that is formed with the end of a lifeline.

The victim, when reached, should be secured in a harness attached to a lifeline or in a harness formed with the end of another lifeline. Rescuers at ground level should hoist the victim from the well before the rescuer in the well climbs out. If it is not possible for the rescuer to climb out, the ground-level rescuers should hoist the rescuer from the shaft with their lifelines.

Rescuers who set up lights to illuminate the shaft of a wet well must be sure the lights are tightly secured. If a lamp falls into the well during the rescue operation it could electrocute victims and rescuers.

POLICE-RELATED SITUATIONS

Police officials expect the cooperation of other emergency personnel when there is a police emergency.

Bomb Threat

In the event of a bomb threat, the flight crew should report the location and give an accurate description of the object to the command post or control point, and this information should then be relayed immediately to the police, fire departments, and rescue units. The information should be relayed by telephone even if a two-way radio is available because radio transmission energy can cause detonation of an electric blasting cap. The object should never be touched or otherwise disturbed. Doors and windows should be opened to minimize primary damage from the blast and secondary damage from fragmentation.

Firearm Emergency

A weapon found at the scene of an emergency must be left in the exact position in which it was discovered. Rescuers should assume the weapon is loaded and in operating order even if it appears otherwise. Police officers should be called.

If the weapon must be moved for any reason before police officers arrive, an air medical crew member should assume responsibility for moving and safeguarding the weapon or should delegate the responsibility to a trustworthy person. Only one person should handle the weapon until it can be turned over to the police officers. If a camera is available, a photograph can be taken of the weapon in place, with reference points, such as doors, windows, furniture, and so on, that will help investigators accurately place the weapon included in the picture. A photograph that shows only the weapon will be useless. The crew member should pick the weapon up by the grips held between his or her fingers. Although this seems inconsistent with the policy of preserving fingerprints, it is the safe way to handle a handgun. Recognizable fingerprints cannot usually be recovered from checked grips. The crew member should not attempt to clear or unload the weapon. The number of live and expended rounds in a revolver, their position in the cylinder, and the status of the round under the hammer all may be important to investigators. When carrying the weapon, the person should keep the barrel pointed in a safe direction, preferably skyward.

EVIDENCE PRESERVATION

Many investigations have been seriously hindered because emergency service personnel inadvertently disturbed or destroyed articles of evidence at the scene of a crime. Investigators look at everything, and even something that seems of little importance may be a valuable piece of evidence to a police officer.

Crime Scene Evidence

The air medical team must keep unauthorized persons from the crime scene, and not touch, kick, or otherwise move anything unless it is necessary during the rescue or during efforts to care for victims. Mental notes of possible clues such as the position of a weapon, overturned furniture, or pooled blood will be helpful. As soon as rescue or emergency care activities are complete, observations can be shared with the investigating officers.

Vehicle Accident Scene Evidence

Among items of significance to accident investigators are tire marks, runoff from radiators and crankcases, blood, broken glass, vehicle trim, motor parts, and even clods of dirt turned up by a vehicle's wheels. To assist police investigators at the scene of a vehicle accident, the flight team should first rope off the crash site so physical evidence can be preserved in place and then keep spectators from picking up or moving pieces of debris.

Police Officer

If responding to assist a wounded or injured officer, the flight team should report to the senior police officer. No one should approach the wounded or injured officer until the police officer-in-charge indicates it is safe to do so. If it will be unsafe to carry out assessment and initial care efforts on the spot, the officer should be moved to a safe place in such a manner that injuries will not be compounded.

SUMMARY

Although the air medical crew may not be directly involved in extrication or rescue activities, crew members should be prepared to help the rescue effort and not endanger themselves so that they are unable to help the injured after they are rescued. Scene management of various incidences should be a component of air medical training programs.

Flight teams can offer additional medical care and rapid transport to those injured in all types of incidents. Only flight teams that have had appropriate training, carry the correct equipment, and have experience performing rescues should be the rescuers. Without the proper equipment and training, the flight rescue crew may find themselves needing to be rescued.

REFERENCES

1. Antosia RE, Partrige RA, Virk AS: Air bag safety, *Annals Emerg Med* 25(6):794-8, 1995.
2. Cooper DC, LaValla PH, Stoffel RC: Search and rescue. In Auerbach P, editor: *Wilderness medicine,* St Louis, 1995, Mosby.
3. Hall HI et al: Surveillance for emergency events involving hazardous substances: United States, 1990-1992, *MMWR CDC Surveillance Summaries* 43(2):1-6, 1994.
4. Karmy-Joes R et al: Bomb-related injuries, *Military Medicine* 159(7):536-9, 1994.
5. Kramer A, Evans J: Ambulance operations and special response situations. In Semonin-Holleran R, editor: *Prehospital nursing: a collaborative approach,* St Louis, 1994, Mosby.
6. Kuner EH, Schlickewi W, Oltmanns D: Protective air bags in traffic accidents: change in the injury pattern and reduction in the severity of injuries, *Unfallchirurgie* 21(2):92-9, 1995.
7. Mellor SG: The relationship of blast loading to death and injury from explosion, *World J Surg* 16(5):893-8, 1992.
8. Sanders MJ: *Mosby's paramedic textbook,* St Louis, 1994, Mosby.

CHAPTER 4

Disaster Management and Triage

COMPETENCIES

1. Delineate disaster criteria based on location, number of victims, and resources available.
2. Identify the safety issues that should be considered by flight crew members when responding to a disaster.
3. Perform disaster triage using a designated system of patient identification.

Disasters represent a serious challenge to helicopter emergency medical services (HEMS) operators and their crews, including the sudden and sometimes unplanned experience of working with agencies that do not routinely work together. Disasters are often a result of a complex series of events that lead to a constantly changing environment and situation. Managing them demands plans that are flexible and adaptive in the face of a frequently chaotic and often emotionally overwhelming situation. By their nature, disasters are unpredictable, unexpected, and certainly unwanted events. Yet responding to a disaster is an aspect of any HEMS operation that must be addressed and carefully planned for before a disaster strikes.

Medical disaster management refers to the medical treatment, prioritization, and disposition/transportation of large numbers of victims during natural and man-made catastrophes. However, disasters are often described in limiting numeric terms, such as mass casualty or multicasualty, and generally refer to victim statistics only.

The development of disaster management principles starts with the operational definition of **disaster** and its related levels of intensity. A particular level of intensity or impact on one community may not be the same from one agency to another. For ground EMS agencies, a disaster incident may vary depending on the location of the incident, resources available, number of victims and their acuity levels, and environmental factors. Use of HEMS responders will be factored by weather, number of victims and their acuity levels, type of ground EMS providers (ALS versus BLS), distance from hospitals, and geography.

Levels of intensity and impact are best illustrated by comparing the response capabilities of rural areas to those of a large urban community. A disaster for one may merely be a busy day for another. Accordingly, the term *disaster* is often vague, and can vary from one locality to another. Often the definition of a disaster is influenced by the extent of media interest, numbers of victims, and the spectacular nature of the event. Assuming large numbers of people are involved, if all injuries are relatively minor, use of the term disaster becomes questionable. In such cases the favored term has become *near disaster.* However, the issue is not what to call the event but whether the local EMS disaster plan was activated. Because of this, there is a more accurate *operational* definition of a disaster. The operational definition is used to aid the decision whether to activate the plan when responders are initially confronted with a possible disaster. Thus the operational definition of a disaster is not what type of incident has occurred, but rather the understanding that a disaster is *any event that overwhelms existing personnel facilities, equipment, and capabilities of responding agencies or institutions.*[3] The development of disaster management principles starts with the understanding of the operational definition and its related levels of intensity.

Interestingly, the AAMS Air Medical Crew National Standard Curriculum cites the definitions of disasters using the ASTM standard F30.03.07.[1] These disaster levels are labeled Level I Emergency Response (Extended Medical Incident), Level II Emergency Response (Major Medical Incident), and Level III Emergency Response (Disaster). Level I incidents can be handled by local resources and facilities. Level II incidents involve large numbers of victims and require multijurisdictional medical mutual aid. Level III incidents result in many casualties, overwhelm local and multijurisdictional resources, and require assistance from state or federal resources.

For emergency planners, an additional variation on these definitions can be used. Rather than using Levels I, II, and III, which essentially refer to numbers of victims, definitions using more common language can be applied. This definition format refers to disasters as **simple** versus **compound** and expands on the concept of multijurisdictional aid. A simple disaster is when a community's physical integrity is not disrupted, roads and communities remain intact, and local resources are enough to manage the incident. These disasters tend to be short-lived and may cover a limited area but could involve overlapping boundaries and jurisdictions. A compound disaster disrupts both the structure and function of a community and requires the assistance of outside agencies, usually state and federal, to manage the incident. Classically this event has multiple or widespread incident sites that may overlap multiple jurisdictions and boundaries and often involves mass casualties and fatalities. Operations, including rescue and recovery, may last several days, weeks, or in extreme cases, months.

It is to this environment of overwhelming numbers of victims and an emotionally charged atmosphere that HEMS providers may be asked to respond. Whether the incident is a 5-victim traffic accident or a jetliner crash (Fig. 4-1), air medical crews must be prepared to interact with local public

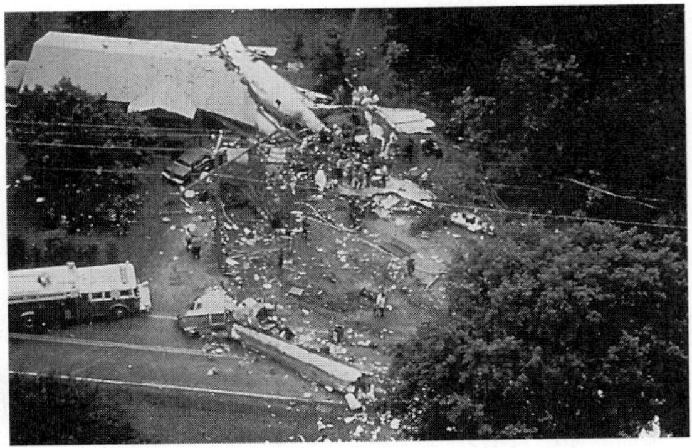

Fig. 4-1 Aerial view of the site of USAir 1016 crash in Charlotte, NC, July 2, 1994. (Courtesy Medcenter Air, Charlotte, NC.)

service agencies and private EMS providers. HEMS transport units must be an integral part of the disaster plan, not just an afterthought. Air medical crew members must extensively train for their roles and responsibilities in the disaster plan. They must know how they are activated to respond and who their command officials are, they must understand their role in the Incident Command System (ICS), and they must have the ability to function in a prehospital care environment.

HEMS organizations must continually update, train, and adjust plans as necessary based on the experiences of others who have responded to multicasualty and mass casualty incidents. Lessons learned by HEMS operators provide valuable information about what went right, what problems were encountered, what component(s) of their plan failed, and what in their training and their plan has been changed because of this understanding.

This chapter reviews the principles of disaster management, triage, incident command, and postincident debriefing. Focus is on the expected roles and responsibilities of air medical crews in disaster operations, regardless of the size and impact of the disaster.

DISASTER MANAGEMENT

The primary concern for HEMS disaster management planners is not the number of victims but rather the development and implementation of a well-researched and prepared disaster plan. The development of a disaster plan starts with an evaluation process known as the **preplan.** The preplan is an honest and unbiased evaluation of the existing resources and capabilities of a particular organization. Community emergency planners, in general, should look at resource issues as they apply to all prehospital care providers (public-sector and private), public service agencies (fire, police), local and state agencies, and finally, local and regional health care facilities. All area HEMS organizations must be identified by type of service (mission profiles), including training and expertise in scene work, level of on-board medical expertise, number and types of aircraft, availability (hours of operation), flight times to different localities, aircraft capabilities for ground and air communication, and emergency dispatch numbers.

Those responsible for developing a HEMS operational disaster plan must take into consideration the normal mission profile of their service, the training and experience in prehospital care operations of their medical flight teams, the normal level of emergency medical and other equipment carried, communication capabilities, and safety-related issues such as protective clothing for flight crews. Deliberation must be given to operating in hazardous environments with uneven terrain, sharp-edged debris, hazardous materials, poor lighting, inclement or hazardous weather conditions, and confined space or structurally impaired areas. Therefore close scrutiny must be given to that part of the preplan assessment that looks at the availability of protective clothing, light sources, crew training for operations in and around hazardous materials, confined space, and hazardous environments.

A lesson in scene safety was learned in the postincident critique of the July 1994 USAir jetliner crash by personnel at Medcenter Air of Charlotte, North Carolina.[5] Arriving in the early stages of the incident, the flight team ended up functioning in a **first responder** role, which is not normally part of Medcenter Air's mission profile. The air medical crew initially worked in and among the wreckage without the benefits of the normal protective gear worn by fire and prehospital care personnel, thereby exposing themselves to increased risks of injury. Other hazards that result from inexperience include arriving at the disaster site wearing unsafe footwear such as high top sneakers. This can result in penetrating foot injuries to flight crews as they walk around and over sharp debris that can penetrate the soles of the shoe. Other injuries include strains, sprains, and fractures of lower extremities. The same hazard issues apply for not wearing leather work gloves and helmets. The most tragic lesson of this type occurred following the April 1995 terrorist bombing in Oklahoma City. A local nurse voluntarily responded to the scene and was killed by falling debris. She had responded wearing only a pair of jeans, a shirt, and sneakers.

Other scene safety issues relate to security, control, and location of landing zones, but most crucially, to control and safety when loading and unloading victims from the aircraft. In the atmosphere of heightened activity and emotions at a large disaster scene, loading and unloading of victims often becomes chaotic. Scene safety must be strictly adhered to. In disasters, EMS pilots will have to deal with additional environmental, communication, and geographic issues not normally encountered as part of a routine scene call. As with the USAir incident, predesignated sites may not always work and alternative landing zones may need to be used when otherwise indicated (Fig. 4-2). This may mean that initial landing zones may be assessed as suboptimum, and aircraft may need to be relocated after touching down at a scene.

Multiple aircraft may be involved in a disaster response or incident. Responding aircraft include those belonging to the military, public service agencies, other HEMS operators, and the media. Preplanning should include a look at organized plans by these groups to work, communicate, and coordinate efforts to avoid any other unfortunate incidents such as midair accidents or collisions. Add the mix of multiple HEMS operations, fire or police aircraft, and a swarm of media helicopters, and it makes for a very crowded sky. In previous large-scale incidents, the FAA has restricted airspace above and around an ongoing incident to prevent such occurrences and to control the presence of unauthorized aircraft. However, this is not always the case in the early stages of the disaster event.

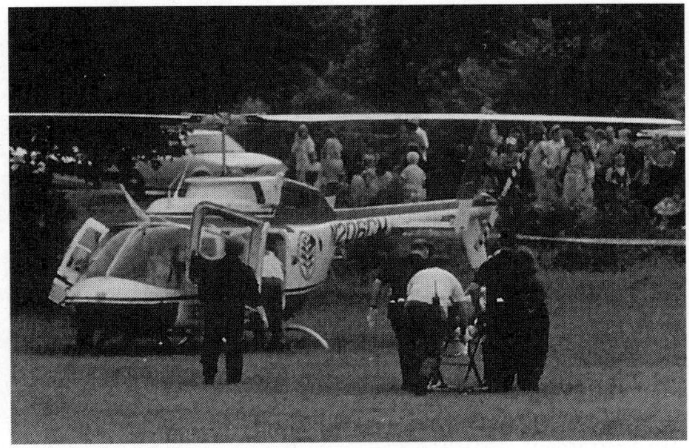

Fig. 4-2 The loading of a USAir 1016 crash victim at the established landing zone. (Courtesy Medcenter Air, Charlotte, NC.)

Another issue to explore during the preplan phase is the need to provide large inventories of medical supplies and be prepared to resupply for protracted disaster incidents. Typically, EMS and HEMS aircraft medical supplies are rapidly exhausted early on. HEMS providers, with local authorities and hospitals, should evaluate their system's ability to bring **disaster packs** or additional caches of medical equipment to the incident site or prearranged localities. This transporting of medical supplies and, possibly, hospital-based medical response teams should be included in the mission profile of HEMS disaster operations. Other secondary uses for HEMS aircraft may include performing aerial scene surveillance to assist local authorities.

Further essential elements in the preplan phase include the vital issues of activation and dispatch of resources and, ultimately, of communications. A strong community disaster plan is one that includes timely activation of all required resources, including notification of those anticipated for response, and alerting of local and regional HEMS providers. The longer the delay in activation of resources, the greater the delay in rescuing, treating, and transporting victims. The best example of being well prepared for emergency response was the 1989 DC-10 crash in Sioux City, Iowa. Emergency responders were given at least a 30-minute warning of the impending crash. Ground ambulances, fire and police units, military rescue, and HEMS were all activated in advance and were in place when the airliner arrived and crashed on airport property. Essentially the disaster came to them with all resources able to respond immediately. Obviously this was an extraordinary case with an extraordinary outcome. The ability of local officials to have a prewarning alarm of an impending disaster, which resulted in an early activation of resources, aided in the overall coordination of rescue efforts and allowed for an instantaneous response to the event. If, however, there is no warning of the event, it is imperative that there be no delays in activating and notifying needed agencies and resources, including hospitals and HEMS providers. Imagine what the response and outcome would have been if the Sioux

City crash had occurred without any warning whatsoever. This is the reality of most disaster responses.

Communications capabilities of HEMS providers are equally as crucial as the issues of early notification, activation, and response. As part of the preplan, helicopter radio capabilities must be evaluated for ground-to-air compatibility with those of fire, EMS, and police ground units, particularly when multiple frequencies and agencies are involved.

A comprehensive preplan looks at internal issues, but also the interface and coordination required with all other responding agencies, including nontraditional ones. Hospital, prehospital, fire, and law enforcement are just some of the agencies to be assessed when developing a well-rounded and flexible HEMS disaster response plan. Once the preplan has been completed, it becomes the working foundation for the development of the operations and disaster plan itself.

THE DISASTER RESPONSE PLAN

Once the preplan is completed, the response plan is developed and put into action through instructional and practical training, with yearly continuing education and practice. Most public service agencies use a system known as the **Incident Command System (ICS)**. It was initially developed for use during multijurisdictional wild fires occurring in Southern California. It allowed fire agencies to develop ongoing letters of agreement and plans to jointly manage catastrophic brush fires while recognizing the need for a lead agency and command structure. Later the ICS was expanded to cover any large-scale event requiring multiple units or agencies, either fire rescue or EMS. Included in the ICS are operational roles for fire, law enforcement, and EMS. The ICS is a management system that allows multijurisdictional agencies to work harmoniously under joint management and control.

Under the ICS, there is one **Incident Commander (IC)** who is responsible for all aspects of the operation. The IC is usually the highest ranking fire or law enforcement officer on the scene (depending on the incident). The highest ranking officer may initially be a fire captain or paramedic, but this job will be delegated to the highest ranking official as that person arrives on the scene, usually a battalion chief or higher ranking officer. The IC is not directly involved with medical operations but rather with the operation as a whole, including search-and-rescue efforts, fire suppression, hazardous materials containment (if necessary), logistics, medical aid, and transportation. The IC delegates others to control each of the separate efforts; for example, the IC would assign the highest-ranking medical person (usually a senior-level paramedic) to medical operations **(medical control)**. This chapter deals exclusively with the medical operation branch under the ICS.

The medical division functions under the operations sector of the ICS. A medical division/branch supervisor or medical control officer (different areas use different titles) coordinates all medical transportation, hospital communications, supply, and medical air operations as they relate to transport of victims, and, in some cases, extrication where medical care is needed.[6] The **medical control officer** serves as the resource and coordinator for division (also known as subsector or branch) leaders/supervisors.

The medical control officer delegates supervisory responsibilities to personnel who are in charge of triage, treatment areas, transportation (ambulance loading and staging), and communications. The **communications supervisor** is responsible for communications with base hospitals or medical control and maintains logs of victim destination. Each branch supervisor has line responsibility and involvement with direct victim care and related issues as previously described. The **ambulance control officer** or **transportation supervisor** works closely with the **air operations supervisor** when requesting HEMS response. The medical control officer also coordinates supply needs and resupply issues, working with branch supervisors as needed. The medical control officer communicates directly with the IC. No other subordinates report to this level of command. All EMS operational requests and considerations must be passed through the medical control officer.

HEMS aircraft take their directions for landing from the air operations supervisor. They will guide in aircraft, establish air-to-ground communications, and secure the landing zone. In smaller operations this task may be performed by someone other than

EMS or fire personnel. It is imperative that someone with a direct line of communication with incoming aircraft have responsibility for this task. Normally, landing zones are kept at a distance from the incident site to minimize rotor wash and maintain control and security. The transportation officer is responsible for dispatching ground vehicles to transport air medical crews if their presence is desired anyplace other than at the landing zone itself.

Depending on local operational plans, air medical crews may either be required to remain with their aircraft and accept victims brought to them for evacuation or asked to report to medical control for further directions. Medical control may request air medical crews to assist in stabilizing victims before air evacuation. Timely air evacuation is a priority once airways are secured. Other procedures may be accomplished in flight depending on aircraft and crew configuration. In either case air medical crews should not self-dispatch to victim care areas, get involved with rescue efforts, or provide direction on where victims will be transported, unless this is part of the local organizational plan.

Once air medical crews are physically separated from their aircraft, a situation may develop in which ambulances arrive at the landing zone ready to transport victims and then find that the only person there is the pilot. This situation has occurred in small and large events across the nation.

Decisions regarding which hospital a victim will be transported to and by what means (ground or air) are made by the transportation supervisor. This individual receives information on patient destinations by the medical control supervisor, who coordinates efforts with local receiving hospitals. It is this very coordinated effort that avoids "relocating the disaster" to area hospitals and reduces the chances of unintentionally overloading one or more of the facilities.

The ICS provides for a coordinated effort among all responding agencies and is only as effective as those who implement and work within it. The primary role of HEMS is that of transportation to and from the scene. Under ICS, added responsibilities of transporting supplies or equipment and additional medical personnel may occur. In rare cases, HEMS aircraft may be used for search and rescue operations or scene surveillance once the primary task of victim transport is completed.

COMMON PROBLEMS IN DISASTER MANAGEMENT

In past years, IMS and HEMS agencies have responded to disasters small and large, simple and compound, and those involving the complicated issues of terrorist events. A pattern of consistent problems, known as the "Five C's" by this author, has emerged as endemic to all disaster events. Disaster planners should use these consistent problems as a guide in anticipating and developing disaster operational plans for HEMS organizations. Understanding what problems continually develop during disaster operations allows planners to mitigate the situation by developing flexible operational disaster plans that take into consideration the variables of such events. The Five C's of disaster management are problems with Communications, Control and command, Collection of resources, Congestion, and Coordination of triage and transportation.

Communications

Communication problems occur as a result of nonfunctioning or marginally functioning communications hardware, inappropriate use or lack of radio frequencies, incompatible frequencies, insufficient numbers of radios and cellular phones, or poor verbal and alternative communications skills by field and hospital personnel. "Ten codes" or coded radio language should always be avoided when dealing with interagency communications, particularly when those agencies normally do not use coded language. Simple language should be used to accurately convey a picture of the incident and its victims, additional resources being requested, and information being passed on. As previously discussed, guide communication from the scene is important. Dispatch centers need immediate information and accurate descriptions of the incident and, in addition, need to know what resources are needed or anticipated. They must be advised whether the disaster is impending (as an inbound crippled jetliner) or is occurring. Historically, in disasters occurring in the United States, communication delays of up to 20 minutes have hindered activation of disaster plans and the timely response of resources, equipment, and manpower. Communication is the foundation on which all of management and operations is built. Without a well-thought-out plan that anticipates communication needs and all contingencies, overall operational plans will fail.

An example of communication difficulties during a HEMS disaster response was experienced by the flight team from Medcenter Air, Carolinas Medical Center, Charlotte, North Carolina. Their post-critique of Medcenter Air's response to the commercial airliner crash of USAir Flight 1016 revealed communication problems that developed immediately on arrival at the scene. The landing zone was located a half mile from the incident site. Ironically, this site had been selected in a previous drill simulating aircraft crashes at the local airport. However, once the flight team was away from the aircraft, they had no way of staying in communication with the pilot, dispatch center, or medical control officer at the hospital. Additionally, after arriving at the crash site, the medical flight crew became separated and were unable to communicate with each other. Drawing from this experience, Medcenter Air is now evaluating the use of alternate communication devices such as handheld radios and cellular phones.

Control and Command

Control and command are only as effective as those persons assigned to leadership positions and those responsible for following their orders. If the command position is not recognized or acknowledged by all involved, then the commander or leader becomes ineffective. This is particularly true when there is a jurisdictional conflict among responding agencies and disputes or conflicts of operational plans develop among the respective organizational heads. Command decisions and plans may fail when there is inappropriate assignment of personnel to job tasks, not taking into consideration the skill, experience, and routine roles of the particular individual or organization. However, even appropriate implementation of the ICS does not guarantee that problems will not develop in the long run.

Congestion

An expectation in any disaster is pedestrian and vehicular congestion, whether it is at the scene or at the hospital. Traffic obstructions can be caused by civilian, media, fire, rescue, and law enforcement vehicles. Additional impediments are caused by onlookers, the media, law enforcement, victims, and rescuers (fire and EMS) alike. This congestion becomes a management problem for the control of ambulance movement and the transport of victims from one area to another, including HEMS landing zones. If a rotor craft is landed too close to an incident, rotor wash can cause havoc and unintentional injuries from flying debris. If the landing zone is too far from the incident, coordinated and timely patient transport from the incident site to waiting aircraft may be hampered.

Collection of Resources

Resources, both personnel and equipment, may create problems either because they are limited or are overabundant. Anticipated resources may or may not appear quickly at the scene. Unrequested responders, volunteers (bystander rescuers), or unauthorized responders may appear at the scene or the hospital. Overstaffing or an excess of available resources complicates issues of congestion, command, and coordination. The greatest error in judgment is to rely on resources that are not yet on the scene, rather than on those that are already available. Those in command must not allow extra personnel to remain in the area when they are not needed for effective operations. These resources can later be used for relief operations, particularly in long-term operations.

Coordination of Triage and Transportation

The process of triage is only effective if those who are the triageurs coordinate their activities and actions. Transportation of victims from the scene to area hospitals and the means of transporting them must not occur as a result of independent decisions and actions by field personnel. The tendency to transport all victims or "relocate the disaster" to one local facility (unless only one exists) should be avoided. Victims need to be divided among existing facilities, taking into consideration transportation times, distance from scene, and the capabilities of the facilities, including whether they have Trauma and Pediatric Centers.

From the moment resources arrive on the scene, communication must be established with local hospitals to determine their patient care capacity and capabilities. Once those capacities are established, victims should be dispersed among all available facilities, determining their destination based on acuity levels, hospital capabilities, and distance/transportation times from the scene. In compound disasters, the hospital themselves may become unusable or diminished in their capabilities. In some cases, hospitals have required emergency evacuations of patients and personnel as a result of structural failure or danger, thus turning them into additional disaster incident sites. All responding field personnel (EMS, HEMS, fire, law enforcement) must be trained in similar triage techniques.

As part of the preplan, area hospitals capable of receiving helicopter transports should have been previously identified. However, air medical crews should not assume that the closest hospital with a helipad or landing zone will automatically receive victims by air. These facilities may be inundated with victims arriving by ambulances or private vehicles because of their close proximity to the incident. Helicopter transport may often take victims to facilities farther from the scene to avoid overwhelming the closest hospitals. Victims benefit both from shortened transport times to these remote health care facilities and from the fact that these centers are less likely to be overwhelmed with victims arriving by ambulance. Thus the staff at these facilities can give more attention to the limited numbers of victims they receive, assuming they have the ability to provide advanced medical care.

TRIAGE

Triage comes from the French verb *trier,* which means "to sort." In medical terms, triage is the process of prioritizing medical care, treatment, and transportation of a number of patients. Its purpose is to sort large numbers of victims, maximize limited resources, and do the most good for those best able to survive. Triage should be based solely on chances for survival and not necessarily the severity of the injury. The process of triage is instituted when existing resources are overwhelmed and medical personnel are unable to render complete care to all of the victims. In other words, the process of triage is to assess the victim's clinical condition as it relates to other victims, assign priority of field treatment, and determine the disposition of that victim.

Triage is used to avoid making decisions that involve the performance of heroic life-saving procedures on those victims who have obvious lethal injuries and are deemed nonviable. This is contrary to routine EMS response where extraordinary care is rendered to the dead and near dead as a matter of course.

A number of triage systems have been developed over the years. Air medical crews should familiarize themselves with the system used in their response area. Historically, patient categorization by triage was based on specific injury types and an assumed diagnosis of injuries, for example, giving priority to a victim with a tension pneumothorax over one with a fractured femur. The process of triage has turned away from the traditional injury/diagnostic approach to the more realistic response to injury and clinical presentation approach, or assessing the patient's hemodynamic status in response to the injury. This approach, called START (Simple Triage and Rapid Treatment) has been gaining popularity since its development in the early 1980s.[7]

START is a way to categorize victims by evaluating three clinical parameters: level of consciousness, respirations, and perfusion. It does not take into consideration the traditional trauma triage criteria of injury type or mechanism of injury. START is a primary triage system and is not meant to be used in secondary or more advanced triage. Its focus is on initial triage efforts during the early phases of a multicasualty or mass casualty incident. It is used to separate higher-priority victims from lower-priority victims and to quickly and efficiently maximize the efforts of limited resources. Secondary triage would take into consideration the types of injures and hemodynamic status of the victim using more advanced assessment techniques. START is useful in hospital settings, especially when the hospital staff is confronted with a sudden onslaught of victims that overloads the facility's capabilities. It usually involves situations where emergency departments are flooded with ambulatory victims who arrive at hospitals by means other than EMS vehicles and who have not had primary triage. This has been the experience of hospitals affected by compound disasters such as earthquakes, tornadoes, and massive explosions.

Triage is based on the victim's potential for survival without the immediate availability of heroic, time-consuming, and extraordinary medical management. Triage via START assesses the victim's clinical condition, as it relates to other victims, assigns priority for field treatment, and determines the disposition of that victim. The most often used terms for triage classifications are **immediate care** (sometimes designated by the color red), **delayed care** (designated by the color yellow), **minor or ambulatory care** (designated by the color green), and **dead** (designated by the color black). This author's preference is the use of both simple descriptive language and color keys.

Some prehospital care systems use numeric categorizations when triaging, traditionally rating victims from 1 to 5 or 0 to 3. Because numbers can be hard to remember and offer no "free association" to memory when the rescuer is under stress, the numeric system has fallen out of favor in lieu of the previously discussed classifications. Therefore the START approach categorizes the victim into one of two primary classifications: immediate and delayed.

A victim classified as immediate care is one who is considered clinically saveable but who required advanced intervention within 1 hour to survive. This category does not include the dead or near dead. A victim categorized as delayed is one who does not fall into the classification of immediate care. This includes victims with significant, severe injuries whose lives are not threatened and whose condition would not deteriorate within 1 hour if otherwise untreated.

The delayed care classification includes those victims with minor injuries (or ambulatory victims) and those with critical injuries who would require extraordinary efforts for survival. If these victims are still alive after all victims classified as immediate care have been treated and transported, then these victims can be given attention and care. Under normal circumstances, victims such as these would be considered the most urgent. However, in disaster operations (events in which resources are overwhelmed), victims such as these would require efforts that exceed the capabilities of those on the scene and would draw resources away from those who are more viable. Thus the essence of what triage accomplishes is the efficient use of limited resources to maximize outcomes for the greater good.

To implement the START system, the triageur assesses the victim's level of consciousness, respirations, and perfusion. It is based on the assumption that the triageur is in an overwhelming situation with limited equipment and resources and thus uses his or her eyes, ears, and senses of touch and smell to assess the victim. Ancillary equipment such as stethoscopes, blood pressure cuffs, and so on may not be available, and the triageur is forced into the "basics." Triage should be accomplished in 15 to 30 seconds so that it can be performed rapidly and succinctly.

Except those who fall into the category secondary to mortal/lethal and nonviable injuries, victims classified as delayed care must have presentations in level of consciousness, respirations, and perfusion that fall within normal parameters. This triage decision is made regardless of injury type and mechanism of injury.

A victim categorized as immediate care is one whose level of consciousness, respiration, or perfusion (at least one of the three) is not within normal parameters. In assessing victims, it is important to note that the level of consciousness parameter is not measured by the Glasgow Coma Scale, but rather is based on a simplified approach of assessing mental activity and consciousness by the victim's ability to follow simple commands. If the victim does not appear awake, alert, and oriented, the level of consciousness is considered "abnormal." However, there is one pitfall with START that was not initially addressed: that of the moribund, nonviable victim. This victim would obviously present as "abnormal" in all three areas and thus technically would be classified as immediate care. However, this victim should not be classified as immediate care because of the extent of injuries and the probability that the victim cannot be saved. To avoid this problem, the triageur should assess pupillary signs on any unconscious, nonresponsive victim to assess for lethal brain injuries. If present, the victim is excluded from immediate care.

In the assessment of respiration status, the issue is again presentation within normal parameters. The triageur would assess the victim for obvious tachypnea, use of accessory muscles, audible adventitious sounds with or without the use of a stethoscope, or respiratory distress. Presence of any of these signs means the victim is categorized as immediate care. This does not include the abnormal respiratory status of a moribund victim with agonal respirations, who would be assigned to delayed care rather than immediate care.

Finally, the triageur would assess perfusion. Assessment of perfusion is a controversial issue. The original START formula called for assessing perfusion by looking only at capillary refill, assuming a blood pressure reading is not feasible. Capillary refill is considered to be of questionable validity when assessing perfusion. However, given the disaster situation and lack of time, equipment, and alternative assessment abilities, capillary refill is used as an assessment tool under the START system. Optimally, capillary refill should be checked by using the mucous membranes of the lower lip rather than distal areas such as fingers and toes.

A capillary refill of more than 2 seconds is considered outside normal parameters and the victim would be assigned to immediate care. However, this does not preclude the triageur from using other assessment techniques such as skin vitals and quality of carotid pulses, as long as the entire triage process does not exceed 30 seconds per victim.

There is one exception to the rules of START. Any patient with penetrating trunk trauma is automatically assigned to immediate care regardless of the presence of three normal assessment parameters. The rationale behind this exception is that the nature of penetrating trauma, particularly high velocity missiles, tends to cause victims to appear well compensated until they suddenly and rapidly deteriorate.

Finally, in addition to familiarizing themselves with and practicing their region's triage system, air medical crews must also acquaint themselves with the triage tags used by local EMS systems. Some triage tags are mini medical records, and others are simply a "filing" system that displays a victim's triage category. Regardless of the systems used, air medical crews will be expected to interact appropriately. There are three major reasons why triage is beneficial in a disaster response[2]:

1. Triage singles out those who need rapid medical care to save life, or, if appropriate, limb.
2. By singling out the minor injuries, triage reduces the urgent burden on medical facilities and organizations. On average, only 10% to 15% of disaster casualties are serious enough to require overnight hospitalization.
3. By providing for the equitable and rational distribution of casualties among the available hospitals, triage reduces the burden on each to a manageable level, often even to "nondisaster" levels.

POSTDISASTER PLANNING

No disaster plan is complete without a postdisaster management or recovery plan. In the past, the short-term and long-term psychologic effects of a disaster on rescuers were ignored or minimized. Fortunately, because of the efforts of such people as Jeffrey Mitchell, PhD, who developed the Critical Incident Stress Debriefing System (CISD) for psychologic recovery and intervention, management personnel are now more aware of the effects of posttraumatic stress (PTS) and **critical incidents** on rescuers and victims alike.[4]

HEMS providers are also potential victims of critical incidents such as disasters and, particularly, death or serious injuries of colleagues involved in aviation accidents. Postincident debriefing is crucial for all members of the HEMS team, including medical crews, pilots, dispatchers, and support personnel to ensure psychologic survival and optimum recovery.[4]

SUMMARY

Disaster drills must continually test and challenge local EMS, fire, and law enforcement agencies, hospitals, and HEMS providers. HEMS have proved to be invaluable, when used wisely, in lessening the overloading of local hospitals with disaster victims and providing valuable scene support.

Air medical crews, pilots, and dispatchers must be trained and updated in their responsibilities during disaster operations to perform maximally and efficiently. EMS systems must include HEMS operations as part of a system-wide approach to disaster management. But it is the responsibility of those HEMS providers to be well versed in triage, scene operations, prehospital medical care, and the ICS to function more effectively.

REFERENCES

1. *Air Medical Crew National Standard Curriculum,* Pasadena, 1988, US Department of Transportation, Samaritan Air Evac and ASHBEAMS.
2. Auf der Heide E: *Disaster response: principles of preparation and coordination,* St Louis, 1989, Mosby.
3. Cohen E: *Disasters! An emergency care workbook,* San Diego, 1983, Idea Inc.
4. Mitchell JT: Stress: development and functions of a critical incident stress debriefing team, *J Emerg Serv* Dec 1988.
5. Daniel M Vaughan, Ruth Pierce, Medcenter Air Carolinas Medical Center, Charlotte, NC.
6. LeSage P: *Fire service field guide: a pocket reference for firefighters and command officers,* inforMed, Los Angeles, 1995.
7. Groth S, et al: Simple triage and rapid treatment: the START system, Hoag Memorial Hospital, Newport Beach, Calif, 1984.

CHAPTER 5

Communications

COMPETENCIES

1. Demonstrate knowledge about radio systems and their use in air medical communication.
2. Use appropriate communication skills before, during, and after air medical transport.
3. Use the appropriate communication device, that is, cellular telephone, aircraft radio, or handheld radio.

Air medical communication encompasses more than use of a radio; rather, it is a total system that permits smooth operation of routine daily flights while ensuring optimal patient care and flight crew safety (Fig. 5-1). No one perfect communications system exists for all air medical programs. The communications system must meet the present and future needs of the program it serves.

COMMUNICATION CENTERS

Planning

Planning for the needs of the communications system should be an integral part of every program's overall strategic planning effort. Each administration must decide very early how highly it values a communications system. Some administrators see it as a costly, nonrevenue-producing entity, whereas others understand not only the intangible value of a first-

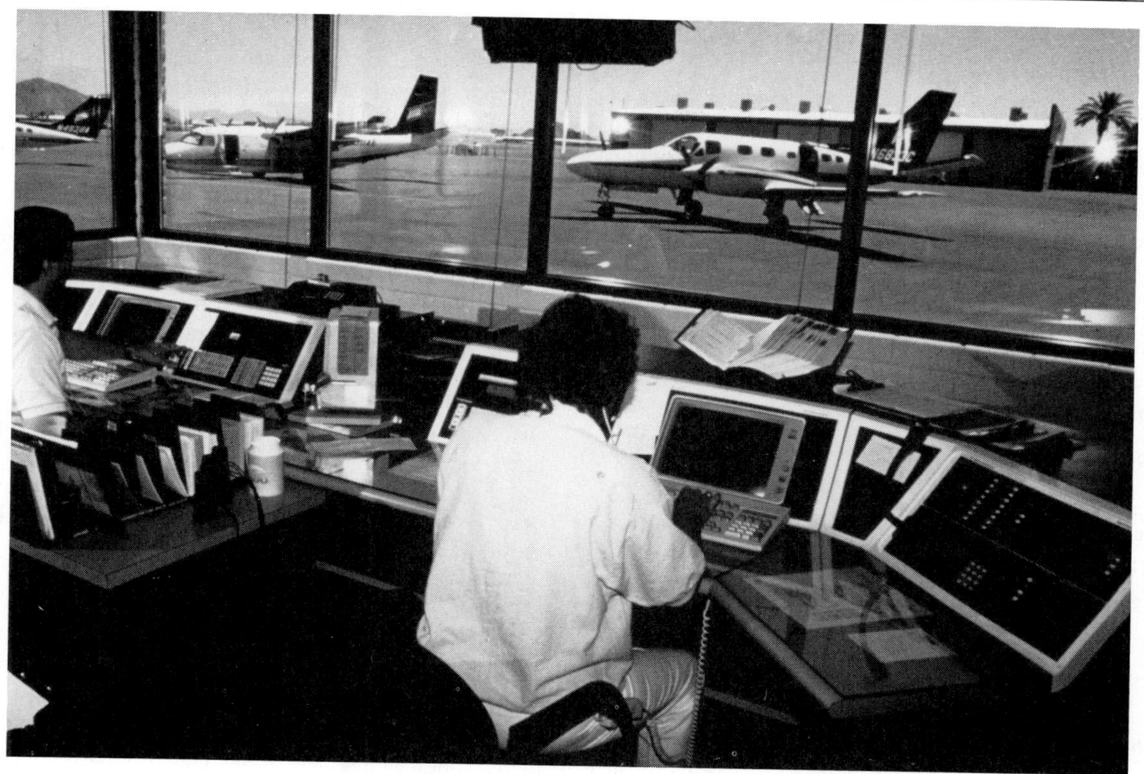

Fig. 5-1 Communications Center, Samaritan AirEvac, Phoenix, AZ. (Courtesy Don B. Stevenson, Phoenix, Ariz.)

rate communications center but the potential it has for saving the lives of an air medical crew. Death benefits, potential liability damages, and legal costs far exceed the cost of installing an elaborate communications center.

Management

Style

Management style plays a critical role in the success of a communications center. With the proactive management style, problems and issues that are likely to occur are addressed before they actually happen, present conditions are continually evaluated, and unanticipated problems are dealt with in a timely, definitive manner.

The reactive management style is not strong on planning and evaluation. With this style, sometimes known as "management by crisis," problems are dealt with only after they occur. In communications centers that operate under this style, little things keep going wrong, details are overlooked, and morale falls, until finally an acute crisis occurs and everyone involved looks around, wondering what happened. In the final step in this sequence, a scapegoat is selected and the problem is fixed in a reactive fashion. Repeated patchwork repairs to any system ultimately result in system degradation and failure.

Support

Administrative support must be available to the air medical communications specialist (ACS) around the clock. The ACS must always have someone to turn to who can make a decision about unusual events or circumstances not covered in the policy and procedures manual.

Similarly, in programs in which medical control is required, the ACS must have a physician available to communicate with the crew if the normal medical control procedure fails for any reason.

COMMUNICATIONS

A major aspect of an air medical communications program is the physical environment of the communications center.[5] Following are some major considerations in the planning process for a communications center.

Location

Whether it is located in a hospital, at an airfield, or within a separate facility, the communications center should be in an area with little pedestrian traffic. Physical inaccessibility and program policy discourage casual visitors.

Seismic Stability

In some areas of the United States, the structural and functional integrity of the facility in the face of a major seismic disturbance is a very real concern and should be discussed with the facility's architect. It should not be taken for granted that seismic stability is part of the design of the facility.

Security

The level of security needed for a given communications center will vary considerably, depending on its location. A steel door with a deadbolt lock should be considered a minimum level of security. Numerous high-technology security systems may be acquired; the level of security attained will ultimately be a function of the budget.

Security does not end with a locked door. Additional security issues are fire alarm and fire suppression systems. Although the communications center may meet current local fire codes, one must remember that most fire codes are minimums for protection, not maximums. It is permissible to adopt stricter safeguards than those required by the code. For more detailed information, one should contact the local or state fire marshal.

Emergency Electrical Power

Each communications center should have its own emergency power supply. Although an independent source of electrical energy is preferable, it is common for hospital-based communication centers to receive emergency power from the hospital's emergency generator.

An electrical generator of sufficient capacity for a given communications center should be located nearby. This generator may be powered by diesel fuel, gasoline, or natural gas, depending on which type of fuel is most economical in a given locale. Consideration should also be given to the use of alternative energy sources abundant in the region, such as sunlight, wind, or hydroelectric power. The technology for these alternative energy sources is available, and it is possible to calculate possible economies for the program when these energy sources are used.

Emergency power must also be instantly available for remote transmitter/receiver sites.

Wiring Access

Each communications center includes enough wiring and cables to stretch the length of several football fields. These wires, which are vital to the operation of the system, should be readily accessible, and the function of each wire should be readily identifiable. This may be accomplished either by running all wiring underneath a raised floor or by terminating all wiring into a utility room behind the wall where the console is located.

Lighting

Whether the communications operations center has the appearance of an office or resembles a combat information center on a ship is a matter of preference. The bottom line is that the ACS is able to clearly see everything that must be done.

It is necessary to have emergency lighting that comes on the instant that power is lost, even if this is only for a short duration.

Heating, Ventilation, and Air Conditioning

Heating, ventilation, and air conditioning systems should be engineered with local geographic weather conditions in mind.[3] These systems not only keep personnel comfortable but help prevent equipment from malfunctioning.

If smoking is permitted in the communications center, an air filtration system is useful, because the by-products of any type of smoke can be harmful to electronic equipment.

Console Layout and Design

Once a custom console is built and installed, it is costly to alter; therefore consoles should be designed carefully, with use of full-scale plans and even cardboard mock-ups. In addition, a console should be designed to be ergonomically functional. The ACS must be able to see and reach all portions of the console without twisting, craning, stretching, or squinting. The seating for a console must roll, swivel, tilt, and be comfortable while providing good lumbar support.

Acoustic Insulation

The amount of insulation required to render the communications center oblivious to the external environment will vary with the location of the center. Enough insulation should be used to deaden the noise from an aircraft engine 100 yards away at ground level. A communications center located deep within a building or above or below ground level will probably not be as sensitive to external street or airfield noise.

Restroom Facilities

Each communications center should be equipped with full restroom facilities including a toilet, sink, and shower. Depending on the schedule and program volume, the ACS may not have the time to go elsewhere to use restroom facilities and certainly should not have to leave the communications center during a tour of duty.

Lounge Areas

It is useful to have a room adjacent to the operations room of the communications center that the ACS may use during slack periods or periods of inclement weather when flights are not being made. This room may contain a couch, chair, coffee table, television, and videocassette player. The ACS should not be in this room while a flight is underway. Whether such a lounge area is available in a given program depends both on policy and space constraints.

The lounge might also contain the kitchen area and/or dormitory area.

Dormitories

The existence of a dormitory depends on program policy, shift schedules, program volume, and the number of personnel on duty. Sleeping while on duty is a controversial topic, and its appropriateness for specific types of personnel must be evaluated by each individual program.

Kitchen Equipment

It is necessary to have a small kitchen and pantry area in each communications center. This area should include a small refrigerator and freezer, a small microwave oven, a coffee maker, and cabinet and counter space.

Storage

A secure storage area should be provided for communications center supplies, backup equipment, and archives. This space should not be shared with other departments.

Decoration

The decor of the communications center should be pleasant, easy to maintain, and in keeping with the character of the organization. It is an excellent idea for the personnel who work in a given area to have input into its decor.

Alternative Sites/Backup Equipment

A worst-case scenario should be prepared by every air medical program, along with a plan of action to deal with such a scenario should it ever occur. Each communications center should be able to continue operations at an alternative site with backup equipment if for any reason the primary communications center becomes inoperable.

Plans should also be made for rapidly repairing or replacing any piece of essential equipment in the communications center.

EQUIPMENT

Selection of equipment for a communications center should be based on the mission of the air medical program, present and anticipated future needs, functions, durability, reliability, expendability, serviceability, and, last but not least, cost. Cost is undeniably the first consideration for many programs.

To make a decision about a given piece of equipment, a program should prioritize these factors, add any others that are applicable, and then determine the most cost-effective choice. The most costly item is not always the best item. However, it is also worth noting that you get what you pay for.

Telephones

Emergency telephone lines should not go through a switchboard; rather, they should be dedicated central office lines, so that if the switchboard fails, the communications center will still have telephone communications. The number of incoming local and wide area telephone service (WATS) lines should be based on the size of the service area and the projected volume of calls. Phone lines can be added relatively quickly when needed.

All calls made with use of emergency phone lines should be recorded, as should any outgoing call pertaining to requests for assistance or notifications.

Telephones today are available with a wide variety of features that may prove useful in a given operation. These features include speed dialing, memory banks of phone numbers, call queuing, hands-free operation, automatic redial, and so on.

Radios

Radios are the key hardware elements in an air medical communications system. The radio frequencies on which a program operates are assigned by the Federal Communications Commission (FCC) on the basis of recommendations by the state chapter of Associated Public Safety Communications Officers, to which it has delegated responsibility for frequency coordination. It is the FCC that issues licenses and assigns call letters. A program's assigned frequencies may be found in several radio bands (upper box).

Included in the ultra-high frequency (UHF) spectrum are the so-called MED channels. MED channels are a set of 10 paired frequencies set aside by the FCC for the exclusive use of emergency medical service (EMS) units. The channels from MED 9 to MED 10 are frequency allocation channels used in metropolitan regions where UHF traffic is high. To use such a channel an EMS unit calls the frequency allocation center, usually located in a fire department or ambulance service communications center, and requests assignment to a channel for the purpose of speaking with a specific hospital. The unit is then assigned an open channel or is told to stand by until one is available (lower box).

RADIO BANDS

VHF high-band FM (148 to 174 MHz_2): The radio signal in this band follows a straight line.

VHF low-band FM (30 to 50 MHz): The radio signal in this band follows the curvature of the earth and has the greatest range.

VHF AM (118 to 136 MHz): This band is typically used for aviation-related communications.

UHF (403 to 941 MHz): These ultra-high frequencies have limited range and are most often used between ground units and base stations. They can be used for air-to-ground and ground-to-air communications for relatively short distances that will fluctuate with the terrain.

MED CHANNEL FREQUENCIES

463.000/468.000 MHz ("MED-ONE")
463.025/468.025 MHz ("MED-TWO")
463.050/468.050 MHz ("MED-THREE")
463.075/486.075 MHz ("MED-FOUR")
463.100/468.100 MHz ("MED-SIX")
463.150/468.150 MHz ("MED-SEVEN")
463.175/468.175 MHz ("MED-EIGHT")
462.950/467.950 MHz ("MED-NINE")
462.975/467.975 MHz ("MED-TEN")

Some programs will have their own private VHF frequency assigned to them. Others may choose to use one of the existing UHF frequencies allocated for EMS use nationally. The same rules and principles apply to use of any of them.

There are several basic types of radio systems, as follows[6]:

1. Simplex system: The simplex system has the ability to transmit in one direction at a time using a single frequency.
2. Full duplex system: The full duplex system has the ability to transmit and receive simultaneously, using two frequencies (typically UHF).
3. Half duplex system: The half duplex system has the ability to transmit or receive in one direction at a time, using two frequencies (typically UHF high band).
4. Multiplex system: The multiplex system has the ability to transmit from two or more sources over the same frequency.

A repeater system is a type of half duplex system that involves a base station "repeater" at an elevated site remote from the communications center. This system is particularly useful in regions with mountainous terrain. A repeater system receives a signal on one frequency and instantly retransmits it on a second frequency to the other radios in the system, thus extending the communications center's range. The process is reversed when the repeater receives signals coming into the base station.

Phone-Radio/Radio-Phone Patch

With a phone-radio/radio-phone patch, special circuits in the radio console permit a radio and telephone to be linked together, one direction at a time, so that the medical crew can speak to a person who is not in the communications center and vice versa. This capability is useful for programs that require voice contact with a medical control physician and for occasions when a member of the medical crew needs to speak to the receiving physician. These optional circuits can be included when the radio console is purchased, or they can be added at a later date.

Programs that use a phone-radio/radio-phone patch have found that radio-like procedures must be used because transmissions are simplex. This presents problems at times when patched through to persons who may not understand the system. Cellular telephones have supplanted this feature in many programs.

Squelch Control

Nearly all radios have squelch control, which is accessed by turning the knob until static is heard and then turning it in the opposite direction just past the point where the static ends. It is best to make this adjustment before using the radio.

Continuous Tone Controlled Subaudible Squelch

Continuous tone controlled subaudible squelch circuits act as a filter to other users of the radio's frequency. Only users of radios with the same tone control frequency setting will normally hear each other. This feature may be disabled when the tone of a transmitting radio is unknown or different or the radio operator wishes to monitor the entire frequency. Private line and channel guard are proprietary names for continuous tone controlled subaudible squelch.

Pagers

Most programs have a need for air medical crews to carry personal pagers. The communications center should have its own paging encoder rather than use pagers that are accessed by dialing a telephone number. Telephone pagers have a lag time of up to several minutes, depending on the volume of pager calls in a given region. Direct encoding will both speed crew response time and result in long-term savings. A variety of pagers are available that can beep, buzz, vibrate, speak, or even display alphanumeric messages.

Recent introduction of two-way paging with use of satellite communications, which will allow voiceless pages to be sent and an acknowledgment to be received with use of data terminals, will no doubt change much of our existing radio communications and paging systems.

An extremely detailed needs assessment should be undertaken by qualified technical personnel before the implementation of any radio system. It is ill advised for a program to purchase a system identical to that of another program on the basis of their satisfaction with it.

Headsets/Microphones/Foot Switches

The use of headsets rather than microphones should be considered in busy communications centers. When used in conjunction with a foot switch, a headset leaves the ACS's hands free, which is particularly desirable in operations in which only one ACS is on duty.

When microphones are used, they should be of the type that filter out background noises. A microphone placed on a bracket or gooseneck fixture attached to the console is preferable because it leaves the desktop space clear. When a headset microphone is used, it should be fairly close to the lips; proximity to the lips will vary because of the varying speech characteristics of different people.

Logging Recorders

All business-related telephone calls and all radio transmissions should be recorded. A program may elect to use an audiocassette logging system, digital audio cassette, VHS audio tape, or a reel-to-reel logging system.

Cassette systems are more suitable for low-volume, low-traffic operations. Cassette loggers typically limit the program to three recorded channels, with a fourth channel allocated for injection of the time signal. Most programs will need a greater capacity than this.

Traditional reel-to-reel loggers are expensive; however, new VHS and digital technology have reduced the cost and size of past generations of reel-to-reel recorders. The tapes for the reel-to-reel system are also expensive, but they are reusable. Currently available technology permits the contents of a 24-hour tape to be compressed and stored on a cassette for future reference. A program might elect to store several days of recording on reels, but this is both costly and creates a storage problem in terms of space.

If the program's budget permits, a dual logger should be purchased. A dual logger provides the redundancy needed in a communications center and permits playback of older tapes while still recording in real time.

Short-term Playback Devices

Short-term playback devices, through the use of either a continuous loop of recording tape or digital technology, record the last several minutes of telephone or radio traffic for review by the ACS when needed. This device enables the ACS to double-check any recent conversation at the touch of a button.

Computers and Peripherals

Computers have become almost indispensable to the well-equipped communications center. What a computer can do for a program is limited primarily by imagination and budget.

Needs should be assessed before any computer system is purchased. First, it should be decided what the program wishes the computer system to do; second, it is necessary to find the appropriate software; and finally, a computer system with the speed and power to accomplish the task should be selected.

Hardware

A suggested starting point for a computer system would be an IBM-compatible computer with a 1.0 gigabyte hard-disk drive, 100 MHz speed, an SVGA color monitor, an enhanced keyboard, and an 80-column print jet or laser printer. A modem for telephone links with other computers is also very desirable, particularly if one wishes to be able to access the scores of electronic databases accessible by computer.

Other devices that may enhance the use of a computer include touch screens, light pencils, a mouse, and a trackball.

Software

A wide variety of software is currently available. The three most used types of software are word processing, database, and spreadsheet programs. Powerful programs that combine all three types of software in one program are available. Whenever possible, it is desirable to use off-the-shelf software that will meet program needs or can be easily modified to meet them. Custom-developed programs usually cost a great deal more because of development expenses, fine tuning, and revisions.

Computer-aided dispatch software is now available commercially through several vendors who track requests for service through charting, charges, and follow-up. These packages are extensive and can be customized for the individual user.

Mobile Data Terminals

Mobile data terminals are small computer terminals that are attached to a radio and have the ability to send data to and receive data from the base station or another mobile data terminal. These systems vary in complexity and require a dedicated radio frequency for their use.

Weather Radar

All pilots have access to Federal Aviation Administration (FAA) Flight Service weather information. While the FAA generally does an excellent job, its reports may not be as up-to-the-minute as desired at a given point in time.

Weather radar display systems are available through several commercial services. These systems may be connected to the National Weather Service radar site in the region by telephone line or computer modem. All weather radar display systems provide displays and printouts of excellent quality. The display should be installed in a place where the pilots have access to it. If the pilot needs an update while airborne, the ACS should also have access to it. This may not be a problem if the aircraft has its own weather radar. If a program has a computer-driven system, the ACS can access the weather report from the communications center. An alternative to the phone line system is to place a remote monitor in the communications center.[2]

Cellular Telephones

Cellular telephone service areas continue to grow rapidly. Cellular telephones may prove invaluable both in the aircraft and as backup equipment in the communications center. Cellular telephones have the distinct advantage of providing a medical crew direct access to medical control or to a receiving facility without going through the troublesome radio-phone patch procedure. These telephones also provide more private conversations; scanners on the market today cannot receive the frequencies on which cellular telephones operate, nor is it legal to modify them to do so.

Fax Machines

A fax machine is an almost indispensable tool in a communications center today, because it enables any needed or requested documentation or information to be sent or received at low cost. For example, if a page has been omitted from a transferred patient's chart and this is not discovered until the patient is en route, a simple phone call to request that the page be faxed can correct this problem in short order. Most hospitals now have at least one fax machine, and some have one in each physician's office. It is also possible to install a circuit card in a computer to enable it to function as a fax machine.

Uninterruptible Power Supply

An uninterruptible power supply is a device that provides steady electrical current to sensitive electronic equipment when there is a power drop-off or surge and serves as a battery backup for a finite period of time until power is restored. It is essential to have an uninterruptible power supply when computers are used for important tasks. These devices can support an operation for periods ranging from a few minutes to several hours. Support for longer periods of time costs more money.

Closed Circuit Television

It may be desirable for the ACS to have access to video scanning of the helipad or hangar ramp. Such scanning serves as a security system and enables the ACS who does not have direct visual contact with the program's parked aircraft to see what is occurring. Television monitors are available that may serve as a computer screen or as a video monitor by pressing a button, thus reducing the cost to the program.

Clocks

Each communications center should have several clocks, which may be analog, digital, or a mix of both types. At least one good quality, battery-operated clock should be available to provide backup during power failures. Air medical crew members should familiarize themselves with the military time system used in aviation. Programs that operate in more than one time zone may wish to keep parallel sets of clocks in operation to avoid confusion in calculating arrival times (box).

Status Board

Every communication center must have a status board that displays, for each aircraft, its assigned N number, the crew on board, and its current status. Any type of board, from a chalkboard to an elaborate electronic device, may be used.

Maps

An aviation sectional map or maps of the program's normal area of operations should be mounted on a wall in the communications center. A compass radial overlay with a center string attached should be affixed to the map, centered over the base of operations. A heavy, dark line radiating from the base operations should be drawn on the map and marked off in 10-mile increments. This map enables the ACS to rapidly obtain a heading and distance to a given point.

There should also be a street map of the metropolitan area around the base of rotary-wing operations as they are called on to proceed directly to the scene. This map should be modified, as previously mentioned.

Topographic maps that show variation in terrain contour and various other maps that may be obtained from state or county highway departments will prove useful in the communications center.

Rolodex

A Rolodex may serve as the primary reference device in an office. It is inexpensive, consumes no energy, and is 100% reliable in operation. Computerized communications centers should have one on hand as part of their backup inventory. Rolodexes are available in several different sizes and configurations.

Cardex

A Cardex is a book similar to a Rolodex in that it has a separate card for each hospital in the service area. Information included in a Cardex should be updated and dated, and each card should include landing zone information and all telephone numbers.

Reference Material

There is no limit to the amount of useful reference material that should be available in the communications center. Available reference materials should include telephone books, aviation material, medical information, hazardous materials data, and anything else thought to be useful by a particular program.

Service Contracts

A service contract should be purchased for all equipment selected for inclusion in a communications center. Service contracts will usually result in long-term savings and more efficient operations be-

24-HOUR CLOCK

AM							
1:00	0100	4:00	0400	7:00	0700	10:00	1000
2:00	0200	5:00	0500	8:00	0800	11:00	1100
3:00	0300	6:00	0600	9:00	0900	Noon	1200
PM							
1:00	1300	4:00	1600	7:00	1900	10:00	2200
2:00	1400	5:00	1700	8:00	2000	11:00	2300
3:00	1500	6:00	1800	9:00	2100	Midnight	2400 (0000)

cause of decreased downtime of equipment. Before any purchase is made it should be determined whether a vendor is able to support the operation with a loaner piece of equipment if the program does not have backup equipment.

POLICIES AND PROCEDURES

A detailed policy and procedures manual is necessary for any organization that wishes to function in a systematic, effective manner. The communications center manual must be a part of the program's overall policy and procedures manual. When the communications center manual is written, it should be carefully integrated with existing policies and procedures to minimize potential conflicting instructions to the ACS.

The manual must cover all aspects of operation that have anything to do with communications. Each segment of the manual should be extremely detailed so that if a question arises about a specific item, it can be resolved by referring to the manual.

A typical communications center manual would include the sections shown in the box and any additional sections that would be appropriate for a particular program.

THE AIR MEDICAL COMMUNICATIONS SPECIALIST

The complexities of organizing a communications system pale with respect to its operation. Beyond dealing with electronic hardware and computer software, the program is faced with one of the most challenging of tasks, dealing with people.

Humans are both the strongest and weakest points in a system. People represent a broad spectrum of personalities and egos, and no two persons are quite the same.

Roles and Responsibilities

The ACS is designated to coordinate requests for aircraft response. The title assigned to the person with the ACS function varies from program to pro-

TYPICAL COMMUNICATIONS CENTER MANUAL

A. Mission statement: A succinct statement of the program's objectives and how they will be accomplished
B. Table of organization: A graphic depiction of how the program's components are related
C. Table of contents: A detailed listing of the contents of each page in the manual
D. Air medical communications specialist: A detailed listing of job descriptions, schedules, training programs, job requirements, and anything else pertaining to the ACS
E. Documentation: Detailed instructions on the use of all forms used by the communications center, whether paper or computerized
F. Equipment: Step-by-step instructions on how to use and troubleshoot potential problems for each piece of equipment used by the communications center; the manufacturer's list of instructions may be inserted as is, or, if they are difficult to understand, they may be rewritten and inserted in simplified form
G. Operational procedures: Detailed instructions on every known aspect of a program's operation as it pertains to communications (typically the largest section of the manual)
H. Quality assurance plan (QA): Components include but are not limited to an in-depth review of ACS performance,* routine preventive maintenance schedules for equipment, and critique sessions held soon after any event in which a communications problem played a role
I. Index: A complete alphabetical listing of the manual's contents

*Performance evaluation of the ACS must be based on written objectives and guidelines, which should be derived from the policy and procedures manual. Areas of evaluation include completeness of documentation, audio review, and procedural accuracy review.

gram. The only limitation is that the FAA uses the term *dispatcher* to designate a person who has a decision-making role regarding whether or not an aircraft takes off. Unless this is the case with a program, another title should be used.

The ACS is responsible for coordinating intra-agency and interagency communications pertaining to any phase of a flight, from a request to hospital admission. The role of the ACS is to serve as a facilitator for the smooth integration of all the resources at the program's disposal, with the dual objectives of program safety and excellent patient care.

Selection

Applicants for ACS positions should be screened as thoroughly as applicants for flight crew positions. Just as all persons who desire to be part of a flight crew are not suited for air medical work, all persons who desire to be an ACS may not be suited to the type of stress inherent in the job.

The decision about whom to hire as an ACS must be determined by each individual program. Certain minimum educational requirements must be met in any case, but some controversy has arisen about background requirements. Areas of controversy include the following:

1. Should the ACS have medical field experience? If so, at what level and how much?
2. Should the ACS have communications center experience? If so, what type(s) of experience are acceptable, and how much experience is necessary?

Neither medical field experience nor communications center experience alone qualifies a person to be an ACS; neither does being a friend or relative of someone employed by the program.

Training

Regardless of the background of the ACS applicant, the person must be trained as an ACS. A curriculum that may be used as a foundation for a program's own curriculum is included in *The AAMS Manual for Air Medical Communications Operations.*[5] Training must be an ongoing process to ensure currency and proficiency.

Testing

The ACS should be tested periodically on all elements of the position. The ACS has the responsibility of knowing everything about the program and being able to use that information at a moment's notice with a high degree of accuracy. In terms of communications procedures, less than 100% accuracy is unacceptable.

Dress Code

The attire that is considered proper for communications personnel is a matter of preference for each program. Consideration should be given to whether anything is gained by the additional expense of uniforms or if civilian attire in certain color combinations is acceptable.

COMMUNICATING

Radios

Language

To effectively communicate within a program, standardized terminology should be used so that meanings are not lost or misinterpreted.

In general, it is preferable to communicate in plain language instead of using various codes; this precludes errors based on the misunderstanding of a garbled, coded transmission. Because of the broad area over which an air medical program operates, it would be extremely difficult to know codes for each of the many jurisdictions in the program's service area.

Speaking

When initiating a radio transmission, an air medical crew member should begin with the name or call sign of the unit being called, followed by the member's own name or call sign. When older radio systems and poorly maintained new systems are used it may be advantageous, when keying the microphone, for the speaker to pause for a second before speaking to allow the radio to reach its maximum output level. This helps prevent the frequent problem of incomplete messages being received. Another cause of this problem is speaking before keying the microphone.

The speaker should talk at a normal rate; yelling into the microphone distorts the transmission. The speaker should know what he or she is going to say before keying the microphone, speak clearly and concisely without irrelevant comments, attempt to control his or her voice level and intonation even when under stress, try to avoid transmissions that reflect disgust, irritation, or sarcasm, and avoid the use of profanity at all times. Radio transmissions are a measure of a program's professionalism, and both the media and a large population of citizens with scanners hear every word that is said on the radio.

It is important that air medical crew members know how to properly operate the two-directional radio-intercom switch commonly found on headset cords in aircraft. Many air crew members have been embarrassed when personal conversations or comments less than socially acceptable were broadcast over a wide area. This is less of a problem in programs that operate pressurized aircraft, in which medical crew members may not be using a headset system.

Intracrew communications are very important. The pilot should keep the medical crew informed of any developments in a clear, complete message that leaves no doubt about what is happening. The following two anecdotes illustrate this point. Although the incidents are somewhat humorous now, the crews involved did not think so at the time. In the first incident, the crew received a badly scrawled note from the pilot, pushed through an opening behind his seat, just as the helicopter began an unexpected banking turn. The note read, "I can't talk." The crew members looked at each other, each thinking that the pilot had experienced a cerebrovascular accident. They were about to become upset when the aircraft resumed straight and level flight. The pilot came on the intercom and explained that he could not talk on the medical radio, that he had spoken to approach control, and that he was returning to base for another aircraft. A more complete written message or advance warning on the intercom could have prevented a tense few moments for the crew.

In the second incident, the pilot of an outbound aircraft observed a transmission chip light blink on. In accordance with company policy he immediately began a descent in preparation for landing. He told the crew "we're going down." The crew went into a not-so-happy mode, prepared themselves for a hard landing, and then began a vigorous discussion over the use of the one pillow on board. A normal landing was made, the mechanic arrived and corrected the problem, and the aircraft returned to its base. Once again, a more complete explanation would have prevented these tense moments.

During a flight the pilot of an airport-based aircraft will communicate with each of the following, in addition to the ACS: ground control, airport tower departure control, air route traffic control center, approach control, airport tower, and ground control again.

Hospital-based rotorcraft may or may not be near an airport but will be in communication with the appropriate segments of the air traffic control system and the program's own communications center. In either case only the pilots should communicate with air traffic control. Aircraft on scene flights will also speak with units already on the scene.

The medical crew should be aware that there are certain times when they should refrain from speaking to the pilot unless absolutely imperative. These times are as follows[4]:

1. During takeoff
2. During landings
3. During instrument approaches
4. In dense air traffic areas

Air crews in programs with multiple aircraft should also be aware that nonessential interaircraft conversations may make it difficult for the ACS to carry on a telephone conversation or to receive an essential transmission from another unit.

If a crew member asks the ACS to make a phone call, he or she should wait a minute or so before transmitting again to avoid interrupting the call.

If either party is having difficulty making a word understood, then that person should spell it using the phonetic alphabet (see the box on p. 72).

Telephone

Often a requesting party's first impression of a program is created by the ACS who answers the phone. A courteous manner combined with comprehensive knowledge of the program will help give the

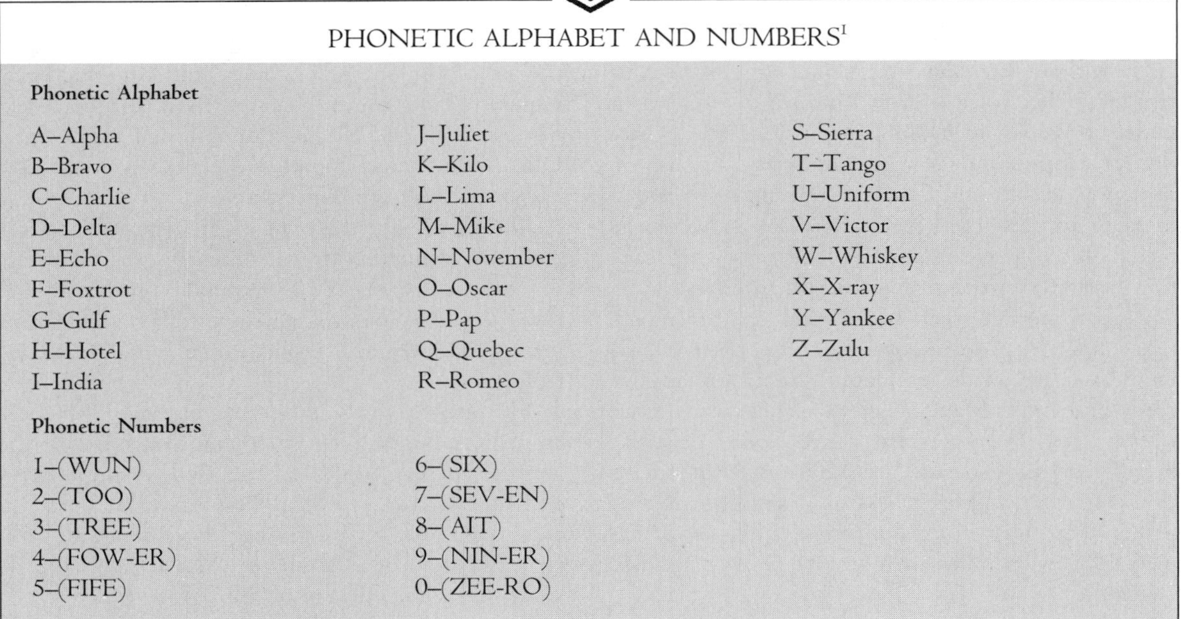

PHONETIC ALPHABET AND NUMBERS[1]

Phonetic Alphabet

A–Alpha	J–Juliet	S–Sierra
B–Bravo	K–Kilo	T–Tango
C–Charlie	L–Lima	U–Uniform
D–Delta	M–Mike	V–Victor
E–Echo	N–November	W–Whiskey
F–Foxtrot	O–Oscar	X–X-ray
G–Gulf	P–Pap	Y–Yankee
H–Hotel	Q–Quebec	Z–Zulu
I–India	R–Romeo	

Phonetic Numbers

1–(WUN)	6–(SIX)
2–(TOO)	7–(SEV-EN)
3–(TREE)	8–(AIT)
4–(FOW-ER)	9–(NIN-ER)
5–(FIFE)	0–(ZEE-RO)

caller the impression that the program is staffed by competent, professional personnel.

Medical Control

Programs that operate with flight nurses or flight paramedics are included under medical control regulations that vary from state to state. Whether communicating with their medical control physician by radio, radio-phone patch, or cellular telephone, the medical crew should follow the medical reporting format used in their region. All reports should be brief and to the point. Any treatment order received should be acknowledged by repeating the order verbatim.

Face to Face

Of particular importance to the success of a program are interpersonal communications among all program personnel. An understanding of the problems and stress inherent to each position tends to foster patience. Cross-orientation sessions between air crew members and communications personnel are useful in creating this understanding. Anyone who works in a program is going to have an occasional bad day, and colleagues must be able to deal with this circumspectly.

Successful working relationships frequently lead to personal friendships. Social events within programs also tend to relieve stress and improve working relationships.[4]

On Paper

In this litigious age, everything that occurs must be documented. "If it is not written down, then it did not happen" is a concept pursued by attorneys who specialize in the field of malpractice.

All forms used by the program should be filled out assiduously. If something does not apply, a line should be drawn through the space or the letters "NA" should be inserted.

When forms to be used in the program are created, an attempt should be made to minimize the number of times that any one piece of information must be written. If the originals do not have separate destinations, forms should be consolidated. Communications forms should have the same flow as those used by the medical crew to make it easier for the medical crew member to write down what the ACS says.

A 6 month supply of most forms should be adequate as long as a new supply is ordered before they run out. All forms should be evaluated periodically to determine if they are still functional.

All written communications from administration should be placed in a file folder or in looseleaf books in reverse chronological order for easy reference. If appropriate, they may be placed in the policy and procedures manual.

With the Media

Local news media usually have a high level of interest in the activities of an air medical program. The ACS must be able to politely but firmly deal with their calls when they interfere with operations. The ACS must be aware of program policy with respect to giving out information and should refer the caller to the appropriate person if this is dictated by policy.

Establishing a good rapport with the local media is essential. Many people have strong negative feelings about certain aspects of the news media. A decision may be reached within a program to notify the media of the types of events in which they usually express interest, time permitting. The flight operation always comes first.

EMERGENCY PROCEDURES

The operational procedures section of the policy and procedures manual should include a subsection dealing with procedures to be followed in the event of any unscheduled event that affects the use of the aircraft or directly involves the aircraft.

Mass Casualty Incidents

The air medical program is undoubtedly a part of any mass casualty incident plan developed in the program's service area. Copies of the program's roles in these situations should be immediately accessible to the ACS.

Unscheduled Events

Detailed contingency plans must exist for various emergencies involving the program's aircraft. These plans must be immediately accessible to the ACS.

Drills

The ACS should participate in practice exercises, both scheduled and unscheduled, relating to various emergencies that might occur. These practice exercises reinforce the ACS's knowledge of the procedures and test the procedures for weak spots.

If a practice exercise that involves a missing or overdue aircraft is held, care must be taken to stop the chain of notification before a flight crew's family is inadvertently notified and caused grief or anxiety.

Critical Incident Stress Management

Each program should have a critical incident stress management plan in place in the event of the loss of an aircraft and its crew. It is imperative that the ACS on duty at the time be included in this plan. The ACS will experience all the same feelings of grief and loss as the other program members, and more. The ACS may believe that he or she could have done something more or failed to do something and thus take on unwarranted feelings of guilt. Unless counseled immediately, this ACS will be lost to the program at some point in the future.

AIRCRAFT RADIOS

Each medical crew member should be familiar with the operation of the radios used in his or her program's aircraft. In some aircraft there may be more than one radio, thus permitting the medical crew to communicate with someone on the ground while the pilot is talking to someone else.

Other aircraft will have one radio and two control heads, one for the pilot and the other for the medical crew. The medical crew member should check with the pilot before using the radio to be certain that he or she has no need of it at the time.

Portable Units

A program may elect to provide medical crew members with portable handheld radios for use on the ground outside the aircraft. These radios are particularly useful for programs that do emergency scene flights, and they are also useful during transfer flights for alerting the pilot to the imminent return of the crew with the patient.

SUMMARY

The communications center of an air medical program is the foundation of a successful venture. Planning and implementation of a communications center must be organized, logical, and cost-effective. The program's mission, philosophy, and resources must be evaluated to ensure quality communications.

REFERENCES

1. *Federal Aviation Administration airman's information manual,* Glendale, Calif, 1989, Aviation Book Company.
2. *Federal aviation for pilots,* Glendale, Calif, 1989, Aviation Book Company.
3. *Fire protection handbook,* ed 16, Quincy, Mass, 1986, National Fire Protection Association.
4. Herron S: Communications. In McCloskey K, Orr R, editors: *Pediatric transport medicine,* St Louis, 1995, Mosby.
5. *Manual for Air Medical Communications Operations Association of Air Medical Services,* Pasadena, Calif, 1989.
6. *Pilot's handbook of aeronautical knowledge,* Washington, DC, 1984, US Department of Transportation.

CHAPTER 6

Flight Safety and Personal Survival

COMPETENCIES

1. Identify safety hazards around the aircraft.
2. Perform a preflight safety check.
3. Execute safety procedures during flight, including securement of equipment, patients, and personnel during flight.
4. Ascertain the location and contents of the flight program's "downed aircraft" policy.
5. Perform basic survival skills including signaling and fire and shelter building.

The majority of the chapters contained in this book contain information written to help the practitioner who performs in the air medical setting provide care for critically ill or injured patients. The information in this chapter is written for the practitioners themselves, who face unique and challenging hazards in the air medical environment. Flight nurses, paramedics, physicians, and pilots are responsible for the care and transport of patients, but these professionals also share a greater responsibility: to function as safety advocates. Flight team members must recognize that their actions affect not only their own safety but also the safety of other crew members or the entire aircraft. With that knowledge in mind, flight team members must develop a safety consciousness that guides their actions. A safety consciousness is developed as a result of training, repetition, and complete familiarity with equipment and procedures. It is only after developing a safety consciousness that flight team members are ready to assume the responsibility of maintaining a secure and protected environment for the patients they transport, other flight team members, ancillary staff, public service personnel, bystanders, and all other persons who interact with the air medical service.

Like other skills, safety advocacy requires time, work, and desire. The role of safety advocate is the most important responsibility of any flight team member because failure to provide the safest environment possible will at some point significantly undermine the ability of flight team members to perform the diverse responsibilities required for patient care.

FLIGHT SAFETY DEFINITION

A discussion of flight safety must begin with a working definition. Flight safety consists of specific practices outlined in a safety plan and incorporated into the daily flight operations with the purpose of reducing or eliminating the risk of severe injury or death to members of the flight team, patients, or ancillary persons operating around or near the aircraft. Unfortunately, not all human endeavors can be totally free of risk. Many work environments present significant risk to those who work in them. However, steps can be taken to assess and prioritize the risk, safety plans can be implemented to address known risk, and an ongoing monitoring program can evaluate the effectiveness of efforts to reduce the risks to an acceptable degree. Over time the work environment will change, which requires flexibility in the safety plan. New information may dictate new approaches to old problems. What must never change is the commitment of the people involved to continually work toward keeping risk at or below an acceptable level.

All persons directly involved in daily flight operations must also define within themselves their personal degree of acceptable risk because, if individuals have serious doubts regarding their personal safety, the stress created by those concerns will ultimately interfere with their job performance.

FLIGHT SAFETY AWARENESS PROGRAM

A strong commitment to safety must begin early in the development of any air medical program. The commitment to safety must be stated clearly in the mission statement of the program and must be supported through the actions of management. Management personnel must provide an open, organized forum for personnel to contribute to the development of safety strategies.[22] One method used to provide an open forum is through the safety committee.[7,11]

The safety committee is composed of various members of the flight program, representing pilots, mechanics, communication specialists, and medical personnel, in addition to administrative staff. The committee establishes a hazard reporting system in which potential hazards in the work environment are reported to individual committee members and are then channeled for further discussion and resolution by the committee. Safety problems are discussed at monthly safety meetings, appropriate action is decided on, and responsibilities to complete the action are assigned. Safety information is reviewed frequently, changes are made as required, and new information is disseminated during regularly scheduled safety meetings at which all members of the program are present.

Statewide and regional safety councils are made up of local programs that work together to address common safety concerns.[16,18] The safety forum allows member programs an opportunity to exchange program policy information on topics such as weather guidelines, communication procedures, and ongoing training. Agreements to provide mutual flight following for member programs are also addressed by state or regional safety committees. One objective of regional or state safety committees should be the elimination of any negative influence caused by competition between programs that operate in the same area.

A successful, comprehensive safety program evaluates training, equipment, policies, and procedures and is strengthened by commitment, teamwork, and open communication by all members of the air medical program.

Role of Program Management

The most important element in accident prevention is a commitment to safety by the program director.[7] Safety is everyone's responsibility; however, the program director is responsible for creating the emphasis on safety. The program director must be familiar with basic Federal Aviation Administration (FAA) regulations and understand the limitations of helicopter operations, such as ceiling and visibility limits. For example, program directors must ensure that standard operating procedures are written in a manner that does not create undue pressure on pilots to complete emergency medical services (EMS) missions. Competition between programs must not be allowed to affect safety. The program director must have an understanding of helicopter design technologies that have a direct influence on occupant safety and must ensure that those technologies are incorporated into helicopters furnished by operators or vendors.

The program director must keep up to date with published industry guidelines and evaluate them for incorporation into the program for which he or she is responsible. This goal requires good communication skills and a willingness on the part of the program director to critically evaluate operating procedures in an effort to constantly improve operations, not just maintain the status quo. Creation of an environment in which safety concerns can be openly and constructively discussed by any flight team member, without fear of punishment, is necessary for participation in and ownership of the safety process by all involved.

Finally, program directors must be willing to commit financial resources for equipment purchases and provide downtime for training, education, and safety seminars.[14] An outreach program to local EMS providers, in which a 1-hour safety presentation is followed by a static display of the aircraft, requires the support of managers, who must budget the necessary persons, time, and financial resources to ensure success.[15]

Although the cost of an ongoing safety program may seem excessive, the cost may one day be measured in other than economic terms if the program is overlooked.

AIR MEDICAL ACCIDENT RATES

The first hospital air medical program was established in 1972. In the following years the air medical industry underwent tremendous growth. With the growth in the industry came the realization that air medical helicopters had an accident rate far greater than that of helicopters engaged in general aviation. From 1980 through 1985 the air medical helicopter industry had an estimated accident rate of 12.34 accidents per 100,000 patients (1.1 patient transport = 1 flight hour). The accident rate for a comparable non-EMS population, such as nonscheduled turbine-powered air taxi helicopter operators, was 6.9 for the same time period.[24] The EMS accident rate was almost double the rate for air taxi operators. In 1982, the worst year on record, the air medical helicopter accident rate climbed to nearly 16 accidents per 100,000 patients transported, compared with the non-EMS air taxi rate of 4.51.[24] In addition, the fatal accident rate among EMS helicopters (5.4) was more than three times that of helicopter air taxis (1.6) for the same period (1980 through 1985).[24] These alarming statistics prompted widespread media coverage and efforts from within the industry to identify causes for the high numbers of accidents.

In 1988 the National Transportation Safety Board (NTSB) released the results of an investigation of 59 EMS accidents that occurred between 1978 and 1986. Of these 59 accidents, 19 were fatal accidents in which 53 persons died. The study reported that of the 53 deaths, 6 were patients, 28 were medical personnel, and 19 were pilots. The study concluded that weather-related accidents were the most common and most serious type of accident experienced by EMS helicopters. Weather-related accidents are also the most easily prevented. Of the 59 accidents, 25% (15 accidents) involved reduced visibility, and 73% (11) of these accidents were fatal. All of the reduced-visibility, weather-related accidents occurred in uncontrolled airspace at low altitude.

Instrument ratings provided no assurance that a noncurrent pilot would be capable of controlling a VFR helicopter under IFR conditions. This conclusion came from information that of the 15 pilots involved in reduced-visibility accidents, 13 had instrument ratings. Although 13 of the 15 pilots had instrument ratings, only 1 was current. A pilot with instrument ratings may not have flown under instrument conditions for many years, and a pilot's instrument skills degrade rapidly with nonuse. The second most prevalent cause of EMS accidents according to the NTSB study was mechanical failure. Mechanical failure accounted for 15 accidents, but only 2 of those accidents were fatal. Ten of the 15 accidents caused no or minor injuries; the 3 remaining produced serious injuries. Twelve of the accidents involved obstacle strikes, 3 of them fatal, and all but 1 occurred during approach or departure.

The NTSB study also found that EMS pilots did not routinely receive initial or recurrent weather-interpretation training. Thirteen of the 15 pilots involved in weather-related accidents received accurate weather briefings before departing on the flight during which the accident occurred. This finding indicated a failure of pilots to understand the weather report or a disregard for the reported information. The study found that weather minimums were often misunderstood by pilots, were regarded as guidelines only by some, or were at times disregarded. Pilot fatigue, often regarded as a factor in EMS helicopter accidents, was identified as an influence in only one accident. The study did find that pilots were often under pressure to accept flights and that the pressure adversely influenced pilot judgment.

The study also found that helicopter design technologies were not being used to their fullest extent. Use of shoulder harnesses with lap belts and appropriate designs of EMS interiors could minimize injuries in a crash landing, improve survivability, and decrease the severity of injuries, but often these improvements were not used in air ambulances. A final conclusion was that competition between EMS helicopter programs had an adverse effect on the programs' operations.

Along with the conclusions of the NTSB study came recommendations. The recommendations were directed to the FAA, to the American Society of Hospital-based Aeromedical Services, which later became the Association of Air Medical Services ASHMBEAMS (AAMS), and to the National Aeronautics and Space Administration (NASA).

FAA Recommendations

The recommendations to the FAA centered around emphasis on improvement of pilot training in areas of poor weather operations and development of procedures for priority handling of calls to flight service stations from EMS pilots requesting weather briefings for patient transfer flights. The study also recommended that interior EMS modifications not compromise the helicopters' safety and that minimum EMS helicopter equipment installation and performance standards be developed. It was recommended that shoulder harnesses be required as standard equipment for all medical personnel and passenger seats. Also, it was recommended that protective clothing consisting of protective helmets, flame- and heat-resistant flight suits, and protective footwear be worn by all air medical crew members. A final recommendation to the FAA was that research be developed and conducted to measure the effect of EMS pilot workload, shift lengths, and circadian rhythm disruptions on pilot performance. The research was also to evaluate current FAA flight time and duty time regulations and their effects on pilots being provided with adequate rest.

ASHBEAMS (AAMS) Recommendations

The NTSB recommended to ASHBEAMS (AAMS) that safety programs be established that were composed of representatives from the program and from local public safety and emergency-response agencies. Program administrators were advised to develop guidelines for specific safety issues dealing with topics such as pilot-in-command, marginal weather operations, and pilot and crew member coordination and communication. Program administrators were also encouraged to provide all air medical flight members with personal protective clothing and equipment to reduce the chances of injury or death in survivable accidents. For each EMS program it was recommended that visual flight rule weather minimums based on local terrain and weather patterns be established and that deviation below the program minimums be prohibited.

NASA Recommendations

The NTSB recommended to NASA that in cooperation with the FAA, NASA should develop and conduct a research program to measure the effect of

EMS pilot workload, shift lengths, and circadian rhythm disruption on pilot performance.

In the years after the 1986 NTSB study the industry has made significant strides in reducing the accident rate. For the years 1987 through 1989 the accident rate per 100,000 flights averaged 4.9,[5] which was still more than double the air taxi operator rate but nonetheless showed notable improvement. In 1990 the industry had no accidents, which made it the safest year on record. By the end of 1991 the industry had posted a 3.1 accident rate per 100,000 flight hours.[28] Despite the dramatic lowering of the accident rate, the most prevalent circumstance contributing to the accident rate continued to be poor weather.[28]

The industry continues to be plagued by weather-related accidents. Efforts must continue to ensure that weather minimums are realistic and safe, and pilots must be supported when they adhere to the minimums. Likewise, efforts must continue to establish weather minimums in areas served by competing programs to prevent first responders from shopping around to find a program willing to transport during poor weather conditions. Training programs that address topics fundamental to EMS pilots, such as weather recognition, night flying, and scene response, must be developed and integrated into an ongoing safety education program. Although much has been done, industry professionals must recognize that much still remains to be done.

National Flight Nurses Position Paper

The National Flight Nurses Association (NFNA) is a professional nursing organization with a membership that includes flight nurses from throughout the United States and Canada, and it is involved in establishing professional practice standards for flight nursing. The NFNA published a position paper in 1988 in which the organization endorsed many of the recommendations of the NTSB study published earlier the same year. The NFNA stated that "available knowledge and technology which could significantly enhance flight nurse's safety in the air medical helicopter environment is not consistently applied and utilized in all air medical transport programs."[25] The NFNA proposed several corrective measures. The proposals dealt with (1) crew scheduling and rest periods, (2) the right of flight nurses to refuse to participate in a flight as a result of concerns for personal safety, (3) the need for programs to develop written protocols for the use of physical and pharmacologic restraints when combative or potentially combative patients are being transported, (4) the need for programs to critically evaluate hot loading and unloading polices and procedures and to ensure personnel assigned to hot load or unload do so only after proper training, (5) the adoption of measures to maximize safety and reduce the potential of serious injury to flight nurses by use of helicopter design changes such as energy-attenuating seats, addition of shoulder harnesses to lap belts at each position in the aircraft, and development and installation of crash-resistant fuel systems in aircraft as soon as possible.

The final position statement dealt with specific in-flight duties to be performed by flight nurses to ensure a safe aviation environment. Identified flight nurse responsibilities included (1) equipment securement during flight, (2) use of seatbelts and shoulder harnesses, (3) proper patient securement within the aircraft, (4) judicious use of night lighting, and (5) isolation of the pilot and controls from potential patient movement.

The NFNA also stated that flight nurses should be active in working with pilots in developing initial and recurrent safety briefings, premission briefings, and postmission debriefings, and that flight nurses should be trained in position-reporting procedures, communication terminology, landing zone safety, helicopter emergency fuel and system shutdown, radio communications, and other aspects of crew member emergency training.

This position paper has been helpful to air medical programs in their efforts to address safety concerns and remains a guide for safety measures in the air medical industry.

PERSONAL SAFETY

Fitness Standards

The air medical environment is physically challenging and requires that air medical crew members maintain a high personal level of physical and emotional fitness. Requirements of each program vary, and no industry-wide formal guidelines exist.[31] However, a common-sense approach would seem to dictate some minimal fitness requirements.

Minimum physical requirements of any nurse wishing to work in the air medical environment should include the ability to wear installed seatbelts and the ability to work within the confined space limitations of individual aircraft. Flight nurses must also have no preexisting conditions that would interfere with their flexibility, strength, or cardiovascular fitness. Flight nurses must not have any condition that would cause altered mental or neurologic function.

Pregnancy

Many women of child-bearing age work in the air medical setting. For those contemplating pregnancy, there is no existing industry standard regarding pregnancy employment policies.[10] The effects of altitude, high noise levels, vibrations, and increased risk for injury in mishaps have been identified as risks to the fetus and may adversely affect maternal health.[19] Further studies are warranted to assess the environmental and physical effects of air medical stressors on the health of the mother and unborn child.

Personal Protective Equipment

The NTSB study of 1988 recommended that air medical personnel who routinely fly EMS helicopter missions wear protective clothing and equipment to reduce the chance of injury or death in survivable accidents.[13] An NFNA position paper also endorsed the use of protective equipment. Protective equipment consists of helmets, fire-resistant flight uniforms, and boots with steel toes and shanks.

Helmets

In the military the use of flight helmets has been shown to protect significantly against head injuries.[8] Despite the obvious advantages afforded to the military by flight helmets, acceptance in civilian air medical programs has not been widespread. Reasons cited for not wearing helmets included high cost, uncertain benefit, and negative public relations.[17] However, a survey performed to determine the public's perception of helmet usage found that patients and family members positively viewed the use of helmets by air medical personnel.[29]

Factors air medical personnel should evaluate when selecting a helmet include choosing a knowledgeable vendor who is familiar with custom fitting helmets. The helmet should be lightweight and should match the center of gravity of the unhelmeted head. Some manufacturers use customized liners that are molded to the individual's head size and fit into the hard outer shell of the helmet, which reduces the cost of a complete helmet for each team member. The helmet's liner must absorb energy and fit comfortably, and the chin strap should hold the helmet firmly in place.

Fire-Resistant Clothing

The goal of fire-resistant clothing is to minimize skin exposure to the intense thermal energy from a postaccident fire. The uniform should be made of a flame-resistant, heat-resistant material, such as Nomex, that is designed to withstand high temperatures for a brief period, usually less than 20 seconds, to enable the wearer to evacuate a burning aircraft.[14] The fabric may reduce the risk or severity of tissue damage but will not prevent thermal injury to the skin.

The fire-resistant flight suit should be worn in combination with cotton, silk, or wool/cotton undergarments that include both briefs and a T-shirt or long underwear.[13] Synthetic materials such as polyester or polypropylene when exposed to flames melt and become embedded into the skin; therefore they should not be worn under the flight suit. The uniform should also fit to allow 0.25 inch of air space between the flight suit and undergarments. Although not specifically recommended by the 1988 NTSB safety study, Nomex gloves can be useful in protecting the hands and should be considered by persons who wear fire-resistant flight uniforms.

Protective Footwear

Footwear is an important consideration for flight nurses, especially for programs that respond to scene work. Boots protect the foot from punctures, lacerations, and thermal injuries and provide stability to the ankle on rough or unlevel ground.

The boot should be constructed of leather that extends several inches above the ankle. The sole should be thick and oil resistant, and the boot should have steel toes and shanks. The boot should also have adequate ventilation to prevent moisture from being trapped. When boots are worn in combination with fire-resistant flight suits, the pant legs should be tucked inside the boot.

Hearing Protection

Noise is a routine hazard faced daily by flight crews in the air medical industry. Long-term exposure to high noise levels is associated with hearing loss, and often the hearing loss goes unnoticed by the person involved.[26] Although sound emission is different for each aircraft, the average sound level is between 90 and 100 dB. The Occupational Safety and Health Administration (OSHA) currently requires employers to provide hearing-conservation programs for employees exposed to time-weighted average sound levels of 85 dB or greater. Hearing protectors, such as earplugs or earmuffs, should be worn during high decibel exposures such as hot loading and unloading or when extreme noise levels exist at scenes. Earplugs are smaller and less expensive, but noise protection varies with fit. Earmuffs offer more uniform protection but are more expensive, are not easily carried or stored, and are less comfortable than earplugs.

PREFLIGHT PREPARATION

Safe performance of duties in the air medical environment begins with education and training. Classroom instruction should include topics such as flight physiology, flight safety, flight communications, stress management, survival training, and legal aspects of air medical transport. When possible, opportunities to practice classroom instruction in the actual environment should be done, such as an exercise in the wilderness to practice survival skills. Safe performance in the air medical environment requires a foundation of knowledge, gained through training and experience, that ultimately builds confidence in the ability to perform safely and effectively.

Aircraft Safety

An introduction to flight safety should begin with an orientation to the characteristics of the particular aircraft in use at the air medical program. Individual aircraft characteristics exist, but only general information will be discussed here.

The wind created by the rotor blades, referred to as *rotor wash,* can exceed 50 mph. In a hover and on the ground during the warm-up or cool-down stage, a rotor wash of approximately 25 mph can occur. This wind becomes a hazard in the form of flying dust, litter, loose clothing, and anything that is not tied down. Personnel should be aware of this and take proper precautions, such as wearing protective glasses to prevent injuries to the eyes. Hats, scarves, blankets, sheets, towels, mattress pads, and loose papers must be secured to prevent them from being blown away. More importantly, objects that are kept secure will be prevented from being pulled into the air intake of the helicopter, damaging the engine, and possibly leading to engine failure.

Rotor wash also increases the risk of windchill to skin. A 25 mph rotor wash with an air temperature of 10° F creates a windchill of −30° F, which can damage exposed skin in minutes. Flight crew members must consider this hazard when flying in cold weather, and must take steps to protect the patient accordingly.

The most obvious hazards of a helicopter are the main rotor and tail rotor blades. These blades turn at approximately 400 rpm, with rotor tips spinning at about 500 mph. At full speed the main rotor blades create a disk that can be seen above the cabin; however, at lower rotor velocity speeds, such as the warm-up and cool-down stages, the blades can "flap" or "sail" with wind gusts. This may allow the blades to drop below shoulder level. The crouch position is advised for anyone approaching or departing an aircraft while the blades are turning.

When a helicopter lands on uneven ground or on a slope, the rotor disk will come closer to the ground on the uphill side. The aircraft should be approached and departed on the downhill side in the crouched position with constant attention paid to the terrain and the rotor blades at all times. At scenes a safety person should be designated to ensure that those loading the aircraft do not inadvertently walk under the tail rotor area. When loading or unloading patients and equipment, the flight crew must take measures to ensure that nothing is carried above the head.

The tail rotor is potentially more hazardous than the main rotor. At greater than 2000 rpm it is nearly invisible. Efforts to reduce tail rotor risk to EMS workers include conduction of routine training sessions with first responders, provision of high-visibility tail rotor lighting on EMS aircraft, use of a helicopter with a fenestron, or installation of high skids under the aircraft to raise the height of the rotor.[9] Flight crew members must always approach the aircraft from the front in full view of the pilot. Those working around the aircraft, such as EMS personnel, must be instructed to remain back from the aircraft after it lands and to approach only after being signaled by the pilot. The safe approach zone is in front of the helicopter and from the sides within the pilot's vision, never from the rear.

The engine exhaust area is another hazardous area that should be avoided. The exhaust coming from the engine is approximately 400° C. The metal pipes in the system should be avoided.

Daily Preflight Procedures

Daily preflight procedures should include an aircraft check to ensure all essential equipment is present, functioning, and properly stored. A daily (or more often, such as at each shift change) preflight briefing should be held during which the pilot, flight team, and communication specialist discuss forecasted weather and any other potential problems that might be encountered during the shift. Opportunities for the crew to conduct postflight briefings should occur, when necessary, to address any safety concern and allow for corrective action.

Helipad Safety

Safety should be a primary focus in design of a hospital helipad. The air medical hospital's helipad should be well planned and designed according to FAA regulations. Considerations include approach and departure routes, the location of the helipad to patient care areas, the size of the helipad, and provision of emergency exits, fire protection equipment,

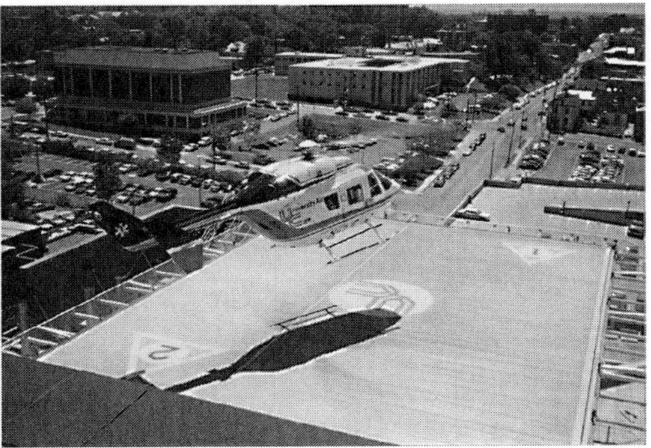

Fig. 6-1 A marked hospital rooftop helipad.

and lighting.[21] In addition, provisions for snow removal and cleaning must be made.

The helipad should be inaccessible to unauthorized persons, and anyone wanting to see the helicopter should be accompanied by a member of the flight crew. All flight crew members should be trained in fire safety and should know the location of fire alarm boxes and extinguishers. Smoking should be prohibited around or near the aircraft. Fig. 6-1 illustrates a marked rooftop helipad.

In-Flight Safety

Securement of Equipment and Patients

In-flight safety is an important responsibility of flight nurses. Responsibility begins with the use of seatbelts and shoulder harnesses during all phases of flight. At times patient needs will require that the shoulder restraint or lap belt be removed; however, the removal should be done only in level flight and only after the need is communicated to the pilot. The safety restraints should then be reapplied as soon as possible.

Flight nurses must develop the habit of always securing equipment such as monitors, intravenous equipment controllers, and equipment and medication boxes to prevent these objects from becoming projectiles and inflicting injuries to the patient or crew (Fig. 6-2). The flight nurse must securely restrain patients during flight to prevent injury, and he or she must ensure that the patient is isolated from the pilot and the controls. Flight nurses have special responsibilities when securing pediatric patients dur-

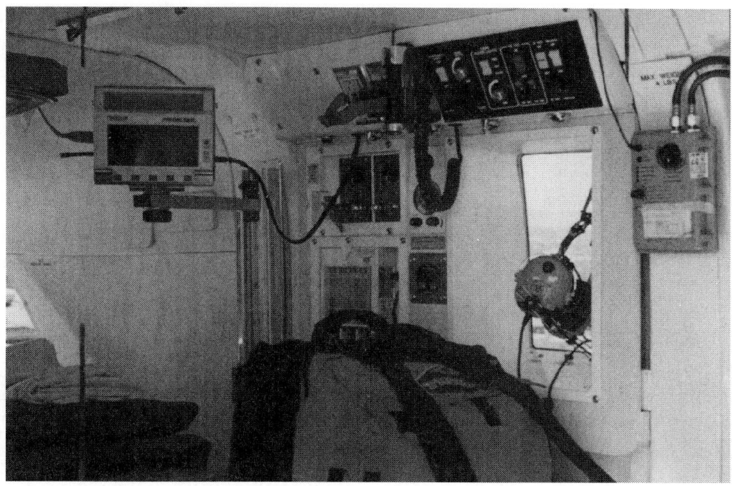

Fig. 6-2 An example of methods that may be used to ensure that equipment is appropriately secured.

ing flight. Infants and small children must not be held during transport. The pediatric patient should be restrained snugly in an infant carrier or car seat that conforms to applicable federal motor vehicle safety standards, and the carrier or car seat should then be restrained to the aircraft stretcher in a rear-facing position. Pediatric immobilization devices are available for those patients who require spinal immobilization.

Combative patients should be evaluated for the use of physical or chemical restraints. Physical restraints should be applied before takeoff. The use of physical or chemical restraints should be guided by program policies that are periodically reviewed and updated.

Other In-Flight Duties

Flight nurses are also responsible for assisting the pilot in command with in-flight duties such as scanning for other aircraft, maintaining a "sterile cockpit" during critical phases of flight, and observing for hazards on approach at scenes or at other unfamiliar landing areas. Other aircraft should be scanned for as an ongoing process, especially when there is no patient aboard. When other air traffic or obstacles are spotted, the flight nurse should report their position by the clock method. The nose of the aircraft is the 12 o'clock position, and the tail is the 6 o'clock position. To ensure that no obstacle goes unnoticed by the pilot, flight nurses should report any obstacle or air traffic even though the pilot may have seen it. Aircraft reporting is helpful to pilots, particularly in areas of congested air traffic. One effective technique for scanning is the front-to-side method.[27] This method involves the flight nurse starting with a fixed point in the center of the front windshield, slowly adjusting his or her vision leftward, returning to the center, refocusing, and then moving the eyes to the right. There are other scanning techniques and selection of one is a matter of preference, but the technique should involve some series of fixations to be successful. When the head is in motion, vision is blurred, and the mind will not register targets as easily.[27]

Observance of a sterile cockpit is a regulation of the FAA (FAR 135.100) that prohibits nonessential communications between the medical crew and pilot during critical phases of flight. The critical phases of flight include all ground operations that involve taxi, takeoff, and landing and all other flight operations except cruise flight.

When approaching unfamiliar landing areas or landing at scenes, flight nurses should be attentive to the radio conversations between the pilot and the on-scene personnel. The flight nurse should understand the landing zone description and look for additional hazards not mentioned in the landing zone briefing. Hazards to look for include wires, trees, vehicles, loose articles, and persons.

IN-FLIGHT EMERGENCIES

An in-flight emergency is often considered only when an accident is reported or has occurred. Training in emergency in-flight procedures should be part of an overall safety program, and proficiency should be demonstrated yearly. Training and retraining will ensure that safety procedures are automatic. During an actual emergency, flight nurses are responsible for (1) confirming with the pilot that an actual emergency exists and assisting as necessary, (2) shutting off the main oxygen supply, and (3) preparing the patient by placing him or her flat and tightening the stretcher straps.[4] As the final step in preparation, the flight nurse should get into the survival position by placing the arms across the chest, forming an X with the forearms, and grasping the shoulder harness, while placing the knees together and the feet approximately 6 inches apart.

Fire Emergencies

Successful prevention of serious injury or death from an in-flight fire requires quick action. Smoke can quickly fill the cabin of an EMS helicopter. The heat and smoke can incapacitate the crew with disastrous consequences. Fire extinguishers should be located within easy reach of the crew. On larger aircraft where the medical crew is separated from the pilot, a fire extinguisher should be located in each compartment. If the fire is electrical, caused by medical equipment plugged into the aircraft power supply, the crew should unplug the equipment, turn off the inverter, turn off the oxygen source, and close the windows and vents to prevent accelerating the fire. If the smoke and heat become excessive, the crew should open windows or doors with discretion, fight the fire aggressively with the fire extinguisher, and prepare for an emergency landing as soon as possible.[20]

Emergency Egress

The actions of the flight crew members immediately after an emergency landing may directly influence their survival. Disorientation and panic will threaten survival.[4] Crew members must make a quick survey to reestablish orientation and assess the condition of the aircraft, other crew members, and the patient. In night conditions or in smoke-filled cabins, orientation can be maintained by use of the hand-over-hand method, wherein an old reference point is kept with one hand while a new one is selected with the other. After a forced landing the main danger is fire. If the pilot has become incapacitated, the fuel switch and master battery switch should be turned off. The position of these switches varies with the aircraft, and flight nurses must be familiar with the procedure for their specific aircraft. After the aircraft has come to a complete stop, the aircraft should be exited by normal means first, jettison doors only if necessary, and forcible means if required.[20] Crew members should meet at a predesignated position a safe distance from the aircraft. After the threat of fire has passed, they should return to the aircraft and assist any persons who were injured during the emergency.

Forced Water Landing

Flight crew members of air medical programs that frequently fly over large bodies of water need to be familiar with emergency egress procedures in the event of a forced water landing. Personal flotation devices should be worn by all flight crew members when missions require flight over water. If the pilot announces an in-flight emergency, the same procedure as outlined in the preceding paragraph should be followed. After the aircraft has made contact with the water, it will usually capsize because helicopters are top heavy as a result of the weight of the engines and transmission. It is important that no attempt be made to exit the aircraft until the blades have completely stopped. Flight crew members should establish a fixed reference point with one hand while finding a new one with the other, jettison the aircraft door after releasing the seat restraints, and maintain a fixed reference orientation with the hands, which is crucial in finding the exits. Air bubbles always travel to the surface, and observing them may help crew members establish orientation; however, poor lighting conditions may prevent adequate visualization of bubbles. Crew members should gently use their arms to push themselves out of the aircraft and avoid kicking to prevent injury to crew members following behind. During surface ascent they should exhale slowly to prevent serious lung damage should they attempt to hold their breath.[30]

Some air medical programs practice emergency egress procedures with an egress simulator.[12,30,32] Wright et al[32] found that egress training can improve the ability of flight crew members to quickly evacuate an aircraft in a forced landing situation, and a training program that focuses on inflight emergencies can increase the flight crew's confidence to deal with these emergencies.

POSTACCIDENT DUTIES

After safely exiting a disabled aircraft, flight team members should meet at a predesignated safe distance from the aircraft until the danger of fire is eliminated. Measures to stabilize the patient and injured crew members should be taken. They should then try to ensure that chances for rescue are optimized.[14]

All EMS aircraft are required by the FAA to carry an emergency locator transmitter (ELT). These transmitters are designed to emit a radio signal when activated that will be received by satellites and relayed to rescue personnel. The radio signal does not pinpoint the position of the aircraft but gives rescuers a general area in which to begin a search. The ELT is activated by an impact exceeding 4 *g* (4 times the force of gravity) and broadcasts on the universal distress channel 121.5. Flight team members should know the location of the ELT and ensure that it has been activated. If an impact does not automatically activate the ELT, it can manually be activated by use of the directions on the front.

After the ELT is checked, the crew's situation needs to be evaluated, and survival priorities must be established. These priorities will largely be determined by the environment in which the forced landing occurred. Immediate goals are to secure a shelter and build a fire. The crew should stay with the aircraft unless a road or building is in sight. After the crew members secure shelter and build a fire, their next priority should be signaling. For a more detailed discussion refer to Survival Principles in this chapter.

Downed Aircraft Procedure

The practice of flight following, in which a communication specialist keeps abreast of the progress of the flight by periodic scheduled communications with the pilot, is a standard operating procedure in all air medical programs. Where distances between the aircraft and base are too great, the pilot makes contact with other programs along the flight path or with airports and asks them to notify the base with flight status reports. Policies and procedures must be in place to aid the communication specialist in the event of an overdue aircraft.

The downed aircraft policy should be a graduated response that outlines the responsibilities of the communication specialist in situations such as the following: (1) an unscheduled landing, which covers any precautionary landing; (2) a missing or overdue aircraft, such as an aircraft that is 15 minutes overdue; (3) aircraft emergency protocol, such as a serious emergency in which the crew is in jeopardy and needs immediate assistance; and (4) aircraft postaccident protocol, such as notification that an aircraft accident has occurred.

Resources that should be used by the communication specialist in assisting in a missing aircraft location include local EMS agencies, state and local police agencies, other nearby air medical programs, airport facilities along the flight path, and the FAA. Administrative personnel must also be notified, and an administrative crisis team must be assembled to assist in incident command. Members of the administrative crisis team should be listed in the procedural policy and should have the following duties: notifying next of kin, establishing a family reception center, providing for stress debriefing, coordinating all press releases, and establishing short- and long-term planning. The response to any disaster requires detailed planning and preparation, with the responsibilities of those involved clearly outlined in a procedural policy that is easily located during an emergency. Periodic review of the procedure and program drills can identify problem areas, and proper revisions can be instituted.[23] Fig. 6-3 contains an example of a downed aircraft policy.

Scene Safety

Air medical assistance at the scene of accidents has become a common occurrence in the prehospital

Rev: 8/1/95

AD [signature] MD SCC FNC [signature] LP ME

University Air Care

Subject: **Accident/Incident Plan**

Policy: University Air Care personnel will follow a defined process for timely and appropriate notification of individuals following identification of an actual or perceived emergency.

Purpose: This plan is a professional approach to dealing with any adversity that may have an effect on the program. It is designed to be a concise, workable guide through any accident or incident involving the University Air Care aircraft and personnel.

Procedure: This plan is a sequenced procedural guide that covers any incident or accident that may occur to a University Air Care helicopter. The protocols listed below are addressed in the pages that follow:

1. **Unscheduled landing protocol** - Any unscheduled (precautionary) landing (e.g., mechanical deficiency, inclement weather, or medical emergency).

2. **Missing/overdue aircraft protocol** - The aircraft is overdue 15 minutes after its estimated time of arrival (ETA).

3. **Aircraft emergency protocol** - A serious emergency in which the crew is in jeopardy and needs immediate help.

4. **Aircraft post accident protocol** - Notification that an aircraft accident has occurred.

In the event of an aircraft mishap, *never* transmit the names of the suspected injured or deceased persons over the radio.

Only the Air Care Program Director and his/her representative or the Medical Center Public Relations Department shall release information to the media. *UNDER NO CIRCUMSTANCES* shall any information be released to any member of the news media, Federal Aviation Administration (FAA), or any other persons unless the information is released by the above-stated individuals.

Fig. 6-3 Downed aircraft policy accident/incident plan. (Courtesy University Air Care, Cincinnati, Ohio.)

setting. Flight teams must be aware of the potentially dangerous situations of landing at unfamiliar locations. The selection and preparation of the landing zone are often the responsibilities of the local EMS agency in charge at the scene, although the pilot has ultimate decision-making responsibility for landing at the site. If the pilot detects a problem with the site, he or she will relay those concerns to the ground guide, and a new site will be chosen. If the concern can be immediately addressed, such as an emergency vehicle too close to the landing zone, steps to correct the concern can be taken, and the site may be used.

Landing zone selection and preparation should be part of an ongoing emergency service education program provided by various members of the flight team. The educational program should include discussion of ground and helicopter communication procedures, hazards such as rotor wash and noise, and the need for eye protection measures. Instructions on hot loading procedures, as well as an aircraft-specific orientation, should also be included.

Predesignated landing zones (PDLZs) are useful in areas of high congestion or in areas in which the terrain prevents a safe landing.[6] PDLZs are selected by local EMS officials, who then consult with the program lead pilot, who schedules an evaluation of the zone. If the zone selection is mutually agreed on, information on the PDLZ is recorded and kept on file in the dispatch center. Potential PDLZs include parks, ball fields, schoolyards, vacant lots, and church or business parking lots. Time of day may be a consideration in use of a particular PDLZ, and any restrictions should be noted in the dispatch file.

When a request from the community EMS agency is received, the communication specialist can transmit the information to the pilot. Included in the information are the coordinates and a written description of the PDLZ, together with any time restrictions. An advantage of PDLZ identification is faster dispatch of the helicopter, especially if the scene is less than 10 minutes away.[6]

Flight team members must also be aware of the dangers encountered in the prehospital setting and should take precautions to prevent themselves from becoming another victim at the scene. Unless specifically trained, flight nurses should not engage in the extrication or rescue effort. The extrication effort should proceed uninterrupted by the flight team, unless airway measures are required and only if the procedure can be done without the rescuer being put in jeopardy. While the extrication of a victim continues, the flight team should prepare the equipment and plan as rapid a departure as possible.

Response to the scene of a violent crime requires special caution. The prehospital setting is becoming more dangerous to emergency care providers. No longer is crime contained to the larger inner cities; it is becoming common in rural areas as well.[3] Flight teams can protect themselves by consulting with law enforcement personnel to ensure the scene is safe. When caring for a victim of a violent crime, flight nurses must try to disturb the scene no more than necessary to preserve evidence.

SURVIVAL PRINCIPLES

Preparation and education are the best means of dealing with the uncertainty and fear associated with survival. Good physical and mental health are essential components of survival. Air medical aircraft should be equipped with a complete survival kit, and all crew members should be instructed in its use. Periodic checking of survival equipment and review of emergency protocols and procedures are essential parts of preflight duties.

Psychologic Preparation

By understanding and dealing with the potential for loss of life or serious injury, the flight nurse can build coping mechanisms that will help in the event of an aircraft emergency or postcrash scenario. Fear, anxiety, anger, and denial can be experienced during the preimpact phase of the emergency. A sound safety program, survival education, and experience will help prepare for a situation that requires survival skills.

Leadership is vital when danger is imminent so that panic and denial can be avoided. To alleviate panic flight crew members should keep busy with tasks or help others. By providing support, comfort, rest, and medical attention to those injured, flight crew members will help all the survivors psychologically.

Those directly or indirectly involved in the incident or accident should be offered counseling after rescue by a qualified mental health professional experienced in critical incident debriefing.

Clothing

In cold-weather environments, measures should be taken to protect all parts of the body because a person's clothing may be the only shelter from the environment and protection against hypothermia. Clothing should protect the wearer against the environment and be comfortable and practical. Tight-fitting clothing, which may restrict movement and circulation during physical exercise, should be avoided. Clothing must be layered for best effect and have proper ventilation to ensure adequate heat regulation.

Warm-weather clothing should protect against the sun. Long-sleeve shirts and pants together with head and eye protection diminish water loss and exposure. Preplanning for a mission in desert terrain should recognize the potential for significant variations in temperature from day to night.

Priorities

Knowledge of the rule of threes when priorities are set will greatly increase the chances of survival in the outdoors. This rule states that the average person can survive 3 minutes without oxygen, 3 hours without shelter in extreme conditions, 3 days without water, and 3 weeks without food.[2,14] Medical concerns and safety are more important in an accident, but once these are addressed, the rule of threes should guide priorities. With the rule in mind, the flight crew's immediate concerns after an accident should be creating or seeking shelter, building a fire, and making appropriate fire signals.[2]

Shelter

The ability to create a shelter is vital and cannot be overemphasized. Warmth and dryness are best achieved when the shelter is kept small and simple. The aircraft and natural shelters require little physical energy and are the easiest to prepare. Shelter provides protection from extremes in environmental temperatures. When formulating a plan for building a shelter, the flight crew should consider the following points: (1) the shelter should be kept as close to the aircraft as possible; (2) the area should be checked for future danger, such as dry stream beds that could flood quickly, avalanche chutes, and steep terrain; and (3) the three basic parts of any shelter are the roof, floor, and walls; if not enough material is available to build a complete shelter, the sequence of priorities is a roof, floor (insulated if possible), windward side, and leeward side. Fig. 6-4 illustrates some general-purpose shelters.

The aircraft provides excellent shelter. If the fuselage of an aircraft is used for shelter, the flight crew should ensure that is supported and will not roll or tilt on the terrain or during adverse weather conditions. Any holes inside the aircraft should be patched with sheets, tarps, or space blankets. All windows or exposed metal should be insulated to prevent heat loss. The flight crew should avoid sleeping or placing the injured on exposed metal or ground.

The flight crew can strip the aircraft of its resources and materials and improvise to meet the survival goal. Below is a partial list of uses for aircraft parts:

1. Battery: signal lights, communications, fire starter
2. Cowling: signal panels, water collection, fire pit, windbreak, shelter
3. Doors: shelter, windbreak, signal panel
4. Fuselage: shelter
5. Engine oil or fuel: fire starter, signal fire
6. Nose spinner: bucket, water collection, tool for snow
7. Seats: insulation, sleeping cushions, fire material, signal material
8. Tires: black smoke signal
9. Vertical stabilizer: shelter supports, signal panel
10. Wings: windbreaks, shelter supports, overhead shade, water collection for dew and rain

The flight team must first consider the length of time and the amount of energy required to build a shelter. Natural shelter provides an alternative that will protect a flight crew member from the environment. The flight crew must be aware of potential dangers when selecting a natural shelter; for example, dead trees or tree limbs that may fall in a strong wind; rock slides; caves with other inhabitants such as bears, skunks, or cougars; and trees or rocks that may conduct lightning.[14] A formation in the earth made of rock, snow, timber, or sand may provide a place in which crew members can burrow. When constructing a shelter, the flight team member must investigate natural resources to discover ventilation and insulation materials available, such as rocks, tree branches, and snow, to incorporate with materials in the aircraft or survival kit. Trapped air with ventilation is an effective insulator, and therefore snow caves are excellent shelters in cold climates. Whether it be a space blanket raised between two trees or an elab-

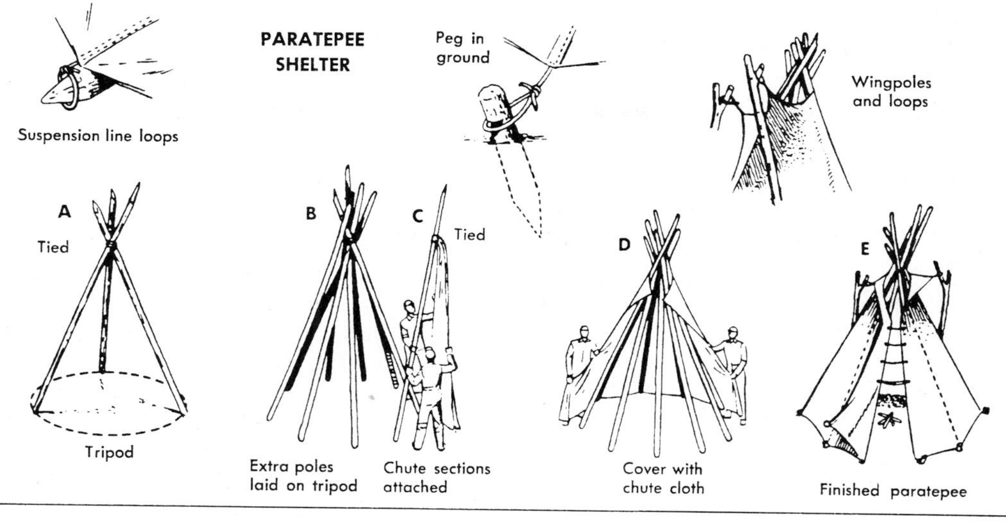

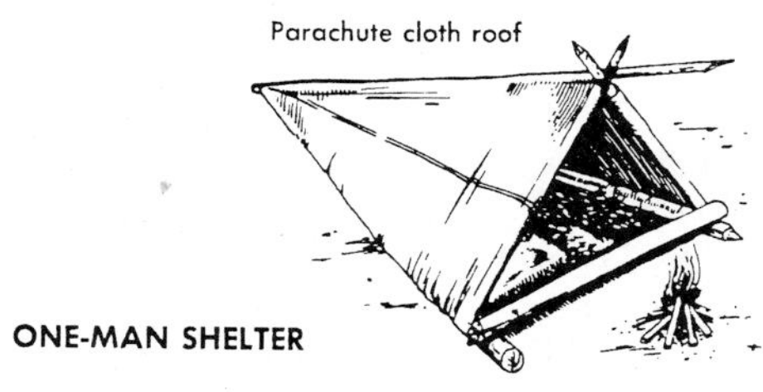

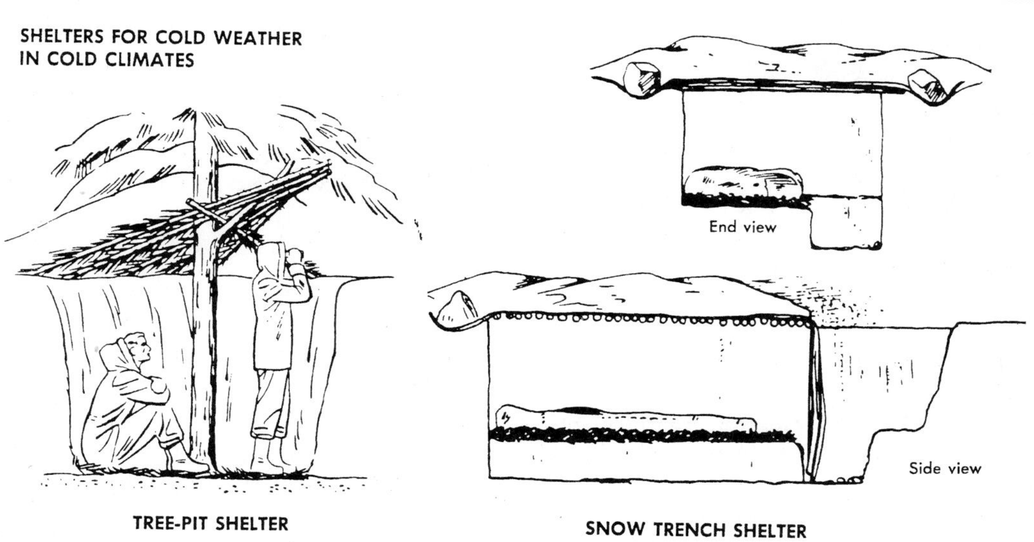

Fig. 6-4 General-purpose shelters. (From Department of the Air Force: *Survival-training education,* AFM 64-3, Washington, DC, 1969, US Government Printing Office.)

orate construction job, the flight crew member should consider the expenditure of energy to build it. Optimally, the shelter should be in sight of the aircraft. The flight crew should keep survival gear in the shelter close to the air medical team members and out of the elements. Diagrams of the steps in shelter building are helpful when they can be applied to a complete program that incorporates aircraft configuration, terrain, climate, and survival equipment available to the flight nurse.

Fire Building

A fire provides warmth, light, and a sense of security. If adequate clothing and shelter are available, a fire may not be needed. When the need is recognized, the crew member should prepare materials and start the fire before dark, considering the placement of the shelter and direction of reflected heat. Once the location of the fire has been chosen, the fire should be contained with some type of boundary. The crew member should gather enough combustible material such as tinder, kindling (small pieces), and large pieces of wood to last through the night. Using the available fire-starting equipment, the crew member should first build the fire with small combustible material and then add larger pieces of wood. Once the fire has evolved, kindling can be added to the tinder. The flight crew should be prepared to use the fire as a signaling tool. Oil or greenery can be added to create effective smoke that can be seen by aerial search and rescue aircraft. There are many methods of fire building and many materials to use (Fig. 6-5). Crew members should be instructed about what fuel is available in the service area and how to use the fire starter available in the aircraft survival pack.

Signaling

Once the basic needs of the flight team have been met, signaling becomes the next priority. The chance of being rescued increases with enhanced visibility. However, signaling must be accomplished without the crew members being further endangered.

The aircraft radio and ELT discussed under Post-accident Duties are the most effective rescue aids. When the aircraft radio is not operational, alternative signaling methods must be used. Smoke is the most effective means by day to signal search and rescue aircraft. Signaling should be one purpose of the survival fire. Other signaling methods are as follows:

1. Smoke: Addition of oil, rubber, or plastic to the fire creates black smoke; addition of green leaves, grass, or water creates white smoke. The flight crew member should pick the color of smoke that will provide the most contrast with the environment.
2. Signal mirror: Reflections off shiny metal objects, cans, or foil can be seen on overcast days. The crew member should practice using a signal mirror by flashing the mirror in the direction of the aircraft when heard, even if it cannot be seen.
3. Flares or flashlight: The flight crew member can signal with a flashlight at night. Flares can be used if they are available in the aircraft.
4. Clothing: Orange parkas, sheets, or other items with bright colors that provide a contrast with the colors of the surrounding nature are useful signals.
5. Whistle: A plastic police whistle will provide ground search and rescue units with easy signaling communication on the ground. Whistles can be used in adverse weather or at night for guidance.[1]
6. Dyes or signal panels: Depending on terrain, the flight crew member can clear an area and lay signal panels in a geometric pattern. Dyes are effective in water and on snow. Fine dyes should be used downwind because they will penetrate clothing and food.

In winter environments, the signal fire should be made on top of a platform. In desert environments, a can with sand and oil can provide a smoke device that will continue to burn for a long time.

Water

Hydration maintenance is crucial in the survival setting. Available intravenous fluids provide electrolyte solutions and some glucose for energy. Air medical crew members should conserve all available water stores by rationing. Crew members must boil water

FLINT AND STEEL

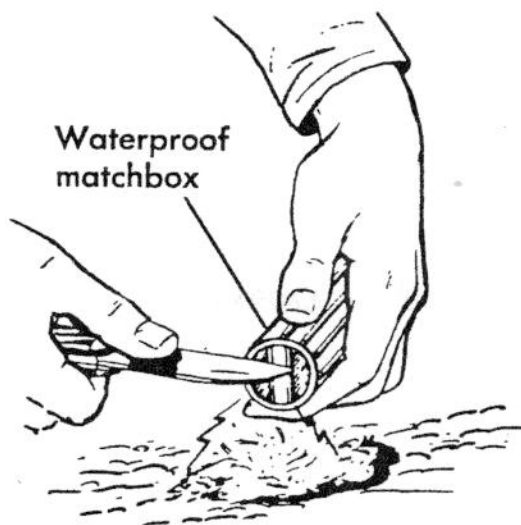

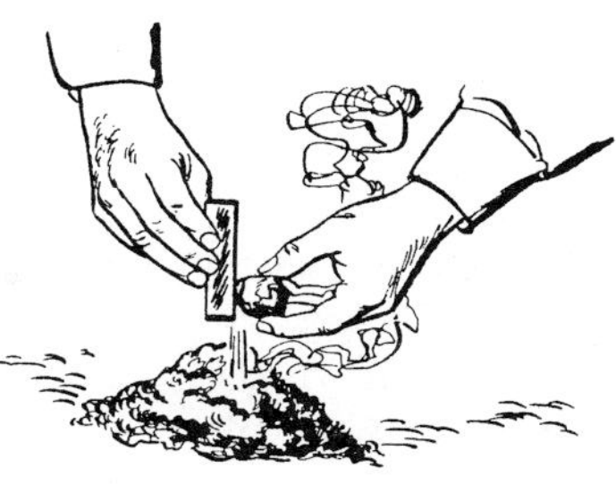

This is the easiest and most reliable way of making a fire without matches. Use the flint fastened to the bottom of your waterproof match case. If you have no flint, look for a piece of hard rock from which you can strike sparks. If no sparks fly when it is struck with steel, find another. Hold your hands close over the dry tinder; strike flat with a knife blade or other small piece of steel with a sharp, scraping, downward motion so that the sparks fall in the center of the tinder. The addition of a few drops of gasoline before striking the flint will make the tinder flame up — FOR SAFETY, KEEP YOUR HEAD TO ONE SIDE. When tinder begins to smolder, fan or blow it gently into a flame. Then transfer blazing tinder to your kindling pile or add kindling gradually to the tinder.

One way to start a fire is with flint and lint ball.

1. Imbed a ¼-inch piece of lighter flint (pyrophoric alloy-large size) in a ½" X ¼" X 2" piece of soft wood or plastic. Flint should be imbedded close to one end and centered.
2. Wind 2- to 3-feet of 8-strand flax (linen) harness maker's thread at the end opposite the flint.
3. To use, unwind about 1 inch of linen, and on a smooth dry surface, scrape the strands of linen into a ball of lint using the sharp edge of a knife.
4. Place lint ball in contact with flint. With the sharp edge of the knife, use pressure and strike a spark directly into the lint ball. Lint will quickly blaze.

One of the distinct advantages of this piece of equipment is its usefulness, even after complete immersion in water. The linen dries very quickly and 5 minutes of air drying after a thorough wetting is sufficient to make it usable.

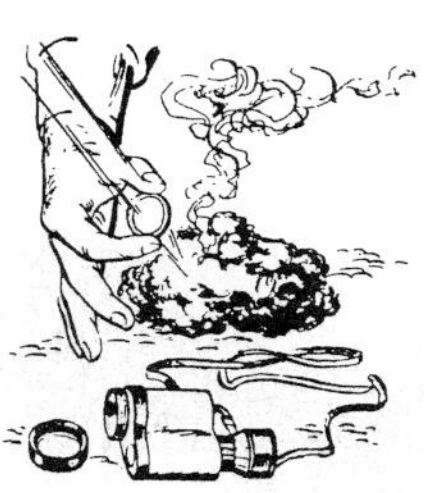

BURNING GLASS

A convex lens can be used in bright sunlight to concentrate the sun's rays on the tinder. A 2-inch lens will start a fire most any time the sun is shining. Smaller lenses will work if the sun is high and the air clear.

ELECTRIC SPARK

If you have a live storage battery, direct a spark onto the tinder by scatching the ends of wires together, to produce an arc.

FRICTION

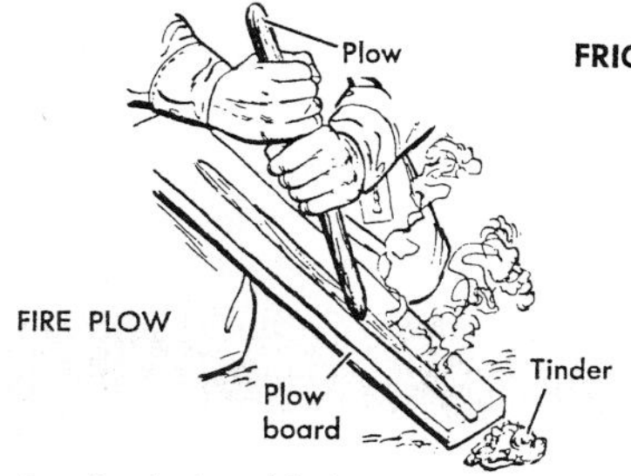

Run plow back and forth in groove with a steady but increasing rhythm until smoke in tinder indicates a spark.

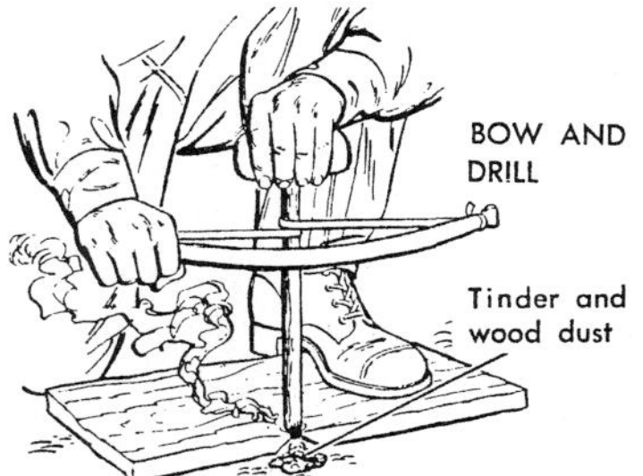

Hand holding drill socket is braced against left shin. Wood dust piles on tinder as drill spins.

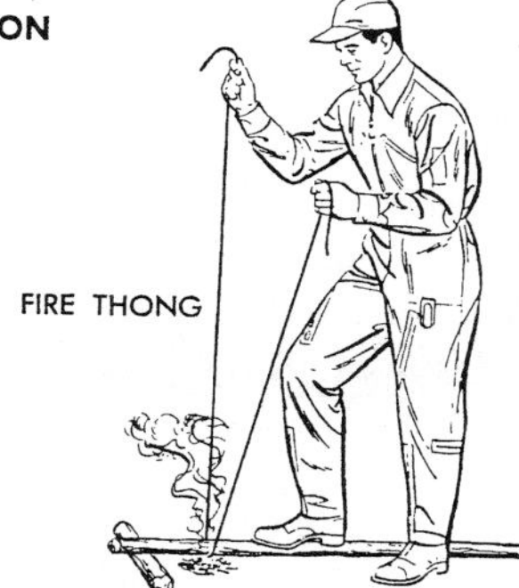

Use a thong of dry rattan or other long, strong fiber, and rub with a steady but increasing rhythm.

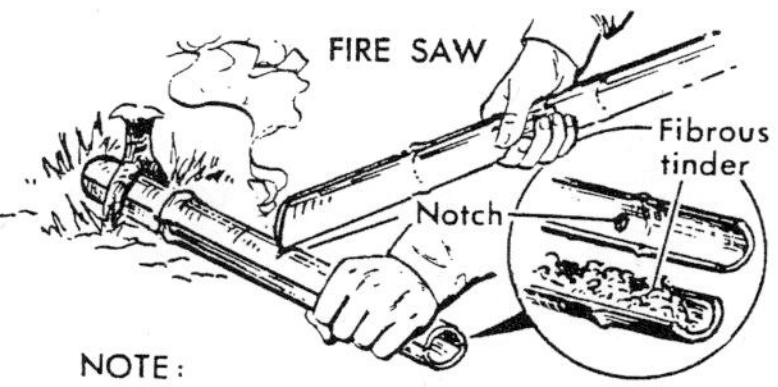

NOTE:

Split bamboo or soft wood makes a good fire saw. Dry sheath of coconut flower is a good base wood.

Fig. 6-5 Fire making without matches. (From Department of the Air Force: *Survival-training education,* AFM 64-3, Washington, DC, 1969, US Government Printing Office.)

or use water-purification tablets to prevent bacterial gastrointestinal infection; vomiting and diarrhea cause large amounts of water loss.

In snow environments, snow should be melted before ingestion to prevent body heat loss. If water is kept in a container, the expansion of the container and its possible rupture if it freezes must be considered; it is better to keep water in a shallow open container for future use. Available water mixed with hot chocolate or instant soup and heated provides a hot meal and liquid.

Food

The need for food is a low priority during a survival situation of fewer than 4 to 5 days. It is vital that the air medical crew recognize depleted energy stores. The psychologic effects of depleted energy stores include personality changes, depression, and diminished problem-solving capabilities.

Specific Environmental Considerations

When flying over water, all flight team members should wear personal flotation devices. Flight team members may consider wearing survival gear and signal devices in a vest system. All personnel should be knowledgeable in the use of these devices. The ability to swim should be mandatory, and open-sea survival should be part of the training received by all flight team members who frequently operate over large bodies of water.

Both rotor- and fixed-wing aircraft should provide seat cushions that can be used as flotation devices. The program safety officer should investigate the availability of open-water survival gear and make specific equipment available when appropriate.

Jettisoning of doors, evacuation of the aircraft, and other emergency procedures should be directed by the pilot. Any available time before the aircraft sinks should be spent on evacuation and gathering of open-sea survival equipment. The crew must be prepared for the aircraft to flip over once it hits the water. Engine weight on rotor aircraft will turn the aircraft upside down.

Once in the water, the flight team can minimize heat loss by using the heat escape–lessening posture (HELP). Team members can achieve this position by bringing the knees up to the chest and putting the arms across the chest. They must use a flotation device with HELP to stay afloat. The surviving flight team members should huddle together to decrease heat loss. The flight team should protect against salt and sun exposure by covering any exposed skin surface. Protection against exposure, care of the raft, and signaling are the primary objectives in open-water survival.

Survival in the Desert

By following basic survival principles with education about heat illness and exposure, the flight team will be better able to survive in desert terrain. Water collection, insect precautions, snakebite treatment procedures, and shelter construction to protect flight team members from the sun are major topics to be covered in a complete desert terrain survival education program. Long-sleeve shirts and long pants should be worn, and complete head, neck, and eye protection is vital.

International Survival Concerns

As flight nurses cross international boundaries, survival concerns need to be addressed. Air medical team members should be aware of climates and terrain that will be flown over and at the final destination of the mission. Recognition of the need for additional survival equipment and food stores should be part of a complete preflight check. Preparation for customs, ports of entry, and passport checks is just the beginning for fixed-wing and rotor aircraft involved in international flights.

In Canada and Mexico complete flight plans are required for entrance into and departure from the country. The ELT and the emergency frequency 121.5 are used in Canada. However, in some countries search and rescue efforts are limited, and in many others they are nonexistent.

Survival Equipment

Survival equipment should be standard on every air medical aircraft. Specific service area, climate, type of aircraft, and time of year are considerations when survival gear is assembled. The survival gear should be assembled and stored in a manner that affords easy access. The box lists items to be included in basic survival kits.

BASIC SURVIVAL KITS

Personal Survival Kit

Waterproof matches
Small flashlight
Sunglasses
Pocketknife
Compass
Parachute cord

Aircraft Survival Kit

Waterproof matches
Candle, dry tinder
Space blanket, tarps, tents, plastic poncho
Nylon cord, rope, duct tape
Mirror, signal flares, plastic whistle, flashlight
Canned smoke
Compass, knife, sunglasses, sunscreen
Water-purification tablets, insect repellant
Foodstuffs, appropriate additional clothing
Cooking kit, drinking cup, toilet paper
Sleeping bag, snowshoes, inflatable raft
Fishing kit, ax or saw, aluminum foil

REFERENCES

1. Air Training Command: *Air Force manual search and rescue survival,* Washington, DC, 1962, Department of the Air Force.
2. Arnold M: Winter survival tactics, *Hosp Aviat* 5(10):14, 1986.
3. Benson K: Violence, trauma, and EMS, *J Emerg Services* 26(4):40, 1994.
4. Bush C: Emergency egress scenarios, *J Air Med Transport* 10(10):35, 1991.
5. Collett HM: Air medical accident rates: a historical look back at causes, *J Air Med Transport* 10(2):14, 1991.
6. Collins MH: Pre-designated landing zones, *Hosp Aviat* 7(6):6, 1988.
7. Cooper LT: An administrator's perspective on managing safety, *J Air Med Transport* 10(3):15, 1991.
8. Crowley JS, Licina JR, Bruckart JE: Flight helmets: how they work and why you should wear one, *J Air Med Transport* 11(8):19, 1912.
9. Dolan J: Keep safe from tail rotor strikes, *J Air Med Transport* 9(2):9, 1990.
10. Drew K: Should a pregnant flight nurse be allowed to fly? *J Air Med Transport* 10(7):11, 1991.
11. Frazer R: Operational quality assurance: a new concept defined, *J Air Med Transport* 10(3):19, 1991.
12. Green B: Egress simulator, *Hosp Aviat* 8(7):28, 1989.
13. Hawkins M: Personal protective equipment in helicopter EMS, *Air Med J* 13(4):1123, 1994.
14. Holleran RS: Prehospital safety. In Holleran RS, editor: *Prehospital nursing: a collaborative approach,* St Louis, 1994, Mosby.
15. Homer S: Development of an air medical outreach program: practical applications, *Top Emerg Med* 16(4):45, 1994.
16. Jones K: Regional air medical safety committees, *J Air Med Transport* 9(9):44, 1990.
17. Kruppa RM: Air medical safety, a follow-up survey, *J Air Med Transport* 8(10):10, 1991.
18. Lillie J, Larsen B: Safety in the '90s, *J Air Med Transport* 10(2):16, 1991.
19. Mason KT: Letter, *Air Med J* 13(6):242, 1994.
20. Mayberry RT: Medical air crew roles and responsibilities during aircraft emergencies, *Aero Med J* 3(4):16, 1988.
21. Militello PR, Ramzy AI: Safety by design, *J Air Med Transport* 9(8):15, 1990.
22. Moon T, Broome R: Air medical safety program, *Top Emerg Med* 16(4):31, 1994.
23. Mrochek P, Sorenson P: Missing aircraft: if disaster strikes, is your program prepared? *Air Med Transport* 8(12): 17, 1989.
24. National Transportation Safety Board: Safety study commercial emergency medical service helicopter operations, National Technical Information Service, NTSB/SS 1988, US Department of Commerce.
25. National Flight Nurses Association: *Improving flight nurse safety in the air medical helicopter environment,* Park Ridge, Ill, July 1988, The Association.
26. Nordberg M: Listen up, *Emerg Med Services* 22(4):35, 1993.
27. PHI Training Department: *Aeromedical crew member training manual,* Lafayette, La, Dec 1994.
28. Preston N: 1991 Air medical helicopter accident rates, *J Air Med Transport* 11(2):14, 1992.
29. Ryan T, Studebaker B, Brennan G: Patient impression of the use of helmets by HEMS personnel, *J Air Med Transport* 11(10):65, 1992 (abstract).
30. Stinson WF: Forced water landing: a practice in survival, *J Air Med Transport* 9(1):23, 1990.
31. Wraa CE, O'Malley JO: Flight nurse physical requirements, *J Air Med Transport* 11(10):17, 1992.
32. Wright AE, Campos JA, Gorder T: The effect of an inflight emergency training program on crew confidence, *Air Med J* 13(4)127, 1994.

CHAPTER 7

Patient Assessment and Preparation for Transport

COMPETENCIES

1. Obtain initial, focused, and comprehensive subjective and objective data through history taking, physical examination, review of records, pertinent laboratory values and x-ray examinations, and communication with other health care providers, including prehospital and referring personnel.
2. Recognize and anticipate critical signs and symptoms related to the patient's illness or injury.
3. Perform critical patient interventions both independently and collaboratively as indicated by the patient's illness or injury.
4. Perform a comprehensive assessment including the collection of subjective and objective data related to the patient's illness or injury for the patient who will be transported by fixed-wing aircraft.
5. Initiate interventions to provide care for the ill or injured patient who will be transported by fixed-wing aircraft related to the effects of this kind of transport.

The first half of this chapter presents an overview of patient assessment and preparation for transport, including identification of the indications for transport; communication; consent for transport; all the factors involved in performing a patient assessment; and steps that must be taken to prepare the patient for transport. The second half of this chapter discusses all issues pertinent to fixed-wing transport.

The transport process begins with identification of the indications for air medical transport. In many cases this step has been initiated by members of the referring agency, such as prehospital care providers or physicians in the transferring hospital.

Communication about the need for air medical transport and the care the patient has received and will require from the flight team is an integral part of preparing the patient for transport. This communication begins before the flight nurse arrives, continues during transport, and concludes with patient follow-up reports to the referring agency.

The issue of consent for transport must be addressed by the flight nurse. Even though most air medical transports are based on implied consent, the flight nurse must be aware of the legal considerations related to consent and transport.

Performing a patient assessment provides the flight nurse with an opportunity to identify patient problems and interventions that will need to be initiated before transport. Patient assessment also allows the flight nurse to prepare for events that may occur during transport.

Patient assessment/preparation for transport is composed of multiple elements, including primary and secondary assessment, performance of critical interventions, and dealing with specific problems such as pain management.

The air medical transport may not always contribute an environment conducive to performing all of the components of patient assessment and preparation. However, the flight nurse must be familiar with all of these components so that he or she can perform the appropriate nursing and collaborative interventions.

INDICATIONS FOR AIR MEDICAL TRANSPORT

Currently no universal agreement exists on the indications for air medical transport. Numerous research studies have identified reasons to transport patients,[6,21,23,33] and national organizations have suggested indications for air medical transport, particularly rotor-wing transport.[2,33] General indications for patient transport include the need for nursing and medical expertise or diagnostic procedures not available at the referring health facility, and a request by the patient's family that the patient be transferred to another facility.

Trauma Patients

Numerous guidelines for air medical transport of trauma patients are available. The reason that air medical transport of trauma patients is commonly accepted is probably related to the history of helicopters, which were first used to transport injured patients from the battlefield and were subsequently used to transport trauma patients in the civilian population (see Chapter 1 for history of air medical transport). In 1992 the National Association of Emergency Medical Services Physicians published extensive guidelines for use of air medical transport.[33] Some indications for the use of air medical transport identified in these guidelines are listed in the box on p. 96.

Scoring systems have also been used to determine indications for patient transport. Some examples of these scoring systems are the trauma revised trauma score, CRAMS score, trauma triage rule, Glasgow coma score, GMR greater than 5 (Glasgow motor score), and vehicular trauma checklist.

Patients with Cardiovascular Emergencies

Even though most of the research related to the indications for air medical transport involves trauma patients, some indications have been recognized for the patient with a cardiovascular emergency. These include the need for cardiac intensive care that is not available at the referring facility, the need for cardiac catheterization, treatment for cardiogenic shock that may include insertion of a balloon pump, mechanical assist devices, experimental medications, and the need for an organ transplant.[9,20]

Pregnant Women and Neonates

Other patients who may be transported by aircraft include pregnant women and neonatal patients. Indications for transport of pregnant women include placenta previa, fetal distress, maternal trauma, prenatal complications, and perimortem delivery. Indications for transport of neonates include the age and weight of the infant and neonatal illness and injury.[3]

Appropriate Patient Transfer

In 1986 the Consolidated Omnibus Reconciliation Act (COBRA) was implemented. This legisla-

INDICATIONS FOR USE OF AIR MEDICAL TRANSPORT

Mechanism of Injury

- Accident speeds greater than 55 miles per hour
- Entrapment
- Death of others in the accident
- Falls greater than 15 feet
- Penetrating injuries to the abdomen, pelvis, chest, neck, or head

Major Burns

- Second- and third-degree burns covering more than 10% of the patient's body surface area in patients less than 10 years of age or more than 50 years of age
- Second-degree burns covering more than 20% of the patient's body surface of patients in any age group
- Third-degree burns covering more than 5% of the patient's body surface for patients in any age group
- Electrical burns
- Lightning injury
- Chemical burns
- Inhalation injury
- Burns to the hands, feet, and perineum
- Patients involved in a serious traumatic event who are less than 12 years of age or more than 55 years of age
- Patients with injuries as a result of nearly drowning, with or without existing hypothermia
- Adult patients with any of the following vital sign changes: systolic blood pressure, less than 90 mm Hg; respiratory rate, less than 10 or more than 35 respirations, per minute; heart rate less than 60 or more than 120 beats per minute or unresponsive to verbal stimuli
- Transport time to trauma center more than 15 minutes by ground vehicle
- Ambulance transport impeded
- Presence of multiple victims
- Time to local hospital via ambulance more than the time to trauma center via helicopter
- Wilderness rescue

tion furnishes guidelines, regulations, and penalties that govern patient transfer and transport. The implications of this law and its recent revisions are discussed in Chapter 35.[12]

When transporting an ill or injured patient, transport services should provide (1) a flight team with the experience necessary to perform an initial assessment and stabilize the patient before and during transport; (2) staff who are capable of using the equipment and technology necessary to deliver care during transport to specific groups of patients, such as the critically ill or injured; and (3) the ability to demonstrate that the transport will make a difference in patient outcome.[1,14]

The American College of Emergency Physicians has developed guidelines for appropriate transfer and transport of ill or injured patients. These guidelines are summarized in the box on p. 97 (*left*). In addition, the American College of Critical Care Medicine has proposed its own recommendations for the transport of critically ill or injured patients. The box on p. 97 (*right*) contains a summary of these guidelines, which address both interhospital and intrahospital transport of patients.

Finally, in 1995, the Emergency Nurses Association (ENA) developed a document that provides guidelines for the transport of ill or injured children. Unlike the documents previously mentioned, this document specifically addresses the needs of the ill or injured child. These guidelines are available from the ENA.

Making the Decision to Transport

Several factors must be considered by referring personnel when they are deciding whether to transport a patient. The first factor to be considered is the appropriateness of transport, which was previously discussed. Identification of a suitable receiving facility is a second factor that must be considered. When choosing a receiving facility, referring personnel must look at the resources available at the receiving facility, such as specialized care staff, equipment, and expertise. The location of the receiving facility is also an important consideration.

Another factor that should be considered when deciding whether to transport a patient involves the

AMERICAN COLLEGE OF EMERGENCY PHYSICIANS GUIDELINES FOR TRANSFER AND TRANSPORT OF ILL OR INJURED PATIENTS

1. The health and well-being of the patient must be the overriding concern when any patient transport is considered.
2. The patient should be evaluated before transfer.
3. The referring personnel should stabilize the patient (to the extent possible) before transport.
4. The patient and patient's family should be informed about the reasons for and the risks of transport.
5. The patient should be transferred to a facility that is appropriate to the medical needs of the patient and that has adequate space and available personnel.
6. The receiving facility must agree to accept the patient.
7. Economic reasons should not be the basis for transferring a patient to a receiving facility or refusing to admit a patient at a receiving facility.
8. Information about the patient's condition and initial care must be communicated to the receiving facility.
9. The patient should be transferred in a vehicle that is staffed by quality personnel and that contains equipment necessary to provide appropriate treatment for the patient who is being transferred.
10. When possible, written protocols and transfer agreements should be in place.

From American College of Emergency Physicians: Principles of appropriate transfer, *Ann Emerg Med* 3:337, 1990.

existence of written policies and agreements between the receiving and referring agencies. Identification of centers that are capable of providing certain types of services and generating triage guidelines could save precious time.

SUMMARY OF AMERICAN COLLEGE OF CRITICAL CARE MEDICINE GUIDELINES FOR THE TRANSPORT OF THE CRITICALLY ILL OR INJURED PATIENT

1. The benefits of transferring the patient should outweigh the risks.
2. The practitioner needs to be aware of the legal implications of patient transfer and transport.
3. Before the patient is transported, physicians and nurses at the referring and receiving facilities should be in contact, a decision should be made about the mode of transportation to be used, and a copy of all medical records relevant to the patient's care should be secured.
4. Accompanying transport personnel should include a minimum of two patient care providers and a vehicle operator. At least one care provider should be a registered nurse.
5. The equipment (including monitors) and medications necessary to manage the patient's airway, breathing, and circulation should be available. Communication equipment used during transport should also be available.
6. Continuous monitoring should take place during transport. At a minimum, ECG monitoring and monitoring of vital signs are required. Patients with specific problems may require additional monitoring, such as capnography and invasive monitoring.

From the Guidelines Committee of the American College of Critical Care Medicine Society of Critical Care Medicine and the Transfer Guidelines Task Force of the American Association of Critical Care Nurses: Guidelines for the transport of the critically ill patient, 1993.

COMMUNICATION

Communication is probably one of the most important components in the preparation of the patient for transport. Communications center operations are discussed in Chapter 5. This discussion will focus on the communication process between personnel at the referring and receiving agencies (either a health care facility or an emergency medical services [EMS] agency).

Communication should begin before the flight team arrives. Written policies, procedures, and triage guidelines should be in place at the referring agency. These documents should address the type of patient that should be transported by air, the care that is required before transport, and steps that need to be taken by the referring agency to prepare for the arrival of the aircraft.

When initial contact has been made by the referring agency, information that should be provided for the flight team includes the patient's chief complaint, indications for air transport, interventions and their effects, and the patient's current condition.[15]

It is important to relay the patient's problem, age, and location so the most suitable flight team can be sent to provide care for the patient. For example, some areas of the United States have flight teams specifically designed to provide care for pregnant women, children, and critical care patients. The equipment required by the patient's illness or injury may influence the nursing skills that may be needed during transport (e.g., an intraaortic balloon pump).

Once the flight team arrives, the nurse or another crew member can obtain any information about the patient directly from the staff at the referring agency. When the flight nurse arrives at the scene, he or she should identify the person in charge and offer assistance.

During the initial assessment and preparation of the patient for transport, the flight nurse communicates with other team members and referring individuals. The communication process is composed of both verbal and nonverbal behaviors, and one's attitude is an important nursing intervention. Thus, the flight nurse should always involve those who have been caring for the patient.

Any laboratory results, x-ray films, or scans should be copied and should accompany the patient. If the patient has any valuables on his or her person, they must be accounted for. Sometimes it is easier to leave valuables with a family member, but this may not be possible. Potential problems may be prevented by recording a list of what was brought with the patient and to whom it was given on arrival at the receiving facility. Clothing or other valuables are sometimes considered evidence and should be treated as such on the basis of evidence protocols.

CONSENT

Patients must consent to treatment. However, it is not always possible to obtain written or verbal consent for air medical transport and for emergency treatment. Consent for air medical transport is usually implied. Implied consent is considered to be given only in an emergency situation, when the patient is incapacitated and is in a life-threatening situation.[12]

Even though the patient's consent is implied, the flight nurse should always explain to the patient and available family members all procedures and the transport process. If family members are available, they may be able to provide consent for treatment. If consent forms are part of the transport documentation, the flight nurse should ensure that they are transported with the patient.

PERFORMING A PATIENT ASSESSMENT

Primary and secondary assessment, identification of patient problems, and initiation of critical interventions provide a framework for preparing a patient for transport. Each of these tasks must be performed in an organized, rapid, and complete manner. It is important to note that patient assessment is a continuous process that occurs before, during, and after transport.

Assessment of the Patient in the Prehospital Care Environment

Assessment of the patient in the prehospital care environment can be an intense challenge. The location of the patient (e.g., trapped in a vehicle) (Fig. 7-1), limited availability of personnel and equipment, and the nature of the illness or injury the patient has sustained present potential barriers to performing prehospital patient assessment.

The environment in which the patient is located poses additional barriers to assessment. Noise, a lack of light and space, vehicle movement and the speed at which the vehicle is moving, and outside weather

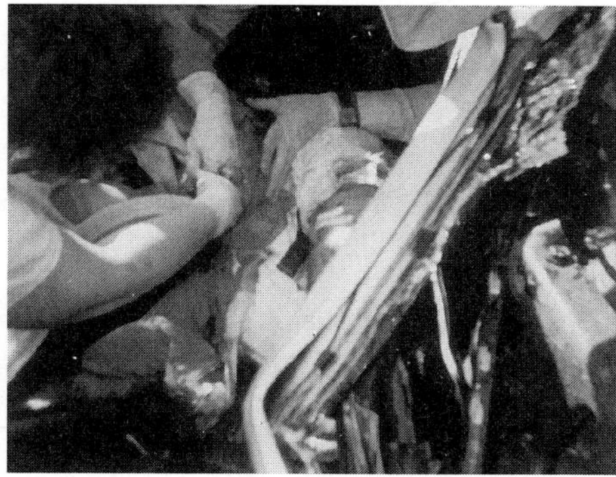

Fig. 7-1 It is difficult to perform a primary and secondary assessment when a patient is trapped in a vehicle. (Courtesy University AirCare, Cincinnati, Ohio.)

can make normal assessment maneuvers such as auscultation difficult to perform.

The type of vehicle used to transport the patient may also pose a barrier to patient assessment. Assessing patients in ground, helicopter, or fixed-wing vehicles can be troublesome. Even though equipment is now more portable, some pieces of equipment are still susceptible to movement and vibrations that could affect their reliability when they are used for patient assessment.

Scene Assessment

Assessment of the patient before he or she reaches the hospital begins with assessment of the scene, whether the nurse will be responding directly to the patient or to another facility. The nurse should assess the surrounding environment for hazards. The box contains a summary of some of the potential hazards that may be encountered.

On arrival at the referring facility, the flight nurse should survey the resources that are available to assist in preparing the patient for transport. Equipment and supplies necessary for patient stabilization may be limited, and thus it may be necessary for the flight nurse to bring additional equipment.

The principles of patient assessment used by the flight nurse are no different than those used when patients are assessed within the walls of a hospital. However, the prehospital environment dictates that the assessment be organized, direct, and rapid. Adaptation and flexibility are necessary when patient assessment is performed outside the hospital. Tight spaces, darkness, noise, and equipment that may or may not be functioning can present challenges in the prehospital care environment.

POTENTIAL ENVIRONMENTAL HAZARDS

Hazards at the Scene

Wires
Uneven ground
Vehicles
Accident itself
People
Signs
Light poles
Water
Loose debris

Hazards at the Referring Facility

Buildings
Wires
People

History

Patient assessment begins with obtaining a history as a primary assessment is being performed. The history of the illness or injury provides a guide for performing critical interventions, preparing the patient for transport, and ongoing assessment during transport.

Generally, the flight nurse is given some information while en route to the patient. However, experience has demonstrated that the situation on arrival may be quite different than that described beforehand.

General Principles of History Gathering

According to Henry and Stapleton,[24] "history is the patient's story of significant events related to and surrounding the present problem." Some general principles should be followed when gathering information related to the patient's illness or injury. One of these principles is that the patient's chief complaint or problem should be identified. If the patient is unable to provide this information, the flight nurse must obtain it from others at the scene (prehospital care providers, police, or bystanders), referring personnel (nurses or physicians), or any persons who may be with the patient. A survey of the scene by the nurse may also provide information. If the patient is unconscious, the nurse should look for medic alert jewelry or information in the patient's wallet or purse.

A common mnemonic used to collect general history information is AMPLE:

A Allergies, alcohol, or substance abuse
M Medications/immunizations for the child
P Past medical history
L Last meal
E Events leading to the emergency
Everything that has been done before the arrival of the transport team

If the patient's chief complaint or problem is related to pain, the PQRST method will be of use when collecting historical information. PQRST[27,29] represents the following:

P Provoking factors: What caused or causes the pain? Does anything relieve the pain or make it worse? What was the patient doing when the pain began?
Q Quality of the pain: Some of the words used to describe the pain may provide the nurse with clues as to the origin of the pain. For example, words such as "burning" or "crushing" are often used by patients to describe chest pain.
R Region and radiation: The patient should be asked to point to the area where he or she feels pain. The nurse should try to determine if there is a pattern to the pain.
S Severity: Numbering, such as from 1 to 10, can be used to describe the severity of the pain.
T Time: The patient should be asked to describe the temporal nature of the pain, such as how long it has been present and when or what time of day it began

The flight nurse may find it difficult to obtain a history in the prehospital care environment because of obstacles such as the patient's inability to communicate because of illness or injury, the lack of witnesses to a particular event, and the absence of family members or significant others at the scene of the illness or injury.

When possible, and particularly when the patient is being transported from a referring facility, as much information as possible should be collected and communicated with the receiving facility. At other times, particularly when patients are transported directly from the scene, this may not be possible. The flight nurse should keep in mind that history may provide as much information about the patient's condition as the primary assessment. History will also alert the nurse to potential problems that may develop during transport.

Trauma History

History gathering is different for the trauma patient than it is for the patient with a medical illness. The mechanism of injury triggers the trauma history. The flight nurse must find out in what manner, when, where, and how the patient was injured. A complete description of the event is often limited. The nurse providing prehospital care should not devote a great deal of time and energy to securing a complete description. However, a general idea of the mechanism of injury will provide clues for potential additional injuries and complications that may occur during transport. The box describes predictable injuries that may occur as a result of motor vehicle crashes.[22,27]

In recent years, instant photographs have been used to provide information about the mechanism of injury. Dickinson, Krett, and O'Connor[16] reported that when photography was used to provide details related to a motor vehicle crash, receiving physicians altered their perceptions about the patient's injuries in 46% of the cases. In addition, the receiving physician upgraded the severity of the motor vehicle crash after viewing the photographs in 22 of 26 cases (85%).

When obtaining the history of a trauma patient, the flight nurse should also gather information that describes the scene of the accident. Did the accident

PREDICTABLE INJURIES RESULTING FROM MOTOR VEHICLE CRASHES

Unrestrained Driver

Head injuries
Facial injuries
Fractured larynx
Fractured sternum
Cardiac contusion
Lacerated liver or spleen
Lacerated great vessels
Fractured patella and femur
Fractured clavicle

Restrained Driver

Caused by a lap restraint
Pelvic injuries
Spleen, liver, and pancreas injuries

Caused by shoulder restraint
Cervical fractures
Rupture of mitral valve or diaphragm

From Neff J, Kidd P: *Trauma nursing: the art and science,* St Louis, 1993, Mosby.

involve multiple victims? Are all of the victims accounted for? If the victims are unable to provide information about additional victims, the presence of schoolbooks, clothing, or toys may suggest that additional victims are present.[10]

History Related to Medical Illness

A patient's medical history begins with the chief complaint or current problem. The PQRST mnemonic previously described can be of assistance when obtaining a medical history. The flight nurse should obtain history related to the present illness, including related signs and symptoms. Significant past medical history and risk factors for a particular disease process (such as smoking and chronic obstructive pulmonary disease) can provide additional pieces of meaningful information.

Information about care initiated before the arrival of the flight nurse must be gathered. These data[22] should include initial physical findings, initial treatments and results, vital sign trends, medications

SUMMARY OF PRIMARY AIRWAY ASSESSMENT

- Airway: patent; maintainable; nonmaintainable
- Level of consciousness
- Skin appearance: ashen, pale, gray, cyanotic, mottled
- Preferred posture to maintain airway (e.g., child with epiglottitis, patient with pulmonary edema)
- Airway clearance
- Sounds of obstruction

given, laboratory results, x-ray findings, ECG findings, intravenous infusions given, intake and output, and status of family notification.

Primary Assessment and Critical Interventions

Primary assessment is based on assessment of the patient's airway, breathing, circulation, neurologic disability, and exposure. During the primary assessment, as patient problems are identified, the flight nurse should initiate any critical interventions on the basis of the patient's illness or injury. The basic steps remain the same whether the flight nurse performs the primary assessment and provides initial patient care at the scene of the injury or illness or at a referring facility.

Airway

The patient's airway is assessed to determine if it is patent, maintainable, or not maintainable. For any patient who is suspected to have a traumatic injury, cervical spine precautions are used while the airway is evaluated. Assessment of the patient's level of consciousness in concert with assessment of the airway status provides the flight nurse with an impression of the effectiveness of the patient's current airway status (box).

If an airway problem is identified, the appropriate intervention should be started. The decision to use a particular intervention will depend on the nature of the patient's problem and the potential for complications during transport. Airway interventions are addressed in Chapter 8.

Supplemental oxygen should be given to all patients before transport. Specific equipment such as a pulse oximeter or CO_2 detector will help provide continuous airway evaluation during transport. The indications and the procedures for use of these devices are included in Chapter 8.

Pharmacologic Adjuncts for Airway Management. Specific pharmacologic agents have been found to be useful in prehospital airway management. These agents include those that provide sedation and amnesia, and neuromuscular blocking agents that facilitate intubation. An in-depth discussion of the use of these medications is provided in Chapters 8 and 18.

Breathing

Assessment of ventilation begins with observing whether the patient is breathing. If the patient is apneic or in severe respiratory distress, immediate interventions are indicated. If the patient is having any difficulty with ventilation, the flight nurse must identify the problem and proceed with the appropriate interventions. Emergent interventions may include decompression with a needle or insertion of a chest tube (box). Ventilation interventions are discussed in Chapters 8 and 21.

Circulation

Palpation of both peripheral and central pulses provides information about the patient's circulatory status. The quality, location, and rate of the patient's pulses should be noted. The temperature of the patient's skin can be assessed along with the pulses. Level of consciousness will help the flight nurse evaluate the patient's perfusion (box).

Active bleeding should be quickly controlled with interventions such as direct pressure. The flight nurse should observe the patient for indications of circulatory compromise. Skin color, diaphoresis, and capillary refill are appraised during circulatory assessment.

Intravenous access is obtained for administration of fluid, blood, and medications. Depending on the patient's location and accessibility of veins, peripheral, central, or intraosseous access may be used.

Disability: Neurologic Assessment

Neurologic assessment includes assessment of the level of consciousness, the size, shape, and response of the pupil, and motor sensory function. A simple method that may be used to evaluate the patient's level of consciousness is the AVPU method:

A Alert
V Responds to verbal stimuli
P Responds to painful stimuli
U Unresponsive

Both the Glasgow and Pediatric Glasgow Coma Scales provide assessment of the patient's level of consciousness and motor function.[18]

SUMMARY OF PRIMARY BREATHING ASSESSMENT

- Rate and depth of respirations
- Cyanosis
- Position of the trachea
- Presence of obvious injury or deformity
- Work of breathing
  - Use of accessory muscles
  - Flaring of nostrils
  - Presence of breath sounds bilaterally
  - Presence of adventitious breath sounds
  - Asymmetric chest movements
  - Palpation of crepitus

SUMMARY OF PRIMARY CIRCULATION ASSESSMENT

- Tachycardia, bradycardia
- Skin appearance: cyanotic, dusky, mottled, pale
- Diminished peripheral pulses
- Skin temperature
- Level of consciousness
- Decreased urinary output (assessment of patients at a referring facility)
- Hypotension
- Dysrhythmia

The flight nurse needs to determine whether the patient has ingested any toxic substances such as alcohol or other drugs. A patient whose mental status has been altered by drugs or alcohol may pose a safety problem during transport; use of chemical paralysis, sedation, or physical restraints may be required.

Exposure

As much of the patient's body as possible should be exposed for examination, keeping in mind the effects of the environment on the patient. Discovering hidden problems before the patient is loaded for transport allows the flight nurse to intervene and prevent potentially disastrous complications. Although exposure for examination has been emphasized most frequently in the care of the trauma patient, it is just as important in the primary assessment of the patient with a medical illness.

The flight nurse should always look under dressings or clothing, which may "hide" complications or potential problems. Intravenous access can be wrongly assumed underneath a bulky cover. Clothing can also hide bleeding that occurs as a result of thrombolytic therapy (box).

Equipment Assessment

Even though the concept of equipment assessment has not been routinely included in previous descriptions of primary assessment, it is an important process that must be performed. Before the patient is transported, the flight nurse should ensure that the patient is wearing an appropriately sized cervical collar, that the chest tube drainage system is functioning, and that the patient is correctly restrained. This assessment of equipment will help avoid problems during transport that could potentially leave the patient at risk for further injury.

SUMMARY OF EXPOSURE ASSESSMENT

- Appropriate tube placement: endotracheal tubes, nasotracheal tubes, chest tubes, nasogastric or orogastric tubes, urinary catheters
- Intravenous access: peripheral, central, intraosseous
- Identification of injury; active bleeding; indication of a serious illness such as pressure of purpura

Secondary Assessment

Whether a secondary assessment can be performed depends on the patient's condition and the amount of time needed for transport. Lack of space in the aircraft, lack of light, and noise may interfere with the flight nurse's ability to perform a secondary assessment during transport.

Secondary assessment involves evaluating the patient from head to toe.[6] The nurse collects patient information by means of inspection, palpation, and auscultation during secondary assessment. Whether the patient has suffered an injury or is critically ill, the flight nurse should observe, touch, and listen to the patient.

Secondary assessment begins with an evaluation of the patient's general appearance. The nurse should observe the surrounding environment and evaluate its effects on the patient. Is the patient aware of the environment? Is there appropriate interaction between the patient and the environment?

Additional systems that should be assessed include the integumentary (color, presence of wounds, temperature); head and neck (deformities, crepitus, pain); eyes, ears, and nose (drainage); thorax and lungs (chest movement, heart and breath sounds); abdomen; genitourinary; and extremities and back (box).

Pain Assessment

Determining the amount of pain the patient is experiencing as a result of his or her illness or injury is an important component of patient assessment. Physiologic indications of pain include tachypnea, controlled respirations, tachycardia, hypotension, hypertension, nausea and vomiting, and diaphoresis. Behavioral indications of pain are crying, protective behavior, guarding, moaning, and self-focusing.

Baseline data are collected about the pain the patient is experiencing so that the flight nurse will be

SUMMARY OF SECONDARY ASSESSMENT[6]

Skin

- Presence of petechia, purpura, abrasions, bruises, scars, birthmarks
- Rashes
- Abnormal skin turgor
- Signs of abuse and neglect

Head and Neck

- Presence of lacerations, contusions, raccoon eyes, Battle's sign, drainage from nose, mouth, and ears
- In the infant, examination of the anterior fontanelle
- Gross visual examination
- Abnormal extraocular movements
- Position of the trachea
- Neck veins
- Swallowing difficulties
- Nuchal rigidity
- Presence of lymphadenopathy or neck masses

Eyes, Ears, Nose

- Lack of tearing
- Sunken eyes
- Color of the sclera
- Drainage
- Gross assessment of hearing

Mouth and Throat

- Mucous membranes
- Breath odor
- Injuries to teeth
- Drooling
- Drainage

Thorax, Lungs, Cardiovascular

- Breath sounds
- Heart sounds

Abdomen

- Shape and size
- Bowel sounds
- Tenderness
- Firmness
- Masses, suprapubic mass
- Femoral pulses
- Pelvic tenderness
- Color of drainage from nasogastric/orogastric tube

Genitourinary

- Blood at meatus
- Rectal bleeding
- Color of urine in catheter

Extremities and Back

- Gross motor and sensory function
- Peripheral pulses
- Lack of use of an extremity
- Deformity, angulation
- Wounds, abrasions
- Equipment is appropriately applied (e.g., traction splints)
- Vertebral column, flank, buttocks

able to evaluate specific pain management interventions during transport.

Scoring Systems

Scoring systems were initially developed to identify patients who were in need of critical care that was not available at referring facilities,[13] such as patients who needed to be transported to a level I trauma center. Scoring systems can be used in the field and for evaluation of patients who may need interfacility support. Scoring systems have most commonly been used for the trauma patient. These systems include the Prehospital Index Score; CRAMS Scale Score; Triage-Revised Trauma Score; and Baxt's Trauma Triage Rule. Little research has been done regarding triage scores and severity scores that can be used for other medical problems.[18]

PREPARING THE PATIENT FOR TRANSPORT

This section will summarize patient preparation for transport. More in-depth discussions about patient preparation are contained in the clinical care sections of this book. The patient is prepared for transport on the basis of information obtained from the primary and secondary assessment, the type of aircraft the patient will be transported in, the amount of time the transport will take, and the potential problems that may develop in relation to the patient's illness or injury during transport. Patient preparation includes anticipatory planning; preparing for potential patient problems makes patient care easier and safer.

During the past 10 years, equipment has evolved that has made it easier to monitor and provide care for the patient during transport. Continenza and Hill[13] recommend that the equipment meet the following criteria:

- It should be useful in the transport setting
- It should be lightweight, portable, and perhaps fulfill several functions (e.g., a monitor with a built-in defibrillator and external pacemaker)
- It should be easy to clean and maintain
- It should have a battery life or power source that will last the length of the transport
- It should have the ability to be used both inside and outside the transport vehicle
- It should be able to withstand the stresses of transport, such as movement, altitude changes, being dropped, water or fluid contamination, weather changes, and use by multiple persons

The box on pp. 106-107 contains a generic list of equipment that may be used when transporting patients by air. The amount and type of equipment carried by each service is dictated by the types of patients cared for.

Airway Management

Patient preparation begins with assessment and management of the patient's airway. The location of the patient may limit the type of airway management the flight team will be able to provide. For example, if a patient is trapped in a vehicle, the flight team may have limited access for airway management.

Factors that may influence the flight nurse's decision about how to manage the airway include the nature of the patient's illness or injury, the amount of time the transport will take, the size of the aircraft, and the positioning of the crew in the aircraft.

If intubation has already been performed, tube placement and security should be evaluated. An unsecured endotracheal tube may inadvertently come out during transport. In addition, movement of the endotracheal tube can cause mucosal damage, induce gagging and coughing, and increase the patient's intracranial or intraocular pressures.[48]

Oxygen should be administered to the patient. When available, additional monitoring equipment such as a pulse oximeter, CO_2 monitor, or apnea monitor should be used for continuous airway evaluation. These monitoring devices are discussed further in Chapter 8.

Ventilation Management

A rapid, focused assessment of the patient's ventilatory status should be performed as the patient is being prepared for transport. If a chest x-ray film has been obtained before arrival, it should be viewed by the flight nurse to determine if any pathology exists. Breath sounds should be auscultated before the patient is placed in the aircraft because of noise interference.

If a pneumothorax is suspected or is present on the x-ray film, appropriate interventions should be initiated. If a chest tube or tubes are already in place, the nurse should check to see whether they are functioning. The drainage system may need to be changed so that it will continue to function during transport.

If a portable ventilator is to be used, the patient's tidal volume, respiratory rate, and FiO_2 must be calculated before the patient is connected to the ventilator. Patients who are dependent on a ventilator may need to spend some time connected to the transport ventilator to ascertain that they are able to tolerate the change.[15] Ventilator use is discussed in Chapter 8.

Circulation Management

Initial care related to circulation management is directed at controlling any active bleeding. Bleeding

EQUIPMENT FOR TRANSPORT

A comprehensive list of equipment that needs to be stocked by air transport services consists of a core set of supplies. The following equipment list serves as a guide, but it must be upgraded for special patient considerations and streamlined in the event of cost constraints.

1. Airway equipment
   - Ambu bags (infant, child, adult)
   - All sizes of masks for ambu bags
   - Simple and complex oxygen masks
   - Nasal cannula
   - Oral and NP airways
   - Nebulizer setup
   - Portable suction unit
   - Tonsil suction
   - Suction catheters in the following sizes: 5/6, 8, 10, 14, and 18 Fr
   - Magill forceps (pediatric and adult)
   - Laryngoscope handles (pediatric and adult)
   - Laryngoscope blades in the following sizes:
     - Miller 0, 1, 2, and 3
     - MAC 2, 3, and 4
   - Spare laryngoscope batteries and bulbs
   - Endotracheal tubes

Uncuffed		Cuffed		Endotrol
2.5	4.0	5.5	7.0	7.0
3.0	4.5	6.0	7.5	8.0
3.5	5.0	6.5	8.0	

   - Stylets
   - Benzoin, adhesive tape, and tracheostomy tape
   - CO_2 detector
   - PEEP valve
   - Pulse oximeter
   - Ventilator and filter and spirometer
   - Cricothyrotomy tray
   - Tracheostomy tubes
   - Needle cricothyrotomy setup
   - Nasogastric tubes in sizes 5 to 18
   - Catheter tip syringe
   - Surgilube
2. Cardiothoracic equipment
   - Cardiac monitor and supplies, including extra batteries
   - Defibrillator and supplies, including adult and pediatric paddles
   - External pacer and supplies
   - Transvenous pulse generator and cable
   - Automatic blood pressure machine
   - Manual blood pressure equipment (pediatric, adult, and obese)
   - Doppler
   - Pressure monitor and transducer and tubing kit
   - MAST pants (?)
   - Thoracotomy tray and drainage system
   - Chest tubes in sizes 12 Fr to 36 Fr
   - Vaseline gauze
   - Needle decompression supplies
   - Pericardiocentesis setup
   - Multiple adapters (Sims, connectors, small and large Y)
3. Intravenous equipment
   - Intravenous solution (? NS, LR, D5W)
   - Blood tubing
   - Minidrip tubing
   - Extension tubing
   - Burratrol set up
   - Intravenous needles (24 to 14 Ga)
   - Butterfly needles (27 to 19 Ga)
   - Intraosseous needles (15 and 18 Ga)
   - Syringes of multiple sizes
   - Intravenous start packs
   - Razors
   - Arm boards
   - Laboratory blood tubes
   - Stopcocks
   - Pressure bag
   - 7 Fr conversion kit
   - Intravenous controllers or pumps and setup
   - Blood products and blood cooler

EQUIPMENT FOR TRANSPORT—cont'd

4. Medications
    - ACLS medications
    - Antianginal agents
    - Antiarrhythmics
    - Anticonvulsants
    - Antiemetics
    - Antihistamines
    - Antihypertensives
    - Diuretics
    - Local anesthetics
    - Narcotics/Narcan
    - Nasal decongestant
    - Paralytic agents
    - Steroids
    - Tocolytics
    - Vasopressor agents
5. Miscellaneous
    - Oxygen
    - Stethoscope
    - Isolation equipment (gloves, masks, goggles)
    - Disposable needle boxes
    - Instruments
        - Bandage scissors
        - Trauma scissors
        - Hemostats
        - Ring cutter
    - Tape
    - Betadine solution
    - Dressing supplies (4 × 4s, Kling, bandages, cravats)
    - Eye shields
    - Burn sheets
    - Burn cable and electrodes
    - Cervical collars
    - Cervical immobilization device
    - Pediatric transport board
    - Car seat
    - Isolette
    - Obstetrics delivery tray
    - Bubble bag
    - Stockinette cap
    - Stuffed toys
    - Emergidose cards
    - Soft/leather restraints
    - Linen, blankets, towels
    - Flashlight
    - Cellular telephone
    - Two-way radio
    - Thermometer
    - Instant camera and film
    - Disposable needle boxes
    - Paperwork
    - Directions and map to receiving facilities

Additional equipment specific to a particular type of service may include the following:

Ambulance

- Immobilization devices (because space and weight are less of a consideration in an ambulance than in a helicopter or fixed-wing aircraft)
- Backboard
- Traction splint
- Vacuum splints

Helicopter

- Ear protection for the patient and crew
- Survival bag stocked with necessary equipment in the event of an emergency landing

Fixed-Wing Aircraft

- Certain bulk supplies (because of extended transport times)
- Intravenous solutions, medication
- Food and drink for the crew
- Patient "comfort kit" (i.e., bedpan, urinal, Foley)
- A more versatile type of ventilator (i.e., allows for patient assist, PEEP, and the like)

can be controlled with direct pressure by applying gauze pads and elastic tape or bandages. Air splints and MAST pants have also been used to help control bleeding. However, the source and cause of the bleeding should be carefully evaluated before transport. Once the patient is "packaged," bleeding can easily be hidden by sheets and blankets.

Intravenous access must be ensured. Whether one or two lines are inserted depends on individual protocols. However, having access to the intravenous line is important for fluid replacement, blood administration, and pain management. Additional methods for access include the insertion of central lines and, in children, insertion of intraosseous lines.

When medications are being infused, intravenous monitors may be used to ensure the appropriate delivery of medication. Medication concentrations and dosages should always be checked before a change is made in the equipment being used. Some flight nurses have found that it is easier to prepare medications with their own equipment and then make any changes in concentration and dosage, particularly when their own equipment requires specific types of tubing.

Foley catheters must be appropriately placed and affixed so that they are not pulled out with patient movement. It is recommended that the catheter bag be emptied before the patient leaves the referring facility. The amount of urine emptied from the bag and its color should be recorded.

If invasive lines such as pulmonary or arterial catheters are in place, the flight nurse will need to check the patency and functioning of these lines. In some cases, transport monitors that offer specific readings during transport may not be available. The lines must be appropriately secured so that their functioning is not impaired. If a transport monitor is available, readings should be taken and recorded before, during, and after transport.

Gastric Decompression

A nasogastric or orogastric tube should be inserted to prevent the potential for aspiration and to provide gastric decompression during transport.[3] This procedure is not generally performed when a patient is transported directly from a scene, but it should be considered, particularly when the patient has undergone bag-valve-mask ventilation.

As with the Foley catheter, the gastric decompression tube must be appropriately placed and secured to prevent it from being pulled out. If the tube is not going to be placed on suction during transport, it should be capped so that it does not spill. When possible, the patient's stomach should be drained before the tube is plugged. The amount of the drainage and its color should be recorded.

When patients are being treated for extensive GI bleeding, such as that seen in the patient with liver disease, a specific type of gastric tube, such as the Sengstaken-Blakemore tube, may be in place. Traction must be maintained so that the tube will continue to function properly. When this tube is present the patient may be at risk for aspiration, asphyxia, gastric rupture, and erosion of the esophageal wall.[28] When this patient is transported, the airway should be secured by intubation, and the flight nurse must be prepared to intervene if any complications occur and to provide continued traction on the tube. The transport of these patients offers a unique flight nursing challenge.

Wound Care and Splinting

Wounds and splinting devices should be surveyed quickly, before the patient is moved. Hidden wounds may cause the patient discomfort and place the patient at risk of bleeding and long-term complications. Improperly placed splints or lack of splinting when indicated may also cause problems.

Several types of splints and splint devices are available to be used for the patient being transported. The flight nurse must be familiar with the type of equipment that is being used. Placement of the splint, potential complications of the device, and when it should be removed are some examples of the kind of information needed. The neurovascular status of the extremity to which the splint is applied should be assessed and documented. Orthopedic and vascular emergencies are discussed in Chapter 15.

Wound care is provided for patient comfort and protection. Dressing the wound will help control bleeding and keep it free of debris. If there is concern about additional bleeding or neurovascular compromise, the wound should be dressed in such a manner that continuous assessment is possible during transport. Any wet dressings are replaced with dry sterile dressings to prevent heat loss during transport.

It is important to keep in mind the need for infection control when tending to the wounds of the patient being prepared for transport. Many patients being transported may have infected wounds that can leave the at risk transport team and anyone else who may need to be transported in the vehicle. Infection control issues are addressed in Chapter 25.

Safety

An entire chapter in this textbook (Chapter 6) has been devoted to safety issues. In this section we will examine the safety measures that must be taken into consideration by the flight nurse when preparing the patient for transport. If the patient is combative, neuromuscular blocking agents and sedation may be indicated to ensure the safety of both the patient and the transport team.

A policy based on guidelines issued by the Food and Drug Administration should be in place regarding the use of restraints.[7] These guidelines include the need to clearly document the need for the use of restraints during transport, follow local and state laws regarding the use of patient restraints, closely monitor the patient in restraints, carefully apply the restraining device(s) and adjust them properly so that they maintain body alignment and are not uncomfortable, and consider restraints to be a temporary solution.

When transporting a child, the child's size, weight, and state laws necessitate that restraint systems appropriate for a child be used. Devices that may be used include care beds, car seats, and transport boards. Any equipment that is used during transport needs to meet both federal and state standards.

Pain Management

Pain management in the prehospital care environment is frequently not given priority consideration.[41] Several factors influence the use or lack of use of pain medications in the field, including the location of the patient, the nature of the patient's illness or injury, the possible masking of symptoms, and the effect of pain medications on the patient's vital signs. Movement, noise, changes in temperature, and fear may be contributing factors that cause or increase the patient's pain during preparation and transport.

Certain patient problems, such as chest pain related to myocardial infarction, have been dealt with outside of the hospital without any difficulty. However, pain management for trauma or other disease states continues to cause controversy.[41]

In 1992 the United States Department of Health and Human Services published its *Clinical Practice Guidelines for Acute Pain Management: Operative or Medical Procedures and Trauma.* The need for appropriate pain management is emphasized in these guidelines. Even though the prehospital management of pain is not directly addressed, these guidelines can easily be applied to the transport process.

The guidelines point out the following[43]:

> The presence of a condition that could eventually result in cardiovascular, hemodynamic, neurologic, or pulmonary instability (e.g., femur fracture, pneumothorax, skull fracture) is not an absolute contraindication to systemic analgesia, although careful titration and monitoring must be provided.

The flight nurse should perform a brief assessment related to the patient's pain. The PQRST mnemonic previously described will help provide the nurse with a baseline description of the patient's pain. If the patient received medication before the flight nurse's arrival, information about the medication used and its effect on the patient should be included in the pain assessment.

Pain medications used for analgesia in the prehospital care environment need to be rapid in onset, short in duration, easy to administer, and easy to store.[41] The intravenous route is the quickest method of administration and has a rapid onset. However, intravenous access may not always be available. Table 7-1 lists medications that may be used to manage pain during air transport.[4,5,32]

Another important point to keep in mind regarding pain management during transport is that many patients have received neuromuscular blocking agents for safe transport, management of specific problems, or both. The flight nurse should pay particular at-

TABLE 7-1

Medications that may be used for sedation and pain management during air medical transport

Medication	Advantages	Disadvantages
Opioids	Analgesia Can be reversed	Respiratory depression Hypotension Addictive
Benzodiazepines	Decreases anxiety Causes amnesia Generally does not interfere with the patient's hemodynamics	Respiratory depression Tachyphylaxis Reversal agent can decrease seizure threshold
Ketamine	Sedation and analgesia Does not cause respiratory depression Amnesia	Increases ICP Can cause hallucinations
Propofol	Sedation and hyponosis Ultrashort acting	Respiratory depression Hypotension

From Barsan W, Jastremski M, Syverud S: *Emergency drug therapy,* Philadelphia, 1992, WB Saunders; Mirski M et al: Sedation for the critically ill neurologic patient, *Crit Care Med* 23(12): 2038, 1995; Benevelli W et al: Safety of fentanyl during transport of trauma patients, *Air Med J* 14(3): 156, 1995.

tention to these patients' needs for sedation and pain management because they are unable to let the flight team know when they are anxious or in pain.

Additional methods that may be used by the flight nurse to help the patient manage pain during transport include the following:

- Distracting the patient; for example, if the patient is alert enough to look out the window, he or she should be allowed to do so; a security object such as a stuffed toy may be of help to a child
- Talking to the patient
- Keeping the patient warm
- Placing the patient in a comfortable position when possible
- Describing everything that is going to occur
- Allowing a family member to accompany the patient
- Using therapeutic touch

PATIENT PREPARATION: THE FAMILY

Any time a family member is ill or injured, a crisis is created in the family. The need to transfer the patient to a distant facility produces additional stress.

At times the flight nurse will not have the opportunity to interact with the patient's family. Family members may not be present at the scene of the illness or injury, or they themselves may be injured. When family members are present, the flight nurse may be able to obtain a pertinent patient history from them.

The flight nurse should ensure that information is provided to the family before, during, and after transport of the patient. Policies and procedures that address when a family member may accompany an injured or ill family member should be in place. A discussion about family needs, how to care for the family, and when transport of a family member is appropriate is contained in Chapter 10.

Documentation

Copies of any relevant documentation from the referring facility or agency should accompany the patient. If the patient was involved in an accident or crash and pictures of the scene are available, they should be brought along by the flight team.

Copies of any laboratory results, x-ray films, scans, and documentation by the referring facility or agency should accompany the patient. If written permission is required for transport, a copy of this document should also be included.

The flight nurse's documentation of his or her initial assessment and preparation of the patient and any interventions that were performed can be done during transport or on completion of the transport. Nursing documentation is based on the specific standards of care for the type of patient being transported. Components of these documents vary depending on the information required by each transport service.

PATIENT ASSESSMENT DURING TRANSPORT

The nature of the patient's illness or injuries and the initial interventions performed will influence the assessment and management needed during air medical transport. Each of the clinical chapters in this textbook addresses the specific care required during transport as a result of the patient's illness or injury. Some general principles of assessment and management during transport include the following:

- Flight nurses should position themselves in the aircraft so that they can effectively manage the patient's ABCs
- Airway equipment, including suction equipment, should be easily accessible
- All intravenous, central, or intraosseous lines should be accessible and functioning
- All tubes and drainage systems should be functioning and should be secured
- If there is any question about cervical spine injury, the cervical spine should be immobilized for transport
- A combative patient should be properly restrained, both physically and with administration of drugs
- All monitors should be placed within the nurse's visual field
- When indicated, wounds and injured limbs should remain exposed for inspection

SUMMARY

Assessment and preparation of the patient to be transported make up the foundation of patient care in the prehospital care environment and during transport of the patient to a location where definitive care can be provided. Primary and secondary assessments provide initial information about the patient's current and potential problems. On the basis of these assessments, appropriate interventions are initiated by the flight team. The box lists some of these flight nursing interventions.[30]

Patient preparation includes not only obvious care but anticipation of what may occur. In the prehospital care environment, resources are limited and anticipatory planning, safety, and prevention are key nursing interventions.

FIXED-WING FLIGHT NURSING

When transporting patients in fixed-wing aircraft, the flight nurse must pay critical attention to preflight preparation because of long periods of time typically spent on the ground and in flight. Fixed-wing aircraft transports usually entail lengthy periods of patient care; thus, it is imperative that the flight nurse obtain detailed preflight information so that

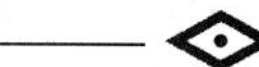

FLIGHT NURSING INTERVENTIONS

Airway management
Electrolyte and acid base management
Drug management
Neurologic management
Respiratory management
Physical comfort promotion
Thermoregulation
Tissue perfusion
Psychologic comfort promotion
Crisis management
Risk management
Lifespan care
Information management

From McCloskey J, Bulechek G: *Nursing interventions classification,* St Louis, 1996, Mosby.

air medical personnel can make appropriate preparations for the transport. The aircraft should not depart to pick up the patient until all preflight preparations are complete. In addition to preparing for the medical aspects of the flight, the logistics and itinerary must be worked out and any other preflight information required by the pilots must be obtained. The flight nurse and pilot(s) should collaborate in gathering this preflight information and in coordinating the entire flight to ensure appropriate quality patient care.

In this section of the chapter, issues encountered by flight nurses in the fixed-wing aircraft transport environment will be discussed. The following topics will be covered: history, flight physiology and stresses of flight, preflight preparation, federal aviation regulations, preparing for patient transport, patient "packaging," in-flight factors influencing patient care, air medical personnel resources, in-flight codes, and safety and emergency procedures. In addition, issues related to international transports and escort flights will be highlighted for flight nurses who transport patients into and out of the United States.

History

The air medical profession has predominantly focused on issues, standards, and safety related to rotor-wing aircraft. The National Flight Nurses Association (NFNA), which was founded in 1981, was established for nurses who typically transported patients in helicopters. The NFNA's focus on the rotor-wing aircraft or helicopter environment was reflected in the organization's initial bylaws and in the 1986 first edition of the *Practice Standards for Flight Nursing.*[34] It was not until the mid 1980s that the NFNA Liaison Committee recognized the need to address issues related to the transport of patients on fixed-wing aircraft, and thus the Fixed-Wing Special Interest Group was formed. This group remains active today.

The Association of Air Medical Services (AAMS) (formerly known as the American Society of Hospital-Based Emergency Aeromedical Services, or ASHBEAMS), established in 1980, also initially focused on helicopter services and issues. The first fixed-wing aircraft committee of this organization, established by the AAMS President's Council to address issues and standards for fixed-wing aircraft programs, was established between October, 1989 and January, 1990. Because the air medical profession has focused primarily on operations, issues, and standards related to rotor-wing aircraft, there has been a slow evolution of standards, documents, and texts related to fixed-wing aircraft air medical transport. An initial set of Recommended Minimum Quality Standards for Hospital-Based Emergency Air Medical Services, established by the AAMS in 1982, included limited fixed-wing aircraft standards. The AAMS' Rotorcraft and Fixed-Wing Standards were revised in August 1992.[37] In addition, the first edition of the *Air-Medical Crew National Standard Curriculum* was published in 1988 by ASHBEAMS (now AAMS), in cooperation with Samaritan AirEvac. Chapter 3 of this publication addresses fixed-wing aircraft safety and orientation.[22]

FLIGHT PHYSIOLOGY

The flight nurse should be aware of cabin pressurization issues and aircraft limitations. Issues of importance to the flight nurse during transport of a patient in a fixed-wing aircraft are briefly highlighted in this section. Flight physiology and the stresses of flight are discussed in detail in Chapter 2. Several of the stresses of flight will be reviewed as they specifically relate to nursing care in the fixed-wing aircraft.

The Gas Laws

Gas laws govern the body's physiologic responses to changes in barometric (atmospheric) pressure, temperature, and volume. These laws become especially critical as the aircraft ascends and descends.

Dalton's Law of Partial Pressure

The pressure of a gaseous mixture is equal to the sum of the partial pressure of the gases in that mixture. However, regardless of altitude, oxygen concentration always remains at 21%.[22] When altitude increases, the barometric pressure decreases, thus causing the amount of available oxygen to decrease as the gas molecules move farther apart.

Fixed-wing aircraft undergo expected decreases in barometric pressures because of the higher altitudes at which they fly. Because change in pressure may result in hypoxia,[35] patients in the fixed-wing aircraft require optimum oxygenation.

Stresses of Flight

Decreased Humidity

The effects of decreased humidity on patients being transported in fixed-wing aircraft must be considered. Not only are in-flight times typically longer in fixed-wing aircraft, but the pressurization of the aircraft further decreases the humidity in the cabin air. To counteract these dehydrating effects, the flight nurse may need to administer humidified oxygen and additional intravenous (IV) fluids and provide mouth care for the patient as needed. Drinking water and other beverages should be available for consumption by the air medical personnel, pilots, any persons who ride along, and patients who are not designated NPO.[39] The flight nurse may need to instill saline solution or ointment in the eyes of comatose patients to protect their corneas. Humidified oxygen should be provided for patients with a tracheostomy.

Gravitational Forces

Acceleration and deceleration, which result from gravitational forces (*g* forces), are noticeably greater in fixed-wing aircraft than in rotor-wing aircraft.[39] Among fixed-wing aircraft, jets are more greatly influenced by gravitational forces than are aircraft driven by propeller or turbopropellor. Because *g* forces are greater on acceleration, positioning of the patient within the aircraft during acceleration may become an issue. Current theory suggests that *g* forces do not usually have a significant effect on most patients, because most patients can compensate for these forces with changes in cardiac output and venous return. In some instances a patient may require positioning with his or her head forward and feet aft. The head-forward position may help to reduce the risk of a transient increase in intracranial pressure during takeoff in the patient with a head injury. This position may also be beneficial in the patient experiencing severe congestive heart failure because it increases venous pooling in the lower extremities.[8]

Cabin Pressurization

In addition to having an understanding of the gas laws, the flight nurse must understand the importance of cabin pressurization at higher altitudes. Smaller fixed-wing aircraft and all rotor-wing aircraft are at a disadvantage because they have no control over the effects of these gas laws. Cabin pressurization is a method of creating an artificial atmospheric pressure or "cabin altitude" in the fixed-wing aircraft. According to the manufacturer's specifications for the type and model of fixed-wing aircraft, there is a maximum pressurization limit or "maximum pressure differential" that is measured in pounds per square inch (PSI).[22]

For example, the PSI for a Cessna Conquest-II 441 aircraft is 6.3, and thus it has a 6.3 maximum pressure differential and can tolerate the difference between the altitude at which it is flying and the cabin pressure. Therefore, the Cessna Conquest-II 441 can fly at an "airplane altitude" of 21,300 feet, and the pilot can adjust the "cabin altitude" pressure to 4000 feet. Another example is a Lear Jet 25B, which has a maximum pressure differential of 8.7 PSI. The Lear's system can maintain a sea level cabin altitude pressure between airplane altitudes of 21,000 to 26,000 feet. If the airplane altitude is at 45,000 feet, the pilot can pressurize the cabin altitude to 8000 feet.[19] It is important to remember that the cabin altitude is usually determined by the destination altitude. The pilot can adjust the cabin altitude between sea level and the maximum pressure differential, depending on the patient's condition and requirements.

The air medical profession should promote the use of pressurized fixed-wing aircraft alone for the transport of patients. In addition to potential complications resulting from physiologic responses to altitude and the stresses of flight, transport of an already compromised patient in an unpressurized aircraft can cause more complications. Cabin pressurization helps to decrease or eliminate some of the stresses.

PREFLIGHT PREPARATION

Preplanning by air medical personnel and the pilot is necessary if the patient transport is to go smoothly. Fixed-wing aircraft flight times are usually much longer than rotor-wing aircraft flight times and may vary greatly from service to service. Fixed-wing aircraft flight times may be as brief as 40 minutes within the state or as long as 3 to 6 hours within a particular region or across the country. In addition, transport distances may range from 150 to 500 miles for a propellor or turbopropellor aircraft to more than 500 miles for a jet. Once the patient transfer has been agreed on by a receiving physician and facility, the flight nurse should begin by obtaining information such as physicians' names, phone numbers, and an accurate account of the patient's diagnosis and condition. This information will, it is hoped, ensure that the skills of the air medical personnel and the medical equipment available during transport are appropriate for the anticipated medical needs of the patient. In addition, logistic information such as patient and luggage weights, the number of family members who will ride along and their weights, and the DNR status of the patient must also be obtained.

Preflight preparation also entails coordination of information with the pilot(s). Issues to be discussed should include location of airports, refueling and restroom stops, weight and balance issues, in-flight times to and from airports, ground ambulance times to referring and receiving facilities, ground unit resources, nutritional and fluid requirements, and disposal of wastes. The flight nurse must take into account in-flight and ground times when calculating the amount of IV fluids, medications, medical supplies, and oxygen that will be needed and when checking to ensure that medical equipment is fully charged.

FEDERAL AVIATION REGULATIONS

Air medical services must actively participate in the daily aviation operations dictated by the Federal Aviation Administration (FAA) to provide safety for all patients and care providers in the air transport environment. The fixed-wing air taxi certificate holder must comply with the appropriate Federal Aviation Regulations (FARs). These regulations pertain to air traffic control, airports, visual and instrument flight rules, and aircraft operations.[11] The majority of air medical services must comply with the appropriate FARs, depending on who possesses the air taxi certificate.

FAR Part 91 pertains to general operating and flight rules for aircraft flying in U.S. air space. FAR Part 135 provides specific rules for air taxi operators and commercial operators. Most air medical services are regulated under Part 135 of the FARs because of the nature of transporting "passengers" or "persons" for compensation or hire.[11] Currently, more than half of the fixed-wing transport programs in operation possess their own FAR Part 135 certificate.[17] A brief explanation of weather minimums, weight and balance, the term *lifeguard,* and ambient temperatures as they relate to FARs will give the flight nurse an understanding of how he or she can assist the pilot in complying with FARs and ultimately with safety.

Weather Minimums–Visual/Instrument Flight Rules

The FARs define explicit weather minimums and rules that must be in effect for an aircraft to operate within consistent safety standards. Under FAR Part 135, air medical services operate under either Visual Flight Rules (VFRs) or Instrument Flight Rules (IFRs).[36] The pilot of a fixed-wing aircraft must comply with the appropriate rules that define flying limitations in adverse weather conditions.

VFRs govern the procedures for conducting flight under visual conditions as interpreted by the pilot. Flight visibility is defined by the distance forward into the visible horizon, and the ceiling (vertical boundary) is the height above the ground or water to the base of the lowest (broken) layer of clouds.[36] FAR Part 91.155 addresses the basic VFR weather minimums that are maintained for the corresponding altitude and class airspace for all aircraft.[11]

IFRs govern the procedures for conducting instrument flight when weather conditions do not meet the minimum requirements for flight under VFRs.[36] IFRs indicate that the pilot intends to navigate by instrumentation for at least a portion of the flight. Most programs that operate with fixed-wing aircraft have the capability to operate under IFRs. However, IFRs pose other limitations, such as the need to land at approved airports when using instrument approaches; complying with restrictions for takeoff, approach, and landing minimums; and having plans in place in case of the need to use approved alternate airports.

Weight and Balance

It is important to meet weight and balance requirements for rotor-wing and fixed-wing aircraft as specified in the Airplane or Rotorcraft Flight Manual. The manual contains aircraft performance data regarding maximum certified gross weights, center of gravity limits, and runway lengths that fixed-wing aircraft will use for takeoff. Because fixed-wing airplanes (depending on the model) have less weight restrictions and more cabin space than rotor-wing aircraft,[40] family members and other persons frequently accompany patients on fixed-wing aircraft transports.

According to FAR Part 91.605, the pilot must ensure that the aircraft is loaded within weight and balance limits at all times.[11] Because the gross weight of the aircraft is predetermined by the Airplane Flight Manual, the pilot is responsible for determining the daily operational weight, which includes the weight of the aircraft, fuel, pilot(s), air medical personnel, and equipment. These calculations must be completed before taking off on a medical transport. Therefore, when in contact with the referring facility, air medical personnel should attempt to obtain the weights of patients and persons who will ride along. The pilot(s) can benefit from early notification of a patient's weight, especially for the patient who weighs more than 300 pounds. The pilot has final authority for weight limitations and may decide that family members or other persons may not accompany the patient. In addition, the pilot may decide to decrease fuel loads, rearrange the seating of passengers, unload unnecessary equipment, leave behind unnecessary passengers and air medical personnel, or depart from an airport with a longer runway.

A second important weight and balance requirement is that aircraft be loaded within the center of gravity range or limitations.[11] Once the maximum weight has been determined, the weight distribution, or where the weight is placed in an aircraft, is critical for aerodynamic performance and safety while the aircraft is in flight.[36] The weight must be properly loaded fore and aft of the center of gravity, according to the manufacturer's Airplane Flight Manual.

Lifeguard Status

Air ambulance services may declare *lifeguard* status for priority flights in the Air Traffic Control system. Lifeguard affords the airplane priority when taking off or landing and should be used with extreme discretion. It is only "intended for those missions of an urgent medical nature" (i.e., when a patient is deteriorating or is in full arrest) when a patient is on board or for the "portion of the flight requiring expeditious handling."[45] Lifeguard status is filed with a flight service station. Although landing and departing time differences are minimal at small airports, lifeguard status often achieves a tremendous time advantage at metropolitan and international airports. An air medical aircraft that is on lifeguard status may be allowed to take off or land ahead of multiple commercial and private aircraft, but this causes delays for these aircraft or extends their holding pattern time, costing thousands of dollars. Therefore, an air medical service must reserve lifeguard status for those times when it is absolutely necessary.

Ambient Temperatures

Several aircraft temperature considerations should be addressed before a flight commences, because temperature can present potential problems in the air medical environment. The first consideration is the amount of time the aircraft will spend on the ground, because air conditioning or heating cannot be left on for more than a few minutes during this time unless an auxiliary power unit is used. Unfortunately, auxiliary power units are usually not available at smaller airports, where most fixed-wing transports originate.

A second temperature consideration is evident at higher altitudes, at which the ambient temperature decreases. As the altitude increases, temperature decreases to the tropopause, which is the location at which the temperature reaches its lowest point and remains constant. The fuselage circumference of most air medical aircraft tends to be relatively small, and insulation of the walls is such that the walls and floor will feel cool.[39] The cumulative effect of all of these factors is often a cooler environment in a fixed-wing aircraft.

A third temperature consideration is encountered when descending into tropical or humid climates. On descent, windows will become fogged and other types of condensation will occur inside the aircraft.

PREPARING FOR PATIENT TRANSPORT

Transferring/Accepting Physician and Facility

The flight nurse must ensure that an appropriate referral is arranged for the fixed-wing transport. Because additional time is usually available to preplan for an interfacility fixed-wing transport, the names of both the referring and accepting physician should be documented for the transfer.

In 1985, Congress enacted the Consolidated Omnibus Budget Reconciliation Act (COBRA), which was amended in July and November 1990. COBRA protects indigent, uninsured patients from being denied access to emergency care by hospitals or from being transferred inappropriately between hospitals on the basis of the patient's inability to pay.[42] This legislation requires that the referring hospital assume liability for the adequacy of stabilization before transport. COBRA also requires documentation before the transfer that the receiving hospital has been verified and that a receiving physician is willing to accept the patient. If a transfer is required for a patient who is not yet stabilized, COBRA states that various conditions are to be met, including the following[42]: "(1) The physician certifies in writing that, in his/her professional opinion, the benefits of the transfer outweigh the risks; (2) the transferring hospital treats the patient within its capacity, which minimizes the risks to the patient; (3) the receiving facility agrees to accept the patient and has available space and qualified personnel to provide appropriate medical treatment; (4) the transferring hospital sends to the receiving facility all medical records (copies) available at the time of transfer; and (5) the transfer is effected through qualified personnel and transportation equipment."

Fixed-wing flight nurses must often validate transfer information from the communications center. It is important that this information be validated because these patients are transferred from towns, cities, and states where air medical personnel are not necessarily familiar with the hospitals and physicians involved in the transfer.

Oxygen Requirements

Determination of in-flight and ground ambulance times from the referring to the receiving facility assists the flight nurse in calculating the amount of oxygen that will be required to meet the needs of the patient. The flight nurse must ensure sufficient oxygen to deliver 1.0 FiO_2 or to operate a ventilator, if needed, for 1 to 1.3 times the entire length of the patient transport.[8] In some patient transports more time is spent on the ground than in flight. Time spent on the ground may be 90 minutes or longer. Therefore, all fixed-wing aircraft should carry a portable back-up oxygen tank in case the main system fails or the ground ambulance has no oxygen available. Some foreign countries do not carry oxygen in their ambulances.

Patient Medical Equipment Requirements

Air medical services are improving fixed-wing aircraft standards by providing dedicated aircraft with custom medical configurations, which allows services to permanently secure ventilators, heart monitors, and other patient medical equipment. Equipment that is required may be based on the mission and the scope of care provided by the air medical service. For example, a service whose mission is critical care for children and adults should have appropriate transport equipment readily available. This may include a heart and hemodynamic monitor, a noninvasive blood pressure (BP) monitor, a pulse generator, IV pumps, a pulse oximeter, an on-board suction device, a transport ventilator, an isolette, and a transport intraaortic balloon pump.

Medical equipment that requires battery power should also have auxiliary power capabilities that can use the aircraft's invertor. The flight nurse should always ensure that the invertor power source on the aircraft and ground ambulance work properly in case batteries should fail. Because many ground ambulances outside the United States do not have invertors, the flight nurse should have spare batteries available.

For example, a critically ill patient in severe cardiogenic shock with severely depressed left ventricular function can be successfully transported by fixed-wing aircraft. Wedige-Stecher[46] reviewed a case report of a patient who required not only intraaortic balloon pump therapy but a left ventricular assist device to take over the left ventricular workload. The patient was transported with all these devices, which gave him his only chance of survival until he was able to receive a heart transplant at a tertiary center. The patient was discharged from the hospital 1 month after the flight. The team coordinator ensured that the proper equipment for the transfer, including the IV pumps and the intraaortic balloon pump, was available and fully charged and that extra batteries were available.

A portable suction unit should also be included in the standard equipment for fixed-wing transports. This unit provides the nurse with back-up equipment should the main suction system fail in the fixed-wing aircraft. The portable suction unit is also valuable during transport once the patient is removed from the aircraft at isolated or foreign airports.

Finally, transport services must comply with their state licensure requirements for air medical aircraft, which include specifications about medical equipment that must be placed on the aircraft. Because these requirements vary from state to state, some aircraft may be required to carry additional equipment according to state regulations.

Patient Care Supplies and Medications

The aircraft must be stocked with adequate medical supplies and medications to provide the nursing care required by the patient. In addition to the required air ambulance equipment, extra supplies may be tailored for the anticipated needs of the patient. For example, if a patient requires breathing treatments while in flight, additional nebulizer setups and extra or multi-vial doses of the medication may be stocked. Also, because an intubated patient may require frequent suctioning, additional saline bullets and sterile suction catheters should be stocked on the aircraft.

Bedding and Linens

Because fixed-wing flights involve longer periods of patient care, comfort becomes a major issue. The traditional fixed-wing aircraft stretcher pads are hard, thin, narrow, and have limited flexibility. The flight nurse can plan ahead and attempt to use bedding, egg crates, or blankets on top of the stretcher to provide extra padding and create a softer surface. If an air mattress is to be used, air must be able to be released to prevent the mattress from rupturing in flight as a result of gas expansion at higher altitudes.

In addition, the flight nurse may stock extra pillows for use in supporting the head, neck, back, and knees, positioning between knees and elbows, and elevating extremities and feet. On longer flights, the nurse must pay greater attention to the patient's position. Patients, especially those who are comatose or paralyzed, may need to be turned to prevent skin breakdowns. The patient may be placed on a "turn" or "draw sheet" so air medical personnel can reposition the patient more easily in flight.

Nutrition and Fluid Requirements

Adequate nutrition and fluids should be provided for all persons on board the aircraft. Depending on the transport time and the time of day, food may be catered for the patient, family, pilots, and air medical personnel. The nurse must choose the proper food or provide a specialized diet (e.g., a low fat or diabetic diet) required by the patient. Proper storage of the food and fluids is necessary. In addition, there should be an adequate stock of fluids, such as juice, and plenty of water for the entire length of the transport. Because of the longer in-flight times, higher altitudes, and stresses of flight, the nurse should provide sources for replenishing energy and preventing dehydration for all persons on board the aircraft. Emphasis should be placed on taking care of oneself in addition to the patient and other passengers during the transport.

Disposing of Contaminated Wastes

All air medical personnel must comply with Occupational Safety and Health Administration (OSHA) regulations regarding occupational exposure to bloodborne and airborne pathogens.[44] The air medical service must have an exposure control plan. Policies, procedures, and equipment must be provided in the plan to comply with these regulations and protect employees from infectious diseases. Infectious diseases and OSHA regulations are discussed in detail in Chapter 25.

Air medical personnel must follow infection control policies by observing universal precautions and stocking extra personal protective equipment, supplies, and cleaning agents for these long flights. Depending on the flight distance and in-flight patient care times, the flight nurse must plan for containing and disposing of contaminated needles, dressings, empty IV fluid bags, and human wastes according to OSHA regulations. A Foley catheter makes it easy to dispose of urine. The nurse must also plan for providing care and properly disposing of wastes should the patient have a bowel movement. Multiple large red isolation bags may be used to dispose of wipes, bedpans, and urinals.

Air medical personnel, pilots, and family members should plan to use restroom facilities before departure and during fuel stops. Although some fixed-wing aircraft have a toilet on board, most do not.

Required Ground Ambulance Capabilities

For fixed-wing transports, the flight nurse can never assume that a particular ground ambulance unit will be available. The nurse must investigate the capabilities and resources of the ambulance that arrives at the airport. If the patient requires various medical equipment, invertor power should be available on the ambulance to power the equipment. The flight nurse should also assess the resources of the ambulance service to determine if it can provide the appropriate basic life support or advanced life support services. In some countries no resources may be available in the ambulance, in which case *all* medical equipment, medications, and oxygen required for the patient must be provided by the flight team.

PATIENT "PACKAGING" FOR TRANSPORT

Preparation

Preparation of a patient for a fixed-wing transport usually requires a thorough assessment, stabilization, and preparation process because of lengthy patient care times. In rare cases the nurse may swoop and scoop the patient, primarily as a result of the patient's condition or when the patient is brought to the transport team at an airport. Most of the time, the flight nurse will provide a rapid assessment at the referring facility and initiate patient care. A preflight plan helps minimize the amount of time spent on the ground before departure.

Loading Considerations

After ground transport to the aircraft, the air medical personnel must plan for transferring the patient into the aircraft and securing the medical equipment. Because most aircraft doors are relatively narrow, the team must make the "patient package" as slender as possible.[38] Once on the aircraft, equipment must be secured according to FAA regulations and placed in a position that will permit continuous assessments while allowing the tubes and catheters to remain patent and accessible.

Numerous companies provide equipment for loading a patient into fixed-wing aircraft. Because there has been an increase in fixed-wing transports, these companies have developed and marketed stands, lifts, slides, and sleds to assist with loading and unloading patients through narrow fixed-wing aircraft doors. These loading devices have significantly eased the loading procedure, but more importantly, they assist with preventing work-related injuries for the pilot and air medical personnel.

Immobilization Equipment

Immobilization devices present unique challenges for loading a patient through a fixed-wing aircraft door and positioning the patient in the aircraft. Standard backboards are too wide to be used for loading patients into many aircraft. For this reason, tapered backboards are suggested. The flight nurse must also prepare for patients who have other immobilization devices, such as a traction splint, in place. Loading the patient on the aircraft may be difficult because of the length of the splint. In addition, positioning the patient can present challenges.

Bulky dressings, splints, and the need to maintain a position of comfort for an injured extremity may make it difficult to transfer the patient smoothly through the aircraft door. In addition, the patient will need to be positioned in the aircraft so the extremity can be supported, while maintaining optimal positioning and allowing access for nursing care.

IN-FLIGHT FACTORS INFLUENCING PATIENT CARE

Limited Space

The fixed-wing aircraft flight nurse must consider several issues that may not be factors in rotor-wing aircraft transport. Space may vary greatly from one aircraft to another. Propellor and turbopropellor aircraft tend to be more spacious than the jet models, which can be extremely important when patients require large advanced life-support equipment or immobilization devices or when family members desire to accompany the patient.

Air Conditioner and Heater

In-flight climate control systems may not meet most caregivers' expectations. The thin walls and floor of the fuselage do not allow much space for thermal insulation. Therefore, the air conditioning may not adequately cool the airplane to the desired temperature on extremely hot summer days, and in the winter, some aircraft cabins may still feel cool when heaters are performing at maximum capacity.

Diversions

Because fixed-wing transport times are often longer than for other types of patient transport, the potential for diversion of the flight is increased. Diversion can be prompted by mechanical problems, weather, or even a significant deterioration in the patient's status.

AIR MEDICAL PERSONNEL RESOURCES

One of the most critical factors for fixed-wing transports is the flight nurse's knowledge of available resources and how these resources can be accessed. The flight nurse must be familiar with medical control policies and procedures. Medical control may be extremely helpful to the nurse involved with political situations, a patient whose condition is deteriorating, cardiac arrests that occur during the flight, interstate transports, and flights outside of the United States. The flight nurse must ensure that the air medical service has policies and procedures in place and must know how to contact his or her medical control to deal with these situations. In addition, the flight nurse must be able to use the resources of the communications center to contact the program director, clinical supervisor, or medical director as needed to assist with patient decisions and coordination of the patient transfer in emergency situations.

Medical Control

Most air medical services receive medical control services from the medical director and the designated medical control physicians. As discussed earlier in this chapter, most fixed-wing aircraft flights are interfacility transports. Therefore, a physician referral has been made to transfer the patient to an accepting physician and facility. Before departing from the referring facility, a nurse may initiate patching to a medical control physician by telephone to discuss a patient's medical condition and request further orders as needed. Once the nurse is in the ground ambulance or in flight, the opportunities for medical patching may be limited for some air medical services.

Radio Communications and Flite Phone

Flight nurses should be familiar with all of the capabilities and aircraft communications of the communications center. The flight nurse should also become familiar with the various nonaviation radio frequencies for contacting the communications center and ground EMS agencies. In addition, air medical services should be encouraged to provide flite phones on the aircraft to initiate medical patching during the flight if the patient's condition deteriorates. It is legal to use flite phones during flight, whereas it is illegal to use cellular phones when airborne. Flite phones are licensed and regulated by the Federal Communications Commission. When a flite phone is available the flight nurse can contact medical control during in-flight medical emergencies.

IN-FLIGHT CODES

A flight nurse faces unique challenges and must use decision-making skills when a patient goes into cardiopulmonary arrest during a fixed-wing aircraft transport. The air medical personnel should be apprised of the patient's current code status. In addition, before transport, the patient and family members accompanying the patient should be made aware of the risks of air medical transport and the potential for diversions should the patient's condition deteriorate.

The flight nurse must address four essential issues if a patient has a full cardiopulmonary arrest during the fixed-wing aircraft transport. The flight nurse must consider the following: (1) the service's policies and procedures for in-flight codes; (2) the decision to return, divert, or continue to proceed to the destination; (3) availability of resuscitation equipment and medications; and (4) endurance of the air medical personnel. After all of these issues have been weighed and deliberated, the flight nurse shall make the final decision in conjunction with medical control.

First, air medical personnel need to be well versed on the air medical service's policies and procedures for full codes on a fixed-wing aircraft transport. Every state has specific laws dealing with terminating resuscitation efforts in the prehospital arena. The program should have policies and procedures in place that relate to patients in full cardiopulmonary arrest and the actions that are required by air medical personnel in consultation with the service's medical control.

In addition, legal aspects of interstate transport may complicate the decision to terminate resuscitation en route or before reaching the destination. Therefore, some air medical services have a policy that a patient cannot be pronounced dead until the aircraft has landed, especially if the transport takes place outside the United States.[25,26]

Second, if the patient deteriorates into a full code during any portion of the transport, the air medical personnel must weigh distance and time factors to decide literally in which direction to transport. This decision may be based on the distance and time it would take to return to the referring facility or to the closest appropriate facility, on the availability of ground ambulances, and on overall patient status. The question for the air medical personnel will be whether to divert the aircraft or continue to the final destination after weighing all these factors.

The third essential issue relates to the service's available resuscitation equipment and medications. This may include oxygen, endotracheal tubes, advanced cardiac life-support medications, fluids, and the battery power on life-support equipment. Given the limited supplies available on fixed-wing aircraft, the flight nurse may be required to make a decision based on the air medical team exhausting all of the resuscitation equipment.

Finally, the endurance of the air medical personnel on the transport should be considered, especially for transports that also require ground times in excess of 90 minutes. The air medical personnel may be required to contact medical control and recommend ceasing resuscitation efforts if the patient does not respond to medical therapy on an extremely long flight.

"Do Not Resuscitate" Orders

Fixed-wing aircraft transport services may provide "Do Not Resuscitate" (DNR) transports at the family's request and not because of medical necessity. These flights are prescheduled with an air medical service, but again, the flight nurse should be familiar with DNR policies and procedures. Because various states have different definitions for DNR patients, services that conduct these types of flights should provide policies and procedures for air medical personnel.

SAFETY AND EMERGENCY PROCEDURES

Safety is the number one priority for the flight nurse. In the fixed-wing aircraft transport environment, a flight nurse should receive initial and annual ongoing education regarding fixed-wing aircraft operations, regulations, and unscheduled aircraft emergencies. According to FAR 91.505 and 135.331, all flight crew should receive emergency training for each aircraft type and model.[11] Because air medical personnel are considered passengers and not "flight crew," an air medical service may not provide all the crew member emergency training requirements. All air medical personnel should receive safety education in potential in-flight emergencies and procedures appropriate for each kind and model of aircraft flown. This will allow the air medical personnel to understand and assist the pilot with various procedures. According to Wright et al,[47] education regarding in-flight emergencies increases the confidence of air medical personnel and pilots and affects their ability to deal effectively with these emergencies before and after the emergency. At a minimum, education should be provided for dealing with the following emergencies: (1) fire during the flight, (2) electrical failure; (3) hydraulic failure; (4) slow or rapid decompression; (5) water ditching, if flying over water; (6) rapid egress procedures; and (7) survival procedures and available equipment. For further review of emergency procedures and survival, see Chapter 6.

INTERNATIONAL TRANSPORT ISSUES

Air Medical Service International Transports

The discussion of air medical transport no longer focuses only on domestic transports. International transports continue to increase for patients who require medical transport from one country to another. Although similarities exist between domestic and international air medical transports, there are many unique differences. This section will focus on some of the issues and obstacles that may be encountered with international transports, such as preflight preparation and logistics, documentation, language barriers, patient locations, ground ambulance times and resources, pilot and air medical personnel duty times, and medical equipment and supplies.[25,26,31]

Preflight Preparation and Logistics

Preflight preparation becomes extremely critical for international air medical transports. As with fixed-wing transports, extensive plans for the logistics must be completed by the entire team with the realization that the flights will often be much longer than other air medical transports. Additional preflight plans must include Customs, Immigrations, international weather briefings, landing permits, refueling stops, ground handling, oxygen requirements, catering arrangements, medical equipment needs, and rest requirements.[31] Inadequate preparations or failure to notify the appropriate authorities will only frustrate the air medical team and create enormous delays. In addition, meticulous attention should be given to obtaining as much accurate patient information as possible to prepare for the medical needs of the patient.[25,26,31] Because international transports of critically ill and injured patients cannot be accomplished by commercial airliners, some air medical services conduct routine international transports. These programs have dedicated jets that are medically configured. To prepare for the worst-case scenario, these aircraft have redundant medical equipment and systems. These jets also offer lavatory facilities and auxiliary power units for maintaining a comfortable cabin environment and charging medical equipment during ground times of the transport.[25] Numerous aviation companies are able to assist an air medical service in preparing for an international transport.

Documentation

Air medical personnel and pilots should always have the appropriate documentation for customs and immigration requirements on their person. This documentation may include passports, driver's licenses, voter registrations, visas, and immunization records.[25,31] International guideline charts are available to explain requirements for different countries.[31] When planning for the flight, the appropriate documentation must also be verified for the patient and any passengers. Frequently the pilot(s) will organize this information when filing the flight plan and making arrangements with customs.

Language Barriers

When attempting to obtain an accurate patient diagnosis and discover the patient's medical condition and care needs, air medical personnel may deal with language barriers from the referring facility, physician(s), and family members that may require the use of a translator. Many long-distance telephone companies now offer translators fluent in multiple languages.[31] In addition, insurance companies that coordinate these international flights have resources available for translating patient information.

It is imperative that the medical director or clinical supervisor and the flight nurse involved with the flight use the necessary resources to obtain patient information that is as accurate as possible, even if this delays the transport.[31] This will ensure that the skills of the air medical personnel and the available medical equipment are appropriate for the anticipated medical needs of the patient. In some cases, when transporting an American citizen back to the United States, the flight nurse may be able to obtain medical information by speaking directly with the patient or family members.

The air medical personnel must also plan for language barriers when arriving at the patient location and during the flight. It may be necessary to request an interpreter at the referring hospital or clinic to translate the medical terms, current treatment, and patient care needs.[31] In addition, the air medical personnel on the flight will benefit from learning specific medical terms and words related to caring for the patient during the flight; for example, terms related to current chest pain status and restroom needs.

Patient Location

International air medical transports may involve patients who are located not only in hospitals but also in clinics, private homes, trailers, hotels, physician's offices, cruise ships or docks, and other locations that may never before have been encountered. It may not be possible to predict how stable the patient will be on one's arrival; therefore, the flight nurse must prepare for the worst-case scenario. Patients arriving at the airport by taxi may have had minimal care. The air medical personnel, being the only provider of advanced life support, will have to initiate medical care.

Ground Transport Times

Preflight planning must include an accurate calculation of the distance and ground times between the patient's location and the airport. Information such as traffic and road conditions may also be sought.[25,26] This information is extremely important for calculating oxygen requirements for ventilatory patients, battery life of equipment, and necessary supplies for the patient during transport.

Ground Ambulance Resources

Whether the patient is transported to the airport or the team is transported to the patient, the resources of the ground unit may be very limited. The ambulance vehicle may be a private car, a taxi cab, a suburban vehicle, a Volkswagen camper, a pickup truck with a camper shell, or an ambulance unit.[26] Some ambulances may be stripped to an empty unit with no oxygen source or suction equipment. Others may be elaborately stocked with supplies and medical equipment. In addition, the skills of the ambulance personnel accompanying the team and patient may vary widely, from a driver with no medical knowledge to emergency medical personnel, nurses, or physicians with varying degrees of skills.

Finally, one must consider the safety issues of the ground transport to and from the airplane. Road conditions, driving skills and compliance with traffic laws, and the inability to secure equipment are a few of the concerns that may be faced during the ground transport. All of these issues contribute additional stresses to international patient transports.

Pilot and Air Medical Personnel Duty Times

Duty and rest times must be considered for each international transport for the pilot(s) and air medical personnel. This is already addressed for the pilot(s) because they must comply with FAR Part 135.267 flight time limitations and rest requirements.[11] Therefore, during the preflight preparation, rest requirements must be calculated into the plan and arrangements made for relief pilots to assume flight duties at appropriate fuel stops or at the destination.

When making preflight preparations, air medical personnel should determine the length of the flight and patient care times and use judgment in scheduling adequate team breaks. Rest for the air medical personnel may be accomplished during the flight with "members of the team sleeping in a rotation where the transport nurse or physician is always awake with the patient."[8] For extremely long transports, the air medical service may send a relief team of air medical personnel to a scheduled fuel stop to assume patient care.

Medical Equipment and Supplies

Just as with preflight preparations for any fixed-wing aircraft transport, it is imperative that the flight nurse ensures that plans are complete for international transports. The flight nurse must be meticulous in planning and arranging for adequate oxygen, medical equipment, batteries, supplies, bedding and linens, nutrition and fluids, and disposal of contaminated wastes. It is important to remember that there is a greater potential for unexpected delays for these transports because of customs coordination, ambulance delays, and refuelling stops. In addition, international transports may be of longer duration than other transports and to destinations with no stock of medical supplies or supplies incompatible with the air medical personnel's equipment. Therefore, the air medical personnel should stock enough medical supplies and medications for twice the predicted time of transport.[31]

Finally, the compatibility of medical equipment with foreign electrical current may need to be considered. The team may need to obtain several types of foreign adapters to convert the current so that monitors and suction units can be properly charged.

ESCORT/MEDICAL ASSIST TRANSPORTS ON COMMERCIAL AIRLINERS

Issues regarding international transport when an air medical service uses a dedicated aircraft have been reviewed. One more form of patient transport, called an *escort flight* or *medical assist transport,* should be discussed. Escorts may be either domestic or international transports. These flights may involve transporting a patient at the basic life support level who requires medical assistance, or a critically ill or injured patient or one who requires advanced life support or extensive nursing care.[31]

With regard to preflight preparation and logistics for this type of transport, the flight nurse should ensure that all arrangements are complete and plan to address several unique obstacles. These issues include not only commercial air carrier regulations, documentation, airline oxygen requirements, oxygen adapters, and electrical power, but also privacy and nonstop flights. Because transporting a patient on a commercial airliner requires coordination that is not under the control of the air medical service, these arrangements may take several days to an entire week to complete.

Commercial Air Carrier Regulations

Regulations for transporting a patient on an airliner vary, depending on the patient's designated level and condition. Many commercial air carriers will allow a stable patient who requires limited nursing care to sit in the first or business class section for transport.[31] On the other hand, transferring a critically ill patient may require the purchase of multiple seats (6 to 12) in the business class section or in the rear coach compartment of the airplane so the litter can be secured. Many airliners have a dedicated patient litter that rests above the folded passenger seats and is bolted to the seat tracks. Special arrangements should be made with each commercial airliner, because each carrier has a different patient litter, loading and securing procedures, and quantity of medical oxygen available. The flight nurse should plan for the logistics of these escorts to ensure that the transport is completed smoothly.

In addition, provisions must be made for transporting medical equipment and supplies in such a way that they are readily available for the patient and yet secured according to the FARs. The equipment also should be organized in such a manner that it can be easily transferred and checked by customs and immigration authorities.

Documentation

The air medical personnel must organize all of the paperwork necessary for the entire transport, including the airline tickets, passports, itinerary, and customs documents. This documentation for the air medical personnel, patient, and family members must be readily available for customs and immigration authorities. Air medical personnel should always keep this paperwork on their person.

Airline Oxygen Requirements

Each air carrier has a different procedure for obtaining oxygen and securing the O_2 tanks. The oxygen tanks routinely provided by most airliners deliver only 2 to 4 L per minute. Therefore, arrangements must be made to have extra oxygen tanks available for patients who require 100% O_2 or a ventilator. A minimum of 24 hours notice is necessary, but it may frequently take several days to make such arrangements.[31] Several airliners do not have the capacity to carry and secure larger oxygen tanks.

Oxygen Adapters

Particular attention should be given to the oxygen adapters and regulators available on each airliner. Most of this equipment is not compatible with air medical transport ventilator fittings. In addition, oxygen flow meters are often irregular. For instance, in some airliners, the O_2 outlet has three prongs.

Electrical Power and Adapters

The commercial air carrier's electrical power sources must be assessed and coordinated to power the medical equipment. A power source may be needed for transport ventilators, heart monitors, intravenous pumps, and suction equipment. As previously mentioned, the appropriate adapters must be obtained to convert the current in these foreign airplanes.

Privacy

Most commercial airliners have various rules pertaining to patients in critical condition. Their presence may offend or upset other paying passengers. Some airlines provide privacy for the patient by installing temporary curtains, but most of the time they are inadequate. Therefore, it may be necessary to bring additional sheets and clothes pins to provide adequate privacy for the patient.

Nonstop Flight

Every attempt should be made to make reservations on a nonstop flight for the patient transport.[31] This eliminates the frustrations of making additional arrangements to get on and off of the airplane, to transfer the patient, and to provide documentation for customs and immigrations officials. In addition, plans must be made to organize all of the medical equipment, patient and family belongings, and luggage of air medical personnel for each transfer.

SUMMARY

Flight nursing is a unique nursing specialty that requires a confident and assertive practitioner who can operate in many uncontrolled environments. Because there is a greater emphasis on the use of advanced technology and skills in flight nursing than in other types of nursing, flight nurses are expected to possess an exceptional level of knowledge and expertise in caring for critically ill and injured patients. The air medical profession continues to evolve into a sophisticated business. Therefore, flight nurses must maintain nursing standards for flight nursing practice.

Although many general principles of practice and patient care principles are identical in the rotor-wing aircraft and fixed-wing aircraft transport environment, differences also exist. First, one must focus on learning safety and emergency procedures to be used in the fixed-wing aircraft. Second, because air medical transport on fixed-wing aircraft requires longer patient care times than other types of transport, the flight nurse must be meticulous in preplanning for the entire flight, coordinating resources, and providing care for all persons on board. As managed care systems and cost containment enter the health care business, the number of air medical fixed-wing aircraft transports will continue to increase. Therefore, flight nurses may expect to expand their practice in the fixed-wing aircraft environment.

REFERENCES

1. American College of Emergency Physicians: Principles of appropriate transfer, *Ann Emerg Med* 3:337, 1990.
2. American College of Surgeons Committee on Trauma: Interhospital transfer. In *Resources for optimal care of the injured patient,* Chicago, 1993, American College of Surgeons Committee on Trauma.
3. Aoki B, McClosky K: *Evaluation, stabilization, and transport of the critically ill child,* St Louis, 1992, Mosby.

4. Barson W , Jastremski M, Syverud S: *Emergency drug therapy,* Philadelphia, 1991, WB Saunders.
5. Benevilli W , Thomas S, Brown D, Wedel S: Safety of fentanyl during transport of trauma patients, *Air Med J* 14(3):156, 1995.
6. Bennet-Jacobs B, Baker P: *Trauma nursing core course,* Park Ridge, Ill, 1995, Emergency Nurses Association.
7. Benson J: *FDA safety alert: potential hazards with restraint devices,* Rockville, Md, 1992, Food and Drug Administration.
8. Brink LW et al: Air transport, transport medicine, *Pediatr Clin North Am* 40(2):452, 1993.
9. Burney R et al: Evaluation of hospital based aeromedical programs using therapeutic intervention scoring, *Aviat Space Environ Med* 6:563, 1990.
10. Campbell J: *Basic trauma life support,* Englewood Cliffs, NJ, 1995, Brady Book.
11. Federal Aviation Administration: Code of Federal Regulations: Title 14, Aeronautics and space, Parts 91 and 135, 1996, US Department of Transportation.
12. Cohn H: Legal issues. In Neff J, Kidd P, editors: *Trauma nursing: the art and science,* St Louis, 1993, Mosby.
13. Continenza K, Hill J: Transport of the critical child. In Blumer J, editor: *Pediatric intensive care,* St Louis, 1990, Mosby.
14. Crippen D: Critical care transportation medicine: new concepts in pretransport stabilization of the critically ill patient, *Am J Emerg Med* 11:551, 1990.
15. DeJarnett R, editor: *Flight nurse advanced trauma course,* Park Ridge, Ill, 1994, National Flight Nurses Association.
16. Dickinson E, Krett R, O'Connor R: The impact of prehospital instant photography of motor crashes on physician perception and patient management in the emergency department, *Prehosp Disaster Med* 7(suppl 1), 1992.
17. Directory of Air Medical Services, *Air Med J* 12(5), 1995.
18. Emerman C, Shade B, Kubincanek J: Comparative performance of the Best trauma triage rule, *Am J Emerg Med* 10(4):294, 1992.
19. Flight Safety International Inc: *Lear Jet 20 Series, pilot training manual,* 1986.
20. Gabram S, Piancentini L, Jacobs L: The risk of aeromedical transport for the cardiac patient, *Emerg Care Q* 2:72, 1990.
21. Haley C, Baker P: *Emergency nursing pediatric course,* Park Ridge, Ill, 1993, Emergency Nurses Association.
22. Hart M: Patient assessment, preparation and care. In US Department of Transportation: *Air medical crew national standard curriculum,* 1988, US Department of Transportation.
23. Hart M et al: Air transport of the pediatric trauma patient, *Emerg Care Q* 3:21, 1986.
24. Henry M, Stapleton E: *EMT prehospital care,* Philadelphia, 1992, WB Saunders.
25. Holdefer WF, Diethelm AG, Tolbert FT: International air medical transport, part I: methods and logistics, *J Air Med Transport* 9(7):6, 1990.
26. Holdefer WF et al: International air medical transport, part II: results and discussion, *J Air Med Transport* 9(8):8, 1990.
27. Kidd P: Assessment of the trauma patient. In Neff J, Kidd P, editors: *Trauma nursing: the art and science,* St Louis, 1993, Mosby.
28. Kitt S et al: *Emergency nursing,* Philadelphia, 1995, WB Saunders.
29. Lee G: *Quick emergency care reference,* St Louis, 1992, Mosby.
30. McCloskey J, Bulechek G: *Nursing interventions classification,* St Louis, 1996, Mosby.
31. McCloskey K, Orr R, editors: *Textbook of pediatric transport medicine,* St Louis, 1995, Mosby.
32. Mirski M et al: Sedation for the critically ill neurologic patient, *Crit Care Med* 23(12):2038, 1995.
33. National Association of Emergency Medical Services Physicians: Air medical dispatch: guidelines for scene response, *Prehosp Disaster Med* 7:75, 1992.
34. National Flight Nurses Association: *Practice standards for flight nursing,* St Louis, 1995, Mosby.
35. Neff JA, Kidd PS, editors: *Trauma nursing: the art and science,* St Louis, 1993, Mosby.
36. US Department of Transportation: *Pilot's handbook of aeronautical knowledge,* Washington DC, 1984, US DTR.
37. Association of Air Medical Services: *Recommended minimum quality standards for rotor-wing and fixed-wing standards,* Pasadena, Calif, 1992, The Association.
38. Schneider C et al: Evaluation of ground ambulance, rotor-wing and fixed-wing aircraft services, *Crit Care Clin* 8(3):543, 1992.
39. Sheehy SB, editor: *Emergency nursing: principles and practice,* ed 3, St Louis, 1992, Mosby.
40. Sheehy SB, Jimmerson CL: *Manual of clinical trauma care, the first hour,* ed 2, St Louis, 1994, Mosby.
41. Stewart R: Analgesia in the field, *Prehosp Disaster Med* 4(1): 31, 1989.
42. United States Code: Consolidation Omnibus Budget Reconciliation Act (COBRA) of 1985 (42USC139dd), as amended by the Omnibus Budget Reconciliation Acts (OBRA) of 1987, 1989, and 1990.
43. US Department of Health and Human Services: Acute pain management: operative or medical procedures, Washington DC, 1992, USDHHS.

44. US Department of Labor, Occupational Safety and Health Administration: Occupational exposure to bloodborne pathogens, 29 CFR part 1910.1030, Washington DC, 1991, OSHA.
45. US Department of Transportation Regulations: *Code of federal regulations and aeronautical information manual,* Newcastle, Wash, 1996, Aviation Supplies and Academics.
46. Wedige-Stecher T: Fixed-wing transport of a patient requiring IABP and left ventricular assist device, *J Air Med Transport* 9(2):6, 1990.
47. Wright A et al: The effect of an in-flight emergency training program on crew confidence, *Air Med J* 13(4): 127, 1994.
48. Zecca A et al: Endotracheal tube stabilization in the air medical setting, *J Air Med Transport* 3:7, 1991.

CHAPTER 8

Airway and Ventilation Management

COMPETENCIES

1. Identify the indications for airway management.
2. Perform an airway and ventilation assessment.
3. Identify the indications and contraindications for specific airway interventions including orotracheal and nasotracheal intubation, surgical cricothyrotomy, and jet ventilation.
4. Describe the functioning of selected ventilators used during transport.
5. Describe the use of neuromuscular blockade for airway management in the critically ill or injured patient.

Airway management is the first priority of patient care and often accounts for the most difficult clinical dilemmas encountered by flight nurses and other emergency personnel. The most common error in airway management is failure to anticipate the need for active intervention in patients at high risk for airway obstruction or respiratory insufficiency.[73] Patients with decreased levels of consciousness, cardiorespiratory disease, head and neck injuries, and major traumatic injuries require quick, decisive airway management, based on a sound knowledge of physiologic and anatomic principles, to stem further progression of a life-threatening condition.

Many skills and equipment are required for control of the airway, but none is more important than the clinical judgment required to recognize that interventions are indicated. In addition to judgment skills, the competent flight nurse must also possess the technical skill to perform an intervention when it is indicated. Judgment skills are developed through experience and practice. Technical performance also can be improved through advanced instruction and practice. Flight nurses must be familiar with alternative options and their risks versus benefits when deciding on a particular airway management technique.

Because of space limitations in most aircraft, securement of an airway during flight can be difficult. Failure of emergency personnel to properly secure the airway before flight can lead to further respiratory decompensation, which can hasten systemic failure and produce a disorderly transport or a situation in which safety may be compromised. Safety must never become a secondary consideration to the flight crew. Therefore it is essential that the airway be fully controlled before air medical transport, even at the expense of additional time at the scene or referring institution.

This chapter describes assessment parameters, interventions, and methods of evaluation for airway control. Therapies to restore breathing and circulation are discussed in later chapters.

PATHOPHYSIOLOGY

Jorden[30] stated "There are six general indications for securing an airway: (1) apnea, (2) upper airway obstruction, (3) airway protection, (4) elevated intracranial pressure requiring hyperventilation, (5) respiratory insufficiency, and (6) impending or potential airway compromise (prophylactic intubation)." Apnea can be the result of cardiac or traumatic arrest and is easily recognized and quickly treated. Upper airway obstruction in the trauma patient is usually caused by the tongue or teeth or by blood. In the nontrauma patient the upper airway may be obstructed by excessive secretions or an edematous epiglottis. Airway protection must be considered for the patient with actual or potential emesis and active bleeding.

A closed head injury produces increased intracranial pressure (ICP) as a result of cerebral edema. Hypoxia and hypercapnia cause cerebral blood vessels to dilate, increasing blood flow and volume, which further escalate the ICP. The resulting brain swelling compromises oxygen and glucose delivery to neurons. Intubation and hyperventilation produce vasoconstriction of cerebral arteries, which prevents further tissue damage. Hyperventilation is the most rapid method of ICP decrease. Elevated ICP tends to develop in pediatric patients with closed head injuries earlier and more frequently than in adults. Therefore intubation and hyperventilation are imperative for the pediatric patient with neurotrauma.

Respiratory insufficiency may be traumatic or nontraumatic in origin and involves disease of the lower airways, where actual gas exchange takes place. Traumatic respiratory insufficiency may result, for example, from a flail segment or pulmonary contusion. Nontraumatic conditions that cause respiratory distress include pulmonary emboli, congestive heart failure, adult respiratory distress syndrome, and status asthmaticus.

Impending or potential airway compromise may be the most difficult situation for the flight nurse to judge. Consideration must be given to the history of illness or injury, therapies used to treat the patient before the flight nurse's arrival, the patient's response to the therapies, and flight time to the receiving agency. A situation in which a patient has sustained burn trauma with an inhalation injury and circumferential burns of the neck and chest should leave the flight nurse with little doubt as to the need for airway control. However, flight nurses frequently find themselves in situations in which the potential for airway compromise is not as obvious. Under these circumstances the flight nurse must rely on subjective and objective assessment parameters and past experience to guide his or her judgment.

ASSESSMENT

Assessment of the airway is a two-part process. The primary survey is quick and crude; the secondary survey is slower and refined. The primary survey begins by assessment of airway patency. If a flight nurse discovers a problem, the assessment stops, and he or she takes immediate actions to establish airway patency. During the secondary survey the flight nurse must determine whether airway patency and an appropriate level of oxygenation can be maintained throughout transport. If in doubt, the flight nurse must initiate appropriate interventions.

Initially, the flight nurse assesses the patient by looking, listening, and feeling for spontaneous respirations. The mouth is opened and observed for obvious injuries and the presence of blood, teeth, the tongue, or foreign bodies obstructing the upper airway. The patient's level of consciousness, if altered, may indicate hypoxia. The patient in the compensatory stage of shock may also have an increase in the rate, rhythm, and depth of respiration, as well as pale, moist skin and tachypnea and tachycardia caused by a stimulation of the sympathetic nervous system. Pallor, rather than cyanosis, is an indicator of shock for both adult and pediatric patients because sympathetic nerve stimulation causes blood to shunt from minor to major organs; the skin is considered a minor organ. Major organs are the heart and brain, and the body will strive to maintain their oxygenation. The patient's general appearance may also provide assessment data. The use of accessory muscles, nasal flaring, and the position the patient assumes should all be noted. The hypoxic patient may attempt to sit upright and may appear anxious and apprehensive and subjectively report shortness of breath.

The neck should be observed for obvious injuries that may produce an expanding hematoma or edema. The position of the trachea and presence of jugular vein distention should also be noted.

The purpose of auscultation is to identify the presence of absent, decreased, or adventitious breath sounds. Absent or decreased breath sounds may be present with a pneumothorax or hemothorax. Adventitious breath sounds will be auscultated if lower airway obstruction is present.

The chest wall should be palpated for tenderness, crepitus, subcutaneous air, and symmetry of movement. Percussion is not a practical tool in the field at a noisy scene. However, in a quiet environment percussion, like palpation, can provide excellent information about the status of the underlying thoracic structures. The normal lung sound is resonant, a hemothorax is dull, and a tension pneumothorax is hyperresonant.

The history of mechanism of injury or progression of illness may also provide subjective and objective data for the flight nurse to use when determining a course of action.

Pediatric patients should be assessed in the same manner as adults. However, children do not have the chronic diseases of adulthood and therefore compensate more efficiently. To the untrained or nonsuspecting eye, the child who appears in mild respiratory distress may be severely ill. Normal pediatric vital signs are demonstrated in Table 8-1. It is essential to recognize bradypnea and bradycardia because these are signs of respiratory failure. Primary cardiac arrest in children is rare. Cardiac arrest is usually caused by respiratory failure, and interventions to support respirations will also sustain the cardiac system. Therefore early and aggressive airway management for children is mandatory.

The child with respiratory insufficiency may demonstrate general signs and symptoms of fatigue, restlessness, irritability, and confusion and may cling to his or her parents in anxiety and apprehension. A weak cry is also typical. Observation may also reveal nasal flaring and substernal, supraclavicular, or intercostal retractions. Skin color is an excellent indicator of oxygenation in children; skin that is pale, with a capillary refill time of greater than 2 seconds, mottled, or cyanotic represents distress in the nontrauma patient. In the pediatric trauma patient cyanosis may not be seen as a result of hypovolemia. Cyanosis is the result of desaturated hemoglobin. Active bleeding will deplete the system of hemoglobin, and cyanosis will not be observed. A fever will be present in children with epiglottitis or pneumonia.

TABLE 8-1

Average vital signs by age

Age (yr)	Pulse range (beats/min)	Respiration range (breaths/min)	Blood pressure (systolic/diastolic in mm Hg)
Newborn	120-160	30-60	80/40
3	80-120	25-30	86/50
5	70-115	20-25	90/52
7	70-115	20-25	94/54
10	70-115	15-20	100/60
15	70-90	15-20	110/64

From Sheehy SB: *Emergency nursing: principles and practice,* St Louis, 1992, Mosby.

Auscultation may reveal expiratory grunting or wheezing and inspiratory stridor. Upper airway problems usually involve a barking cough or stridor whereas wheezing and grunting breath sounds are associated with lower airway disease or obstruction. Diminished breath sounds may be present even in the face of a nontraumatic event.

If arterial blood gas results are available, children should maintain a PaO_2 greater than 80 torr while breathing room air. With supplemental oxygen, a child with a normal cardiovascular system should demonstrate a PaO_2 of more than 100 torr.

Examination of the traumatized child will yield findings similar to those previously discussed. However, palpation, percussion, and a high index of suspicion are necessary for a thorough examination. The chest wall and mediastinal structures are more mobile in children than in adults. Children can withstand severe blunt chest trauma without sustaining rib fractures, but the heart and lungs may be severely contused. Likewise, the child with a tension pneumothorax may have a shift of the mediastinal structures much faster than an adult would. Interventions for the child with chest trauma are discussed later. It is crucial for the flight nurse to recognize that any sign or symptom of respiratory compromise warrants aggressive airway management in children.

INTERVENTION

In the patient with a history of trauma, all airway interventions must be accomplished, and cervical spine immobilization must be maintained. The airway should be opened, all blood or emesis suctioned, and foreign bodies removed. The tongue may be displaced from the oropharynx through placement of an airway adjunct or by use of a modified jaw thrust. If the patient's mandible is not intact, the tongue can be protracted directly by traction with a towel clip, suture, or clamp. An oropharyngeal airway, when properly positioned, rests in the lower posterior pharynx. For an adult it is inserted backward until it reaches the posterior wall of the pharynx and then is rotated into the proper position. This method of insertion is contraindicated for the pediatric patient because rotation of the rigid plastic device may cause dental or soft palate injuries. Instead, the oropharyngeal airway should be inserted with a tongue depressor.

With either method of insertion, proper position must be confirmed by assessment of airflow and efficacy of ventilation. An incorrectly placed oropharyngeal airway may worsen or create an airway obstruction where none existed by the tongue being pushed posteriorly against the pharyngeal wall or the epiglottis being pushed against the laryngeal opening. The use of an oropharyngeal airway may induce vomiting in a conscious patient; therefore, it should be used only in unconscious patients. Head tilt must be maintained despite the presence of an oropharyngeal airway.[56]

Nasopharyngeal airways may be used in patients with marginal stupor or coma who need assistance in maintaining an open airway. However, nasopharyngeal airways should be avoided for any patient with suspected head or facial trauma. Like that of the oral airway, the nasal airway's tip lies in the posterior pharynx behind the tongue. Selection of the appropriate size of nasal airway is important because traumatic insertion may cause severe epistaxis or adenoid bleeding, especially in children. Lubricant use will facilitate its insertion. The airway is inserted with the beveled edge along the nasal septum. When the left nostril is used, the nasopharyngeal airway must be inserted upside down to maintain the beveled edge against the septum and then rotated once the airway tip is in the posterior pharynx. If significant resistance is met, the other nostril should be tried. The appropriate size for both the oral and nasal airways is obtained by comparison of the length of the airway device to the distance from the nares or mouth to the angle of the mandible.

Ventilatory assistance must be initiated immediately for the apneic patient and for the patient with severe hypoventilation. In preparation for intubation respirations can be assisted by a pocket or bag valve–mask device. Supplemental oxygen can be delivered through either device. At a flow rate of 10 L/min, an FiO_2 of approximately 50% can be delivered through a pocket mask. The bag-valve mask with a reservoir can deliver an FiO_2 of 90% to 100% at flow rates of 10 to 15 L/min. All masks should be transparent so that emesis can be immediately identified, the airway promptly suctioned, and assisted ventilations resumed.

Esophageal, nasal, and oral intubations are noninvasive measures available to the flight nurse to gain control of the airway. Invasive measures include transtracheal ventilation and cricothyrotomy.

Esophageal Intubation

The technique of esophageal intubation began during the late 1960s and has been in use primarily in the prehospital setting since that time. Criticisms of the earlier esophageal obturator airways (EOAs) led to refinements in the esophageal airway that are frequently encountered by flight teams today in areas in which medical personnel are not trained in endotracheal intubation techniques or when attempts at endotracheal intubation are unsuccessful. Contraindications to the use of the esophageal airway follow: (1) age less than 16 years or height under 5 feet, (2) presence of a gag reflex, (3) conscious or semiconscious patient, (4) known or suspected esophageal disease or injury, and (5) known or suspected caustic ingestion. The presence of maxillofacial injuries is considered to be a relative contraindication to the use of esophageal airways.[27,45,55,59]

The original EOA developed in 1968 is a two-part device—a mask and tube. The tube is approximately 37 cm long, open at the top, and blind at the bottom. An inflatable cuff lies above the blind end. Several holes are near the top portion of the tube, and when the tube is inserted, these holes lie in the oropharynx. The tube attaches to the mask through an opening at the lower end of the mask. Steps for insertion of the EOA are described in the following box. A tightly sealed facemask and the cuffed end of the blunt tube theoretically prevent air from escaping through the mouth and into the stomach. If the chest does not rise, the tube should be removed immediately because it may have passed into the trachea. If placement is correct, air is forced into the tube from an external source and enters the trachea because the distal inflatable obturator cuff effectively seals off the esophagus. Achievement of a tight seal on the facemask and ventilation of the patient require two people. With removal of the EOA, vomiting will occur. Therefore, before the EOA is removed, the patient must be tracheally intubated for airway protection.

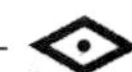

STEPS FOR INSERTION OF THE EOA

1. Position the patient. Nontrauma patient: flex head forward. Trauma patient: maintain in-line traction.
2. Preoxygenate with high-flow O_2.
3. Grasp the lower jaw and tongue with the thumb and index finger and pull forward.
4. Blindly insert the tube into the mouth. The tube will follow the natural curvature of the pharynx and pass into the esophagus.
5. Advance the tube until the mask forms a tight seal on the face.
6. Do not use force to pass the tube. If resistance is met, withdraw the tube slightly, improve the tongue/jaw lift, and readvance slowly.
7. Test for tube placement by auscultation of bilateral breath sounds and observation of symmetric chest wall movement.
8. Inflate the tube cuff with 30 ml of air.

A later modification of the EOA, the esophageal gastric tube airway (EGTA), is essentially an EOA with a lumen that allows passage of a 16-gauge gastric tube for removal of gastric contents and relief of gastric distention. However, the EGTA also requires two people for optimal ventilatory assistance. There are several disadvantages to the EOA and EGTA. First, the airway may be completely obstructed with both devices if the trachea is inadvertently intubated.[77] Second, during transport it is difficult for a tight facemask seal to be obtained and for adequate ventilation to be maintained, and esophageal and gastric ruptures have been reported.[8]

The pharyngeotracheal lumen airway (PTLA)[41] (Fig. 8-1) is a further modification of the esophageal airway device and was quickly followed by the Esophageal Tracheal Combitube[16,27] (Fig. 8-2). Both devices are double tubes inserted the same way as described for the EOA. The double-tube system allows for either tracheal or esophageal intubation without

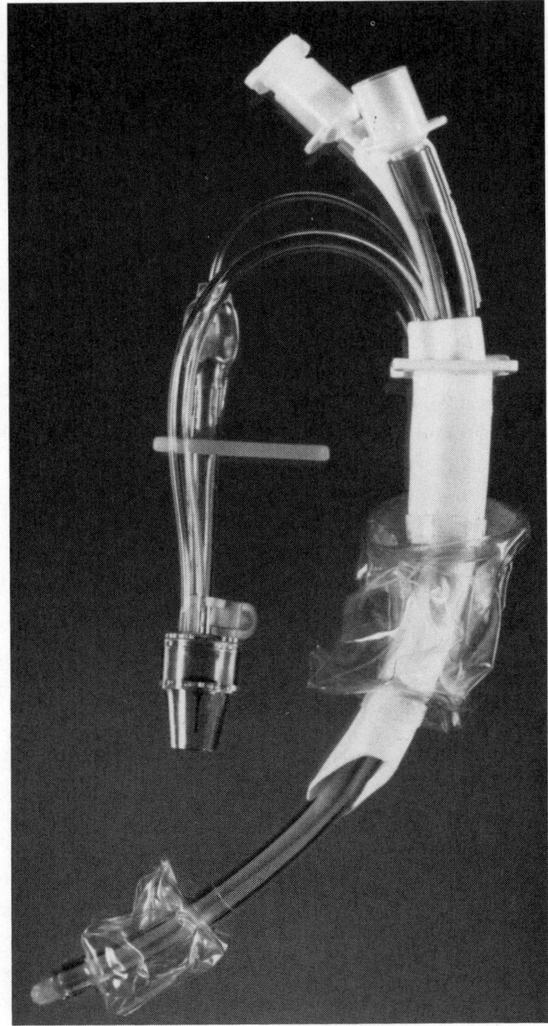

Fig. 8-1. Pharyngeotracheal Lumen Airway. (Courtesy Respironics, Inc, Monroeville, Pa.)

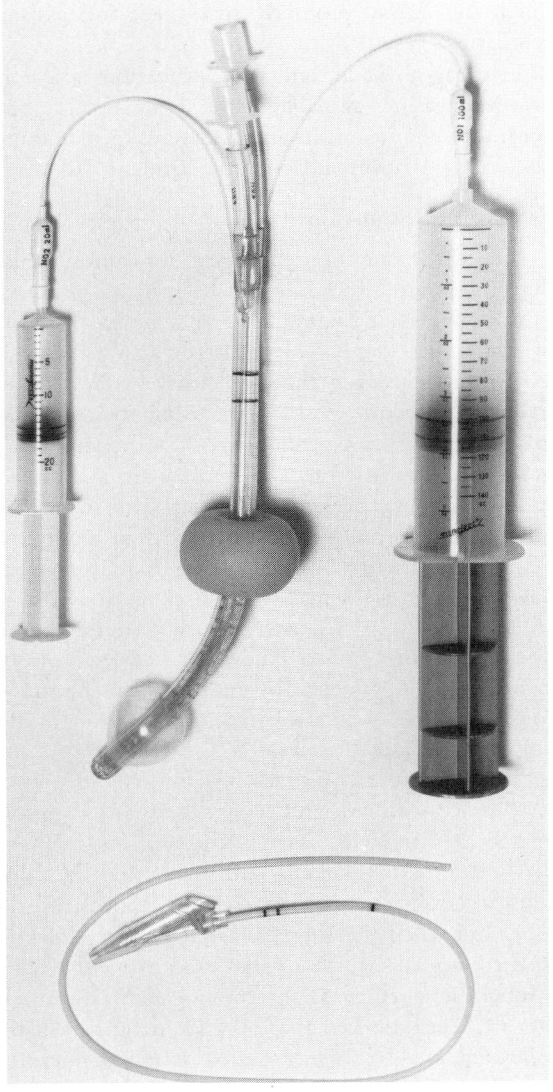

Fig. 8-2. Esophageal Tracheal Combitube. (Courtesy Sheridan Catheter Corp, Argyle, N.Y.)

ventilatory compromise. Both devices also incorporate double-balloon systems that serve as airway seals. The distal balloon, which holds 15 to 20 ml of air, seals the esophagus and prevents gastric regurgitation or, in the event of tracheal intubation, aspiration. The proximal balloon is inflated with 100 to 140 ml of air and is designed to be positioned between the base of the tongue and the soft palate so that the mouth and nasopharynx will be sealed off and the escape of air through the mouth will be prevented. The pharyngeal balloon may also tamponade oral bleeding and prevent aspiration of blood into the trachea. Both devices require only one person to manage them.[16,41] The PTLA is a definite improvement over the EOA or EGTA but still has some significant disadvantages. The oropharyngeal balloon does not prevent aspiration of teeth or other oral debris, and the oropharyngeal balloon can migrate out of the mouth anteriorly, partially dislodging the airway. Also, endotracheal intubation around the PTLA is difficult because of the residual air in the oral balloon.[3]

Neiman[41] compared blood gas measurements achieved between the PTLA and traditional endotracheal tube (ETT). Frass et al[16] conducted a similar comparison using the Esophageal Tracheal Combitube. Both devices demonstrated adequate oxygenation. However, endotracheal intubation offers several advantages over esophageal airway management techniques. Endotracheal intubation provides a route for administration of most resuscitative drugs and a route for tracheal suctioning. Direct laryngoscopy during intubation may allow visualization of foreign bodies in patients who aspirate them and allow for their removal before intubation.[3] Pons[45] described the many issues that have for years surrounded the use of esophageal intubation devices. He concluded his article by stating that "airway control in the emergency department means tracheal intubation, not esophageal; airway management in the field should mean the same."[45]

Tracheal Intubation

Intubation of the trachea involves the passage of an ETT through the nose (nasotracheal) or mouth (orotracheal) into the trachea. Tracheal intubation provides protection against aspiration, allows for controlled and precise ventilation, and is a method of drug administration. In addition, intubation protects the airway in situations of progressive airway closure caused by epiglottitis, inhalation burns, soft tissue trauma or infections, and other obstructive conditions. It is superior to esophageal intubation for airway management.[54]

Complications of oral and nasal endotracheal intubation can be both significant and disastrous (see box on p. 134. Unsuccessful intubation or a missed inadvertent esophageal intubation may lead to prolonged hypoxia resulting in long-term injury or death. If the patient cannot be intubated, other means of oxygenation and ventilation must be substituted. Pulse oximetry during intubation can help prevent oxygen desaturation during multiple intubation attempts and should always be available. Intubation predisposes the patient to a number of harmful physiologic responses, including laryngospasm, bronchospasm caused by airway irritability or aspirated secretions, hypertension, and dysrhythmias unrelated to hypoxia.[54,74] In addition, intubation may be the single most potent stimulus for ICP increase. An unrecognized right main stem bronchus intubation is a complication that may lead to inadequate ventilation and left lung atelectasis.

The ability to perform advanced airway maneuvers must begin with knowledge of normal anatomy. Knowledge of the anatomic structures is especially important when structures are only partially visible or are displaced as a result of injury. Familiarity with the anatomic differences between the adult and child is equally important.

The Larynx

Endotracheal intubation entails manipulation of the anatomy to allow passage of an ETT through the larynx either blindly or through direct visualization with a laryngoscope. An understanding of the relationship of the cartilages of the larynx and their relative positions will help the flight nurse to perform intubation faster and more confidently.

The larynx, or voice box, is an intricate arrangement of nine cartilages, three single and six paired, connected by membranes and ligaments and moved by nine muscles. From above it attaches to the hyoid bone and opens into the laryngopharynx, and on the inside it is continuous with the trachea. In an adult it extends from the level of the fourth to the sixth cervical vertebrae.

The three single cartilages form the basic boxlike structure of the larynx and provide the major external landmarks. The thyroid cartilage, commonly known as the Adam's apple, is formed by the fusion of two curving cartilage plates and is typically larger in men than in women because of the growth-stimulating influence of male sex hormones during puberty. The ring-shaped cricoid cartilage is sandwiched between the thyroid cartilage above and the first tracheal ring. Because the cricoid cartilage is a

COMPLICATIONS OF INTUBATION

Early Complications Occurring During the Intubation Procedure

1. Neck
   Cervical strain: subluxation/dislocation, fracture, neurologic injury
2. Mouth
   Soft tissue injury resulting in abrasion and hemorrhage involving lips, tongue, buccal mucosa, pharynx
   Temporomandibular joint subluxation/dislocation
   Dental injury
3. Airway/respiratory
   Arytenoid: dislocation, avulsion
   Vocal cord: spasm, avulsion, laceration
   Pyriform sinus perforation resulting in pneumothorax, pneumomediastinum
   Tracheal and bronchial rupture
   Right main stem bronchus intubation, with atelectasis and respiratory compromise
   Bronchospasm
4. Gastrointestinal
   Esophageal: intubation, perforation
   Vomiting and aspiration
5. Cardiovascular
   Hypertension, tachycardia, bradycardia, dysrhythmia
   Cardiac arrest, interruption of CPR

Late Complications Occurring After Tube is in Place

1. Airway/respiratory
   Tube obstruction: secretions, blood, kinking
   Accidental extubation, endobronchial intubation
   Vocal cords: ulceration
   Trachea: ulceration, ischemic necrosis
   Pneumothorax, pneumomediastinum
   Aspiration, atelectasis
   Cough resulting in increased intrathoracic, intracranial, intraocular pressures
2. Gastrointestinal
   Esophageal intubation
   Tracheoesophageal fistula
3. Cardiovascular
   Tracheoinnominate artery fistula
4. Infections
   Sinusitis, pneumonia, tracheobronchitis, mediastinitis, abscess

From Dauphinee K: Orotracheal intubation; nasotracheal intubation, *Emerg Med Clin North Am* 6(4):7110, 1988.

complete ring, the tracheal diameter does not narrow during cricoid pressure.[17] The cricoid cartilage is connected to the thyroid cartilage by the cricothyroid membrane and is the desired location for a cricothyrotomy.[37] The upper free edge of the cricothyroid membrane forms the vocal cords. Because of the attachment of the vocal cords to the cricoid ring, downward pressure on the cricoid ring helps to bring the vocal cords into view when they are hidden behind the tongue.[17] The third single cartilage is the epiglottis, a spoon-shaped structure that prevents anything other than air from entering the tracheal inlet. The epiglottis is a major visual landmark during intubation (Figs. 8-3 and 8-4).

The most important paired cartilages of the larynx are the arytenoids. The arytenoids are pyramid shaped and anchor the vocal cords in the larynx. The vocal cords look pearly white because of their avascular nature. At rest the vocal cords lie partially separated or abducted. Excessive secretions or aspiration stimulates the airway and activates the defense reflexes. Laryngospasm, or spasmodic closure of the vocal cords, is the most severe form of airway closure and can totally prevent ventilation and the passage of an ETT.[79] If a tube is forced through the cords with excessive pressure, an arytenoid can actually be dislocated and permanent hoarseness can result.[79] The remaining two pairs of cartilages, the cuneiform and corniculate, form the posterior wall of the larynx. Committing these structures to memory will assist the flight nurse in quickly identifying the glottic opening, and when the opening is obscured from view, the ETT can be steered into position with the structures in view as reference points.

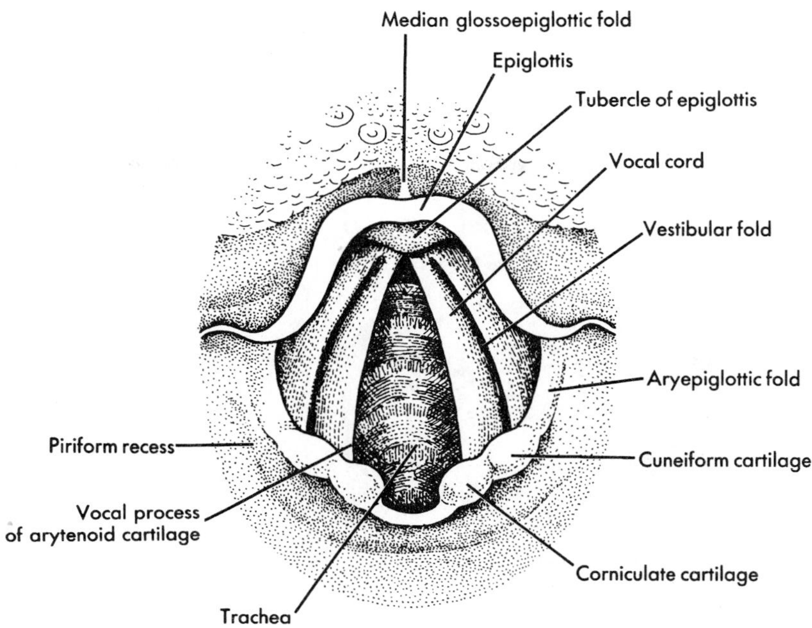

Fig. 8-3. Laryngoscopic view of the airway. (From Rosen P et al: *Emergency medicine: concepts and clinical practice,* vol 1, ed 3, St Louis, 1992, Mosby.)

Orotracheal Intubation

Orotracheal intubation is the most common method of airway management for all age groups. In children orotracheal intubation is used almost exclusively.[14] It is a safe procedure that involves psychomotor skills that are easily mastered. There are few, if any, true contraindications to orotracheal intubation in the emergency setting. However, during circumstances in which major facial and neck trauma prevents recognition of landmarks or during isolated mandibular trauma in which the temporomandibular joint may be immobile, the orotracheal route becomes much more difficult and may necessitate a surgical airway. Other conditions that might dictate a surgical airway include circumstances in which there is significant bleeding in the oral pharynx or supraglottic area and in patients with epiglottitis in whom landmarks are obscured or passage of a tube is impossible.[54] Again, these conditions are considered relative, not absolute, contraindications. Another relative contraindication for oral intubation is the patient with a suspected unstable cervical spine injury. Oral intubation may be acceptable if strict in-line cervical spine immobilization is maintained.[34,48] Trauma to the teeth, soft tissues of the mouth, posterior pharynx, or vocal cords caused by improper use of the laryngoscope blade are complications of oral intubation.

In the adult the narrowest portion of the airway is the glottic opening, the space between the true vocal cords. In children the narrowest portion is at the cricoid cartilage below the vocal cords. In the child it is possible for the flight nurse to see the tube pass through the vocal cords but to be unable to pass the tube through the cricoid ring. If this situation occurs, a smaller tube should be chosen; an ETT should never be forced down a child's airway.[47]

The choice of blade, straight or curved, is left to the personal preference of the intubator, although the straight blade is recommended in obese patients and in patients with a short, muscular necks. In these persons the airway is located more forward, and curved blades often do not provide an adequate view.[75] Patients with receding chins also tend to have an anterior larynx, which may make intubation more dif-

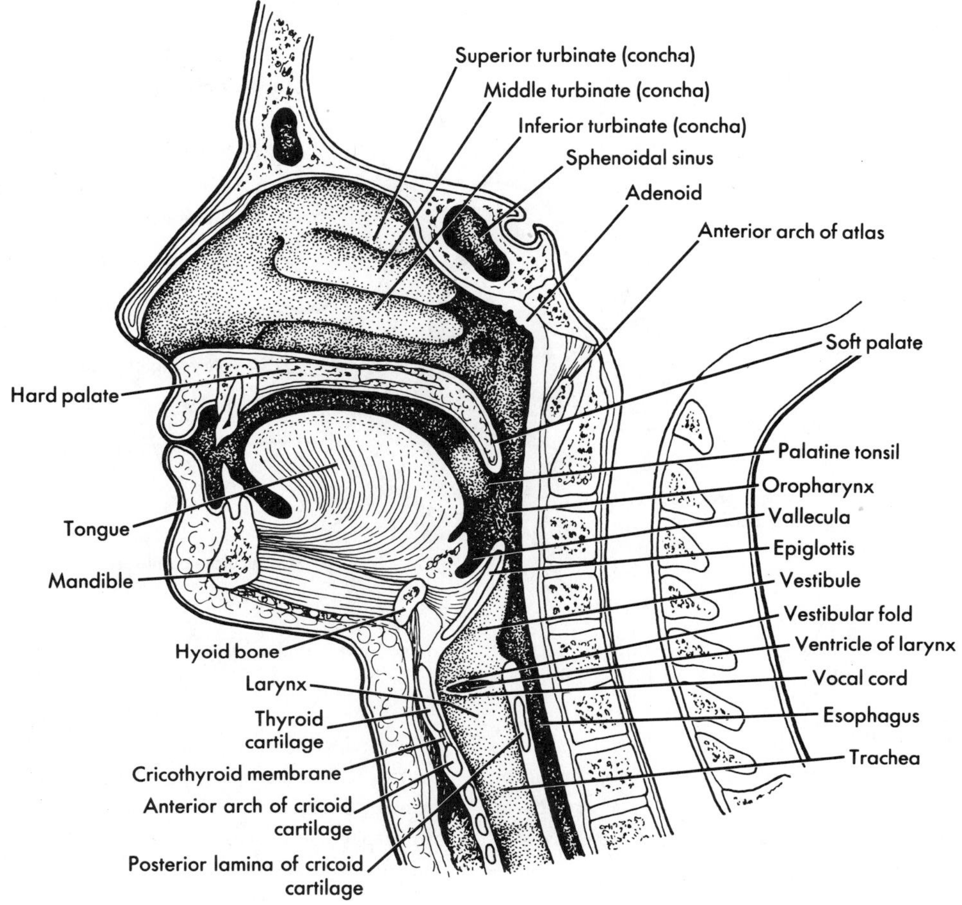

Fig. 8-4. Sagittal view of the airway. (From Rosen P et al: *Emergency medicine: concepts and clinical practice,* vol 1, ed 3, St Louis, 1992, Mosby.)

ficult with a curved blade.[76] The adult size blade is a no. 3 or 4. Steps for orotracheal intubation are included in the box on p. 137.

Selection of the appropriate size tube is an important consideration in patient intubation. In general, the largest tube possible should be selected. This will minimize airway resistance, assist in suctioning, and minimize the need for excessive inflation of the tube cuff, which can cause mucosal damage. The cuff pressure should be at minimal occluding volume. At pressures greater than 25 mm Hg, mucosal ischemia starts to occur. A persistent air leak in the balloon is often caused by a faulty valve at the pilot balloon. To correct this condition without reintubating, the flight nurse should attach a stopcock to the balloon, reinflate the balloon, and close the stopcock.[54] The average adult female airway can accommodate a 7- to 8-mm tube (the size refers to the inside diameter of the tube), and the average male airway, an 8- to 9-mm tube. The pilot balloon should be tested for leaks and lubricated before insertion.

Preoxygenation is an important step that is frequently terminated prematurely. The procedure requires a tight seal on the facemask and use of a bag-valve-mask device with reservoir to deliver the highest FiO_2 for 3 to 5 minutes. If done correctly, preoxygenation will supersaturate the patient and allow for as much as 5 to 8 minutes of apnea. Pulse oximetry should be available to aid in oxygen desaturation detection. If CPR is being performed, it should not be interrupted for more than 15 seconds for any single intubation attempt,[54] but frequently, unforeseen obstacles prolong the procedure. With proper preoxygenation, the flight nurse has more than adequate time for intubation to occur in a very deliberate, nonhurried, and controlled environment rather than in a state of panic.

The Sellick maneuver, digital pressure over the cricoid cartilage exerted posteriorly, can assist with intubation in two ways and is useful in both oral and nasal intubation. First, it improves visualization of the glottic opening by pressing the larynx downward and perhaps into the field of view. Cricoid pressure forces the cricoid ring against the vertebral column and effectively seals the esophagus, preventing the aspiration of passively regurgitated gastric contents or swallowed blood. In general, gastric emptying ceases when a person sustains significant trauma, and a patient is considered to have a full stomach if he or she has eaten within 6 hours of sustaining trauma or receiving anesthesia.[17] If the patient actively vomits, the assistant should immediately release the cricoid pressure and actively suction the patient's airway. Cricoid pressure may occasionally prevent the passage of a tube if the posterior pressure is too great or if the pressure is over the thyroid cartilage and not the cricoid ring. This is especially true in the pediatric patient because of the child's pliable airway structures. If difficulty is encountered, the assistant should release part or all of the pressure.

Insertion of the tube through the relaxed cords should continue until the cuff is just past the cords. To ensure the tip of the tube is above the carina, the tube is placed so that the teeth are approximately at the 21-cm mark on the tube for women and at the 23-cm mark for men.[59] With completion of the intubation, the laryngoscope is gently withdrawn, the cuff is inflated with 5 to 10 ml of air, and placement of the tube is confirmed. Tube placement confirmation begins with auscultation of breath sounds in

STEPS FOR OROTRACHEAL INTUBATION

1. Position the patient. Nontrauma patient: Flex the neck forward and extend the head backward, creating a "sniffing" position. Trauma patient: Maintain in-line traction.
2. Preoxygenate the patient.
3. Hold the laryngoscope in the left hand and open the patient's mouth with the right hand.
4. Insert the blade into the right side of the mouth, sweep the tongue to the left, and advance to the appropriate landmarks. The Miller (straight) blade tip goes beyond the epiglottis; the MacIntosh (curved) blade tip enters the vallecula.
5. Pull the laryngoscope blade at a 45-degree angle; avoid twisting the laryngoscope handle. Visualize the epiglottis and vocal cords. Apply cricoid pressure.
6. Insert the ETT from the right corner of the mouth and watch the tube pass through the vocal cords. Use the largest tube possible. Remove the stylet.
7. Inflate the tube cuff with 5 to 10 ml of air or to minimal occluding volume. (Minimal occluding volume is determined by placing the hand over the mouth and noting cessation of air leak with ventilation.) Capillary flow pressure in the tracheal mucosa is approximately 25 mm Hg, so cuff pressure should be less than that.
8. Confirm tube placement by auscultating bilateral breath sounds over the chest and axilla and by noting a lack of gurgling over the epigastrium. Observe for symmetry of chest wall motion. For a child observe the cardiac monitor for the maintenance of an appropriate pulse rate and improvement in the patient's color.
9. Secure the tube in place.

the right and left chest areas and over the stomach. A number of adjuncts are available to assist in confirmation of tube placement and are discussed later in this chapter.

Once intubated and oxygenated, previously hypoxic patients may have an increased level of consciousness and may become combative. In a patient's confusion his or her first priority is extubation. Soft restraints and a bite block may be in order. An oral airway may be used as a bite block to prevent the patient from biting down on the ETT. The bite block should be secured in place separately from the ETT. If the bite block and the ETT are secured together, the patient may inadvertently extubate himself or herself by lodging the tongue behind the oral airway and pushing it and the ETT out.

ADVANTAGES OF NASOTRACHEAL INTUBATION VERSUS THE OROTRACHEAL TECHNIQUE

1. Tube is more easily secured and hence is less likely to be dislodged.
2. More comfort during awake intubation and on the patient awakening.
3. Easier insertion in a patient with impaired neck or jaw motion.
4. No danger of the patient biting the tube.
5. Facilitates surgery to the oral cavity.
6. Favored in patients in whom laryngoscopy is difficult or contraindicated.
7. Useful in patients in whom neuromuscular blockade is hazardous.

From Dailey R et al, editors: *The airway: emergency management,* St Louis, 1992, Mosby.

Nasotracheal Intubation

Nasotracheal intubation is often referred to as a blind procedure because the larynx is not visualized as in the orotracheal method. For successful performance of the blind method of tracheal intubation, the patient must have spontaneous respirations, although the use of a lighted stylet in an apneic patient can facilitate the nasotracheal route. In addition to the patient having spontaneous respirations, the nasotracheal method also requires a relatively quiet environment, which could make it a difficult procedure at a noisy scene. In general, the nasotracheal technique requires more time than the orotracheal technique[44] but also offers many advantages over the orotracheal technique (box).

Nasotracheal intubation is a relatively easy procedure that is usually well tolerated by patients. The technique is especially useful in dyspneic patients because they have breath sounds that are easily heard and their glottis tends to remain open. For trauma patients the procedure can be performed with no movement of the cervical spine and can be performed on a patient who is sitting. Therefore the nasotracheal method can be a useful procedure in the trauma patient who needs airway management but who is still trapped upright within the vehicle. Also, the patient cannot bite the tube, and the tube is easily secured in place so mouth care is also easily provided. A disadvantage of blind nasal intubation is that upper airway bleeding induced by this technique can obscure visualization during subsequent attempts at direct laryngoscopy should the blind technique fail.

The only absolute contraindication to the standard blind nasotracheal technique of intubation is apnea or near apnea.[44] Other contraindications to nasotracheal intubation are considered relative, and they include (1) a suspected basilar skull fracture (may risk cranial intubation) or other closed head injury; (2) acute epiglottitis; (3) severe nasal or maxillofacial fractures; (4) upper airway foreign body, abscess, or tumor; and (5) anticoagulation therapy or other blood-clotting abnormalities causing epistaxis. There are disadvantages that are not contraindications to the procedure that should be noted. Nasotracheal intubation puts the patient at risk for the development of meningitis or encephalitis. Special consideration must also be given to the patient for whom bacteremia would be detrimental, such as the immunocompromised patient or the patient with a cardiac valve abnormality or prosthesis.

The most common complication of nasotracheal intubation is hemorrhage. Traumatic intubation may cause epistaxis through abrasion of the nasal mucosa or rupture of a nasal polyp. Bleeding can be minimized by use of a tube 1 mm smaller than would be used orally. Use of a vasoconstrictive agent to the nasal mucosa, such as topical phenylephrine, lubrication of the tube well, and avoidance of excessive pressure will also help prevent excessive bleeding. In the awake patient it is also advisable to provide nasopharyngeal anesthesia with lidocaine or Cetacaine, and aqueous lidocaine gel may be used to lubricate the tube.[44] In children the relatively large size of the tonsils and adenoidal tissue may produce severe bleeding if ruptured. Perforation and dissection of the posterior pharyngeal wall have also been reported.[9] Steps for nasotracheal intubation are included in the box.

The proper head position in the patient being nasotracheally intubated is the sniffing position with a bit less extension than when an oral intubation is performed. Extreme extension creates a more acute angle for the tube to pass through the larynx and makes the procedure more difficult. However, if cervical spine injury is suspected, the head and neck must be maintained in the neutral position. The beveled edge of the tube should be introduced against the nasal septum of the nostril chosen. The tube is advanced through the nose and into the pharynx with continuous forward pressure and gentle rotation. If the nasal passage appears to be obstructed, the other nostril may be used, or the tube may be substituted with a smaller one. The tube must never be forced. The intubator must listen and feel for air movement through the tube as the tube enters the pharynx and is advanced toward the glottis. Cricoid pressure may also be helpful. As the tube approaches the glottis, breath sounds will be heard maximally. On inspiration the tube is advanced through the cords. Tube position is then verified as described earlier.

Several devices are available to aid placement of the nasotracheal tube. The Endotrol tube is specifically designed for nasotracheal intubation and for use in patients with an anterior larynx. The Endotrol tube has a ring on the upper portion that directs the tip anteriorly when traction is applied to the ring. Should cord spasm develop, a topical anesthetic may be sprayed onto the cords through the tube. Another device used to aid placement of the nasotracheal tube is the airway whistle or BAAM (Beck Airway Airflow

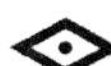

STEPS FOR NASOTRACHEAL INTUBATION

1. Assess nasal patency. Alternately occlude each naris, listen to air passage, and ask the patient or family members about past medical problems.
2. Anesthetize the nasal passage with lidocaine and a vasoconstrictor such as phenylephrine. Cetacaine to the posterior pharynx may also be used.
3. Position the patient. Nontrauma patient: may sit upright or assume a sniffing position with a bit less extension than for oral intubation. Trauma patient: maintain in-line traction.
4. Provide supplemental oxygen.
5. Lubricate the tube liberally.
6. Introduce the tube perpendicular to the floor for the supine patient or to the bed for the upright patient.
7. Point the bevel of the tube toward the nasal septum. (If the left naris is used, the tube is inserted backward.)
8. Gently pass the tube and listen to breath sounds through the end of the tube as it is advanced. Occlusion of the opposite naris may make the breath sounds louder.
9. Just proximal to the glottis, the breath sounds become maximal. Take care not to touch the cords prematurely so as not to induce laryngospasm and cough.
10. Quickly advance the tube on inspiration into the trachea. An assistant should apply the Sellick maneuver (cricoid pressure) to help align the glottic opening.
11. Confirm the tube position by auscultating breath sounds and observing symmetric chest wall motion and ensure that the patient is unable to speak.
12. Secure the tube in place.

STEPS FOR USING THE LIGHTED STYLET

1. Position the patient. Nontrauma patient: flex the neck forward and extend the head backward, creating the sniffing position. Trauma patient: maintain in-line traction.
2. Preoxygenate the patient.
3. The lighted stylet should be checked to ensure its light is bright enough by directly looking at the light. If the light is not uncomfortable to the eyes, it should be discarded and a new one used.
4. The lubricated stylet is inserted into a transparent ETT, and the light is positioned at the tip of the ETT, but not beyond.
5. The distal end of the ETT is then bent at a slightly greater than 90-degree angle.
6. The intubator kneels or stands on either side of the patient at the level of the shoulders, facing the patient.
7. For the oral technique lift the tongue or the tongue and jaw, pulling the epiglottis anteriorly and clearing the supraglottic area for introduction of the tube stylet. Slide the tube down along the tongue and lift the glottis in a "soup ladle" motion. For the nasal technique use the lighted stylet with a directional tip tube such as the Endotrol tube. The tube stylet is inserted with the beveled edge against the septum after applying a topical anesthetic and phenylephrine.
8. As the tube stylet is advanced, observe for the transilluminated glow in the midline. If the tip is off midline, a dim glow will be observed. If the glow is extremely dim or cannot be seen, the epiglottis has not been elevated and is probably covering the glottic opening. Correct by lifting forward on the jaw, tongue, or both.
9. When a bright midline glow is observed, the tube stylet is advanced until the glow is located at the sternal notch.
10. Carefully remove the stylet without dislodging the tube. Secure the tube.
11. Confirm proper tube placement in the usual manner.

Monitor). The whistle is attached to the standard 15-mm endotracheal connector and amplifies the patient's breathing as the tube is being advanced through the posterior nasopharynx. As the tube is advanced further, the sound increases in intensity. Deviation from the airflow tract will result in a decrease or loss of the whistle sound, indicating a need for tube redirection. Once intubation is complete, the airway whistle is removed. An air medical program evaluated the BAAM airway whistle and found that it was easy to use even in the noisy in-flight environment and had the added advantage of protecting the intubator against contact with blood, vomitus, and sputum during the intubation procedure.[32] A technique for using the BAAM airway whistle combined with the controllable-tip ETT during blind oral intubation and digital intubation has also been described.[7]

Lighted Stylet

An optional method of endotracheal intubation is the use of the lighted stylet. Referred to as the *transillumination method,* it uses a rigid wire stylet with a lightbulb at the distal end and is powered by a small battery source in the proximal end. The technique relies on the transillumination of the neck tissue to guide the placement of the ETT. The lighted stylet was originally designed to aid in the blind nasotracheal method of intubation; however, design modifications have now been made to allow use in both orotracheal or nasotracheal methods.[78] The brighter transilluminated glow from the trachea is easily distinguished from the dull or absent glow should the esophagus be intubated. Medical personnel can also use the lighted stylet to accurately position the ETT of an intubated patient by adjusting the stylet so that the transilluminated glow is at the level of the sternal notch. The tube is then slid to align proximally with a point that will also align the light with the distal tip of the ETT[61] (box).

Verdile[67] described the advantages of the transillumination method in prehospital care as follows: (1) rapidity of intubation, an average of 20 seconds; (2) ability to intubate without manipulation of the head and neck; and (3) low incidence of complications. Vollmer et al[69] published similar results.

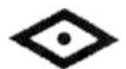

STEPS FOR DIGITAL ORAL INTUBATION

1. Position the patient. Nontrauma patient: flex the neck forward and extend the head backward, creating a sniffing position. Trauma patient: maintain in-line traction.
2. Preoxygenate the patient.
3. Select the appropriate size ETT in the usual manner. Insert an intubation stylet and bend the tube stylet in an open J configuration. Lubricate the tube.
4. Kneels or stand on either side of the patient at the level of the shoulders, facing the patient.
5. With gloved hands insert the fingers of the nondominant hand along the patient's tongue, pull the tongue forward, and "walk" the fingers down to palpate the epiglottis with the middle finger. If the epiglottis is not palpated, pull forward on the tongue.
6. The tube stylet is then slid along the left side of the mouth, with the medial aspect of the middle finger and the volar aspect of the index finger used to guide the tube tip in the direction of the epiglottis. Keep the index finger above the tube and the tube tip in contact with the middle finger.
7. Hold the tube against the epiglottis with the index finger and slip the tube distally toward the glottic opening.
8. As the tube enters the glottic opening, resistance will increase. At this point hold the tube firmly and withdraw the stylet slightly. Advance the tube through the cords and then completely remove the stylet.
9. Confirm proper tube placement in the usual manner.

Digital Intubation

Digital intubation, or tactile orotracheal intubation, was the original method of intubation beginning in the mid-1700s.[67] With the invention of the laryngoscope the technique became obsolete. Although not the method of choice, digital intubation can be helpful when other conventional methods have failed. The technique is useful in comatose patients with head and neck trauma, in obese patients or those with short, muscular necks, and in patients with severe bleeding or excessive secretions that prevent direct visualization by laryngoscopy. The digital technique may also be useful in cramped spaces, such as ground or air ambulances in which space is limited, or in situations in which equipment such as a laryngoscope or suction apparatus is lacking or has failed.[60]

Digital intubation requires that the patient be completely unconscious and that the mouth can be opened widely without fear of the patient biting. In an air medical program this technique has been used with remarkable success in children and neonates, despite their small mouth openings.[19] It relies on the ability of the intubator to guide the tip of the tube through the glottic opening using the middle and index fingers of the nondominant hand (box).

PEDIATRIC MANAGEMENT

Successful management of the pediatric airway begins with the knowledge that anatomic differences in children require adaptations to the techniques described earlier for proper care to be provided. Fortunately, the differences slowly diminish as a child ages. Not only does the clinician have to be familiar with anatomic differences but the child's fear or apprehension can complicate treatment efforts. Even the routine act of supplemental oxygenation with a nasal cannula or mask can become a challenge in an awake child because of the child's fear of having something in his or her nose or wrapped around his or her face. The child should be prepared by being talked to and comforted as much as possible. This step is important to the child and to the adult.

The indications for intubation are the same for the pediatric patient as for the adult. Complications are also similar in both populations. The most common complications of orotracheal intubation for all age groups include dental trauma and esophageal and right main stem bronchus intubations that go unrecognized. The most common cause of unsuccessful pediatric intubation is operator inexperience.[14] Although the complications appear to be many and severe, benefits of orotracheal intubation far outweigh the disadvantages. Orotracheal intubation is considered the gold standard of airway control and should be a skill mastered by all flight nurses.

There are anatomic differences in the upper and lower airways of the infant who is 1 year or younger, the child who is 1 to 8 years old, and the older child or adolescent who is 8 to 16 years old. As the child approaches 8 years of age, the larynx closely resembles that of the adult in structure and position. However, the overall size remains less than that of the adult. An infant's head is much larger in proportion to the rest of the body and results in a natural sniffing position. In infants and some young children the sniffing position is too pronounced, and the flight nurse may need to place a towel under the infant's shoulders to raise the rest of the body and straighten the airway, thereby improving airflow. The infant is also an obligate nose breather, and secretions or edema in this area can cause airway compromise. Infants and small children also have tongues that are large in relation to the size of their oropharynges, which makes the tongue, as it is in the adult, the most common cause of airway obstruction. The relatively small size of children's mouths also makes intubation more difficult. Because of the small size of the pediatric airway, minimal edema can create a life-threatening obstruction. An infant's airway, normally 4 mm in diameter, will decrease to 2 mm with 1 mm of circumferential edema caused by secretions or trauma caused by intubation. By comparison, the adult airway, normally 8 mm in diameter, will decrease to 6 mm with 1 mm of circumferential edema. The result is only a 25% decrease in diameter as compared with a 50% decrease in the infant with an equal amount of swelling.[79] The vocal cords of a young child are more pliable than those of the adult and are easier to damage, resulting in potential obstruction. Additionally, the larynx is more anterior in the young child, which leads to more frequent intubation of the esophagus.

Lungs can easily be overdistended and barotrauma induced by overzealous rescue attempts. Ventilation should be limited to the amount of air needed to cause the chest to rise. Excessive volumes exacerbate gastric distention and increase the risk of pneumothorax.[1] When possible, a self-inflating bag-valve ventilation system should be used, optimally with a pop-off valve. Resuscitation bags are available for neonates (delivering volumes of 500 to 600 ml) and adults (delivering volumes of 1.0 to 1.5 L). An oxygen reservoir should be used to enhance the oxygen concentration.[1] Initial respiratory rates used for controlled ventilation should approximate normal spontaneous respiratory rates based on age.[14]

The proper ETT size can be determined in several ways. It can be approximated by the size of the child's little finger or nares. A more precise method to ensure proper ETT size is as follows:

Newborn: Preterm = 3.0
Full-term = 3.5

$$\text{Then: } \frac{\text{Age (years)} + 16}{4} =$$

Internal diameter of ETT (mm)

ETT depth (cm) in orally intubated children (or adults), tube measured at lip line = Tube size × 3

Pediatric tubes are cuffless, which prevents subglottic stenosis and ulceration, and they range in size from 2.5 to 6.5 mm. Cuffless tubes are recommended in children younger than 8 years of age[14] because the cricoid cartilage is the narrowest portion of the trachea, and if the proper size tube is used, it serves as a physiologic cuff. A tube that is too large will not pass through the cricoid cartilage. A tube that is too small will not provide total airway protection.

The anatomic differences between the pediatric and adult airways are illustrated in Fig. 8-5. The anatomic differences can be summarized as follows[18]:

1. A child's larynx lies more cephalad than an adult's.
2. A child's epiglottis is at an angle of 45 degrees to the anterior pharyngeal wall, whereas an adult's lies parallel to the base of the tongue.
3. A child's epiglottis is large, stiff, and U-shaped, whereas an adult's is flattened and more flexible.
4. The infant's or child's larger tongue and the position of the hyoid bone depress the epiglottis.
5. The cricoid ring is the narrowest portion of the child's airway.

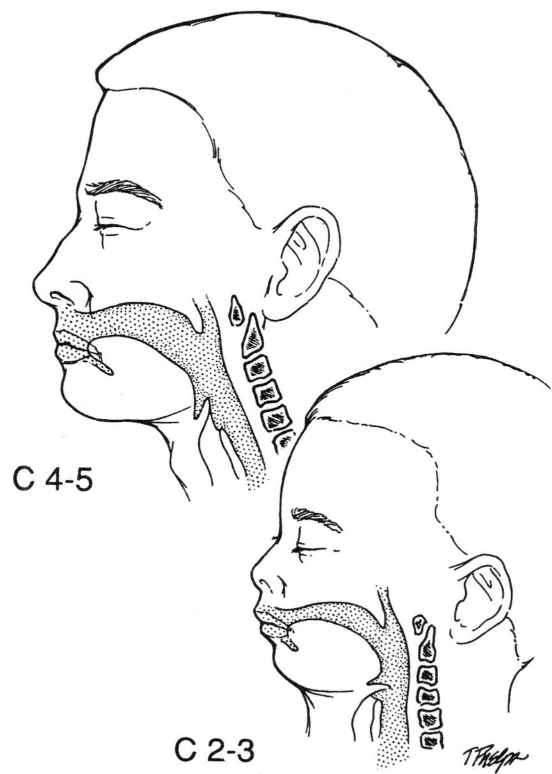

Fig. 8-5. Comparative anatomy of the adult and infant airways. (From Nichols DG et al, editors: *Golden hour—the handbook of advanced pediatric life support*, ed 2, St Louis, 1996, Mosby.)

The use of a Miller (straight) blade permits easier cord visualization. A straight blade is inserted beyond the epiglottis, which is lifted up along with the tongue and jaw. If the blade is inserted too far and landmarks are not easily recognized, the blade should be gently backed out, and the glottic opening will often "pop" into view. Inability to recognize the epiglottis increases the likelihood of tracheal intubation. Pediatric Miller blades range in size from 0 to 2. The 0 blade is used for the premature and small newborn, and the Miller 1 is used for the larger newborn to age 2 years. A Miller 2 or the MacIntosh 2 is used in children older than 2 years. For the child older than 12 years, the MacIntosh 3 is frequently used.[14]

During intubation, it is beneficial to assign an assistant the task of observing the cardiac monitor for heart rate. In young infants the cardiac output is very rate dependent, and bradycardia is universally associated with hypotension.[14] A heart rate of less than 100 beats/min in a neonate, less than 80 beats/min in an infant, and less than 60 beats/min in a child constitutes bradycardia. Should this be observed, the intubation attempt is aborted, and oxygenation by bag-valve mask is initiated. Atropine should be administered to all children and adolescents receiving succinylcholine to block vagal stimulation.

Tube placement is confirmed by auscultation with observation and palpation. Breath sounds are transmitted readily, although the child's thorax and abdomen make it hard to judge tube placement. Therefore along with auscultation the flight nurse should observe the symmetric rise and fall of the chest wall, monitor for maintenance of heart rate, and check the patient's color for improvement. The chest wall should also be palpated for symmetry of movement.

ETT depth is generally three times the inside diameter of the tube size. This rule of thumb applies to premature infants and to adults when the appropriate size tube for the patient's age is in place.[14] Once placed, the tube should be well secured with tape and tincture of benzoin. The use of tracheostomy tape should be avoided because it may kink the tube or reduce the tube's diameter if secured too tightly. Because the tube is cuffless and the child's trachea is so short, movement of the child's head may lead to a main stem intubation or to extubation. As with the adult, assessment of tube placement should occur after each patient transfer—for example, after the child is loaded into the aircraft before liftoff.

A part of airway management for children is the placement of a nasogastric tube. A child's stomach is relatively larger than an adult's and may contain food and a significant amount of air. Children tend to swallow air when crying (aerophagia). If full, the stomach may impinge on the diaphragm and decrease vital capacity. If a postintubation chest radiograph is available, the tip of the ETT should be at the T_2 to T_3 vertebral level or at the level of the lower edge of the medial aspect of the clavicle.[1]

INVASIVE AIRWAY MANAGEMENT

With competent airway management skills, rarely will the need to establish a surgical airway be encountered. However, the likelihood is good, particularly for flight nurses who frequently care for trauma victims, that at some time the skill will be needed. Because of the relatively infrequent opportunity to gain experience, there can be reluctance to attempt the procedure when the clinical situation clearly dictates the need. Reluctance to perform the procedure, and the delay that results, can add additional urgency to a situation that necessitates swift action. Flight nurses must be knowledgeable in the techniques of invasive airway management: needle cricothyrotomy and surgical cricothyrotomy.

Cricothyroidotomy is a procedure used to gain airway control that requires a surgical incision through the cricothyroid space. A needle cricothyrotomy (also called *transtracheal ventilation* and *percutaneous transtracheal ventilation*) is a method of airway control that uses a needle through the cricothyroid space and therefore requires less surgical skill than a cricothyroidotomy. Needle cricothyrotomy is generally accepted as the preferred surgical airway maneuver in children 8 years and older. Palpation and identification of landmarks of the neck may be difficult in children, and identification of the cricothyroid membrane may be especially difficult in infants. An additional complicating factor is that the laryngeal prominence does not develop until late childhood and adolescence.[33] However, Barkin and Rosen[1] have said that surgical cricothyrotomy can be performed in patients older than 3 years, and Walls[71] states that surgical cricothyrotomy is absolutely contraindicated in children 5 years old and relatively contraindicated for children younger than 10 years old, depending on the expertise of the health care provider. The procedure is a technically difficult one in children. The goal is to avoid damage to the cricoid cartilage, which in children is the only circumferential structure supporting the larynx and upper trachea (Fig. 8-6).

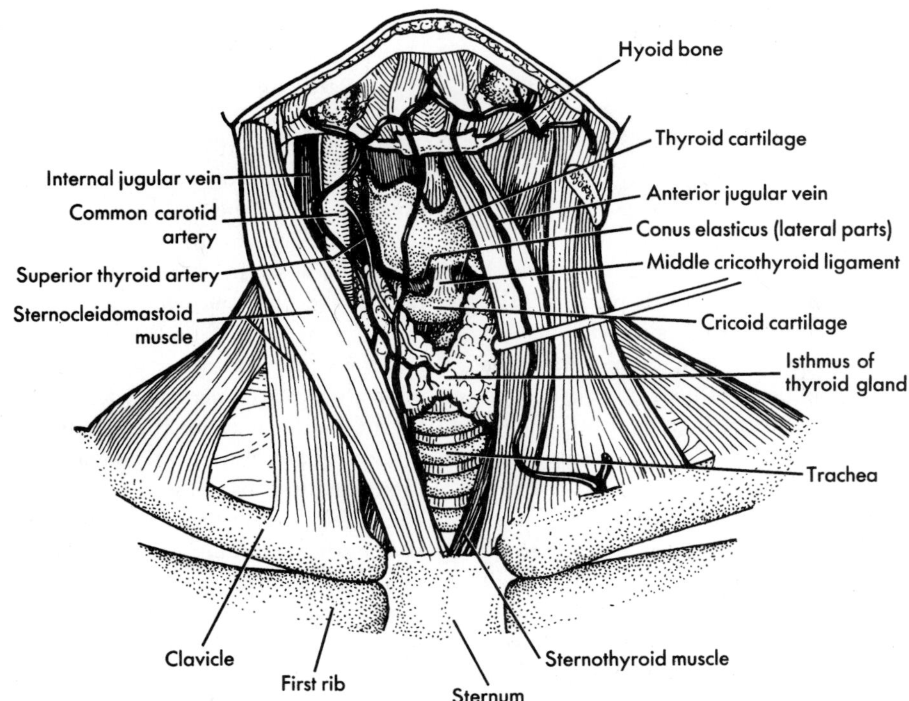

Fig. 8-6. Anterior aspect of the neck with relative anatomic structures. (From Rosen P et al: *Emergency medicine: concepts and clinical practice,* vol 1, ed 2, St Louis, 1988, Mosby.)

Indications for the establishment of a surgical airway include (1) the inability to gain airway access by other means and (2) complete upper airway obstruction. Airway inaccessibility during orotracheal or nasotracheal intubation may be the result of trauma, which can cause abnormal anatomy or profuse bleeding and thereby obscure visualization of the glottic opening. Upper airway obstruction may be the result of a foreign body, mass lesion, or edema. Edema can be caused by infection, caustic ingestion, allergic reaction, or an inhalation injury. Suspected cervical spine fracture is recognized increasingly less frequently as an indication for cricothyrotomy.[37] There are also a number of contraindications to surgical airway maneuver. However, these are considered relative contraindications and include (1) the inability to locate the correct landmarks for puncture, (2) gross infection over the puncture site, (3) primary laryngeal injury, and (4) patient younger than 3 to 5 years.

Needle Cricothyrotomy

Needle cricothyrotomy involves the insertion of an over-the-needle cannula through the cricothyroid membrane into the trachea. Steps for this procedure are included in the box above right. The use of a kink-resistant catheter, 14- or 16-gauge cannula, is recommended. The needle is removed, and the cannula is left in place. Commercially available cannulas are designed with side holes in addition to the distal port and incorporate a flange that aids securement of the catheter. The additional holes decrease pressure-related mucosal damage. The cannula must then be connected to an oxygen-delivery device capable of delivering short bursts of oxygen from a high-pressure source of 50 psi. This method of ventilation is known as *translaryngeal jet ventilation,* and it provides emergency oxygenation and ventilation.[62] The ventilatory rate should be from 12 to 20 breaths per minute with an insufflation time of about 1 to 2 seconds.

Frequently described is an alternative method to the use of the jet ventilator in which the connector from a no. 3 ETT is connected to the cannula, which is then connected to a resuscitation bag. This technique meets oxygen requirements. However, ventilation cannot be achieved, and respiratory acidosis quickly results.[62] The respiratory acidosis that results generally limits ventilation in this manner to approximately 30 minutes. The use of a resuscitation bag is at best a temporary measure, whereas jet ventilation is considered a true-positive pressure-ventilation technique. Another advantage of jet ventilation is that aspiration of airway secretions is prevented as the high airway pressures escape proximally through the open glottis. Normally, air flows passively from the lungs, up through the larynx, and out the mouth. With upper airway obstruction, normal airflow is not possible, and provision for exhalation must be made or barotrauma will occur. A Y connector can be placed onto the cannula after its insertion.

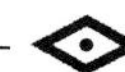

STEPS FOR NEEDLE CRICOTHYROTOMY

1. Stabilize the patient's head in a neutral position.
2. Identify the cricothyroid membrane and prepare the skin.
3. Stabilize the cricoid and thyroid cartilages with the nondominant hand.
4. Insert a 12- or 14-gauge over-the-needle intravenous catheter into the membrane at a 45-degree angle caudally (toward the feet). On passage into the trachea, the needle is removed, and the cannula is advanced caudally.
5. The hub of the needle is connected, preferably to a jet ventilator capable of delivering oxygen at a pressure of 50 psi. Otherwise, the connector is removed from a 3.0-mm ETT and attached to the intravenous catheter. It is then connected to a bag-valve mask. This method is temporary until other means of airway securement can be achieved.

Surgical Cricothyrotomy

Surgical cricothyrotomy is an invasive procedure that should be governed by protocols. Steps for surgical cricothyrotomy are detailed in the box on page 146. Under circumstances in which the anatomy of the neck is distorted, the trachea can be identified by

STEPS FOR SURGICAL CRICOTHYROTOMY

1. Stabilize the patient's head in a neutral position.
2. Identify the cricothyroid membrane and prepare the skin.
3. Stabilize the cricoid and thyroid cartilages with the nondominant hand.
4. Make a vertical incision 5 to 7 cm through the skin.
5. Identify the cricoid membrane and insert the tracheal hook. Use the tracheal hook, now in the nondominant hand, to stabilize the thyroid. Apply upward traction (45-degree angle) on the inferior margin of the thyroid cartilage.
6. Use the tip of a no. 11 blade to create a horizontal incision through the cricoid membrane. Avoid insertion of the blade too deeply and injury of the posterior wall of the trachea or the esophagus.
7. Insert a Trousseau dilator and spread vertically to enlarge the diameter of the cricoid space. Mayo scissors may be used to help enlarge the space in the transverse direction.
8. Remove the tracheal hook.
9. Place a cuffed ETT or tracheostomy tube through the dilator.
10. Remove the dilator. Secure the tube and verify proper position in the usual manner.

slow advancement of a needle connected to a syringe through the skin and attempted aspiration of air. Once air has been aspirated, signaling entrance into the trachea, the needle and syringe should be left in place and cut down over the needle. If the incision is too small, identification of the structures will be more difficult. A vertical incision over the midline is recommended for minimization of bleeding. The nondominant hand should be used for grasping and stabilization of the larynx until the tracheostomy hook can be inserted. If a tracheostomy hook is not available, one can be made by removal of the cannula

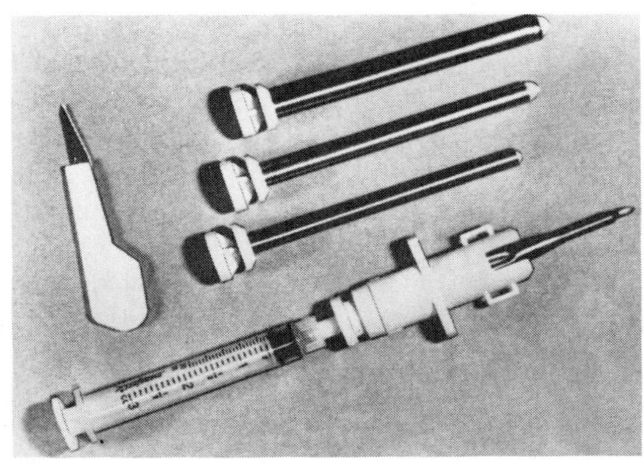

Fig. 8-7. NuTrake. (Courtesy International Medical Devices, Inc, Northridge, Calif.)

from a 16- or 14-gauge catheter and bending of the needle into a hook about 0.25 inch above the tip with a hemostat. After the skin incision has been made and the cricoid membrane identified, the membrane should be incised, and the tracheostomy hook should be inserted through the membrane and used to stabilize the inferior border of the trachea. The diameter of the cricothyroid space is enlarged by insertion and spreading of a Trousseau dilator. Once the dilator is in place, the hook is removed to prevent puncture of the balloon of the tracheostomy tube. A cuffed 6.0-mm ETT or a Shiley tracheostomy tube is placed through the dilator, and the dilator is then removed. The balloon is inflated, and the tube is checked for correct position in the usual manner.

A number of cricothyrotomy devices have been marketed. One such device, the NuTrake, is shown in Fig. 8-7. A small knife is provided for the initial incision. A trocar is then blindly inserted through the cricothyroid membrane and into the trachea until the housing unit rests on the skin. The opening through the membrane is gradually enlarged through a series of insertions of progressively large obturators. The smallest obturator is 4.5 mm, and the largest is 7.2 mm. A PediaTrake device (Fig. 8-8) contains airways with internal diameters of 3, 4, and 5 mm. Both devices come as kits, providing for good organization of equipment. An evaluation of the NuTrake found placement by an untrained operator

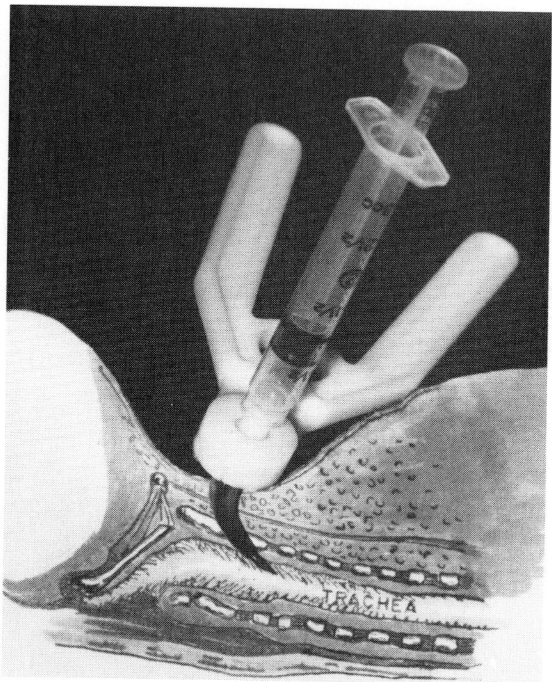

Fig. 8-8. PediaTrake. (Courtesy International Medical Devices, Inc, Northridge, Calif.)

"surprisingly difficult" and recommended training before use.[4] Because both devices are blindly inserted, potential damage to the surrounding neck structures must be considered before use.

RAPID-SEQUENCE INDUCTION

Rapid-sequence induction refers to a specific method of inducing general anesthesia while securing active airway control.[57] The procedure calls for preoxygenation of the patient with 100% oxygen and cautious avoidance, when possible, of positive-pressure ventilation, which results in gastric distention. Cricoid pressure and medication for sedation and analgesia, followed by a neuromuscular blocking agent (NMBA), are then used to facilitate intubation. If the situation warrants, paralysis may be maintained by administration of a longer acting NMBA. Before the use of NMBAs a brief neurologic assessment should be performed.

NEUROMUSCULAR BLOCKING AGENTS

The use of NMBAs to achieve intubation and to facilitate ventilation has proved effective in the emergency department and the prehospital, and it enhances the safety of patients transported by air.* However, one study of trauma patients transported by air did indicate that intubation and neuromuscular blockade are associated with hypothermia and stressed the need for flight teams to take protective measures to guard against this complication.[23]

All NMBAs work at the level of the neuromuscular end plate, disrupting neurotransmitter (acetylcholine) function and preventing effective contraction of skeletal muscle (Fig. 8-9). These agents do not produce analgesia, anesthesia, or amnesia, and reports of patients with total recall and pain perception who were paralyzed without sufficient anesthesia during operations and procedures exist.[42,49,68] Therefore it is essential to sedate the patient before and during extended periods of paralysis. Clinically, neuromuscular blockade may result in hyperkalemia, regurgitation, and aspiration of gastric contents, and it is also associated with a risk of globe rupture in patients with ocular trauma.

NMBAs can be classified in three ways: type of block produced (depolarizing versus nondepolarizing), duration of action (ultrashort, short, intermediate, long), and structure (acetylcholine-like, benzylisoquinolinium compound, aminosteroid compound).[12]

Succinylcholine

Succinylcholine is the only ultrashort-acting NMBA and the only depolarizing agent in common clinical use.[12] Despite having more adverse effects than nondepolarizing agents, succinylcholine remains the agent of choice for rapid-sequence induction because of rapid onset of paralysis (30 to 60 seconds) and short duration of action (4 to 6 minutes). If the flight nurse is unable to intubate a patient who receives succinylcholine, the patient can be bag-valve mask supported for the relatively short time until spontaneous respirations return. A nondepolarizing

*References 10, 22, 31, 46, 53, 64.

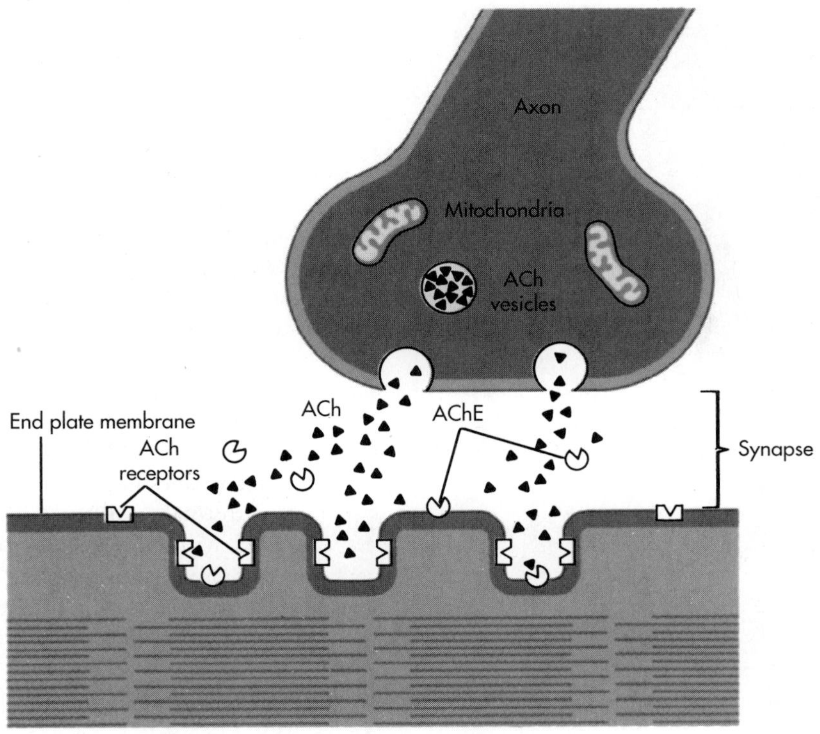

Fig. 8-9. Disruption of acetylcholine function by neuromuscular blocking agents. (From Clark JB, Queener SF, Karb VB: *Pharmacologic basis of nursing practice,* ed 4, St Louis, 1993, Mosby.)

agent given for rapid-sequence induction has the disadvantage of longer onset of action (2 to 5 minutes) and a longer duration (12 to 40 minutes) before return of spontaneous respirations.[12] Nondepolarizing agents such as vecuronium will work almost as rapidly if given in higher doses. However, the patient will be unable to assist with respirations for 30 minutes or more.

Succinylcholine is associated with several potential complications including the following: hyperkalemia; increases in intracranial, intraocular, and intragastric pressure; cardiac dysrhythmias; and pseudocholinesterase deficiency.[12,57,65] The hyperkalemia associated with succinylcholine, which can approach or exceed life-threatening levels, is of greater consequence in patients who have had burn or massive muscle trauma 2 to 3 days previously, and patients may continue to be at risk for 2 to 3 months.[57] Bradydysrhythmia is a complication that frequently is associated with succinylcholine use, especially in young children, but may also occur in adults. Pretreatment with atropine 0.015 mg/kg is advised in children to prevent bradycardia,[57] and pretreatment with lidocaine 1.5 mg/kg in patients with suspected head injury has been shown to attenuate the rise in ICP associated with endotracheal intubation.[40] In patients who have sustained significant skeletal fractures, the fasciculations (irregular muscle contractions produced by depolarization of the muscle membrane before complete cessation of muscle activity) caused by succinylcholine can cause additional injury at the fracture site. Administration of a defasciculation dose of a nondepolarizing agent can prevent this complication.[57,72] Succinylcholine will also cause the release of a small amount of histamine into the systemic circulation and can result in bronchospasm, which can be a concern but not a contraindication in patients with chronic obstructive pulmonary disease or asthma.[57]

The only absolute contraindication to succinylcholine use is in situations in which a cricothyrotomy would be difficult or impossible. Examples include (1) children younger than 2 years, (2) patients with massive neck swelling or trauma in which landmarks are obscured; or (3) cases in which ventilation and intubation would be difficult, such as epiglottis or upper airway obstruction.

Nondepolarizing Agents

Nondepolarizing agents are used to extend the time of paralysis after intubation. Pancuronium was the first nondepolarizing NMBA to be used, beginning in the 1960s, and was used exclusively until the mid-1980s when the newer agents atracurium and vecuronium were marketed. In the 1990s mivacurium and rocuronium were introduced.[12] The new nondepolarizing agents were developed to produce onset of paralysis more rapidly but have a duration of activity shorter than that of pancuronium, and they prevent tachycardia and increased peripheral vascular resistance, which occur with the use of pancuronium. All of the new agents produce fewer cardiovascular effects and have a predictable recovery profile.

NMBAs are now administered in intensive care units for extended periods to (1) facilitate mechanical ventilation by promoting ventilator synchrony, (2) control movement of patients with severe hemodynamic instability, (3) control muscle rigidity in tetanus, (4) immobilize severely agitated patients who have received maximum sedation and pain medications but who continue to be a danger to themselves, (5) facilitate a motionless state in patients with gaping and unstable surgical incisions; and (6) decrease intracranial pressure in patients with head injuries.[15] Table 8-2 lists the NMBAs. After the introduction of these agents in intensive care units, case reports began to describe prolonged weakness and muscle atrophy in patients who received NMBAs for 24 to 48 hours or longer. The drugs most often implicated were pancuronium and vecuronium, and patients at greatest risk were those with kidney or liver dysfunction.[12] This side effect of NMBAs has been shown to be prevented by monitoring of the degree of blockade with a peripheral nerve stimulator, thereby avoiding overdos-

TABLE 8-2

NMBAs

NMBAs	Intravenous dosage (mg/kg)	Onset (min)	Duration (min)	Comments
Depolarizing				
Succinylcholine	Adult dose: 1.0-1.5 Pediatric dose: 1.5-2.0	1.5-2.0	4-6	Pretreat with atropine in children and adolescents; many adverse effects
Nondepolarizing				
Pancuronium	00.04-0.01	3-5	60-100	Stimulate heart rate and cardiac output; no histamine release
Atracurium	0.4-0.5	2-3	20-45	Metabolism independent of kidney or liver function; histamine release
Rocuronium	0.5-1.0	1-2	20-40	Shortest onset of all nondepolarizing NMBAs; no histamine release
Vecuronium	0.1	2-3	20-40	Minimal cardiovascular effects; no histamine release
Mivacurium	0.15-0.25	2-3	12-20	Shortest duration of all nondepolarizing NMBAs; histamine release

age, which has been implicated as a cause of prolonged weakness.[15]

A peripheral nerve stimulator is a device that delivers an electric current to one of several peripheral nerves (the ulnar nerve is the most widely used) through pregelled electrodes placed over the skin. The muscle response to nerve stimulation is then observed. The muscle response to nerve stimulation is also dependent on the type of test. There are three test modes of stimulation, but the "train of four" (TOF) is the best and most common method of peripheral nerve stimulator monitoring to assess the level of neuromuscular blockage.[15] TOF stimulation involves initiation of four electrical stimuli during a 2-second period (2 Hz). An unparalyzed patient will have no fatigue and will have four equal twitches when tested at this frequency. As paralysis increases, the number of twitches will decrease because of fatigue at the neuromuscular junction. Blockade is quantified by a count of the number of thumb adductions or twitches. Four twitches correlate with approximately 75% receptor blockade; three twitches, 80%; two twitches, 85%; and one twitch, 90%. When all four twitches are absent, 100%, or total neuromuscular blockade, is assumed to be present.[15] The frequency of TOF monitoring is recommended every 4 hours during active titration and every 8 hours during maintenance infusion.[15] It is important to note that thus far all reports of prolonged weakness have been in intensive care unit patients receiving long-term administration of these agents. Monitoring with a peripheral nerve stimulator has not yet been identified as beneficial in patients receiving short-term neuromuscular blockade.

Reversal of Neuromuscular Blockade

On rare occasions prolonged paralysis after the administration of NMBAs presents a problem in patient evaluation or treatment, and the need to reverse the agent arises. Pharmacologic reversal of these agents is possible. However, in most situations it is safer and easier to allow normal drug metabolism and excretion to clear the neuromuscular agent.[64] Succinylcholine has no known reversal agent. The patient's respirations must be supported during the duration of action time (4 to 6 minutes), after which the drug will undergo normal metabolism and muscle action will return.

TABLE 8-3

Drugs used to reverse NMBAs

Drug	Dosage
First-line drug combination	
Neostigmine	0.05 mg/kg (not to exceed 5 mg) and atropine 0.015 mg/kg
Given by slow intravenous push	
Repeat dose not recommended	
Second-line drug combination	
Pyridostigmine	0.2 mg/kg and atropine 0.015 mg/kg
Given by slow intravenous push	
Repeat dose not recommended	
Or	
Edrophonium	0.5 mg/kg and atropine 0.007 mg/kg
May repeat 10 min after initial dose (mixed thoroughly in same syringe)	

From Syverud SA: Muscle relaxants. In Barsan WG, Jastremski MS, Syverud SA, editors: *Emergency drug therapy*, Philadelphia, 1991, Saunders.

Reversal of the nondepolarizing agents involves administration of drugs that inhibit acetylcholinesterase. This allows the local concentration of acetylcholine molecules to rise. The reversal agents include neostigmine, pyridostigmine, and edrophonium (Table 8-3).[12,64] The administration of these anticholinesterase-inhibiting drugs causes a strong parasympathetic response consisting of cardiovascular effects, bronchoconstriction, and increased glandular secretions. The cardiovascular effects are of greatest concern and include bradycardia, heart block, and cardiac arrest.[12] These effects can be countered by administration of anticholinergic agents such as atropine or glycopyrrolate, given in conjunction with anticholinesterase inhibitors.

The protocol for endotracheal intubation with succinylcholine is included in the following box. The next box illustrates the protocol for the use of prolonged paralysis before air transport. Both protocols have been used successfully in the University of Cincinnati air medical program, University Air Care, and serve as examples.

PROTOCOL FOR RAPID SEQUENCE INDUCTION WITH SUCCINYLCHOLINE

1. Assemble required equipment: bag-valve mask connected to an oxygen source, suction, appropriate size ETTs, laryngoscope blades and handle, cricothyrotomy tray, medications.
2. Ensure patency of the intravenous site.
3. Place patient on cardiac monitor and pulse oximeter. When possible, assign someone to watch the monitors during the procedure and have them notify the nurse or physician if any dysrhythmia should occur.
4. Perform a brief neurologic assessment while allowing the patient to breathe 100% oxygen through the mask or assist ventilations as indicated.
5. Premedicate as follows:
   Fentanyl 50 to 100 μg intravenous push for sedation of a patient with a head injury and a Glasgow Coma Scale score less than 13.
   Midazolam *(Versed)* 2 to 2.5 mg slow intravenous push for patients without head injuries or those with Glasgow Coma Scale scores greater than 13.
   Atropine 0.01 mg/kg intravenous push for pediatric and adolescent patients.
   Lidocaine 1 mg/kg for ICP management in patients with head injuries, central nervous system injuries, hypertensive crises, or cardiac instability.
6. Administer succinylcholine 1.5 mg/kg by intravenous push.
7. Apply cricoid pressure to occlude the esophagus until intubation is successfully completed.
8. After fasciculations stop (if they occur), demonstrate adequate patient relaxation by ventilation with the bag-valve mask. Jaw relaxation and decreased resistance to bag-valve mask indicate that the cords are paralyzed and intubation may proceed.
9. Perform endotracheal intubation. If unable to intubate during the first 20 seconds, stop and ventilate the patient with the bag-valve mask for 30 to 60 seconds. If inadequate relaxation is present, give a second dose of succinylcholine 1 to 1.5 times the initial dose. If repeated intubation attempts fail, ventilate the patient's lungs with the bag-valve mask until spontaneous respirations occur or consider an alternative airway such as cricothyrotomy.
10. Treat bradycardia occurring during intubation first with oxygen and ventilation. If that does not work, administer atropine 0.5 mg by intravenous push.
11. Once intubation is completed, inflate the cuff and confirm ETT placement. Apply an end-tidal CO_2 detector for additional confirmation.
12. Release cricoid pressure and secure ETT.

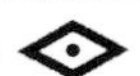

PROTOCOL FOR USE OF NMBAs IN PATIENTS AFTER ENDOTRACHEAL INTUBATION

1. Ensure ETT is functioning and is in proper position above the carina. Be sure the patient is receiving supplemental oxygen.
2. Assemble required equipment: bag-valve mask, suction, medications.
3. Airway equipment should be readily available in the event of an inadvertent extubation during the use of these drugs.
4. Ensure patency of the intravenous site.
5. Place patient on cardiac monitor and pulse oximeter.
6. Sedate the awake patient and manage his or her pain with fentanyl and/or midazolam in accordance with the Glasgow Coma Scale.
7. Give vecuronium 0.1 mg/kg intravenous push.
8. If inadequate relaxation occurs, repeat 25% of the initial dose.
9. Ensure adequate sedation and pain management are maintained in the patient receiving NMBAs during transport.

RESPIRATORY ADJUNCTS

In-flight evaluation of airway interventions occurs under less than optimal conditions. Aircraft may be noisy and dimly lit. Traditional auscultation is extremely difficult, and poor cabin lighting may interfere with the normal visual cues of assessment.[21,24] Parameters used for evaluation include the level of consciousness, stability of vital signs, observation of the patient's color, and symmetric rise and fall of the chest wall. Several pieces of equipment may assist with evaluation and provide objective data.

End-Tidal CO_2 Detection

The disposable end-tidal CO_2 detector Easy Cap (Fig. 8-10) assists proper ETT placement by incorporating a nontoxic, chemically treated indicator that changes color in the presence of carbon dioxide.[6] The device can reliably function for up to 2 hours

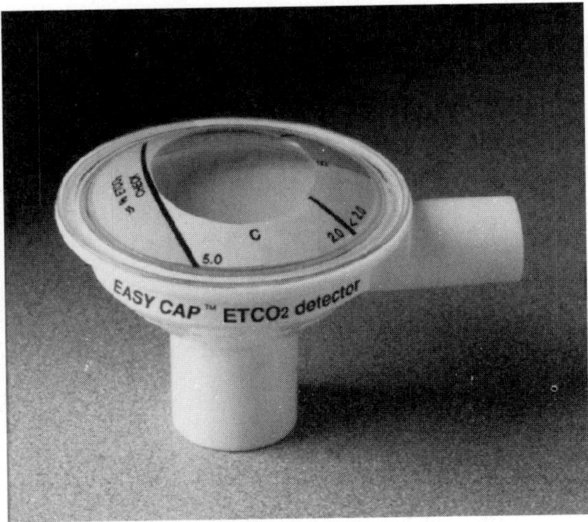

Fig. 8-10. Easy Cap end-tidal CO_2 detector. (Courtesy Nellcor Puritan Bennett, Inc, Pleasanton, Calif.)

and is not affected by environmental temperature extremes. With early use of the Easy Cap it was thought that patients in cardiopulmonary arrest may not have enough perfusion to generate a color change in the device. Recent investigations have concluded that when used during cardiopulmonary resuscitation in patients with low end-tidal carbon dioxide levels, the device should produce a detectable color change.[28] Hayden et al[20] found in a study of 566 prehospital intubations of patients in cardiac arrest that a color change occurred in 95.6%, with only 1 false-positive result. In addition to verifying endotracheal placement after intubation, the Easy Cap device can also be used to monitor tube placement while in flight.[6] If the indicator becomes contaminated with pulmonary secretions or comes in contact with medications administered through the ETT, the indicator will no longer function. The device may be removed from the ETT after administration of medications given through the ETT for at least six breaths, or until fluids are no longer visible, and then replaced with no loss of function.[6] Pedi-Cap (Fig. 8-11), a new, smaller detector, is now available and is designed for neonates and children who weigh up to 15 kg. It provides 2 hours of continuous service. The adult

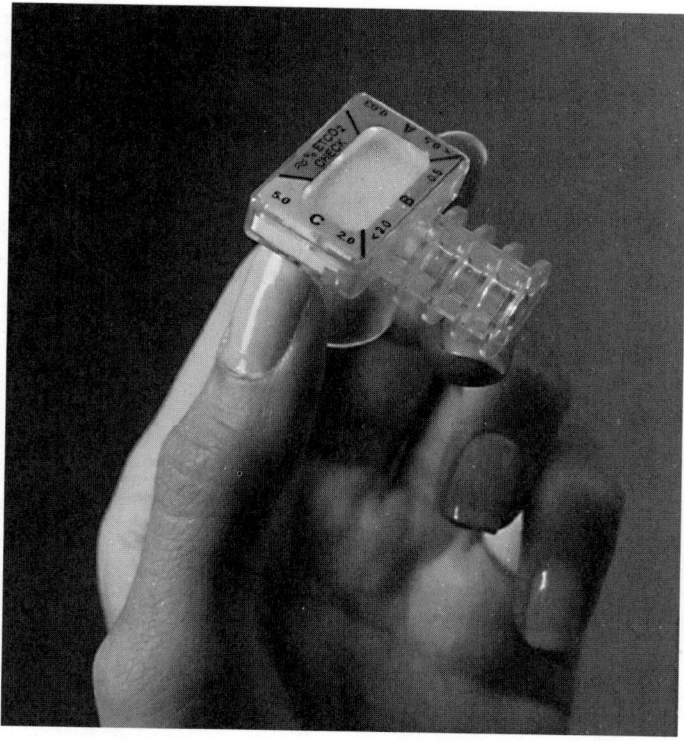

Fig. 8-11. Pedi-Cap Pediatric end-tidal CO_2 detector. (Courtesy Nellcor Puritan Bennett, Inc, Pleasanton, Calif.)

model is not recommended in patients who weigh less than 15 kg.

Capnography

Capnography is the measurement of end-tidal CO_2 volumes with each breath by use of infrared light absorption by placement of a sensor between the breathing circuit and the ETT. The instrument works by emitting an infrared light beam through a sensor located immediately distal to the ETT. As carbon dioxide is exhaled, the CO_2 molecules absorb the infrared light. The instrument then measures how much light was absorbed, thereby determining the concentration of CO_2.[63] The data are then displayed in digital or wave form or both. Fig. 8-12 shows two such instruments. The graphic wave form, called a *capnogram,* displays levels of CO_2 over time. Capnometry refers to the numeric display. Normal end-tidal CO_2 volume is a close indicator of the arterial pressure of carbon dioxide, and the difference between these two parameters, known as the *CO_2 gradient* (P[a-ET]CO_2) has been reported to be less than 6 mm Hg in normal patients.[66]

Capnography technology has been in use during the last decade in the operating room for assessment of the respiratory status of patients during surgery, for detection of hyperventilation or hypoventilation, and for detection of equipment problems. The value of capnography to the flight team is its ability to confirm proper ETT placement, to indicate situations in which the ETT has become displaced, and to detect disruption of the ventilator circuit.[43] However, as with any piece of equipment, caution should be exercised when capnography is used to ensure the clinical picture matches the readings. Carbon dioxide present in

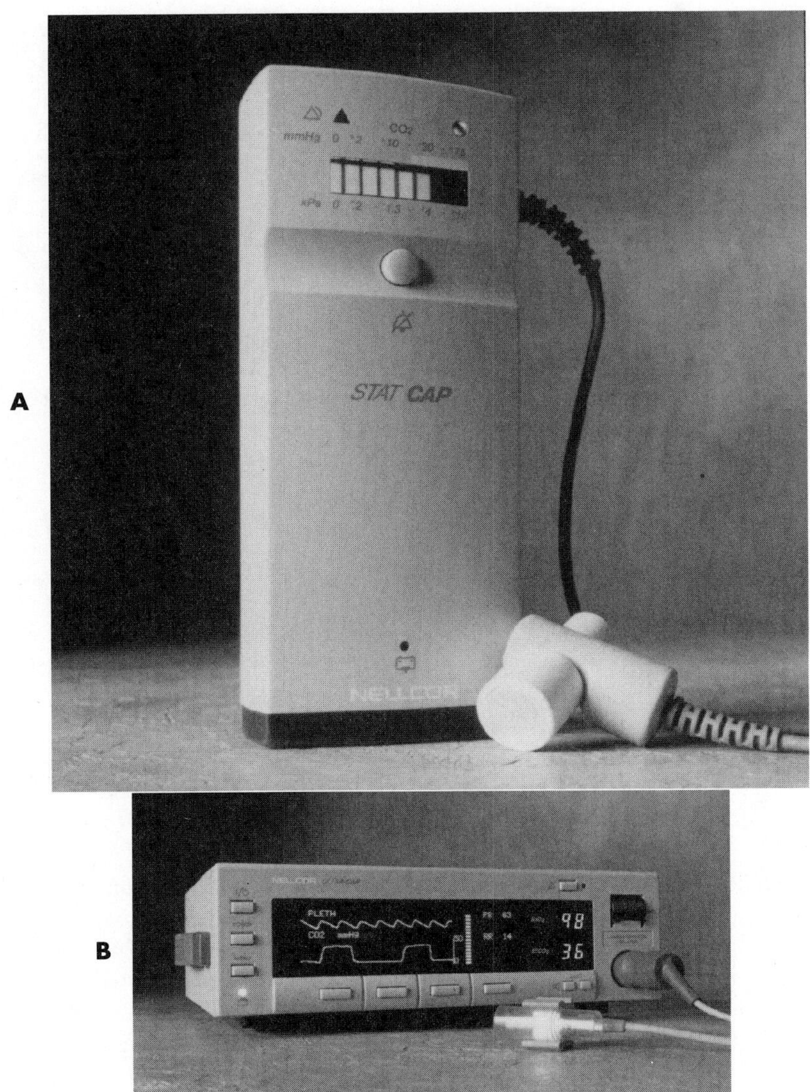

Fig. 8-12. CO_2 indicators. **A,** Stat Cap airway CO_2 indicator. **B,** Ultra Cap combination capnograph and pulse oximeter. (Courtesy Nellcor Puritan Bennett, Inc, Pleasanton, Calif.)

the exhaled gas indicates that alveolar ventilation has transpired but does not necessarily mean that the ETT is in the trachea. A tube positioned in the pharynx will also provide normal readings.

Continuous capnography has been used during blind nasotracheal intubation in spontaneously breathing patients. The posterior displacement of the tip of the tube to the larynx was recognized promptly by the use of continuous capnography. Likewise, when the tube was repositioned for entry into the trachea, the capnograph monitor displayed the presence of CO_2.[63]

Recent advances in technology have allowed smaller, more durable instruments for prehospital use. Thus far, capnography has just begun to be assessed in the air medical setting. As technology continues to progress, the likelihood increases that capnography use will become a standard of care in the air medical environment.

Pulse Oximetry

In the emergency department or intensive care unit health care providers rely on arterial blood gases or, more specifically, the partial pressure of oxygen tension (PaO_2) drawn on an intermittent basis to guide therapy. Pulse oximetry provides a reliable and continuous evaluation of oxygenation.

Oxygen in the blood is dissolved in the plasma or is bound to hemoglobin. The oxygen dissolved in the plasma is referred to as the *partial pressure of oxygen* (PO_2). The normal value of oxygen dissolved in the arterial blood (PaO_2) is measured in millimeters of mercury or torr. In children and adults this value ranges from 80 to 100, with higher values expected in the pediatric population. The PO_2 accounts for 1% to 2% of the total oxygen content.

The portion of oxygen bound to hemoglobin is referred to as *oxygen saturation* (SO_2). In arterial blood the normal value of oxygen saturation (SaO_2) ranges from 95% to 97.5%. The SO_2 accounts for 98% or more of the total oxygen content.

The relationship between the PaO_2 and SaO_2 is displayed in Figure 8-13, the oxyhemoglobin dissociation curve. If one value is known, the other can be estimated. It is important to note that the relationship is not a linear one. The upper portion of the curve demonstrates a compensatory mechanism of the body; in a normal healthy adult, more oxygen than necessary is carried. A drop in the PaO_2 from 100 to 80 mm Hg shows a minimal change in the SaO_2. The steep portion of the curve demonstrates a rapid decline in SaO_2 with small decreases in PaO_2. When the SaO_2 falls below 90%, there is a rapid decline in the oxygen content.

Pulse oximetry continuously monitors the SaO_2 value. A sensor device is placed across a pulsating arteriolar bed, such as the toe, nose, or finger. Fig. 8-14 illustrates two types of pulse oximeters. The sensor houses a light source and photodetector device. The pulse oximeter processes the light absorption to determine SaO_2 values. The successful use of an oximetry device is dependent on proper placement of the sensor device. It should be positioned such that the light source and photodetector are in direct alignment. The patient's skin at the placement site should be clean and dry. The ability to obtain a pulse at the site of placement is also important. The accuracy of pulse oximetry may be affected by clinical conditions such as hypotension or hypothermia, or during vasopressor therapy secondary to vasoconstriction. McGuire and Pointer[36] studied the use of the pulse oximeter in the field, and Jones et al[29] studied its use in the emergency department. Both described a good correlation between SaO_2 and PaO_2 values as measured by arterial blood gas monitoring. Both also recommended treatment of patients with SaO_2 per pulse oximeter of 91% or less (SaO_2 of 91% correlates with a PaO_2 of 65 torr). This value (91%) is below normal, but both studies found that patients who have this level may not display obvious signs and symptoms of hypoxia.

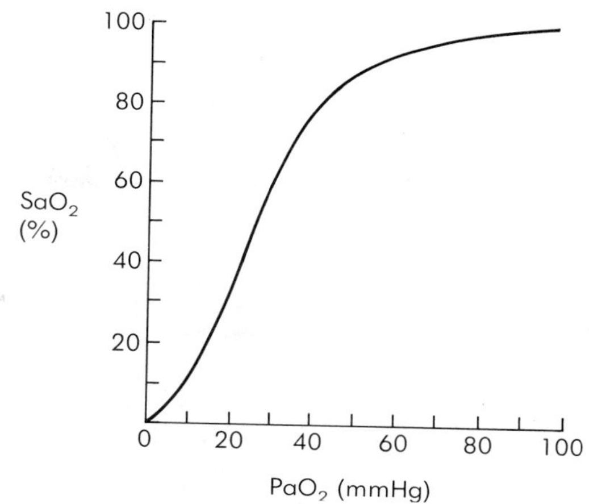

Fig. 8-13. Oxyhemoglobin dissociation curve.

The accuracy and efficacy of pulse oximetry in the air medical setting have also been established.[11,38,50,58] The value of this device to the flight nurse lies in its ability to act as an early warning system. A low SaO_2 is detected much earlier than by clinical observation, permitting expeditious and

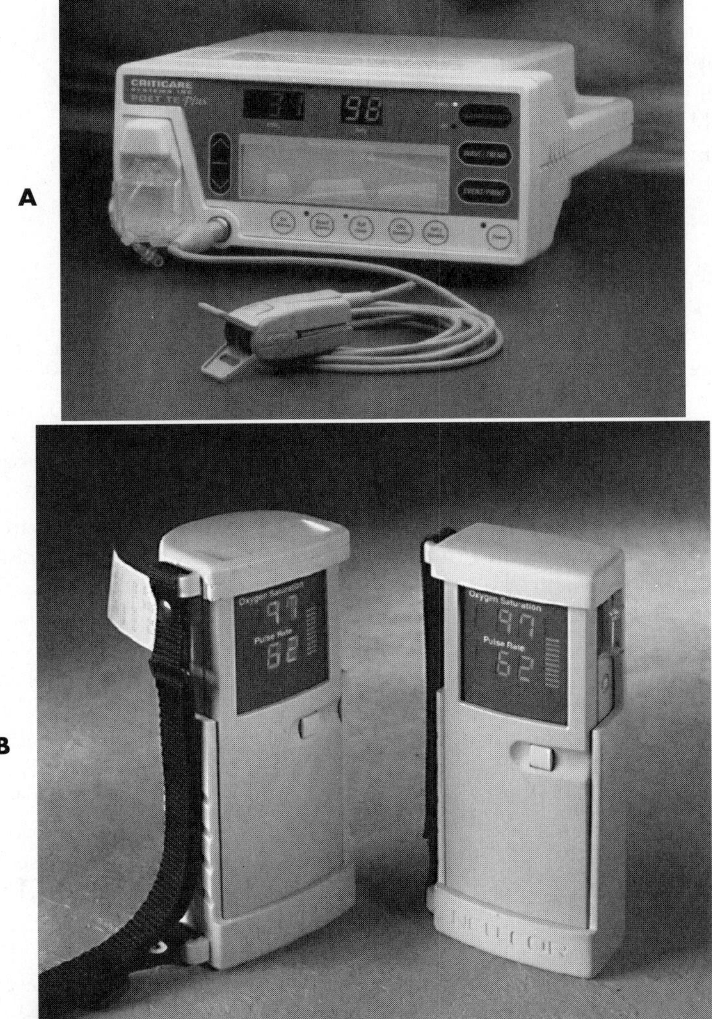

Fig. 8-14. Pulse oximeters. **A,** Poet TE Plus combination capnograph and pulse oximeter. (Courtesy of Criticare Systems Inc, Milwaukee, Wis. Reprinted with permission.) **B,** N-20 portable pulse oximeter. (Courtesy Nellcor Puritan Bennett, Inc, Pleasanton, Calif.)

aggressive interventions. Continuous pulse oximetry monitoring improves the recognition and management of hypoxemia during emergency endotracheal intubation,[35] and during flight it offers visual reassurance to the flight team that airway management is having its intended effect. If oxygen saturation measured by pulse oximetry suddenly changes, a repeat airway assessment should be performed to determine the cause, and corrective action should be taken.

Pulse oximetry has also been found to be useful in determination of systolic blood pressure in the air medical setting by application of an appropriate size blood pressure cuff on the same arm as the pulse oximetry probe. The cuff is inflated until the pulsatile display on the pulse oximeter is obliterated. The manometer reading at the point of obliteration is recorded as the systolic blood pressure.[39]

Transport Ventilators

Once the airway is controlled, ventilations can be assisted with either a bag valve–mask device or a ventilator. In recent years, the market has been flooded with transport ventilators. In 1985 Branson et al[5] provided a description and performance evaluation of several models. They recommended that air and ground ambulance ventilators be "compact, light-weight, fuel efficient, flexible, user friendly, durable, and require little maintenance." This statement still reflects the requirements of ventilators. Of these criteria fuel efficiency and flexibility deserve the greatest consideration.

Most transport ventilators are oxygen-powered devices. Thus, when selecting one to purchase or deciding which patient should be placed on a ventilator, medical personnel should consider the amount of oxygen on board the aircraft. Fig. 8-15 shows two models of transport ventilators.

A

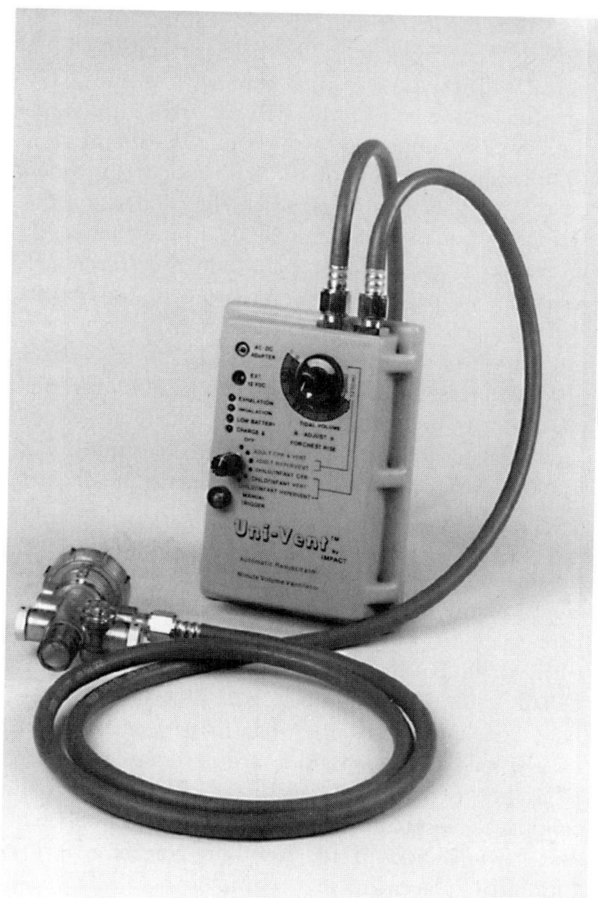

B

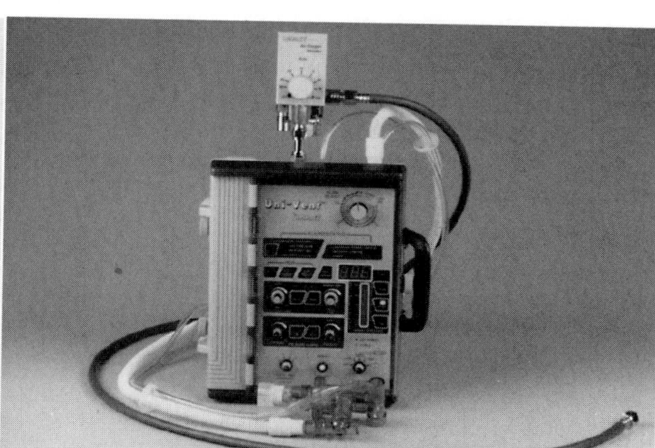

Fig. 8-15. Transport ventilators. **A,** Uni-Vent Model 706 automatic resuscitator. **B,** Uni-Vent Model 750 transport ventilator. (Courtesy Impact Medical Co, West Caldwell, N.J.)

Flexibility is a must. The majority of ventilators manufactured for the prehospital setting are capable of providing ventilation for both adults and children. Some of the more sophisticated models are capable of providing a wide range of ventilatory modes and therefore are useful in meeting the requirements of patients with routine tidal volume and rate settings. In addition, they can meet the demands of the critically ill patient with special ventilatory needs such as control, assist-control, and synchronized intermittent mandatory ventilation operating modes. Many are PEEP compensable and use comprehensive alarm systems for continuous system self-checks. Ventilators with electronic circuitry also have the added benefit of being unaffected by changes in altitude.

The use of ventilators versus manual ventilation remains controversial, particularly in the initial treatment of patients with obvious chest trauma or in patients who have potential chest injuries. Ventilators eliminate the ability to "feel" lung compliance, which can indicate a pneumothorax is developing or can signal an obstruction in or displacement of the ETT.[51]

Even in the hands of skilled operators, the risk of unintentional hyperventilation and acute respiratory alkalosis is a common problem during manual ventilation, according to Hurst et al.[25] Hyperventilation and the associated alkalosis may precipitate coronary vasospasm and lead to arrhythmias. In patients with head injuries requiring hyperventilation to control ICP, additional ischemia at the injury site may occur if $Paco_2$ levels fall below 25 torr because of manual ventilation that is too vigorous. Transport ventilators have been shown to be useful in preventing the negative effects of unintentional hyperventilation.[25]

Transport ventilators have the additional benefit of allowing both members of the flight team to continue patient care unencumbered by the need to manually ventilate the patient after initial ventilator setup. A sensible policy is for a transport ventilator not to be used for patients with potential chest injuries, such as from trauma scenes, and to use transport ventilators for patients with head injuries or for other critical care transports.

When using a transport ventilator, a flight nurse should calculate tidal volumes at 10 to 15 ml/kg and then check them using a spirometer, especially in children to prevent the risk of barotrauma.[13]

ESOPHAGEAL INTUBATION DETECTION

Assessment of ETT placement is a routine maneuver after intubation. The potentially catastrophic consequences of an undetected esophageal intubation stress the importance of the ability to recognize and correct the situation should it occur. Observations such as chest movement, breath sounds, epigastric auscultation and observation, reservoir bag compliance, and tube condensation are some of the more commonly prescribed methods of tube position assessment. However, each of these methods at times may prove inaccurate.[2]

A tool for detection of esophageal intubation has recently been marketed. The detector consists of a 60-ml syringe fitted with a standard 15-mm ETT adaptor on the end of the syringe. After intubation, the device is connected to the ETT, and the plunger is pulled back. Because of the rigid support provided by the cartilaginous rings, when the plunger of the syringe is pulled back, air will be aspirated without resistance if the ETT is placed in the trachea. If resistance or negative pressure is encountered when the plunger is pulled back, the esophagus has been intubated. The esophagus readily collapses when a negative pressure is applied because, unlike the trachea, it has no cartilaginous support. The syringe aspiration technique of verifying ETT position was found to be accurate in both the emergency department and the prehospital setting.[26]

A further modification of the plunger device incorporates a self-inflating bulb fitted with an ETT adaptor. The bulb is squeezed before it is connected to the ETT. If the bulb self-inflates, tracheal intubation is signaled. If the bulb remains deflated, esophageal intubation is indicated. Studies have concluded that prior bag-mask ventilation or esophageal ventilation does not interfere with the reliability of the self-inflating bulb in detecting esophageal intubation.[52] The self-inflating bulb has also been shown to be useful in correct identification of placement of the Esophageal Tracheal Combitube.[70]

AIRWAY MANAGEMENT CASE STUDY

The University of Cincinnati Air Medical Team was dispatched to a motor vehicle collision 30 miles south of Cincinnati on a major interstate highway. The collision involved an elderly couple returning from a weekend trip from Knoxville, Tennessee. A car driven by a 72-year-old man collided into the rear of a stopped semitrailer. The driver's 71-year-old wife was in the front passenger seat. The couple were riding in a late-model, full-size General Motors car that was not equipped with air bags. The flight team arrived in a BK-117, which was capable of transporting two patients, 21 minutes after being dispatched. Additional information from the scene indicated that the driver of the semitrailer was not injured and that no skid marks were noted from the car. The initial responders were volunteer firefighters and basic emergency medical technicians.

The scene commander reported that the female patient had just been extricated but that the male patient remained entrapped. The team was directed to the 71-year-old woman, who was initially evaluated moments after extrication. She reportedly was wearing a seat belt with shoulder restraint. A cervical collar was in place, and the patient was immobilized on a backboard. The initial assessment revealed the following information.

Airway: Patient was awake but somewhat confused. Oxygen was in place and being delivered by nonrebreather mask. The upper airway was clear and free of blood or vomitus.

Breathing: Respiratory rate was 28 breaths per minute, with bilateral equal chest expansion noted. The anterior ribs were tender to palpation but no subcutaneous air or crepitus was noted.

Circulation: Skin was pale with 1+ radial pulses bilaterally. Capillary refill was 3 seconds.

Deficit: Movement and sensation were noted in all extremities. Pupils were midrange, round, and reactive bilaterally. Bilateral cataracts were noted. Her Glasgow Coma Scale score was 13 (E_4, V_4, M_5).

Extremities: No upper extremity fractures were noted. She reported tenderness over her right clavicle and shoulder area, presumably from the shoulder restraint. Her pelvis was stable. A midshaft femur fracture was noted on the right.

The patient was placed on a cardiac monitor, and atrial fibrillation was observed with a ventricular rate of 116 beats/min. A large-bore intravenous line was established with normal saline solution. The initial blood pressure was 112/72 mm Hg. Pulse oximetry was 99%. One team member continued assessment of Mrs. K while the second team member evaluated Mr. K. Information was radioed to the pilot to configure the aircraft for a two-patient transport after shutting down. Time needed to reconfigure for two patients is about 5 minutes after shut down.

Mr. K remained trapped in the car. Primary survey revealed the following.

Airway: Patient was unresponsive to verbal stimuli and moaned weakly to painful stimuli. Airway was clear and patent. High-flow oxygen was being delivered by a nonrebreather mask. A cervical collar was in place.

Breathing: Respirations were slow and deep at 12 breaths per minute. The patient's position in the car precluded further examination.

Circulation: His skin was pale, no radial pulses were palpable, and a rapid, strong carotid pulse was noted.

Deficit: No movement to pain was noted.

Mr. K obviously needed tracheal intubation for airway protection and hyperventilation for a suspected head injury. Discussion between the flight team surrounded whether Mr. K should be intubated in the car by the blind nasotracheal method or whether intubation could be delayed until after he was extricated from the car. The incident commander reported that Mr. K would be free from the wreckage in 3 to 5 minutes. The flight team elected not to interrupt extrication efforts because of the short time until extrication and because Mr. K's position in the car appeared as if it might complicate intubation attempts. Extrication efforts continued, and Mr. K was removed on a long backboard. After Mr. K was removed from the car, a repeat primary examination revealed the following.

Airway: Airway was patent. No blood or vomitus was noted. Dentures were seen but could not be removed.

Breathing: Respirations were deep and regular. Rate was 10 to 12 breaths per minute. Palpation of the chest revealed crepitus on the right, with subcutaneous air noted in the area of the right axilla. There was obvious deformity to the right clavicle.

Circulation: Skin color was pale with absent radial pulses bilaterally. Carotid pulses were palpable. Capillary refill was absent in all extremities.

Deficit: Painful stimuli elicited only moans. Pupils were round, equal at 4 mm bilaterally, and sluggishly reactive. His Glasgow Coma Scale score was 4 (E_1, V_2, M_1).

The flight team had anticipated the need for emergent intubation, and equipment was ready. Cardiac monitor was applied and revealed a sinus rhythm with a rate of 96 beats/min. Initial pulse oximetry was 90% on high-flow oxygen by nonrebreather mask. An emergency medical technician reported a blood pressure of 90/60 mm Hg. An intravenous line of normal saline solution was established. Attempts to remove Mr. K's dentures were again unsuccessful because his jaws were clenched. The flight team prepared for rapid-sequence induction intubation. Lidocaine 100 mg and succinylcholine 100 mg were given by intravenous push while cricoid pressure was maintained and 100% oxygen was used to gently assist ventilations. Pulse oximetry improved to 94% with assisted ventilations. Mr. K was then orally intubated with an 8.0-mm ETT on the first attempt while strict cervical spine alignment was maintained. Breath sounds were auscultated bilaterally and an end-tidal CO_2 monitor indicated proper ETT placement with good exchange of carbon dioxide. Mr. K's color did not improve significantly, and breath sounds were diminished on the right. A needle thoracostomy was performed on the right side, and air was noted on entrance into the pleural space. No blood was returned. The needle was left in place, and manual hyperventilation was begun.

While Mr. K was being secured to the flight stretcher, Mrs. K was loaded into the aircraft. Mr. K's secondary examination was deferred, and he too was loaded into the aircraft. In flight Mrs. K remained awake and reported leg and shoulder pain. She remained normotensive, and her pulse oximetry remained at 99% while she was on a nonrebreather mask.

Mr. K's color improved, and his pulse oximetry was 96% with continued manual hyperventilation. His systolic blood pressure was 130 palp. Intravenous fluids were decreased to guard against further aggravation of his head and lung injuries.

Mr. K was unloaded at the University of Cincinnati and transported immediately to the Center for Emergency Care where a trauma team was standing by. Mrs. K was unloaded after the aircraft was shut down, and she also was evaluated in the Center for Emergency Care.

Mr. K's evaluation revealed that ribs 3 and 4 on the right were fractured and that he had pneumothorax and a pulmonary contusion. A no. 36 chest tube was inserted on the right. A right clavicle fracture was also noted. Results of peritoneal lavage were negative. A head computed tomography scan revealed a rim subdural hematoma and a large parietal contusion. Mr. K was admitted to the neurosurgical intensive care unit for continued evaluation and treatment. His condition continued to spiral downward, and he died 1 week later.

Findings on Mrs. K's chest, abdominal, and pelvic radiographic films were negative. A midshaft femur fracture was identified on the right. Findings of head and abdominal computed tomography scans were negative. Mrs. K was taken to the operating room for open reduction and internal fixation of the right femur and was admitted to the surgical intensive care unit for 24 hours. She was then discharged to an orthopedic unit for continued postoperative care and was discharged home 1 week later.

REFERENCES

1. Barkin RM, Rosen P: *Emergency pediatrics: a guide to ambulatory care,* ed 3, St Louis, 1990, Mosby.
2. Birmingham PK, Cheney FW , Ward RJ: Esophageal intubation: a review of detection techniques, *Anesth Analg* 65:886, 1986.
3. Birnbaumer DM, Biemann JT: Esophageal airways. In Dailey R et al, editors: *The airway: emergency management,* St Louis, 1992, Mosby.
4. Bjoraker DG, Kumar NB, Brown AC: Evaluation of an emergency cricothyrotomy instrument, *Crit Care Med* 15(2):157, 1987.
5. Branson RD et al: Ventilators for aeromedical transport, description, and performance evaluations, *Hosp Aviat* 4(11):13, 1985.
6. Campbell RC et al: Evaluation of an end-tidal carbon dioxide detector in the aeromedical setting, *J Air Med Transport* 9(11):13, 1990.

7. Cook RT, Stene JK, Marcolina B: Use of a Beck Airway Airflow Monitor and controllable-tip endotracheal tube in two cases of nonlaryngoscopic oral intubation, *Am J Emerg Med* 13(2):180, 1995.
8. Crippen D, Olveey S, Graffis R: Gastric rupture: an esophageal obturator complication, *Ann Emerg Med* 10(2): 370, 1981.
9. Dauphinee K: Orotracheal intubation; nasotracheal intubation, *Emerg Med Clin North Am* 6(4):699, 1988.
10. DeGarmo B, Dronen S: Pharmacology and clinical use of neuromuscular blocking agents, *Ann Emerg Med* 12(1): 48, 1983.
11. DeJarnette R et al: Pulse oximetry during helicopter transport, *Air Med J* 12(4):93, 1993.
12. Dickens MD: Pharmacology of neuromuscular blockade: interactions and implications for concurrent drug therapies, *Crit Care Nursing Q* 18(2):1, 1995.
13. English DK: Ventilators. In Dailey R et al, editors: *The airway: emergency management* St Louis, 1992, Mosby.
14. Feaster WW: Oral endotracheal intubation: pediatric perspective. In Dailey R et al, editors: *The airway: emergency management,* St Louis, 1992, Mosby.
15. Ford EV: Monitoring neuromuscular blockade in the adult ICU, *Am J Crit Care* 4(2):122, 1995.
16. Frass M et al: The esophageal tracheal combitube: preliminary results with a new airway for CPR, *Ann Emerg Med* 16(7):768, 1987.
17. Frezer SJ: Cricoid pressure: how, when and why, *AORN J* 45(6):1374, 1987.
18. Haines M: Pediatric intubations, case presentation, and review, *Aero Med J* 2(2):28, 1987.
19. Hancock PJ: Finger intubation, *Air Med J* 13(10):421, 1994 (abstract).
20. Hayden SR et al: Colormetric end-tidal CO_2 detector for verification of endotracheal tube placement in out-of-hospital cardiac arrest, *Acad Emerg Med* 2:499, 1995.
21. Hightower DP et al: Red cabin lights impair air medical crew performance of color-dependent tasks, *Air Med J* 14(1):75, 1995.
22. Holleran R: The use of neuromuscular blocking agents in acute airway management: implications for the flight team, *J Air Med Transport* 9(5):6, 1990.
23. Holleran RS, Davis K, Storer D: Neuromuscular blockade and intubation: association with hypothermia in the air medical trauma patient, *Air Med J* 13(11-12):483, 1994.
24. Hunt RC et al: Inability to assess breath sounds during air medical transports by helicopter, *JAMA* 265(15): 1982, 1991.
25. Hurst JM et al: Comparison of blood gases during transport using two methods of ventilatory support, *J Trauma* 29(12):1637, 1989.
26. Jenkins WA, Verduke VP, Paris PM: The syringe aspiration technique to verify endotracheal tube position, *Am J Emerg Med* 12(4):413, 1994.
27. Johnson JC, Aterton GL: The Esophageal Tracheal Combitube: an alternate route to airway management, *J Emerg Med Services* 16(5):29, 1991.
28. Jones BR, Dorsey MJ: Sensitivity of a disposable end-tidal carbon dioxide detector, *J Clin Monit* 7(3):268, 1991.
29. Jones J et al: Continuous emergency department monitoring of arterial saturation in adult patients with respiratory distress, *Ann Emerg Med* 17(5):463, 1988.
30. Jorden RC: Airway management, *Emerg Med Clin North Am* 6(4):671, 1988.
31. Krisanda T et al: Succinylcholine as an airway management adjunct in a suburban ALS system, *Ann Emerg Med* 22(5):923, 1993 (abstract).
32. Krishel S, Jackimcuzk K, Balazs K: Endotracheal tube whistle: an adjunct to blind nasotracheal intubation, *Ann Emerg Med* 21(1):33, 1992.
33. Mace SE: Cricothyrotomy, *J Emerg Med* 6(4):309, 1988.
34. Majernick T et al: Cervical spine motion during orotracheal intubation, *Ann Emerg Med* 15(4):417, 1986.
35. Mateer JR et al: Continuous pulse oximetry during emergency endotracheal intubation, *Ann Emerg Med* 22(4):675, 1993.
36. McGuire TJ, Pointer JE: Evaluation of a pulse oximeter in the prehospital setting, *Ann Emerg Med* 17(10):1058, 1988.
37. Melick C, Rosen P: Cricothyrotomy and tracheotomy. In Dailey R et al, editors: The airway: emergency management, St Louis, 1992, Mosby.
38. Melton JD et al: Occult hypoxemia during aeromedical transport: detection by pulse oximetry, *Prehosp Disaster Med* 4:114, 1989.
39. Mohler J, Hart SC: Use of a pulse oximeter for determination of systolic blood pressure in a helicopter air ambulance, *Air Med J* 13(11-12):479, 1994.
40. Murphy M: Increased intracranial pressure. In Dailey R et al, editors: *The airway: emergency management,* St Louis, 1992, Mosby.
41. Nieman JT et al: The pharyngeotracheal lumen airway: preliminary investigation of a new adjunct, *Ann Emerg Med* 13(8):591, 1984.
42. Parker M et al: Perception of a critically ill patient experiencing therapeutic paralysis in an ICU, *Crit Care Med* 12(1):69, 1984.

43. Peterson C, Budd R, Balazs K: Comparative evaluation of three end-tidal CO_2 monitors used during air medical transport, *J Air Med Transport* 11(2):7, 1992.
44. Pointer JE: Nasotracheal intubation. In Dailey R et al, editors: *The airway: emergency management,* St Louis, 1992, Mosby.
45. Pons PT: Esophageal obturator airway, *Emerg Med Clin North Am* 6(4):693, 1988.
46. Redan J et al: The value of intubation and paralyzing patients with suspected head injury in the emergency department, *J Trauma* 31(3):371, 1991.
47. Reed J: Orotracheal and nasotracheal intubation, *Emerg Care Q* 3(3):1, 1987.
48. Rhee KJ et al: Oral intubation in the multiply injured patient: the risk of exacerbating spinal cord damage, *Ann Emerg Med* 19(5):511, 1990
49. Roberts DJ, Clinton JE, Ruiz E: Neuromuscular blockage for critical patients in the emergency department, *Ann Emerg Med* 15(2):152, 1986.
50. Rose WD, Laird SL: Evaluation of the pulse oximeter and end-tidal CO_2 detector during aeromedical transport, *J Air Med Transport* 10(11):75, 1991 (abstract).
51. Rouse MJ, Branson R, Holleran R: Mechanical ventilation during air medical transport, *J Air Med Transport* 11(10):5, 1992.
52. Salem MR et al: Use of the self-inflating bulb for detecting esophageal intubation after esophageal ventilation, *Anesth Analg* 77(6):1227, 1993.
53. Sayre M, Weisberger I: The use of neuromuscular blocking agents by air medical services, *J Air Med Transport* 11(1):7, 1992.
54. Scott J: Oral endotracheal intubation. In Dailey R et al, editors: *The airway: emergency management,* St Louis, 1992, Mosby.
55. Shea SR, MacDonald JR, Grouzinski G: Prehospital endotracheal tube airway or esophageal gastric tube airway: a critical comparison, *Ann Emerg Med* 14(2):102, 1985.
56. Sheehy S: Basic life support. In Sheehy S, editor: *Emergency nursing: principles and practice,* St Louis, 1992, Mosby.
57. Simon B: Pharmacologic aids in airway management. In Dailey R et al, editors: *The airway: emergency management,* St Louis, 1992, Mosby.
58. Smith SB et al: Introduction of pulse oximetry in the air medical setting, *J Air Med Transport* 10(11):11, 1991.
59. Stemper CL: Advanced life support. In Sheehy S, editor: *Emergency nursing: principles and practice,* St Louis, 1992, Mosby.
60. Stewart R: Digital intubation. In Dailey R et al, editors: *The airway: emergency management,* St Louis, 1992, Mosby.
61. Stewart R: Lighted stylet. In Dailey R et al, editors: *The airway: emergency management,* St Louis, 1992, Mosby.
62. Stewart R: Manual translaryngeal jet ventilation. In Dailey R et al, editors: *The airway: emergency management,* St Louis, 1992, Mosby.
63. Stock MC: Capnography for adults, *Crit Care Clin* 11(1): 219, 1995.
64. Syverud S et al: Prehospital use of neuromuscular blocking agents in a helicopter ambulance program, *Ann Emerg Med* 17(3):236, 1988.
65. Syverud SA: Muscle relaxants. In Barsan WG, Jastremski MS, Syverud SA, editors: *Emergency drug therapy,* Philadelphia, 1991, WB Saunders.
66. Szaflarski NL, Choen NH: Use of capnography in critically ill adults, *Heart Lung* 20(4):362, 1991.
67. Verdile VP: Digital and transillumination intubation, *Emerg Care Q* 3(3):77, 1987.
68. Vitello-Cicciu JM: Recalled perceptions of patients administered pancuronium bromide, *Focus Crit Care* 11:28, 1984.
69. Vollmer TP et al: Use of a lighted stylet for guided orotracheal intubation in the prehospital setting, *Ann Emerg Med* 14(4):324, 1985.
70. Wafai Y et al: Effectiveness of the self-inflating bulb for verification of proper placement of the Esophageal Tracheal Combitube, *Anesth Analg* 80(1):122, 1995.
71. Walls RM: Cricothyroidotomy, *Emerg Med Clin North Am* 6(4):725, 1988.
72. Walls RM: Rapid-sequence intubation in head trauma, *Ann Emerg Med* 22(6):1008, 1993.
73. Walter FG, Lowe RA: Airway management. In Hamilton G et al, editors: *Emergency medicine: an approach to clinical problem solving,* Philadelphia, 1991, WB Saunders.
74. Whitten CE: Complications: inserting an endotracheal tube, *Emerg Med* 22(7):89, 1990.
75. Whitten CE: Difficult intubation: tricks to remember, *Emerg Med* 22(1):85, 1990.
76. Whitten CE: Preintubation evaluation: predicting the difficult airway, *Emerg Med* 21(9):107, 1989.
77. Yancey W et al: Unrecognized tracheal intubation: a complication of the esophageal obturator airway, *Ann Emerg Med* 9(1):18, 1980.
78. Yealy D, Paris P: Recent advances in airway management, *Emerg Med Clin North Am* 7(1):83, 1989.
79. Young GP: Clinical airway anatomy. In Dailey R et al, editors: *The airway: emergency management,* St Louis, 1992, Mosby.

CHAPTER 9

Shock and Coagulopathies

COMPETENCIES

1. Describe the pathophysiology of shock and selected coagulopathies.
2. Perform a complete assessment of the patient who is in shock.
3. Recognize the signs and symptoms of selected coagulopathies.
4. Identify the supportive care required by the patient who is in shock.
5. Describe the treatment of selected coagulopathies.

Shock has been described as the "rude unhinging of the machinery of life." Shock is the manifestation of cellular insufficiency. No matter what the etiology of shock, the common denominator of all shock states is the amount of oxygen consumed by the cells.[8] Shock is divided into three major phases: a compensatory stage, a progressive stage, and an irreversible stage.[87]

Shock can result from alterations in circulating volume, cardiac pump function, and peripheral vascular resistance.[87] Shock causes a myriad of physiologic changes in the nervous, respiratory, renal, and gastrointestinal systems.[16]

Alteration in circulating volume, particularly hemorrhage, is one of the most common causes of shock and one frequently encountered by air medical teams. One complication of hemorrhage is the development of a coagulopathy. Dilutional effects of massive transfusions, continued bleeding, and hypothermia are some of the causes of coagulopathy seen by flight nurses.[7,28,44]

Disseminated intravascular coagulation (DIC) has been called the most important coagulopathy encountered by emergency care providers.[44] DIC is a secondary complication of such disease states as shock from traumatic injury, abruptio placentae, and anaphylaxis.[38,40]

This chapter discusses the etiology, pathophysiology, and initial management of shock. It also includes a discussion about coagulopathies because they are common complications related to the management of shock.

ETIOLOGY[18,19,27,46,54,62,80]

The multiple etiologies of shock are summarized in the box.

ETIOLOGIES OF SHOCK

- *Hemorrhagic:* Acute blood loss from an internal or external vascular injury.
  - *External:* Penetrating trauma, amputation, and open fractures
  - *Internal:* Injury (splenic, liver) fractures—particularly pelvic, body tissue injury, bleeding from other internal source such as gastrointestinal (GI) tract, and esophageal varices
- *Hypovolemia:* Fluid loss such as from third spacing, burn injury, vomiting, diarrhea, diabetes mellitus, diabetes insipidus, and diuresis
- *Neurogenic:* Spinal cord injury, alteration in vascular tone from drugs, food, plants, and venom
- *Anaphylaxis:* Allergic reaction to a foreign substance including drugs, food, plants, and venom
- *Obstructive:* Obstruction of blood flow (e.g., from a tension pneumothorax or cardiac tamponade)
- *Cardiac:* Pump failure that may result from a myocardial infarction, valvular malfunction, septal defect, right-sided infarct, or direct injury to the heart such as a myocardial contusion
- *Sepsis:* Infectious agent causing the shock cascade, shock secondary to sepsis now the most common cause of death in the intensive care unit (ICU), most common responsible bacteria *Escherichia coli, Klebsiella,* and staphylococci

PATHOPHYSIOLOGY

As previously stated, shock is the manifestation of cellular metabolic insufficiency. The amount of oxygen available for tissue consumption has been defined as oxygen delivery (DO_2). The body tissues do not extract all the oxygen available to them so that the body does have some reserve.[87]

The amount of oxygen extracted from tissues for metabolism has been defined as *oxygen consumption (VO_2)*. Oxygen consumption is calculated by determining the differences between the amount of oxygen delivered to the tissues and the amount of oxygen returned to the right side of the heart. Oxygen consumption depends on cardiac output, hemoglobin, SaO_2, and venous oxygen saturation (SVO_2). The normal VO_2 is 180 to 250 ml/min.[78,87]

When blood flow is diminished because of blood or fluid loss or redistribution of the circulating blood flow, the delivery of oxygen to the tissues is diminished. When enough oxygen to meet the needs of the body tissues is not available, an oxygen debt results. Oxygen debt has been described as the difference between tissue oxygen demand and oxygen consumption.[78,87]

Shock has been divided into three specific stages. These are the compensatory stage, the progressive stage, and the irreversible stage. No matter what the origin of shock, a decrease in available oxygen triggers cellular responses, which in turn affect all body systems.

Cellular Response

A reduction in the amount of available oxygen causes an alteration in cellular metabolism, resulting in a cascade of significant cellular changes and leading to injury and death if interventions prove ineffective or are too late. Figs. 9-1 and 9-2 illustrate the cellular and micropathophysiologic changes that occur during cellular ischemia.[78]

Body Systems Response

The lack of available oxygen to the cell initiates a cellular response as discussed that results in body system changes. As demonstrated in Fig. 9-3, the immune system reacts by the activation of a complement cascade that eventually release cytokines such

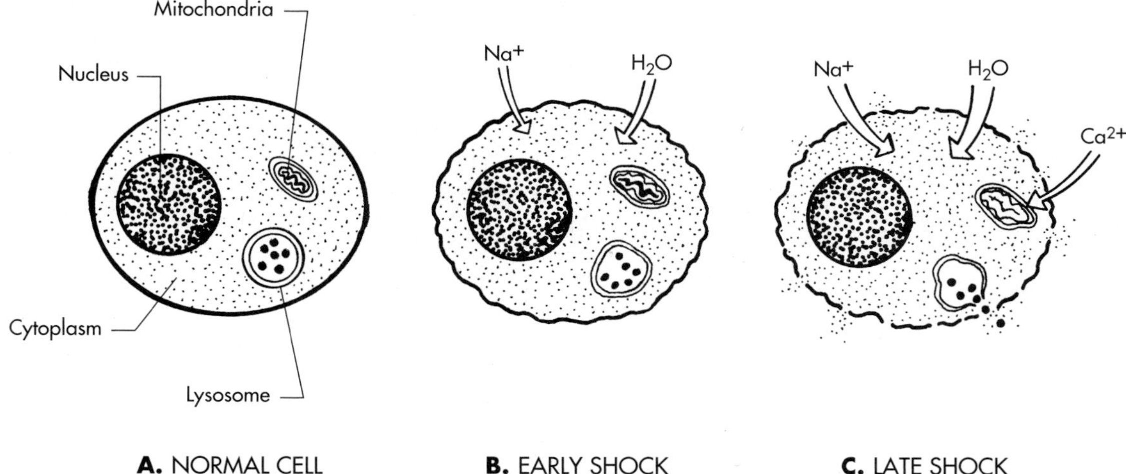

Fig. 9-1. A, Normal cell. **B,** Massive amounts of water and sodium enter the cytoplasm, causing blebs to develop. **C,** Calcium changes in the mitochondria causing destruction; lysosomes rupture, spilling proteolytic enzymes into the cytoplasm; the cell wall loses integrity, and the cell dies. (Redrawn from Kitt S et al: *Emergency nursing,* Philadelphia, 1995, Saunders.)

as tissue necrosis factor (TNF) and interleukin I (IN-I). These cytokines are key in the production of cellular toxins such as arachidonic acid, thromboxane, and leukotrienes. These substances lead to bronchoconstriction, platelet aggregation, capillary permeability, and vasoconstriction or vasodilation.[75,78]

Fig. 9-4 summarizes the other system changes associated with the hypoxia of shock that result in some of the classic signs and symptoms of shock. These include altered mental status, changes in skin color and temperature, and a decrease in or an absence of urinary output.[75,78,87]

Regardless of the source of shock, if it is not quickly recognized, the concomitant changes occurring in blood pressure, flow, and volume and the alterations in oxygen transport causing hypoxia will lead to tissue hypoxia, organ dysfunction, multiple organ failure, and death.[3,18,45,57]

The flight team must always be wary of the causes of shock and the subtlety of its signs and symptoms in its early stages. Research demonstrates that shock needs to be treated and reversed as soon as possible to prevent additional injury and eventual death.[5,9,68]

STAGES

Compensatory

During the compensatory phase of shock, the body attempts to compensate for the stress that has been caused by a specific illness or injury. One compensatory mechanism is stimulation of the baroreceptors, which causes a decrease in vagal tone and an increase in sympathetic discharge. The results of this mechanism are some of the classic signs and symptoms of shock, including an increase in heart rate, force of myocardial contractility, and venous and arterial vasoconstriction. This stage of shock is reversible.

Progressive

If the presence of shock goes unrecognized or the cause of it is not managed, the shock cycle will continue to progress. The initial insult that caused shock will continue to activate vicious cycles of compensatory mechanisms that, if not appropriately managed, will lead to death. During this phase the effects of tissue hypoxia and anaerobic metabolism are experienced.[35]. Cytokines such as TNF and the interleukins, especially I and 6, initiate the pathophys-

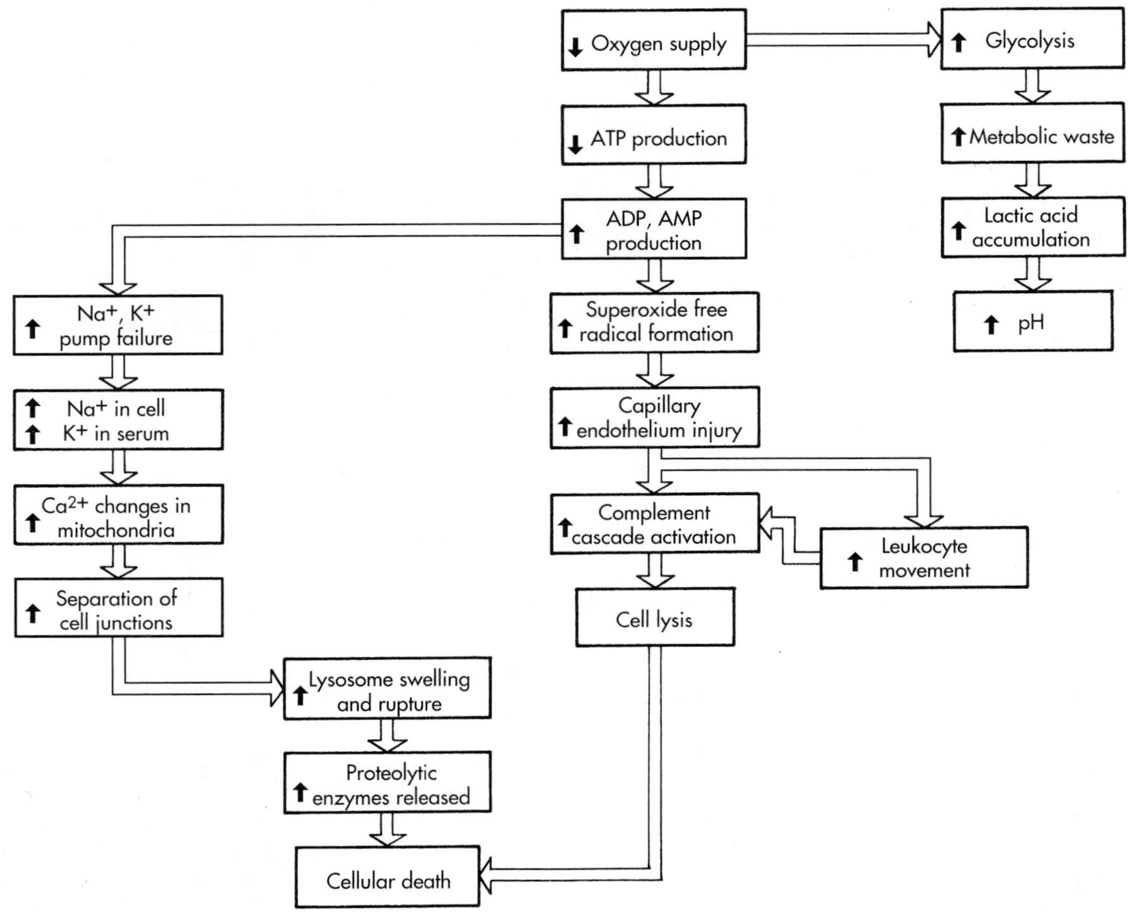

Fig. 9-2. Micropathophysiologic changes occurring during cellular ischemia. *ATP,* Adenosine triphosphate; *ADP,* adenosine diphosphate; *AMP,* adenosine monophosphate; *Na^+*, sodium ion; *K^+*, potassium ion; *Ca^{2+}*, calcium ion; *pH,* logarithm of the reciprocal of the hydrogen ion concentration. (Redrawn from Kitt S et al: *Emergency nursing,* Philadelphia, 1995, Saunders.)

iologic changes that may eventually lead to multiple organ failure.

Irreversible

In the irreversible stage of shock the body becomes refractory to treatment. In the final stages of shock the patient may still be alive but treatments such as fluid resuscitation, antibiotic administration, and ventilatory management become ineffective (Fig. 9-5). The reason this occurs is unknown.

Systemic Inflammatory Response Syndrome

In 1992 a new description for the shock cascade was proposed. The body's response to a clinical insult that causes shock or systemic inflammatory response syndrome (SIRS) was at first related more directly to septic shock, but as research continues, SIRS is probably involved in the first phase of shock.[8,13] Moore et al[56] proposed that this model can be easily applied to the management of the trauma patient and that unrecognized and undertreated shock after in-

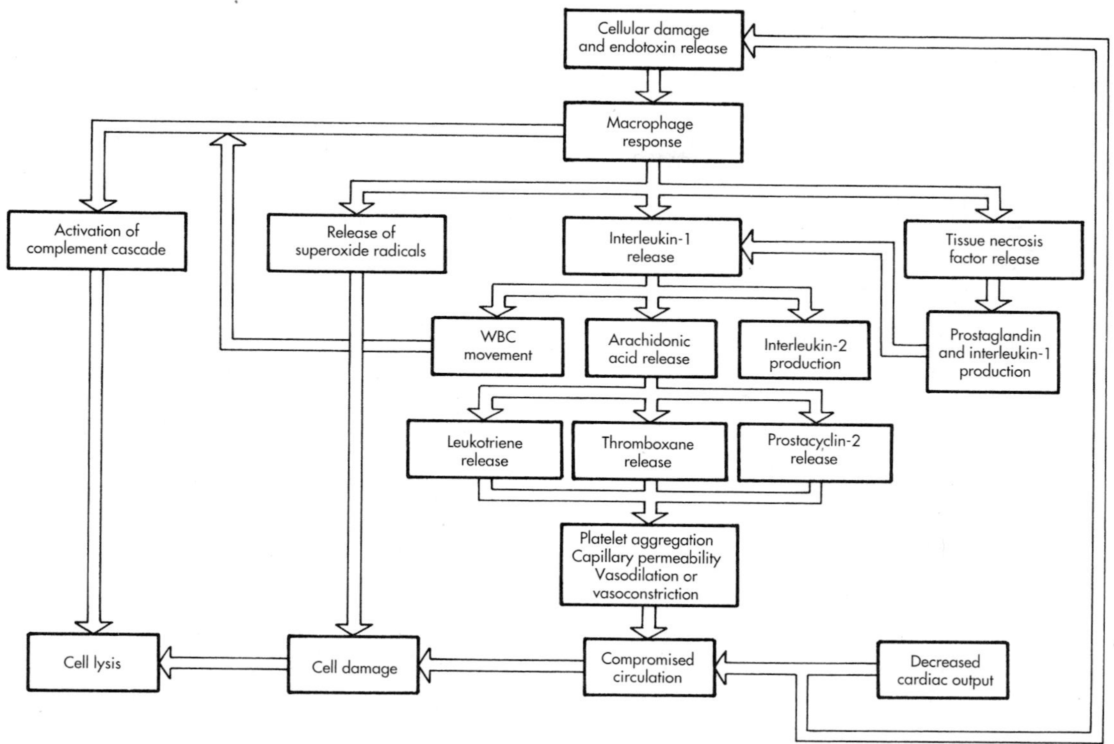

Fig. 9-3. Cascading response of the immune system in shock. (Redrawn from Kitt S et al: *Emergency nursing*, Philadelphia, 1995, Saunders.)

jury contribute to the occurrence of multiple organ failure and eventual death.

The pathophysiology of shock and current research emphasize the need for the flight team to recognize the presence and act quickly to prevent further injury. This may be through fluid resuscitation, blood administration, use of selected medications such as vasoactive drugs, and rapid transport to definitive care.[71]

PATIENT ASSESSMENT AND SHOCK MANAGEMENT

The management of the patient in shock begins with the recognition that the patient is in shock. Early recognition of shock directly affects the morbidity or mortality of the patient. Shock can be diagnosed early based on history and clinical signs such as weak and thready pulse, cold and clammy skin, pallor, and cyanosis. Simultaneous goals of therapy include the following[91]:

1. Correction of the initial insult by hemostasis, pericardiocentesis, treatment of arrhythmias, or antibiotics
2. Maintenance of vital organ function such as cardiac output, arterial blood pressure, and urinary output
3. Correction of secondary consequences such as hypovolemia, acidosis, hypoxemia, and DIC
4. Identification and correction of any aggravating factors manifested by evidence or suggested by a history of preexisting disease

Complete assessments and general therapy are accomplished almost simultaneously and should proceed as shown on p. 170.

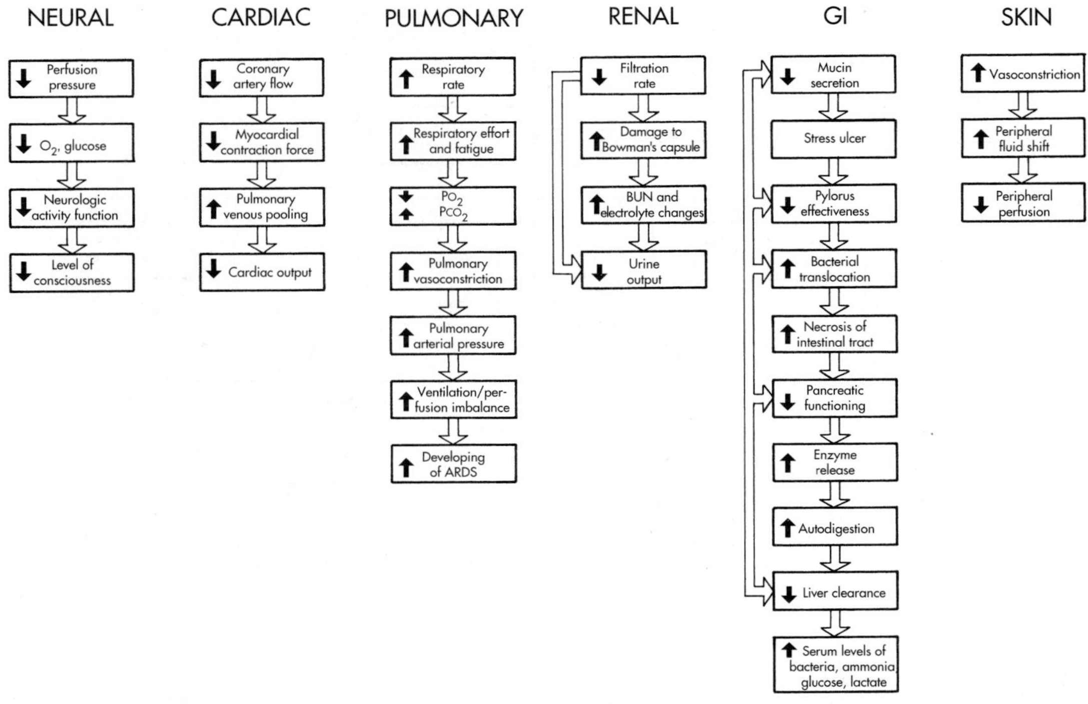

Fig. 9-4. Major organ system changes that occur from hypoxia associated with shock. *O_2*, Oxygen; *PO_2*, partial pressure of oxygen; *PCO_2*, partial pressure of carbon dioxide; *ARDS*, adult respiratory distress syndrome; *BUN*, blood urea nitrogen. (Redrawn from Kitt S et al: *Emergency nursing*, Philadelphia, 1995, Saunders.)

Correction of Hypoxia

The goal of correcting hypoxia during the initial resuscitation of the patient in shock is to correct the oxygen deficit that has occurred. The air medical team should use high-flow oxygen delivery systems, intubate or perform cricothyrotomy when necessary, and provide mechanical ventilation[82]. Respiratory muscle effort is the major site of oxygen expenditure for the resting patient and may place undue metabolic demands on the heart. Assisted ventilation providing maximal sedation and neuromuscular blockade may be necessary for the transport of a critically ill patient.

Fluid Resuscitation

Fluid resuscitation has become one of the most controversial topics in shock management over the past 6 years. As previously stated, research has questioned some of the previously common methods used to manage the patient in shock in prehospital and transport environments.[11,12,51]

The purpose of volume resuscitation is to restore oxygen transport and cellular uptake of needed oxygen, militate against the oxygen debt accumulation, repay a preresuscitation oxygen deficit, and prevent the complications of SIRS and the development of multiple organ failure. The prehospital and transport management of fluid resuscitation must pay careful attention to the long-term consequences of any intervention.[87,88]

Recent studies have shown that hypotension may be a protective mechanism. Unless the source of the bleeding can be adequately managed in the prehospital care environment, aggressively resuscitating a patient may do more harm than good. Increasing the blood pressure of a shock patient increases the risk

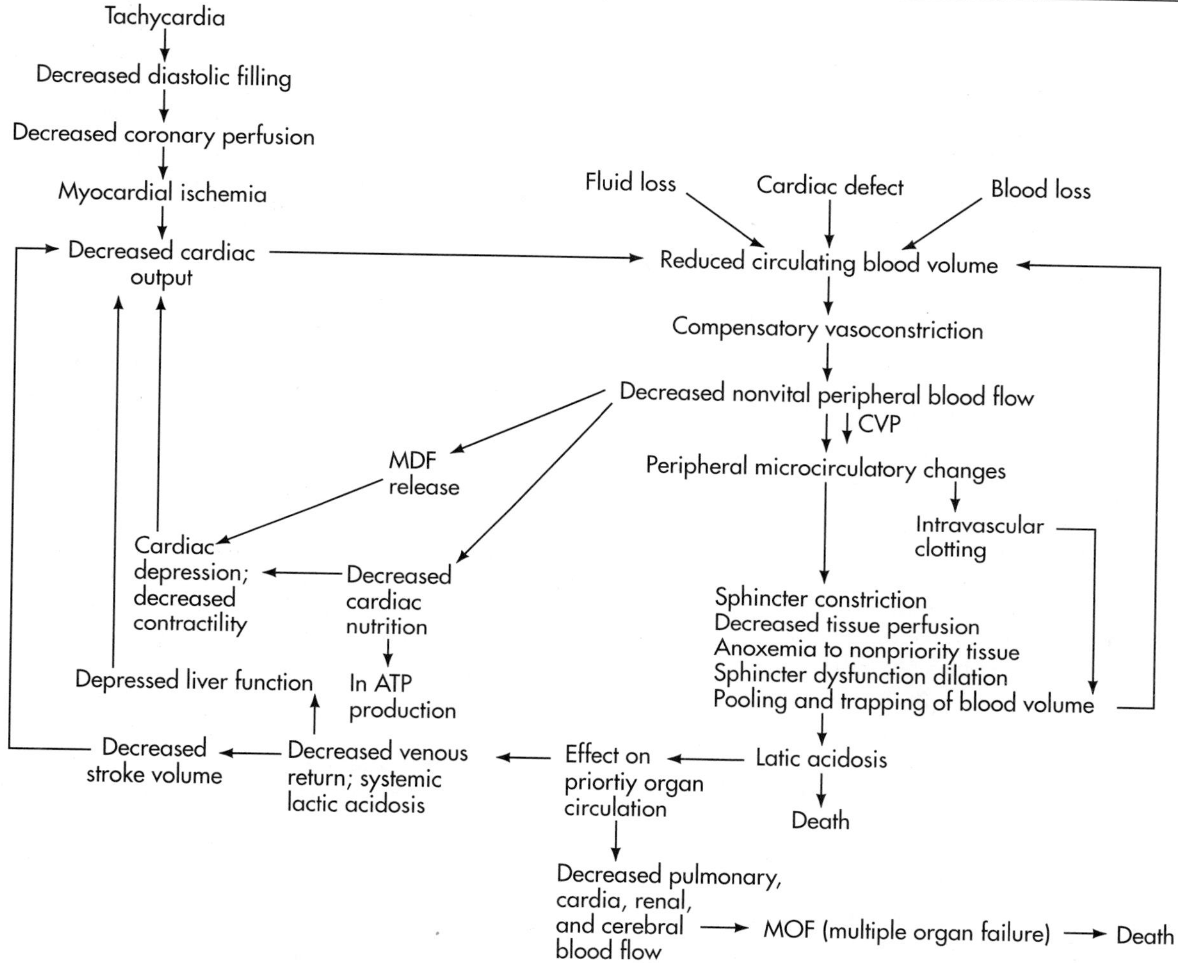

Fig. 9-5. Compounding factors in irreversible shock.

of bleeding, may dislodge formed clots, and depending on the resuscitation fluid, dilutes circulating volume and increases clotting time. Crystalloids and colloids do not carry oxygen, which is one of the primary fuels cells need to survive.*

The amount of fluid required by the shock patient—particularly those in hemorrhagic or hypovolemic shock—depends on the amount of intravascular volume depletion. During resuscitation the flight nurse needs to monitor the patient closely for sufficiency of volume replacement. The patient's blood pressure, pulse rate, level of consciousness, and urinary output (when available) provide parameters that can be monitored during transport. These parameters also supply the flight nurse with indications of a fluid overload.[72]

Multiple fluids have been used for resuscitation, including lactated Ringer's, normal saline, hypertonic saline, Hetastarch, and plasmanate. In hemorrhagic

*References 8, 10, 11, 17, 25, 29, 47, 50, 53, 59, 84.

STEPS IN INITIAL ASSESSMENT OF PATIENT IN SHOCK

1. Assess or establish airway, administer oxygen.
2. Stop hemorrhage, then inspect for wounds.
3. Measure BP, pulse, respiratory rate and depth, and temperature.
4. Assess mental status for consciousness (calculate Glasgow Coma Scale [GCS] value), alertness, confusion, pupillary response, motor response, and ability to follow commands.
5. Assess skin and skeleton; note abnormalities, deformities of skeleton, and weakness.
6. Assess perfusion: pulses, capillary refilling, cyanosis, conjunctiva, and temperature of the extremities.
7. Assess for jugular vein distended (JVD), or jugular vein flat.
8. Initiate intravenous access and follow appropriate fluid resuscitation protocol.
9. Apply cardiac monitor; treat lethal dysrhythmias.
10. Check urinary catheter; monitor output every 30 to 60 minutes.
11. Check invasive monitoring lines, hemodynamic manipulation with fluid, and pharmacologic therapy.
12. Assess laboratory studies of complete blood count (CBC) and levels of arterial blood gases (ABGs), potassium, calcium, magnesium, and other electrolytes.
13. Assess findings from x-ray examination, computerized axial tomography (CAT), arteriographic study, and other invasive and noninvasive diagnostic studies.

shock, blood and blood products are required for resuscitation. However, some flight programs do not carry O negative blood with them. Regardless of which fluids are chosen for resuscitation, the patient needs to be monitored closely for the effectiveness of resuscitation and the potential complications that may occur.*

*References 12, 25, 29, 31, 41, 42, 53, 58, 66, 72, 77.

The complications of massive fluid resuscitation include hypothermia, coagulopathy, metabolic derangements such as hypocalcemia and hypokalemia, organ dysfunction, and extravascular fluid shifts. These may lead to the development of ARDS adult respiratory distress syndrome (ARDS), sepsis syndrome, acute renal failure, DIC, pneumonia, multiple organ failure, and death.[67,81]

Pneumatic Antishock Garment

One of the most common methods once used in the management of the injured patient in shock was the application of pneumatic antishock garments (PASGs) or military antishock trousers (MAST). As the original name *MAST* suggests, this device was found to be of great use during the Vietnam War. However, little research had been done related to their effectiveness and the potential complications that could occur once they have been applied.[20,86]

Mattox et al[51] published a landmark study in 1989 that demonstrated several important points about the use of PASGs (box). This study and other animal model studies proved that PASGs did work, but their application in certain patient populations may actually increase patient morbidity and mortality.[51]

Currently, the Basic Trauma Life Support Course[18] recommends that the indications for the applications of PASG in the prehospital environment include external hemorrhage that can be controlled (PASG possibly being used initially until fluids are replaced), severe shock with no palpable pulses (nonpenetrating injury), and isolated spinal shock and as an air splint in pelvic fractures or bilateral lower extremity injuries.[18] Continued use of PASG can lead to the development of decubiti and other stasis injuries.[2,22]

Correction of Acidosis

Any respiratory component of acidosis can be corrected by proper ventilation. Sodium bicarbonate administration should be based on arterial pH measurements because overcorrecting can lead to alkalosis, which will shift the oxyhemoglobin dissociation curve to the left, decreasing oxygen delivery to the cells.[4,83,91] The flight nurse must also keep in mind that sodium bicarbonate is incompatible with many fluids and vasoactive medications.

SUMMARY OF 1989 MAST STUDY[51]

1. PASG application does not increase the length of prehospital time.
2. PASG does increase blood pressure.
3. PASG does not decrease the length of time in the emergency department, operating room, or hospital.
4. When PASG was applied, an overall increased mortality was seen for all patients.
5. Patients with prehospital time greater than 30 minutes and PASG application did not have better survival rates.
6. Patients with thoracic injuries had a greater chance of dying before arrival at the hospital if PASG was applied.
7. Patients with major abdominal injuries did not have an overall better survival rate if PASG was applied.

Pharmacologic Management

The pharmacologic management of shock depends on the source of the shock. For example, usually little need exists for pharmacologic agents in traumatic hemorrhagic shock. The primary therapy is administration of fluids, blood, and blood products. However, once the primary therapy has been initiated, pharmacologic management may be indicated if the patient does not improve.

Commonly used medications in the management of shock include inotropic agents, vasopressors, vasodilators, antibiotics, and steroids. The box contains a summary of some of the medications that may be used in shock management and indications for their use. Because dosages depend on the age, size, and severity of the patient's condition, the flight nurse needs to be familiar with the indications, dosages, and side effects of these medications.[43]

MEDICATIONS USED IN THE MANAGEMENT OF SHOCK

Antibiotics	Morphine sulfate
Dobutamine	Nitroglycerine
Dopamine	Sodium nitroprusside
Epinephrine	Steroids

Other Interventions

As summarized in the box on p. 164, multiple causes of shock exist. When the blood flow is obstructed as in cardiac tamponade and tension pneumothorax, the patient will exhibit signs and symptoms of shock. Critical interventions in obstructive shock include pericardiocentesis and thoracic decompression. Although some disease states may induce a pericardial tamponade or tension pneumothorax and contribute to obstructive shock, the most common causes of these life-threatening maladies are blunt and penetrating thoracic trauma.[18,21,30]

Pericardiocentesis is indicated for the patient in shock when blunt or penetrating trauma to the chest (particularly the sternum) has occurred and the patient is hypotensive and has bradycardia, distended neck veins, and muffled heart sounds.[18,21,30]

Needle decompression or chest tube insertion is indicated when the patient is in shock and experiencing severe respiratory distress, hypotension, bradycardia, jugular vein distention, and tracheal deviation. When the patient is intubated, difficulty ventilating this type of patient should alert the flight nurse to the potential of a tension pneumothorax, once again in the patient with a history of blunt and penetrating trauma.[18,21]

Other interventions that may be used in the management of shock are the mechanical devices used to assist circulation or increase tissue perfusion. Some of these devices include intraaortic balloon pumps (IAB), left ventricular assist devices (LVAD), and extracorporeal oxygenation devices (ECHMO). The uses of these types of equipment require special skills and significant preparation.[23]

Clinical Monitoring

Depending on the time, location, and initiation of interventions, the patient in shock may not have clinical monitoring devices in place. Multiple methods may be used to monitor the patient in shock, including hemodynamic and SVO_2 monitors. The box contains a summary of some of these clinical monitors.[15,19,33]

CARDIOPULMONARY AND METABOLIC MEASUREMENTS IN SHOCK

Arterial BP
Pulse rate and rhythm and, by calculation, the rate-pressure product
CVP and/or PCWP
CO and by calculation:
- CI stroke index
- Systemic vascular resistance
- Left ventricular stroke work index
- Right ventricular stroke work index
- Pulmonary vascular resistance
- Contractility estimation by plotting left ventricular end diastolic pressure against CO

Arterial blood PO_2, PCO_2, pH, and by derivation or secondary measurement:
- Arterial oxygen content
- Mixed venous O_2 tension
- Physiologic shunt
- Arteriovenous oxygen content difference
- Oxygen consumption
- Alveolar arterial oxygen content difference

Hemoglobin concentration
Urine flow and by secondary measurement:
- Specific gravity
- Urine-to-plasma creatinine concentration ratio
- Urine sodium concentration

Arterial blood lactate
Mental status
Electrolyte concentrations in plasma

Modified from MacLean A: *Ann Surg* 201(4):408, 1985.
BP, Blood pressure; *CVP,* central venous pressure; *PCWP,* pulmonary capillary wedge pressure; *CO,* cardiac output; *CI,* cardiac index.

Central venous and Swan-Ganz catheter pressures provide an index of the status of absolute and relative blood volume, the need for fluid replacement, and the effects of interventions. Accurate serial measurement of heart rate and rhythm, respiratory rate, cardiac filling pressure, cardiac output, tissue perfusion indices, and end-organ function (mental state and UO) must be done when possible.[24,49,73,79,91]

Regardless of the types of clinical monitor being used, the flight nurse needs to ensure that they can be used during transport. All ports, intravenous lines, and monitors need to be secured and accessible. If invasive monitors are being used, the flight nurse should document an initial reading once equipment has been changed and according to transport protocols or as the patient's condition indicates during transport.[33]

TREATMENT PROTOCOLS FOR LOW BLOOD VOLUME

Hemorrhage

Description

Circulation can be compromised in various ways. Failure of circulation occurs either locally or systemically, resulting in shock. Systemic circulation failure is caused by inadequate blood volume or a pump defect. The first of three types of inadequate volume is hemorrhage, or loss of plasma and red cell mass from the vascular system. Hemorrhage is either internal or external: The amount depends on the vessel, the extent of damage, and the ability to form and maintain a clot. The effect of hemorrhage depends on the preexisting state of the cardiovascular, respiratory, renal, and hematologic systems.[68]

Normal blood volume is approximately 7% of the ideal adult body weight (approximately 70 ml/kg) and 80 to 90 ml/kg in children.[26] In hemorrhage a graded physiologic response is based on the percentage of blood volume lost acutely. The clinical symptoms progress as blood loss increases.

The blood pressure sometimes does not change until 30% to 40% of the total blood volume is lost. Specific attention should be paid to pulse rate, respiratory rate, skin circulation, pulse pressure, and the patient's mental status.[26]

Intrathoracic and intraabdominal bleeding (cavitary hemorrhage) are well recognized as causes of hypovolemia in trauma. Significant losses from noncavitary losses (pelvic fracture, skin laceration, and multiple long-bone fractures) may result in a 20% to 50% total blood loss, placing the patient into a severe shock state.

An isolated, closed femur fracture can result in up to 2½ L of blood lost in the fracture hematoma. In pelvic fractures, 40% to 50% of the total blood volume may be lost. The mortality rate in pelvic fracture is 6.4% to 15%; however, 42% to 70% of the deaths are attributed to blood loss. These patients require aggressive resuscitation.

Noncavitary blood losses contribute to additional loss of blood in 85.2% of patients with intraabdominal or intrathoracic hemorrhage. Blood losses will occur in 2 to 5 hours after the injury, so air medical crew members should be alert for delayed hypovolemia.

Treatment requires tamponading of the bleeding and supporting and splinting fractures. Fluid management includes administering crystalloid and blood. Knowing that severe blood losses can occur with noncavitary losses is essential for early recognition to ensure proper treatment and prevent wasted time in searching for cavitary hemorrhage.[60,62,63]

Indicators

A history of any of the following factors should lead to suspicion of hemorrhage:

- Trauma to the thorax, abdomen, pelvis, or an extremity
- Melena or hematochezia
- Hematemesis
- Hemoptysis or epistaxis
- Vaginal bleeding
- Surgery

Predisposing Conditions

The following conditions can predispose to hemorrhage:

- Anemia
- Hemoglobinopathies
- Thrombocytopenia
- Liver disease
- Any hemorrhagic diathesis, hemophilia, and DIC
- Neoplastic disease
- Peptic ulcer disease
- Alcoholism
- Atherosclerosis
- Sepsis
- Surgery

Causes

Internal Hemorrhage

- Pleural cavity hemorrhage: intrathoracic vessel trauma, dissecting aortic aneurysm, ruptured varices, fracture
- Peritoneal cavity hemorrhage: liver, spleen, or any artery trauma; abdominal aneurysm; tumor; arteritis; volvulus; strangulated ovarian cyst
- Retroperitoneum hemorrhage: tumor, trauma fracture, ectopic pregnancy; soft tissue extremity trauma, fracture, venipuncture; skin trauma, purpura
- Bladder hemorrhage: tumor, transurethral prostatectomy
- Cavity hemorrhage: complication of surgery

External Hemorrhage

- GI tract hemorrhage (associated with hematemesis): inflammatory gastritis, peptic ulcer disease (PUD), esophagitis, tumor of esophagus, stomach
- Endotracheal hemorrhage: esophageal lacerations, foreign body ingestion, abdominal trauma
- Vascular hemorrhage: varices, aneurysms, mesenteric occlusion, hematologic disease
- GI tract (associated with hematochezia): ulcerative colitis (inflammatory), shigellosis (infectious), amebiasis, tumor, vascular hemorrhoids, volvulus, mesenteric occlusion; Meckel's diverticulum (congenital)
- Respiratory tract hemorrhage: trauma, inflammation, infection, vascular lesions, infarction of lung, bleeding in an abscess, ruptured aortic aneurysm, bronchiectasis
- Vaginal hemorrhage: pregnancy, abortion, abruptio placentae, placenta previa, lacerations from delivery, cervical and endometrial cancer, dysfunctional uterine bleeding

Fluid Loss

Description

The second of the three major types of inadequate volume is fluid loss. This occurs in conditions with a reduced blood volume and hemoconcentration because of water loss and unusually high solute loss.

The usual modes of fluid loss are vomiting, diarrhea, excessive sweating (fever, heatstroke), excessive urination, and loss from body surface area of denuded skin. (The management of burns and burn shock is discussed in Chapter 16.)

Indicators

A history of the following would indicate low blood volume due to fluid loss. In addition, hematocrit levels and CVP values are good indicators of fluid loss:

Burns
Diarrhea, vomiting, excessive urination, sweating
Poorly controlled diabetes, lowered insulin usage with polyuria
Exposure to environment for prolonged time with decreased food and water supply
Fever
Ascites
Extensive surgery
Diuretic use or abuse

Predisposing Conditions

A patient with any of the following conditions could be predisposed to low blood volume caused by fluid loss:

Age: very young or very old
Surgery: GI resections, hyposectomy, extensive resections
Diabetes mellitus
Adrenal insufficiency
Drugs: diuretic therapy
Hyperthyroidism
Regional enteritis, ulcerative colitis
Liver disease
PUD
Malnutrition, anemia
Peritonitis, pelvic inflammatory disease
Neoplasia
Diabetes insipidus

Examples of causes of excessive fluid loss are urinary fluid loss with hyperglycemia in diabetes, excessive use of diuretics, and addisonian crisis and burns. Children and older adults are more susceptible to dehydration because their supply of fluids depends on their ability to communicate their need for fluid to others. Comatose patients are at high risk. In addition, patients with nasogastric suction, vomiting, diarrhea, sickle cell disease, calcemic nephropathy, and surgical fistulas are at risk.

Abnormal Peripheral Distribution

Description

Loss of blood volume can be caused by vasomotor dysfunction with sequestration of blood in the resistance circuit or venous capacitance bed. The absolute blood volume does not change, but an increase in vascular space results in a decrease of effective blood volume and tissue perfusion. Vasomotor dysfunction results in (1) high or normal arterial resistance with expanded venous capacitance (pooling) or (2) low arterial resistance with arteriovenous shunting.

Septic Shock

Sepsis, a very common cause of shock, is defined as the systemic response to an infection. Each year, thousands of people die of sepsis in the United States.[37,39] In 1992, septic shock was reclassified and defined as sepsis-induced hypotension despite adequate fluid resuscitation with lactic acidosis, oliguria, and acute alteration in mental status.[1,2,68,69,85]

Early in the course of sepsis, the patient has fever, hyperventilation, respiratory alkalosis, increased cardiac output, and decreased systemic peripheral vascular resistance (SPVR). This is often referred to as *warm* or *hyperdynamic shock.* Regional perfusion does not meet metabolic needs, and eventually the patient becomes hypodynamic, hypovolemic with a decreased cardiac output, peripherally vasoconstricted, hypotensive with a narrow pulse pressure, and oliguric. Blood is pooled in the venous capacitance bed and lost from fever, vomiting, diarrhea, and third spacing of fluids.

As shock progresses, multiple organ failure occurs. After the flight nurse obtains appropriate blood cultures and cultures of other potential infection sites, appropriate antibiotic therapy should be started.

Proper management includes hemodynamic invasive monitoring. Treatment should include increasing cardiac output and oxygen delivery, improving tissue perfusion, and decreasing tissue hypoxia. Increasing cardiac output to 50% or greater than normal improves survival. Arterial lactate levels measure severity of perfusion failure. The goal is to decrease lactate levels by 50% over 24 hours.[32]

In most cases, vigorous fluid resuscitation will reverse the perfusion failure. Hemodynamic monitoring of the pulmonary capillary wedge pressure (PCWP) and cardiac output is essential. Fluid challenges of 250 ml may be given every 15 minutes until the increase in PCWP no longer boosts the cardiac output.

If prominent signs of vasoconstriction exist, air medical personnel should consider vasodilators. Sodium nitroprusside and phentolamine will decrease PVR and increase cardiac output. β-Adrenergic drugs may be useful, such as low-dose dopamine, and dobutamine.

Several research protocols are currently being used in the management of sepsis. Flight nurses need to be familiar with the prescribed treatment being used by critical care researchers in their service area.

Neurogenic Shock

Neurogenic shock is a result of an injury or insult to the reticular activating system and spinal cord. In the presence of major brainstem dysfunction or spinal cord injury, hypotension without tachycardia or cutaneous vasoconstruction may be of neurogenic cause. Vasoactive drugs should not be administered until volume is restored. Many times, if no blood loss has occurred, hypotension may be resolved by placing the patient flat or in a slight Trendelenburg position if no injury to the cervical spine has occurred as confirmed by medical personnel. Respiratory insufficiency is common, and ventilatory support should be implemented as necessary.[23,26,61]

The treatment of spinal shock includes appropriate immobilization for transport and initiation of pharmacologic management for hypotension. Vasoactive drugs such as dopamine may be needed to maintain peripheral vasoconstriction. If the flight nurse transports the patient within 8 hours of the injury, methyl prednisone should be started to decrease the effects of inflammation on the spinal cord. The initial dose of methyl prednisone is 30 mg/kg over 15 minutes followed 45 minutes later by a maintenance infusion of 5.4 mg/kg over 23 hours.

The flight nurse must also ensure that the patient is kept warm because spinal cord injury leaves the patient poikilothermic. In addition, the nurse must be sure no pressure is being exerted on the patient's skin that may cause further injury because the patient is insensitive to it.

Anaphylaxis

Anaphylaxis is an acute systemic allergic reaction as a result of the release of chemical mediators after an antigen-antibody reaction. It is mediated by immunoglobin E (IgE), which rests on the surface of mast cells and basophils in the body, especially along the respiratory and GI tracts. With a reaction occurs the formation and release of histamine, the kinins, and the slow, reactive substance of anaphylaxis. These cause three major effects: (1) vasodilation, (2) smooth muscle spasm, and (3) increased vascular permeability with edema formation[39,78] (Fig. 9-5).

Anaphylactoid reactions (not mediated by IgE) have identical signs and symptoms and are caused most often by drugs such as iodinated x-ray contrast, procaine compounds, and fluorescein. In either reaction, the sooner the onset, the more severe the reaction is likely to be.

Patients experience a sense of impending doom; pruritus, especially of the palms and feet; and sudden headache. Adverse reactions may occur quickly and affect all systems[78]:

Respiratory: upper airway edema; angioedema of hypopharynx, epiglottis, larynx, and trachea; asthma; stridorous breathing with supraclavicular, suprasternal, and intercostal retractions

Cutaneous: flushing, pruritus, urticaria, and angioedema

Cardiovascular: arrhythmias and electrocardiogram (ECG) abnormalities, probably caused by decreased coronary perfusion and oxygenation; vasodilation and hypotension possibly occurring with or without other symptoms from venous pooling or increased capillary permeability and water loss into the interstitial space

Neurologic: sudden loss of consciousness, seizures, cerebral anoxia secondary to airway obstruction, and decreased blood pressure

Rarely, GI spasm of smooth muscle leading to cramps, diarrhea, sudden and explosive involuntary defecation, and vomiting with potential for aspiration

Genitourinary: incontinence and laborlike pains in female uterus

Death from upper airway obstruction, vomiting and aspiration, bronchospasm, and vascular collapse

Management. Treatment for patients with anaphylaxis is as follows:

For some stings and bites, compression dressings may be applied to decrease the progress of the toxin. If the injection site is on an extremity, the nurse should apply a tourniquet proximal to the site.

Epinephrine—Administration of 1:1000 epinephrine subcutaneously dilates bronchial smooth muscle, causes vasoconstriction, and decreases vascular permeability.

Dosage:

Adult: 0.3 ml and 0.3 ml at site, repeating every 15 to 20 minutes, 4 to 5 times, if needed

Child: 0.005 ml/kg, repeating every 15 to 20 minutes if needed

For severe reactions a 1:10,000 epinephrine solution (5 ml) may be given intravenously and repeated every 5 to 10 minutes.

Antihistamine (Diphenhydramine)—An antihistamine will compete with the binding sites.

Dosage: 50 to 100 mg by mouth or intravenously in severe reactions

The nurse should administer oxygen, monitor the patient, and administer IV saline or crystalloid.

The nurse should secure the airway by intubation or cricothyrotomy.

The nurse should initiate cardiopulmonary resuscitation.

Administration of steroids is also needed.

Unexpected anaphylaxis with a rapid clinical course may result in a swift recovery or death. There is little time to act; early recognition is therefore essential.

Obstructive Shock

Description. Circulation can be compromised and the patient become hypotensive and hypoxic because of direct failure of the heart muscle or compression or obstruction. The result of this pathophysiologic process may be a pericardial tamponade or tension pneumothorax.

Cardiac tamponade and tension pneumothorax, once recognized, are easily reversible mechanical obstructions to cardiac output. Cardiac tamponade occurs when blood or effusion accumulates in the closed pericardial sac. The heart is unable to fill, the central venous pressure rises, blood pressure and pulse rate decrease, and heart sounds may be muffled (Beck's triad). Needle pericardiocentesis is the treatment of choice.

Tension pneumothorax results in a complete collapse of one or both lungs with compression on mediastinal vessels and organs. Air under tension may be evacuated by needle or chest tube insertion.

Indicators. A history of any of the following may indicate the potential for mechanical obstruction resulting in hypotension and hypoxia:

Chest pain
Dyspnea
Syncope
Trauma to the chest

Predisposing Conditions. Predisposing conditions include the following:

Blunt or penetrating trauma
Preexisting pulmonary disease such as chronic obstructive pulmonary disease or asthma
Cardiomyopathy
Bacterial endocarditis

COAGULOPATHIES

One of the common complications of shock is the development of coagulopathies and DIC, particularly as the result of massive blood loss and fluid resuscitation. In addition, the presence of a preexisting condition such as hemophilia or the patient's taking of a medication such as Coumarin that interferes with coagulation poses further challenges in patient care.

Hemorrhage is a common component of the clinical picture for many patients transported by air. Most patients who are bleeding have normal clotting mechanisms, and when normal measures taken to control bleeding are not effective, a coagulopathy, or bleeding disorder, may be suspected. Diagnosing a specific coagulopathy in the transport environment is difficult or impossible, but an index of suspicion should be raised in certain cases based on the flight nurse's assessment of the patient, the available history, and an evaluation of laboratory findings that may be available if the patient is transported between facilities. Some patients will have an established history of an inherited coagulopathy, whereas others may be expected to have a bleeding disorder or tendency toward such a disorder based on their current disease process. Confirmation of that suspicion will require more extensive laboratory testing than is available in most community hospitals and is best determined by consultation with a hematologist or an internist in a medical center with experience and facilities to properly evaluate and care for the patient.

A *coagulopathy* is defined as "any disorder of blood coagulation."[34,36,44,89] This is a broad categorization of a variety of disorders that interfere with the ability of the body to control hemorrhage. Some coagulopathies are inherited disorders, whereas others are acquired and unrelated to genetic tendencies. Coagulopathies can be primary disorders or secondary to an underlying disease. Of the 12 clotting factors (box), clotting factor may be deficient, or another stage of the clotting cascade may not function normally. Some coagulopathies are life threatening; others are so mild as to go undetected until late in life. Approximately 80,000 deaths in the United States occur each year from bleeding disorders of acquired or congenital origin.[7]

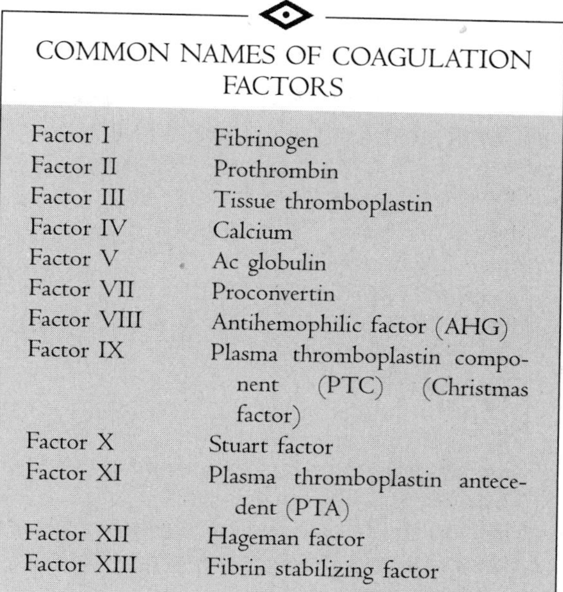

COMMON NAMES OF COAGULATION FACTORS

Factor I	Fibrinogen
Factor II	Prothrombin
Factor III	Tissue thromboplastin
Factor IV	Calcium
Factor V	Ac globulin
Factor VII	Proconvertin
Factor VIII	Antihemophilic factor (AHG)
Factor IX	Plasma thromboplastin component (PTC) (Christmas factor)
Factor X	Stuart factor
Factor XI	Plasma thromboplastin antecedent (PTA)
Factor XII	Hageman factor
Factor XIII	Fibrin stabilizing factor

Incidence

Some coagulopathies are hereditary in origin. The famous "bleeders" of history have been victims of hemophilia. Any deficiency of 1 of the 12 clotting factors may cause a clotting disorder, but the most commonly seen hereditary coagulopathies are hemophilia A, hemophilia B, and von Willebrand's disease.

Hereditary Coagulopathies

Hemophilia A

Of all the hereditary coagulopathies, hemophilia A, sometimes called "classic hemophilia," is the most common. About 70% to 90% of "hemophiliacs" have hemophilia A. It is seen in 1 to 2 of every 10,000 people in the United States.[64] The gene is found on the X chromosome and is transmitted as a sex-linked recessive trait; therefore nearly all its victims are male. Female carriers (heterozygotes) pass the gene to one-half their daughters, who then also become carriers, and to one-half their sons, who will have the disease. Males with the disease (hemizygotes) pass the gene to all of their daughters, who become asymptomatic carriers; sons are normal. Of hemophilia patients, 30% have no family history of the disease.

Hemophilia B

Also called "Christmas disease," hemophilia B is similar to hemophilia A. About 9% of those with

DIC-RELATED DISEASE STATES

Obstetric

Abruptio placentae
Amniotic fluid embolism
Toxemia of pregnancy
Hydatidiform mole
Retained dead fetus
Septic abortion

Infection

Bacterial: gram-negative or gram-positive septicemia
Rickettsial: Rocky Mountain spotted fever
Viral: varicella, rubella, arboviruses, influenza A
Parasitic: *Plasmodium falciparum* malaria
Fungal: histoplasmosis

Trauma

Trauma with shock
Head injury
Burns
Anoxia
Heatstroke

Malignancy

Metastatic carcinoma: pancreas, lung, breast, stomach, prostate, colon
Acute promyelocytic leukemia

Shock States

Cardiac arrest

Miscellaneous

Aortic aneurysm
Snakebite
Transfusion reactions
Anaphylactic drug reactions
Prostatic surgery
Lung surgery
Extrocorporeal circulation

inherited coagulation defects have this disease. It is 15% as frequent as hemophilia A and is found in approximately 1 of every 100,000 persons in the United States.[64] Like hemophilia A, it is found almost entirely in males as a sex-linked recessive trait.

von Willebrand's Disease

This form of hemophilia occurs in 5 to 10 of every 1,000,000 persons in the United States. It is found in both genders because it is inherited as an autosomal dominant trait.[7,34]

Acquired Disorders

Coagulopathies may also be acquired rather than inherited. Acquired disorders occur much more commonly than inherited ones.[7,34] These bleeding disorders are secondary to another disease process or therapy. Although many varieties exist, the types most likely to confront the flight nurse are described in the following sections.

Vitamin K Deficiency

Vitamin K must be present in the blood for clotting to occur. It is obtained by the body through the diet and produced by intestinal bacteria. Vitamin K levels may be deficient due to poor diet or sterilization of the gut from antibiotic therapy. Patients at risk include the postoperative patient with oral intake who is on an extended course of antibiotic therapy.

Hepatic Coagulopathy

Liver disease is one of the most common causes of coagulopathy. Because 11 of the 12 clotting factors are synthesized in the liver, patients with liver dysfunction, particularly those with severe cirrhosis, are deficient in those factors. In addition, vitamin K deficiency often contributes to the coagulopathy because patients with liver disease are unable to store vitamin K at optimum levels.

Disseminated Intravascular Coagulation

DIC is a complex disease that has been found at autopsy in 3% to 10% of cases.[6] It is a secondary response to many diseases, including some infections, malignancies, and obstetric complications.[44] Braunwald[14] stated that sepsis is one of the most common disorders associated with DIC. The box lists many of the disease states for which DIC may be a further complication.

Robbins[14,44] stated that 50% of DIC patients are obstetric patients, and 33% have terminal cancers. DIC appears to result from the entrance of substances into the blood that cause accelerated clotting, thus the variety of primary diseases (see box) with which it has been associated.

Drug-Induced Coagulopathies

A variety of medications can either enhance or inhibit clotting. Drug-induced coagulopathies may be the most commonly seen cause of abnormal bleeding.[65] However, a few of these medications alone will cause significant problems without accompanying platelet or clotting-factor deficiency.[55]

Massive Transfusions

Another cause of bleeding that can be seen by air medical personnel is the dilutional effect of massive transfusions. Banked blood is deficient in clotting factors and platelets, and hemorrhage may occur in the patient who has received large volumes of crystalloid or banked blood without attention to clotting factors or platelet replacement. Those at risk include patients with major trauma, GI hemorrhage, or obstetric complication.

NORMAL PHYSIOLOGY

Hemostasis, the arrest of bleeding, is an extremely complex process. The normal coagulation process is a balance between uncontrolled bleeding and generalized thrombosis or clotting. (Fig. 9-6 summarizes the coagulation process.) The flight nurse needs some understanding of the coagulative process to be adequately prepared for patients with actual or potential coagulopathies.

At least four components are necessary for normal clotting to take place: (1) blood vessels, (2) platelets, (3) clotting, and (4) fibrinolysis, or clot dissolution.[74] If any one of these components malfunctions or is deficient, a coagulopathy will result. Nearly every conceivable aspect of these four components has been known to malfunction. A few disorders are seen much more frequently than others—the remaining bleeding disorders are rather rare.

Blood vessels are composed of connective and smooth muscle tissue lined with endothelial cells.

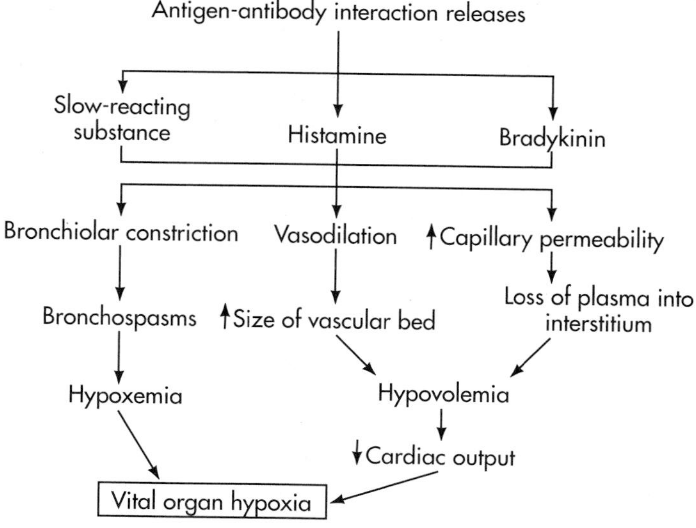

Fig. 9-6. Pathophysiology of anaphylactic shock.

Vessel walls serve as an important protective barrier to contain and protect the circulating blood. If injured, the vessel constricts at the site of injury through a reflex nervous system response. This decreases blood flow and slows bleeding. In addition, after blunt trauma, blood flowing into the injured tissue creates a hematoma, which decreases blood loss by mechanical pressure, tamponading the ruptured vessel.

The second and third components, platelets and clotting factors, interact to form the clot. Platelets, also known as *thrombocytes,* are actually cell fragments from larger cells called *karyocytes,* which are formed in the bone marrow. When a blood vessel is injured, collagen is exposed in the connective tissue. Collagen is oppositely charged to the circulating platelets, causing platelets to be attracted to the injured site. The platelets adhere to exposed tissue and vessel walls, but they also stick or aggregate to one another, forming a platelet plug. Platelets then rupture as they plug the damaged vessel wall, releasing incomplete thromboplastin, also known as *clotting factor III.* Clotting factor III reacts with calcium, called *factor IV,* and several other blood factors to help form the permanent clot. The platelet plug is adequate to stop minor bleeding at least temporarily, but more severe bleeding also requires the interaction of coagulation factors to form a stable fibrin clot.

Collagen exposed at the injured site activates factor XII, which stimulates other reactions, eventually forming thrombin, enhancing the aggregation of platelets. Thrombin also converts fibrinogen, factor I, which is present in plasma, into fibrin, an insoluble protein of densely intertwined threads that catch erythrocytes and platelets.

After the clot has served its purpose in stopping the hemorrhage, the fibrin clot is dissolved by the fibrinolytic system. This process, known as *fibrinolysis,* begins within 24 hours after clot formation. Plasminogen, a serum globulin found in the clot, is activated by substances in the blood and becomes plasmin, a proteolytic enzyme that digests proteins, including fibrin, fibrinogen, and factors V and VIII. This prevents the permanent thrombosis of the injured blood vessel.

PATHOPHYSIOLOGY

Hereditary Coagulopathies

Hemophilia A

The hemophilias are the most common hereditary bleeding disorders, and hemophilia A is the most prevalent of the hemophilias. The deficiency in this disease is factor VIII, also known as *antihemophilic factor,* with severity of symptoms closely related to the level of factor VIII in the blood. Platelet plug formation is normal; however, deficiency of factor VIII impairs the capacity to form a stable fibrin clot. The disease is almost always discovered by age 5, although mild cases may not be recognized until after trauma or surgery as an adult.[74]

Between acute episodes of bleeding, hemophiliacs may be without symptoms unless they are anemic from previous blood loss. Medical attention will be sought for hemarthroses (bleeding into joints), hematuria, and epistaxis. Bleeding can also occur into deep tissues. Mucosal bleeding is unusual, as is GI bleeding, unless peptic ulcer disease is also present. Trauma is often the cause of bleeding, and that bleeding may occur or reoccur 8 hours or even 1 to 3 days after the injury and continue for days or weeks.

Bleeding is particularly dangerous when pressure is exerted on organs, vessels, or nerves. It can be life threatening when it is intracranial, lingual, laryngeal, retropharyngeal, pericardial, pleural, or simply exsanguinating. CNS hemorrhage is the leading cause of death of hemophiliacs and should be taken seriously.[65] CNS bleeding may occur spontaneously unrelated to trauma or a specific lesion.

A long history of severe or poorly controlled hemophilia may leave the patient severely handicapped with permanent joint damage resulting from hemarthroses, causing fibrous or bony ankylosis. Hemophiliacs may also suffer complications secondary to the treatment process. Multiple blood product transfusions or factor-concentrate infusions can result in liver disease, hepatitis, and HIV.

Hemophilia B

Hemophilia B is very similar to hemophilia A. It is a hereditary disorder with the same genetic pattern, affecting primarily males. Hemophilia B is caused by a deficiency of factor IX activity. This results in prolonged partial thromboplastin (PT) times. Clinical symptoms and bleeding are the same as in hemophilia A, as is the risk to the patient's life.

von Willebrand's Disease

von Willebrand's disease is a result of two defects: defective platelet adherence and decreased levels of factor VIII. Platelets occur in normal numbers but do not adhere to the subendothelial collagen of the capillary wall to form the platelet plug. Therefore bleeding is prolonged. von Willebrand's disease is usually milder than hemophilia A or B. Bleeding is mostly from skin or mucous membranes rather than deep bleeding into tissue or joints. Easy bruising, epistaxis, dental bleeding, menorrhagia, and GI bleeding are the usual clinical manifestations.[65]

Acquired Coagulopathies

Bleeding disorders that are acquired are seen more often by the flight nurse than inherited coagulopathies.

Vitamin K Deficiency

Factors II, VII, IX, and X are vitamin K dependent, requiring the presence of vitamin K to function normally.[55] The body acquires vitamin K from leafy green vegetables in the diet and as a by-product of intestinal bacteria. If these sources are not available to the body, a deficiency will result in 2 to 4 weeks. Hemorrhage from vitamin K deficiency can occur in patients receiving antibiotic therapy for extended periods while taking nothing by mouth because antibiotics may "sterilize" the gut, eliminating the bacterial source of vitamin K. Intestinal malabsorption and liver disease can cause bleeding from vitamin K deficiency. Hemorrhagic disease of the newborn is also a vitamin K deficiency caused by a lack of vitamin K–producing intestinal flora and the immaturity of the liver.[14]

Hepatic Coagulopathy

Liver disease is a common cause of coagulopathy. It is most often seen in patients with severe hepatic cirrhosis but also occurs with other acute and chronic liver diseases. Any patient with severe liver dysfunction is at risk for hemorrhage. All coagulation factors except VIII are synthesized in the liver by hepatocytes. Therefore patients with liver disease will be deficient in those factors. However, before bleeding occurs, liver disease is usually advanced and easily recognized by other signs of the disease.

Other factors may contribute to bleeding tendencies in the patient with liver disease. A vitamin K deficiency may result from intestinal malabsorption, poor dietary habits, or the anorexia associated with liver disease. Further coagulopathy is often present because of low platelet count and platelet dysfunction. Finally, liver disease results in increased proteolytic activity in the blood, probably because the liver has a decreased ability to remove these proteolytic substances from circulation. The clinical picture is very close to that of DIC, which may also develop.

Disseminated Intravascular Coagulation

DIC has been called the most important coagulopathy in the emergency department.[65] This life-threatening disorder is actually a secondary complication of a broad spectrum of diseases (see box on p. 178). It may have a variety of causes, including the entry of foreign protein into circulation or massive vascular injury, as occurs in crushing trauma. Whatever the cause, the result is that the coagulation and fibrinolytic systems are out of control. Platelets and coagulation factors are consumed by this abnormal clotting. Thrombin formation overwhelms its inhibitor system, further accelerating clotting and activation of fibrinogen. Fibrin is deposited in the microvasculature of many organs, resulting in poor tissue perfusion and eventual focal necrosis of tissue. Organ failure may result. Later the fibrinolytic system loses fibrin and impairs thrombin formation, and clots wash away. In summary, platelets, clotting factors, and fibrinogen are consumed so quickly that the body is unable to replace them and maintain hemostatic levels. This creates a clinical picture of petechiae, peripheral cyanosis, GI bleeding, vaginal bleeding, prolonged bleeding, ecchymoses, hematomas, bleeding from surgical or invasive procedure sites, and signs of organ injury.

Drug-Induced Coagulopathies

Coumarin. The coumarins, primarily dicoumarol and warfarin, are medications frequently prescribed. Coumarin interferes with the action of vitamin K, causing a deficiency with resultant bleeding. Levels of prothrombin and factors VII and X are particularly decreased. Inappropriate dosage levels, need for dosage adjustment, or intentional overdosage by the patient can be the cause of the coagulopathy.

Heparin. Heparin has several actions, the most important of which is the inactivation of thrombin. With the inactivation of thrombin, fibrinogen is not converted to fibrin (insoluble protein threads that strengthen clots). Heparin also interferes in the action of factors IX, X, XI, and XII, resulting in bleeding at single or multiple sites.

Other Medications. Aspirin affects platelet function and may cause bleeding. Aspirin blocks an enzyme called *cyclooxygenase,* which results in a decrease in platelet aggregation and decreased vasoconstriction. The clinical manifestations of aspirin-induced platelet dysfunction are minimal unless the patient also has an underlying coagulation defect such as von Willebrand's disease or other platelet or coagulation disorders.[55]

Thrombolytic therapy has become a common method of management for myocardial infarction and is being evaluated in the treatment of a pulmonary embolus and nonhemorrhagic stroke. A serious complication of this therapy is bleeding.

These medications work by causing clot dissolution by specific mechanisms such as binding to fibrin and activating plasminogen to form plasmin, which in turn dissolves fibrin clots, fibrinogen, and other clotting factors. Even though some drugs are clot specific, their mechanisms of action leave the patient at risk for bleeding from puncture sites, from procedures such as intubation, and into specific places such as the brain or GI tract. Patients with previous histories of medical or surgical problems that can leave them at risk for bleeding are particularly vulnerable.[43] Other medications may interfere with platelet and clotting functions, but symptoms are generally mild and easily treated (box).

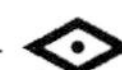

DRUGS CAUSING DECREASED PLATELET NUMBER OR FUNCTION

Drug-Induced Thrombocytopenia

Alcohol
Antibiotics (sulfa, rifampin)
Aspirin
Cytotoxic agents
Digitoxin
Diphenylhydantoin
Estrogen
Gold salts
Heparin
Heroin
Nonsteroidal antiinflammatory drugs (NSAIDs)
Para-aminosalisylic acid
Phenylbutazone
Phenytoin
Quinidine, quinine
Streptokinase
Thiazides
t-PA

Drug-Induced Decreased Platelet Function

Aspirin
Clofibrate
Dextran
Dipyridamole
NSAIDs (indomethacin)
Sulfinpyrazone

Massive Transfusions

Patients receiving large quantities of banked blood over a short time experience coagulopathies because of a dilutional effect. Banked blood becomes deficient in platelets and factors V and VII after storage at 4° C for 48 hours or longer. An estimated 10 to 12 units or more of blood given in a 24-hour period will cause coagulopathies if platelets or fresh blood are not also given to increase platelet and clotting-factor levels.[52] The flight nurse must help prevent this type of coagulopathy from reaching clinically significant proportions.

ASSESSMENT

Physical Assessment

As with any other physical assessment, the flight nurse should first evaluate the airway, breathing, and circulation (the ABCs). Once any necessary interventions have been undertaken to support those systems, attention can be given to a more detailed physical assessment.

Hemorrhages, ecchymoses, and hematomas nearly always result from identifiable local trauma. However, as the flight nurse continues to assess the patient, certain observations indicate that a coagulopathy may be present. Some of these red flags include the following[74]:

1. Bleeding at multiple sites or in several body systems concurrently
2. "Spontaneous" deep hematomas or hemarthroses
3. Unusually prolonged bleeding after local injury
4. Disproportionately large hemorrhage after a minor insult
5. Late bleeding that follows a period of apparently normal hemostasis after surgery or trauma
6. Inability to find an organic cause for hemorrhage in a specific area or an organ system

The flight nurse must be careful not to overlook the obvious. Many patients with previously diagnosed coagulopathies wear an identification tag such as the Medic-Alert tag as a necklace or bracelet, others carry a card identifying their specific disorder, and some carry a treatment protocol at all times. This kind of documentation saves valuable time in directing the flight nurse's assessment and care delivery.

During the assessment the flight nurse examines the skin and mucous membranes for signs of bleeding and notes petechiae, purpura, ecchymoses, and hematomas. Oozing from IV or IM injection sites or hematomas or ecchymoses around those sites may be significant. The flight nurse looks for gingival or other mucous membrane bleeding; hematuria or GI bleeding may be part of the pattern indicating coagulopathy. Joint deformities or stiffness may be present from previous hemarthroses. CNS bleeding is a life-threatening occurrence that is easily missed, and headache or other CNS signs should be aggressively pursued. The flight nurse also should look for signs of liver, renal, or splenic disease or infection.

Any bleeding that is unusual or does not stop with direct pressure as expected should raise the flight nurse's suspicion a coagulopathy is present. Identifying a specific coagulopathy based on physical assessment, particularly in the transport environment, is almost impossible. However, characterizing the signs and symptoms of some of the major categories of coagulopathies is useful.

Bleeding typical of a coagulation defect, such as the hemophilias, is large-vessel bleeding, often intramuscular, with large, deep hematomas and hemarthrosis. Crippling joint deformities may be present from previous hemarthrosis.

In hemophilia the platelet plug forms normally, but coagulation, which should follow, is defective. Therefore the platelet plug may initially control bleeding. Later, delayed onset of bleeding may occur, or there may be rebleeding after initial control of hemorrhage. In general, coagulation factor deficiencies are less responsive to local pressure than platelet abnormalities.

Bleeding in DIC usually occurs at multiple sites, such as an oozing around IV or venipuncture sites or frank bleeding from mucosa. Purpura and ecchymosis may be present. The patient is often in shock.

Platelet defects, as in aspirin-induced bleeding or other types of thrombocytopenia, is manifested as small-vessel bleeding. Spontaneous bleeding occurs into the skin, such as petechiae, purpura, or numerous overlapping ecchymoses. Bleeding may be mucosal. Bleeding after trauma is more immediate than in clotting-factor deficiencies, and it usually stops with local pressure. Bleeding does not reoccur hours or days later, as does the pattern seen in clotting-factor disorders.

History

A thorough history is extremely important in patients with suspected coagulopathies. The patient with a known coagulopathy may be more knowledgeable and expert about needed clinical management than the average nurse or physician. Family history of a coagulopathy may also guide in the assess-

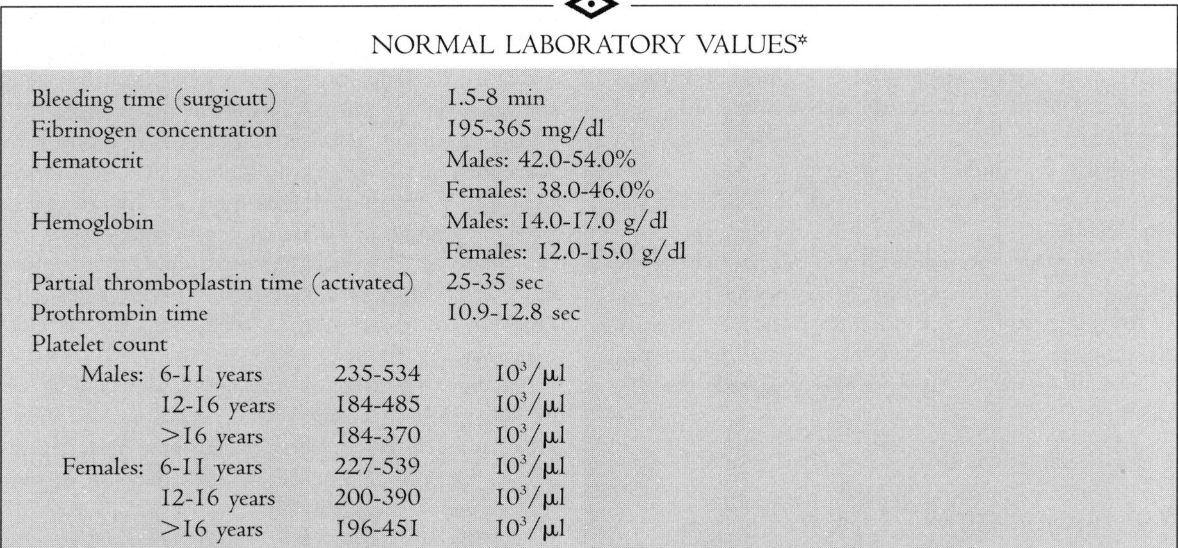

NORMAL LABORATORY VALUES*

Bleeding time (surgicutt)			1.5-8 min
Fibrinogen concentration			195-365 mg/dl
Hematocrit			Males: 42.0-54.0%
			Females: 38.0-46.0%
Hemoglobin			Males: 14.0-17.0 g/dl
			Females: 12.0-15.0 g/dl
Partial thromboplastin time (activated)			25-35 sec
Prothrombin time			10.9-12.8 sec
Platelet count			
Males:	6-11 years	235-534	$10^3/\mu l$
	12-16 years	184-485	$10^3/\mu l$
	>16 years	184-370	$10^3/\mu l$
Females:	6-11 years	227-539	$10^3/\mu l$
	12-16 years	200-390	$10^3/\mu l$
	>16 years	196-451	$10^3/\mu l$

*Normal values vary among laboratories depending on reagents used and the method and instrumentation employed.

ment; however, this information should be substantiated by accompanying clinical signs and symptoms of the disease.

The patient's medical history may include unusual bleeding from the umbilical stump after birth and bleeding after dental extractions, trauma, or surgical procedures. A history of hemarthrosis, frequent epistaxis, or menorrhagia is significant. The flight nurse should question the patient about taking anticoagulants or other drugs that affect platelet function. A history of liver disease or other organ system failure is significant, as is evidence of infection or DIC-associated factors.

Laboratory Values

Frequently, laboratory values are included in the patient's medical record received during an interfacility transport. These values should be referred to when the flight nurse undertakes the initial evaluation of the patient's condition (box).

Table 9-1 lists possible diagnoses based on results of the most readily available blood tests that evaluate coagulation and fibrinolysis. A definitive evaluation and diagnosis of the patient will require further laboratory testing at the receiving medical center.

In general, the intrinsic pathway is measured by the PTT. The extrinsic pathway is evaluated by the PT (Fig. 9-7).

A platelet count will reveal thrombocytopenia but will not establish that platelet function is normal. Bleeding time, another widely available screening test, is increased in significant thrombocytopenia or platelet dysfunction disorders such as von Willebrand's disease. Fibrinogen concentration does not measure fibrinolysis directly but can suggest it when evaluated in conjunction with the other tests described.

INTERVENTIONS AND TREATMENT

Diagnosis of a specific coagulopathy is difficult or impossible in the transport environment. Emergency interventions appropriate for patients experiencing acute effects of a coagulopathy are primarily supportive.

The first priority is airway management. This may be required if there is evidence of obstruction caused by bleeding or hematomas in the pharyngeal or laryngeal areas. Airway obstruction worsens as bleeding continues into the airway. An enlarging hematoma caused by bleeding into the soft tissues could com-

TABLE 9-1

Laboratory evaluation of coagulopathies

Abnormal tests	Possible diagnoses
Plat or Plat BT	Idiopathic thrombocytopenic purpura, drug reaction, bone marrow depression
Plat, PT, PTT, Fib	DIC, liver disease
BT	Platelet dysfunction, mild von Willebrand's disease, salicylates, uremia
BT, PTT	von Willebrand's disease
PT	Factor VII deficiency (rare)
PTT	Hemophilia, heparin
PT, PTT	Vitamin K deficiency, coumarin drugs, liver disease, heparin, factor V, X, II, or I deficiency
Fib	Decreased fibrinogen (rare)
Fib, PT, ± PTT	DIC, primary fibrinolysis
All normal	Normal hemostasis, factor XII deficiency, allergic vasculitis, scurvy, dysproteinemia, etc.

Plat, Platelet count; *BT,* bleeding time; *PT,* prothrombin time; *PTT,* partial thromboplastin time; *Fib,* fibrinogen concentration.

pletely obstruct the airway. Endotracheal intubation may be necessary to preserve the airway. Nasal intubation should be avoided because of a high likelihood of serious epistaxis. Supplemental oxygen should be delivered to most hemorrhaging patients. Pulse oximetry may assist in this area.

The next priority is to stop ongoing major hemorrhage. Patients who are continuing to hemorrhage should be treated similarly to any bleeding patient the flight nurse may encounter. Direct pressure with a sterile dressing helps control bleeding. Raising the bleeding part above the patient's heart decreases hydrostatic pressure and slows bleeding. Pressure must be held for a much greater time than for the patient with normal coagulation mechanisms.

Volume replacement of shed blood is important. Initial replacement with up to 2 L of lactated Ringer's solution is recommended. If assessment indicates the need for additional volume replacement, blood products should be considered if available.

The patient should be protected from additional trauma such as bumped elbows during loading and unloading from the aircraft. The flight nurse should minimize needle sticks, and prolonged pressure should be applied to venipuncture sites. IM injections especially should be avoided because of the risk of intramuscular hematoma. Intubation, catheterization, and other invasive procedures should be undertaken gently with good technique and only when indicated by the patient's condition.

Medications that depress platelet function should be withheld until medical consultation is available. Anticoagulants should also be withheld, with the exception of heparin in the case of DIC. This is an accepted therapy appropriate in some situations to control the clotting system that is out of hemostatic balance.

Infusion of fresh whole blood, fresh frozen plasma, or platelets may be started at the referring hospital in an attempt to raise clotting factor or platelet levels. This is a useful therapy but is rather inexact when undertaken before complete laboratory evaluation. Only the specifically indicated blood component should be given because of the risk of autoimmunization and the possible transmission of infectious disease.[90] Whole blood transfusions are rarely indicated for correction of coagulopathy. The volume of whole blood necessary may result in fluid overload.

Fresh frozen plasma can be infused to increase clotting-factor levels in deficient patients. A unit of fresh frozen plasma raises any clotting-factor level 2% to 3% in the average-size adult. Fresh frozen plasma is not recommended if PT and PTT times are less than one and one-half times normal. Fresh frozen plasma is a useful method for correcting warfarin-induced hemorrhage when the seriousness of the patient's condition does not allow time for correction by simply discontinuing warfarin therapy or administering vitamin K.

Platelets can also be infused to correct bleeding caused by low platelet counts (thrombocytopenia) or deficiencies in platelet function. One unit of platelets should raise the platelet count by at least 5000 in

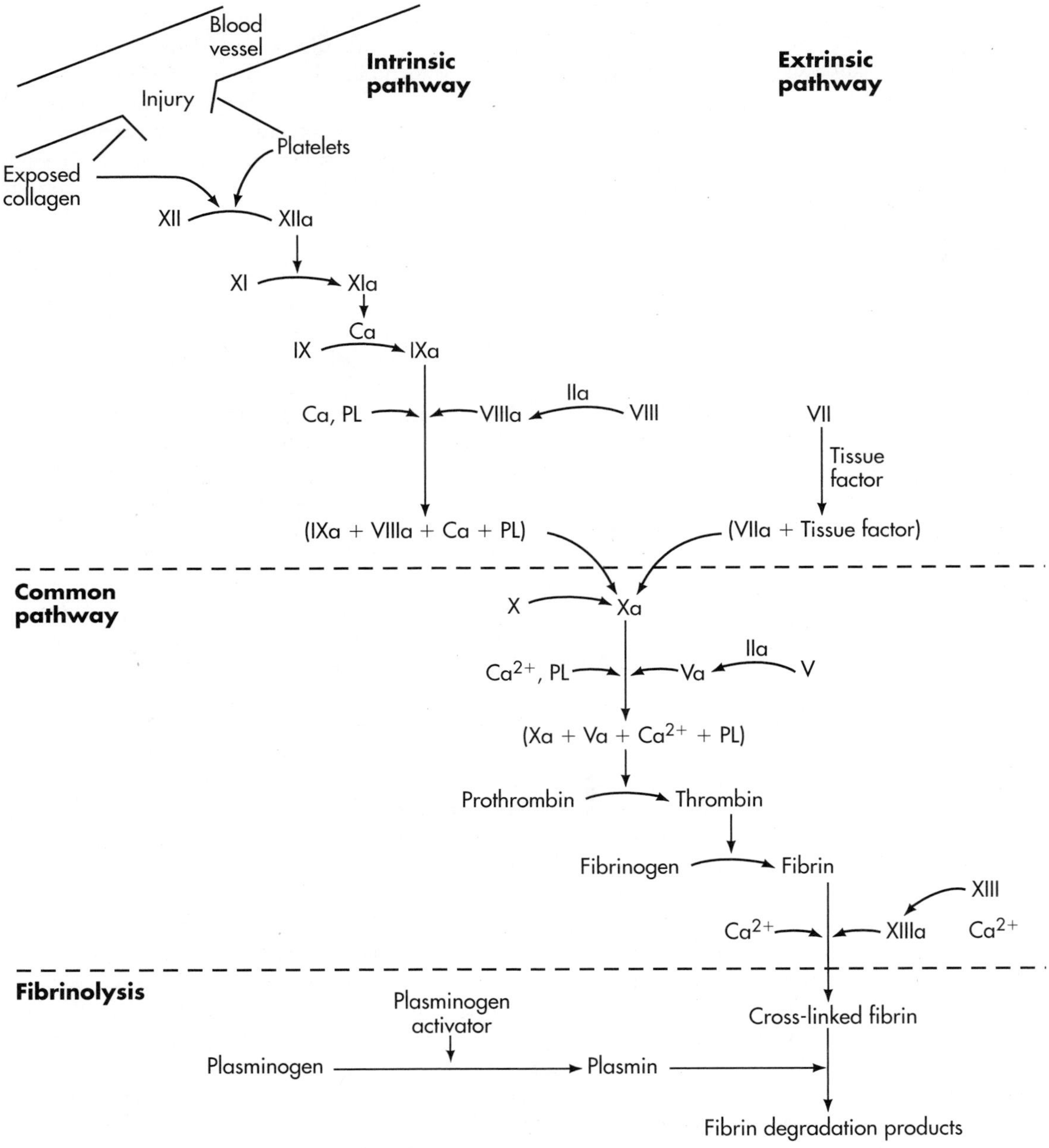

(1) Factors in the intrinsic pathway are present in circulating blood.
(2) The extrinsic pathway depends on the release of thromboplastin from damaged cells.
(3) "a" refers to the activated form of the designated factor.
(4) Ca = calcium. PL = phospholipid

Fig. 9-7. Coagulation and fibrinolytic system.

the average adult. The decision to infuse platelets depends on clinical parameters in addition to platelet count. Patients who are clinically stable may require platelet counts for less than 10,000 to 20,000/μL. Patients undergoing invasive procedures generally should have a platelet count of 50,000/μL. However, patients with coagulation defects, hemorrhage, sepsis, or other unstable conditions may require higher platelet counts.

Specific treatment of certain disorders bears comment. Hemophilia A patients should be treated early and aggressively for any bleeding episode. Standard treatment involves infusion of a factor VIII replacement. Cryoprecipitate is a frozen form of factor VIII concentrate. Most patients use factor VIII concentrate supplied in powder form. A single dose corrects minor bleeding, but severe hemorrhage may require continuous infusion for up to several weeks.

Hemophilia B is clinically indistinguishable from hemophilia A but requires treatment with either fresh frozen plasma or a concentrate enriched in the deficient factor IX.

von Willebrand's disease is treated similarly to hemophilia A, often with cryoprecipitate.

Vitamin K deficiency should be treated with parenteral replacement. IM injection is preferred, but 2.5 to 10 mg is sometimes given intravenously in a slow, diluted infusion. An attempt should be made to correct the cause of the deficiency. Emergency treatment of hemorrhage with fresh frozen plasma should correct the clotting defect, at least temporarily.

Emergency treatment for hepatic coagulopathies includes administration of vitamin K. Fresh frozen plasma infusion replaces all known coagulation factors and is safer and more complete therapy than prothrombin complex replacements. For patients with thrombosis, treatment by anticoagulation with heparin can be dangerous because heparin metabolism is unpredictable in cirrhosis. Severe bleeding may result.

DIC is treated by an attempt to correct the underlying cause. Once this is eliminated, DIC will resolve. Any significant bleeding or thrombosis requires immediate treatment. Fresh frozen plasma and cryoprecipitate are recommended to replace clotting factors. Platelet concentrates are given to increase the platelet count.[14] Heparinization is a controversial treatment of the thrombosis seen in DIC. The clotting cascade is out of control in DIC, and clotting factors are rapidly consumed, resulting in uncontrollable hemorrhage. Heparin reduces thrombin generation and prevents the further consumption of clotting factors. The risk is that heparin may cause further bleeding.

SUMMARY

The management of the patient who is in shock or may be suffering from the complications of coagulopathy is based on early recognition, swift and appropriate treatment, and rapid transport. Regardless of the cause, uncontrolled shock leads to fatal derangement. The early diagnosis of shock requires consideration of the history of the precipitating incident, the patient's medical history, and sometimes subtle signs exhibited by patients while compensatory mechanisms manage to maintain blood pressure and cardiac output.

An improved understanding of the pathophysiologic signs of shock helps the flight nurse recognize patients with shock and potential or actual bleeding disorders. Although definitive diagnosis and treatment are generally not possible during transport, early recognition enhances the patient's chances for timely treatment. Supportive measures routinely practiced by flight nurses help stabilize the patient in shock until further evaluation and treatment become available at the tertiary receiving facility.

SHOCK AND COAGULOPATHY CASE STUDY

The flight team was requested to the scene of a multiple car accident. Because several injuries were reported to the dispatcher, both aircraft were sent to the scene. Information received by the flight team during transport related that there were 5 victims of a MVC. One vehicle had broadsided another on the driver's side, and one car had been pushed into a ditch. The victims ranged in age from 4 to 30 years of age.

On arrival of the flight team, they were directed to the children who had both been restrained in the back seat of the broadsided vehicle and appeared to be the most severely injured. The parents of the children had received only minor injuries. Both were quite concerned about their children and wanted the flight team to know that both children had a history of von Willebrand's disease.

The first child, a 7-year-old boy, was alert and oriented. He had an actively bleeding laceration on his forehead, a rapidly expanding bruise on his abdomen in the shape of the lap belt, and other small abrasions and lacerations. Direct pressure was applied to control the bleeding from the laceration. His vital signs were BP 100/62, a pulse rate of 130, and a respiratory rate of 28. The child was placed in spinal immobilization, 100% oxygen was applied by face mask, and an intravenous line of normal saline was initiated. Because the child's peripheral pulses were decreased, the flight nurse initiated a fluid bolus of 20 ml/kg. The child was packaged for transport and rapidly taken to the emergency department at the children's hospital.

The second child attended by the second flight team was a 4-year-old girl. Her airway was being maintained with a bag-valve-mask and 100% oxygen. Intubation had been attempted by the rescue squad without success because the child's teeth were clenched. She was bleeding orally from the intubation attempt. She was responding only to pain with a Glasgow Coma score of 7, and her pupils measured 3 mm in diameter and were equal and both reactive.

Her color was pale, and she was cold and clammy. Her peripheral pulses were weak, and she had a heart rate of 160. Peripheral access had been attempted but was unsuccessful. The flight team initiated an intraosseous needle in the child's right tibia. Because of the potential for airway complications during transport, the child was intubated with a 5.0 uncuffed endotracheal tube using rapid sequence induction. Drugs administered included atropine, fentanyl, and succinylcholine.

The child was placed in spinal immobilization and a fluid bolus of 20 ml/kg of normal saline initiated. She was prepared for transport and placed in the helicopter. There was no obvious sign of external bleeding, but her abdomen was bruised, distended, and firm.

During transport, her pulse rate continued to increase to 180. Her peripheral pulses remained weak. The flight team started 1 U of O-negative packed red cells and continued repeating the fluid bolus. The child was hot off-loaded at the children's hospital and immediately evaluated by the trauma team.

Both children suffered liver injuries, and the girl also had a small splenic injury and moderate closed head injury. The young boy was treated with bed rest and given cryoprecipitate. His sister remained intubated for management of her head injury. Her abdominal injuries were treated the same as her brother's. Both children made a full recovery.

Even though the flight team was provided information about the children's medical history, it did not alter the care these children received for their injuries and consequent shock. Early recognition of their shock, airway management and delivery of oxygen, control of external bleeding, fluid and blood administration were all provided for them before and during transport. One of the most important roles the flight team played in the care of these children was rapid transport to definitive care.

REFERENCES

1. Ackerman M: The systemic inflammatory response, sepsis, and multiple organ dysfunction, *Crit Care Nurs Clin North Am* 6:243-250, 1994.
2. Ali J, Qi W: Fluid and electrolyte deficit with prolonged pneumatic anti-shock garment application, *J Trauma* 38(4):612, 1994.
3. Alspach JG, Williams SM: *Core curriculum for critical care nursing,* ed 3, Philadelphia, 1985, Saunders.
4. American Heart Association: *Textbook of advanced cardiac life support,* Dallas, 1994, The Association.
5. Anderson HL III et al: Extracorporeal life support for respiratory failure after multiple trauma, *J Trauma* 37(2): 266, 1994.
6. Angelica A, Todaro A: Action stat! Reversing acute dehydration, *Nurs 93* 23(6):33, 1993.
7. Bang N: Hematology/oncology. In Ayers S, Grenvik A, Holbrook P, Shoemaker W , editors: *Textbook of critical care,* Philadelphia, 1995, Saunders.
8. Barone J, Snyder A: Treatment strategies in shock: use of oxygen transport measures, *Heart Lung* 1:81-85, 1991.

9. Battistella F, Wisner D: Combined hemorrhagic shock and head injury: effects of hypertonic saline (7.5%) resuscitation, *J Trauma* 31(2):182-187, 1991.
10. Behrman S et al: Microcirculatory flow changes after initial resuscitation of hemorrhagic shock with 7.5% hypertonic saline/6% dextran, *J Trauma* 31(5):589-600, 1991.
11. Bickell W et al: Immediate versus delayed fluid resuscitation for hypotensive patients with penetrating torso injuries, *N Engl J Med* 331(17):1105-1109, 1994.
12. Bickell WH et al: Resuscitation of canine hemorrhage hypotension with large volume isotonic crystalloid: impact on lung water, venous admixture, and systemic arterial oxygen saturation, *Am J Emerg Med* 12(1):36, 1994.
13. Bone R: Sepsis, sepsis syndrome, and the systemic inflammatory response syndrome (SIRS): Gullivar in Laputa, *JAMA* 273:155-156.
14. Braunwald E: *Harrison's principles of internal medicine,* ed 10, New York, 1987, McGraw-Hill.
15. Bridges EJ, Woods SL: Pulmonary artery pressure measurement: state of the art, *Heart Lung* 22(2):99-107.
16. Brown KK: Septic shock: how to stop the deadly cascade, *Am J Nurs* 94:20-27, 1994.
17. Brown KK: Critical interventions in septic shock, *Am J Nurs* 94:21-26, 1994.
18. Campbell JE: *Basic trauma life support, advanced prehospital care,* ed 3, 1995, Brady.
19. Cardona VD et al: *Trauma nursing: from resuscitation through rehabilitation,* ed 2, Philadelphia, 1994, WB Saunders.
20. Cayten CG et al: A study of pneumatic anti-shock garments in severely hypotensive trauma patients, *J Trauma* 34(5):728-735, 1993.
21. Chameides L, Hazinski MF: *Textbook of pediatric advanced life support,* Dallas, 1994.
22. Chang FC et al: PSAG: does it help in the management of traumatic shock? *J Trauma* 39(3):453, 1995.
23. Chikanori T et al: Effects of mild Trendelenburg on central hemodynamics and internal jugular vein velocity, cross sectional area flow, *Am J Emerg Med* 13(3):255, 1995.
24. Anxiety in the critical care setting, *Crit Care Nurse* Aug 1994 pp 2-16.
25. Cohn SM, Farrell TJ: Diasprin cross-linked hemoglobin, resuscitation of hemorrhage: comparison of a blood substitute with hypertonic saline and isotonic saline, *J Trauma* 39(2):210, 1995.
26. Committee on Trauma: *Advanced trauma life support manual,* Chicago, 1984, American College of Surgeons.
27. Committee on Trauma: *A guide to the evaluation and treatment of serious head injuries,* Chicago, 1983, American College of Surgeons.
28. Committee on Trauma: *A guide to the initial therapy of shock,* Chicago, 1983, American College of Surgeons.
29. Cross J et al: Hypertonic saline fluid therapy following surgery: a prospective study, *J Trauma* 30(6):817-826, 1989.
30. Cummins RO: *Textbook of advanced cardiac life support,* Dallas, 1994, American Heart Association.
31. Dabich MA, Wade CE: A review of the efficacy and safety of 7.5% NaCl/6% dextran 70 in experimental animals and humans, *J Trauma* 36(3):323, 1994.
32. Darling GE: Multi-organ failure in critical patients, *Can J Surg* 31(3):172, 1988.
33. Darls EK, Schroeder JS: *Techniques in bedside hemodynamic monitoring,* ed 4, St Louis, Mosby.
34. Ebb D, Bray G: Bleeding disorders in children. In Ayers S et al, editors: *Textbook of critical care,* Philadelphia, 1995, Saunders.
35. Epstein CD, Herning RJP: Oxygen transport variables in the identification and treatment of tissue hypoxia, *Heart Lung* 22(4):328-343, 1993.
36. Ertel W et al: Release of anti-inflammatory mediators after mechanical trauma correlates with severity of injury and clinical outcome, *J Trauma* 39(5):879-887, 1995.
37. Fisher J: *The plague makers,* New York, 1994, Simon and Schuster.
38. Gaedeke MK: Action stat! Disseminated intravascular coagulation, *Nurs 94* 24(7):53, 1994.
39. Guyton AC: *Textbook of medical physiology,* ed 8, Philadelphia, 1991, Saunders.
40. Hudak C et al: *Critical care nursing,* ed 4, Philadelphia, 1986, Lippincott.
41. Jacobs L: Timing of fluid resuscitation in trauma, *N Engl J Med* 331(17):1153-1154, 1994.
42. Jones S, Nesper T, Alcoulmre E: Prehospital intravenous line placement: a prospective study, *Ann Emerg Med* 10:1039-1043, 1990.
43. Keen J: *Critical care and emergency drug reference,* St Louis, 1994, Mosby.
44. Keenan A: Hematologic emergencies. In Kitt S et al, editors: *Emergency nursing,* Philadelphia, 1995, Saunders.
45. Klein AR: *Emergency nursing core curriculum,* ed 4, Philadelphia, 1994, Saunders.
46. Kokiki J: Septic shock: a review and update for the emergency department clinician, *J Emerg Nurs* 19(2):102-105, 1993.

47. Kowalenkno T et al: Improved outcome with hypotensive resuscitation of uncontrolled hemorrhagic shock in a swine model, *J Trauma* 33(3):349-353, 1992.
48. Maclean LD: Shock: a century of progress, *Ann Surg* 201(4):407, 1985.
49. Marthay MA, Chatterjee K: Bedside catheterization of the pulmonary artery: risks compared with benefits, *Ann Intern Med* 109(10):826, 1988.
50. Martin R et al: Prospective evaluation of preoperative fluid resuscitation in hypotensive patients with penetrating truncal injury: a preliminary report, *J Trauma* 33(3): 354-362, 1992.
51. Mattox K et al: Prospective MAST study in 911 patients, *J Trauma* 30(8):1104-1112, 1989.
52. May HL: *Emergency medicine,* New York, 1984, Wiley.
53. Mazzoni M et al: The efficiency of iso- and hyperosmotic fluids as volume expanders in fixed-volume and uncontrolled hemorrhage, *Ann Emerg Med* 19(4):350-358, 1990.
54. McQuillan K: Initial management of traumatic shock. In Cardona V et al, editors: *Trauma nursing,* Philadelphia, 1994, Saunders.
55. Mills J: *Current emergency diagnosis and treatment,* ed 2, Los Altos, Calif, 1985, Lange Medical.
56. Moore E et al: The post-ischemic gut serves as a priming bed for circulating neutrophils that provoke multiple organ failure, *J Trauma* 37:881-887, 1994.
57. Moore F, Moore E, Peterson V: Inflammatory models of multiple organ failure, *Trauma Q* 12(1):47-58, 1995.
58. Oman KS: Use of hematocrit changes as an indicator of blood loss in adult trauma patients who receive intravenous fluids, *J Emerg Nurs* 21(5):395-400, 1995.
59. Owens TS et al: Limiting initial resuscitation of uncontrolled hemorrhage reduces internal bleeding and subsequent volume requirements, *J Trauma* 39(2):200, 1995.
60. Pedowitz RA, Shackford SR: Noncavitary hemorrhage producing shock in trauma patients: incidence and severity, *J Trauma* 29(2):219, 1989.
61. Pettijean ME et al: Thoracic spinal trauma and associated injuries: should early decompression be considered? *J Trauma* 39(2)368-372, 1995.
62. Price S, Wilson LM: *Pathophysiology: clinical concepts of disease process,* ed 5, St Louis, 1996, Mosby.
63. Querin JJ, Dixon LS: Twelve simple sensible steps to successful blood transfusions, *Nurs 90* 20(10):68-75, 1990.
64. Rifkind R et al: *Fundamentals of hematology,* ed 3, Chicago, 1986, Year Book Medical.
65. Rosen P: *Emergency medicine concepts and clinical practice,* St Louis, 1992, Mosby.
66. Rottman S, Larmon B, Manix T: Rapid volume infusion in prehospital care, *Prehosp Disas Med* 3:225-230, 1990.
67. Rueden K, Dunham CM: Sequelae of massive fluid resuscitation in trauma patients, *Crit Care Nurs Clin North Am* 6:463-472, 1994.
68. Russell S: Hypovolemic shock: is your patient at risk? *Nurs 94* 24(4):34-39, 1994.
69. Russell S: Septic shock: can you recognize the clues? *Nurs 94* 24(4):40-46, 1994.
70. Samuels D, Bock H: *Air medical crew national standard curriculum,* Pasadena, Calif, 1988, ASHBEAMS.
71. Sayre MR: What's new in the treatment of hemorrhagic shock, *J Air Med Transport* 10(5):20-25, 1991.
72. Schmoker JD et al: Hypertonic fluid resuscitation improves cerebral oxygen delivery and reduces intracranial pressure after hemorrhagic shock, *J Trauma* 31(12):1607-1613, 1991.
73. Schrieber TL, Miller DH, Zola B: Management of myocardial infarction shock: current status, *Am Heart J* 117(2):435, 1989.
74. Schwartz GR: *Principles and practices of emergency medicine,* ed 2, Philadelphia, 1986, Saunders.
75. Schwartzberg S: Cytokines: experimental and clinical studies, *Trauma Q* 22(1):7-15, 1995.
76. Schultz SC et al: Use of base deficit to compare resuscitation with lactated Ringer's solution, haemacel, whole blood, and diasprin cross linked hemoglobin following hemorrhage in rats, *J Trauma* 35(4):619-626, 1993.
77. Schultz SC et al: The efficacy of diasprin cross-linked hemoglobin solution resuscitation in a model of uncontrolled hemorrhage, *J Trauma* 37(3):408, 1994.
78. Selfridge-Thomas J: Shock. In Kitt S et al, editors: *Emergency nursing,* Philadelphia, 1995, Saunders.
79. Shatney CH: Initial resuscitation and assessment of patients with multisystem blunt trauma, *South Med J* 81(4): 501, 1988.
80. Sheehy SB: *Emergency nursing: practices and principles,* ed 3, St Louis, 1992, Mosby.
81. Sommers M: Rapid fluid resuscitation: how to correct dangerous deficits, *Nurs 90* 20(1):52-59, 1990.
82. Spearing-Bolgiano C: Administering oxygen therapy: what you need to know, *Nurs 90* 20(6):47-51, 1990.
83. Stark JL: Interpreting BUN/creatine levels: it's not as simple as you think, *Nurs 94* 24(9):58-61, 1994.
84. Stern S et al: Effect of blood pressure on hemorrhage volume and survival in a near-fetal hemorrhage model incorporating vascular injury, *Ann Emerg Med* 22(2):155-163, 1993.

85. Talan D: Recent developments in our understanding of sepsis: evaluation of antiendotoxin antibodies and biological modifiers, *Ann Emerg Med* 22:1871-1890, 1993.
86. Valedi MH: Pneumatic anti-shock garment-associated compartment syndrome in uninjured lower extremities, *J Trauma* 38(4):616, 1995.
87. Vary T, Kearney M: Pathophysiology of traumatic shock and multiple organ failure. In Cardona V et al, editors: *Trauma nursing,* Philadelphia, 1994, Saunders.
88. Vassar MJ et al: Prehospital resuscitation of hypotensive trauma patient with 7.5% NaCl vs 7.5% NaCl with added dextran: a controlled trial, *J Trauma* 34(5):622, 1993.
89. Whitney J: Wound healing. In Cardona V et al, editors: *Trauma nursing,* Philadelphia, 1995, Saunders.
90. Willis JL: Use of blood components, *FDA Drug Bulletin* 19:14-15, 1989.
91. Wyngaarden JB, Smith LH Jr: *Cecil's textbook of medicine,* ed 18, Philadelphia, 1988, Saunders.

CHAPTER 10

Patient Care Issues

COMPETENCIES

1. Performs a focused assessment of the needs of families before, during, and after transport.
2. Initiates nursing interventions to meet the needs of the family.
3. Participates in the development and implementation of protocols for "pronouncing patients dead in the field."

Patient care during air medical transport is generally focused on meeting the physiologic needs of an acutely ill or injured patient. However, other issues such as attending to the patient's family and dealing with issues related to death and dying must also be considered by the flight nurse before, during, and after transport.

Although flight teams are accustomed to air transport, they should not forget that this is a new and often frightening experience for family members of a seriously ill or injured person. The flight nurse should consider care of the family to be an extension of patient care and not an additional task that needs to be accomplished. The support that health care professionals provide to the patient's family during the initial stages of the patient's crisis can be invaluable. Contact with the flight team or emergency department (ED) employees may be the family's first interaction with medical personnel in this emergency. How the family perceives the response of these health care providers can be the impetus to either healthy or ineffective coping. Ideally, early interventions aimed at decreasing the family's stress should be performed to prevent the breakdown of the family structure.

Death is an inherent part of flight nursing. Some patients die before transport, and the role the family may play in this dying process can make patient care particularly arduous for the flight team. Whether to allow the family to be present during resuscitation attempts is an issue that has been gaining attention from both health care professionals and the public.

Finally, patients who die before transport can present the flight nurse with the complex challenge of deciding when and when not to try and resuscitate and transport the patient. Research has documented that the outcomes of patients who undergo cardiac arrest before reaching the hospital are dismal, and patient transport is expensive.[7,8] Currently, flight programs make "no-transport" decisions on the basis of a number of factors.

This chapter contains information relating to care of the patient's family, the presence of the family while attempts are made to resuscitate the patient, and transport when the patient has died. These issues present the flight nurse with a number of patient care challenges in addition to the challenge of meeting the acute physical needs of the patient.

FAMILY ISSUES RELATING TO TRANSPORT OF THE PATIENT

Family members of critically ill or injured patients are already under stress,[1] and the need to transport the patient on a fixed-wing aircraft or helicopter adds to the level of stress they experience.[12] Decisions concerning care must be made quickly, and the patient's family members often feel uninformed and unsure, especially if they have limited medical knowledge. Because time is a factor, the family has no opportunity to elicit medical information and request second opinions.

Family members may feel uncomfortable about relaying concerns about the transport to medical personnel. Some such concerns are related to the medical treatment rendered or even the safety of air transport. The family members may feel anxious because they will be separated from the patient for the duration of the transport. The family may also feel out of control if there are unknown entities surrounding the flight. How the person was injured or the events that led to the injury may not be known. They may not understand information concerning the medical diagnosis. The patient may be transported to a receiving hospital unknown to the family and located in an area unfamiliar to them. The referring physician, the flight team, and the receiving physician may all be unknown by the family. Any of these circumstances can cause the family to feel out of control.

Because most patients who are transported by air have injuries or illnesses that are sudden and unplanned, family members usually do not have time to prepare for the emergency. If they have never been exposed to this type of crisis, they may not have the coping skills needed to effectively manage the stress entailed.

Referring Facility

The flight team should make every effort to speak with the patient's family before leaving the referring facility. This interaction may be as simple as an introduction, such as "Hi, my name is Jane Doe and I am the flight nurse who will be with your family member during the flight." During this interaction the flight team can assess the family for abnormal stress reactions (discussed in Chapter 38). The team can then alert personnel at the receiving hospital's social or pastoral service department if it appears that the family may need their assistance. The flight nurse can also take this opportunity to determine the family's plans for traveling to the receiving hospital and get an estimate of their time en route. Family members should be notified of the aircraft's intended destination, and they should be told where to report once they arrive at the hospital. If necessary, directions to the receiving hospital can be given to the family; some flight programs provide individual maps for this purpose.

It is appropriate for the flight team to pause before leaving the institution to allow family members to say goodbye to the patient; this is especially important if the patient's injuries are life threatening, because if this is the case, the family may not have another opportunity to speak to the patient before he or she dies. In this author's experience, the opportunity to say goodbye to the patient is greatly appreciated by the family. In most cases, depending on the severity of the patient's injuries, the transport can be delayed for a few minutes without negatively affecting the patient's outcome. These simple interactions between the family and the flight team are invaluable in helping to alleviate the family's stress.

Fultz[9] conducted a study to identify the information needs of family members regarding air medical transport. The information needs rated as very important by family members included what was wrong with the patient, why the patient had to be flown to another facility, and where the patient could be found at the receiving hospital. The box below lists important needs that most family members perceived as being unmet.[9] The results of this research are important; flight programs should use this information as a guide when providing care to the family to better care for the needs of the patient's family.

Receiving Facility

Information concerning the patient's family members should be communicated to the receiving hospital to facilitate continuity of care. The social services department of the receiving hospital can be alerted to cases in which their services may be especially needed. Personnel at receiving hospitals will want to know whether the family plans to travel to their hospital. Because large distances must sometimes be covered by ground, an estimated time of arrival is useful. Knowing the family's plans can be helpful in case the patient's condition deteriorates and consent to perform particular procedures is needed. The hospital may need to know the family's wishes for treatment if the patient's condition is life threatening. Organ procurement issues can be considered if the staff knows when and if the family intends to arrive. These issues are particularly important if the patient is a minor.

Family members frequently leave the referring facility as soon as the decision is made to transfer the patient, and they may arrive at the receiving hospital ahead of the patient. In this case the referring nurse can notify the receiving hospital of the family's departure for their facility. If the receiving hospital is aware of the family's intended time of arrival, they can direct the family to the appropriate area within the hospital.

FAMILY NEEDS OF PATIENTS TRANSPORTED BY HELICOPTER

Family members of patients requiring helicopter transport perceived that they lacked the following:

1. The opportunity to see the patient before he or she was put in the helicopter
2. Information about who would take care of the patient in flight
3. Information about the safety of air transport
4. Directions to the receiving hospital
5. Knowledge about how the patient fared during the flight

From Fultz JH et al: Air medical transport: what the family wants to know, *J Air Medical Transport* 431, Nov/Dec 1993.

Transporting Family Members

Family members frequently ask if they can travel to the receiving facility in the helicopter or fixed-wing aircraft. In this era, patients and families are more assertive in making their requests known to the medical community. The decision to transport a family member must be made by the medical crew and the pilot. The personal feelings of a team member should not interfere with making a decision that is best for the patient and family. The entire transport team should provide input, but the pilot is responsible for making the final determination. Safety for the entire team is the primary factor on which to base this decision; second, transporting family members should not interfere with patient care.

Other factors the team may take into consideration when deciding whether to transport members of the patient's family are the patient's age, the seriousness of the patient's condition, other transportation available to the family, and the length of the transport time. The following box provides examples of inclusion and exclusion criteria for transporting family members in the aircraft.

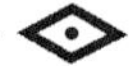

EXAMPLES OF INCLUSION/EXCLUSION CRITERIA FOR DETERMINING WHETHER FAMILY MEMBERS SHOULD ACCOMPANY A PATIENT DURING AIR MEDICAL TRANSPORT

Inclusion of family members during air medical transport may be desirable in the following cases:

1. The referring facility is far from the receiving facility and the family has no other means of transportation
2. The patient is near death and the family wishes to be with the patient during his or her last moments
3. The patient is a child and it would be beneficial for a parent to accompany the child
4. The family and the patient both strongly want the family to accompany the patient

Exclusion of family members during air medical transport may be desirable in the following cases:

1. Inclusion of the family member will interfere with patient care
2. The family member is overly anxious and poses a danger to the safety of the transport
3. The family member's weight exceeds permissible parameters
4. The LZ is walled in on three sides and thus the pilot must do a vertical lift for take-off
5. A crew member has a concern with taking the family member
6. Marginal weather
7. The family member has a fear of flying
8. The distance by ground between the two facilities is short
9. The patient is not stable and requires extensive care

Prepared by JM Williams, Cincinnati, Ohio, 1996.

Some aircraft are not capable of carrying an additional passenger because of performance factors or space limitations. Aircrafts that have the capability of carrying extra passengers also have limitations, including engine power, effects of weather on equipment performance, and the amount of weight the aircraft can safely carry.

Parents often ask if they can accompany their child on the transport. It is important to determine whether the presence of the family member will pose an in-flight safety problem because of an inappropriate level of anxiety. All family members will exhibit some anxiety, and thus it should not rule out the possibility of the person going on the transport. The determination must be made on the basis of whether inclusion of the family members will interrupt the pilot's duties if they sit in the front or interfere with care to the patient if they sit in the back. It cannot be stressed enough that if transporting the family member in any way jeopardizes safety or care, the person should not be transported.

The flight team may want to exclude the family from the transport when the weather is marginal. It may be necessary for the pilot to divert around bad weather to remain flying under visual flight rules. A precautionary landing or a diversion into an airport with use of instrument controls may be a real possibility in bad weather. Diversions or precautionary landings require extra concentration on the part of the pilot; thus it could interfere with flying if the pilot had to explain what was happening or calm a worried passenger.

Once the determination is made that family members can be transported, they will require a safety briefing by the pilot. The family member should be directed to the aircraft for the briefing while the patient is being prepared for the transport; this will give the pilot an appropriate amount of time to conduct the safety briefing. The extra passenger can be belted in the seat and be ready for lift off. If this is done before the patient reaches the aircraft, the transport will not be delayed.

Edgington[5] conducted a survey of all air medical programs in North America concerning whether family or friends are taken on transports. The results demonstrated that 60% of the programs carry extra passengers. The helicopter programs that carried family members did not advertise that they did so, and they transported them on less than 5% of their flights. Extra passengers were taken more frequently on transports of children. Fixed-wing aircraft programs transported family members on 35% to 95% of their flights. One fixed-wing aircraft program located in the Midwest claimed to carry family members on almost every flight. A program located in the West indicated that offering to transport family members was important because their transferring sites were so remote that the family refused to consent to the transfer unless they were allowed to accompany the patient.[5]

Forty percent of the programs surveyed did not transport family members. The following box summarizes the reasons that influenced the decision by these programs not to transport family members. Of the programs surveyed, the ones that carry extra passengers listed the benefits of transporting family members. The next box lists some of these benefits. Problems with the transfers were rare; only three problems were listed. On one flight a child experienced respiratory arrest and the parent was asked to assist in ventilation. In the other two cases, the passengers experienced air sickness. One program in Oregon has a preflight screening form to determine a prospective rider's suitability for transport. The form included questions about whether the potential passenger had had "recent alcohol or drug consumption, inner ear problems, pregnancy, back or joint trouble, and recent blood donation or dental work."[5]

The flight team must make a split-second decision as to whether the family can be transported with the patient. Experience helps to make this decision process easier. No specific rules exist for including or excluding the family. Each situation must be assessed separately. In many instances, family members will not be allowed to accompany the transport team. The possibility of transporting family members should not automatically be ruled out by the flight team because at times it is appropriate and it would be good if the team made an effort to include the family. If family members ride in a helicopter there may be some increased emotional difficulty for the transport team. However, the benefits to the patient and family when emotional support is provided far outweigh the emotional risks to the transport team.

REASONS FOR DECIDING NOT TO TRANSPORT FAMILY MEMBERS

- Liability concerns
- Lack of useful load on the aircraft
- Exposure of the family to invasive medical procedures
- Operator restrictions
  - Lack of insurance for passengers
  - Prohibition by the program's operations manual
- Concerns about a lack of time to properly brief family members
- Concerns about increased stress for the medical team as a result of having a family member on the aircraft

From Edgington BH: Transporting the family and other concerned parties aboard air medical aircraft, *J Air Med Transport* Feb 11-13, 1992.

BENEFITS OF TRANSPORTING A FAMILY MEMBER

- The family member may provide emotional support for the patient
- The family member will be available to sign releases for further treatment and to fill in gaps in the patient's medical history
- The family member may be able to act as a translator
- Organ procurement questions can be resolved more quickly
- The medical team may have the opportunity to explain the patient's prognosis and disposition to the family

From Edgington BH: Transporting the family and other concerned parties aboard air medical aircraft, *J Air Med Transport* Feb 11-13, 1992.

FAMILY PRESENCE DURING RESUSCITATION

Having family members present while attempts are made to resuscitate a patient is an emotionally charged topic that is gaining the attention of health care practitioners and the public. Whether families should be allowed to view a resuscitation is a topic of controversy among the medical community. Providing emotional support for family members can be difficult. Before health care providers determine the stance they will take on this issue, they should familiarize themselves with the literature, discuss the issue with others who have participated in a resuscitation attempt with family members present, and ask themselves the following question: "If my child or family member needed to be resuscitated, would I want to be there?" The box below lists other questions that practitioners should consider when dealing with this issue. A major point to keep in mind is that in most situations, the risks to the health care provider in emotionally supporting the family do not outweigh the benefits that are provided for the family.

QUESTIONS TO BE CONSIDERED BY HEALTH CARE PROVIDERS WHEN EVALUATING WHETHER FAMILY MEMBERS SHOULD BE ALLOWED TO BE PRESENT DURING RESUSCITATION ATTEMPTS

1. How do you feel about allowing family members to participate in a resuscitation attempt?
2. Have you ever facilitated family participation in a resuscitation attempt?
3. Have you ever experienced a situation in which family members participated in a resuscitation attempt?
4. What, if anything, makes you feel uncomfortable about participation of family members in a resuscitation attempt?
5. What, if anything, would make you feel more comfortable about participation of family members in a resuscitation attempt?

From Emergency Nurses Association: *Presenting the option for family presence,* Park Ridge, Ill, 1995, The Association.

The mission statement or philosophy of most institutions is probably amenable to having family members present during a resuscitation attempt. The practice standards of the National Flight Nurses Association state that the flight nurse should possess the skills to effectively communicate with the patient's family.[14]

The Emergency Nurses Association (ENA) has issued a position statement in support of the option of family members being present during invasive procedures or resuscitation attempts.[6] The ENA believes that allowing family members to be present during resuscitation attempts facilitates the grieving process. The ENA also believes that families have a right to be together and that this allows the patient and family members to support each other.[6]

The vision of the American Association of Critical Care Nurses (AACN) is that they will work toward a patient-driven health care system in which critical care nurses make their optimal contribution. The AACN interviewed many nurses who indicated that listening and learning from patients and families is the key to accomplishing this vision. The information obtained from patients and families could then be used to challenge conventional care and ultimately change individual practice. The AACN realizes that activities that alter both the system and individuals are necessary for this vision to come true. The AACN wants nurses to look at the hospital experience "through the patient's eyes," which, they realize, requires enormous effort.[10]

Although nurses have historically professed to be patient and family advocates, very little research supports this statement. When Gorden[10] interviewed Dracup, she cited her previous study on family visitation issues, which found that nurses and families were not in concert with each other. Dracup and Beau examined whether nurse's perceptions of family needs were similar to the actual needs of the families. The results of their survey demonstrated that nurses did not always know what the family wanted. The recommendation was made that nurses continually ask family members what they want, instead of assuming they know what the family wants. Dracup discussed two other issues with Gorden: first, families want to visit patients more frequently in the intensive care unit, yet 80% of hospitals continue to successfully restrict visiting hours; and second, regarding the issue of family members being present during resuscitation attempts, being in the room during a code or when the patient dies is far less upsetting for some persons than sitting alone and frightened in a waiting room or living with the haunting memory that a husband, wife, or child had died alone.[10]

When family members are encouraged to become involved in the situation, they feel supported, useful, and have a sense of some control. When this happens, the nurse-family relationship is enhanced. Family members who are frustrated and angry because they do not know what is happening to the patient are actually harder to manage and take more time than those who are kept informed. Nurses must keep in mind that family members may not feel comfortable expressing their feelings, especially if they think these feelings are contradictory to the nurse's feelings. Asking family members what is best for them will help the flight nurse attain the goal of being a family advocate. Most family members like to be involved in every aspect of the patient's life except when it comes to hospitalization.

At one time, the issue of whether a father should be allowed in the delivery room during the birth of his baby was controversial; many health care professionals voiced their opposition and resisted this change in policy. Currently, fathers, siblings, and extended family members are often present in birthing rooms. Fathers are even allowed in the operating room when a cesarean section is being performed. This routine practice is not questioned today, and families and health care providers have adjusted to this change in practice. It would be unheard of today for an obstetric nurse to deny a family member access to a mother giving birth. It appears that it may be just a matter of time before it will be common practice for family members to be present during a resuscitation attempt; it is hoped for the family's benefit that this process of change will begin sooner rather than later.

Family Presence Program

Foote Hospital in Michigan[3] is a pioneer in the family presence program. The Foote Hospital program was initiated because of two instances in which family members refused to leave the patient during a resuscitation attempt. After these two instances occurred, a survey was sent to the families of patients who had been resuscitated in the Foote Hospital ED. The survey asked if they would have wanted to be present during the resuscitation attempt of their family member if they had been given the opportunity. Seventy-two percent of the respondents indicated that they would have liked to have been present. These results demonstrated to the staff at Foote Hospital that there was a need for a formalized family presence program.[3]

Foote Hospital approached the issue by developing a formalized program. Initially a chaplain or social worker provides the family with information about the condition of the patient and determines if the family would like to view the resuscitation attempt. During the time that the chaplain or social worker is with the family, the medical personnel are performing any necessary invasive procedures required by the patient. After the invasive procedures have been completed, the chaplain or social worker accompanies the family into the resuscitation room and stays with them to provide support and information. Because the medical staff has very little responsibility for providing support to the family, they can then keep their attention focused on the resuscitation. If further invasive procedures are needed, family members are asked to step out of the room.[3]

The nurses at Foote Hospital, who were informally surveyed before the program was initiated, had two main concerns: that the family would interrupt patient care and that outward expressions of grief by family members would make it difficult for nurses to perform their job. They also had a fear that they would be observed doing or saying something that would upset the family.[2] The following box lists reasons that health care providers give for not wanting family members to be present during resuscitation attempts. Stress for the family is another concern cited by nurses.

The literature confirms that family members have a desire to be present during resuscitation attempts and that this process helps them in their grief work.[3] After Foote Hospital's program was established, a survey revealed that three out of four staff members

REASONS GIVEN BY HEALTH CARE PROVIDERS FOR EXCLUDING FAMILY MEMBERS DURING RESUSCITATION ATTEMPTS

- The family may disrupt or interfere with patient care
- Outward expressions of grief by family members might make it difficult or impossible for staff members to control their own emotions
- The experience may be too traumatic for the family

From Emergency Nurses Association: *Resolution 93-02: family presence at the bedside during invasive procedures and/or resuscitation,* Park Ridge, Ill, 1993, The Association.

supported the program. They believed that the program benefited the family even if it was emotionally harder for the staff. Follow-up research with family members who were present during resuscitation attempts demonstrated that the program was successful and that it helped them in their grief process. Many family members commented that they were glad to be able to see that everything possible was done for their loved one. One family member commented that he was glad to be able to say goodbye before the person died.[3]

Implications for Flight Nursing Practice

Both physicians and nurses have opinions on the issue of whether family members should be present during a resuscitation attempt. Most beliefs on this issue are at opposite ends of the spectrum; few people have middle-of-the-road opinions. Many of those who oppose family presence have admitted that they have never participated in a resuscitation attempt with a family member present. Their feelings are based on what they perceive might happen instead of on reality. Persons who have experience with resuscitation with family members present generally state that they believe it is good for the family and that they only occasionally have problems with the family.

Anecdotes from the Foote Hospital program recount families who have actually been involved in the decision to end a resuscitation attempt. The family was witness to the attempt and was able to say, "Yes, everything was done for my family member. Everyone worked very hard and it is obvious that the attempts to save the life were futile."[3] This scenario would never happen if family members were left alone in a waiting room and were not informed about what was happening. Difficulty in grasping the reality of the unknown hinders the grieving process.

Some health care providers are more comfortable with providing emotional care than are others. Some nurses allow family members to visit patients for extended periods of time, whereas others restrict visits to the exact amount of time mandated by the facility or even less. Some doctors take the time to talk to the patient's family members and keep them updated, whereas others avoid contact with the family. If family presence programs are to be successful, everyone's needs must be addressed. Physicians and nurses who find it difficult to provide emotional care will have the most difficult time adjusting to this change. Helping them with the transition will be essential.

Campbell et al.[2] found that nurses and physicians differ on how they handle death. Nurses tend to view death more as a natural part of life and associate it with positive terminology, such as rebirth, tranquility, and victory. Physicians, who tended to view death negatively, used words such as unsafe, alone, forgotten, and cold to describe the experience. Gender was not differentiated in this study. An argument could be made that gender instead of the profession of the respondents was the factor that led to different attitudes toward death, because the majority of nurses are women and the majority of physicians are men. In addition, male nurses have been influenced in their education mainly by female professors, and female physicians have been influenced mainly by male professors. Historically, women take a different approach to interpersonal and emotional events than do men. In general, men are much more uncomfortable handling and discussing issues surrounding death than are women. When this is taken into consideration, it appears that in general nurses are best equipped to be patient and family advocates and to assist physicians in determining what is best for the family. Nurses should be the family's voice when communicating with physicians and, if necessary, they should create the atmosphere necessary to have family members present.

Flight nurses and emergency personnel, because of the nature of their work, are exposed to situations in which family members may be in close proximity during the resuscitation process. Flight nurses have a wealth of information on this topic that comes from personal experience, and they should relate these experiences to other health care providers. Flight nurses should be on the forefront of supporting family presence; this support can play an important role in changing practice.

If family members are to be allowed in the resuscitation room, the code scenario of hospitals will have to change. The code scenarios of flight teams would be a good example for them to follow. When flight teams resuscitate a patient outside of the helicopter or fixed-wing aircraft in the presence of prehospital care providers or referring hospital personnel, the code is conducted in a professional manner. Because flight team members are never on their "own turf" the care they provide is open for scrutiny by all bystanders. Less noise and chaos are generally present during a resuscitation attempt by a flight team than in a hospital simply because fewer people are present. Flight nurses can attest to the fact that a code can be successfully run with fewer people than are used in a hospital. Speaking in normal, calm tones during a code seems to have a calming effect on those present; thus simply decreasing the noise level during a resuscitation attempt will lessen the degree of chaos.

One factor the flight team must consider when giving emotional care to the family outside of the hospital is the lack of ancillary support services, such as social services or pastoral care. The flight team must adjust to this lack of support services and find other innovative ways to provide care to the family without jeopardizing patient care.

Birth and death are both private life processes that belong to the patients and their families. Health care providers do not have the right to interfere in either of these processes. People should be able to die with peace and dignity with their families at their sides.

Although not everyone is prepared to view resuscitation attempts, the literature supports the fact that many persons wish families to be present when attempts are made to resuscitate a family member. It is also well documented that being present at resuscitation attempts is helpful for their grief work. Flight nurses should be patient advocates in the true sense of the word by asking the family what they want and by helping them to achieve their goals.

TO TRANSPORT OR NOT TO TRANSPORT

During the past several years, the cost of air medical transport and appropriate utilization of services have become important issues that many flight programs have learned to deal with. Deciding when to transport patients who have sustained cardiac arrest, whether as a result of trauma or a medical problem, continues to be one of the most difficult dilemmas faced by flight programs. Research has demonstrated that survival rates of patients who have out-of-hospital cardiac arrests range from 1.9% to 5%. Many survivors sustain severe neurologic injury, and the quality of their life is impaired.[7,8,11]

Data from a 10-year period of transporting patients who required cardiopulmonary resuscitation during air medical transport indicated that only 1.9% of these patients survived. The injuries sustained by the patients ranged from those resulting from motor vehicle crashes to gunshot wounds to the head. The only intervention provided by the flight team that was not provided by emergency medical services was the administration of blood. The average cost of each flight was $2671.[7]

In a study from the University of Louisville,[8] researchers found that six patients, or 2.4% of patients with traumatic arrest, survived. The air medical costs for these patients averaged $2600. The researchers concluded that patients with cardiac arrest who have obvious severe brain injury and those who have been in arrest for longer than 30 minutes should not be resuscitated.[8]

Whether to transport a patient who may be "dead" in the field remains a difficult decision and has profound ethical implications. Air medical transport illustrates one example of a technological imperative or the "unquestioning impulse to use any available technologic intervention."[4] The public also has come to expect both emergency medical services and flight programs to come to the rescue of all who need medical assistance, which attaches additional pressure to the decisions that must be made related to the transport of a patient who is in full arrest.

An ethical practice model suggested by Drought and Liaschenko[4] may serve as a framework for making the decision of whether to transport or pronounce the patient dead and not transport. The practice model is based on the practice account of morality and is composed of the following: (1) the practice knowledge is obtained from dealing with concrete problems, not abstract or hypothetical situations (e.g., the knowledge that patients who sustain blunt cardiac arrest in the field have less than a 1% chance of surviving has been obtained from actual cases); (2) the knowledge that is obtained from practice is shared with other practitioners, such as the fact that multiple studies have demonstrated that the survival rate of patients who have an out-of-hospital arrest is less than 5%[7,8,11]; (3) this knowledge has implications for all types of transported patients; and (4) it is dynamic, that is, research is continuous to describe the problem.[4]

The flight nurse must always be critical when making an ethical decision related to the transport of patients who have sustained cardiac arrest. In other words, "critical" means being thoughtful and reflective of the means, goals, and implications of this practice.[4] The flight nurse must consider the feelings of those who have been caring for the patient, the wishes of the patient's family, if present, and whether everything has truly been "done" for the patient.

Education, critical examination of the facts, and evaluation of one's personal values related to death and dying will help the flight nurse and other team members develop guidelines and make difficult decisions. Case presentations, literature reviews, and the use of clinical guidelines are some methods that may be used to make moral practice decisions. Fig. 10-1 presents a protocol that is used to pronounce patients dead in the field. As pointed out by Mattox,[13] "both society and trauma resuscitators [must] accept that the patient who has a fatal injury [should] die with dignity, not being subject to extensive and expensive resurrection techniques."

BEREAVEMENT AFTER SUDDEN DEATH IN THE FIELD

When patients are pronounced dead in the field or are not transported from a referring facility, their families may not be able to benefit from support services available when patients are taken to the receiving facility. Family members often have many questions after the death of a loved one. If family members are at the scene, the flight team should make an attempt to interact with them. If at all possible, the family should be encouraged to view the patient's body at the scene.

The initial shock experienced by family members may prevent them from knowing what questions to ask. The flight team can talk to the family about the facts that led up to the incident and explain the possible injuries that caused the death. Family members often do not remember what was said to them as much as they remember the attitude of the person who was talking to them. Table 10-1 lists interventions that health care professionals may use in their initial responses to crises.

Common responses of family members to the death of a patient are anger and hostility. These feelings are the result of a lack of control, frustration, and helplessness over the events surrounding the illness and death. Expressed anger often disguises underlying fears and anxieties that need to be addressed. Angry persons often discourage health care professionals from helping them, thus leaving them feeling lonely and isolated. Rando[15] believes that if the family accepts the death surround, the grief experience will be more quickly resolved and the feelings of anger, hostility, and guilt will be diminished.[15]

Flight teams can help the family to understand that the advanced care that their team delivered was the best care possible. The public may not be aware that the flight team is capable of providing the same care that would have been delivered in an ED; they may be under the impression that the best care possible is that which is given in the hospital. They may believe that the role of the flight team is to provide

UNIVERSITY OF CINCINNATI HOSPITAL
UNIVERSITY AIR CARE NURSING

Policy Page 1 of ____

Policy: Pronouncing Patients Dead-Scene

File: p-10-a	**Date Originated:** 11/86
Revised: 5/90	**Reviewed:** 4/92, 4/94, 4/95

Previous Reviews/Revisions: 11/86 - 11/91

Precautions:

Responsibility:

Equipment:

Purpose:
To provide guidelines for the pronouncing dead of patients by the University Air Care Flight Physician at the scene of an accident, injury, or illness.

Procedure:

A. Due to the presence of a physician on the University Air Care Team, a patient may be pronounced dead in the field in the following circumstances:
  1. If in the judgment of the University Air Care Physician the patient is clinically dead with no chance of survival.
  2. The requesting agency, rescue personnel, and family members *if and when present* are comfortable with the decision to terminate resuscitative efforts.
  3. There are no medical-legal contraindications to pronouncing the patient dead in the field, such as in homicide or suicide cases.

B. The following are specific situations that if present would generally prohibit pronouncing a patient dead in the field:
  1. Rescue personnel have been working diligently to save the victim's life and feel that the patient should be transported to a higher level of care.
  2. Invasive surgical procedures such as chest tube insertion have been accomplished by the University Air Care Team.
  3. Advanced skills for establishing an adequate airway such as endotracheal intubation and cricothyrotomy may be necessary to determine the likelihood of survival for a patient. These procedures do not preclude pronouncing a patient dead in the field but if accomplished should cause the University Air Care Team to carefully consider all the factors associated with pronouncing a patient dead in the field.
  4. A patient **may not** at any time be pronounced dead in the aircraft or on the helipad.
  5. In the event that a flight nurse is flying without a physician, they **cannot** pronounce a patient dead.
  6. Whenever there is a question as to whether a patient should be pronounced dead in the field, contact should be made with the Emergency Medicine Faculty.

Reviewed by: ______________________________

____
Senior Administrator, Patient Care Services

Fig. 10-1. Example of a protocol used in an air medical program when it is necessary to pronounce a patient dead.

TABLE 10-1

Interventions for initial family responses to crisis

Family responses	Interventions
Anxiety, shock, fright	Giving information that is brief, concise, explicit, and concrete Repetition of information and frequent reinforcement; encourage families to record important facts in writing Ascertain comprehension by asking family members to repeat the information they have been given Encourage or allow ventilation of feelings, even if they are extreme Maintain constant, nonanxious presence in the face of a highly anxious family Inform the family as to the potential range of behaviors and feelings that are within the "norm" for crisis Maximize control within the hospital environment as much as possible
Denial	Identify the purpose that denial is serving for family (e.g., is it buying them "psychological time" for future coping and mobilization of resources?) Evaluate the appropriateness of the use of denial in terms of time; denial becomes inappropriate when it inhibits the family from taking necessary actions or when it is impinging on the course of treatment Do not actively support denial but neither dash hopes for the future (e.g., "It must be very difficult for you to believe your son is nonresponsive and in a trauma unit") If denial is prolonged and dysfunctional, more direct and specific factual representation may be essential
Anger, hostility, distrust	Allow for ventilation of angry feelings, clarifying the thoughts, fears, and beliefs that are behind the anger; let them know it is "OK" to be angry Do not personalize the family's expression of these strong emotions Institute family control within the hospital environment when possible (e.g., arrange for a set time[s] and set person[s] to give them information about the patient and answer their questions) Remain available to families while they vent these emotions Ask families how they can take the energy in their anger and put it to positive use for themselves, for the patient, and for the situation
Remorse and guilt	Do not try to "rationalize away" guilt for families Listen, support their expression of feeling and verbalizations (e.g., "I can understand how or why you might feel that way; however . . .") Follow the "howevers" with careful, reality-oriented statements or questions (e.g., "None of us can truly control another's behavior"; "Kids make their own choices despite what parents think and want"; "How successful were you when you tried to control ___________'s behavior with that before?"; "So many things have happened for which there are no absolute answers.")
Grief and depression	Acknowledge the family's grief and depression Encourage family members to be precise about what it is they are grieving and depressed about; give grief and depression a context Allow the family appropriate time for grief Recognize that grieving is an essential step for future adaptation; do not try to rush the grief process Remain sensitive to your own unfinished business and, hence, comfort/discomfort with the family's grieving and depression

From Kleeman KM: Families in crisis due to multiple trauma, *Crit Care Nurs North Am* 1(1):25, 1989.

Continued.

TABLE 10-1 cont'd

Interventions for initial family responses to crisis

Family responses	Interventions
Hope	Clarify with family members what their hopes are, individually, and with one another Clarify with families what their worst fears are in reference to the situation; are the hopes/fears congruent? Realistic? Unrealistic? Support realistic hope Offer gentle factual information to reframe unrealistic hope (e.g., "With the information you have or the observations you have made, do you think that is still possible?") Assist families in reframing unrealistic hope in some other fashion (e.g., "What do you think others will have learned from ________ if he doesn't make it?" "How do you think ________ would like for you to remember him/her?")

rapid transport and that the gold standard of care is provided in the hospital.

The flight nurse is responsible for giving medical care to the victim and emotional care to the family. If at all possible, the flight team should assist the prehospital care providers in talking with the family. Because of the nature of air medical operations, it is not always possible for the team to stay at the scene and assist the family. If the team cannot stay, the flight nurse's assessment of the family may be an impetus for initiating a referral for follow-up. If the base station is associated with a hospital, the social service department may be able to assist with the follow-up. The flight team may get involved with this follow-up at a later date by calling the family and repeating some of the medical information that the family either did not understand or were not capable of comprehending at the time of the patient's death.

SUMMARY

Emotional care of the family is an important aspect of flight nursing. Flight nurses may need additional education or awareness of their potential impact in this area. Flight nurses should not become so accustomed to helicopter transport that they forget what this means to the family.

Because the staffs of flight programs are exposed to many critical and deadly situations, they must be aware of their own needs. Internal staff support is essential. Flight teams may at times need critical incident stress management by a more formalized team (see Chapter 38).

In the future, flight teams may develop critical pathways that ensure that family members receive care after the sudden death of a loved one. If flight programs currently have innovative programs that are especially helpful to the families of patients, this information should be disseminated in the air medical literature or at national conferences. To continue the exemplary care that is rendered by flight nurses, care of the patient's family must be provided.

PATIENT CARE ISSUES CASE STUDY

A 60-year-old woman with an inferior wall myocardial infarction was to be transported by helicopter for a cardiac catheterization and possible angioplasty. The patient was at a referring facility, and the decision to transport was made suddenly. The patient's family members were at home and were unaware of the impending transfer. The referring hospital contacted the patient's husband, who then contacted other members of the patient's family.

When the flight team went to the patient's room to prepare her for transport, they found that she was extremely anxious about the impending catheterization. To make matters worse, she was terrified of flying.

As the flight team was preparing the patient for transport, the telephone in her room kept ringing. The intensive care nurse believed that the patient should not take the time to talk with the family members who were calling because it would delay her impending transfer. The flight nurse suggested that because the team was not ready to leave, the patient would have time to talk with her family without causing any delay in transport.

The flight nurse encouraged the anxious woman to speak with her family. Her family members expressed concern about the need for transfer and the seriousness of her condition. The phone conversations did not delay the transport and had a calming effect on the patient. She became much more interactive with the flight team.

During the flight, the patient kept her eyes closed and appeared calm. Her husband met her at the receiving facility. He was very concerned about his wife's condition and her fear of flying.

The flight nurse explained to the husband the interventions that had taken place before transport and their effects on his wife during the transport. He was grateful that she was able to speak to their children before transport and was surprised that she tolerated the flight without incidence.

REFERENCES

1. Caine RM: Families in crisis: making the critical difference, *Focus Crit Care* 6:184, 1989.
2. Campbell TW, Abernethy V, Waterhouse GJ: Do death attitudes of nurses and physicians differ? *Omega* 14(1): 43, 1983.
3. Doyle CJ et al: Family participation during resuscitation: an option, *Ann Emerg Med* 16:673, June 1987.
4. Drought TS, Liaschenko J: Ethical practice in a technological age, *Crit Care Nurs Clin North Am* 7(2):297, 1995.
5. Edgington BH: Transporting the family and other concerned parties aboard air medical aircraft, *J Air Med Transport* 11(2):11, 1992.
6. Emergency Nurses Association: *Family presence,* Park Ridge, Ill, 1993, Emergency Nurses Association.
7. Falcone RE et al: Air medical transport for the trauma patient requiring cardiopulmonary resuscitation: a 10-year experience, *Air Med J* 14:197, 1995.
8. Fulton R, Voigt W, Hilakos A: Confusion surrounding the treatment of traumatic cardiac arrest, *J Am Coll Surg* 181:209, 1995.
9. Fultz JH et al: Air medical transport: what the family wants to know, *J Air Med Transport* 12(11-12):431, 1993.
10. Gorden S: Inside the patient-driven system, *Crit Care Nurse* (supplement 3-28), June 1994.
11. Jecker N: Ceasing futile resuscitation in the field: ethical considerations, *Arch Internal Med* 152(2):3035, 1992.
12. Kleeman KM: Families in crisis due to multiple trauma, *Crit Care Nurs Clin North Am* 1(1):25, 1989.
13. Mattox K: "Ideal" post traumatic parameters, *J Trauma* 34(5):734, 1993.
14. National Flight Nurses Association: *Flight nursing practice standards,* St Louis, 1995, Mosby.
15. Rando T: *Grief, dying and death: clinical interventions for care givers,* Champaign, Ill, 1984, Research Press Co.

CHAPTER 11

Trauma

COMPETENCIES

1. Demonstrate the ability to perform the following assessment skills: scene assessment, primary assessment, and secondary assessment.
2. Recognize the need for and perform the following interventions as needed to transport the trauma patient safely: airway control and ventilation, chest decompression, spinal immobilization, fluid resuscitation.
3. Demonstrate knowledge of trauma triage criteria.

The incidence of traumatic injuries is epidemic in our society today. Trauma is the leading cause of death in persons younger than 44 years.[4] Trauma is surpassed by only cancer and atherosclerosis as the major cause of death in all age groups.[1] It is estimated that more than 60 million injuries occur in the United States annually, and 145,000 people die of their injuries.[1] Disability from injury outweighs mortality by three to one.[1] A sign of the current epidemic of violence in the United States is the rise in firearm-related injuries. In 1991 firearm injury was the second most frequent cause of death in persons aged 15 to 34 years, with 38,317 fatalities.[23]

Particularly hard hit from injuries are males between the ages of 15 and 24 years. Motor vehicle crashes represent the primary injury cause. In fact, death in this age group is five times greater from motor vehicle crashes than from cancer and nine times greater than from heart disease[17] (see box). Reasons for this disproportionately high involvement of 15- to 24-year-old males are many, but lack of driving experience and alcohol consumption are pri-

DEATHS PER 100,000 POPULATION BY CAUSE, 15- TO 24-YEAR-OLDS	
Motor vehicle crashes	36.1
Suicide	12.9
Other accidents	12.3
Homicide	12.1
Cancer	5.4
Heart disease	2.8
Birth defects	1.2
Cerebrovascular disease	0.8
Pneumonia/influenza	0.6
Chronic obstructive pulmonary disease	0.5
Anemias	0.3
Other	10.9

mary contributors. It is difficult for most 15- to 24-year-olds to imagine a lethal or disabling injury happening to them, and therefore they feel no fear about attempting things that place them at a very high risk for injury.

The fact that trauma primarily affects young people has major implications for our society. For every death three persons experience a nonfatal injury.[30] Permanent impairment often prevents persons who have undergone trauma from returning to their preinjury daily routines. Extensive rehabilitation is required to assist patients with adjustments that must be made in their daily living and prepare them for returning to the work force, school, or home.

Costs associated with these trauma injuries are staggering. Approximately 40% of health care dollars are expended annually because of trauma.[1,23] These costs include not only the acute-care dollars but also the follow-up medical care and rehabilitation, indirect work loss from accidents, insurance administration costs, and litigation costs.[25] Private insurance monies are rapidly exhausted, and reimbursement according to the federal government prospective payment system (diagnosis-related groups) does not adequately cover expenses incurred.

PREVENTION

Traumatic injuries are the most preventable public health problem today. Once considered a chance occurrence beyond human control, an accident is now viewed as an interaction that could have been prevented, and injury is now viewed as resulting from exposure to identifiable and correctable environmental hazards.[37] Public awareness of the vastness of the trauma epidemic is inadequate, as evidenced by the very nature of its frequency. Injuries and fatalities, such as those from motor vehicle crashes, are so commonly reported (or even not reported) by the media that these events seem unremarkable. By continuing to believe that accidents are inevitable or beyond human control, the public avoids responsibility.[13,39]

Two approaches to injury prevention follow: (1) education or persuasion targeting human behavior or perception modification, and (2) enactment of laws or regulations aimed at the person at risk or the agent, vehicle, or physical environment. The diverse abilities of the air medical crew member make him or her an optimal health care provider to participate in injury-prevention education.

INJURY DYNAMICS

One of the most important factors that has positively influenced the morbidity and mortality of trauma patients during the last decade is air medical transport, because the time from the accident to initiation of definitive care is the key to patient survivability. The addition of sophisticated aircraft with highly trained air medical personnel has brought critical care management outside the trauma center to the rural hospital or the scene of the accident.

The transport of the multiply injured patient requires in-depth nursing knowledge and skills, as well as expert prioritization and organization skills. Trauma patients treated at the scene of an accident require unique care interventions not performed by other nursing specialties. A thorough understanding of the mechanisms of injury and the kinematics of trauma are essential for any air medical crew member caring for injured patients. These principles will provide a direction of care.

History

One of the first steps the flight nurse takes in caring for a multiply injured victim is to elicit a history of events preceding and following the accident. With hospital transfers this is most commonly obtained from other nurses, physicians, and family members, but a history obtained at the scene of an accident involves many additional reporters, including law enforcers, firefighters, and paramedics. When the flight nurse is responding at the scene of the accident, an aerial view of the situation helps begin the history—the nurse has the advantage of evaluating the entire scene, the damage sustained to the vehicles or the buildings, the extent of impact, and the objects flung or blown out of the central area of impact.

On the ground, life-threatening injuries are always a flight nurse's top priority, and obtaining a detailed history may be impractical in certain cases. However, the importance of a thorough history is vital to direct the nurse in the patient's care. Because time is a critical factor for the survivability of the trauma patient, the history should be obtained while the flight nurse is gaining access to the patient or while he or she is simultaneously performing the primary assessment. If the patient has an altered level of consciousness, the only history obtained may be from the hospital or emergency personnel present, who may not be going to the receiving hospital. Hence it is important for the flight nurse to learn to elicit the history while concurrently assessing the patient. Important information to elicit in the history includes time of the accident, mechanism of injury, any alteration in the patient's level of consciousness, and the patient's past medical history and current medications.

A further detailed history may be obtained from the patient during the secondary survey as time and patient condition allow and can be routinely performed in the aircraft during transport.

Mechanism of Injury

Injuries occur when external forces are applied to the body. The type and amount of injuring force and the tissue response to that force determine the extent of injury.[2,8] When the body's tissue cannot withstand any additional force, destruction occurs, as evidenced by the common injuries seen in the multiply injured patient: fractures, lacerations, and ruptured internal organs. A complete understanding of a force and the way it is applied is necessary to predict potential injuries and thus adequately care for the injured patient.

Newton's first law of motion states that a body at rest tends to remain at rest, and a body in motion tends to remain in uniform motion until acted on by an outside force. When the body contacts an object, energy is transferred, and damage occurs.

Force is a result of energy transference, which can be explained by the laws of physics:

1. Energy can be neither created nor destroyed; it can change form.
2. Kinetic energy (KE) =
$$\frac{\text{Mass} \times \text{Velocity}^2}{2}$$
3. Force = Mass × Acceleration

Because energy is neither created nor destroyed, it is transferred, and its transference is dependent on the mass of the object times the speed squared over a common denominator of 2. For example, an automobile weighing 3000 pounds is traveling at 40 miles/hr when it strikes a telephone pole.

$$\text{KE} = \frac{3000 \times 40^2}{2}$$

The kinetic energy transferred in this impact to both objects is 2,400,000 units.

The same force is applied to destruction of the body. Energy is transferred from the automobile to the human being. Several factors determine the amount of energy the human being absorbs, including the following:

1. The amount of energy absorbed by the objects that initially collide (the telephone pole and the automobile, for example)
2. The amount absorbed by protective factors, such as seatbelts, helmets, padded steering wheels, dashboards, and airbags

The forces involved in the impact will cause varying degrees of destruction. The more slowly the force is applied, the less energy transference and the lower the degree of destruction. The extent of injury is also dependent on which body parts receive the impact.[7,28] For example, the skull can take more force before damage occurs than can the abdomen.

Force can be delivered by compression, acceleration, deceleration, and shearing.[28]

Compression: Direct compression or pressure on a structure is the most common type of force applied. The amount of injury sustained is dependent on the length of time of compression and the area compressed.[24,28]

Acceleration/deceleration: Acceleration is the increase in the velocity of a moving object. Deceleration is the decrease in velocity of an object.[7] In an automobile accident the body is thrown forward (acceleration) by the impact and decelerates as it comes in contact with the steering wheel, seatbelt, or dashboard. The internal organs also accelerate and decelerate, causing destruction to the tissues and vasculature.

Shearing: Shearing forces occur when the tissues, organs, or both are pushed ahead. The most common mechanism causing a shearing injury occurs when a pedestrian is run over by a vehicle. As the vehicle grabs a part of the body, the area is pushed forward until it can no longer take the force, and it tears. Degloving routinely occurs from shearing forces.

TABLE 11-1

Characteristics of strains

Type	Reaction	Examples
Tensile	Stretching	Bony fractures, aortic tears
Shearing	Movement of tissue in opposite directions	Brain injuries, lacerations/avulsions
Compressive	Crushing force	Compartment syndrome, ruptures

The viscoelastic properties of tissues in the body help to absorb energy. When the energy delivered is below the limit of injury, the energy will be absorbed and cause no damage. When the forces applied deliver more energy than the body can absorb, strains occur.[7] Strains may be classified as tensile, shearing, or compressive. Table 11-1 displays the characteristics and examples of each strain.

KINEMATICS OF TRAUMA

Patterns of injury have been identified by evaluation of the type of accident that has occurred and the amount of force generated. Although all patients should be evaluated individually, certain injuries are common to certain accidents. Prediction of these injuries is referred to as kinematics. Age, preventive measures taken, and velocity are factors in the alteration of injury patterns, and the flight nurse should consider them when evaluating a patient.[21]

Blunt Injuries

Motor Vehicle Crashes

Motor vehicle crashes account for more deaths of victims up to 50 years of age than cancer, heart disease, or stroke. During a lifetime, a person is likely to be in an automobile crash once every 10 years and has a 33% chance of having a disabling injury.[32] The extent of injuries for a particular motor vehicle crash depends on the type of collision that occurs and the position of the occupant in the vehicle. It is important to remember that in all motor vehicle crashes the body will travel through the car at the same speed the automobile was traveling before it crashed.[15,19]

Head-on Collisions. As an automobile collides with another automobile or with any object head-on, energy is transferred to the vehicle. The front of the vehicle routinely stops less than ½ second after impact. The rear of the automobile continues to move forward until all the energy is dispersed. Although the front end of the car is destroyed, it is the rear of the vehicle that causes the destruction by its continued forward movement.[27] The same principle of injury occurs with the body during a head-on collision. The initial impact occurs in the front of the vehicle. The unrestrained driver will hit the steering wheel with the thorax; the head may hit the windshield, and the knees contact the dashboard (Fig. 11-1). Predictable initial injuries from initial impact are fractured ribs, pneumothorax or hemopneumothorax, concussion, skull fractures, patella and femur fractures, dislocated hips, and acetabular fractures. The progression of injury proceeds, as will the automobile, and the person's internal organs will be thrown from the rear forward until all energy is dispersed. Common injuries include ruptured spleens (direct compression from the steering wheel), lacerated livers (stretching of hilum until the tensile strength is exceeded), and ruptured thoracic aortas (heart and aorta are forcibly thrown forward, stretched, and then compressed against the ribs).

The restrained driver in a head-on collision has much of the energy absorbed by the seatbelt. The seatbelt may impose a load 20 to 50 times as great as the body weight. The only portion of the human body capable of incurring this load is the pelvis.[31] Unless the patient has the belt properly applied securely over the pelvis, direct compression of the abdomen may occur. The first indicator of these injuries is often the presence of abrasions over the abdomen from the belt. Other injuries associated with seatbelt use include sternal fractures, breast injuries, and lumbar vertebral body fractures.[33] As seen with abdominal seatbelt injuries, abrasions, ecchymosis, or both are important indicators. Lap belts should be worn with a diagonal shoulder strap to stop forward movement of the upper body. Diagonal straps worn alone can cause severe neck injuries, including decapitation.[28] Safety improvements have also been added to vehicles made after 1968, such as energy-absorbing steering columns, which have helped decrease the severity of injuries.[20]

Air bags are available to cushion forward motion only. They are very effective in the first collision, but because they deflate immediately, they are not effective in multiple-impact collisions.[28]

Rear-end Collisions. An automobile hit from behind rapidly accelerates, causing the car to move forward under the patient. Predictable injuries are to the back (T12-L1 is the most common area of injury), legs (femur, tibia/fibula, and ankle fractures), and neck (cervical strain, C2 fracture caused by hyperextension) if the head restraint is not in the proper position.[16] If the automobile undergoes a second collision by striking the car in front of it, the predictable head-on injuries also need to be evaluated.

Side Impact. An automobile hit on the side will routinely cause lateral injuries to the patient. An un-

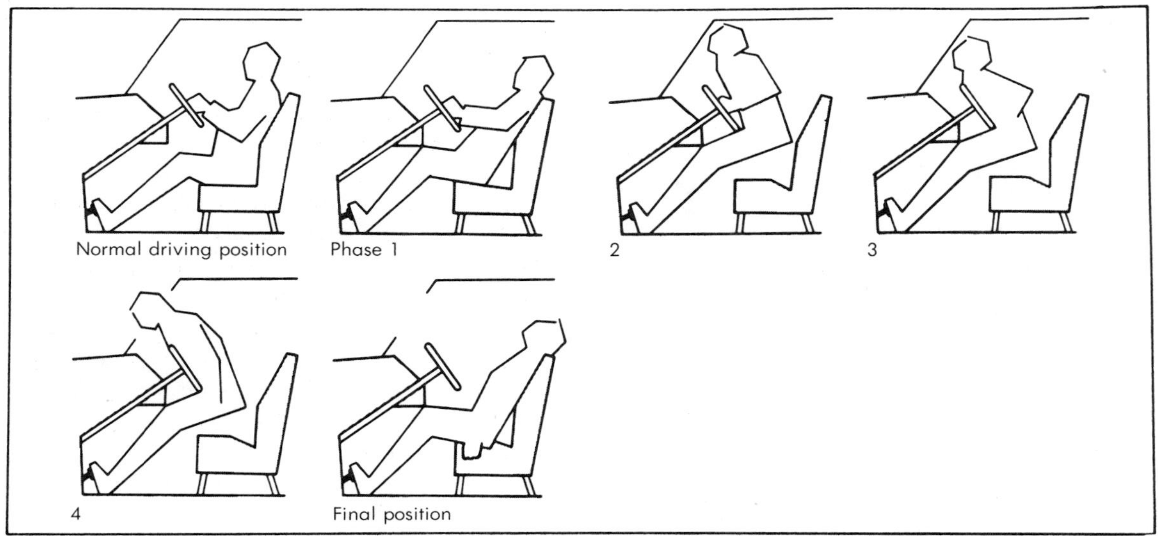

Fig. 11-1. Phases of movement of the unrestrained occupant during frontal collision.

restrained driver hit on the side will sustain initial injuries to the left clavicle, ribs, femur, and tibia/fibula. Abdominal injuries, such as ruptured spleens, are seen in these crashes, usually because of the fractured lower lateral ribs, but also because of direct compression on the abdomen.[28] Secondary injuries occur when the patient is propelled to the other side of the car, which causes injuries to the opposite side.

Rollovers. Predictable injuries caused by vehicle rollovers are more difficult to define. The unrestrained patient tumbles inside the vehicle, and injury occurs to the areas of the body that are hit. The flight nurse should always care for these patients judiciously and realize the potential for multiple-system injuries.

Motorcycle Crashes

Because the motorcycle offers minimal or none of the initial energy transference, energy is directly absorbed by the rider, and injuries are substantially more severe than with motor vehicle crashes. The predicted injuries during a motorcycle crash, like those during a motor vehicle crash, depend on the type of collision that occurs.

Head-on Collisions. To accurately predict injuries involving the motorcycle rider, it helps to understand the design of a motorcycle (Fig. 11-2). The center of gravity is located in front of the driver's seat. As the cycle strikes an object head-on, the rear (or lighter portion) tips upward from the weight under the handlebars, which prevents the driver, who is

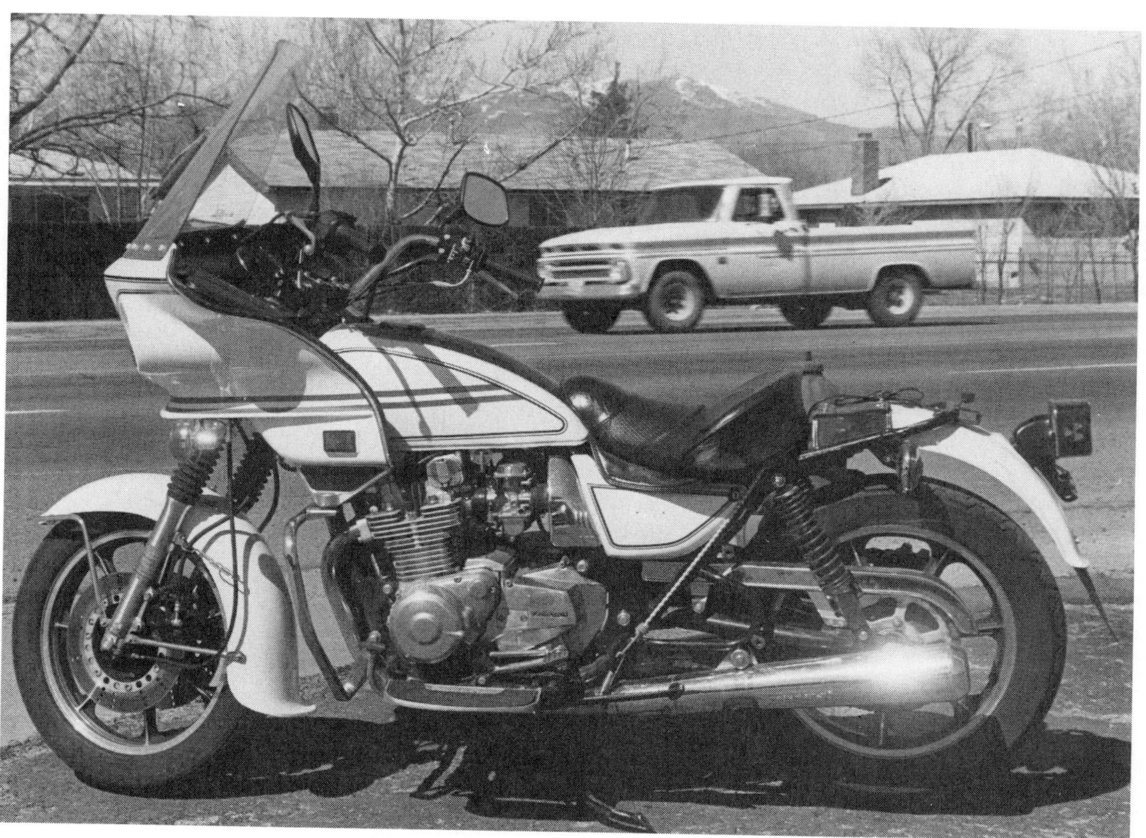

Fig. 11-2. Construction of a motorcycle places the center of gravity in front of the driver's seat. Head-on collision will cause the cycle to tip up and throw the occupant over the front.

propelled over the handlebars, from total ejection. Associated injuries with this type of crash are fractured femurs, tibias, and fibulas (from the handlebars); chest and abdominal injuries (from direct compression against handlebars or tire); and head and neck injuries (from impact with the tire or any object in front of the cycle). Any motorcycle crash can cause the rider to be ejected, but it is most common during head-on collisions. As with ejection from any vehicle, the head acts as the missile. Suspicion of and intervention for major head and cervical spine injuries is imperative with any ejected patient.

Side Impact. Injuries associated with the side-impact motorcycle crash are related to the body parts crushed between the cycle and the second object. Most commonly seen injuries involve the leg and foot on the impact side. Open fractures of the femur, tibia/fibula, and malleolus are predictable.

Laying down the Motorcycle. Motorcycle riders have learned the technique of laying down the bike and sliding off the side before colliding with another object. The energy transference is a result of sliding away from the bike. Commonly seen are abrasions of the affected side. Fractures may occur if the patient hits the road hard or comes in contact with another object. Preventive clothing, such as leather jackets, pants, and gloves, will absorb more energy than average clothing and in this type of impact may prevent abrasions from occurring.

Falls

Falls from heights greater than 15 to 20 feet are associated with severe injuries. In predicting injuries associated with falls, flight nurses should understand the following:

1. The average roof of a one-story house is approximately 15 feet off the ground; a two-story fall would be approximately 30 feet.
2. With a fall greater than 15 feet, adults will usually land on their feet. Below 15 feet, adults will land as they fell, that is, if the person falls head first, he or she will land on his or her head.
3. Because small children have proportionally larger heads, no matter what the distance, they will tend to fall head first.
4. The wounding in vertical deceleration is derived by the following equation:

$$W = \frac{KE \times K}{TA}$$

Wounding *(W)* is related to the kinetic energy *(KE)* of the body divided by the time of deceleration *(T)* and the area of the body through which the energy is dissipated *(A)*.[7]

It is important for the flight nurse to estimate the distance fallen. Second, it must be determined what the patient landed on. A soft landing surface such as dirt or sand will absorb much more energy than a hard surface such as concrete.

Three predictable injuries are seen in falls. The forces involved are deceleration and compression. The first injury, calcaneus fractures, is caused by compression of the feet on impact. Then, as the energy dissipates after impact and the top of the body pushes down toward the point of impact, compression fractures to T12-L1 are seen. Finally, the body moves forward, and the patient puts both arms out to complete the fall; bilateral wrist fractures ensue.

Penetrating Trauma

All objects that cause injury from penetration deliver the same two types of force: crushing and stretching.[17] Depending on the velocity of the penetrating object, the wound can be small or massive.

Stab Wounds

Stab wounds are considered to be low velocity and produce their major damage by crushing the tissues as the penetrating object enters. An object that is narrow at the beginning and thicker at the end will crush the tissues as it enters and stretch them apart as the thicker part is inserted.[27] The area of injury for stab wounds is typically localized to the area of insertion. The penetrating instrument might remain embedded in the patient or might have been removed; embedded penetrating objects should be stabilized with bandages for transport and not removed (Fig. 11-3).

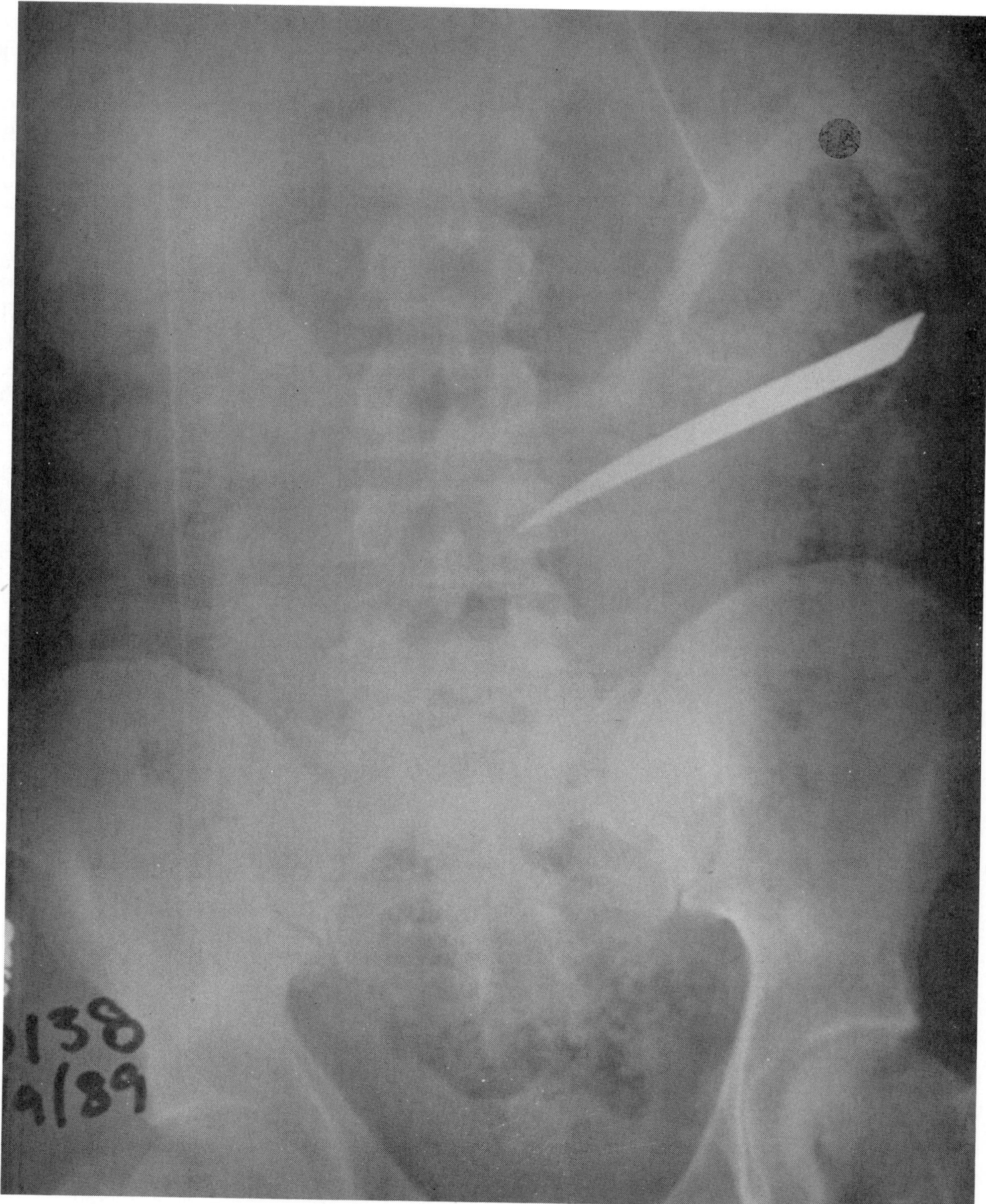

Fig. 11-3. Knife with the handle broken off embedded in a patient. Object was discovered when the x-ray was taken.

Gunshot Wounds

Wounding from bullets can have four causes: (1) direct contact by the missile, (2) crushing force in the immediate vicinity of the missile, (3) temporary cavity formation, and (4) collapse of the temporary cavity.[3]

The degree of wounding depends on the amount of energy transferred from the bullet to the body. The type of weapon used, the type of bullet, the distance at which the weapon was fired, and the body part penetrated are key factors in wound severity.[29]

Firearms can be handguns, rifles, and shotguns. The barrel length of the gun affects bullet velocity. The longer the barrel, the higher the bullet velocity.[12] Handguns therefore are considered low-velocity firearms. Doubling the velocity of a missile will quadruple the kinetic energy transferred to the body. In general, missiles from weapons that travel at speeds higher than 2000 ft/sec are said to be high velocity. The degree of deformation by the penetrating missile is influenced by the following factors:

Yaw and tumbling: Yaw is deviation up to 90 degrees of the bullet from a straight path,[38] and tumbling is rotation of the bullet 360 degrees. Both cause increased tissue crush and stretching.

Deformation of a bullet when striking tissue: Certain missiles are constructed of soft lead and flatten on impact. Other bullets have hollow points that cause a "mushrooming" effect on impact; hollow-point bullets are also known as **expanding bullets.** The increased diameter of these bullets increases tissue destruction.[27]

Fragmentation: Each fragmented portion of the missile causes damage in its path. Increased velocity increases the potential of fragmentation.[27]

Explosive effect: Explosive bullets are intended to cause massive damage with a single shot. The bullet is composed of black powder and lead shot. On impact, detonation of the powder causes explosion and disintegration of the bullet casing, further propelling the lead shot.[35]

The closer to the target the bullet was fired, the greater the amount of kinetic energy transferred to

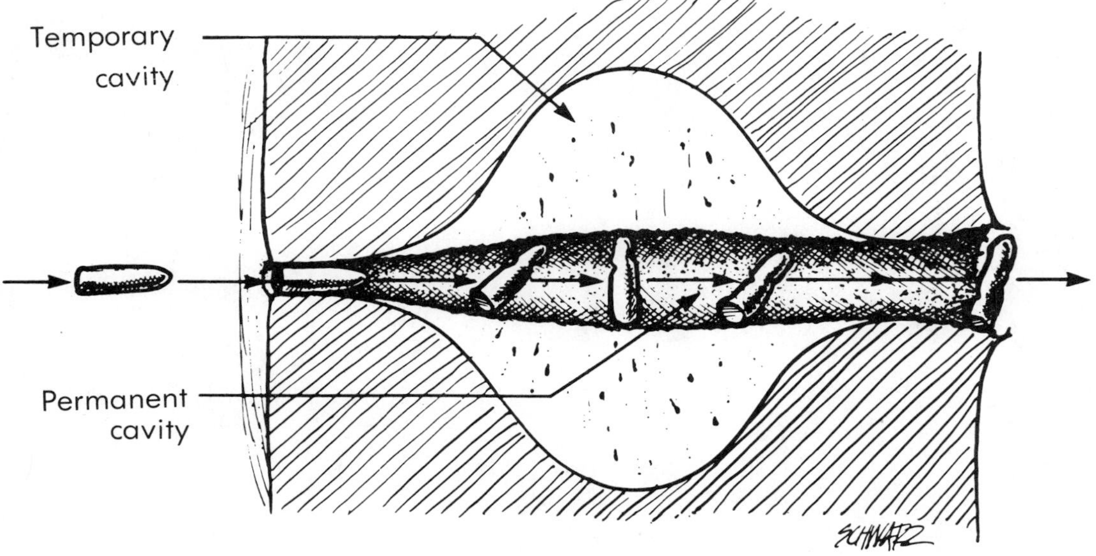

Fig. 11-4. Effects of yaw and temporary and permanent cavitation from a missile. Permanent cavity is caused by necrotic muscle tissue. Temporary cavity is caused by stretching of soft tissue. (From Weiner SL, Barrett J: *Trauma management for civilian and military positions,* Philadelphia, 1986, WB Saunders.)

the tissues. For that reason, firing distance is important to ascertain during the history taking.

Cavitation occurs with all penetrating objects. The permanent cavity is formed from the crushed tissue produced by the object. Temporary cavity formation occurs from transfer of kinetic energy from the missile to the tissue. The velocity, size, shape, and ballistic behavior of the missile and the biophysical properties of the tissue determine the extent of the temporary cavity.[34] As a missile strikes tissue, temporary cavitation occurs forward of and lateral to the missile. Relatively elastic tissues, such as lung, bowel wall, and muscle, tolerate the stretch of the temporary cavity much better than the solid, nonelastic organs, such as the liver and spleen.[18] Past literature has estimated temporary cavity formation as large as 30 to 40 times the missile diameter.[5] Recent studies have indicated that temporary cavitation is usually no more than 10 to 14 times the missile diameter for high-velocity missiles[18,26] (Fig. 11-4).

PATHOPHYSIOLOGIC FACTORS

Multiple trauma causes severe stress to the human body and is associated with a flux of hormones and physiologic reactions. The degree of metabolic and hormonal changes depends on the severity of injury, the effectiveness of resuscitation, and the preinjury condition of the patient.[30] The pathophysiologic analysis of traumatic injuries is discussed in detail in the individual trauma chapters that discuss specific traumas. In general, metabolic response to injury in the early phase differs from that in the late phase.

The early phase occurs during resuscitation and lasts for 24 to 48 hours after injury. During this time, sodium retention occurs, extracellular fluid is depleted, metabolic rate is decreased, and body weight gain occurs because of excess fluid volume. The greater the severity of injury, the longer the period of fluid retention. Increased catecholamine output, increased cortisol levels, and decreased insulin secretion occur in the initial phase. Additionally, vasopressin, renin, angiotensin, and aldosterone levels are increased.

The late metabolic phase of injury, which begins approximately 48 hours after injury, displays an increase in metabolic rate and body weight loss. Glucose reserves are rapidly exhausted, and fat serves as the primary energy substrate. Body proteins are broken down, and protein catabolism occurs.

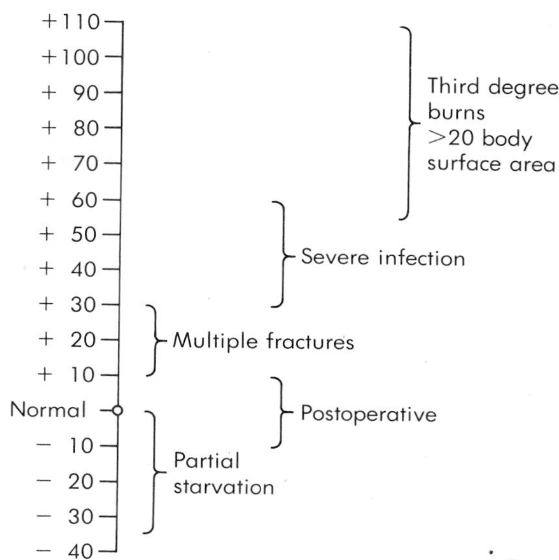

Fig. 11-5. Effects of injury, sepsis, and nutritional depletion on resting energy exposure. (Modified from Richardson JD, Polk HC, Flint LM, editors: *Trauma clinical care and pathophysiology,* Chicago, 1987, Year Book Medical Publishers.)

Hormonal changes associated with the late phase are an elevated insulin level and increased catecholamine, glucagon, and cortisol levels. The catabolic effect seen in this phase is caused by glucagon and cortisol combining with the catecholamines.[11,30]

Fig. 11-5 displays the effects of injury, sepsis, and nutritional depletion on resting energy exposure in the postoperative trauma patient with no complications.[30]

PRIMARY AND SECONDARY ASSESSMENT

When developing a systematic approach for assessing the trauma patient, flight nurses must intervene in life-threatening injuries, discover occult injuries, and prioritize care. In the prehospital setting scene evaluation is very important and includes an assessment of safety. Every team member is responsible for recognizing all possible dangers and ensuring that none still exists. No one should become a victim. The flight nurse should evaluate the scene and if necessary move the patient to a safe area before initiating treatment. The flight nurse is challenged by many factors while attempting to perform a detailed assessment. Three of the most common factors are time, noise level, and the inability to fully disrobe a patient. It is the responsibility of the flight nurse to evaluate each patient situation individually to determine the best approach for the assessment. For example, the flight nurse transporting a patient by rotocraft from the scene of the accident may routinely perform the primary assessment on the scene, load the patient, and do the secondary assessment in the aircraft, thus avoiding delay in definitive care. However, the auscultation of breath sounds and bowel sounds is not possible during the helicopter flight and thus should be performed before liftoff and out of the normal assessment sequence.

Primary Assessment

The focuses of the primary assessment are evaluation of the airway, breathing, and circulation and intervention when life-threatening conditions are identified. The primary assessment should be performed quickly and in the following order of priority: (1) airway and cervical spine stabilization, (2) breathing and ventilation, (3) circulation with hemorrhage control, (4) disability (neurologic status), and (5) exposure (the patient is undressed).

Airway

A secure, patent airway is the first priority for the flight nurse. While the airway is being assessed, the patient's cervical spine should not be moved. The patient's airway should be assessed for patency. Basic maneuvers should be instituted, including suctioning and opening of the airway with a chin-lift or jaw-thrust technique. A patient with head injuries or facial fractures risks losing his or her airway, and the flight nurse should always be prepared to manage the airway before it occludes. Frequent suctioning is often indicated, and the equipment should be at hand. Endotracheal intubation allows for optimal control of the airway, and in the trauma patient the nasotracheal route is primarily indicated to avoid hyperextension of the neck, which occurs with oral intubation. The flight nurse must be able to recognize the indications for intubation and apply the form of airway management that is optimal for the situation and clinical condition.

Breathing

The majority of life-threatening injuries are in the chest and affect breathing (see the following box). Recognition of these injuries is imperative to effectively manage ventilation. Once a patent airway is established, the flight nurse must determine the effectiveness of air exchange. The rise and fall of the chest alone are not sufficient for the flight nurse to determine the status of breathing. The flight nurse should assess the rate of ventilation, use of accessory muscles, and presence of circumoral cyanosis. If spontaneous breathing is absent, the air medical crew begins positive-pressure ventilation through a bag-valve device. For patients who do not require a bag-valve mask, high-flow oxygen through a nonrebreather mask is effective to augment ventilations. All multisystem trauma patients should receive supplemental oxygen during transport, regardless of whether they are symptomatic.

Circulation

Evaluation of circulation is accomplished by pulse assessment. A quick palpation of radial pulses may be sufficient for the flight nurse to determine effective circulation, but consistent evaluation of the fol-

INDICATORS OF IMMEDIATE LIFE-THREATENING CHEST INJURY

1. Open pneumothorax
2. Flail chest
3. Massive hemothorax
4. Tension pneumothorax
5. Cardiac tamponade
6. Penetrating cardiac wounds
7. Air embolus

lowing pulses is recommended to adequately determine circulation: radial, brachial, femoral, and carotid. Absent pulses dictate the need for initiation of chest compressions. Cardiac monitoring should be initiated at this time.

Patients who need immediate surgical intervention may best be treated by the flight nurse performing airway, breathing, and cervical spine control on the ground and gaining venous access in the air. This process allows minimal delay for the patient requiring immediate surgery. The concept that an intravenous line is supportive, rather than restorative, care to the patient is important to remember. Unlike intubation and ventilation of the patient, an intravenous line cannot correct the problem. It only provides supplemental fluid until the underlying condition is corrected. A patient in hypotensive shock may need immediate surgery, and extra time taken, especially at the scene, for lines to be initiated only adds to the delay of definitive care for that patient.

Before moving on to the secondary assessment, the flight nurse should judiciously check the patient for any uncontrolled hemorrhage. Active bleeding is controlled by direct pressure.

A quick neurologic examination with the components of the Glasgow Coma Scale is performed at this first assessment stage.

Secondary Assessment

The optimal initial step in the secondary assessment is for the patient to be completely disrobed. As mentioned earlier, this is often impractical in the prehospital setting. Baring of the chest is essential for evaluation of life-threatening injuries, and exposure of the abdomen is crucial for proper examination, and both should be done in all trauma patients. All restrictive clothing, such as belts, should be removed or cut away. When the patient is exposed for assessment, attention must be given to keeping him or her warm; blankets should cover body areas not being examined at the time.

The secondary assessment proceeds in a systematic fashion from head to toe to reveal all injuries the patient has sustained. During this assessment, the nurse strictly adheres to assessment of the patient and does not intervene for specific injuries. To avoid missed injuries, the flight nurse must develop a routine when performing the secondary assessment. Inspection, auscultation, palpation, and information the patient offers are key to performing this assessment. When proficient, the flight nurse can perform the secondary assessment in approximately 60 seconds. It is easy to focus on obvious injuries during this assessment, but the challenge is to discover occult injuries that may have an adverse affect on the patient's morbidity or mortality.

After completing the secondary assessment, the flight nurse can focus on the patient's specific injuries to determine their severity and to intervene when necessary, for example, by splinting an extremity.

The primary and secondary assessments, along with the treatment of life-threatening injuries, are the most important aspects of trauma care the flight nurse can deliver. They direct the priorities of care during flight and for the staff at the receiving hospital and are the cornerstone for optimal outcome of the patient with multiple injuries.

SCORING OF TRAUMA PATIENTS

Numeric scoring for determination of the severity of injuries is common practice today. Scoring provides a potential outcome classification for trauma patients, through either single-system injuries, multisystem injuries, or the patient's physiologic condition. A variety of injury-severity scores exists; none of them is 100% accurate, and their questionable reliability should be considered with their use. Two common prehospital scoring systems and accepted retrospective scores are discussed in the following subsections.

Prospective Scoring

It has long been a goal of emergency response personnel to develop a numeric score to determine the severity of a patient's injuries at the accident scene. Use of such a score would mean rapid verification of trauma patients and appropriate triage to a trauma center; thus appropriate resources could be used, and morbidity and mortality could be significantly improved. Numerous prehospital scoring indexes have been developed, and two have gained national support.

		Rate	Codes	Score
A. Respiratory rate		10-24	4	
Number of respirations in 15 seconds: Multiply by 4		25-35	3	
		>35	2	
		<10	1	
		0	0	A. ______
B. Respiratory effort		Normal	1	
Retroactive: Use of accessory muscles or intercostal retraction		Retractive	0	B. ______
C. Systolic blood pressure		≥90	4	
Systolic cuff pressure: Either arm, auscultate or palpate		70-89	3	
		50-69	2	
		>50	1	
No carotid pulse		0	0	C. ______
D. Capillary refill				
Normal: Forehead or lip mucosa color refill in 2 seconds		Normal	2	
Delayed: More than 2 seconds capillary refill		Delayed	1	
None: No capillary refill		None	0	D. ______
E. Glasgow Coma Scale		Total GSC points	Score	
1. Eye opening				
Spontaneous	______ 4	14-15	5	
To voice	______ 3	11-13	4	
To pain	______ 2	8-10	3	
None	______ 1	5-7	2	
		3-4	1	E. ______
2. Verbal response				
Oriented	______ 5			
Confused	______ 4			
Inappropriate words	______ 3			
Incomprehensible sounds	______ 2			
None	______ 1			
3. Motor response				
Obeys commands	______ 6			
Purposeful movements (pain)	______ 5			
Withdraw (pain)	______ 4			
Flexion (pain)	______ 3			
Extension (pain)	______ 2			
None	______ 1			
Total GCS points (1 + 2 + 3)	______		Trauma Score ______ (Total points A + B + C + D + E)	

Fig. 11-6. Components of the Trauma Score.

TABLE 11-2

Revised Trauma Score variable break points

Glasgow Coma Scale score	Systolic blood pressure (mm Hg)	Respiratory rate (breaths/min)	Coded value
13-15	>89	10-29	4
9-12	76-89	>29	3
6-8	50-75	6-9	2
4-5	1-49	1-5	1
3	0	0	0

Trauma Score

The Trauma Score is a physiologic index that is comprised of five categories: systolic blood pressure, respiratory rate, respiratory expansion, capillary refill rate, and score on the Glasgow Coma Scale (Fig. 11-6). The score is a number between 1 and 16. Associated with each score is a probability of survival for that score. The lower scores are associated with higher mortality rates. To increase reliability of outcome predictions, the Revised Trauma Score has been developed. The Revised Trauma Score includes the Glasgow Coma Score, systolic blood pressure, and respiratory rate (Table 11-2), but both capillary refill rate and respiratory expansion have been removed because of their subjectivity.[3] The major limitation to the Trauma Score remains the fact that it measures physiologic response; as long as the patient compensates, the score will not accurately reflect his or her condition. The Trauma Score has a sensitivity rate of approximately 80%, and therefore 20% of patients with severe injuries will not be identified with this score.[6]

CRAMS Score

The CRAMS score is also used in the prehospital setting. The CRAMS scale involves assessment of the following areas: circulation, respiration, abdomen and chest, motor, and speech. Each area is graded either 2 (normal), 1 (a deviation from normal), or 0 (absent or none). The highest possible score is 10, which indicates an uninjured patient. The major drawback to the CRAMS score is the need for an actual hands-on assessment for scoring of the abdomen and chest section.[26]

ABBREVIATED INJURY SCALE

0 No injury
1 Minor
2 Moderate
3 Severe
4 Serious
5 Critical
6 Maximum, virtually unsurvivable

For all prospective scales only acute injuries should be scored. A person with paraplegia involved in a motor vehicle accident will have only additional injuries scored, not the previous paraplegia.

Retrospective Scoring

Attachment of a numeric score to each diagnosed injury is the concept of retrospective scoring.

Abbreviated Injury Scale

The Abbreviated Injury Scale (AIS), published by the American Association for Automotive Medicine, categorizes injuries into six body regions (head, neck, thorax, abdomen, spine, and extremity and external) and assigns an individual score to each injury (see the box above). Scores are integers from 1 to 6, according to severity. The lower the score, the less

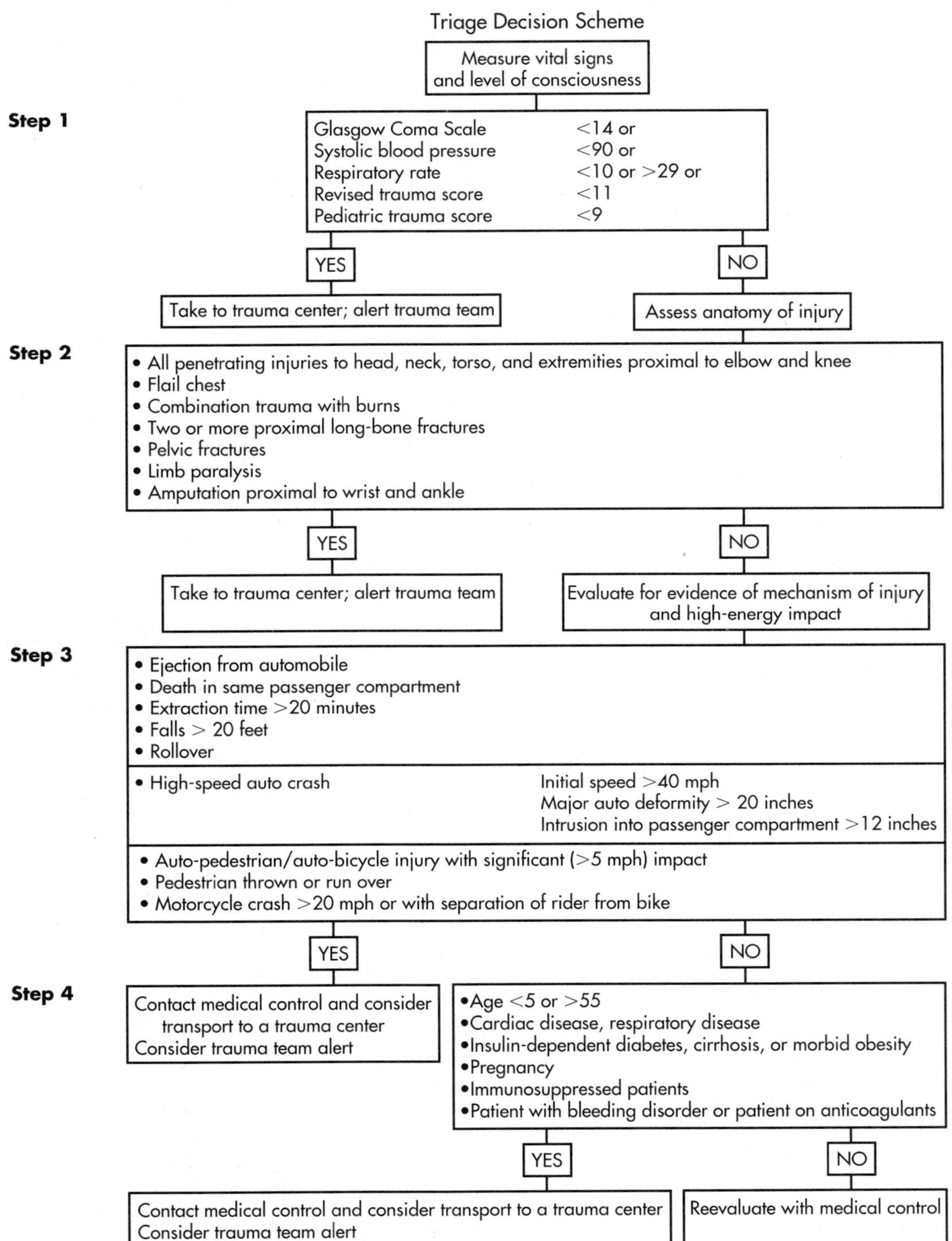

When in doubt take victim to a trauma center

Fig. 11-7. Trauma triage decision-making. (From Committee on Trauma, American College of Surgeons: *Resources for optimal care of the injured patient,* 1993, American College of Surgeons.)

severe the injury.[14] The AIS method was designed to determine severity of motor vehicle injuries. In the 1985 revision of the AIS, penetrating injuries were addressed in all body regions, but the scale is still considered more sensitive to blunt injuries.[13,14] The AIS allows determination of individual injury severity but does not take into account multisystem injuries.

Injury Severity Score

The Injury Severity Score (ISS) quantifies multisystem injury by use of the AIS scores. The ISS is determined by adding of the squares of the highest AIS scores in the three most severely injured body systems. The ISS is a number between 1 and 75, with 1 being a minor injury and 75 being largely nonsurvivable. A patient who receives a score of 6 in any AIS category is automatically scored as having an ISS of 75. It is widely accepted that any patient with an ISS greater than 15 is a major trauma patient.

TRISS

The TRISS method ties together the Trauma Score, ISS, age, and type of injury to determine the probability of survival for the patient.[6,9]

With the focus on percent of mortality, the injury scoring systems have yet to address the probable morbidity associated with physiologic response and actual injuries.

FIELD TRIAGE

Determining appropriate triage to a trauma center is a necessary skill for flight nurses in many parts of the United States today. Proper identification of patients who meet trauma center criteria is routinely based on physiologic criteria such as a blood pressure lower than 90 mm Hg, anatomic criteria such as two long-bone fractures, and a field triage score such as the Revised or Pediatric Trauma Score.[1] Fig. 11-7 displays the standard field triage criteria to a trauma center.

TRIAGE PATIENT TRANSPORT

Care of the multiply injured patient during transport is aimed at maintaining adequate airway, breathing, and circulation; continued stabilization; and constant monitoring of the patient. The success of the transport depends on the flight nurse's ability to anticipate the patient's progression and expect the unexpected.

The number one trauma-related cause of death is central nervous system injury.[28] Expected care by the flight nurse may include hyperventilation and administration of mannitol to decrease intracranial pressure. Problems anticipated by the experienced flight nurse for patients with central nervous system injuries include ineffective airway (if the patient is not intubated) and potential for vomiting with aspiration.

Exsanguination is a common cause of prehospital trauma mortality. Rapid transport to a trauma center for definitive treatment is imperative. The initiation of large-bore intravenous lines may also be indicated during transport.

SUMMARY

The flight nurse provides a critical level of knowledge and expertise of care for the multiply injured patient in the prehospital setting. By understanding the kinematics of trauma, performing a thorough assessment, and delivering care in an organized manner, the flight nurse will have a positive effect on decreasing the morbidity and mortality of such patients.

MULTIPLE-TRAUMA CASE STUDY

The flight team was dispatched to a multiple-victim scene 15 miles from the hospital. It was reported that two victims were dead and two others were severely injured. The rescue squad performed the initial care practice at the advanced level. On arrival at the scene, the flight nurse's aerial view of the scene revealed a single car that had been split in half. Two victims were being attended to by rescuers, and two bodies lying near the wreckage were covered with sheets.

On the basis of the report the flight team received before arrival, they began preparation to transport two victims in the aircraft. Both viable patients had been thrown from the vehicle over the guardrail. Patient 1 was a 15-year-old girl whose left leg had been amputated above the knee. She had multiple abrasions and lacerations on her face and chest. Her Glasgow Coma Scale score was 7 (eye opening, 1; verbal response, 1; motor, 5). She was pale and diaphoretic. She had a palpable femoral pulse of 130 beats/min and a respiratory rate of 8 breaths/minute. Patient 2 was a 16-year-old girl who was awake, screaming, and not following any commands. Her right leg had been amputated above the knee. Her vital signs included a radial pulse of 100 beats/min and a respiratory rate of 28 breaths/minute. Both girls were immobilized on backboards with cervical collars and head blocks. Each had one intravenous line in place.

The flight team elected to intubate the first patient because of her low Glasgow Coma Scale score and her advanced level of shock. Rapid-sequence induction was initiated, and the patient was intubated without difficulty. A palpable systolic pressure of 70 mm Hg was ascertained. A second intravenous line was started, and O-negative blood was infused. The patient was loaded into the aircraft. The second patient was quickly assessed, and oxygen by 100% mask was placed. Soft restraints were applied as a precaution. The patient's blood pressure was 120/80 mm Hg, and the flight nurse decided not to start an additional line. Both patients were prepared for transport and secured in the aircraft.

During the 15-minute transport to the trauma center, the first patient remained hypotensive and tachycardic. No additional neuromuscular blocking agent was administered. The patient received 2 ml fentanyl for agitation. The second patient remained stable. Both patients were hot off-loaded on arrival at the trauma center. Both patients were admitted to the shock resuscitation unit, and a report was given to the resuscitation team.

REFERENCES

1. American College of Surgeons: *Advanced trauma life support student manual,* Chicago, 1993, American College of Surgeons.
2. American College of Surgeons: *Hospital and prehospital resources for optimal care of the injured patient,* appendixes A through J, Chicago, 1993, American College of Surgeons.
3. Copes W: Major trauma outcome study: letter to MTOS participants, Aug 11, 1988, American College of Surgeons.
4. Baker SP, O'Neill B, Karpf R: *The injury fact book,* New York, 1992, Oxford.
5. Barach E, Tomlanovich M, Nowak R: Ballistics: a pathophysiologic examination of the wounding mechanisms of firearms: part I, *J Trauma* 26(3):225, 1986.
6. Boyd CR, Tolson MA, Copes WS: Evaluating trauma care: the TRISS method, *J Trauma* 27(4):370, 1987.
7. Cardona VD, editor: *Trauma nursing: from resuscitation through rehabilitation,* Philadelphia, 1988, WB Saunders.
8. Centers for Disease Control and Prevention—Biomechanics and Injury Control, Division of Injury, Epidemiology and Control: Personal communication, Feb 1989.
9. Champion HR et al: A new characterization of injury severity, *J Trauma* 30(5):539, 1990.
10. Champion HR, Gainer PS, Yackee E: A progress report on the Trauma Score in predicting a fatal outcome, *J Trauma* 26(10):927, 1986.
11. Civetta JM, Taylor RW, Kieby RR, editors: *Critical care,* Philadelphia, 1988, JB Lippincott.
12. Cloonan CC: Management of gunshot wounds in the emergency department, *Trauma Q* 4(1):27, 1987.
13. Conroy C: Trauma as a public health issue, *Trauma Q* 1(3):69, 1985.
14. Copes WS et al: The Injury Severity Score revisited, *J Trauma* 28(1):69, 1988.
15. Daffner RH et al: Patterns of high-speed impact injuries in motor vehicle occupants, *J Trauma* 28(4):498, 1988.
16. Dejarnette R: *The flight nurse advanced trauma course,* Thorofare, NJ, 1994, Slack.
17. Fackler ML, Bellamy RF, Malinowski JA: The wound profile: illustration of the missile-tissue interaction, *J Trauma* 28(1 suppl):S21, 1988.
18. Fackler ML, Malinowski JA: The wound profile: a visual method quantifying gunshot wound components, *J Trauma* 25(6):522, 1985.
19. Fleming A, editor: *Occupants,* Washington, DC, 1988, Insurance Institute for Highway Safety.
20. Holleran RS: *Prehospital nursing: a collaborative approach,* St Louis, 1994, Mosby.
21. Jacobs B, Baker P: *Trauma nursing care course,* Emergency Nurses Association, 1995, Park Ridge, Ill.
22. Janzon B: *High-energy missile trauma: a study of the mechanisms of wounding of muscle tissue,* Göteborg, Sweden, 1983.
23. Kizer K et al: Hospitalization charges, costs, and income for firearm-related injuries at a university trauma center, *JAMA* 273(22):1768, 1995.
24. Lau IV et al: Biomechanics of liver injury by steering wheel loading, *J Trauma* 27(3):225, 1987.

25. MacKenzie EJ et al: Functional recovery and medical costs of trauma: an analysis by type and severity of injury, *J Trauma* 28(3):281, 1988.
26. Mattox K, Moore EE, Feliciano DV, editors: *Trauma,* Norwalk, Conn, 1988, Appleton & Lange.
27. McSwain NE Jr, Kerstein MD, editors: *Evaluation and management of trauma,* Norwalk, Conn, 1987, Appleton-Century-Crofts.
28. National Association of Emergency Medical Technicians: *Prehospital trauma life support student manual,* ed 3, St Louis, 1994, Mosby.
29. Ordog GJ et al: Civilian gunshot wounds: determinants of injury, *J Trauma* 27(8):943, 1987.
30. Richardson JD, Polk HC, Flint LM, editors: *Trauma clinical care and pathophysiology,* Chicago, 1987, Year Book.
31. Sato TB: Effects of seat belts and injuries resulting from improper use, *J Trauma* 27(7):754, 1987.
32. Sleet DA: Motor vehicle trauma and safety belt use in the context of public health priorities, *J Trauma* 27(7): 695, 1987.
33. Sumchai A, Eliastam M, Werner P: Seatbelt cervical injury in an intersection type vehicular collision, *J Trauma* 28(4):498, 1988.
34. Suneson A, Hansson H-A, Lycke E: Pressure wave injuries to rat dorsal root ganglion cells in culture caused by high-energy missiles, *J Trauma* 29(1):10, 1989.
35. Sykes LN Jr, Champion HR, Fouty WJ: Dum-dums, hollow-points and devastators: techniques designed to increase wounding potential of bullets, *J Trauma* 28(5):618, 1988.
36. Trunkey DD: Trauma care at mid-passage—a personal viewpoint: 1987 AAST presidential address, *J Trauma* 28(7):889, 1988.
37. Waller JA: Injury as disease. *Accid Anal Prev* 19(1):13, 1987.
38. Wiener SL, Barrett J: *Trauma management for civilian and military physicians,* Philadelphia, 1986, WB Saunders.
39. Zuidema GD, Rutherford RB, Ballinger WF, editors: The management of trauma as a public health issue, *Trauma Q* 1(3):69, 1985.

CHAPTER 12

Neurologic Trauma Emergencies

COMPETENCIES

1. Provide a baseline neurologic assessment and ongoing serial evaluations of the trauma patient
2. Provide life-sustaining and supportive care with appropriate and aggressive interventions to patients with neurologic trauma to achieve maximum potential for recovery
3. Review the importance of safety for the patient and crew during transport of the patient with neurologic trauma
4. Provide aggressive airway support for the patient with neurologic trauma

Traumatic neurologic emergencies with which air medical crews may have to contend involve disorders of both the central and the peripheral nervous systems. In one way or another the vast majority of these disorders will ultimately affect the respiratory system and thus airway management will be crucial. However, depending on the patient's condition, specific treatment may be instituted that will lessen the impact of emergencies with which the flight nurse will have to contend. The ultimate result may be a progression to coma, often in association with increased intracranial pressure (ICP) or a spinal injury. Therefore it is essential that the flight nurse understand the causes of increased ICP and the neurologic syndromes discussed later in this chapter. Because of the extensive nature of this topic, we have categorized types of neurologic traumatic emergencies and listed by headings the components and management issues as they relate to flight nursing.

HEAD INJURIES

Head injury statistics are staggering. Each year, approximately 2 million head injuries occur in the United States, 140,000 deaths result from head injuries, and 50,000 to 70,000 people are permanently disabled as a result of head injuries. Two thirds of those who sustain head injuries are under the age of 30 years. Costs incurred to care for a head-injured person over the course of his or her lifetime range from $4.1 to $9 million. Severe head injuries are responsible for 9.6 million lost work days and 6.6 million days of hospitalization per year. In general, 20% of all head injuries are classified as major and potentially life threatening.[19,41,42,47]

Head injuries make up 15% of all injuries that occur as a result of motor vehicle accidents and are the major cause of accidental death.[19] Obviously, prevention of head injuries is the long-term solution to this enormous problem.

The outcome for a patient with head injuries may be determined by the severity of the injury and the time elapsed before the patient receives adequate medical attention; thus there is a need for rapid evaluation, assessment, and transfer of the patient to an appropriate-level care facility by the flight nurse. The flight nurse must possess a knowledge of the basic principles of pathophysiology of head injury in order to apply appropriate diagnostic and therapeutic methods and perform a thorough and ongoing systemic evaluation of the patient.

When trauma to the head occurs, the hair and scalp provide some dampening effect on impact. However, the brunt of the blow is delivered to the skull, which has enough elasticity to be flattened or indented when struck with a blunt object. The maximum depression occurs instantly and is followed within a few milliseconds by several oscillations. A severe blow to the skull actually causes a generalized deformation by flattening in the direction of the impact, with a corresponding widening of the diameter at right angles to the impact line.[4,12]

The skull travels faster under impact than does the brain. Although the brain is often contused by the unbending skull at the site of impact, severe brain injuries occur when the brain is hurled against the skull's rough, bony prominence, the crista galli, the major sphenoid wings, or the petrous bones. It is not uncommon for the frontal and temporal poles to be injured. The undersurface of the temporal poles and, less often, the occipital poles are contused or pulped as a result of the unbending skull. Similar damage can also be caused by the edges of the relatively unyielding falx and tentorium. So-called coup lesions develop in opposite areas of the brain on impact.[12,42]

Damage may result from direct injury or may be secondary to compression, tension, or shearing forces caused by the particular injury. In addition, secondary complications result from the head injury. Ischemia and cerebral edema may ensue. There seems to be an immediate increase in ICP on impact; however, there is also a secondary increase several minutes after the injury. The increase in ICP at the time of impact results from acceleration and deceleration of the head and deformation of the skull, the former being more significant than the latter.[3,12,20]

During impact, cerebral spinal fluid may offer some protection to the brain. However, this protective layer is insufficient in the subarachnoid space around the frontal and temporal lobes, the most frequent sites of contusion.[42]

Types of Head Injuries: Pathologic and Clinical Considerations

Head injury may exist in isolation; however, various combinations of injuries usually occur. Each component contributes in a different degree to the overall severity and outcome of the injury.[22]

Skull Fracture

The skull is composed of three layers: an outer layer, a middle cancellous layer, and an inner layer that is one-half as thick as the outer layer and contains grooves that have large vessels. Whether a fracture actually occurs in the area of impact depends on the type of injury. The more concentrated and focused the impact tends to be, the greater the likelihood of a fracture.

Approximately 70% of skull fractures are linear.[17] A linear skull fracture produces a line that usually extends toward the base of the skull. Impact can produce a single linear fracture or multiple fractures, referred to as *linear stellate fractures,* that radiate from the compressed area. Although linear fractures may look benign, they can cause serious complications. One such complication is infection. If the fracture line is open a few millimeters at the time of impact, debris such as hair, dirt, and glass may travel into the cranial vault. Linear fractures may also lead to epidural hematoma if the fracture line crosses a groove in the layer of the skull that houses the middle meningeal artery. Another complication occurs when the dura, which is strongly attached to the skull, tears at the fracture site.

Diastatic and Basilar Skull Fractures. Diastatic fracture involves a separation of bones at a suture line or a marked separation of bone fragments; both are usually visible on skull x-ray films. Facial fracture may also play a role in head injuries. A blow to the lower jaw when the jaw is closed can cause the mandibular condyles to displace upward and backward against the base of the skull, leading to a concussion or a basilar skull fracture. Another type of facial fracture, which may or may not involve the cranium, is an orbital blow-out fracture, which usually involves the floor of the orbit and is caused by blunt impact to the orbit and its contents.

Basilar skull fractures can occur when the mandibular condyles perforate into the base of the skull, but they most often result from extension of fractures of the calvaria. Many basilar skull fractures are impossible to see on an x-ray film. Basilar fractures often produce Battle's sign (an oval-shaped bruise over the mastoid) or "raccoon eyes" (ecchymotic areas around the eyes).

Depressed Skull Fracture. The presence of depressed elements of a fracture may warrant specific diagnostic and therapeutic measures. If the depressed fracture is closed, the rationale for surgical correction is to evacuate any local mass if present, repair any dural lacerations to prevent cerebral herniation through the defect, and correct any cosmetic disfigurement caused by the depression. In general, if the depression on the tangential view of the skull is greater than the thickness of the skull, the dura is probably lacerated and surgery is recommended. Depressions of a lesser degree, unless over the forehead, rarely require surgical exploration.

A compound depressed skull fracture usually requires surgical debridement. If the injury has been caused by a blow to a static head, the patient's level of consciousness is frequently well preserved, and there may be no neurologic deficits. When a blow has been sustained to a moving head, consciousness is impaired.

Skull fractures can be the source of various complications, including intracranial infections, hematomas, and meningeal and brain tissue damage. Approximately 3% of all skull fractures are associated with *pneumocephalus,* which is defined as the presence of air within the cranial vault.[4] Traumatic pneumocephalus may occur if the frontal, ethmoid, or sphenoid sinuses or the mastoid processes are fractured. Air that has entered the skull will locate in the epidural, subdural, subarachnoid, interventricular, or intercerebral space. Pneumocephalus seldom produces symptoms unless it is under tension and thus produces compression of the underlying brain tissue. The incidence of pneumocephalus and cerebral spinal fluid rhinorrhea with sella turcica fractures is small, but there is a high incidence of infection if this condition is present. There may be associated palsies of the oculi motor, trochlear, trigeminal, or abducens nerves.[29]

In general, temporal bone fractures can cause pneumocephalus if dural tearing occurs in conjunction with injury to the eustachian tube, the middle ear, or the mastoid process. The patient may have sensory neurologic hearing loss, otorrhagia, or cerebral spinal fluid rhinorrhea in the presence of a temporal bone fracture.

Hemorrhage

Subdural Hematoma. Subdural hematoma is a collection of blood between the brain surface and the dura. It may occur as a result of a contusion or laceration of the brain with bleeding into the subdural space, tearing of the veins that bridge the subdural space, or an extension of an intercerebral hematoma through the brain surface into the subdural space. Subdural hematoma might be unassociated with skull fracture.[39]

Subdural hematomas are classified as acute, subacute, or chronic, depending on the time elapsed between the injury and the appearance of signs and symptoms of neurologic dysfunction. As with other types of head injury, the time course of development and the degree and rate of neurologic dysfunction depends on many factors. As a general rule, if dysfunction occurs within 24 hours, the hematoma is acute; if it occurs between 2 and 10 days, it is subacute; and if it occurs after 2 weeks, the hematoma is chronic. This particular classification is partially pathologic. The location of the hematoma and the amount of mass effect play important roles in determining the timing of surgical intervention.

Elderly patients may have larger subdural hematomas with slowly developing symptoms because they have larger potential subdural spaces as a result of cerebral atrophy. In contrast, symptoms may be displayed rapidly and marked increases in intercranial pressure may develop in a younger patient with a small subdural space.

Subdural hematomas generally occur in children under the age of 2 years. Signs and symptoms include a bulging fontanelle and a large head (because of separation of the sutures) and retinal hemorrhages (because of increased ICP). In the infant patient a shocklike state may also develop because a relatively large blood volume loss may be caused by a subdural hematoma.

Acute subdural hematomas are usually associated with a high morbidity and mortality, reflecting the usually severe nature of the associated injuries and the not-infrequent association of rapidly rising ICP resulting from the mass effect and development of cerebral edema. Two separate related pathophysiologic problems are cerebral contusion and edema and the presence of blood in the subdural space. The computed tomography (CT) scan is very valuable in determining whether surgery is indicated. If the major problem contributing to the patient's poor neurologic status is the mass effect, then surgical intervention is necessary. If the major problem is the cerebral injury, then corrective treatment should be directed toward treating increased ICP.

Both of these groups of patients are treated with intensive medical therapy (muscle paralysis, hyperventilation, and mannitol) to maintain an ICP of less than 20 torr. The major objective in the treatment of patients with acute subdural hematoma is the control of cerebral edema and elevated ICP, whether or not surgical decompression is performed. The primary objective of surgical decompression is to correct the brain displacement and herniation. Historically the result of treatment of patients with acute subdural hematomas is poor, with mortality rates as high as 90%. The morbidity and mortality rate can be significantly reduced with evacuation of the hematoma within 4 hours, as reported by Seeling in 1981; a reduction from 90% to 30% was obtained.[39]

Epidural Hematoma. Epidural hematomas are classified as acute or subacute. An acute epidural hematoma that is arterial in origin generally produces symptoms within a few hours. Subacute epidural hematomas are venous in origin and take a longer time to produce symptoms. These hematomas are associated with linear skull fractures in 90% of patients, but they may also occur as a result of blunt injuries in which there is no evidence of fracture.[4] The classic symptoms displayed by a patient with an epidural hematoma are transient loss of consciousness, recovery with a lucid interval during which the patient's neurologic status returns to normal, and the secondary onset of headache and a decreasing level of consciousness. As a result of the initial injury, the middle meningeal artery may tear, causing traumatic unconsciousness. Spasm and clotting then occur in the middle meningeal artery, and the bleeding stops. During the next several hours the artery gradually bleeds and a hematoma is formed, stripping the dura from the inside of the skull. Once a headache with a decreasing level of consciousness becomes obvious, the secondary rise in ICP has already occurred, and distortion of the brain with significant mass effect occurs. Because compensatory mechanisms of the inner cranial space have already been exhausted, the patient's neurologic status rapidly deteriorates. The patient experiences a downhill course, usually with dilatation of the ipsilateral pupil because of third-nerve compression by the herniating temporal structures, progressive unconsciousness with weakness or decerebration of either the contralateral extremities or the ipsilateral extremities, Cheyne-Stokes respirations, and, if no treatment is initiated, loss of pupillary reflexes, caloric responses, bradycardia, and death. It is thus extremely important to identify the epidural hematoma in the earliest possible stage, when a headache and drowsiness are the only complaints, and to transfer the patient for immediate neurosurgical intervention.[23] The classic history and clinical progression, however, is only seen in one third of patients with epidural hematomas. Another third are unconscious from the time of injury, and the final third are never unconscious. In children, bradycardia and early papilledema may be the only warning signs.[4,26]

The best diagnostic test is the CT scan, and surgical evacuation is used to treat the patient with acute epidural hematoma. The flight nurse may need to use medical management to control rapidly progressive intracranial hypertension so as to gain the time needed to reach the operating department and evacuate the clot. Endotracheal intubation, muscle paralysis, hyperventilation, and use of osmotic agents may all be necessary. The flight nurse plays a key role in the outcome of these patients through continued observation, early recognition of changes in neurologic status, and rapid intervention with use of the described measures to prevent herniation syndrome. Most patients with epidural hematomas make a rapid recovery after early evacuation of the clot.

Intracerebral Hematoma. Movement of one section of brain tissue over or against another section causes tears in blood vessels, which leads to contusions or intracerebral hematomas. Most intracerebral hematomas are found in the frontal and temporal lobes, usually very deep, and are associated with necrosis and hemorrhage. The anatomic relationship between these areas and irregularities of the skull have already been discussed. Intracerebral hematomas are readily identified on the CT scan. The clinical picture may vary from no neurologic defect to deep coma; however, two clinical patterns should be recognized. Patients with slowly accumulating frontal and temporal hematomas frequently demonstrate a rather slow deteriorating rate of consciousness with minimal focal signs during a 24- to 48-hour period. These hematomas must be identified early because a sudden change in ICP precipitated by a seizure or suctioning may produce herniation. The second usual clinical pattern is demonstrated by patients with delayed hemorrhage. These patients show progressive recovery of consciousness during a 10- to 14-day period and then headaches may suddenly develop, followed by rapid neurologic deterioration. The exact pathology of this delayed hemorrhage is not clear, but it is probably a new hemorrhage and not the sudden expansion of preexisting hematoma.

Large solitary intracerebral hematomas should be evacuated, as should a delayed hemorrhage. Mortality after surgery for traumatic intracerebral hematomas has been reported to be greater than 42%. The primary problems related to these patients are the degree of cerebral injury and the intensive monitoring and management required for long periods.[4,25]

Closed Head Injury

Concussion. The term *concussion* applies to injuries that result in transient alterations of consciousness. There have been reports of deaths when prolonged apnea ensues, but recovery is the rule. No specific neurologic abnormalities are present, although a postconcussive syndrome may follow even minor injuries.

Cerebral Contusion. Cerebral hemorrhagic contusions frequently occur in patients, particularly adults, after head injury. Of the patients who die as a result of head injury, 75% have contusions at autopsy. Hemorrhagic contusions are infrequently seen in children, but areas of localized decreased density on a CT scan may represent nonhemorrhagic contusions or possibly local ischemia.[21]

Generally, no surgical intervention is recommended for cerebral contusions, because brain matter cannot be removed in areas of the brain that control motor, sensory, or visual functioning. If, however, the contusion occurs over the frontal or temporal lobes, with significant edema and shift, it is feasible to remove contused portions of the brain surgically. When a temporal lobe contusion is present and signs of herniation are seen, surgical excision of the temporal lobe may be beneficial. Generally, patients with contusion are treated by controlling elevated ICP medically.[13]

Penetrating Injuries

Gunshot Wounds. When a person is shot at close range, there may be evidence of smoke on the skin. When the muzzle of the gun is somewhat farther from the scalp but still close, there may be evidence of powder burns. A bullet striking the skull can cause great destruction of the underlying brain tissue.

Although some of the energy of impact may be dissipated by the shattering of bones and soft tissues, the impact on the brain after a bullet penetrates the skull is still great. The bullet's ability to destroy tissues is directly related to its kinetic energy at the moment of impact. The degree of damage to the brain depends primarily on the muzzle velocity of the bullet and the distance between the gun and its target.

A bullet that passes through the head produces a larger defect on the inner table of the skull than that produced on the outer table. High-velocity bullets cause extensive injury to the brain and cranium. The entrance wound is usually smaller than the exit wound, but there may be a great deal of variation in their sizes. Multiple linear fractures that radiate from either the entrance or exit wound are common. Some fractures may be far away from the trajectory of the bullet, particularly in thin bones. The flight nurse should describe the wounds but not attempt to determine whether they are entrance or exit wounds.

Injuries to the major cerebral arteries, veins, or venous sinuses can occur during any of the bullet's intracranial passages. Cerebral injuries cause an immediate but transitory increase in ICP. The eventual ICP depends on the degree of intracranial bleeding, which may be profuse even in the absence of injury to major vessels. Secondary cerebral edema causes a delayed increase in ICP. Damage to the hemisphere causes loss of autoregulation, falling cerebral blood flow, an increase in cerebral blood volume and ICP, and, eventually, brain death.

Intracranial hematomas are frequently associated with penetrating wounds to the brain. If the bullet passes close to or transverses the ventricle, an intraventricular hematoma may result.

Infection is seen often in injuries caused by shell fragments because these fragments are more likely than bullets to carry dirt, hair, and bone fragments into the brain. Infections develop most often from retained bone fragments, improper closure of the scalp and dura, and delay of definitive surgery beyond 48 hours.

Stab Wounds. Whenever the skull has been penetrated there is a risk of intracranial infection. The injury should be managed so as to minimize that risk. All patients with penetrating injuries should receive tetanus prophylaxis.

Most stab wounds are caused by assaults with sharp instruments such as knives, scissors, and screwdrivers or when the patient (often a child) falls on a stick or sharp toy. It is best to transport a stab-wound patient with the object immobilized, secured, and left in place.

If the penetrating object has been removed, it may be difficult to determine exactly where penetration of the skull occurred, particularly if entry occurred at the eyelid or sclera. When the patient arrives at the hospital, the area of injury is explored and debrided, as with an open injury.

Physical Assessment: Head Injury

Examination of a patient who is unconscious requires integration of information from several systems: mental status, the pupils, other cranial nerves, the motor system, and respiratory function (see Table 19-1, Physiologic disturbance correlated with anatomic level of lesion).

Mental Status

The best indicator of ICP, especially from a mass lesion, is a patient's progression (that is, deterioration) from consciousness to unconsciousness as noted by the flight nurse during assessment of mental status. Consciousness is a mental state in which the person is stimulated by the environment and can react appropriately to it. A useful way of quantitating the conscious state is to divide it into alert, lethargic, or obtunded stages (see box).

The *alert* patient readily responds to the examiner, although, depending on the state of the central nervous system (CNS) injury, there may be some confusion, speech disturbance, and motor deficits. The **lethargic** patient appears to be drowsy or asleep but can be aroused easily and can respond reasonably appropriately to the examiner's questions, although if

STAGES IN PROGRESSION FROM CONSCIOUSNESS TO UNCONSCIOUSNESS

Conscious State

Alert: Patient responds readily but may have some confusion, speech disturbance, or motor deficit.

Lethargic: Patient appears drowsy or sleepy but can be aroused to respond to questioning.

Obtunded: Patient is extremely drowsy, is difficult to arouse, and rarely answers in complete sentences.

Unconscious State

Stuporous: Patient does not verbalize appropriately or coherently; may moan and groan or utter monosyllables.

Comatose: Patient gives no evidence of awareness.

left alone, he or she will slowly return to an apparent sleep state or certainly lack attentiveness. The **obtunded** patient is extremely drowsy, arouses with greater difficulty than a lethargic patient, rarely answers in complete sentences, and certainly does not volunteer information. In fact, during the active questioning period the examiner may have to repeatedly stimulate the patient to gain attention.

Deterioration beyond the obtunded level results in the unconscious state. This state may be classified as either stupor or coma.

The **stuporous** patient does not verbalize appropriately or coherently. Two distinct levels of activity can characterize this state. The patient in a lightly stuporous state may moan and groan in response to stimulation or may utter an occasional recognizable monosyllabic word, often a slang or curse word. The patient who is in a light stuporous condition will respond to pain by moving all extremities, unless there is a primary motor system injury, and will appear to crudely localize the site of the pain. However, a patient who is in a deeply stuporous state will not appear to localize and protect against pain. The patient who is in true coma may have decorticate posturing, decerebrate posturing, or flaccid motor response.

In examining the pattern of motor response it is important to be aware of the possibility of primary motor system injury. For example, a left cortical lesion or a lesion in the left internal capsule may cause a contralateral hemiparesis that even in the awake patient may distort the motor response.

The **comatose** state roughly divides into three levels of reflex motor activity: **decorticate posturing, decerebrate posturing,** and **flaccidity,** to use clinically descriptive terms rather than more precise neurophysiologic descriptions. The patient in a decorticate state is unconscious and gives no evidence of awareness. Painful stimulation causes extensor rigidity in the lower extremities combined with a flexor posture of the upper extremities. Depending on the extent of the underlying damage to the motor system, this posturing may occur spontaneously or after painful stimulation and may be more prominent on one side than the other. Decerebrate posturing is exhibited by extensor rigidity in all four extremities. The patient who is flaccid has no motor response to painful stimulation.

For consciousness to be present, a stimulus must be presented to the CNS and must pass through the brain stem (with the exception of visual stimulation) to the diencephalon. From there the stimulus must reach the cerebral cortex, where it is recorded. The patient must have sufficient cortical function so that the stimulus can excite associations through memory, which will let the patient acknowledge the presence of the stimulus and make use of that stimulus to relate appropriately to the external environment.

For example, when an intracranial mass lesion develops after head trauma and unconsciousness does not initially result, the patient may be expected, as the mass lesion increases, to progress systematically through the various levels and stages just described. The mass lesion may be a hematoma or a significant cerebral edema. A patient with a head injury resulting in a primary upper brain stem lesion might be unconscious and would immediately evidence a comatose state without having ever experienced cortical or diencephalic deterioration. A person who survives a near-drowning or delayed cardiopulmonary resuscitation may have severe bilateral cortical injury and may not progress significantly. A person who experiences a spontaneous hemorrhage in the brain stem, particularly in the region of the pons or midbrain, would be expected to become suddenly comatose with no evidence of an orderly progression through the stages noted previously.

Examination of the Pupils

The pupils are innervated by both the parasympathetic (third-nerve) and the sympathetic systems, with the former causing constriction and the latter causing dilatation. The size of the pupil will depend on the degree to which each system is influencing the pupil at the time of examination. The normal pupil will constrict promptly to light. Examination of the pupils consists of assessment of the relative size of the two pupils and their reactivity to light. Injury to the parasympathetic system will result in pupillary dilatation. Injury to the parasympathetic system may occur within the midbrain at the origin of the parasympathetic contribution to the third nerve, or it may occur outside the brain stem where the third nerve exits and proceeds forward beneath the brain into the region of the cavernous sinus. The sympathetic innervation begins in the posterior hypothalamus, descends the length of the brain stem and cervical cord, and exits in the lower cervical upper thoracic area, where it proceeds up the neck in the cervical sympathetic chain to the base of the skull and then out to the orbit where innervation occurs. Injury to the sympathetic system results in pupillary constriction because of the actions of the unopposed third nerve. The sympathetic system can be injured within the CNS anywhere along its pathway and during its course through the chest and neck. Because of the relatively small size of the structures involved, it is unlikely that lesions within the brain or brain stem will affect either the parasympathetic or the sympathetic systems unilaterally. Therefore, it can be assumed that if bilateral pupil abnormalities are seen, the nerve supply to the pupils has been affected by a lesion within the brain or brain stem. For example, bilaterally small pupils may very well be caused by a lesion within the brain stem that affects both descending sympathetic tracts. On the other hand, a unilateral affected pupil can be expected to be caused by a lesion of the tracts outside the brain or brain stem (extraaxial). A unilaterally dilated pupil may be caused by compression of the third nerve by a herniating temporal lobe after it has exited the midbrain and as it crosses the floor of the skull. A unilateral small pupil resulting from sympathetic denervation will react more sluggishly to light. Bilaterally dilated and fixed pupils are generally caused by global hypoxia or by bilateral temporal lobe herniation from central cerebral edema with bilateral third-nerve compression. Bilaterally constricted pupils may be caused by central herniation of the posterior hypothalamus at the site of origin of the sympathetic fibers through the tentorial notch or by bilateral involvement within the brain stem, such as from a pontine hemorrhage. Midbrain lesions that affect the parasympathetic bilaterally will yield pupils that are in midposition and are nonreactive to light. It is helpful to examine other cranial nerves because they can reveal the competency of brain stem function.

Brain Stem and Cranial Nerve

The integrity of the brain stem can be evaluated by examining certain cranial nerves, especially those related to conjugate gaze. In the patient who is awake, conjugate gaze is controlled by visual input through the complex system that coordinates the function of the extraocular muscles by way of cranial nerves III, IV, and VI. In the patient who is unconscious, however, visual input gives way to vestibular input to control conjugate gaze. This is best evaluated by examining the oculocephalic or oculovestibular reflexes.[36]

The oculocephalic reflex is demonstrated by stimulating the vestibular system through movement of the head in reference to the neck. While the patient lies supine on the ground, stretcher, or bed, the assessing nurse opens the patient's eyelids. Under normal circumstances the eyes should stare at the sky or ceiling. The nurse then rotates the head briskly but gently to one side or the other. Under normal circumstances the eyes may momentarily remain in their position in the orbits but will immediately track conjugately to the side opposite the direction of the movement so that the eyes will be directed once again toward the sky or ceiling. If conjugate activity cannot be observed, for example, if one eye tracks and the other one does not or if neither eye tracks, this signals an abnormality and suggests a disturbance of the brain stem. This maneuver should never be performed in a patient with a head injury or multiple trauma until the cervical spine has been determined to be without injury.

The oculovestibular reflex is demonstrated by cold caloric stimulation, in which cold saline solution is irrigated into the external auditory canal. In a few seconds the eyes will conjugately deviate to the side of the irrigation and remain in that position from several seconds to several minutes. If this response is not seen an abnormality is present in the brain stem involving the medial longitudinal fasciculus, the vestibular system, or both. The flight nurse should not perform this maneuver on a patient with head injury until the possibility of a basal skull fracture involving the temporal bone has been excluded.

The midportion of the pons may be evaluated by the presence or absence of the corneal reflex. The corneal reflex can quickly be assessed by lightly touching the cornea with the corner of a soft gauze dressing and observing whether a blink reflex occurs.

Motor Examination

The motor system is best examined in conjunction with an examination of the patient's mental status. The awake patient can be asked to perform certain motor tasks, such as moving his or her legs or gripping. If the patient is unconscious, motor activity in response to pain is a good way to determine the level of unconsciousness, as previously described.

Respiratory Pattern

Most patients with significant head injuries will hypoventilate early after the injury. Later the respiratory pattern may vary, depending on the level of the lesion. Patients with decorticate posturing often demonstrate an accompanying Cheyne-Stokes pattern of respiration in which there is a regular crescendo-decrescendo change in the volume of inspiration, with the rate remaining rather regular. The patient with decerebrate posturing may exhibit central neurogenic hyperventilation. Patients with brain stem lesions may have varying rates and depths of respiration, and an ataxic element is often noted. With lower brain stem lesions the rate becomes more irregular, more shallow, and less frequent, until medullary lesions result in respiratory paralysis. It is often necessary for the flight nurse to intubate the patient for respiratory control.

The respiratory patterns of patients in a metabolic coma will be dictated by the cause of the coma. Patients with intrinsic metabolic lesions that lead to conditions such as diabetic ketoacidosis or hepatic coma may demonstrate a driven hyperventilation; patients who have ingested opiates will have a much more shallow respiratory pattern with a decreased frequency, depending on the drug level. Naloxone hydrochloride may be used in a dose of 0.4 to 2 mg intravenously as an opiate antagonist and to confirm the presence of opiate ingestion before obtaining a blood sample for drug level. However, naloxone should not be used to treat known drug ingestion. Instead, tubes should be inserted and the airway managed until the drug has cleared and respiratory activity returns to normal. Use of naloxone in greater than recommended doses has been reported to produce cardiovascular instability.

The Glasgow Coma Scale

The Glasgow Coma Scale (GCS), as shown in Table 12-1, is widely used to measure the severity of coma in patients and is therefore an indicator of prognosis. However, eye opening response may not be accurately assessed in the patient with severe maxillofacial injuries whose airway is being mechanically supported. In addition, in a patient with a contralateral mass lesion, the best motor response may not depict progressing hemiparesis. When examining a patient it is best merely to record the GCS results in the narrative record that goes to the receiving health care providers.

Reexamination

Successful acute management of the comatose patient depends on frequent examination of the patient to determine his or her level of neurologic function and rate of deterioration. The information provided in Table 19-1 can be helpful in this analysis.

When the flight nurse sees the comatose patient for the first time, he or she should initiate a complete neurologic examination to establish a baseline. Findings during subsequent examinations will provide the flight nurse with an understanding of the intracranial injury. When a focal mass lesion such as a hematoma or focal contusion develops in a patient, he or she will steadily progress in depth of coma through the various levels depicted in Table 19-1. For example, when the initial examination of a patient results in findings compatible with a diencephalic level of coma, the coma will be determined to have deteriorated to a midbrain level if the patient is subsequently found to have decerebrate posturing, midposition pupils, and central neurogenic hyperventilation. If the insult is unilateral, hemiparesis and an ipsilateral dilated pupil will be seen before bilateral motor signs of herniation are seen. If the patient initially shows signs of coma resulting from a primary brain stem injury—a static lesion—a further deterioration in the level will not be demonstrated within the next few hours, other than what would normally be seen with a developing mass lesion. Finally, if the patient does not have a significant head injury but rather on initial examination is found to have a suppressed level of consciousness because of a metabolic disorder, such as drug intoxication, the examinations over time will demonstrate a pattern of what appears to be multilevel involvement, depending on the sensitivity of the system being examined to the drug concentration in the blood.

Interventions and Treatment

Airway and Ventilation

The flight nurse's highest priority is establishing an adequate airway, especially for supine, unconscious patients or patients with high-level spinal cord injury. Not only must the airway be maintained, but ventilation must be adequate; the rate and quality of respiration must be carefully observed. The nose and mouth should be cleared of blood and mucus. Any clinical signs of upper airway obstruction or respiratory difficulties should prompt immediate endotracheal intubation or, if necessary, a surgical airway and mechanical ventilatory support. Rapid sequence intubation will facilitate intubation and minimize increases in ICP.[2] Care must be taken to maintain cervical spine immobilization while gaining access to the

TABLE 12-1

The Glasgow Coma Scale

CIRCLE THE APPROPRIATE NUMBER AND COMPUTE THE TOTAL

Best eye-opening response:	______ Right ______ Left	
	Never	1
	To pain	2
	To verbal stimuli	3
	Spontaneously	4
Best verbal response:		
	No response	1
	Incomprehensible sounds	2
	Inappropriate words	3
	Disoriented and converses	4
	Oriented and converses	5
Best motor response:	______ Right ______ Left	
	No response	1
	Extension abnormal (decerebrate rigidity)	2
	Flexion abnormal (decorticate rigidity)	3
	Flexion withdrawal	4
	Localizes pain	5
	Obeys commands	6
	Total: ______ **3-15**	
Neurologic evaluation:	Record on Glasgow Coma Scale sheet. Repeat evaluation frequently. A score of 15 is normal; below 7 indicates coma; 3 signifies brain death. **Vital signs:** Level of consciousness Glasgow Coma Scale Pupillary size and reactivity Right ______ Left ______ Focal weakness Present ______ Absent ______	

airway. A nasogastric tube should be inserted with care to prevent aspiration pneumonia, particularly when the patient has a basilar skull fracture.

Respiratory distress may be caused by pulmonary injury, airway obstruction, or aspiration. Increased arterial partial pressure of carbon dioxide ($PaCO_2$) increases blood flow and results in cerebral edema. Controlled hyperventilation should therefore be used to maintain $PaCO_2$ at approximately 30 mm Hg and arterial partial pressure of oxygen (PaO_2) at more than 80 mm Hg. Because no equipment is currently available to directly monitor ICP during transport, the flight nurse should monitor other parameters that indirectly control ICP. Pulse oximetry and end-tidal CO_2 ($ETCO_2$) devices are readily available and function well in the air medical environment.[26,35]

On arrival at the hospital, approximately 35% of comatose patients with severe head injuries are hypoxic ($PaCO_2$ <80 mm Hg), 15% are hypotensive (systolic pressure below 95 mm Hg), and 10% are apneic.[20] Because these abnormalities will result in cerebral ischemia and secondary brain injury,[11,26] the flight nurse should strive to correct hypoxia and hypotension while maintaining mild hyperventilation.

Fluid Administration

Skilled flight crews should transport the patient without delay to an optimal care hospital where CT scanning and neurosurgical care are available.[44] Intravenous access, 16 gauge or larger, with isotonic fluid administration at a rate of approximately 80 to 100 ml per hour (in the absence of hypovolemia) should be instituted. If the patient is not intubated, oxygen should be administered by nonrebreather mask at high flow rates, and if the patient requires intubation, oxygen should be administered at a concentration of 100% with mild hyperventilation.

Monitoring

Repeated assessment of the patient's pupils, eye openings, and motor and verbal responses during transport is mandatory. The flight nurse should monitor the patient's blood pressure, pulse, temperature, and respiratory status (pulse oximetry and $ETCO_2$) and be prepared to administer diuretics such as mannitol and furosemide (Lasix) should there be a progressive neurologic deterioration consistent with a mass lesion, suggesting tentorial herniation.[27]

Cerebral edema can be temporarily reduced with controlled hyperventilation and administration of osmotic diuretics, such as mannitol. Mannitol is the most common diuretic used because it is not metabolized and is nontoxic and easily administered. The average dose is 1 to 1.5 g per kilogram given in an intravenous bolus. Because large volumes of urine may be excreted, a urinary catheter must be in place. This loss of fluid may further compromise an unstable systemic circulation, and thus osmotic diuretics should not be used if hypovolemia is present. Repeated use may cause fluid and electrolyte disassociation that may be severe. The use of osmotic diuretics should be reserved for cases in which herniation syndrome is thought to be developing after trauma, when a mass lesion is suggested, when there is a decreasing level of consciousness, when hemiparesis is present, when the patient has a dilating pupil, or when there is evidence of increased ICP in the patient with rapid decrease in loss of consciousness and bilaterally dilated pupils.[1,7,10,42,46]

If the patient is restless or agitated, hypoxia should be suspected until a specific cause can be found. Most patients with head injuries have sustained other injuries that will cause pain. Even in the patient who is inattentive or stuporous, hypoxia rather than pain should be considered the cause of restlessness until this is proved otherwise.

The intubated patient who is restless or who resists ventilatory support is increasing his or her ICP, which may be extremely critical. These patients should be subdued with pharmacologically appropriate doses of paralytic agents.[7] If paralytic agents are used, it is important to closely monitor the patient's temperature for the presence of hypothermia, because of the inability of the patient to shiver, or for evidence of malignant hyperthermia, particularly in children.

Seizures that develop during transport should be promptly treated because they produce hypoxia and cause increased ICP; diazepam, administered intravenously in 5 to 10 mg doses, may be used effectively. Prophylactic use of antiepileptic medications may also be considered.[43,49] Unconscious patients or

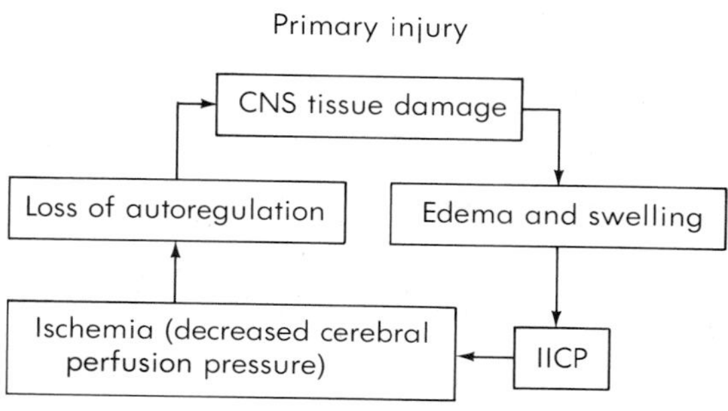

Fig. 12-1. Sequence of pathophysiologic events installed by primary injury.

those who have a depressed level of consciousness associated with seizure activities should be intubated for maximal control of the airway. Because having an adequate airway is of paramount importance, the airway should be secured immediately.

In general, hypertension and bradycardia may develop in patients who have increased ICP. Hypotension and tachycardia are not signs of intracranial injury, except in a patient who is herniating. However, small children may become hypovolemic from scalp lacerations associated with head injuries and should be monitored and treated accordingly with volume replacement.

Patients with head injuries may lose their cerebral autoregulation (Fig. 12-1). If this is the case, cerebral perfusion is directly related to mean systemic arterial pressure. Thus hypotension may lead to underperfusion, and hypertension may lead to vascular congestion and mass effect. Both extremes should be avoided.

Hyperthermia also increases ICP, and thus normal body temperatures should be maintained with the use of acetaminophen suppositories or cooling techniques. Shivering should be controlled because it increases ICP.

SPINAL CORD INJURY

The flight nurse should perform a baseline evaluation of the patient with a spine injury before transfer and should monitor the patient closely for changes in neurologic status during the transfer process. All trauma patients are suspect for spine injury and should be treated accordingly.[38] These patients should be transferred supine on a firm surface with the spine in good alignment.[40] Studies suggest that logrolling of patients with spine injuries is destabilizing at the fracture site and should be avoided if possible. A scoop stretcher may be used to transfer the patient onto the rigid helicopter or fixed-wing aircraft stretcher in such a way as to avoid the torsion effects produced by the logrolling maneuver.[24]

When appropriate and delineated by established guidelines, patients with cervical spine injury may be transported in traction. Proper equipment such as a spring-loaded scale system is necessary, because use of hanging weights is inappropriate in the air medical setting. Traction may be applied with the use of a halter or cranial tongs.[9,30,31,37] Spring-loaded cranial tongs are the most common device used for cervical traction in the emergency setting.[45] With proper training, the flight nurse may apply the cranial tongs and traction before the transfer. If skull fractures over the insertion site preclude the application of cranial tongs, traction may be applied with the use of a halter.[30] More advanced cranial tongs that are compatible with scanning by CT and magnetic resonance systems are now being produced.

Etiology and Incidence

The incidence of spinal cord injuries (SCIs) that result in paralysis or debilitating weakness as a consequence of trauma to the spinal cord has been analyzed statistically in many different ways in many different countries. Studies reported in the Head and Spinal Cord Injury System Data Bank show that the occurrence rate is about 30 to 40 new cases per million population per year.

The age distribution of acute SCIs peaks in the 15- to 24-year-old age group. Frequency decreases in the middle-age group, with a second peak occurring at about the age of 55 years.[19] The incidence in women is lower for all age groups. Traffic accidents continue to be the most frequent cause of SCIs in all age groups. Among children, 65% of cases of SCI are caused by traffic accidents. Motorcycles and bicycles cause 10% to 12% of SCIs. Excessive consumption of alcohol is a factor in one third of cases involving accident victims with SCIs.[19]

More than half of work-related SCIs are caused by falls, and falls are the primary cause of SCIs in the home, particularly among the elderly, who fall down steps, from chairs, or off ladders.[5]

Approximately 7% of SCIs are caused by accidents that occur during sporting and recreational activities, and these SCIs most commonly occur as a result of diving into shallow water. The increasing number of women involved in sports is reflected in the rise of injuries for that group.[19]

Initial Assessment

Management of spine trauma begins with the realization that the patient may have an unstable spine. Whether at the accident scene or at a local referring hospital, the flight nurse should conduct a rapid, thorough primary and secondary assessment of the patient with an SCI before he or she is transferred. This assessment will provide a baseline for serial assessments and will reveal additional injuries and commonly associated complications, such as aspiration, neurogenic shock (bradycardia and hypotension), and poikilothermy.[14,32]

Airway

The patient's airway should be checked for patency and cleared of foreign matter or secretions. While maintaining alignment of the spine, the upper airway should be opened with use of the modified jaw-thrust maneuver to allow spontaneous or assisted ventilation.[1]

Breathing

Breathing may be absent or inadequate in patients with high cervical cord injury (C-4 or above), resulting in loss of both diaphragmatic and intercostal phrenic nerve intervention and paralysis of these respiratory muscles. In such cases assisted ventilation with a bag-valve mask or pocket mask or tracheal intubation with oxygen supplementation is indicated.[1] Rapid sequence intubation with judicious spine immobilization may be required for airway and ventilation control.[16,33] Whatever method is used, the flight nurse must ensure proper, consistent alignment of the entire spine. In cases of significant facial trauma, it may be necessary for the flight nurse to perform a needle or surgical cricothyrotomy to gain airway access and to provide ventilatory support.[6]

Circulation

As with all critically injured patients, intravenous access is mandatory for patients with SCIs. Intravenous lines may be inserted on the scene or en route, depending on the patient's condition, distance of transfer, and existing protocols. Isotonic solutions such as lactated Ringer's solution or normal saline solution are preferred, with the rate and volume of infusion based on the patient's cardiovascular response. In the absence of hemorrhage, maintenance fluids are indicated to minimize pulmonary complications. Neurogenic shock may be present in patients with cervical or high thoracic spine injury. Interruption of sympathetic outflow below the level of injury results in loss of autoregulation, a decrease in vascular tone, and inability of the heart to increase its intrinsic rate. With passive vasodilation and a normal or bradycardic state, the patient becomes hypotensive.[49] The flight nurse should differentiate this shock state from hypovolemia and infuse crystalloids accordingly. In the absence of hypovolemia, the patient with an SCI can be considered "normotensive," with a blood pressure of 80 to 90 mm Hg. If the patient is hemodynamically unstable, administration of low-dose dopamine (3 to 5 mg/kg per minute) may be considered. If severe bradycardia develops ($<$40/min), atropine should be considered for maintenance of normal hemodynamic function. Hypovolemia must be ruled out before vasopressor therapy is begun.[1,49]

This sympathetic block or injury-induced sympathectomy produces poikilothermy. In this state the patient loses the ability to vasodilate and sweat in hot environments and the ability to vasoconstrict and shiver in cold environments. Thus the patient's core body temperature will often reflect the environment and must be considered if warming or cooling techniques are withheld.[33,49]

Vasovagal reflex with tracheal suctioning must also be considered for these patients. Preoxygenation is important to prevent vagal stimulation and severe bradycardia, which could lead to cardiac arrest.[33]

Secondary Assessment

Once the primary survey has been completed, life-threatening situations have been addressed, and the patient has been stabilized, the flight nurse can perform a secondary assessment, which includes performing a baseline neurologic evaluation, obtaining a history of the incident and of allergies, medications, previous illnesses or injuries, and the time of the patient's last meal, and completely exposing and examining the patient. Data about the mechanism and time of injury are valuable. To help expedite the transfer, this information can be obtained during the head-to-toe assessment.

Examination of the patient with an SCI should be performed with the patient maintained in a neutral position and the entire spine immobilized. A sensory and motor assessment will help the flight nurse determine the level and extent of injury. Autonomic function such as anal sphincter control can be assessed, and if sacral sparing is present the injury should be considered incomplete.[1]

The flight nurse should visually inspect and palpate the cervical spine area to determine the presence of deformity, crepitus, pain, and muscle spasm, which is frequently associated with cervical spine injury.[1] A second air medical member should maintain the patient's head in a neutral position during this inspection.

Lower Spine Injuries

The patient should be asked to wiggle his or her toes. If the patient can move the toes of both feet, he or she should be asked to raise each leg slightly, one at a time. The patient's legs should not be raised if the prior examination revealed no movement or association. If the patient shows any obvious weakness, it must be assumed that he or she has sustained an injury to the spinal cord.

Cervical Spine Injuries

The patient should be asked to wiggle his or her fingers. If the patient can do so, he or she should be asked to raise each arm one at a time. Again, substantial active movement of the upper extremity should be avoided if evidence exists of obvious fractures of the spine or extremity. The flight nurse should ask the patient to squeeze his or her fingers with both hands. In addition, the flight nurse should ascertain the patient's dominant hand and cross over, matching the flight nurse's dominant hand to the patient's dominant hand. The strength of the patient's grasp should be similar. If the patient cannot move his or her fingers and arms or has obvious weakness, it should be assumed that the patient has an SCI in the cervical region.[17]

Sensory Examination

The presence of a sensory deficit confirms the suspicion of a cord or nerve-root injury. The flight nurse should test the patient's ankles and wrists and ask the patient if he or she can feel the touch. In the event that the patient cannot feel the touch in one or more places or if he or she reports numbness and/or tingling, it can be assumed that the patient has sustained an SCI.[17]

Neurologic Examination of the Unconscious Patient

The condition of an unconscious patient's spinal cord should be checked by pricking the skin lightly on the soles of the feet or ankles with a sharp object. If there is no spinal cord damage, the painful stimulus triggers an involuntary muscle reflex and the extremities will move, unless the patient is in a profound coma. If the cord is damaged, there may be no such reaction. The lack of response to pinpricks in the upper extremities indicates damage to the spinal cord in the cervical region. Failure of only the lower extremities to respond indicates an SCI in the thoracic or lumbar regions.[17]

The degree of functional loss with sudden spinal cord transection depends on the level of the injury. The higher the injury, the more function lost. Complete sudden cord transection results in complete flaccid paralysis below the level of injury, areflexia (spinal shock) below the level of injury, urinary retention, and, occasionally, in the male patient, priapism.

Incomplete sudden cord transection results in varying degrees of paralysis and sensory loss below the level of injury, areflexia (below the level of injury), and varying degrees of bladder or bowel paralysis. The box may be used as a guide for evaluation of muscle strength and motor function.

MUSCLES TO BE TESTED FOR EVALUATION OF MOTOR STRENGTH

Actions to be Tested	Muscles	Cord Segment
Abduction of the arm	Deltoid	C-5
Flexion of the forearm	Biceps	C-5, C-6
Extension of the forearm	Triceps	C-7
Flexion of digits 2, 3, 4, and 5	Flexor digitorum and profundus	C-8
Opposition of metacarpal of thumb	Opponens pollicis	C-8, T-I
Hip flexion	Iliopsoas	L1-2
Knee extension	Quadriceps femoris	L3-4
Dorsiflexion of foot	Deep peroneal	L-5
Dorsiflexion of big toe	Extensor hallucis longus	L-5
Plantar flexion of foot and big toe	Gastrocnemius flexor	S-I

Interventions and Treatment

The patient with an SCI frequently has association trauma and therefore may have varying degrees of stability.[17] Judicious airway assessment and management is required for the patient with an SCI, when there are injuries in the cervical region. In the absence of hypovolemia, intravenous fluids should be monitored closely and maintained at a rate that will prevent pulmonary overload. On the basis of local protocols and ongoing research, the flight nurse may administer pharmacologic agents, such as high-dose methylprednisolone and GM-I ganglioside.[18,28,34]

Classification of Cervical Spine Injuries by Mechanism of Injury

Flexion Injuries

Anterior subluxation (see box above) is a flexion lesion characterized by disruption of the posterior ligament complex (Fig. 12-2). Because the anterior longitudinal ligament remains intact and the disk is not completely disrupted, this lesion is stable at the time of injury and is difficult to see radiographically.[15]

Physicians disagree on whether bilateral interfacetal dislocations result from hyperflexion or a combined flexion and rotary force. Unilateral and bilateral interfacetal dislocations involve soft-tissue injury of the posterior ligament complex, and tomograms frequently reveal an unstable injury with a high incidence of cord damage.[8,15]

The stability of a simple wedge fracture depends on associated posterior ligament disruption. This flexion injury usually results from a compressive force on the anterior portion of the vertebral body with stretching of the posterior ligament complex. These fractures are generally in the mid or lower cervical segments and are considered stable fractures because of maintenance of posterior and anterior ligaments and the integrity of the interfacetal points.[15]

"Teardrop" hyperflexion fracture dislocations are seen as a result of diving or traffic accidents and falls. This type of fracture is extremely unstable because the vertebra is displaced posteriorly as the person strikes an object, and displacement disrupts the apophyseal joint capsule disk below. The anterior margin of the vertebra fractures in a teardrop-shaped fragment, and the fractured vertebra remains displaced posteriorly. While often severe, the degree of neurologic deficit depends on the severity of hyperflexion compression. Patients who sustain "teardrop" flexion fractures frequently have acute anterior cervical cord syndrome. Immediate quadriplegia, loss of anterior cord senses (pain and temperature), and retention of posterior cord senses (position, motion, and vibration) results.[15]

Flexion-Rotation Injuries

Fractures resulting from flexion-rotation are characterized by the displacement or fracture of one or more vertebrae. Fractured vertebrae may produce a

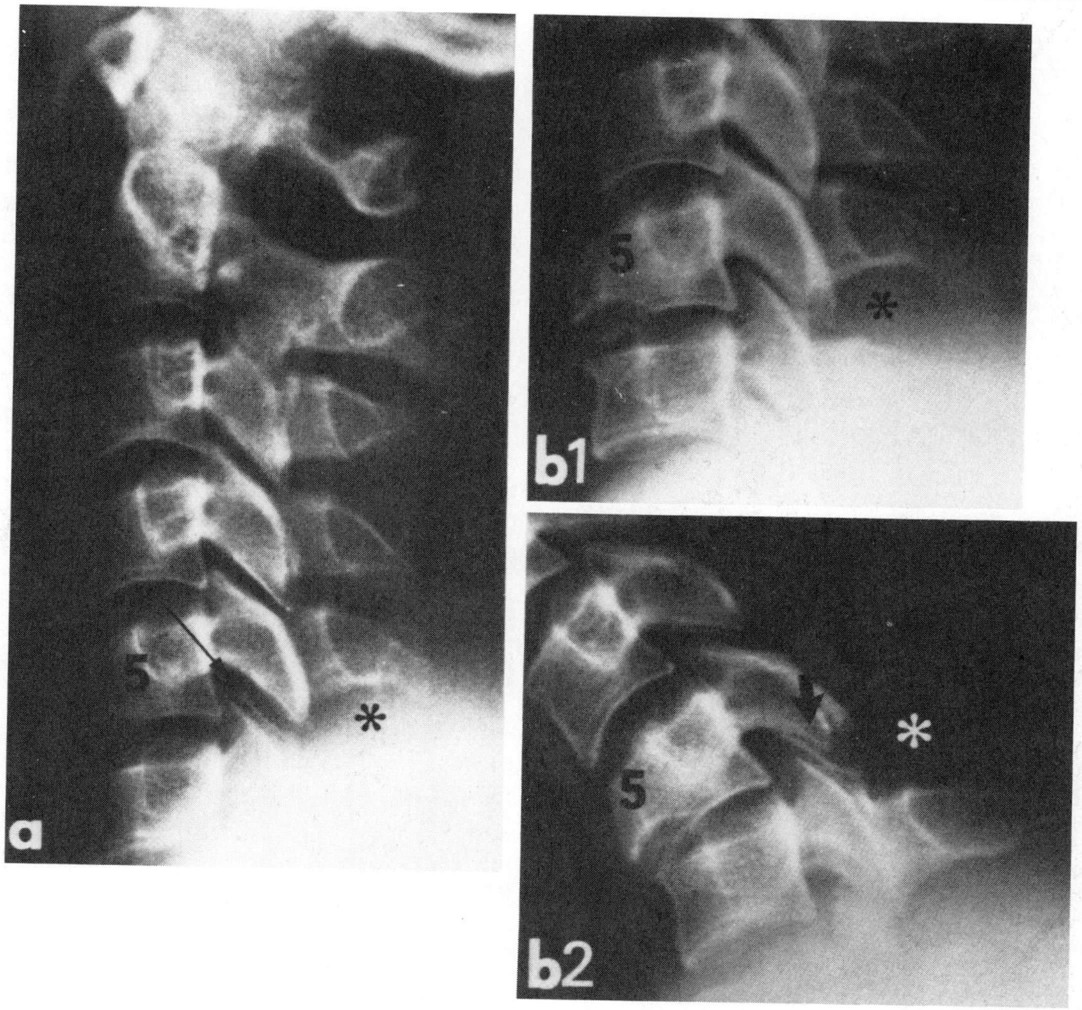

Fig. 12-2. Anterior subluxation of C-5 on C-6 associated with a wedge fracture of C-5. (From Harris JH Jr, Edeiken-Monroe B: *The radiology of acute cervical spine trauma,* Baltimore, 1987, Williams and Wilkins.)

unilateral facet dislocation with corresponding nerve-root compression. Severe distraction forces may cause an anterior displacement of the upper cervical body greater than 50%, which can result in bilateral locked facets and major cord injury, such as quadriplegia.[15]

Extension-Rotation Injuries

Pillar fractures, usually caused by motor vehicle accidents and falls, are the most common "combined" injury of the cervical spine. The mechanism of injury results in force concentrated on the apophyseal joints of the mid and lower cervical segments and resultant vertical fractures of a lateral mass. A distraction of the fracture elements is probably caused by rebound flexion of the head and neck.[15]

Vertical Compression

Compression cervical spine injuries include the "Jefferson" fracture of the atlas and the bursting fracture of the lower cervical vertebrae. Compression

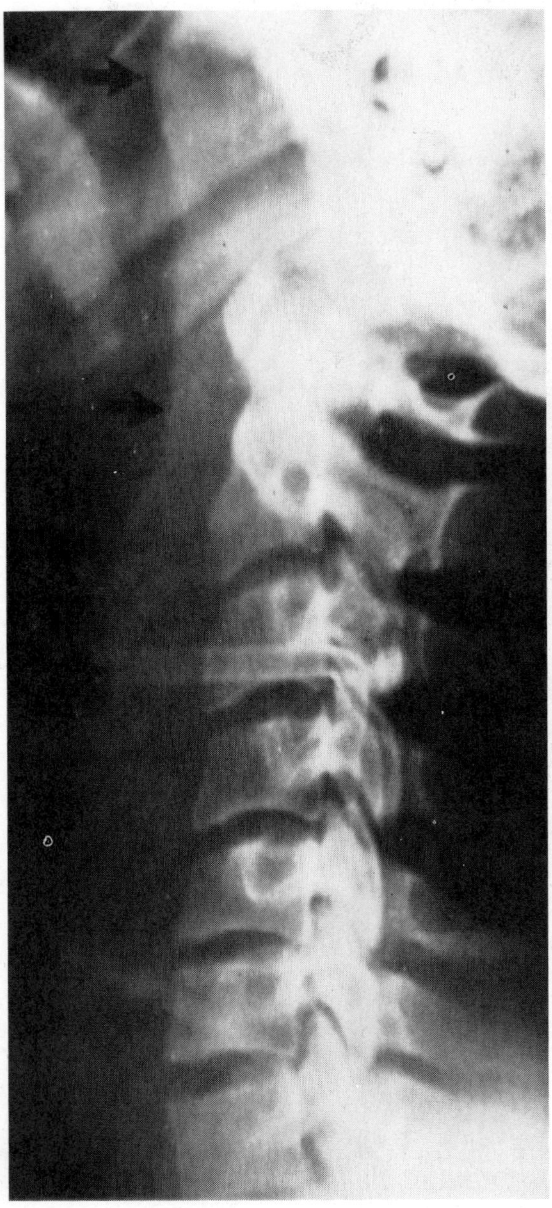

Fig. 12-3. Hyperextension dislocation characterized by intact cervical vertebrae and diffuse prevertebral soft tissue swelling *(arrows)* extending throughout the cervical region and into the nasopharynx. (From Harris JH Jr, Edeiken-Monroe B: *The radiology of acute cervical spine trauma,* Baltimore, 1987, Williams and Wilkins.)

fractures of the cervical spine are uncommon because the injury must occur from force transmitted vertically through the skull and occipital condyles of the spine at the precise moment the spine is straight.[15]

Extension Injuries

Most hyperextension injuries result from contact with a windshield or other structure in the interior of an automobile. The National Crash Severity Study reported that nearly all severe neck injuries are sustained by unrestrained occupants of automobiles. Research has shown that occupants of the front seat who wear lap-shoulder belts sustain significantly fewer serious or fatal neck injuries. Extension injuries can be of three types. The extension "teardrop" fracture is a rare extension injury that involves the anterior corner of the axis. This type of fracture is usually associated with degenerative arthritis of the cervical spine. The hangman's fracture is an unstable, bilateral fracture of the pedicles of the axis. This fracture is often associated with dislocation of the C-2 or C-3 cord segment and prevertebral soft-tissue swelling.[15] Hyperextension fracture-dislocation injuries are associated with direct force backward or a backward and upward force without an axial loading force. The typical hyperextension-dislocation injury is accompanied by the following triad of signs: (1) midface skeletal or soft-tissue injury; (2) varying degrees of central cord syndrome; and (3) a lateral cervical spine radiograph that appears normal with the exception of diffuse prevertebral soft-tissue swelling[15] (Fig. 12-3). This type of extension injury is believed to be responsible for the quadriplegia in the rare patient whose cervical spine films appear normal. The probable mechanism of injury is cord compression between the posterior vertebral body, lamina, and ligamentum flavum during extension.

Thoracic Spine Injuries

Injuries to the thoracic and lumbar spine vary in severity from muscle strains and ligamentous strain to fractures of the vertebral body, fractures of the dorsal elements, dislocation of the facets, and complex combination fracture dislocations. The spinal cord and the nerve roots may be injured by an encroachment into the spinal canal. Patients with stable compression fractures may sustain concomitant injury to the spinal cord, and patients with grossly unstable comminuted fractures may escape neurologic injury. In general, however, the more comminuted, displaced, and unstable the spine fracture, the greater the likelihood of severe cord damage.[5]

Direct injuries to the spine and the spinal cord may occur as a result of a direct blow, such as from a falling tree limb or other heavy object, a stab wound, or a gunshot wound. Most injuries are caused by indirect trauma to the vertebral column resulting from energy generated by forces applied to the head, shoulders, trunk, or pelvis. These forces may contain an axial load as the main force with varying degrees of lateral bending, flexion, extension, or torsion. The thoracic and lumbar spine are most commonly injured by the kinetic energy produced by the person's body traveling through space and a sudden deceleration of the shoulders, upper trunk, or buttocks against an immovable object, with the vector of forces concentrated in an area of the thoracic or the lumbar spine. The most common area is that of the thoracolumbar junction, with specific patterns of vertebral body fractures and dorsal-element dislocation at T-11 and T-12, rotational-flexion fractures of both body and dorsal elements at T-12-L-1, and bursting fractures of the body of L-1. Fractures of the midthoracic spine usually occur at the T-5 or T-6 level.[48]

The most common site of lumbar fractures is L-2 or L-3. A specific type of flexion-distraction injury occurs when a person is restrained by a seatbelt and experiences sudden deceleration, which causes sudden flexion and distraction centered at the midlumbar spine. Patients with these fractures often escape spinal cord cauda equina damage, and the fracture may be overlooked in the presence of head injury or associated small intestinal injuries. Any person who has pain after being in an automobile accident in which he or she wore a seatbelt must be examined specifically for the presence of a spinal fracture.

The thoracic spine is protected from injury by the rib cage, the sternum, and the chest wall. These bony structures permit little flexion and extension motion of the upper and midthoracic spine; however, there is a normal rotation motion. The lumbar spine allows for more flexion, extension, and lateral motion because it lacks the above mentioned supporting structures.[48]

Midthoracic spine injuries are usually caused by acute flexion, rotation, and axial load forces at the midthoracic region, resulting in either a simple compression fracture of the vertebral bodies or a complex fracture dislocation in which the vertebral body and the dorsal elements are fractured.

Most injuries at the thoracolumbar junction are caused by a combination of flexion, rotation, and axial load. An injury that is centered at T-11-T-12 frequently causes a dislocation without fracture of the posterior facets and a slice fracture through the upper portion of the T-12 vertebral body.

Rotational forces are commonly associated with fracture dislocations of T-12-L-1 level. If the injury has more of an axial load than a rotational force, the body of L-1 suffers a burst injury. In this type of injury the posterior elements of the lamina, spinous process, and facet joints may be intact or may also be fractured.

SUMMARY

The management of all neurologic traumatic emergencies includes rapid assessment, airway management, and serial examinations throughout the assessment and transfer phases. Upon completion of the transfer, it is important that the receiving physician be provided with a thorough report of events, including the time of the incident, the mechanism of injury or preceding events, care rendered by the referring facility and flight crew, response of the patient to care initiated, the past medical history of patient, and observed changes in the patient's condition. This thorough report will provide the receiving physician with information to guide his or her management and ensure continuity of care for the patient with the best possible chance for a positive outcome.

NEUROLOGIC TRAUMA CASE STUDY

The flight crew received a request to transport a patient from a rural referring hospital located 85 miles from their base hospital. Information received from their communications center was as follows: The patient was a restrained driver in a one-vehicle rollover. Paramedics on the scene reported no loss of consciousness and no hypotension. The referring hospital emergency department reports a C6-C7 subluxation with spinal cord involvement.

On arrival at the referring hospital, the following assessment was made by the flight crew:

Respiratory: Spontaneous respirations were present and equal bilaterally at 16/min, trachea midline, chest expansion equal. There was no evidence of chest trauma. The patient was receiving O_2 through a nonrebreather mask at 15 L/min with a saturation of 98%.

Cardiovascular: Radial and pedal pulses were present at a regular rate of 84/min. Cap refill was less than 3 seconds, and the patient's skin was warm and dry to touch. IVs × 2 established before arrival were patent. The patient's temperature was 37.2° C.

Neurologic: The patient was awake, alert, oriented to person, place, and time, and had a Glasgow Coma Scale score of 15. The patient had neck pain, paresthesia of the hands and fingers, and hyperesthesia of the right hand (extremely painful to touch). The patient's pupils were PERRL at 2 to 3 mm, and cranial nerves II through XII were grossly intact. Reflexes were 2+ throughout except for triceps, which were 1+.

Gastrointestinal: The patient's abdomen was soft, nondistended, and nontender. NG tube patent to low suction.

Genitourinary: Foley to dependent drainage.

Extremities: There was no evidence of trauma, and the patient moved all extremities spontaneously. Grips were weak bilaterally.

Allergies: NKDA

Medical history: Negative

Medications: None

X-ray findings available at the referring hospital showed a C6-C7 subluxation. The patient was transferred to the helicopter stretcher via a scoop stretcher and secured. The flight nurse then prepared for insertion of Gardner Wells tongs. The procedure was explained to the patient and consent was obtained. The scalp was prepped in the usual manner and anesthetized with 1% lidocaine. Gardner Wells tongs were then placed and 15 lbs of traction applied with use of a spring-loaded scale and stretcher-mounted system. Solu-Medrol 30/mg per kg was administered during a 15-minute period as per protocol. The patient was then transferred to the helicopter, boarded, and secured.

A neurologic examination after application of traction and before departure revealed reduction in neck pain and paresthesia of the left hand. Right-hand hyperesthesia persisted.

IN FLIGHT

The flight nurse initiated a Solu-Medrol infusion of 5.4 mg/kg per hour and maintained Ringe's lactate solution at a TKO. Heart monitoring showed normal sinus rhythm. Vital signs monitored every 15 minutes revealed blood pressure of 120-130/76, pulse of 60 to 70 per minute, and a respiratory rate of 16. O_2 saturation remained 96% to 98% on a nonrebreather mask at 15 L/min.

Radio contact was established and the flight nurse report included a request for neurosurgery consultation in addition to the general surgery trauma team assessment.

The patient was transferred to the emergency center of a level one trauma center for evaluation and treatment. Cervical traction was maintained throughout transfer and continued via conventional hanging weights in the emergency center when transfer from helicopter stretcher via scoop stretcher was completed.

Results of laboratory studies were as follows:

Hct 46, Hgb 15.7
Serum chemistry WNL
PT, PTT WNL
Amylase WNL
BAL 0

Radiologic studies revealed the following:

Chest	Clear
Cervical	Anterior displacement of C6 on C7, no fracture of bony abnormality
Thoracic spine	Clear
CT cervical spine	Fracture of the left lateral mass of C7 with involvement of the process and extension through the transverse foramen

The patient was admitted to the neurosurgical intensive care unit and remained in cervical spine traction.

CURRENT RESEARCH AREAS IN NEUROLOGIC TRAUMA EMERGENCIES

Researchers continuously pose questions and seek answers in an effort to positively influence the outcome of the patient with neurotrauma. It is the flight nurse's responsibility to prepare for the future by participating in research and incorporating the results into his or her practice. Listed below are some of the areas of ongoing research.

Effects of Controlled Mild Hypothermia

Marion DW et al: The use of moderate therapeutic hypothermia for patients with severe head injuries: a preliminary report, *J Neurosurg* 79(3):354, September 1993.

Nikas DL: Commentary on effect of mild hypothermia on uncontrollable intracranial hypertension after severe head injury, *AACN Nurs Scan Crit Care* 4(1): 13 Jan-Feb 1994.

Shiozaki T et al: Effect of mild hypothermia on uncontrollable intracranial hypertension after severe head injury, *J Neurosurg* 79(3):363, September 1993.

Effects of Mannitol on Cerebral Blood Flow

Davis M, Lucatorto M: Mannitol revisited, *J Neuroscience Nurs* 26(3):170, June 1994 (review).

Gigliuto CM, Stone KE, Algus M: The use of mannitol in the medical ICU, *NJ Med* 88(1):48, January 1991.

Harada K et al: Effect of rapid mannitol infusion on middle cerebral artery blood flow velocity and pulsatility index—a transcranial Doppler ultrasonography study in monkeys, *Brain Nerve* 45(7):649, July 1993.

Hickey JV: *Neurogenic pulmonary edema: the clinical practice of neurological and neurosurgical nursing,* ed 3, Philadelphia, 1992, JB Lippincott.

Monitoring Modalities

Mark K: Retrograde jugular catheter: monitoring SaO_2, *J Neuroscience Nurs* 26(1):48, 1994.

Martin NA, Thomas KM, Caron M: Transcranial Doppler: techniques, applications, and instrumentation, *Neurosurgery* 3:761, 1993.

Muizelaar JP, Schroeder ML: Overview of monitoring of cerebral blood flow and metabolism after severe head injury, *Can J Neurol Sci* 21(2):S6, May 1994 (review).

Sheinberg M et al: Continuous monitoring of jugular venous oxygen saturation on head-injured patients, *J Neurosurg* 76:212, 1992.

Neuroprotective Agents

Bullock R: Opportunities for neuroprotective drugs in clinical management of head injury, *J Emerg Med* 1(suppl 11):23, 1993.

Muizalaar JP: Cerebral ischemia—reperfusion injury after severe head injury and its possible treatment with polyethyleneglycal-superoxide dismutase, *Ann Emerg Med* 22(6):1014, June 1993 (review).

Sen S et al: Alpha-phenyl-tert-butyl nitrone inhibits free radical release in brain concussion, *Free Radical Biol Med* 16(6):685, June 1994.

Neurogenic Pulmonary Edema

Hickey JV: *Neurogenic pulmonary edema: the clinical practice of neurological and neurosurgical nursing,* ed 3, Philadelphia, 1992, JB Lippincott.

Chemotherapeutic Agents in Spinal Cord Injury

Hill MG: Commentary on past and current clinical studies with GM-1 ganglioside in acute spinal cord injury, *ENA's Nurs Scan Emerg Care* 3(6):10, November-December 1993.

Nayduch D, Lee A, Butler D: High dose methylprednisolone after spinal cord injury, *Crit Care Nurse* 14(4):69, August 1994.

Oman KS: Commentary on methylprednisolone for acute spinal cord injury, *ENA's Nurs Scan Emerg Care* 3(1):11, Jan-Feb 1993.

Prevention

Hunt L: Ocular injuries from driver's air bag, *Insight* 20(1):18, April 1995.

HOSPITAL COURSE

The patient continued to move all extremities well, but reported hyperesthesia and decreased strength in the right hand. The patient was initially evaluated for halo application; however, a follow-up x-ray film revealed continued subluxation, and thus operative correction was opted.

Cervical spine flexion and extension x-ray studies revealed mild anterolesthesis of C6 on 7 and widened facet joints consistent with ligamentous injury. The patient underwent an anterior cervical disectomy with fibular allograft fusion and caspar plating. Findings during surgery were a stretch and partial tearing of the posterior longitudinal ligament at the C6-C7 level.

The patient, who was active military, was discharged to rehabilitation at a military base with no neurologic deficit.

One month after injury, the patient showed improvement in paresthetic numbness (the paresthetic numbness in his left hand has improved and almost resolved and the paresthetic numbness in his right hand remains slight) and improved strength (strength in bilateral grips is nearly equivalent, with perhaps trace attenuation in the right grip strength as compared to the left; deltoid biceps, triceps, and span challenges demonstrate good and symmetric strength), and x-ray films show good alignment.

Three months after injury the patient was working with weights and completing repetitions with use of light weights. He had full range of motion of his neck without complaints of pain and a normal neurologic examination, except for some dysesthesia in the ulnar aspect of his right hand and arm with some decreased grip strength.

DISCUSSION

The mechanism of injury, patient assessment, and radiologic findings were sufficient for the flight nurse to use Gardner Wells tongs. On the basis of protocol, the patient was transported with cervical spine traction to reduce the risk of further deficit and to provide a more definitive approach to caring for the patient with potential spinal cord injury.

Cervical subluxation with neurologic deficits suggests spinal cord compromise. Although in this case the patient had minimal neurologic deficit, it must be emphasized that patients with any deficit are at risk for deterioration in the degree or level of deficit. Because of the posterior longitudinal ligamentous injury, this patient was at risk for further subluxation with any manipulation of the spine during transport, which could include seizure activity, vomiting, or muscle spasm at the injury site.

Definitive management of cervical spine malalignment is traction for realignment and stabilization. With the use of a stretcher-mounted traction system and Gardner Wells tongs, this patient could be transported in cervical traction, thus initiating definitive management before and during transfer to the neurosurgeon. It is supported by the division of neurosurgery at this university that aggressive early management with traction and steroids will provide optimal conditions for maximum recovery of the patient with spinal cord trauma.

REFERENCES

1. Advanced Trauma Life Support Course for Physicians, American College of Surgeons Committee on Trauma, ATLS/ACS, Chicago, 1993.
2. Anderson L, Rose W, Edmond S: Analysis of intubations: before and after establishment of a rapid sequence intubation protocol. Scientific Abstract, 15th Annual Air Medical Transport Conference, Detroit, Michigan, October 17-21, 1994.
3. Baker S, O'Neill B, Karpf R: *The injury fact book,* Lexington, Mass, 1984, Lexington Books.
4. Becker DP, Gardner S: Intensive management of head injury. In *Neurosurgery,* vol 2, St Louis, 1985, McGraw-Hill.
5. Bohlman HH, Ducker TB, Lucas JT: Spine and spinal cord injuries. In Rothman RH, Simeone FA, editors: *The spine,* vol 2, Philadelphia, 1982, WB Saunders.
6. Chen FH, Fetzer JD: Complete cricotracheal separation and third cervical spinal cord transection following blunt neck trauma: a case report of one survivor, *J Trauma* 35(1):140, 1993.
7. Chestnut RM, Marshall LF: Management of head injury: treatment of abnormal intracranial pressure, *Neurosurg Clin North Am* 2(2):267, 1991.
8. Cooper PR, Chalif DJ: Fractures and dislocations of the upper cervical spine, *Contemp Neurosurg* 5(16):1, 1983.
9. Crutchfield WG: Skeletal traction for dislocation of cervical spine: report of a case, *Southern Surgeon* 2:156, 1933.
10. Davis M, Lucatorto M: Mannitol revisited, *J Neurosci Nurs* 26(3):170, 1994.

11. Fessler RD, Diaz FG: The management of cerebral perfusion pressure and intracranial pressure after severe head injury, *Ann Emerg Med* 22(6):998, 1993.
12. Gennarelli T, Thibault L: Biomechanics of head injury. In *Neurosurgery*, vol 2, St Louis, 1985, McGraw-Hill.
13. Gennarelli TA et al: Diffuse axonal injury and traumatic coma in the primate, *Ann Neurol* 12:564, 1982.
14. Geisler FH: Acute management of cervical spinal cord injury, *Trauma Q* 4(3), May 1988.
15. Harris JH Jr: *The radiology of acute cervical spine trauma*, Baltimore, 1987, Williams and Wilkins.
16. Hastings RH, Wood PR: Head extension and laryngeal view during laryngoscopy with cervical spine immobilization maneuvers, *Anesthesiology* 80(4):825, 1994.
17. Hickey J: *The clinical practice of neurological and neurosurgical nursing*, ed 2, Philadelphia, 1985, JB Lippincott.
18. Hill MG: Commentary on past and current clinical studies with GM-1 ganglioside in acute spinal cord injury, *ENA's Nurs Scan Emerg Care* 3(6):10, 1993.
19. *Injury in America: a continuing public health problem*, Chicago, 1985, National Academy Press.
20. Jennett B, Teasdale G: *Management of head injuries*, Philadelphia, 1981, Davis.
21. Keller TS, Schneider RC: Craniocerebral trauma. In *Correlative neurosurgery*, ed 3, vol 2, Springfield, Ill, 1982, Charles C Thomas.
22. Manifold S: Craniocerebral trauma: a review of primary and secondary injury and therapeutic modalities, *Focus Crit Care* 13:33, 1986.
23. Marshall LE: Surgical treatment of extracerebral lesions in head injury. In Pitts LH, Wagner FC Jr, editors: *Craniospinal trauma*, New York, 1990, Thieme Medical.
24. McGuire RA et al: Spine instability and logrolling maneuver, *J Trauma* 27:525, 1987.
25. Miller JD: Head injury and brain ischemia, *Br J Anesthesiol* 57:120, 1985.
26. Morris M, Kinkade S: The effect of capnometry on manual ventilation technique, *Air Med J* 14(2):79, 1995.
27. Muizelaar JP, Schroder ML: Overview of monitoring of cerebral blood flow and metabolism after severe head injury, *Can J Neurol Sci* 21(2):S6, 1994.
28. Nayduch D, Lee A, Butler D: High-dose methylprednisolone after acute spinal cord injury, *Crit Care Nurse* 14(4):69, 1994.
29. Neave V, Weiss M: Neurological evaluation of a patient with head trauma: coma scales. In *Neurosurgery*, vol 2, St Louis, 1985, McGraw-Hill.
30. Neville S, Watts C: Cervical spine fractures: a method of management by traction during transport, *J Aeromed Healthcare* May/June 22-23, 1985.
31. Neville S et al: Use of traction in cervical spine fractures during interhospital transfer by aircraft, *J Spinal Disord* 3(1):67, 1990.
32. Nikas D: Pathophysiology and nursing interventions in acute SCI, *Trauma Q* 4(3), May 1988.
33. Norwood S, Myers MB, Butler TJ: The safety of emergency neuromuscular blockade and orotracheal intubation in the acutely injured trauma patient, *J Am Coll Surg* 179(6):646, 1994.
34. Oman KS: Commentary on methylprednisolone for acute spinal cord injury, *ENA's Nurs Scan Emerg Care* 3(1):11, 1993.
35. Peterson C, Budd R, Balazs K: Comparative evaluation of three end-tidal CO_2 monitors used during air medical transport, *J Air Med Transport* 11(2):7, 1992.
36. Popp A, Bourke R: Pathophysiology of head injury. In *Neurosurgery*, vol 2, St Louis, 1985, McGraw-Hill.
37. Prolo DJ, Hanbery JW: Cervical stabilization-traction board, *J Am Med Assoc* 224(5):615, 1973.
38. Saboe LA et al: Spine trauma and associated injuries, *J Trauma* 31(1):43, 1991.
39. Seeling JM et al: Traumatic acute subdural hematoma: major mortality reduction in comatose patients treated within four hours, *N Engl J Med* 304:1511, 1981.
40. Smith M, Bourn S, Larmm B: Ties that bind—immobilizing the injury spine, *J Emerg Med Serv* 14(4), April 1989.
41. Sullivan TE et al: Closed head injury assessment and research methodology, *J Neurosci Nurs* 26(1):24, 1994.
42. Tabaddor K: Nonoperative management of head trauma, *Contemp Neurosurg* 2(26):1, 1980.
43. Temkin NR, Dikem SS, Winn HR: Management of head injury, posttraumatic seizures, *Neurosurg Clin North Am* 2(2):425, 1991.
44. Ward JD: Management of head injury: prehospital care, *Neurosurg Clin North Am* 2(2):251, 1991.
45. Watts C: Trauma to the cervical spine, *Mod Med* 101, April 1986.
46. White RJ: Acute evacuation and management of head injury. In Najarian JS, Delaney JP, editors: *Emergency surgery: trauma-shock-sepsis-burns*, 153, Chicago, 1982, Year-Book Medical.
47. White RJ, Likavec MJ: Current concepts: the diagnosis and initial management of head injury, *N Engl J Med* 327(21):1507, 1992.
48. Whiteside TE Jr, Shah S: On management of unstable fractures of thoraco-lumbar spine, *Spine* 1:99, 1976.
49. Yablon SA: Posttraumatic seizures, *Arch Physical Med Rehabil* 74(9):983, 1993.

CHAPTER 13

Thoracic Trauma

COMPETENCIES

1. Perform a thoracic assessment identifying indications of thoracic injury.
2. Identify signs and symptoms of life-threatening thoracic injuries, including a tension pneumothorax, a hemothorax, and a flail chest.
3. Initiate appropriate interventions for a thoracic injury, including needle decompression, open chest wound treatment, and flail segment stabilization.

Thoracic injuries present a demanding challenge to the flight nurse. Approximately 25% of all trauma deaths involve thoracic injuries. Thoracic injury remains second only to central nervous system injury as the leading cause of all trauma deaths.[1] In the pediatric population, with the exception of lung contusions, serious injuries to vital thoracic structures are associated with a mortality rate of more than 50%.[7] An understanding of the severity and mechanism of injury, management concerns of specific thoracic injuries, and special flight considerations aids the flight nurse in providing care during transport.

Thoracic trauma is classified by either the mechanism of injury or the degree to which the injury is life threatening. Classification of thoracic trauma by mechanism of injury encompasses two categories: blunt and penetrating traumas. Blunt trauma is associated with motor vehicle accidents, compression injuries, falls, and assaults. Penetrating trauma occurs as a result of gunshot wounds, stab wounds, and impalement. Thoracic injuries may also be categorized as life-threatening or potentially life-threatening conditions. Life-threatening thoracic conditions are airway obstruction, tension pneumothorax, massive hemothorax, open pneumothorax, flail chest, cardiac tamponade, aortic rupture, and myocardial rupture. Potentially life-threatening conditions are myocardial contusion, pulmonary contusion, aortic disruption, tracheobronchial disruption, esophageal rupture, and diaphragmatic disruption. Because many of the thoracic injuries are life threatening, transport by air to a regional trauma center or tertiary care setting may be indicated.

Special considerations for in-flight care of the patient with thoracic trauma relate to altitude changes and gas expansion. As previously discussed (Chapter 2), gases expand with increasing altitude. Because of the expansion of gases with increased altitude, a patient with an untreated pneumothorax or a nonfunctioning chest tube may be at great risk for a tension pneumothorax developing.[14] As part of the flight nurse's anticipatory planning and managing of care, the effects of how changes in altitude may affect a patient with thoracic injuries must be considered.

The greatest threat in the management of a patient with specific thoracic injuries is hypoxia.[5] After thoracic injury, the contributing causes of hypoxia may be decreased blood volume, failure to ventilate the lungs, ventilation-perfusion mismatches, or pressure changes within the intrapleural space. The ABCs of resuscitation (maintenance of airway, breathing, and circulation) serve as a framework for management of each specific injury. The ABC framework assists in quick detection of life-threatening injuries and implementation of rapid interventions. Airway obstruction is discussed in Chapter 8.

LIFE-THREATENING THORACIC INJURIES

Tension Pneumothorax

Etiologic Factors

Both blunt and penetrating thoracic trauma cause tension pneumothorax, or it can occur as a complication of treatment of an open pneumothorax. Air progressively accumulates under pressure, and the flap of the injured lung acts as a one-way valve; air is allowed to enter the pleural space on inspiration but not allowed to escape on expiration.

Pathophysiologic Factors

Ventilation is inadequate because the air entering the pleural space increases the intrapleural pressure with each inspiration. This causes collapse of the ipsilateral lung and a mediastinal shift to the opposite side, leading to compression of the contralateral lung (Fig. 13-1). Perfusion becomes inadequate because of decreased venous return to the heart as a result of the increased intrapleural pressure and shift of mediastinal structures.

Assessment

The mechanism of injury is important for the flight nurse to establish a high index of suspicion. The patient will exhibit severe respiratory distress, dyspnea, and cyanosis. Agitation and anxiety are common.[11,17] Clinical evidence of shock may be present. Breath sounds will be either decreased or absent over the involved hemithorax. The trachea should be assessed because a shift to the unaffected side occurs as intrapleural pressure increases. As air passes into the tissues, subcutaneous emphysema can be palpated. Jugular venous distention occurs because of the increased intrapleural pressure. Constant observation of the patient's chest excursion is important during transport because auscultation is next to impossible.

Interventions

The immediate lifesaving intervention is rapid decompression of the pleural space. To release the intrapleural pressure, the flight nurse should place a large-bore needle into the pleural space, specifically into the second intercostal space, two finger breadths lateral to the sternal border on the affected side. The flight nurse should then place the needle superior to the rib margin to avoid the intercostal artery. The anterior site is used for avoidance of the internal mammary vessels.[11,17] If a tension pneumothorax is present, the air within the pleural space will force the plunger out of the syringe attached to the needle.

The needle thoracostomy should be converted to a tube thoracostomy as soon as possible. A single chest tube is acceptable for a pneumothorax, hemothorax, or hemopneumothorax.[13] In addition, intra-

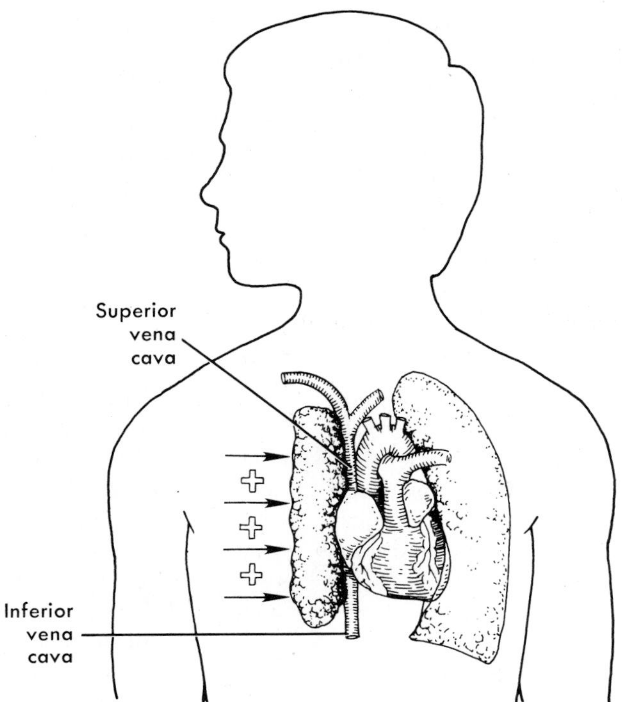

Fig. 13-1. Tension pneumothorax. (From Sheehy SB: *Emergency nursing: principles and practice,* ed 3, St Louis, 1992, Mosby.)

venous access and fluid resuscitation should be done. Supplemental oxygen is indicated because hypoxia is a real threat.

Evaluation

Constant reevaluation of the patient's cardiopulmonary status is warranted. If a chest tube is placed and a persistent air leak occurs, the presence of a tracheobronchial disruption must be considered.

Massive Hemothorax

Etiologic Factors

Massive hemothorax develops as a result of blunt or penetrating injuries of intrathoracic organs or laceration of an intercostal artery. The rapid and massive accumulation of blood and fluid in the pleural space can result in severe hemodynamic compromise.

Pathophysiologic Factors

The compliant lung offers little resistance to a large amount of blood becoming sequestered in the pleural space (Fig. 13-2). Hypovolemic shock results. Compression of the ipsilateral lung occurs from the accumulation of blood, and a mediastinal shift can occur from compression of the contralateral lung. In this way ventilation-perfusion mismatches happen.

Assessment

The mechanism of injury is vital to the initial assessment of the patient suspected of having a massive hemothorax. Because of the decrease in blood volume, manifestations of shock appear. Altered mentation, decrease in blood pressure, increase in heart rate, and signs of peripheral vasoconstriction are common. Breath sounds are decreased or absent

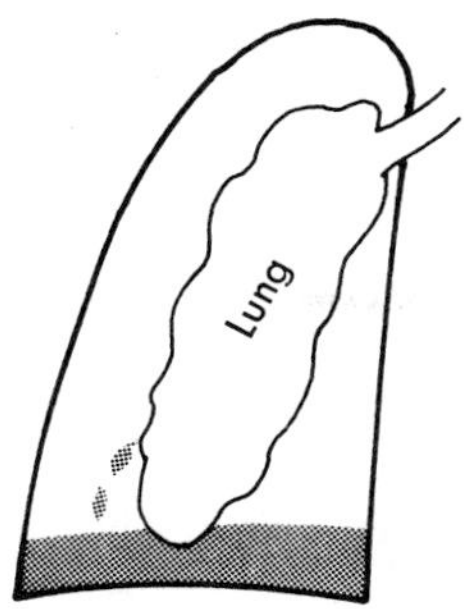

Fig. 13-2. Hemothorax. (From Sheehy SB: *Emergency nursing: principles and practice,* ed 3, St Louis, 1992, Mosby.)

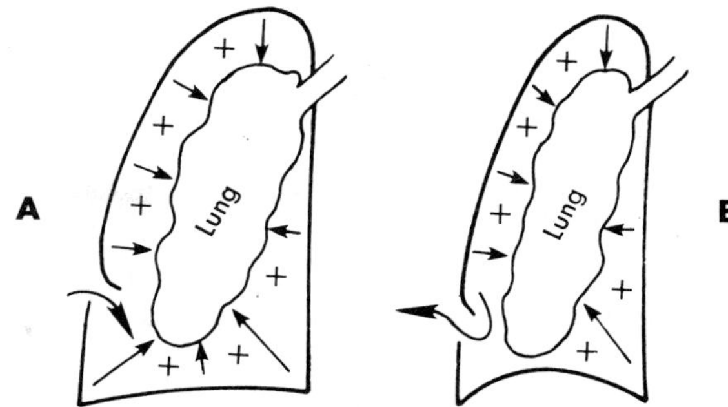

Fig. 13-3. Sucking chest wound. **A,** Inspiration. **B,** Expiration. (From Sheehy SB: *Emergency nursing: principles and practice,* ed 3, St Louis, 1992, Mosby.)

over the involved hemothorax, and chest excursion on the affected side is decreased. Unlike with cardiac tamponade, the trachea is in the midline, and the neck veins are flat.[19]

Interventions

Restoration of lost blood volume is of first importance, and an initial response is to achieve intravenous access with at least two large-bore catheters and to administer crystalloids or colloids (Chapter 9). Supplemental oxygen should be administered. Endotracheal intubation may be required. Emergent management involves placement of a tube thoracostomy.

In cases of massive hemothorax the flight nurse may consider autotransfusion. The use of autotransfusion in thoracic trauma patients has been greatly debated because of the potential effect of anticoagulants and abdominal contaminants.[3,15] Flight nursing considerations related to autotransfusion are transport delay during supply setup and space limitation during transport. In situations of prolonged transport times, isolated chest trauma, conflicting religious beliefs, or cross-matching difficulty, autotransfusion may serve as a bridge until definitive care is provided. The need for surgical intervention, a thoracotomy, is based not only on the initial amount of chest tube drainage, hemodynamic status, and fluid resuscitation amounts, but also on the location of chest-wall penetration or the rate of ongoing blood loss (200 ml/hour).[3,15]

Evaluation

The air medical crew member constantly reassesses the ventilatory status of the patient and monitors the parameters of the patient's response to volume replacement.

Open Pneumothorax

Etiologic Factors

An open pneumothorax, or sucking chest wound, is caused by a penetrating object. Air enters the pleural space through the opening or defect in the chest wall (Fig. 13-3).

Pathophysiologic Factors

If the diameter of the chest-wall defect is greater than the diameter of the patient's trachea, air will move through the chest wound rather than through the trachea and airways. The defect in the thoracic wall leads to an equilibration of atmospheric and pleural pressure. The result is loss of the negative intrathoracic pressure, which leads to respiratory insufficiency. Air in the pleural space promotes collapse of the ipsilateral lung and a mediastinal shift to the unaffected side. The mediastinal shift and loss of normal negative intrathoracic pressure produce decreased venous return to the heart and cardiac insufficiency.

Assessment

A penetrating thoracic trauma should lead the flight nurse to closely assess the thorax to determine whether a sucking chest wound is present. The patient will be in respiratory distress, with tachypnea and grunting, and as air enters and leaves the pleural space through the chest-wall defect, the flight nurse will hear a sucking noise during respiration. Clinical manifestations of shock occur as a result of intermittent obstruction of venous return.[11,17]

Interventions

In the prehospital setting the wound should be covered, but not sealed, with an occlusive dressing. A dressing taped on three sides creates a flutter-valve effect; air is prevented from entering the chest on inspiration but is not prevented from leaving the chest on expiration. If an occlusive dressing is used and a defect in the lung exists, a tension pneumothorax may develop because the air is not allowed to escape from the pleural space.

If a tension pneumothorax develops, the flight nurse should immediately remove the occlusive dressing. The patient may require the placement of a chest tube to treat the underlying lung defect.[14] If the patient's ventilation and oxygenation continue to deteriorate, the flight nurse should immediately prepare to intubate. Maintenance of intravenous access is also imperative as a route for volume resuscitation and medication administration.

Evaluation

Evaluation must consist of continuous monitoring of the patient's cardiopulmonary status. Assessment parameters for expanding pneumothoraces are limited during flight because of the background noise levels. Astute evaluation of the patient's chest pain, tachycardia, increasing dyspnea, tracheal deviation, and development of subcutaneous emphysema prompts the flight nurse to begin hemodynamic compromise.[1,14]

Flail Chest

Etiologic Factors

A flail chest usually occurs as a result of blunt thoracic trauma. Multiple rib fractures cause separation of a portion of the rib cage and loss of stability of the chest wall. The flail segment usually involves the anterior or lateral chest wall because the posterior chest wall is protected by heavy posterior muscles and the scapula.

Pathophysiologic Factors

Paradoxical chest movement interferes with the normal "bellows" function of the thoracic cage, causing inadequate gas exchange. Progressive respiratory insufficiency is caused by the underlying pulmonary contusion. The instability of the chest wall and the pain from the fracture sites lead to hypoventilation and subsequent hypoxemia.

Assessment

Observation of chest excursion is important; however, the paradoxical movement may not be obvious except in cases of severe flail. The flail segment moves in the opposite direction from the rest of the thoracic cage during respiration, moving inward during inspiration and outward during expiration (Fig. 13-4). Initially, the flail may not be obvious because of spasms of the muscles in the thoracic wall. The patient is also in respiratory distress, with cyanosis, grunting, and use of accessory muscles, and will report severe chest pain on the involved side.

Interventions

At first the flight nurse acts promptly to stabilize the flail segment and increase the effective tidal volume. Internal stabilization with an endotracheal tube and controlled mechanical ventilation should be done as soon as possible. In conjunction with controlled mechanical ventilation, use of continuous positive airway pressure (CPAP) or positive end expiratory pressure (PEEP) also aids in internal stabilization. External stabilization techniques include application of firm, gentle pressure over the flail segment, placement of the patient injured side down if his or her condition allows, and placement of small sandbags over the flail segment (Fig. 13-5). And, of course, the patient needs intravenous access and supplemental oxygen.

Evaluation

Constant reassessment of the patient's cardiopulmonary status is vital to treatment of the patient with a flail chest. Mentation, skin color, and SaO_2

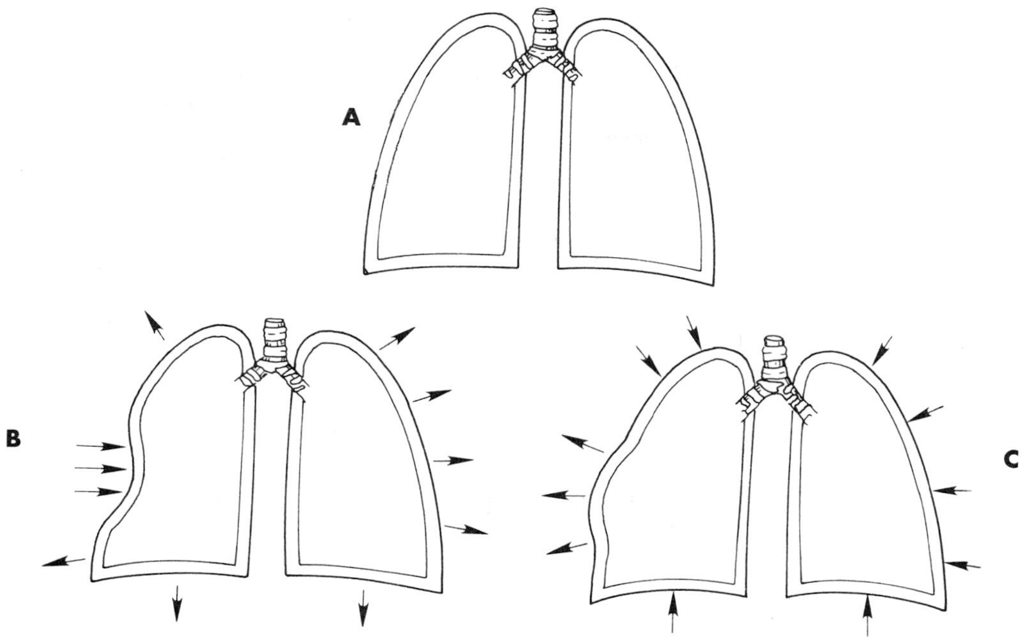

Fig. 13-4. Flail chest. **A,** Normal lungs. **B,** Flail chest on inspiration. **C,** Flail chest on expiration. (From Sheehy SB: *Emergency nursing: principles and practice,* ed 3, St Louis, 1992, Mosby.)

measurements, in addition to vital signs, are parameters to monitor. Pain control cannot be accomplished until the patient's condition is fully evaluated.

Acute Cardiac Tamponade

Etiologic Factors

Acute cardiac tamponade occurs when blood accumulates in the pericardial sac (Fig. 13-6) as a result of blunt and penetrating cardiac trauma.

Pathophysiologic Factors

The hemodynamic effects of cardiac tamponade depend on how quickly fluid (blood) accumulates in the pericardial sac; rapid accumulation of blood (from 150 to 250 ml) may be fatal because the normal pericardial sac contains 20 to 50 ml of pericardial fluid. If the accumulation is slow, the fibrous pericardium stretches and can accommodate several liters of fluid without hemodynamic consequences. The main hemodynamic consequence is a decrease in diastolic filling because of increased intrapericardial pressure. Once the diastolic filling decreases, stroke volume and cardiac output fall. Central venous pressure increases as a result of increased intrapericardial pressure.

Assessment

The patient with acute cardiac tamponade will show signs of decreased cardiac output, such as altered mental status, cool, clammy skin, tachycardia, and a falling arterial blood pressure. Venous hypertension also occurs, as evidenced by marked neck-vein distention (unless the patient is hypovolemic) and rising central venous pressure. Distant, muffled heart sounds may not be detectable in the field. Pulsus paradoxus is a fall in the systolic blood pressure greater than 15 mm Hg during normal inspiration.

Interventions

The patient needs a patent airway and supplemental oxygen. Intravenous access and continuous as-

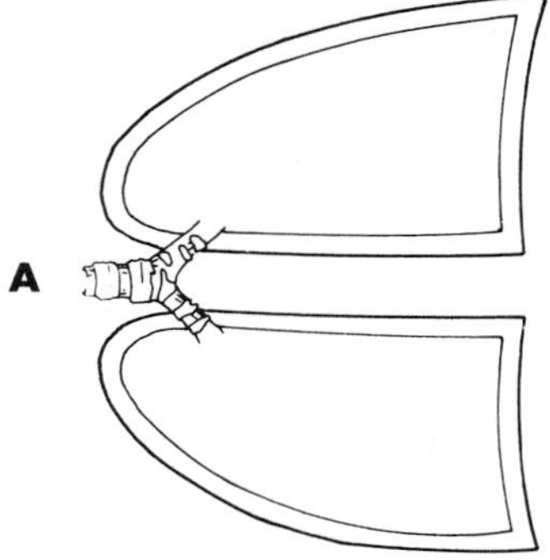

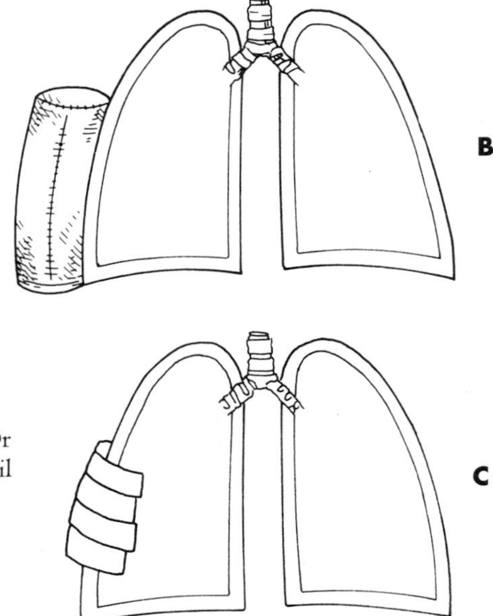

Fig. 13-5. Therapeutic interventions and options for flail chest. **A,** Place patient with flail side down. **B,** Or place patient in semi-Fowler position and sandbag flail segment. **C,** Or tape flail segment. (From Sheehy SB, Barber J: *Emergency nursing: principles and practice,* ed 2, St Louis, 1985, Mosby.)

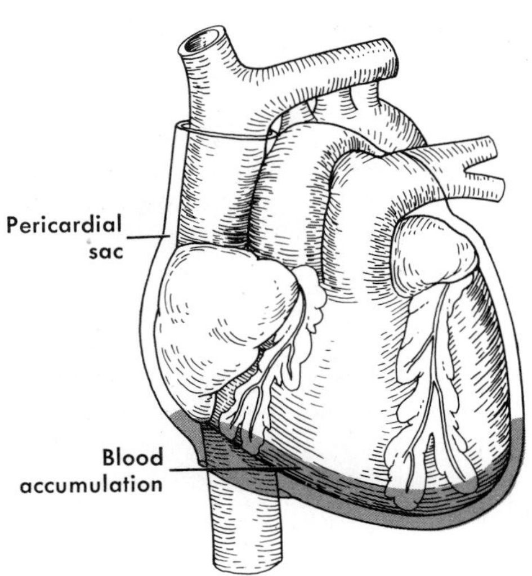

Fig. 13-6. Cardiac tamponade. (From Sheehy SB: *Emergency nursing: principles and practice,* ed 3, St Louis, 1992, Mosby.)

sessment for signs of decreasing cardiac output are necessary.

The initial treatment of a patient with suspected cardiac tamponade is a rapid intravenous fluid bolus.[14] This measure improves filling pressures and temporarily improves cardiac output until pericardiocentesis can be performed. The emergent treatment of choice is pericardiocentesis (Fig. 13-7).[20] The flight nurse places a needle into the pericardial sac and may withdraw as little as 15 to 20 ml of blood to improve the patient's condition. Pericardial blood will generally not clot because it has been defibrinated by heart motion. Pericardiocentesis is extremely challenging for the flight nurse to perform during flight because of the confined environment and air turbulence.

Because the long-term survival rate is less than 10%, aggressive interventions offer the best chance for patient survival. Failure to diagnose and repair aortic injuries within 24 hours of the patient's arrival results in mortality rates of 25% to 40%.[9] The transesophageal echocardiogram has been used as a rapid, accurate, and safe method of aortic transection identification.[18,21] During transport the flight nurse may

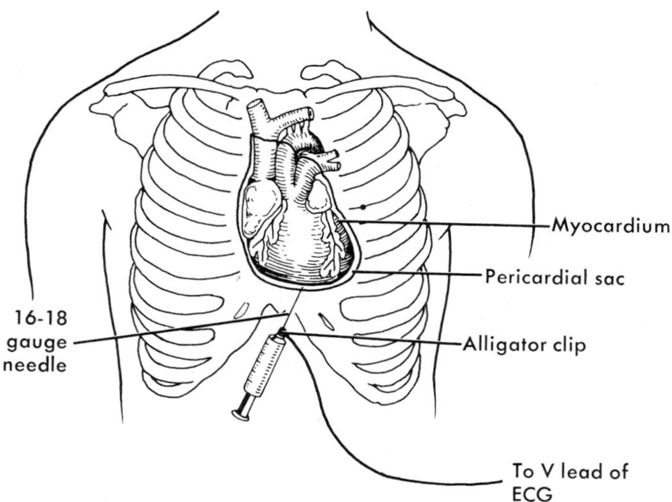

Fig. 13-7. Pericardiocentesis. (From Sheehy SB: *Emergency nursing: principles and practice,* ed 3, St Louis, 1992, Mosby.)

use β-blocker medication as a means to decrease cardiac output and limit the extent of aortic tear. Once complete rupture occurs during flight, the flight nurse cannot do anything to avert the patient's death. Definitive care often consists of an immediate exploratory thoracotomy.

Evaluation

When a trauma patient continues to deteriorate even with aggressive management, the flight nurse should consider acute pericardial tamponade.

Aortic Rupture

Etiologic and Pathophysiologic Factors

Aortic rupture occurs as a result of blunt or penetrating trauma, and death occurs immediately in 80% to 90% of patients, although when the rupture or transection occurs in only the medial and intimal layers, the intact adventitia may prevent exsanguination temporarily.

Assessment

The patient may not show any external signs of chest trauma. Severe chest and midscapular pain is not uncommon. If conscious, the patient will report dyspnea. Hypertension in the upper extremities is caused by a periaortic hematoma, partial aortic occlusion, or stretching of the cardiac plexus; a harsh systolic murmur can be auscultated along the precordium. If a chest x-ray has been done (before interfacility transport), findings that promote a high index of suspicion on the part of the flight nurse are (1) widening of the superior mediastinum, (2) loss of aortic knob shadow, (3) fracture of the first rib, (4) depression of the left main stem bronchus, (5) deviation of the trachea to the right, (6) pleural capping, and (7) deviation of the nasogastric tube in the esophagus.[8]

Interventions

The ABCs of resuscitation are necessary because it is impossible to prevent patient death if complete rupture occurs in flight. An immediate exploratory thoracotomy is necessary.

Myocardial Rupture

Etiologic and Pathophysiologic Factors

Rupture of the heart is the most lethal of blunt thoracic injuries.[16] Death occurs as a result of exsanguination. However, 61 reported cases of survival of nonpenetrating rupture of the myocardium have been reported; the majority were men who had been involved in motor vehicle accidents.[22]

Assessment and Interventions

Absent vital signs are key indicators that a fatal event has occurred. Resuscitation efforts are those used for any traumatically injured patient.

POTENTIALLY LIFE-THREATENING INJURIES

Myocardial Contusion

Etiologic Factors

Blunt trauma is the mechanism that produces myocardial contusion. The compression of the heart between the sternum and vertebrae occurs as a result of motor vehicle accidents, falls, or blows to the chest.

Pathophysiologic Factors

Lesions may vary from small areas of petechiae to large contusions and necrosis of the myocardium. Bleeding and edema occur at the site of injury.

Assessment

The patient should be suspected of having a myocardial contusion if the injury is highly suspicious. The patient may be completely asymptomatic or may report chest pain that is characteristically identical to that of angina or acute myocardial infarction. Sinus tachycardia is common, and cardiac arrhythmias may occur. Patients at risk are those who have abnormal initial electrocardiogram findings with ST-T segment changes.[8] Use of cardiac enzymes as a diagnostic tool in patients with suspected myocardial contusions has been found to be of little value.[2]

Interventions

Management is similar to that for a patient who has sustained an acute myocardial infarction. Supplemental oxygen, intravenous access, and prophylactic lidocaine are part of the treatment regimen. Recent studies question the efficacy of intensive care unit monitoring and lengthy hospitalization for patients with simple myocardial contusions.[4,10]

Pulmonary Contusion

Etiologic Factors

Pulmonary contusion occurs as a result of blunt thoracic trauma. It is not uncommon to have a pulmonary contusion associated with a flail chest.

Pathophysiologic Factors

Intraalveolar hemorrhage and edema occur as a result of blunt injury to the lung parenchyma. The alveolar-capillary integrity is lost, and interstitial hemorrhage and edema occur. Systemic hypoxemia is caused by decreased lung compliance and ventilation-perfusion mismatches.[13]

Assessment

The patient has a history of blunt thoracic trauma and usually demonstrates dyspnea and tachypnea. Tachycardia and anxiety, which may be caused by the stress of injury or hypoxemia, are also not uncommon. Rales and rhonchi are auscultated over the injured area. If arterial blood gas reports are available, hypoxemia can be determined. Maximum changes are seen in the chest x-ray from 48 to 72 hours after the injury.[5]

Interventions

Adequate ventilation with an aggressive pulmonary toilet is necessary. Supplemental oxygen should be administered. Endotracheal intubation is necessary when the Po_2 is lower than 60 mm Hg on room air or lower than 80 mm Hg with supplemental oxygen. Intravenous fluids, if not needed for resuscitation of other injuries, should be restricted. Corticosteroid use is controversial.

Diaphragmatic Rupture

Etiologic Factors

Herniation of abdominal viscera into the chest occurs when there is a traumatic defect in the diaphragm produced by blunt or penetrating trauma to the upper abdomen or lower thorax. If the injury occurred at the time the diaphragm was contracting strongly, a large avulsion tear will result. The vast majority of diaphragmatic ruptures occur on the left side because the liver protects the right hemidiaphragm.[1,22]

Pathophysiologic Factors

Herniation of abdominal contents into the thoracic cavity causes compression of the ipsilateral lung and displacement of mediastinal structures. Cardiopulmonary insufficiency results, causing significantly reduced respiratory efficiency. The herniated viscerae are compressed, causing gastric or intestinal obstruction and/or ischemia and gangrene.

Assessment

The patient may initially be asymptomatic or in severe distress. Abdominal or chest pain radiating to the shoulder may be present; dyspnea and cyanosis are also common signs. A paralytic ileus may accompany the injuries, so detection of bowel sounds may not be possible in the thorax cavity. Breath sounds will be decreased or absent on the side of the herniation. The abdomen will be markedly scaphoid. There will be a mediastinal shift to the unaffected side.[1,5,22]

Interventions

Ventilation must be maintained, generally with an endotracheal tube and mechanical ventilator. The flight nurse undertakes intravenous access and routine resuscitative measures, and immediate surgery for repair is indicated.

Tracheobronchial Disruption

Etiologic Factors

Tracheobronchial disruption occurs most often from blunt trauma. Penetrating thoracic trauma is a less common cause.

Pathophysiologic Factors

Air passes through the tear into the pleural space or the mediastinum. In the pleural space it produces a pneumothorax; in the mediastinum it causes mediastinal emphysema. The patient's airway may be maintained initially because the tracheobronchial cartilage holds the lumen open.

Assessment

Hemoptysis, respiratory distress, and subcutaneous or mediastinal emphysema (or both) are present. A pneumothorax with a persistent air leak or failure of a lung to reexpand after tube thoracostomy should lead the flight nurse to suspect a tracheobronchial disruption. A tension pneumothorax may be the first visible sign of the problem.

Interventions

The flight nurse performs immediate endotracheal intubation with placement of the tube below the level of injury, accompanied by bronchoscopy and chest tube placement as soon as possible.[1,14]

Esophageal Perforation

Etiologic Factors

The most common cause of esophageal perforation is iatrogenic traumatic instrumentation, although penetrating trauma, ingestion of a foreign body, or blunt trauma also can be causes.[12,23]

Pathophysiologic Factors

Gastric contents and bacteria leaking into the mediastinum can lead not only to mediastinitis but to fatal, systemic toxicity. Perforation also results in massive fluid loss, leading to hypovolemic shock.

Assessment

The location of the perforation will determine the clinical signs and symptoms. Subcutaneous emphysema, dyspnea, dysphagia, fever, hematemesis, and shock are common observations.

Interventions

Intravenous access, nasogastric tube placement, antibiotic administration, and immediate surgery are the interventions of choice for esophageal perforation.

SUMMARY

Transportation of a patient with a traumatic thoracic injury requires anticipatory planning to have all necessary equipment available. The flight nurse's prompt recognition and treatment of thoracic traumatic injuries may reduce mortality and morbidity, especially ensuring patency of the airway and performing specific measures for blunt or penetrating injuries.

THORACIC TRAUMA CASE STUDY

A single-victim motor vehicle accident was reported. The patient was a 24-year-old, semiconscious male driver who appeared to have fallen asleep, run off the road, and collided with a tree. There was no indication at the scene that he had been drinking alcohol. On the flight nurse's arrival at the scene, the patient was being placed in an ambulance.

The primary survey completed and reported by the ground emergency medical service personnel revealed that the patient had an open airway, was having slightly labored breathing, and had a weak, palpable pulse. He had no gross bleeding. There were multiple minor lacerations and abrasions.

The secondary survey, performed by the flight nurse on arrival at the scene of the accident, showed the following:

Vital signs: BP: 164/110, HR: 96, RR: 36
Pupils: PERL
Airway: Open
No obvious deformities of skull or face
C-collar remains in place from extrication
GCS = 9
Chest expansion asymmetric
Neck veins distended
Trachea deviated to the left
Minor abrasions to chest and back area. Small puncture wound, distal to the right scapula
No other wounds or abnormalities noted
No abdominal wounds or distention noted
No obvious deformity to extremities

The air medical crew then initiated the following interventions.

The patient's head, neck, and back were immobilized with a KED on a long board.
Emergency medical service personnel initiated two large-bore peripheral intravenous lines in each arm while the secondary survey was being conducted.
High-flow oxygen was established.
Recognizing the signs of a tension pneumothorax, the flight nurse placed a 10-gauge needle between the second and third intercostal spaces anteriorly in the midclavicular line on the right side. A rush of air was heard after needle insertion.
Breathing was reassessed, and dyspnea began to subside.
Breath sounds were clear on the left side and absent on the right.
Distention in the neck veins began to subside.
The patient was secured and transported.
Vital signs were monitored in flight.

Outcome

The patient was received in the emergency department of the area trauma center by the trauma team and was reassessed by the trauma surgeon, who ordered cervical, skull, chest, and abdominal x-rays; blood gases; laboratory analysis; and an ECG. Cervical, skull, and abdominal x-ray findings were normal. Blood gas levels, laboratory values, and ECG findings were within normal limits. Chest x-ray revealed a pneumothorax of the right side and a small-caliber bullet in the right chest cavity. The patient was transferred to the operating room where a chest tube was inserted and the bullet removed. It was theorized that the bullet entered the back, puncturing the lung. An internal flap formed, prevented the resulting pressure from being released, and caused the tension pneumothorax. The patient's hospital stay was uneventful, and he was released.

REFERENCES

1. American College of Surgeons Committee on Trauma. Thoracic trauma. *Advanced trauma life support student manual.* Chicago, Ill, 1993, American College of Surgeons.
2. Biffl WL et al: Cardiac enzymes are irrelevant in the patient with suspected myocardial contusion, *Am J Surg* 168(6):523, 1994.
3. Blansfield J: Emergency autotransfusion in hypovolemia, *Crit Care Nurs Clin North Am* 2(2):195, 1990.
4. Christensen MA, Sutton KR: Myocardial contusion: new concepts in diagnosis and management, *Am J Crit Care* 2(1):28, 1993.
5. Church T: Thoracic trauma. In Lee G, editor: *Flight nursing principles and practice,* St Louis, 1991, Mosby
6. Cohn SM et al: Exclusion of aortic tear in the unstable trauma patient: the utility of transesophageal echocardiography, *J Trauma* 39(6):1087, 1995.
7. Cooper A: Thoracic injuries, *Semin Pediatr Surg* 4(2):109, 1995.
8. Daleiden A: Clinical manifestations of blunt cardiac injury: a challenge to the critical care nurse, *Crit Care Nurs Q* 17(2):13, 1994.

9. Feczko JD et al: An autopsy case review of 142 nonpenetrating (blunt) injuries of the aorta, *J Trauma* 33(1): 846, 1992.
10. Fildes JJ et al: Limiting cardiac evaluation in patients with suspected myocardial contusion, *Am Surg* 69(9):832, 1995.
11. Herron H, Falcone RE: Prehospital decompression for suspected tension pneumothorax, *Air Med J* 14(2):69, 1995.
12. Klygis LM et al: Esophageal perforations masked by steroids, *Abdom Imaging* 18(1):10, 1993.
13. Kshettry VR: Chest trauma, assessment, diagnosis, and management, *Clin Chest Med* 15(1):137, 1994.
14. National Flight Nurses Association: *Thoracic trauma. Flight nurse advanced trauma course student manual,* 1995.
15. Nichols CG, Larson RE, Schmidt EW, editors: *A practical approach to emergency medicine: autotransfusion,* Boston, 1993, Little, Brown.
16. Pevec WC, Udekwu AO, Peitzman AB: Blunt rupture of myocardium, *Ann Thorac Surg* 48:139, 1989.
17. Rutter KM: Action stat! Tension pneumothorax, *Nursing* 25(4): 1995.
18. Saletta S et al: Transesophageal echocardiography for the initial evaluation of the widened mediastinum in trauma patients, *J Trauma* 39(1):137, 1995.
19. Schrader KA: Penetrating chest trauma, *Crit Care Nurs Clin North Am* 5(4):687, 1993.
20. Sheehy SB, Barber J: *Emergency nursing: principles and practice,* ed 2, St Louis, 1985, Mosby.
21. Shively BK: Transesophageal echocardiography in the diagnosis of aortic disease, *Semin Ultrasound CT MR* 14(2): 106, 1993.
22. Sukul DM, Kats E, Johannes EJ: Sixty-three cases of traumatic injury of the diaphragm, *Injury* 22(4):303, 1991.
23. Tucker JG, Kim HH, Lucas GW: Esophageal perforation caused by coin ingestion, *South Med J* 87(2):269, 1994.

CHAPTER 14

Abdominal and Genitourinary Trauma

COMPETENCIES

1. Perform an abdominal assessment.
2. Identify signs of abdominal trauma.
3. Provide appropriate treatment for the patient with an abdominal injury.

Regionalized trauma care has drastically reduced the incidence of death after injury. However, despite improvements in prehospital, resuscitative, surgical, and critical care, unrecognized abdominal injury remains a preventable cause of death after injury.[2] In a retrospective review of 22,577 patients admitted to six trauma centers, significant preventable errors were made in 1032 (4%). Of the total errors 53.4% occurred in the resuscitative phase. Failure to evaluate the abdomen was the single most common error identified in the study.[10] Additional studies acknowledge errors in the resuscitative phase, including inappropriate or delayed diagnosis of intraabdominal injuries, that can lead to preventable trauma deaths.[15]

Exsanguination is one of the most common causes of death from trauma. Because patients with abdominal trauma may have severe hemorrhage, rapid air transport can significantly reduce the mortality and morbidity from both blunt and penetrating abdominal injuries. Four common causes of massive bleeding in trauma patients include external injury, massive hemothorax, retroperitoneal injury (e.g., pelvic fracture, renal laceration, or major vessel lesion), and intraperitoneal injury (e.g., liver, spleen, or major vessel laceration).[38] The likelihood of significant intraabdominal injury is high when a patient has hypotension in the field, a major chest injury, or pelvic fracture.[47]

Patients with genitourinary injuries alone are not usually in danger of life-threatening hemorrhage. Shock and time elapsed between injury and arrival in the operating room are the major factors affecting survival of abdominally injured patients, and these factors can be ameliorated by intervention of trained air medical personnel able to recognize life-threatening injuries, initiate treatment, and rapidly transport the patient by air.

Although genitourinary trauma alone is not immediately life threatening, air medical transport can significantly affect the recovery time and reduction of complications resulting from injuries. Many level III facilities are not equipped to diagnose and treat specific genitourinary injuries. Air medical transport may be appropriate when a delay in ground time diminishes the chances of full recovery from renal, bladder, and genital injuries.

Immediate laparotomy and surgical stabilization at any outlying hospital may be a lifesaving measure for level I trauma patients admitted initially to a level III facility, especially when the transport time to a level I center is lengthy. Once the massive hemorrhage or other life-threatening abdominal injury is stabilized surgically, the patient may be transported to a level I center for further evaluation. Factors contributing to the decision to transport are based on the need for additional care and technology not available at a referring hospital.[12,20,25,35]

ABDOMINAL TRAUMA

Anatomy of the Abdomen

The abdomen contains several major organs of the body responsible for digestion, nutrition, and elimination of toxins and waste from the body. Because the spleen filters aged red blood cells and one of the functions of the liver is to eliminate toxic waste from the bloodstream, both organs are vascular in nature. The spleen, liver, and vascular system of the abdomen are the primary sources of exsanguination during abdominal trauma.[38] Injuries to the hollow abdominal organs, such as the small and large intestine, can result in abscess formation, wound infection, and sepsis, especially if trauma to the intestine remains undiagnosed for a period of time. When injuries to the abdomen occur, they may have a large impact on morbidity and mortality.

The abdominal cavity includes all structures and organs between the respiratory diaphragm and the urogenital diaphragm. This space is divided into three compartments: the first, and largest, is the peritoneal cavity; the second is the space within the pelvic structure; and the third is the retroperitoneal space. The peritoneal cavity contains the diaphragm, spleen, liver, stomach, transverse colon, and most of the small intestine and mesentery.

The bony structure of the pelvis contains the rectum, bladder, iliac vessels, and female reproductive organs; the penis and scrotum are located outside the abdominal cavity below the urogenital diaphragm.

The retroperitoneal space is separated from the abdominal cavity by the posterior peritoneum and therefore is not always accessed by peritoneal lavage. Injuries in this area may be difficult to diagnose and are easily overlooked. The organs contained in this space are the aorta, vena cava, distal esophagus, kidneys, ureters, and portions of the duodenum, pancreas, colon, and rectum.

Knowledge of the basic anatomy of the abdomen and position of the organs is crucial because identification of organs possibly injured by blunt or penetrating trauma helps the air medical crew provide the treatment necessary for those injuries when preparing for or effecting the patient's transport.

Classification of Injuries

Abdominal trauma can be blunt or penetrating depending on the mechanism of injury. Blunt trauma is caused by any type of force being exerted on the abdomen as the result of falls, motor vehicle accidents (MVAs), bicycle and motorcycle accidents, or any force striking the abdomen.[1,6] As the body receives an impact, the organs in the abdominal cavity continue moving forward; vessels and tissues tear away from their attachment points.

Patients have fewer fatal injuries with the increased use of seat belts, motorcycle and bicycle helmets, child restraint seats, and air bags, and with enforcement of alcohol restraints. However, the majority of blunt abdominal injuries (50% to 75%) are the result of MVAs.[13,16] The use of seat belts decreases the possibility of multisystem injuries, but improper placement across the abdomen rather than the pelvis, loose application, or use of only lap belts can result in visceral trauma. The abdominal organs most frequently injured by blunt trauma are the liver, spleen, and kidney, although hollow-organ (intestinal) injury can occur. Abdominal injuries among air bag–protected occupants occur less frequently than head, chest, and lower extremity injuries. However, abdominal injuries may be occult, and deformation of the steering wheel is an indicator of an increased likelihood of internal injury.[3,41]

Trauma is classified as penetration when an object such as a knife or bullet enters the abdominal cavity, and anything that has penetrated the abdomen and remains in place may be designated as an impaled object. Penetrating injuries of the abdomen are caused by gunshot wounds (GSWs) or stab wounds. The degree of injury of GSW patients depends on the caliber of the gun and its distance from the patient. High-velocity weapons and close-range shotguns cause more destruction to abdominal organs than do low-velocity weapons. However, bullets from low-velocity weapons can deflect off organs and bony prominences and create extensive injuries that are not easily recognized on initial examination. In stab wounds the length of the knife or object, depth of penetration, and angle at which it was inserted determine the amount of injury. The major organs involved in penetrating injuries are the liver, small bowel, colon, stomach, and vascular structures. The large size and anterior position of the liver and bowel in the abdomen make them particularly vulnerable to penetrating trauma.

Objects found impaled in the patient on arrival of the flight crew should be left in position and stabilized for flight. Removal of the object may cause further injury or increase bleeding. If placing the patient into the aircraft is not possible because of the size and position of the object, it may have to be cut off while still in place within the abdominal cavity. The object should be moved as little as possible. In some instances the trauma surgeon must be transported to the scene to assist in the shortening or removal of the object.[43]

Patient History

The history of the injury and the physical examination should be obtained before transport because the information is important to the air medical crew when they assess and stabilize a patient for transport. The trauma surgeon may use the information when deciding the degree of injury and whether surgery should be performed soon after arrival at the emergency center. When possible, a past medical history, including medications, allergies, illnesses, and events leading up to injury, should be obtained from the patient, family, or referring hospital. It is also helpful to know whether the patient has used alcohol or drugs, has a head or neck injury, has psychiatric problems, or has underlying medical conditions (i.e., cardiovascular disease or coagulapathies).[13] Initial vital signs and level of consciousness, intake and output, and treatments done before the arrival of the air medical crew, as well as any changes in assessment of treatments in flight, should be reported to the trauma team at the receiving trauma center.

When a patient with blunt abdominal trauma is transported from a pedestrian accident or MVA, important information to obtain from the prehospital personnel at the site are the time of injury, probable speed of impact, damage to the vehicle (steering wheel, direction of impact on the vehicle), patient's position in the vehicle, and restraint devices used. When time permits, brief inspection of the damage to the vehicle by the flight nurse may provide more information on possible patient injuries. In patients injured from falls, the height of fall and position of impact will help point to the type of injuries involved. The history of assault victims should include the type of instrument that struck them.[20]

When a patient with a GSW is transported, information on the type and caliber of gun, number and location of wounds, and distance the victim was from the assailant should be determined whenever possible. In stab-wound patients the size and length of the object and number of wounds should be ascertained. Although internal bleeding is difficult to measure in penetrating injuries, the amount of blood lost at the scene should be noted for determination of the fluid replacement needed and indication of the degree of injury.

Physical Examination

The physical examination is the most important procedure for diagnosis of abdominal injury. It is effective in detection of any blood loss into the peritoneal cavity or peritoneal irritation. Examination of the abdomen should be as thorough as possible. When a trauma patient who is in hemorrhagic shock is transported from a scene of accident or assault, the only assessment that time may permit is palpation for distention and tenderness. The abdominal assessment should include inspection, auscultation, and palpation before interfacility transport, especially when time and distance are great. Serial abdominal assessments should be done throughout transport because peritoneal irritation and accumulation of blood in the peritoneal cavity may not produce symptoms immediately.

The abdomen should be fully exposed to allow the flight nurse to inspect for contusions, abrasions, deformity, hematoma formation, open wounds, and penetrating injuries. An ecchymotic discoloration around the umbilicus (Cullen's sign) can indicate intraabdominal or retroperitoneal hemorrhage. When it is possible to examine the patient's back, the flight nurse should look for any obvious signs of trauma that would indicate an abdominal or genitourinary injury. Flank bruising may signify retroperitoneal hematoma formation from trauma to the kidneys, major blood vessels, or other organs contained in that space.

Auscultation should be done primarily in a quiet, controlled area because bowel sounds are difficult to hear in the noisy air transport environment. Absence of bowel sounds can be an important indicator of an ileus and abdominal injury, and assessment of bowel sounds before an interfacility transfer may alert the flight nurse to the possibility of abdominal injury. Inspection and palpation of the abdomen are doubly important because hearing bowel sounds in the noisy prehospital environment is difficult and taking the time to listen for bowel sounds at the scene when rotor noise makes hearing difficult does not alter patient treatment during transport and may delay liftoff. An abdomen that is tender and distended on palpation needs immediate attention; rapid transport with continual observation of vital signs and level of consciousness should be instituted. The major causes of a distended abdomen are gastric dilatation and rapid intraabdominal bleeding. Tenderness on palpation with involuntary guarding or rebound tenderness is indicative of peritoneal irritation. Subjective reports of abdominal pain by a trauma patient should always be addressed. Because head-injured patients with a decreased level of consciousness are unable to identify abdominal pain, detection of a distended abdomen on palpation without any obvious signs of trauma may be the only indication of intraabdominal trauma.

The perineum should be visually inspected for any injuries to the genitals, urethra, or rectum. Perineal hematoma formation can be caused by a retroperitoneal hematoma, pelvic fracture, or direct peritoneal trauma.

Diagnostic Procedures

Specific diagnostic procedures may have been done by a referring facility before arrival of the flight crew. Review of laboratory values such as hemoglobin and hematocrit levels can indicate hemorrhage in the patient and alert the flight nurse to the patient's need for blood transfusion. X-ray films can provide information on diagnosis of ruptured hollow abdominal organs or location of foreign objects. Results from testing of peritoneal lavage fluid may indicate intraabdominal bleeding or trauma to the intestine. Review of results of these diagnostic tests by the flight nurse before or during transport may help him or her determine patient treatment in flight.[44,45]

Laboratory test results that may be of benefit are initial hematocrit level, white blood cell count, blood type and crossmatch, and urinalysis. Baseline tests from outlying hospitals are important to the level I trauma surgeon because changes in laboratory values drawn at the receiving hospital may help diagnose abdominal and genitourinary injury.

X-ray examination of the abdomen may have been done. When viewing abdominal x-ray films for trauma, the flight nurse should direct his or her attention to the diaphragms, loops of distended bowel, psoas shadow, and any free subdiaphragmatic air. Free air in the peritoneal space indicates hollow-organ injury. Loss of the psoas shadow may indicate blood accumulation in the peritoneal space. Foreign bodies may be seen on abdominal films of penetrating injuries.

Peritoneal lavage is usually done at a level I trauma center; however, physicians in outlying hospitals may elect to do this procedure before deciding to transport a patient.

Diagnostic Peritoneal Lavage

Diagnostic peritoneal lavage (DPL) should be done only after the stomach has been decompressed with a nasogastric tube and the bladder decompressed with a Foley catheter. DPL is contraindicated in patients who are alert and can give accurate histories. Patients with obvious intraabdominal trauma requiring surgery should not be subjected to DPL. DPL performed early after an injury can miss hollow viscera and require that patients be observed for 24 hours despite negative findings.[47]

Computed tomography (CT) of the abdomen is another diagnostic procedure used as an adjunct to peritoneal lavage for the adult trauma patient and for monitoring purposes in children. CT is effective in demonstrating solid viscus injuries such as spleen or liver lacerations, the presence and quantity of hemoperitoneum, and retroperitoneal injuries such as renal lacerations or hematomas associated with pelvic fractures. CT is helpful in decreasing the number of unnecessary laparotomies.[17] DPL and CT are the primary diagnostic modalities in the evaluation of patients with suspected blunt traumas. DPL is fast and accurate but is associated with complications. CT is also accurate but requires patients to be stable and transportable. Ultrasound is reliable in detecting free intraperitoneal fluid and may be used in place of DPL and CT.[32] Laparoscopy and thoracoscopy are also used as diagnostic modalities in blunt and penetrating abdominal trauma.

Ultrasonography is being used with increasing frequency in the United States. In patients with hemodynamically unstable conditions, it provides a rapidly available evaluation of the expected amount of free intraperitoneal fluid or of a solid-organ lesion with acceptably high accuracy. Ultrasonography has proved to be a reliable, cost-efficient, and noninvasive modality in primary evaluation and follow-up of patients with blunt abdominal trauma. In addition, patients are not exposed to radiation or contrast media.[28] Laparoscopy and thoracoscopy are also used as diagnostic modalities in blunt and penetrating abdominal trauma.

Patient Assessment, Treatment, and Transport

In many cases injury is not limited to the abdomen, particularly in patients with blunt-trauma injuries. Once the primary assessment is completed and the patient stabilized, the secondary examination should be done for determination of any other injuries.

In addition to the usual airway and breathing assessment and management, signs and symptoms of cardiovascular system collapse, such as hypotension, delayed capillary refill, and decreased level of consciousness, are important indicators of abdominal injuries. Patients with visceral injuries have the potential for sudden onset of severe hypovolemic shock because of the vascular nature of many organs in the abdominal cavity and the space for occult blood accumulation. Rapid recognition of the possibility of major abdominal injury is of paramount importance. Rapid transport after initial stabilization should be the goal when a patient is in hemorrhagic shock or has impending exsanguination.

Patients in severe shock or near exsanguination exhibit a decreasing level of consciousness as hypoxia increases and pale to mottled skin that is cold, clammy, and possibly profusely diaphoretic (see box). Mucous membranes may be pasty white, and capillary refill is delayed or absent. When no obvious external bleeding is present, the flight nurse should examine the abdomen. If the abdomen is distended and rigid with no bowel sounds, the flight nurse should suspect intraabdominal bleeding. The conscious patient will report severe abdominal pain. If the abdomen is tautly distended, pressure will be exerted on the diaphragm, causing potential shortness of breath and tachypnea. The patient will be tachycardic and hypotensive; a blood pressure reading may not be obtainable even with a weak brachial pulse. If the blood pressure does not respond to fluid administration, exsanguination is a real possibility. The

SYMPTOMS OF NEAR EXSANGUINATION

- Decreasing consciousness
- Pale-to-mottled skin that is cold, clammy, and possibly diaphoretic
- Pasty white mucous membranes
- Delayed or absent capillary refill
- Distended and rigid abdomen with no bowel sounds
- Potential shortness of breath and tachypnea
- Tachycardia and hypotension
- Unobtainable blood pressure reading
- Blood pressure that does not respond to fluid administration
- Reports of severe abdominal pain

survival of an exsanguinating patient may depend on the amount of time it takes for him or her to be admitted to surgery.

Not all patients with abdominal injuries display all the symptoms described above. Varying degrees of these symptoms, such as abdominal tenderness without initial distention, decreased but not absent bowel sounds, and tachycardia without hypotension, should alert the flight crew to the possibility of exsanguination.

Initial stabilization at the scene when transport time will be short should consist of airway management, 100% oxygen delivery, and spine immobilization. For the abdominally injured patient, two large-bore intravenous lines of crystalloid fluid should be inserted without delay. The second intravenous line can be started in flight as needed. Blood-pump tubing and pressure infusers on the intravenous fluids will help rapidly infuse fluids when hypotension occurs. Low blood pressure is a late sign of shock. Therefore hypotension without other symptoms of poor tissue perfusion such as pallor, decreased capillary refill, and tachycardia does not necessarily indicate shock. A cardiac monitor should be applied for assessment of tachycardia, cardiac irritability, or both. The likelihood of significant intraabdominal injury is high when a patient has hypotension in the field, a major chest injury, or pelvic fracture.[47]

Much controversy exists in the medical field today regarding the use of the pneumatic antishock garment (PASG) for hypotensive patients. After his extensive literature review on MAST use, McSwain[33] recommended that, because of the possibility of compartment syndrome occurring with the use of the MAST suit, the pants should be inflated until the Velcro begins to crackle. Further inflation should be done cautiously while its effect on blood pressure is monitored. Altitude changes can increase the pressure exerted by the MAST on the patient's body; however, time should not be consumed with constant checking or adjusting of the pressure.

Hospital-to-hospital transfers, either by fixed-wing or rotor-wing aircraft, may incur a longer patient transport time. Patient management should include all the treatment instituted for the short-scene-call transport. In addition, a nasogastric tube should be inserted for suspected intestinal injury, gastric distention, or aspiration. If massive external or internal hemorrhage is occurring, the referring hospital may have type-specific or O-negative blood infusing or ready to send with the patient. If the report before liftoff indicates hypovolemic shock, the air medical crew should request that the referring hospital have blood ready for transport on the patient's arrival. For some patients, blood transfusion before arrival at the level I trauma center can be the factor that decreases morbidity and mortality. Hypothermia caused by massive intravenous fluid resuscitation can have a negative influence on patient outcome; therefore warming of intravenous fluids for the administration of many liters of fluid, or at least use of fluids from an emergency department instead of cold fluids in the aircraft, can be important. The goals of air medical transport are rapid patient stabilization and transport to the nearest facility capable of treating the abdominally injured patient.

SPECIFIC ABDOMINAL ORGAN INJURIES

Diaphragm

Incidence and Mechanism

Blunt injury to the diaphragm, resulting in rupture or partial tear, occurs when a tremendous force is applied to the abdomen. The left diaphragm is injured more often than the right because the liver absorbs the impact of the force on the right side. If a right-sided tear has occurred, liver injury will probably accompany it. Spleen injuries often occur with left-sided diaphragmatic trauma.[13,50] Diaphragmatic tears can occur without herniation of bowel into the chest cavity. If an intestinal herniation into the pleural space does occur, intestinal strangulation may develop. A penetrating injury of the diaphragm should be suspected when a knife wound occurs at or below the nipple line anteriorly or at the inferior border of the scapula posteriorly.[8]

Assessment and Symptoms

The flight nurse may not be able to diagnose a diaphragmatic tear that has not resulted in bowel herniation. Further diagnostic procedures may be necessary for him or her to ascertain a diaphragmatic tear. Physical examination of the patient with a diaphragmatic hernia may reveal absent or reduced breath sounds on the affected side. Bowel sounds may be heard in the chest cavity when intestinal contents have herniated into the pleural space. Respiratory distress may accompany intestinal herniation. If stomach contents are returned when a needle thoracostomy is performed for a believed tension pneumothorax, diaphragmatic hernia should be suspected. When a chest x-ray has been done, it may indicate intestinal herniation by the presence of stomach contents or a curled nasogastric tube in the chest cavity. Diaphragm injuries missed on diagnostic examination may result in intestinal incarceration or strangulation that occurs weeks to months later. Associated mortality is high.[13]

Treatment

Specific treatment for a known or suspected diaphragmatic tear with possible herniation should focus on airway management, oxygenation, and ventilation because of the potentially decreased lung capacity. Intubation and ventilation should be done when respiratory failure occurs. A nasogastric tube inserted for transport will reduce the possibility of aspiration and gastric dilatation, especially for patients with herniation.

Liver and Spleen

Incidence and Mechanism

The spleen is the most commonly injured organ in blunt abdominal trauma; the liver is second, and they frequently are injured at the same time. In both spleen and liver trauma, early deaths are the result of hemorrhage or other injuries; late deaths result from infection. The mortality rate for liver injuries is 13%, with a higher percentage of deaths occurring from penetrating injury.[14] Penetrating injuries that occur below the nipple level of the thorax or in the upper abdominal cavities may involve the liver or spleen.

The mechanism of injury for liver trauma is direct trauma to the liver itself, causing fractures in the organ, or deceleration forces that may avulse hepatic veins from the inferior vena cava and diaphragm attachments. Tears in the hepatic, arterial, and portal venous vessels from compressive or shearing forces can result in rapid bleeding. The biliary duct system and hepatic vasculature are injured more often in penetrating injuries of the liver than in blunt injuries.

Assessment and Symptoms

Both the liver and spleen are vascular in nature. Patients with blunt and penetrating injuries can have symptoms that vary from slight tachycardia with abdominal guarding to profound shock and a distended, taut abdomen when intraabdominal hemorrhage is occurring. A distended abdomen may indicate severe bleeding from either the liver or the spleen. When these patients are assessed, inspection and palpation of the abdomen should be done to locate contusions, abrasions, and pain. Other injuries, such as rib and scapula fractures, are associated with spleen and liver trauma. The amount of force involved in blunt abdominal injuries and the mechanism of injury and location of wounds in penetrating trauma are important indicators of spleen and liver injury.

Subjective symptoms of spleen injury may be localized tenderness in the left upper quadrant. Referred shoulder pain (Kehr's sign) from left hemidiaphragm irritation can also be present, but it is rarely seen. Localized abdominal pain from liver injuries will occur in the right upper quadrant.

The gallbladder is rarely injured in blunt abdominal trauma because it is protected within the liver itself. The flight nurse may not easily recognize gallbladder rupture because symptoms and diagnostic findings may not appear for several days to weeks.

Treatment

Because exsanguination may be the cause of death immediately after the accident in spleen and liver trauma, specific treatment in these injuries should focus on hemodynamic status. To maintain tissue perfusion and blood pressure when hypotension and shock are present, the flight nurse should inflate the PASG, run intravenous lines wide open with pressure infusers attached, and institute rapid transport. Relay of information to the trauma center when obvious intraabdominal hemorrhage is present can prepare the trauma team for immediate care of the patient.

If the patient had initial surgery at an outlying hospital and infection and liver dysfunction occur, the flight nurse may transport the patient to a facility with resources better equipped to treat patients with complications. The spleen serves as a defense against infection by filtering old blood cells and bacteria and is a source of immunoglobulins. The long-term complications of spleen injury, which may be the reason for air transport, are caused by infection, particularly when a splenectomy has been done. Because of the many functions of the liver, complications of liver injury can include coagulopathy problems, nutritional and immune deficiencies, and drug regulation.

Pancreas and Duodenum

Incidence and Mechanism

Both the pancreas and duodenum lie within the retroperitoneal space; they are in intimate proximity to each other and usually are injured together. Both are well protected and constitute less than 3% to 12% of all abdominal injuries.[13] Mortality and morbidity from pancreatic and duodenal injuries occur more frequently from secondary complications of infection, pseudocyst or fistula formation, gastrointestinal tract malfunction, and chronic pancreatitis. Injury in blunt trauma should be suspected when direct force is applied to the left upper quadrant, as in steering wheel and bicycle handlebar impalement. Injury is caused by compression of these organs against the vertebral column. Injuries to both the pancreas and duodenum occur more frequently from penetrating than from blunt trauma.

Assessment and Symptoms

Symptoms of isolated, blunt pancreatic and duodenal injuries may be difficult to observe. If duodenal digestive juices and blood are contained within the retroperitoneal space, the patient may not have many abdominal symptoms. Assessment of the patient will usually show tenderness over the area of the pancreas and absence of bowel sounds. The patient may be hemodynamically stable, with symptoms associated only with peritonitis (such as abdominal tenderness or guarding), or may have no symptoms at all. These injuries are difficult to diagnose, but the flight nurse can help with the diagnosis by accurately reporting the history and mechanism of injury to the receiving physician. If peritoneal lavage was done at the referring hospital, results may be diagnostic when amylase is present, but a lack of amylase in the peritoneal fluid does not rule out pancreatic injury because of the retroperitoneal position of the pancreas.

Treatment

The transport treatment for these patients includes a high index of suspicion for injury when the patient has vague abdominal symptoms after trauma. Treatment should include any procedures necessary for patient stabilization and supportive care if the patient's respiratory and cardiovascular status remains stable. If duodenal injury is suspected, nasogastric tube insertion will reduce the gastric and duodenal juices' infiltration of the peritoneal space. Outlying hospitals may transfer these patients several days after injury when isolated pancreatic and duodenal symptoms occur.

Colon and Small Intestine

Incidence and Mechanism

Colon and small-intestine damage occurs more frequently in penetrating than in blunt injuries, and in most cases the liver, spleen, or other organs are also injured.[13] Colon injuries are caused by penetrating missiles or stabbings 90% of the time. The small intestine is the most commonly injured organ in penetrating injuries, presumably because of the volume it occupies in the abdomen.[14] Blunt injury to the small intestine occurs with crushing of the bowel against the spinal column. Improper use of the seat belt, steering wheel impact, or a blunt object applied to the abdomen can produce this crushing effect. If a victim has a transverse bruise across the lower abdomen from a lap belt, rupture of the small intestine should be considered.[13] Bowel evisceration may occur with penetrating trauma, and bowel contents should be covered with sterile saline solution during transfer.

Assessment and Symptoms

The same thorough assessment for abdominal trauma should be done in suspected cases of intestinal injury. The flight nurse should inspect the location of all entrance and exit sites of patients with GSWs and the entrance wounds of stabbing victims. Examination of the back, buttocks, and perineum is important because wounds to these areas are easily overlooked. Documentation of the locations of wounds should be as accurate as possible. Evisceration of the bowel may be found with penetrating injuries; the color and size of protruding bowel should be noted on the initial examination.

Symptoms of isolated colon injury are associated with peritoneal irritation from blood or feces free in the peritoneum. Pain on palpation with guarding may be present, and symptoms of fever and leukocytosis may increase with time elapsed since injury. Fecal material may be present in the peritoneal lavage fluid when colon disruption has occurred. Abdominal x-ray films may reveal free air in the peritoneum or a loss of the psoas shadow.

Symptoms of small-bowel injury include tenderness, patient reluctance to change positions, rebound tenderness, and guarding. In small-intestinal injuries, peritoneal lavage may demonstrate turbid or bile-stained fluid, an elevated white blood cell count, or presence of amylase. X-ray films may reveal free air in the peritoneum or a small-bowel ileus.

Treatment

Because most injuries of the intestine are associated with other more immediate life-threatening injuries, transport management should be prioritized accordingly. While airway and cardiovascular systems are being stabilized, saline dressings should be applied to any eviscerated bowel or dry dressings to any open wounds. The amount of blood loss at the scene should be noted. When hypotension is refractory to fluid administration and the PASG leg compartments are fully inflated, the abdominal compartment can be inflated even if eviscerated bowel is present.

Most complications of bowel injuries occur later in the patient's course of recovery. The major factors related to morbidity and mortality are sepsis, abscess formation, wound infection, and intraabdominal peritonitis.

Gastric and Esophageal Trauma

Incidence and Mechanism

Gastric and esophageal injuries are uncommon because the esophagus and stomach are well protected within the upper abdominal cavity. The abdominal esophagus is 2 to 4 cm long and lies within the retroperitoneal space, anterior to the aorta. The pliability of the stomach reduces its chances of injury in blunt trauma, although a full stomach is more likely to rupture. The majority of esophageal and gastric injuries are caused by penetrating trauma.

Assessment and Symptoms

Symptoms of gastric and esophageal trauma are signs of peritoneal irritation, such as pain and guarding. Nasogastric tube drainage may show evidence of blood, and that may indicate gastric rupture in the absence of other obvious sources of bleeding, such as facial trauma, in which the patient may have swallowed blood. Review of the abdominal x-ray film at the referring hospital may show free air in the peritoneum, indicating disruption of the intestinal tract, which may involve the esophagus, stomach, or both.

Treatment

Diagnosis of gastric and esophageal trauma injuries will most likely be confirmed after arrival at the trauma center. Transport treatment of these patients is similar to that of any other trauma patient with life-threatening injuries. If a gastric rupture is suspected, a nasogastric tube should be carefully inserted for long transports. Time of last food consumption can be useful information to the trauma surgeon, especially in an unconscious patient.

Abdominal Vascular Injuries

Incidence and Mechanism

Injuries to the abdominal arterial and venous systems occur more frequently with penetrating trauma than with blunt trauma. A five-year retrospective study of 530 MVA fatalities revealed that aortic injuries occurred in 18% of victims. The typical victim was a male driver with an elevated blood alcohol level, who was involved in a head-on collision.[49] Compression or deceleration forces applied to the abdomen can result in avulsion of small vessels from the larger vessels from which they branch, and intimal tears within the vessel itself may occur. Intimal tears can result in thrombosis formation, whereas vessel avulsion tears can result in exsanguination. Penetrating injuries of vascular tissue cause lacerations and free bleeding. The major vessels frequently injured are the aorta, inferior vena cava, and the renal, mesenteric, and iliac arteries and veins. Vascular system injury is the primary cause of death in patients who sustain GSWs and stab wounds to the abdomen. Mortality is high, even when patients are not in shock at presentation.[18]

Assessment and Symptoms

A patient with no obvious active external bleeding source who experiences severe shock shortly after injury probably has arterial injury. Bleeding is profuse, and rapid fluid replacement may not be able to maintain blood pressure and tissue perfusion when intraabdominal arterial lacerations are present. When vein, liver, or spleen injuries produce hypovolemia, fluid replacement can usually maintain tissue perfusion if it is given rapidly. If fluid administration of 3 L or more does not reverse hypotension, an arterial injury should be suspected.[13] Patients with abdominal vascular injuries may present as or become the exsanguinating patient described earlier depending on the degree of intraabdominal bleeding and the time elapsed since injury occurred. With arterial injuries the femoral pulse on the affected side may be absent. Major abdominal vein injuries can also produce profound shock, but it may occur up to 30 minutes after the injury instead of immediately. Bleeding from venous injuries may be self-controlled by direct pressure of the abdominal organs or abdominal pressure itself, limiting the possibility of early exsanguination.

Treatment

With abdominal vascular injuries, when exsanguination is imminent, rapid transport to a level I trauma center is critical to patient survival.

Complications after survival of the initial abdominal vascular injury include continued bleeding from vascular reconstruction areas or disseminated intravascular coagulation that develops from massive blood transfusions, liver ischemia, or profound shock. Thrombosis formation can occur and cause tissue ischemia to the kidneys or gastrointestinal tract. When renal or visceral veins are involved, pulmonary embolism can develop. If initial surgical stabilization occurred at a level III facility, the flight nurse may transport the patient with the complications that followed the initial insult.

TRAUMA IN SPECIAL POPULATIONS

Trauma to the Pregnant Patient

The pregnant trauma patient presents a unique challenge to the air medical flight crew. Physiologic and anatomic changes that occur during pregnancy alter the symptoms and diagnostic parameters of injured pregnant women. Failure to recognize these changes in the early assessment of the pregnant trauma patient can result in delayed diagnosis and treatment of hypovolemia and hypoxia, which ultimately affects maternal and particularly fetal survival. Because two lives are at risk with the traumatized pregnant patient, assessment and treatment should be directed at both, but because the primary cause of fetal death is maternal death, the mother's life ultimately takes precedence.[13] To ensure the best possible chance of maternal and fetal survival, the air medical crew should properly stabilize the pregnant trauma patient at the scene or referring facility and air transport her to the nearest level I facility capable of treating both her and the fetus.

Incidence and Mechanism

Trauma is the leading cause of non-obstetric-related maternal deaths and is responsible for between 3% and 46% of maternal deaths, depending on geographic location. MVAs are the leading cause of maternal mortality in nonurban areas. In urban areas maternal mortality from violence is the leading cause of death. The incidence of death is higher in younger women, minority groups, and women during the earlier months of pregnancy.

Injuries resulting from blunt trauma to the abdomen from either MVAs or any other form of nonpenetrating trauma usually occur within the gravid uterus in pregnant women. When seat-belt use is documented in the pregnant trauma patient, it is important to note the type of seat belt used. Seat belts with shoulder harnesses are recommended during pregnancy. Lap belts can increase intraabdominal and intrauterine pressure, thereby increasing the likelihood of fetal injury. When direct pressure for any reason is applied to the gravid uterus, the flexible uterus may conform while the rigidly attached placenta separates and abruption occurs. Uterine rupture and placental abruption are uncommon, but both should be considered in pregnant patients who have undergone blunt abdominal trauma.[13]

The fetus can suffer a variety of direct injuries as a result of blunt trauma. These injuries range from skull fractures to abdominal and chest trauma. When a maternal pelvic fracture is present, fetal skull fractures are commonly seen, especially in the last trimester when the baby's head is in the pelvic ring.[13]

Falls are not likely to result in major injury to the fetus if the mother does not have major fractures, contusions, or head injury; the fetus is well protected in the amniotic fluid.

GSWs are the most frequent cause of penetrating injury to the pregnant patient. Stab wounds do occur but result in less injury. Whereas stab wounds create a single entry into the abdomen, bullets move with force and can produce more damage as they travel within the abdominal cavity. The extent of injuries to the pregnant uterus and fetus during penetrating trauma depends on the length of pregnancy and uterine size.

A number of changes occur during pregnancy that make treatment of the pregnant trauma patient unique:

1. Cardiac output, heart rate, and respiratory rate are increased.
2. Physiologic anemia occurs because the plasma volume increases at a greater rate than the red cell mass.
3. Respiratory alkalosis can be present because of the increased respiratory rate.
4. The diaphragm is elevated at least one intercostal space during late pregnancy.
5. Supine hypotension may occur after 20 weeks' gestation when the gravid uterus causes compression of the vena cava in the supine position.
6. An electrocardiogram may show left axis deviation with flattening or inversion of the T wave in lead III.
7. Blood pressure may be slightly lower during the second trimester but returns to normal near term.

Assessment and Symptoms

Because early pregnancy is likely to be unrecognized during the trauma evaluation, menstrual history should be included as for any female patient of childbearing age. Routine pregnancy testing is advocated in female patients.[13] If the patient is known to be pregnant, the gravidity and parity history should be obtained. Vaginal bleeding, preterm labor, or other problems associated with pregnancy that were present before the injury should be noted.

Compounding the difficulty in determination of hypovolemia is the normally increased heart rate of the pregnant patient and the slightly decreased blood pressure during the second trimester. In addition to these changes, uterine perfusion decreases by 10% to 20% with maternal hemorrhage because blood volume is shunted away from the uterus to preserve maternal blood pressure. The combination of increased plasma volume, tachycardia, and slight hypotension in the normal pregnant woman and physiologic shunting of blood away from the uterus to preserve maternal blood volume when hypovolemia is present may result in a delay of maternal signs of hypovolemic shock, such as tachycardia, hypotension, and poor perfusion. Decreased uteroplacental perfusion caused by shunting places the fetus at risk. Early assessment of fetal heart rate is essential because decreased fetal movement and increased fetal heart rate can indicate imminent maternal shock before it is apparent in the mother. A fetal heart rate above 160 beats/min when maternal trauma is present is an early sign of fetal distress, whereas fetal bradycardia is a later sign. When fetal bradycardia occurs, the fetus has already been significantly stressed, which may be the result of decreased volume of maternal circulation. Fetal distress develops primarily from decreased uterine blood flow and hypoxia. When the patient is being transported from a hospital setting, the flight nurse must review the fetal monitor strip for any decelerations or indications of fetal distress.

Any type of maternal chest injury can be detrimental to the mother and especially to the fetus. The elevated diaphragm during a normal pregnancy increases the possibility of atelectasis and hypoventilation caused by fractured ribs. Dilutional physiologic anemia decreases the oxygen-carrying capacity of the blood; therefore fetal hypoxia can ensue. Maternal hypoxia causes decreased perfusion of the uterus, and the decreased fetal circulation can add to any fetal distress already present.

Abdominal assessment may be difficult during the later stages of pregnancy. The abdomen is already distended with the gravid uterus, and bowel sounds are normally diminished. The hemoperitoneum may be hidden behind or within the uterus. Abdominal pain must be distinguished from contractions. Placental separation may present as a rigid, painful abdomen, and the uterus can actually increase in size as bleeding continues. Vaginal bleeding may or may not be present with placental separation. Vaginal examination should be avoided when bleeding is present, but the amount and color of vaginal bleeding observed should be documented. Serial assessments of the abdomen and perineum should be done during transport so that the flight nurse can observe for evidence of intraabdominal bleeding, vaginal bleeding, and onset of labor. Inspection of the abdomen for contusions, abrasions, or obvious trauma may identify the possibility of internal bleeding when signs of hypovolemia are absent.

Treatment

The priorities in treatment of the pregnant trauma patient are diagnosis and treatment of hypovolemia and hypoxia before the symptoms can be seen in the mother. Once the maternal trauma patient exhibits hypotension and respiratory compromise, the fetus has already been stressed. Fetal survival depends on aggressive maternal care.

Management of the pregnant patient's airway requires the same considerations as for other trauma patients. Because of the potential for fetal hypoxia with even a small change in the maternal oxygenation, 100% supplemental oxygen should always be provided in flight regardless of the mother's condition. This is especially true when altitude changes can add to the compromised oxygenation. Intubation should be done early rather than late in the pregnant trauma patient. Any signs of respiratory compromise such as poor blood gas levels or a decreased level of consciousness should be aggressively treated with oxygenation and intubation. Waiting until obvious respiratory failure occurs submits the fetus to unnecessary risk. When adequate maternal tissue perfusion is present, the use of pulse oximetry provides a good method for oxygen saturation monitoring in flight.

Nasogastric tube insertion protects the patient from aspiration. The elevated abdominal contents during pregnancy decrease gastric emptying and increase pressure on the stomach. Early gastric emptying may prevent complications of vomiting and aspiration.

The flight team should not hesitate to perform a needle thoracostomy or chest tube insertion when clinical signs of pneumothorax are present. When a chest tube is inserted during the later stages of pregnancy, the tube should be placed at the third or fourth intercostal space because of the elevated diaphragm.

Hypotension should be treated before symptoms are seen in the maternal trauma patient. Once the normal signs of hemorrhagic shock appear in these women, fetal survival may be unlikely. Two large-bore intravenous lines should be inserted, and pressure infusers should be applied to the crystalloid fluid. For adequate uteroplacental perfusion and reduced fetal anoxia, the pregnant patient requires more fluid replacement than the nonpregnant trauma victim. Overhydration is preferable to fetal demise in a pregnant patient who is presumed to be stable. Lactated Ringer's solution instead of normal saline solution should be used in the pregnant trauma patient because Ringer's solution has been proved to be more effective in restoration of fetal oxygenation than other fluids.

Application of a PASG and inflation of the lower legs can be done safely in the pregnant trauma patient. The major complication of leg inflation in the pregnant woman can be increased pressure on the engorged and possibly torn pelvic veins, which may result in increased blood loss. Abdominal compartment inflation is appropriate in major maternal pelvic fractures when maternal and fetal death are imminent or fetal demise has occurred. If inflation of the PASG does not improve the patient's condition or if it causes deleterious effects, it should be deflated.

Supine hypotension can have a significant impact on an already compromised fetus. In the trauma patient, spinal immobilization is necessary for transport. To reduce the effects of compression of the vena cava by the gravid uterus, the flight nurse can tilt the backboard to the left side. Placement of a towel, pillow, or blanket under the right hip can be sufficient to move the uterus to the side, and manual displacement of the uterus to one side is also possible. If maternal hypotension is present, correction of supine hypotension during fluid replacement can be an important influence on fetal survival.

When the flight nurse suspects abruptio placentae, he or she should immediately initiate rapid fluid resuscitation, oxygen administration, and transport. Hypovolemic shock and fetal distress will quickly ensue. Disseminated intravascular coagulation (DIC) complications can occur, especially if fetal demise has occurred. The best treatment for patients with DIC is delivery of the fetus.

Uterine rupture should be treated similarly to placental separation. Fetal parts may be felt easily in the abdominal wall, and the top of the uterus may be difficult to define. Shock, abdominal pain, and lack of fetal heart tones will also be found on examination. The lifesaving treatment for the mother is immediate laparotomy at a level I facility where perinatal tertiary care is also available.

Labor can be a complication of trauma during pregnancy. Regular contractions with cervical dilation are considered premature labor when gestation is less than 37 weeks. Treatment of hypovolemia and hypoxia should be done rapidly if labor is suspected. Precipitous delivery in the patient with a depressed level of consciousness can be avoided if the onset of labor is continuously assessed. Contractions lasting longer than 40 seconds and occurring every 7 to 10 minutes should be treated as labor. If, in the flight nurse's judgment, the patient is unlikely to deliver during transport, treatment of labor should consist of observation of contractions and fetal heart rate only. Tocolytic agents can be initiated for contraction reduction when regular uterine activity is present in the absence of uteroplacental injury, after fluid resuscitation and oxygenation have been initiated, and after the patient demonstrates adequate renal perfusion. The flight nurse administers magnesium sulfate; the usual dosage is a 6-g bolus followed by a 3-g/hour drip, unless pregnancy-induced hypertension or impaired renal function is present. In an outlying facility with a long transport time, imminent delivery, or abruptio placentae, the decision to deliver the fetus before transport may be necessary to increase the chance of maternal and fetal survival. When possible, ethical and medicolegal issues such as delivery of the fetus before transport should be discussed with the patient, family, referring physician, colleagues of the air medical crew, and the air medical crew director before decisions are made.

Survival of both mother and child depends on the care rendered before arrival at the trauma center. Treatment of hypovolemia and hypoxia should be the first priority. Time from injury to arrival at a level I trauma center and whether the appropriate team is available immediately to treat the injuries and deliver the baby are important to maternal and fetal morbidity and mortality.

Abdominal Trauma in Pediatric Patients

Trauma continues to be the leading cause of death in children. Injuries occur more frequently in boys, and for both genders the incidence is increased during the summer months. Abdominal trauma in children includes both blunt and penetrating trauma.

Blunt trauma is responsible for 80% to 95% of all pediatric trauma.[22] Blunt trauma leaves minimal evidence of the underlying injury and is difficult to assess in the unconscious child.[22] Management of blunt trauma in children can be quite complex because head injuries are present in 80% to 85% of victims.[9] The most commonly injured organs in pediatric abdominal trauma are the liver and spleen. Pancreatic and duodenal injuries are less frequent and usually are associated with specific mechanisms of injury, such as child abuse and lap-belt injuries.[9] Nonsurgical management of liver, spleen, and pancreatic injuries without duct involvement is common in children as long as the child is monitored closely and has ready access to surgery. Hemodynamic instability beyond the resuscitation period may require interhospital transport if the child is not already at a pediatric trauma center.[42]

Children can experience blunt abdominal trauma when subjected to child abuse. The mechanism of injury is bursting of the abdominal viscera from compression against the spine. Abdominal injury during child abuse may be further complicated by a time delay between initial insult and treatment. Frequently there is a delay before parents bring a child in for evaluation. The child may have hypovolemia and peritonitis as a result of the delay.[22] When sepsis and shock are present, the mortality and morbidity increase. Children do not incur vascular injury to the abdomen from blunt trauma as frequently as adults, but when venous vascular trauma is present, mortality is high.

Blunt abdominal injuries are also associated with specific injury patterns in children.[9] Lap-belt complex describes injuries sustained by children restrained in a motor vehicle by lap belts only. Rapid acceleration or deceleration against the belt results in sharp flexion of the lumbar spine and a rapid rise in intraabdominal pressure and may result in rupture of the small bowel and lumbar spine injury. This type of injury should be suspected in the presence of seatbelt ecchymosis. Bicycle accidents that cause children to be thrown against handlebars can cause duodenal and pancreatic injuries.[9] Intraabdominal trauma should be suspected when there are no plastic or foam coverings on the metal ends of handlebars.

Several anatomic differences between adults and children exist that make children more vulnerable to blunt injury. Abdominal organs are closer to the surface of the body because children have less muscle and adipose tissue; consequently even lower energy impacts may cause injury.[9] Abdominal trauma is frequently the cause of significant blood loss in pediatric trauma patients, and children with Pediatric Trauma Scores of 8 or less are considered to be at increased risk for trauma-related mortality.[46]

In assessing children it is important for the flight nurse to remember that serious injury may be present with little or no outward indication.[9] Abdominal distention, absence of bowel sounds, increasing abdominal girth, and hemodynamic instability indicate the possibility of an abdominal injury. Injured children require an organized, properly equipped team approach to emergency management. Knowledge of the anatomic and physiologic differences that predispose the child to certain injuries is crucial.

Penetrating injuries account for 5% to 20% of pediatric injuries; however, because of the increased use of weapons, this number is increasing.[9] Reported injury patterns differ in some urban areas from those of the nation in general, with as much as one third of reported deaths resulting from homicide and with an equal number dead on arrival.[48]

It is vital that prehospital transport teams be knowledgeable of the regional location of pediatric trauma consultants and level I pediatric trauma centers. Evaluation of an emergency medical system's response to pediatric survivors of a jet liner crash on Long Island revealed limited pediatric training of prehospital personnel that resulted in inadequate triage and transportation to facilities equipped to give a higher level of care. Deficiencies in the regional disaster plan included failure to do the following: (1) recognize that children have special needs requiring referral; (2) improve the training of prehospital personnel in pediatric emergency care; (3) classify injured children according to appropriate triage criteria; (4) recognize and use tertiary care pediatric centers for treatment of injured children; and (5) designate appropriate centers for care of injured children.[46]

Abdominal Trauma in Elderly Patients

Major advances in health care have made it possible for a greater number of persons to live to advanced age and thereby be exposed to the same risk of injury as the younger segment of the population.[21] Trauma is the fifth leading cause of death in the elderly and accounts for 25% of yearly trauma fatalities.[11] Although injury accounts for only 2% of deaths in persons older than 65 years, the injury rate per 100,000 population is actually higher in the elderly than in younger persons. Mortality varies among the elderly population, with a higher mortality rate in persons older than 80 years and a significantly lower rate in those between the ages of 65 and 79 years.[11]

The elderly have physiologic changes that make them more vulnerable to injury, and when they deteriorate, they do so more quickly. In the event of an unreliable history, typical age-related diseases such as cardiovascular disease, hypertension, or diabetes mellitus may be assumed.[13] Altered mental status or cognitive or sensory impairment should be considered as evidence of brain injury until proved otherwise. In general, evaluation of the elderly patient should be conducted in a fashion similar to that for other adults. Mortality and morbidity rates are higher in elderly trauma patients, and aggressive treatment is recommended to decrease complications, such as multiple-organ failure, that occur during the hospital stay.[11,37] Literature on geriatric trauma is limited and offers an area wide open for research.

GENITOURINARY TRAUMA

Genitourinary trauma includes injuries to the kidney, bladder, ureters, urethra, and genitalia and is not usually immediately life threatening, as are the abdominal injuries previously discussed. Because of the position of the urinary and reproductive system within the abdominal cavity, a high index of suspicion for trauma in the genitourinary organs should be maintained when regions of the abdomen and back are injured. The American College of Surgeons Advanced Trauma Life Support Course emphasizes the transport of trauma patients from outlying hospitals without delay for urologic studies. Expeditious treatment of other, more life-threatening injuries at a level I trauma center may be crucial to patient survival. Delay of transport for urologic studies may not alter treatment in transport and could increase the chance of death.[2,30]

Renal and Ureter Trauma

Incidence and Mechanism

Renal trauma is frequently associated with abdominal injury; the kidney is the third most commonly injured abdominal organ.[9,27] Injuries sustained from blunt mechanisms such as MVAs, falls, contact sports, and assaults account for 70% to 80% of all renal trauma, and 5% of patients may eventually lose renal function.[19] Blunt injuries sustained from sudden acceleration/deceleration result in the stretching of the ureters and renal arteries and veins with the weight of the kidney. Contusions are generally from a direct blow to the flank. Of all renal and ureter blunt traumas, 85% are minor contusions, and the remaining 15% consist of renal vascular injury, deep cortical lacerations, or shattered kidneys.[19,29]

Penetrating injuries are usually caused by GSWs or stabbings to the back or abdomen, with an 80% incidence of associated injury in other abdominal organs.[6,39] Low-velocity bullet injuries are more common than high-velocity bullet injuries (79% versus 8%), and their damage is typically parenchymal laceration. Often a high-velocity GSW injury results in nephrectomy because the kidney explodes from the impact or passage of the bullet.[1,19,36]

Most renal injuries (80% to 85%) are minor and consist of contusions and minor lacerations; 10% are major and extend into the medulla, collecting system, or both, with the possible result of extravasation of urine (Fig. 14-1). Vascular injuries occur in 1% to 3% of renal injuries, and retroperitoneal hematoma formation is likely.[4,34]

Ureteral injury, although rare, is generally a result of penetrating trauma such as GSWs or stab wounds. Rapid-deceleration accidents may avulse the ureter from the renal pelvis.[4,31]

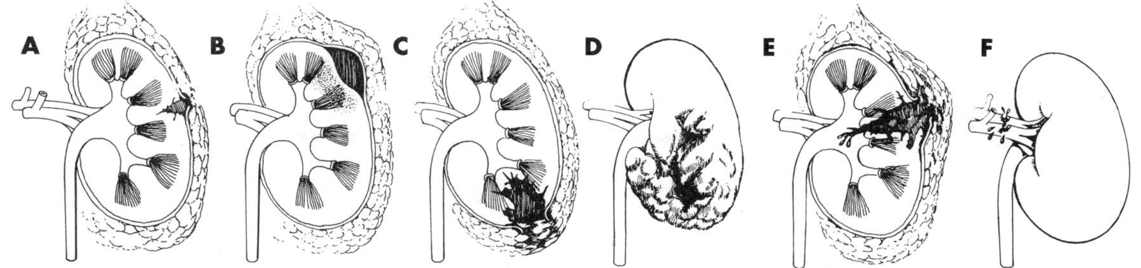

Fig. 14-1. Renal injuries classified by severity. **A** and **B**, Minor injuries. **C**, **D**, **E**, and **F**, Major injuries. (Adapted from Blaisdell W, Trunkey D, McAninch J: *Trauma management,* vol 2, New York, 1982, Thieme.)

Assessment and Symptoms

On secondary assessment any contusions, abrasions, or stab penetrations to the back and flank area should alert the flight nurse to the possibility of renal trauma. The patient may also have subjective symptoms of flank pain. Kidney damage should always be suspected with gunshot injuries to the abdomen. Hematuria is a marker for both renal and extrarenal abdominal injuries after blunt trauma. All patients with gross hematuria should be evaluated after transfer for both renal and associated abdominal injuries. In addition, patients in shock or with a history of shock and microscopic hematuria after blunt trauma should also be suspected of having abdominal injuries. Studies show that patients with microscopic hematuria but no shock do not demonstrate any major renal injury and are treated successfully without surgical intervention.[23]

Treatment

Because renal injuries are not immediately life threatening, the flight nurse should give supportive care and identify the patient's risk for kidney injury when other life-threatening injuries are absent. If a Foley catheter is in place, the air medical crew should transport with gravity drainage and monitor urine output. Ureter injury will probably not be diagnosed until full evaluation is completed at the trauma center; therefore no specific intervention exists for air transport. At the receiving hospital surgery may be indicated for major kidney injuries, ureteral tears, or renal vascular damage, although current literature indicates that the trend in treatment is toward nonsurgical management.[24,40]

Bladder and Urethral Trauma

Incidence and Mechanism

Blunt trauma to the bladder is most commonly associated with pelvic fractures (90% of cases of bladder rupture have associated pelvic fractures). Because the bladder lies within the pelvic girdle, bone fragments from the pelvis can penetrate the bladder. Rupture can also occur when a direct blow to the lower abdomen occurs with a distended bladder. Rupture can cause extravasation of urine into the peritoneal cavity. If diagnosis is not established immediately and urine is sterile, no symptoms may be noted for several days; if the urine is infected, immediate peritonitis and acute abdominal pain will develop.[31]

Urethral injuries are associated with bladder rupture and pelvic fractures and occur more often in men than in women. The most severe urethral damage is usually caused by shearing forces at the level of the prostate gland during pelvic fracture; the urethra may be torn near the prostate gland. Straddle injuries caused by bicycle, horse-riding, or gymnastic accidents, as well as direct penetrating trauma, may cause injuries to the lower or more external urethra.

Assessment and Symptoms

Identifying patients at risk is the best way for the flight nurse to determine bladder and urethral injuries in the field. Subjective symptoms in common with both bladder and urethral injuries are lower abdominal pain, groin tenderness, and inability to void. Hematuria will most likely be present with bladder trauma. Shock in these patients is usually associated with other visceral or vascular injuries. Blood at the meatus is the single most important sign of urethral injury.

Treatment

Transport treatment of patients with bladder and urethral injuries should emphasize a high index of suspicion for their injuries; life-threatening injuries should take priority. A Foley catheter should not be inserted when blood is found in the urethral meatus. With a urethral tear, further damage can occur if a catheter is improperly inserted, although a prolonged transport time and a distended, painful bladder are indications for careful, controlled insertion of a Foley catheter in these patients. Autonomic hyperreflexia is a serious complication of a prolonged distended bladder that causes hypertension, bradycardia, and increased intracranial pressure.[26] The flight nurse should keep these symptoms in mind when transporting a patient with a diagnosed urethral tear and inability to void. When a ruptured bladder is suspected or diagnosed, transport should be accomplished without delay. The diagnosis will be confirmed at the trauma center by retrograde cystography in bladder trauma or retrograde urethrogram in the urethral injury.

Genital Trauma

Incidence and Mechanism

Genital trauma is more common in men than in women. The female reproductive tract is well protected within the pelvic bony structure; consequently, injuries are infrequent with either blunt or penetrating trauma. Bone fragments from a pelvic fracture may pierce the uterus, vagina, or other female organs. Injuries to the exterior female perineum from straddle accidents can result in hematoma formation. Ninety percent of female genital injuries are to the uterus.[39] In men, penetrating trauma to the penis or scrotum is most often caused by a GSW. Urethral disruption may accompany these injuries. Other causes of blunt injury are MVAs, industrial accidents, and assault. Of scrotal injuries, 50% are caused by blunt trauma, and patients usually have contusions, hematomas, avulsions, lacerations, or testicular rupture at presentation.[19]

Assessment and Symptoms

Assessment of the patient with genital injuries includes a thorough history and a visual inspection. Respect for dignity should always be maintained. Reports of the event may be embarrassing for the patient, and the flight nurse must be careful to listen without judgment, although discrepancies between history and mechanism of injury should be noted. On physical examination the flight nurse should visually inspect the perineal area for hematoma formation anywhere on the perineum, scrotum, or penis. If the scrotum is swollen and painful, ruptured testes should be suspected. Rectal injury can also be identified when the perineal area is examined, and the flight nurse should look for any obvious trauma and document any lacerations or avulsions, including the presence and amount of vaginal bleeding. Menstrual history is important for female patients if they are able to provide that information.

Treatment

Unless bleeding is profuse, injuries to the genitals are not immediately life threatening. Treatment for transport should consist of saline dressings to avulsions and lacerations, particularly those to the scrotum. Ice packs to both scrotum and penile hematomas help reduce swelling and pain; direct pressure should be applied to the areas of penile injury. In the case of penile or scrotum amputation, the parts should be transported in saline dressings on ice, and the flight nurse should ensure that the tissue is not in direct contact with the ice, which could cause further tissue damage.

Vaginal bleeding is difficult to control, and pressure dressings should be applied if possible. Exsanguination can occur with major vaginal tears because of the rich blood supply. When severe bleeding and shock are present, rapid transport to the nearest facility capable of treating gynecologic injuries should be the first priority. If objects are impaled in the genitalia, they should be left in place and immobilized.[7] The success rate of repair to genital injuries is high, and even penile reimplantation has been successful with microvascular surgery.[5,31]

SUMMARY

The initial treatment for all patients, including pregnant trauma patients, with suspected abdominal and genitourinary injuries from blunt or penetrating trauma should include all procedures done for any trauma victim, such as airway control and ventilation, oxygenation, emergency treatment of life-threatening chest injuries, volume replacement and restoration of tissue perfusion, and stabilization of any fractures. The airway should be protected with intubation when needed, and breathing should be supplemented with 100% oxygen, ventilation, or both when the patient's condition warrants it. The patient's circulation should be monitored by assessment of the pulse, blood pressure, and capillary refill. For blood-volume restoration two large-bore intravenous lines should be established as soon as possible with crystalloid fluid, specifically lactated Ringer's solution. This fluid should be rapidly infused for severe hypovolemia and hemorrhagic shock by use of blood tubing and pressure infusers. The PASG should be applied and inflated as hypotension and shock dictate. The flight nurse should insert a nasogastric tube, which should be placed on low constant suction for long flights to decrease gastric dilation and reduce the possibility of aspiration. In particular, patients with diaphragmatic herniation or gastrointestinal tract injuries or who are pregnant should have a nasogastric tube inserted for transport.

Exsanguination, one of the major causes of death in trauma victims, can take place quickly in the abdominally injured patient because of the vascular nature of the abdominal organs and the large peritoneal space for blood accumulation. Calculation of the amount of lost blood is difficult in abdominal trauma patients because the abdomen can sequester large volumes of blood before signs of abdominal distention occur. The primary duties of the flight nurse when transporting patients with abdominal trauma should be recognizing and arresting profound shock and exsanguination by decreasing the blood loss from the intravascular space, replacing circulatory volume, and maintaining tissue perfusion.

Once immediately life-threatening injuries are stabilized, a secondary survey should include assessment for any fractures, major lacerations, and perineal trauma, and initial treatment should be instituted for those injuries present. If bowel evisceration has occurred, a normal saline-soaked dressing should be applied.

Any trauma resulting in hematoma formation to the male or female external genitalia should be treated with ice and pressure dressings. When lacerations are present on the male genitalia, wet saline dressings should be applied, and when bleeding of the penis and scrotum is present, pressure dressings should be applied. Vaginal bleeding should be observed, and a pressure dressing should be applied to the perineum when bleeding is profuse.

Renal and ureter trauma requires little intervention in flight by the flight nurse. When renal trauma has been diagnosed before transport, urine output should be monitored. Urethral tears should be diagnosed and treated with cautious Foley catheter insertion only when necessary for transport.

Flight nurses play a significant role in transporting the patient with abdominal or genitourinary injuries after initial surgical stabilization has been done. Complications that may be the reason for transport of post-surgery trauma patients are generally caused by infection. Sepsis, wound infection, and abscess formation are complications that follow intestine, pancreas, liver, and spleen injuries. Interventions for transport of patients with sepsis or wound infections should be directed toward supportive care and continuation of treatments already instituted. DIC can be a complication of liver injuries and abruptio placentae. Patients with DIC should be observed for any source of bleeding, and fluid resuscitation should be instituted if massive hemorrhage and hypovolemic shock occur.

Air transport reduces the time from injury to definitive treatment. Alerting the trauma center of the patient's condition through radio contact can provide the trauma team with valuable information, which also reduces delay of treatment of specific life-threatening injuries, thereby increasing the patient's chances of survival.

In review, the major contributing factors to the mortality of the abdominally injured patient are exsanguination and resulting hemorrhagic shock. The primary role of the flight nurse is to identify and manage life-threatening conditions of the airway, cervical spine, respiratory system, and cardiovascular system, and to provide rapid transport to the appropriate facility where the patient will receive definitive care. Patients should receive specialized treatment of their injuries with the least amount of time delay, thereby enhancing their chances for a full recovery.

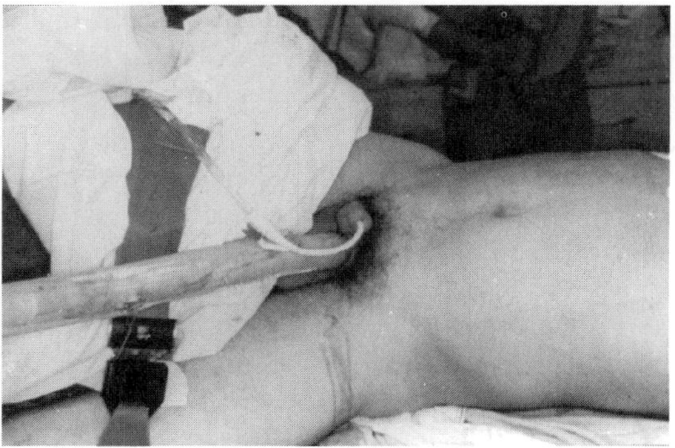

Fig. 14-2. Injury resulting from a logging accident.

ABDOMINAL AND GENITOURINARY TRAUMA CASE STUDY

An air medical team was requested for an interhospital transfer from a rural facility that was 25 minutes away by rotor-wing aircraft. The patient was a 31-year-old man who had been involved in a logging accident. The patient was the driver of an articulated tractor that was pulling felled pine trees. The tractor drove over a tree, which snapped and projected up and into the operator's cage. This resulted in the top portion of the pine tree being impaled into the driver's left scrotum, passing through his abdomen, and exiting through the left flank region (Fig. 14-2).

The time of injury was 10:00. The local emergency medical service arrived on the scene at 10:10, and extrication was completed at 10:30. The patient's Glasgow Coma Scale score was 15; respiratory rate, 28 breaths per minute; heart rate, 80 beats/min; and blood pressure, 100/P mm Hg. A decision was made to "load and go," and the patient arrived at the referring hospital at 10:50. Air transport was requested at 10:54. A liftoff delay occurred from a prior mission. The air medical crew arrived at the referring facility at 11:40.

On arrival at the referring hospital, the patient was awake and alert and reported loss of sensation to the right lower extremity. Vital signs were stable. Two large-bore IV lines were established, and lactated Ringer's solution was infused. IV antibiotics, analgesics, and tetanus were administered.

When the flight team arrived at the hospital, the patient was taken to the emergency department. He was positioned on his left side with his right leg elevated. The exposed portion of the impaled tree limb was approximately 2 inches wide and had been cut back to approximately 30 inches to facilitate transport. The patient was awake, alert, and oriented with a patent, natural oral airway. Circumoral cyanosis was noted. The patient was receiving supplemental oxygen through a nasal cannula at 2 L/min. No respiratory distress was apparent, and breath sounds were clear bilaterally with adequate symmetric chest expansion. Radial pulses were palpable, and capillary refill was within normal limits. The flight nurse was unable to palpate bilateral femoral pulses. Blood pressure was 104/80 mm Hg, and the cardiac monitor revealed a normal sinus rhythm with a rate of 84 beats/min and a respiratory rate of 24 breaths per minute. The patient had decreased sensation in the right leg but was able to move all extremities. His skin was warm and pale, and his lower extremities were cool and mottled. No external bleeding was noted. Reported hemoglobin level was 15.8, hematocrit 47.7, and WBC 17,000. Two large-bore IV lines were in place, and lactated Ringer's solution was infused. The patient had received 1.5 L of IV fluids before the air crew's arrival.

The patient's abdomen was flat, rigid, and tender to palpation. A Foley catheter was already in place with a sufficient quantity of clear, yellow urine.

The patient was given supplemental oxygen by a nonrebreather mask at 15 L/min. The patient was transferred onto the aircraft litter and remained positioned on his left side with his right leg elevated. He was transferred into the aircraft, and the litter was secured on the secondary patient platform to allow clearance of the tree limb.

In flight, the patient's neurologic status remained unchanged. His vital signs remained essentially stable except for one episode of tachycardia. The IV fluid rate was increased at that time, and the patient responded well to the fluid challenge. He reported severe pain, and orders were obtained from medical control for 2 mg morphine sulfate by IV push at 12:15. The patient received moderate relief with the pain medication.

Patient report was given by radio to medical control. The trauma team was alerted and was standing by on arrival at the trauma center. A trauma protocol was enacted, and the patient was immediately transferred to the operating room. The patient underwent surgery to remove the impaled tree limb and exploration and repair of the following: laceration of the left scrotum, laceration of the left flank, retroperitoneal injury, laceration of the right hypogastric vein, laceration of the inferior vena cava, laceration of the right hypogastric artery, and transection of the distal ileum. The patient had an uncomplicated hospital course and spent 5 days in the intensive care unit and 2 days on a ventilator and was discharged after a total hospital stay of 15 days.

REFERENCES

1. Acton CH et al: Bicycle incidents in children—abdominal trauma and handlebars, *Med J Aust* 160:344, 1994.
2. American College of Surgeons: Abdominal trauma. In *Advanced trauma life support program for physicians,* Chicago, 1993, American College of Surgeons.
3. Augenstein JS et al: Occult abdominal injuries to airbag protected crash victims: a challenge to trauma systems, *J Trauma* 38:502, 1995.
4. Blaisdell W , Trunkey D, McAninch J: *Trauma management,* vol 2, Urogenital trauma, New York, 1985, Thieme-Stratton, Thieme Verlag.
5. Bourn M, Bourn S: Genitourinary emergencies: a prehospital perspective, *Emerg Med Clin North Am* 6:379, 1988.
6. Boyd CR, Tolson MA: Mechanisms of abdominal trauma: implications for initial care, *Emerg Care Q* Feb 1988, p. 22.
7. Boyd CR et al: Penetrating abdominal trauma and the basics of ballistics, *J Air Med Transport* Jun 1991, p. 6.
8. Buckman RF et al: Major bowel and diaphragmatic injuries associated with blunt spleen or liver rupture, *J Trauma* 28:1317, 1988.
9. Cox SA: Pediatric trauma: special patients/special needs, *Crit Care Nurs Q* 17:51, 1994.
10. Davis JW et al: An analysis of errors causing morbidity and mortality in a trauma system: a guide for quality improvement, *J Trauma* 32:660, 1992.
11. DeMaria EJ: Evaluation and treatment of the elderly trauma patient, *Clin Geriatr Med* 9:461, 1993.
12. Emergency Nurses Association: *Standards of emergency nursing practice,* ed 2, St Louis, 1991, Mosby.
13. Feliciano DV, Marx JA, Sclafani SJA: Abdominal trauma, *Patient Care* 26:44, 1992.
14. Feliciano DV, Rozycki GS: The management of penetrating abdominal trauma, *Adv Surg* 28:1, 1995.
15. Fisher RB, Dearden CH: Improving care of patients with major trauma in the accident and emergency department, *BMJ* 300:1560, 1990.
16. Fossum RM, Descheneaux KA: Blunt trauma of the abdomen in children, *J Forensic Sci* 36;47, 1991.
17. Freshman SP et al: Secondary survey following blunt trauma: a new role for CT scan, *J Trauma* 34:337, 1993.
18. Goins WA, Anderson BB: Abdominal trauma revisited, *J Natl Med Assoc* 83:883, 1991.
19. Guerriero WG: Etiology, classification, and management of renal trauma, *Surg Clin North Am* 68:1071, 1988.
20. Jacobs LM et al: Prehospital advanced life support: benefits in trauma, *J Trauma* 24:8, 1984.
21. Jones JS et al: Geriatric training in emergency medicine residency programs, *Ann Emerg Med* 21:825-9, 1992.
22. Keen TP: Nursing care of the pediatric multitrauma patient. In Olson CM et al: Stabilization of patients prior to interhospital transport, *Am J Emerg Med* 5:33-9, 1987.
23. Knudson MM et al: Hematuria, as a predictor of abdominal injury after blunt trauma, *Am J Surg* 164:482, 1992.
24. Lebet RM: Abdominal and genitourinary trauma in children, *Crit Care Nurs Clin North Am* 3(3):433, 1991.
25. Leicht MJ et al: Rural interhospital helicopter transport of motor vehicle trauma victims: causes for delays and recommendations, *Ann Emerg Med* 15:450, 1986.
26. Levy JB et al: Nonoperative management of blunt pediatric major renal trauma, *Urology* Oct 1993, p. 418.
27. Lowe MA et al: Risk factors for urethral injuries in men with traumatic pelvic fractures, *J Urol* 140:506, 1988.
28. Lucciarini P et al: Ultrasonography in the initial evaluation and follow-up of blunt abdominal injury, *Surgery* 114:506, 1993.

29. Macfarlane MT: *Trauma, urology,* Baltimore, 1994, Williams & Wilkins.
30. Maull KI et al: Retroperitoneal injuries: pitfalls in diagnosis and management, *South Med J* 80:1111, 1987.
31. McAninch JW: Injuries to the genitourinary tract. In Tanagho EA, McAninch JW , editors: *Smith's general urology,* Norwalk, Conn, 1992, Appleton and Lange.
32. McKennay M et al: Can ultrasound replace diagnostic peritoneal lavage in the assessment of blunt trauma? *J Trauma* 37:439, 1994.
33. McSwain NE: Pneumatic anti-shock garment: state of the art 1988, *Ann Emerg Med* 17:506, 1988.
34. Monstrey SJM et al: Renal trauma and hypertension, *J Trauma* 29:65, 1989.
35. Moylan JA: Impact of helicopters on trauma care and clinical results, *Ann Surg* 28:139, 1988.
36. O'Connell KJ et al: Comparison of low- and high-velocity ballistic trauma to genitourinary organs, *J Trauma* 28:139, 1988.
37. Pellicane JV, Byrne K, DeMaria EJ: Preventable complications and death from multiple organ failure among geriatric trauma patients, *J Trauma* 33:440, 1992.
38. Phillips GR, Kauder DR, Schwab CW: Massive blood loss in trauma patients, *Postgrad Med* 95:61, 1994.
39. Richardson D et al: *Trauma: clinical care and pathophysiology,* Chicago, 1987, Year Book.
40. Rossi D et al: Management of intra-abdominal organ injury following blunt abdominal trauma in children, *Intensive Care Med* 19(7):415, 1993.
41. Rutledge R et al: The cost of not wearing seat belts: a comparison outcome in 3396 patients, *Ann Surg* 217: 122, 1993.
42. Schafermeyer R: Pediatric trauma, *Emerg Med Clin North Am* 11:187, 1993.
43. Shorr RM et al: Selective management of abdominal stab wounds: importance of the physical examination, *Arch Surg* 16:1141, 1988.
44. Spirnak JP: Pelvic fracture and injury to the lower urinary tract, *Surg Clin North Am* 68:1057, 1988.
45. Taylor GA et al: Hematuria: a marker of abdominal injury in children after blunt trauma, *Ann Surg* 208:688, 1988.
46. van-Amerongen RH et al: The *Avianca* plane crash and emergency medical system's response to pediatric survivors of the disaster, *Prehosp Disaster Med* 92:105, 1993.
47. Wachtel TL: Critical care concepts in the management of abdominal trauma, *Crit Care Nurs Q* 17:34, 1994.
48. Weesner CL et al: Fatal childhood injury patterns in an urban setting, *Ann Emerg Med* 23:231, 1994.
49. Williams JS et al: Aortic injury in vehicular trauma, *Ann Thorac Surg* 57:726, 1994.
50. Worthy SA et al: Diaphragmatic rupture: CT findings in eleven patients, *Radiology* 194:885, 1995.

CHAPTER 15

Orthopedic and Vascular Emergencies

COMPETENCIES

1. Perform neurovascular assessment of an injured extremity.
2. Apply a splint appropriately.
3. Identify and treat potential complications related to orthopedic and vascular injuries.

A simple fracture or dislocation can become a devastating injury, resulting in severe, permanent disability. Even a moderate sprain, if inadequately treated, can result in an unnecessarily extended disability and can lead to recurrent injuries.

The hands of a pianist, the elbow of a pitcher, the legs of a dancer are all vital to each of these people. Although musculoskeletal injuries are rarely fatal, they often result in long-term disability that accounts for millions of dollars lost to the economy each year.[10] The first care provided to a patient with a fracture, dislocation, or severe sprain will often determine the ultimate results occurring as a consequence of the injury.[7] The flight nurse can often prevent permanent disability with a prompt temporary measure such as splinting. This is especially true in patients with multiple traumas when more definitive management must be postponed until life-threatening injuries have been taken care of adequately.

MUSCULOSKELETAL SYSTEM

A flight nurse's basic understanding of the composition and function of the musculoskeletal system is essential to proper management of orthopedic emergencies, and ultimately to the welfare of the patient as a whole. The musculoskeletal system is composed of bones, ligaments, muscles, joints, and tendons, blood vessels, and nerves. The function of the musculoskeletal system is to allow movement, provide support, and protect internal organs.[6]

Bone is a living structure with its own neurovascular innervation and capacity to heal. Bone is a specialized connective tissue with a calcified collagenous intercellular substance and is either cancellous or compact. The calcium content of bone depends on many factors such as parathyroid hormone and estrogen, dietary intake, and stress. An acid–base balance with a slight decrease in pH can cause bone demineralization.[6]

DEFINITION OF AN ORTHOPEDIC EMERGENCY

An orthopedic injury—a trauma to the axial skeleton—is rarely considered an emergency. However, it does require urgent care. In terms of orthopedic involvement with underlying organs, emergencies can exist. An example is the fracture and/or dislocation of the knee or elbow. Not only are these extremely painful injuries, but they can cause permanent damage to nerves and vessels distal to the injury if not taken care of immediately. Table 15-1 lists various orthopedic injuries with their possible complications.

CLASSIFICATION OF ORTHOPEDIC INJURIES

When force is applied to a limb, the energy of the impact dissipates to deform supporting structures. If there is an excessive amount of force, more than one structure in the line of force may be damaged.[5] This type of stress to the axial skeleton and its supporting structures can cause various types of injuries, including fractures, dislocations, sprains, tendon injuries, and strains.

Fractures

A fracture is defined as any break in the continuity of the bone or cartilage, and it may be complete or incomplete, depending on the line of fracture through the bone.[7] Fractures generally are classified as *closed* or *open.* If the skin is unbroken, the fracture is technically closed, regardless of the number of fractures, but if the skin is broken, the fracture is open, even though it may be simple and minor in nature. An open fracture is the more serious because of the risk of infection. Fig. 15-1 illustrates nine different types of fractures as defined by their radiographic appearance.

Fractures of the long bone may produce steady, slow bleeding and can result in 750 ml of blood loss

TABLE 15-1

Urgent complications of orthopedic injuries

Injury	Possible Complications
Clavicle fractures	Brachial plexus compression or damage; pneumothorax or hemothorax
Humerus fractures	Injury to brachial artery or radial nerve
Pelvic fractures	Injury to bladder, urethra, rectum
Distal femoral shaft fractures	Femoral or popliteal vessel injury
Proximal tibia fractures	Compression of the anterior tibial compartment; tibial nerve injury
Clavicular head dislocation	Compression of trachea, subclavian, and carotid arteries
Posterior elbow dislocation	Compression of brachial artery
Posterior hip dislocation	Aseptic necrosis of the femoral head and sciatic nerve damage
Knee dislocation	Compression of the popliteal vessel
Ankle dislocation	Compression of the pedal artery

From Perdue P: Abdominal injuries and dangerous fractures, *RN* 44(7):35-37, 84, 1981.

TYPE OF FRACTURE	DEFINITION
Transverse 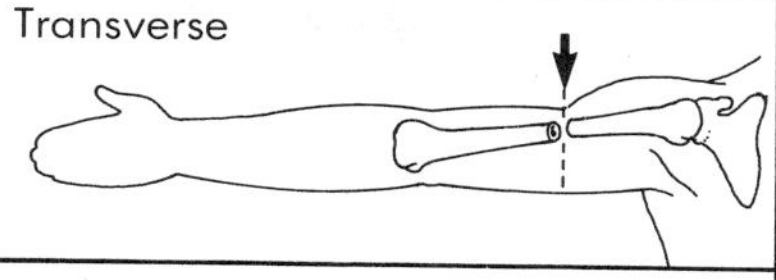	Usually produced by angulating force; once the fragments are aligned and immobilized, stability is assured
Oblique 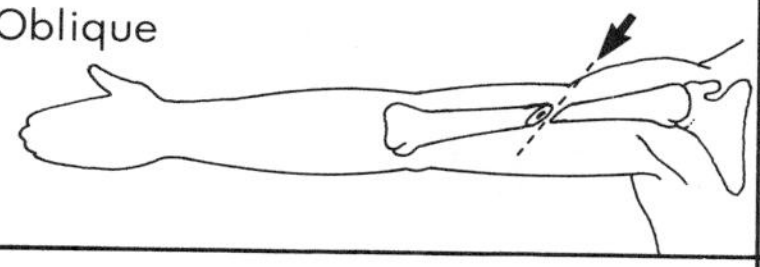	Fragments tend to slip by one another unless traction is maintained
Spiral 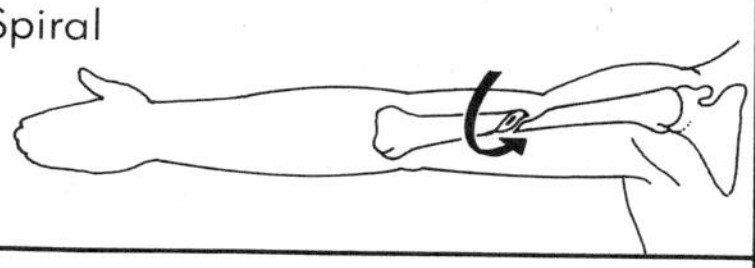	Produced by twisting or rotary force; reduction difficult to maintain
Greenstick 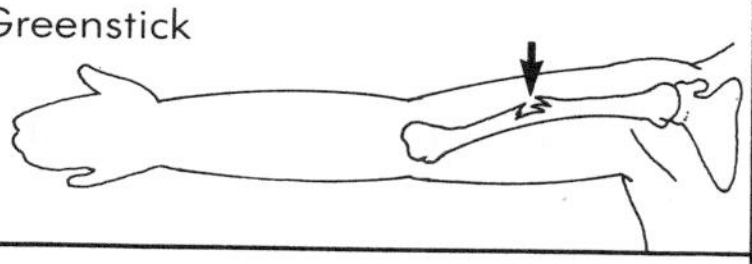	Caused by compression force in long axis of the bone; often seen in children under age of ten
Compression 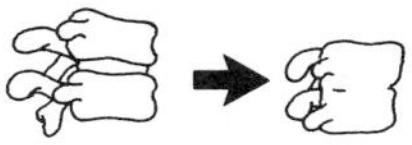	Usually produced by severe violence applied to cancellous bone, such as the spine
Comminuted 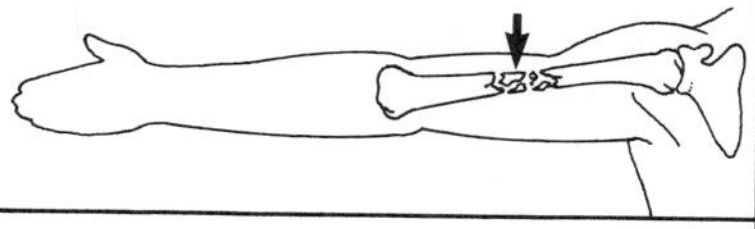	Always more than two fragments
Impacted 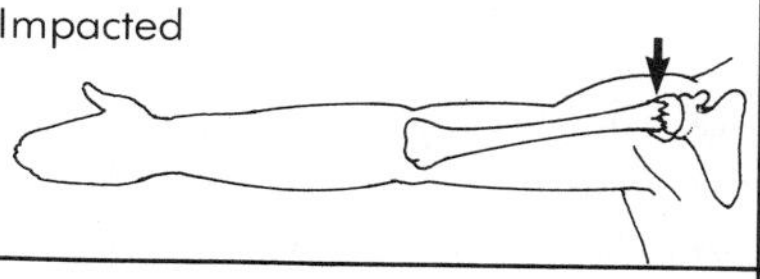	Produced by severe violence, driving bone fragments firmly together
Avulsion 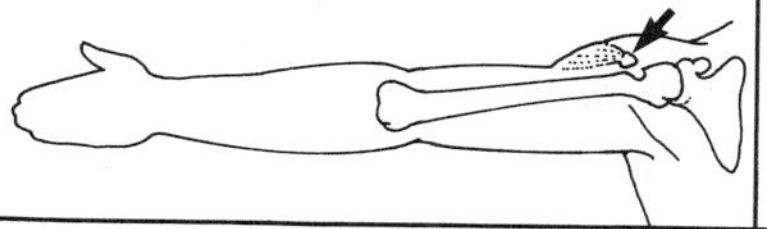	Produced by forcible contraction of a muscle which pulls off a fragment of bone
Fracture dislocation 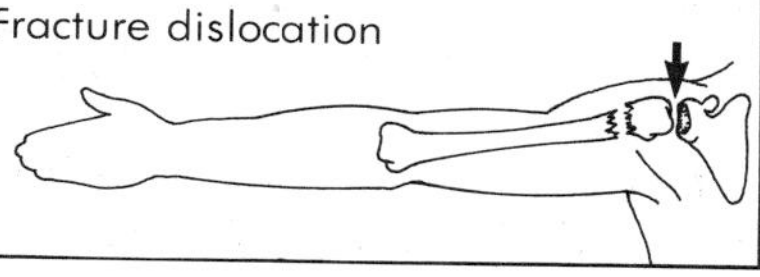	In addition to fracture there is a subluxation or dislocation of the joint

Fig. 15-1. Fractures according to their radiographic appearance.

from the humerus or tibia and 1500 ml of blood from each femur.[7] These patients must be watched closely for shock, and the long-bone fracture should be immobilized for comfort. Another risk associated with fractures, even uncomplicated ones, is that of fat embolism, which can cause varying degrees of respiratory distress, including respiratory failure. Signs and symptoms of fat embolism are petechial rash, diffuse pulmonary infiltrates, hypoxemia, confusion, fever, tachycardia, and tachypnea. Patients at highest risk of fat embolism are those with long-bone fractures of the lower extremity.[3]

Dislocations

A dislocation is the displacement of the normal articulating ends of two or more bones. A *complete* dislocation causes a tearing of the ligaments. A dislocation may also be described as *compound* when the joint is exposed to the outside air. Joints that are frequently dislocated are shoulders, elbows, fingers, hips, and ankles. Less frequently seen are dislocated wrists or knees. A dislocation is referred to as *subluxated* when the displacement is incomplete.

Sprains

A sprain is a partial tearing of a ligament caused by a sudden twisting or stretching of a joint beyond its normal range of motion. Sprains can vary in severity, and the more seriously injured ligaments will resemble a fracture or dislocation because they all present with pain, swelling, discoloration, and impaired movement. No deformity occurs as with dislocation, but an x-ray is required to rule out a fracture. Diagnosing a sprain without radiographic confirmation is dangerous, and treatment should always include proper splinting and referral for definitive care. Two common areas for sprains are the knee and the ankle. A sprained ankle is caused by a sudden twisting inward of the foot.

Strains

A strain is an injury to the muscle from overexertion or overextension. This may cause intense pain, some swelling, and decreased movement. Strains are usually seen in backs and arms and are rarely serious.

MECHANISMS OF ORTHOPEDIC INJURIES

There are multiple mechanisms that may cause injury to the musculoskeletal system. These include motor vehicle collisions (one of the most common); falls, particularly to the elderly; sports, such as football and soccer; and routine activities such as cleaning around the house. Bones, muscles, ligaments, and their surrounding nerves and blood vessels can be injured by either accelerating or decelerating forces. It is important to remember that when a force is applied to the musculoskeletal system that causes an injury, the surrounding tissue and organs may be injured along with the bones and muscles.[6,11]

The following describes some of the common mechanisms of injury and their resultant trauma.

Head-On Collisions

In a head-on motor vehicle collision the occupant can follow either a down-and-under pathway or an up-and-over one. In the down-and-under pathway, the occupant slams his or her knees into the dashboard, and that part of the body comes to a fairly rapid stop. The result can be a dislocation of the knee or a fracture along the shaft of the femur. More commonly, however, the pelvis continues its forward motion and the person sustains a posterior fracture or dislocation of the hip. Usually the upper body will also continue forward, with the chest hitting the steering wheel.

In an up-and-over pathway, the body goes up and over the steering wheel, with the head slamming into the windshield. After the head is stopped, the trunk continues forward, causing a hyperflexion, hyperextension, or crushing injury of the cervical spine.

Rear-Impact Collisions

In a rear-impact collision, the vehicle is hit from behind, and the energy of the impact is transferred forward. This transfer of energy will also occur with all parts of the body that are in contact with the car. But the head, in the absence of a headrest, will snap back, and there will be an energy transfer at vertebra C-3 or C-4, producing whiplash-type injuries, which are basically sprains and strains of the ligamental supporting structures in that area.

Lateral-Impact Collisions

Lateral-impact collisions generally produce injuries in three areas of the body, all from the side. The first point of impact is the chest. The upper part of the chest will be pushed in as the shoulder is rotated back out of the way. The second point of injury is the pelvis. The greater trochanter receives the initial impact, and the head of the femur will be driven in that direction. The pelvis can also be fractured as it is pushed in, or the head of the femur can be driven through the acetabulum and into the retroperitoneal space. The third point of injury is the head and neck. As with rear-impact collisions, the body is in motion, and the head stays in position. The resulting injury is to the contralateral supporting structures of the neck. And again, these usually are not fractures, but rather they are tears and strains of the ligamental supporting structures.

Rotational Collision

In a rotational collision, the vehicle will rotate around the fixed point of impact. As a result the occupant will sustain a combination of injuries that occur both in a head-on collision and a lateral-impact collision.

Rollover Collision

In a rollover collision, it is difficult to predict the type and extent of injuries. Unrestrained occupants will bounce around like pellets in a can, striking various structures in the car.

Motorcycle Accidents

With motorcycle accidents, injuries sustained are associated with those of head-on collisions and with angular collisions, such as lateral impacts or not-quite-head-on collisions. Also, the rider can receive ejection injuries.

In a head-on collision, when the motorcycle hits, it will tilt up and the rider will be thrown forward, hitting his or her head, chest, or abdomen on the handlebars. If the rider's feet stay on the pegs, the energy will be absorbed in the midshaft of the femur, probably producing bilateral femur fractures.

In an angular collision, the motorcycle often falls on the rider, crushing the lower leg and often causing open fibular and ankle fractures. In an ejection collision, the rider is thrown free of the motorcycle, and the type and extent of the injuries depend on what part of his or her body collides with what object.

Falls

Falls are a common mechanism of musculoskeletal injury for both the young and the old. Falls can result in injuries to extremities and more serious injuries such as pelvic fractures. It is important to consider injuries such as cervical and lumbar spine trauma that may be concurrent with falls.[6,11]

HEALING OF ORTHOPEDIC INJURIES

There are three main stages of repair. In the first stage, a hematoma forms within the first 48 hours. The bone ends and the surrounding soft parts (endosteum, marrow, reticulum, bone chips, periosteum, and extraskeletal tissue that has been lacerated) are bound together by the interlacing mesh of the fibrin formed from the clotted blood always present at the site of a fracture.[1] The second stage is marked by consolidation or callus formation that restores continuity between fragments. Perivascular connective tissue cells, round cells, and fibroblasts infiltrate the fibrin scaffolding working in a circular motion toward the center to begin the formation of granulation tissue. This mass of cells and tissue then becomes more organized and creates a sleeve of callus, thereby stabilizing the fragments.[1] After about 6 weeks, cartilage is replaced by bone, and at the completion of this stage the fragments are united. Stage 3 occurs with the use and action of normal stresses over a period of months by the provisional callus being removed by remodeling. The dead ends of fragments are resorbed, cancellous bone is replaced by compact bone, and the union is complete. This process may take a year or more, but the cast can be removed at the end of stage 2.

The rate of union varies from bone to bone and depends on many factors. The healing of fractures is primarily a local phenomenon. A good blood supply to the fragment, adequate proximity of fractured surfaces, and adequate immobilization are the most important prerequisites for healing. However, severe, prolonged negative nitrogen balance, excessive steroids, and a severe lack of vitamin C can impair bone healing. Wound contamination associated with open fractures must also be considered as an impairment to adequate bone repair.[10] Advanced age, diseases such as cancer, osteoporosis, and diabetes, and a disturbance of metabolism should be considered factors affecting the patient's chances of survival, and not factors that might interfere with the healing process.[1]

ASSESSMENT OF AN ORTHOPEDIC INJURY

In patients with multiple trauma, musculoskeletal injuries are rarely life threatening. Thus before assessing possible fractures, the nurse should evaluate associated injuries. The evaluation should begin with attention to airway, breathing, and circulation (the ABCs). Only when the patient has been fully evaluated and is judged stable should an attempt be made to treat an injured limb. The flight nurse should periodically reassess the patient to make sure that vital functions remain stable.[5] To properly document a musculoskeletal assessment, certain orthopedic terms must be used. The box lists common orthopedic terms.

Assessment and monitoring of the trauma patient has four purposes: (1) to monitor the patient's response to the injury, (2) to evaluate the patient's response to treatment, (3) to identify underlying pathologic conditions, and (4) to provide early warnings of complications.[5] To adequately provide this assessment data, a good history is very important. This information can be obtained by talking to the first respondents on the scene or by reading the medical record. As previously discussed, injuries can often be anticipated by knowing the mechanism of injury and the circumstances under which it was sustained.

Open fractures produce greater blood loss and risk of infection than closed fractures, and so demand more immediate attention. However, closed fractures must be carefully monitored too.[13] The examination for fractures should be organized by body areas, observing first for obvious deformities. If conscious, the patient should be asked to try to move each extremity. If there is a fracture or dislocation, movement or attempted movement is almost always painful or extremely limited with a dislocation. Range of motion, or lack of it, needs to be recorded. Finally, the extremities should be palpated proximally to distally, evaluating for pain, displacement, crepitus, and decreased or absent pulses. The flight nurse should press down on the iliac crests to determine

COMMON ORTHOPEDIC TERMS

Abduction: movement of a body part away from the body's midline
Adduction: movement of a body part toward the midline
Ankylosis: decreased range of motion caused by stiffening of the joint
Dorsiflexion: movement of the hand or foot upward
Eversion: movement of the ankle outward
Extension: movement of the joint to open it or maximally increase its angle
External rotation: outward rotation
Flexion: bending of the joint
Hyperextension: extension past neutral
Internal rotation: inward rotation
Inversion: movement of the ankle inward
Kyphosis: round back; increased flexion of the spine
Lordosis: swayback; increased hyperextension of the spine
Plantar flexion: movement of the foot downward
Pronation: movement of the forearm to place the palm downward
Rotation: movement of one bone turning on another
Scoliosis: lateral curvature of the spine
Supination: movement of the forearm to place the palm upward
Torsion: twisting of the bone on its axis
Valgus: deformity causing an outward turning of the foot or toe (e.g., genu valgus or knockkneed)
Varus: deformity causing an inward turning of the foot or toe (e.g., genu varus or bowlegged)

pelvic stability[5] and on the sternum and rib cage to determine stability of the ribs.

The classic signs of musculoskeletal trauma include deformity, localized swelling, pain, pallor, diminished or absent pulses, paresthesia, and paresis or paralysis.[5] If the patient is conscious, the flight nurse can ask whether the pain is increasing or decreasing and its exact location. Increased swelling, nerve compression, and infiltrated IVs, as well as the actual fracture, can cause an increase in pain. Peripheral pulses (especially those distal to the fracture site) should be checked bilaterally for pressure, strengths, and quality. Paresthesia can be easily checked in the conscious patient by touching or pinching the affected extremity and assessing for altered sensation. Capillary refill needs to be monitored and skin temperature noted.[13] Paralysis at the time of the injury or ensuing paralysis on repeated examination is of great importance in determining definitive care. Also, joints above and below the fracture site or point of injury need to be evaluated. Neurovascular status assessments of the affected extremity should be done frequently, but especially before and after transport.

Children require special consideration in evaluation for musculoskeletal injuries. Because their bones are more flexible than those of adults, greater force is often required to cause a fracture than would be necessary in an adult. Therefore, a child who has sustained even minor rib fractures must be assumed to have sustained serious internal injuries. The flight nurse should suspect a splenic and/or diaphragmatic injury in a child with low rib fractures. Children are also likely to receive avulsion fractures because of their flexible skeletons.[5]

MANAGEMENT OF ORTHOPEDIC INJURIES

Careless handling of a patient with an injury to the musculoskeletal system may convert a simple problem into a much more serious one. The closed wound may become an open one, a clean wound may become grossly contaminated, or blood vessels and nerves may be seriously injured. There are five basic principles for managing fractures and/or dislocations: (1) avoid unnecessary handling, (2) immobilize, (3) apply clean dressings to wounds, (4) control hemorrhage with direct pressure, and (5) check for the "5 p's" distal to the injury—pain, pulselessness, paresthesia, pallor, and paralysis.[6,8]

Wound Management

Local wound care is initiated by assessing the wound for evidence of severe hemorrhage, debris, and the presence of bone ends protruding through the skin. These findings should be noted on the chart, and a dry, sterile dressing should be applied. So that circulation is not further impaired, there should be no attempt at wound cleansing or pulling the bones back beneath the skin. Severe hemorrhage is generally controllable by direct pressure over the wound or over the arteries just proximal to the wound.[6] Good wound care is as important to the positive outcome of a patient as is good splinting. This technique should not be overlooked. Tetanus status should be noted at some point during patient care.

Splinting

Good emergency care rendered to a patient with any type of orthopedic injury will decrease his or her hospital stay, speed recovery, and lessen the chance of serious complications. Because the extent of injury is difficult to assess initially, it is always best to assume a fracture is present and immobilize it until further evaluation can be made by x-ray.

The primary objective of splinting is to prevent motion of fractured bone fragments or dislocated joints and thereby prevent the following complications:

1. Laceration of the skin by broken bones, which can increase the risk of contamination and infection
2. Damage to local blood vessels causing excessive bleeding into surrounding tissue, ischemia, and even tissue death
3. Restriction of blood flow to an area as a result of pressure of bone ends on blood vessels
4. Damage to nerves by inadvertent excessive traction, contusion, or laceration resulting in possible permanent loss of sensation and paralysis[15]

5. Damage to muscles with possible subsequent necrosis, scarring, and permanent disability[15]
6. Increased pain associated with movement of bone ends[15]
7. Shock
8. Delayed union or nonunion of fractured bones or dislocated joints

Some basic principles of management for any type of orthopedic injury must be considered in splint application. First is to splint the patient's fracture immediately. A fracture, dislocation, or sprain should be splinted or traction applied before the patient is moved or transported. Second, pulse, color, pain, and sensation distal to the injury always need to be assessed before and after splinting. Third, if a fracture is open, the flight nurse should stop the bleeding and dress the wound before applying a splint. No attempts to push the protruding bone back inside should be made. Fourth, with some very important exceptions, a severely angulated fracture should be straightened before splinting to lessen the chance of further damage to vessels and nerves around the fracture site.[15] A fracture or dislocation of the spine, shoulder, elbow, wrist, or knee should not be straightened. The dislocated joint should be splinted above and below the injured site in the position that it is found. For angulated fractures, overlying clothing should be cut or torn away. One should be as gentle as possible because bone ends can break through the skin just from rough handling. The extremity should be gently but firmly grasped by placing one hand just below the fracture site and the other hand farther down the extremity. If possible, someone should apply countertraction by holding the patient in place while a steady downward pull is being exerted. The angle of fracture should not be forcibly changed. The flight nurse should maintain traction until the splint is properly applied. With a traction splint on a lower extremity, manual traction should be continued until the splint has been properly applied. Finally, the splint should be applied firmly but in a way that does not interfere with circulation, and the flight nurse should be sure that it is padded sufficiently to prevent pressure points.

The flight nurse must address certain considerations, including the size of the aircraft, the aircraft's configuration, and altitude as it relates to the use of splints, when splinting a patient's injuries and preparing the patient for transport.

Soft Splint

A soft splint is one that has no inherent rigidity, such as a pillow or a rolled blanket. Both can provide considerable support when wrapped around an injured part and bandaged.

Rigid Splint

A rigid splint has inherent rigidity. It is placed along the side, front, or back of the injured extremity, and when used correctly, it will immobilize the fracture. Examples of rigid splints include backboards, metal splints, ladder splints, hinged splints, cardboard splints, and the pneumatic antishock garment. Rigid splints are effective only when they are long enough to allow the entire fractured bone to be immobilized, are padded sufficiently, and are secured firmly to an uninjured part.[15]

When using a rigid splint, the flight nurse immobilizes the joints above and below the fracture site. Therefore, a rigid splint must be long enough to extend over joints and immobilize the entire fractured bone. Many things, such as rolled newspapers or pieces of wood, can be used to make a rigid splint. Whatever is used, however, must be long enough, strong enough, and well-padded enough to do the job (box).

With various other types, depending on the site of the fracture, a rigid splint can be contoured to fit the extremity. For example, wire ladder splints can be bent, cardboard can be cut and taped to the desired form and shape, or a pillow splint can be used with rigid board support.

When using a rigid splint to immobilize a dislocated joint, the flight nurse will immobilize the bones above and below the joint. Because one should never try to straighten or reduce a dislocation, many times it is necessary to improvise a splint because of the odd shape of an extremity with a dislocated joint.

Traction Splint

Traction splints are also rigid splints. However, they are not used to reduce a fracture but rather to align it and immobilize the bone to prevent further

GENERAL PRINCIPLES OF SPLINTING

- Expose and examine the injured extremity. Look for a wound, tenting of the skin, or obvious discoloration that may indicate the presence of or potential for an open fracture.
- Support the body part.
- Remove jewelry and constrictive items of clothing.
- Assess and document sensory and circulatory status before immobilization. If there is no palpable distal pulse, medical control may recommend applying gentle traction along the long axis of the extremity (distal to the injury) until the distal pulse is palpable.
- Immobilize the extremity so that the splint includes the joints above and below the fracture or the bones above and below the dislocation. Avoid excessive movement of the body part. (Movement may increase bleeding into the tissue space, increase the risk of fat embolism, or convert a closed fracture to an open fracture.)

NOTE: Immobilization requires a minimum of two rescuers.

- When applying splints to the hand or foot, leave the fingers or toes exposed to provide for inspection and evaluation of neurovascular status.
- Reevaluate and document sensory and circulatory status after immobilization. If a nerve or pulse deficit develops after splinting, remove the splint and place the extremity in its original position.

From Sanders MJ: *Mosby's paramedic textbook*, St Louis, 1994, Mosby.

damage during movement and transportation.[15] The traction splint immobilizes by a steady longitudinal traction pull exerted on the injured extremity. Traction splints should not be used on an injury to an upper extremity because of the danger of further damage or of impeding the circulation. Examples of traction splints are the Thomas half-ring, the Hare traction splint, and the Sager splint. Traction splints immobilize by pulling on the distal portion of the entire extremity below the fracture. When applying a traction splint, the flight nurse watches the patient for signs of pain or relief in his or her face and uses that as a guide for the proper amount of traction.

Splinting Fractures of the Upper Extremities

Fractures of the clavicle usually occur at the middle and distal thirds of the bone from a blow to the shoulder. Pain, swelling, and deformity are generally evident. Supporting the arm in a sling and binding it against the chest with a swathe will sufficiently immobilize the fracture. However, injuries that occur in motor vehicle collisions may fracture the bone more medially, pushing it into the thoracic outlet and possibly injuring the long, subclavian artery or vein or the brachioplexus. The pulmonary and neurovascular injuries then become first priority.[6,7]

Fractures of the upper end of the humerus may or may not involve the shoulder joint. There will be pain and tenderness, but severe angulation is less commonly observed. The goals in treating humeral fractures are to maintain shoulder function and achieve fracture union. These goals can best be achieved by treating the problem as a soft tissue injury that happens to involve bone.[7] If there is gross deformity at the fracture site, the arm should be splinted in the position found with padded boards and pillow splints. In most cases, however, there will be little gross angulation and the arm may be splinted with a sling and swathe.[15]

Fractures of the midshaft of the humerus endanger the radial nerve. The flight nurse can check for damage to the radial nerve by observing the patient's ability to spread his or her fingers. If there has been damage, there will be pain on movement and tenderness at the fracture site. If angulation is present, the flight nurse should use gentle, constant traction, apply a sling, and, with traction still being held, place a padded board along the outer border of the humerous. A swathe is applied around the sling, the padded board, and the injured arm, binding the arm to the chest. A fracture without angulation may be splinted in the same manner.

Fractures of the elbow endanger the radial, ulnar, and median nerves, and the brachial artery. The flight nurse should check for pulse, movement, and sensation (Fig. 15-2). The fracture should be splinted in

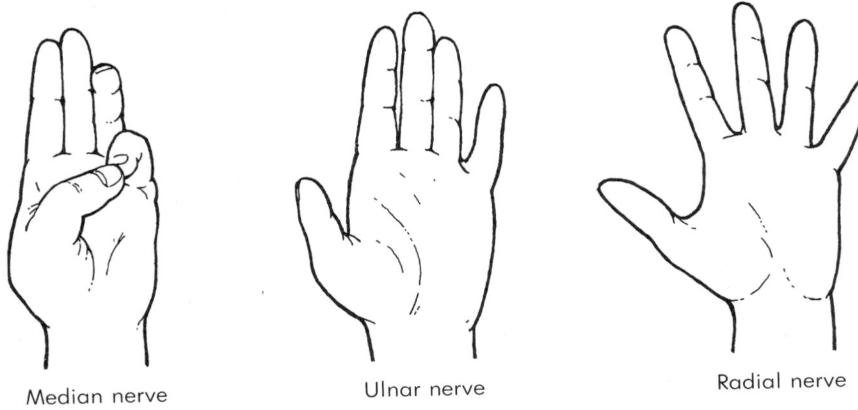

Fig. 15-2. Testing for neurologic function in the upper extremities.

the exact position found, using a rigid splint above and below the fracture. If possible, the arm should be bound to the side to offer additional support.

After gentle traction has been applied to any severe angulation of a fracture of the radius or the ulna, a rigid splint should be applied, immobilizing both the elbow and the wrist.

Fractures of the wrist without angulation should be splinted in the same manner as the radius and the ulna. Those fractures with severe angulation, however, should be splinted in the position found.

Severe hand injuries often involve both soft tissue and bone injury. In most cases, the hand should be splinted in the position of function, with the fingers slightly bent and a bulky fluff dressing in the palm of the hand. A rigid splint should also be used to immobilize the wrist.

Splinting Dislocations of the Upper Extremities

With a shoulder dislocation, the normal rounded appearance of the shoulder is flattened. There are basically two types of shoulder dislocations: anterior and posterior. Most dislocations are anterior. In the anterior dislocation, the patient will hold his or her arm away from the body, and there will be a bony prominence in the front of the shoulder.[4] A pillow splint, and frequently the help of a second person to hold the arm, can best obtain maximum stability without changing the deformity. With a posterior dislocation, there is little evident deformity, and the arm is held against the chest or abdomen. A sling and swathe are all that is necessary to maintain position. A rare inferior dislocation (the humerus is dislocated downward from the shoulder) may cause the patient to hold his or her arm above the head. The flight nurse splints it in the position found. All of these patients should be transported in a sitting position.

A dislocated elbow may appear as a posterior or anterior dislocation. With a posterior, the more common, the arm is flexed. A long splint with the flexion maintained should be applied. A sling will help to maintain stability. This patient should also be transported in a sitting position. With an anterior dislocation, the arm is extended and the joint immovable because of pain. Again, the flight nurse will splint in the position found.

A dislocated wrist is most often a Colles' fracture, occurring just proximal to the joint. A dislocated wrist will have an obvious deformity, and a well-padded splint should be used. The index finger is the most commonly dislocated finger, with the deformity being obvious and the fingertip slightly cyanotic and cold. A splint is all that is needed to help control pain. Immobilization is all that is needed for both injuries.

Splinting Fractures of the Lower Extremities

Fractures of the hip and proximal femur are anatomically divided into two types: fractures of the neck of the femur (transcervical) and fractures through the trochanters (intertrochanteric). Both appear the same clinically, with pain and swelling around the hip, pain on hip motion, and various degrees of shortening and external rotation.[15] The fractured hip is best splinted with pillows in the position found. In assessing a hip injury, there may be associated injuries to the knee, sciatic nerve injury, and ipsilateral femoral shaft fractures.

With fractures of the shaft of the femur there is a strong contraction of the gluteus medius muscle, which has a tendency to pull the proximal fragment of the femur outward as the adduction causes bowing at the fracture point.[7] These fractures should be splinted immediately with a traction splint and kept in the splint until definitive orthopedic care is rendered. Femoral shaft fractures can cause extensive blood loss that can lead to hypovolemic shock, so an IV also should be initiated in these patients.[6,7]

Fractures of the knee should be splinted as they are found, with no attempt made to correct any angulation. Checking for and reporting changes in pulse, movement, and sensation is especially important with any type of knee injury. Fractures of the patella are recognizable as swelling of the anterior knee with little or no resistance to extension of the joint. The flight nurse should splint this kind of fracture with a rigid splint and the patient's knee in extension.

Fractures of the tibia and/or fibula are also best managed with a rigid splint after the application of traction to correct severe angulation. The splint should immobilize both the ankle and knee joints and is best when carried as high as the groin. Great care must be taken with these fractures to prevent penetration of bone ends through the skin.[15]

Severely angulated fractures of the ankle should be straightened by traction applied to the heel and forefoot. A rigid splint should then be applied to immobilize the foot and ankle. If there is any question of a sprain or fracture, the injury should be splinted until a diagnostic x-ray can be made. Another method that can be used to splint some injuries is the application of PASG.

A PASG is very effective in the splinting of both long-bone and pelvic fractures and should not be overlooked by the flight nurse when considering size and configuration of an aircraft.

Splinting Dislocations of the Lower Extremities

Differentiating between a dislocated hip and a fractured hip is often impossible, although with a dislocated hip the patient's thigh is sometimes flexed to some extent and turned slightly inward. Treatment for either one is the same. The flight nurse should splint, using pillows and sandbags, in the position found. Because of the close proximity of the sciatic and femoral nerves, an immediate neurologic assessment of the affected limb is of utmost importance (Fig. 15-3).

Dislocations and fractures of the knee are treated the same. Any resistance to attempts to straighten an angulation indicates that it should be splinted in the position found, again paying heed to pulse, movement, and sensation. A rigid splint, preferably a padded board, should be used.

Ankle dislocations rarely occur without associated fractures and should be aligned and splinted exactly the same as ankle fractures. Dislocation of the foot is rare but generally involves more than one joint. It also should be treated the same as fracture of the foot. Toe dislocations are innately stable and need no splinting.[7]

Whenever possible after splinting a dislocation or a fracture, the flight nurse should elevate the affected extremity and apply ice to the injured part. This makes the patient more comfortable and augments the splinting.

PELVIC FRACTURES

A pelvic fracture can be one of the most serious injuries a patient with multiple injuries can sustain. The major cause of death is hemorrhage from arteries and veins torn by the fracture or dislocation.

The most common form of pelvic fracture results from a severe external force directly on the pelvis or from an indirect force transmitted upward along the shaft of the femur. Minor fractures of the pelvis include breaks of individual bones without a break in the continuity of the pelvic ring. These fractures are relatively stable and rarely require hospitalization. Major pelvic fractures are generally fractured in at least two separate places, and there may be a separation of one or both sacroiliac joints. These fractures are commonly seen in patients with multiple traumas.

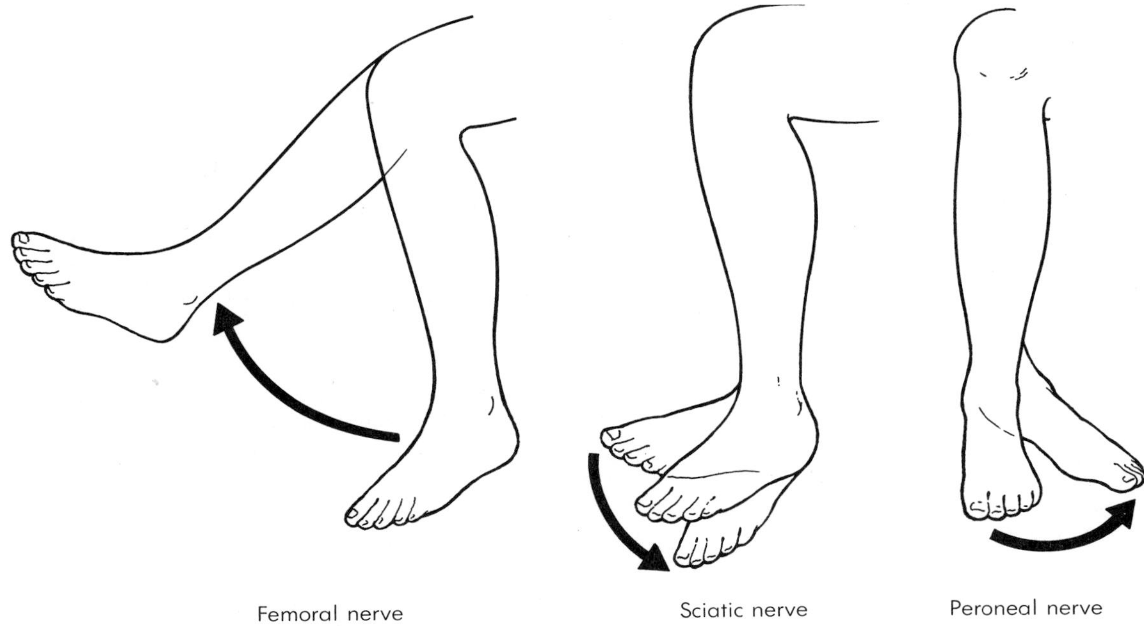

Fig. 15-3. Testing for neurologic function in the lower extremities.

Approximately 60% of pelvic fractures should be considered major injuries because of the complications of injury to the structures lying within the pelvis.[4] Besides the danger of damage to the major vessels within the pelvic girdle, fractures of the pubic ramus may lacerate the urethra, fractures of the brim of the pelvis may disrupt the ureters, and the bladder itself may rupture.[7] Open fractures of the pelvis occur when there is a direct communication between fracture fragments and a laceration of the skin, vagina, or rectum. This is an uncommon fracture caused by a high-velocity injury, and there is subsequent massive hemorrhage with a 50% mortality rate. Even small amounts of blood on vaginal and/or rectal examination should indicate the possibility of an open fracture.[4]

Control of bleeding is a top priority.[4,7] Approximately 500 ml of blood loss from each fracture can be expected,[4] so a large-bore intravenous line must also be placed for possible blood transfusion.

Patients with pelvic injuries should also be catheterized, unless urethral injury is expected. The indicating symptoms of urethral injury include blood at the meatus, the urge to void but the inability to do so, and in men, a prostate that is positioned high. Many patients with a pelvic injury will have hematuria.

Forces powerful enough to cause pelvic fractures can cause other serious injuries. Associated injuries should be identified from the knee to the chest.

VASCULAR EMERGENCIES

The first crude vascular repair was performed by Hallowell over two centuries ago, and the basic suture techniques as we know them today, including the use of autografts and homografts, were well worked out by the end of the first decade of this century. However, application of these techniques did not occur until the Korean War. Today's relatively optimistic outlook toward peripheral vascular injuries is the result of a variety of innovations including rapid transportation, availability of blood and antibiotics, abandonment of mass tourniquet techniques, a better appreciation of the true nature of certain forms of vessel injury (penetrating, blunt, and fracture-associated injuries), recognition of the importance of fracture stabilization, and many diagnostic and surgical advances.

A major amount of persistent bleeding, either apparent externally or manifested by shock, a hematoma, or a falling hematocrit level demands serious consideration for exploration and hemostasis.

Vascular Examinations

Vascular abnormalities can be discovered by careful observation, palpation, and auscultation. This examination can be done rapidly and is the basis for immediate treatment.

The patient's general appearance and description of pain is helpful because most arterial obstructions or ruptures are accompanied by severe pain distal to the site. Bilateral arm blood pressures are necessary to rule out an occluded arm.

The flight nurse should next make a comparison of pulses. This is done by simultaneous or rapid sequential palpation of the temporal, carotid, radial, femoral, popliteal, and pedal or dorsalis pedis pulses.

Auscultation over hematomas with associated arterial or venous injuries may make early diagnosis of an arteriovenous fistula possible. Rounds of turbulence are indicative of communication between an artery and a vein.

Observation of the skin for pallor, cyanosis, sweating, venous collateral engorgement, and edema is important for distinguishing between arterial and venous injuries. Temperature changes on the same extremity or differences in paired extremities may be indicative of impaired circulation. Assessment of capillary refill can also signify circulatory integrity.

Movement and sensation must be observed because traumatic injuries are frequently accompanied by nerve injuries; major arteries and nerves are closely associated anatomically. However, it is vital to note pulses because neurologic deficits will occur as a result of acute obstruction with severe ischemia.

Comparison of Arterial and Venous Conditions

Arterial and venous injuries are pathologically different, and the flight nurse must be constantly alert during the examination to differentiate between the two. A number of signs and symptoms must be assessed.

An arterial injury will be manifested by continuing copious hemorrhage from an open wound. The hemorrhage may be concealed and appear in the form of a rapid accumulating hematoma. There may be neurologic manifestations, either motor and sensory or spinal cord (produced by acute aortic thrombosis). The patient will report severe pain distal to the site. The temperature of the affected area will be cool, and the color will be pale, blotchy, and/or cyanotic. Blood pressure in the affected extremities will differ, capillary filling will be poor, and pulses will be absent or diminished.[2,9] The flight nurse must be alert to potential arterial injury with any fracture, especially fracture dislocation.

With venous injury comes potential for major hemorrhage, either from an open or a concealed wound, but bleeding tends to be less severe because of the low pressures involved. There will be edema. Pain will be general and local along the course of the vein. Temperature in the affected area can be either cool or warm, and color may be mottled and show patchy areas of cyanosis. Neurologic manifestations will be paresthesias distal to the site and sweating. Generally, capillary filling will be good, although it can be impaired. Pulses may be diminished because of spasm or impalpable because of edema.[2,9] Pulses are the most important indicator of vascular injury.

Primary Care of Vascular Injuries

The most important indication for treatment following vascular injury is external hemorrhaging. This should be controlled initially with direct pressure over the site of injury or the artery proximal to the site (the pressure point). The site should also be immobilized and elevated, if possible. Only after all of this has been done and is ineffective should the use of a tourniquet be considered. The tourniquet should be 3 to 4 inches wide (a blood pressure cuff works well) and should be tightened only enough to stop the bleeding. The prolonged application of a tourniquet gravely jeopardizes the success of reconstructive surgery and may make amputation necessary.

Shock must be combatted and volume replaced; therefore large-bore IV lines must be placed. Pulse rate and blood pressure must be closely watched and, if possible, CVP monitoring, urinary output, and hematocrit levels observed.

Finally, expeditious diagnosis and treatment are of paramount importance in any acute vascular injury. The viability of the extremity or organ may depend on the speed with which diagnosis, primary care, and definitive care are undertaken. Although it is recognized that the "golden hour" period is only relative, the results of treatments do correlate well with this concept.

TRAUMATIC AMPUTATIONS

Complete traumatic amputations of extremities occur from time to time from various kinds of trauma, such as motor vehicle collisions, entanglements in farm or industrial machinery, or crushes caused by heavy objects or falls. Excellent emergency care of the patient and the severed extremity will likely result in a successful reimplantation.

A primary assessment must first be made of the patient, and any life-threatening conditions must be addressed. Hemorrhage should be controlled with dry, sterile pressure dressings, and the extremity should be elevated and immobilized. As with any vascular injury, a tourniquet should only be used as a last resort. If bleeding is not a problem, then the flight nurse should flush the wound with crystalloid solution depending on the local protocols, apply a dry, sterile dressing and a mild pressure gauze wrap to the extremity, and immobilize and elevate the extremity. The flight nurse then should flush the amputated part with crystalloid solution, wrap it in a dry, sterile gauze or towel (if unavailable, use a clean sheet), and place it in a plastic bag or container. Then the severed part is put in another container and cooled by another plastic bag containing ice. Dry ice should not be used because it increases necrosis. As with any acute vascular injury, the expediency with which the patient and amputated part reach definitive care directly correlates with the success of reimplantation.

SUMMARY

In most cases, orthopedic and related vascular injuries are not life threatening; however, the long-term outcome for patients who sustain these injuries is greatly influenced by the initial care that they receive. The flight team should approach orthopedic and vascular emergencies with these goals in mind: (1) minimize the complications associated with fractures, both open and closed; (2) decrease complications of immobility caused by these injuries; (3) facilitate the general management of more definitive care; and (4) help to preserve and restore complete function of the affected extremity.[12]

ORTHOPEDIC VASCULAR TRAUMA CASE STUDY

The flight team was called to the scene of a farm accident. An 82-year-old man fell off his tractor and was run over by the back tires. He remained in the field for over an hour before he was found.

When the flight team arrives, they find the patient lying on the ground. He is awake and alert, complaining of intense pain in his chest, right leg, and abdomen. The patient is pale and diaphoretic. There is an open fracture of the right leg, which is severely deformed. His blood pressure is 80 by palpation, his pulse rate is 128, and his respiratory rate is 22. The patient's cervical spine has been immobilized. There is no palpable pulse in his right foot.

The patient's airway is clear and his breath sounds are present and equal on both sides. One-hundred percent oxygen has been applied by face mask. An intravenous line is initiated and the patient is given 2 ml of fentanyl so that his right leg can be splinted. The leg is reduced with little difficulty and a pulse can be palpated. A dry sterile dressing and a pneumatic splint are applied. The patient is given a 200-ml fluid bolus of normal saline, but he remains hypotensive. Compression of the patient's pelvis causes him additional discomfort. The patient is secured to the stretcher and placed in the aircraft.

During transport, the patient continues to complain of pain in his chest and leg. A unit of O-negative blood is infused. The patient is transported to the trauma center.

REFERENCES

1. Committee on Trauma, American College of Surgeons: *Advanced trauma life support course instructor manual,* Chicago, 1993, ACS.
2. Fahey VA, Racelis MC: Vascular emergencies. In Kitt S et al, editors: *Emergency nursing,* Philadelphia, 1995, Saunders.
3. Farrell J: The trauma patient with multiple fractures, *RN* 48(6):22-25, 1985.
4. Harrahill M: Open pelvic fracture: the lethal injury, *J Emerg Nurs* 20(3):243-245, 1994.
5. Heckman JD: Looking beyond the trees to the forest, *Consultant* 22(2):133-146, 1982.
6. Jacobs B, Baker P: *Trauma nursing core course,* Park Ridge, Ill,1995, Emergency Nurses Association.
7. Jagmin MG: Musculoskeletal emergencies. In Kitt S et al, editors: *Emergency nursing,* Philadelphia, 1995, Saunders.
8. Lower J: Maxillofacial trauma, *Nurs Clin North Am* 21(4): 611-628, 1986.
9. Mabee JR: Compartment syndrome: a complication of acute extremity trauma, *J Emerg Med* 12(5):651-656, 1995.
10. Maher AB: Early assessment and management of musculoskeletal injuries, *Nurs Clin North Am* 21(4):717-727, 1986.
11. McSwain N: To manage multiple injury consider mechanisms, *Emerg Med* 16(4):56-76, 1984.
12. Pashley J, Wahlstrom NL: Polytrauma: the patient, the family, and the health team, *Nurs Clin North Am* 16(4): 721-727, 1981.
13. Perdue P: Abdominal injuries and dangerous fractures, *RN* 44(7):35-37, 84, 1981.
14. Rodts MF: An orthopedic assessment you can do in 15 minutes, *Nurs 83* 13(5):65-73, 1983.
15. Sanders MJ: *Mosby's paramedic text,* St Louis, 1994, Mosby.

CHAPTER 16

Burn, Electrical, and Lightning Injuries

COMPETENCIES

1. Calculate percentage of total body surface area burned using both the *rule of nines* and the Lund and Browder charts.
2. Calculate appropriate fluid replacement amounts and rates of administration.
3. Prioritize the care of patients who have received thermal, chemical, or electrical burns.
4. Describe appropriate escharotomy sites.

BURN INJURIES

Incidence and Causative Factors

Approximately 2 million people are victims of burn injuries annually; 100,000 result in hospitalization and 10,000 in death. For adults, there are 12 deaths per 1 million population, and for children, there are 39 deaths per 1 million population. The majority of victims are children and elderly and disabled people, whose death rates are five times greater than those of other groups.[3,20,26,57] Most (68%) significant burns occur in the home, and most of the remainder (24%) occur in industrial settings.[3]

Etiology and Epidemiology

A burn wound is an injury caused by the interaction of an energy form (thermal, chemical, electrical, or radiation) and biologic matter (Fig. 16-1).[3] Most burns are thermal: flame burns, scalds, or contacts with hot substances. Frostbite is often included in this category; however, no current statistics are available regarding its incidence.

Chemical injuries occur when the source of energy contacted is capable of causing tissue necrosis. Examples of necrosis-causing chemicals include strong acids, which cause coagulation necrosis from protein

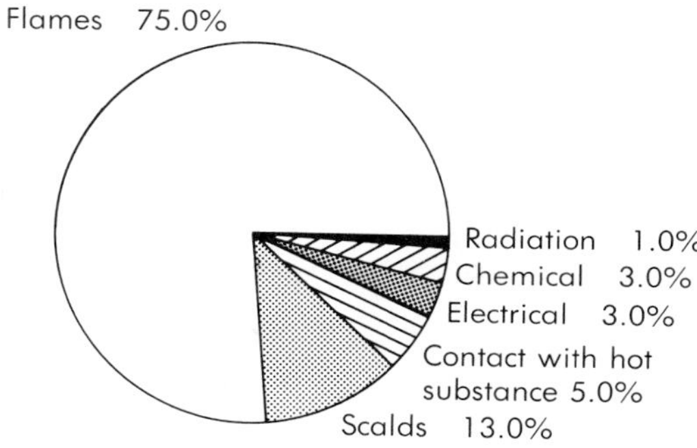

Fig. 16-1. Causes of burn injuries.

precipitation, or alkalis, which cause liquefaction necrosis.

Electrical burns occur when contact is made with a high-voltage current. The current itself is not considered to have any thermal properties while traveling through material of low resistance; however, the potential energy of the current is transferred into thermal energy when it meets resistance with biologic tissue and is dispersed throughout that tissue. This action is accomplished primarily by conduction.

Radiation injuries can be caused by both ionizing and nonionizing radiation. Radiation injuries make up a very small percent of burn injuries.[15,20,25]

Pathophysiology of Burn Wounds

The causes of burns vary, but the local and systemic responses are generally similar. The extent of the injury is influenced by three factors: (1) the intensity of the energy source, (2) the duration of exposure to the energy source, and (3) the conductance of the tissue exposed. The relationship between the duration of exposure to and intensity of the energy source is significant in determining the magnitude of the injury. Increased intensity with increased exposure causes increased amounts of tissue damage. Conductance can be affected by the presence of hair, water content of the tissues, and thickness and pigmentation of the skin.[3,15]

To better understand the pathophysiology of burn wounds, the flight nurse must know the anatomy and functions of the skin. Skin is composed of two layers, the epidermis and the dermis. The epidermis, the outer layer, consists of the basement layer of cells that migrate upward to become surface keratin. The inner layer, the dermis, consists of collagen and elastic fibers and contains hair follicles, sweat and sebaceous glands, nerve endings, and blood vessels. Beneath the cutaneous layers is a layer of subcutaneous tissue consisting primarily of connective tissue and fat deposits; this layer overlies muscle and bone.[34]

The primary functions of skin include (1) regulation of body temperature through dilation and constriction of the dermal and subcuticular vessels in response to environmental temperature, (2) protection against injury and bacterial invasion, (3) prevention of body fluid loss, and (4) sensory contact with the environment. When a burn injury occurs, it interrupts and compromises these functions.[34]

Responses of the body to thermal injury consist of varying degrees of tissue damage, cellular impairment, and fluid shifts. Locally, there is a brief initial decrease in blood flow to the area, followed by a marked increase in arteriolar vasodilation. A concurrent release of vasoactive substances from the burned tissue causes increased capillary permeability. These combine to produce intravascular fluid loss and wound edema.

Hypoproteinemia resulting from the increase in capillary permeability aggravates edema in the nonburned tissue.[50] Insensible fluid loss from the burn wound increases the basal metabolic rate and, along with fluid shift, leads to hypovolemia.

Many other physiologic responses to burn injuries can compromise patient outcome. With the decrease in circulating plasma is an increase in hematocrit.[15] This in turn can cause hemoglobinuria, when the hemoglobin is filtered through the kidneys, and can contribute to renal failure. Increased peripheral vascular resistance leads to a decrease in venous return to the heart, decreased cardiac output, impaired tissue perfusion, and a decrease in renal perfusion, which can also contribute to renal failure.[27]

A decrease in splanchnic blood flow occurs, which increases the occurrence of mucosal hemorrhages in the stomach and duodenum. There may also be increased risk of sepsis from bacterial translocation owing to diminished mucosal barrier function in the intestine. Burns on more than 20% of the body surface area (BSA) can also experience the problem of adynamic ileus, which can be of special concern for the patient being transported by air at high altitudes.[51]

Decreased immune responses increase the patient's susceptibility to infection. This requires the flight nurse to take extra precautions to prevent further injury to the burn victim through exposure to contaminated environments. Precautions include covering the burn wound with a dry, sterile dressing and in the case of a large burn wound, placing the patient on one dry, sterile sheet and covering him or her with another, with blankets added over the sterile sheets as needed. Wet dressings should not be used because they provide an open pathway for bacteria. Additional measures that can help to decrease the contamination of the burn wound are to wear gowns, gloves, and masks to form a reverse isolation.

Assessment

The assessment of the patient with burn injuries, as with any traumatically injured patient, begins with the ABCs of the primary assessment. Burn wounds are often very dramatic in appearance and can lure the flight nurse's attention away from more immediate life-threatening problems. Evaluation of the burn wound itself, including size and depth of the injury and fluid resuscitation needs, is done in the resuscitation phase between the primary and secondary surveys.

The subjective assessment includes obtaining a history as thorough as circumstances permit. The history should include the mechanism and time of the injury and a description of the surrounding environment, such as injuries incurred in an enclosed space, the presence of noxious chemicals, the possibility of smoke inhalation, and any related trauma. Information regarding tetanus immunization status should also be obtained with the history.[2,15,20,23,50]

The objective assessment of the burn injury itself includes assessment of burn size and depth, associated inhalation injuries, and calculation of fluid resuscitation needs. The size of a burn wound is most frequently estimated by using the *rule of nines* method, which divides the body into multiples of 9% (Fig. 16-2). A more accurate as-

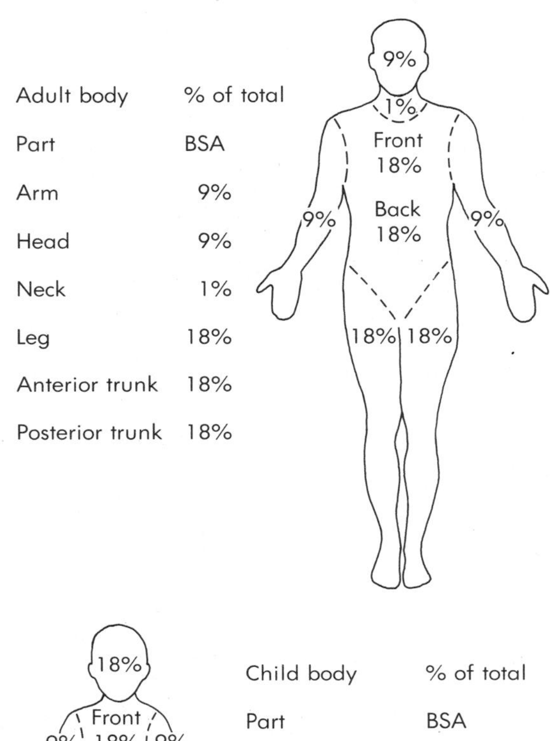

Adult body	% of total
Part	BSA
Arm	9%
Head	9%
Neck	1%
Leg	18%
Anterior trunk	18%
Posterior trunk	18%

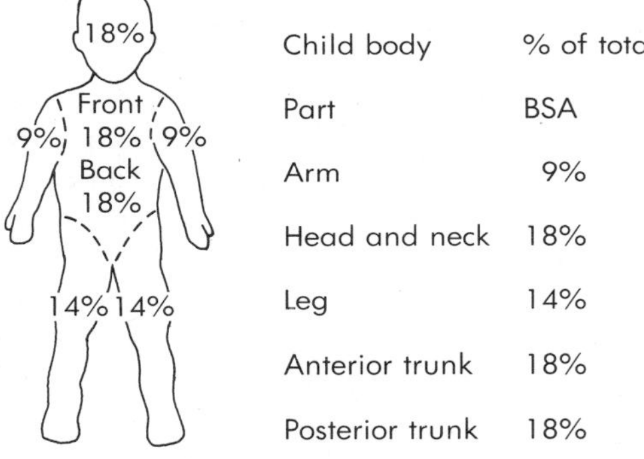

Child body	% of total
Part	BSA
Arm	9%
Head and neck	18%
Leg	14%
Anterior trunk	18%
Posterior trunk	18%

Fig. 16-2. The rule of nines.

sessment can be made of the burn injury, especially for pediatric patients, by using a Lund and Browder chart, which takes into account changes brought by growth (Fig. 16-3). For estimating scatter burns, a fairly accurate approximation can be made using the patient's palm to represent 1% of the total BSA and visualizing that palm over the burned area.[25,45]

Because the depth of a thermal burn wound is determined primarily by the temperature of the

Age	0-1	1-4	5-9	1-14	15
A—½ of head	9 ½%	8 ½%	6 ½%	5 ½%	4 ½%
B—½ of one thigh	2 ¾%	3 ¼%	4%	4 ¼%	4 ½%
C—½ of one leg	2 ½%	2 ½%	2 ¾%	3%	3 ¼%

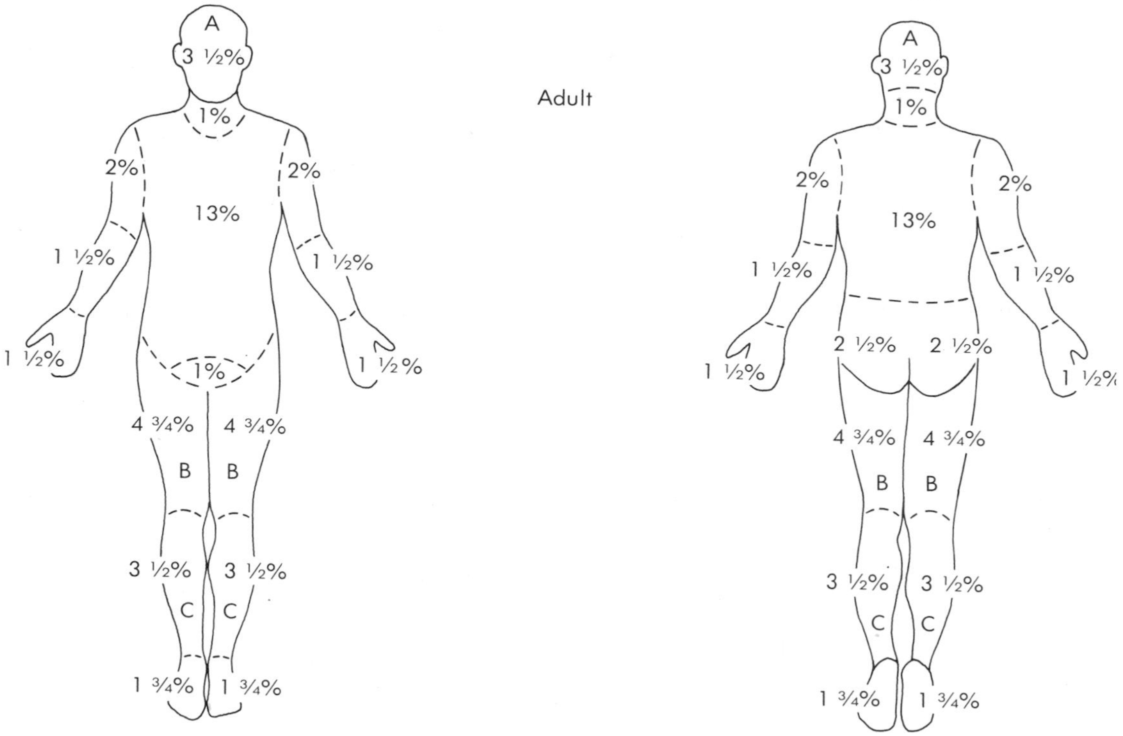

Fig. 16-3. Lund and Browder method for calculating percentage of burned body surface area.

burning agent, the duration of exposure, and the conductance of the tissue involved, estimation of injury depth is difficult initially.

Burn wounds typically present in a "bull's-eye" pattern, with each ring representing a different zone of intensity. A superficial partial thickness injury or a first degree burn involves the epidermis and is represented by the outermost ring, the *zone of hyperemia.* This type of injury is usually red in appearance, is painful, and heals in 7 to 10 days.

A deep partial-thickness injury, or second degree burn, involves the epidermis and dermis. It is seen as the middle ring and is called the *zone of stasis,* which is potentially viable tissue despite the heat injury. This wound is characterized by reddened skin that is wet or blistered, is very painful, and generally heals in 14 to 21 days.

Full-thickness injuries are the center ring, called the *zone of coagulation.* These injuries encompass third degree wounds, consisting of both dermal layers and extending into the subcutaneous tissue, and fourth degree wounds, which extend into muscle and bone. Full-thickness injuries are charred and leathery in appearance or white and waxy, with thrombosed vessels that are easily visible under the surface. They are painless because of destruction of sensory nerves, and there is no epithelial growth for healing. These wounds require grafting.[3,11,34,43,50]

Fluid Resuscitation

The goal of initial fluid resuscitation is to restore and maintain adequate tissue perfusion and vital organ function, in addition to preserving heat-injured but viable tissue in the zone of stasis.[11,15] Fluid needs are based on the size of the patient and the extent of the burn. The two most common formulas for estimating fluid needs are the Parkland formula, which is 4 ml/kg/% BSA burned, and the Modified Brooke formula, which is 2 ml/kg/% BSA burned.[3,15,43] These have been combined and presented as the Consensus formula of 2 to 4 ml/kg/% BSA burned.[45] All of the formulas call for one-half of the total amount to be given over the first 8 hours from the time of the injury and the second half to be given over the following 16 hours.

There is some controversy over the most appropriate fluid to be used in burn resuscitation. There are proponents of various combinations of hypertonic and isotonic solutions, crystalloid and colloid. Choice of fluid will largely be a matter of local opinion and current research.*

Taking into account the increased evaporative water loss in the formula for fluid resuscitation for pediatric patients, the Shrine Burn formula calculates 2000 ml × the total BSA + 5000 ml × the total BSA burned for the first 24 hours after the injury. This formula also calls for one-half of the total amount to be given over the following 16 hours. This formula is widely used by the Shrine Burn Centers. Emphasis in pediatric fluid resuscitation is shifting to the minimum amount necessary to maintain vital organ function. There is also current research suggesting that children tolerate rapid initial volume infusion, with half of the calculated volume given over 4 hours and the remainder given over 20 hours, a formula that differs somewhat from the adult regimen.[12,26,41,55]

*References 12, 28, 29, 41, 46, 55.

Monitoring the effectiveness of fluid resuscitation is a very important part of patient management. The parameters most easily available during air medical transport are vital signs, mental status, and urinary output.

Vital Signs

Vital signs are not the most accurate method of monitoring a patient with a large burn because of the pathophysiologic changes that accompany such an injury. Blood pressure may be difficult to ascertain because of increasing generalized edema. An invasive monitoring device may not be accurate because of the peripheral vasoconstriction caused by release of vasoactive mediators such as catecholamines. Pulse may be somewhat more helpful in monitoring the appropriateness of fluid resuscitation. Presence of more than a mild tachycardia or a persistent tachycardia is evidence of hypovolemia. The flight nurse should be careful not to overlook young, otherwise healthy adults whose normal resting heart rate may be in the 40 to 60 beats-per-minute range. A heart rate of greater than 70 beats per minute may not indicate the underlying volume deficit for this type of patient.[6]

A decrease in level of consciousness not associated with trauma may also be indicative of hypoxia or hypovolemia. This problem should be alleviated with appropriate adjustments in ventilatory and circulatory support. If the level of consciousness does not improve with increased hydration and oxygenation, other problem sources such as carbon monoxide poisoning or electrolyte imbalance should be suspected and investigated.[11,43]

Urinary output is perhaps the most accurate method of evaluating the effectiveness of fluid replacement. Adults should have an hourly output of 30 to 50 ml.

The urinary output in children should be maintained at 1 to 2 ml/kg/% BSA burned for children under 30 kg. Oliguria is an indication of inadequate fluid volume and should be easily corrected by increasing the rate of fluid administration. When this is ineffective, and fluid volume needs have been accurately assessed and administered, an osmotic diuretic such as mannitol can be given to avoid acute renal failure.[11,45,55]

Inhalation Injuries

There are three types of identifiable inhalation injuries: asphyxiation from carbon monoxide poisoning; supraglottic injury, which is primarily thermal in nature; and infraglottic injury, which is primarily chemical. Inhalation injuries are the primary cause of death at the scene of the burn injury and contribute significantly to the overall morbidity and mortality of burn patients.[20]

Carbon monoxide intoxication occurs when the affinity for carbon monoxide to hemoglobin is markedly greater than that of oxygen; therefore, the carbon monoxide binds with the available hemoglobin to form carboxyhemoglobin and causes hypoxia. The signs and symptoms of carbon monoxide poisoning include pink to cherry-red skin, tachycardia, tachypnea, headache, dizziness, and nausea. It is diagnosed by measuring carboxyhemoglobin levels. Levels of 0% to 15% rarely cause symptoms and may be normal, especially for a heavy smoker. Levels of 15% to 40% cause varying amounts of central nervous system disturbances such as confusion and headache. Levels greater than 40% can cause mental obtundation and coma.[11,43] Any patient with suspected carbon monoxide injury should be given 100% oxygen.[11,43] The treatment of carbon monoxide poisoning is discussed in both the Pulmonary and Toxicology chapters in this text.

Supraglottic injury can be suspected when facial burns, singed facial hair, or carbonaceous sputum are present. Other signs and symptoms of upper airway injury include presence of redness or blistering in the posterior pharynx, stridor, wheezing, bronchorrhea, or any other sign of respiratory difficulty. Absence of these indications initially does not exclude the possibility of inhalation injury because upper airway edema may not be present until after the onset of fluid resuscitation.[14,25]

Infraglottic injury is often more difficult to ascertain because the injury is progressive in nature. It is caused by the inhalation of the particulate by-products of combustion. It is manifested by an increase in both pulmonary vascular resistance and pulmonary capillary permeability, which causes pulmonary edema. The primary symptom is hypoxemia that is resistant to oxygen therapy.[35]

Inhalation injuries are unpredictable in onset. Any patient with suspected inhalation injuries should be closely observed for 24 hours for onset of respiratory complications.

Treatment

Transport of a burn victim requires an orderly, prioritized approach. Equipment and supplies should be organized in advance when possible to expedite assessment and stabilization of the burn victim.

Even though supplies and equipment vary between air medical programs, depending on protocols and primary service populations, little is required beyond the standard emergency medical supplies to provide quality burn care. The possible additions might include sterile sheets to cover the burn wounds and a pulse oximeter to monitor oxygen saturation during transport.[11]

Management of the burn victim begins with the ABCs of the primary survey, including airway, breathing, and circulation with a brief baseline neurologic examination. While doing assessments and making interventions for life-threatening problems in the primary survey, the flight nurse should take precautions to maintain cervical spine immobilization.[45]

If intubation is required, the nasotracheal route is the preferred approach.[45] Intubation should be accomplished early because it may become impossible with the onset of edema after the initiation of fluid replacement. It is more difficult to assess for dyspnea in an aircraft because of the noise and vibration, so the flight nurse should learn to rely on other parameters for assessing respiratory status.[25,33]

Securing an endotracheal tube may be difficult because tape, which is most often used, will not adhere to burned skin. Several alternatives are available, such as the use of cotton twill ties or suturing or stapling the tube to the nose or lip.[11,43,50,51]

The resuscitation phase follows the primary survey. At this point the flight nurse's first priority is to stop the burning process. This may require copious irrigation of the burn wound, as in the case of chemical burns, or simply removing clothing and jewelry from the patient. It is important to protect the patient from further injury. The second priority is to administer 100% oxygen, preferably humidified.[33]

Humidified oxygen helps to keep the airway moist, inhibiting the inspissation of material that could produce atelectatic areas in the lung.

Two IV lines should be initiated peripherally with a 16-gauge catheter or larger. The fluid of choice for initial resuscitation is variable, but crystalloid is the most common.[11,25,28,29,45] Ideally, lines should be placed in nonburned areas but may be placed through the burn if they are the only veins available for cannulation. Intravenous lines should be sutured in place if there is any danger of their being dislodged because venous access may not be available peripherally after the onset of generalized edema. Blood should be obtained for initial lab studies when IV lines are initiated if that has not already been done.[15,43] Vital signs are the next step in readying the patient for transport. The PASG may be applied before transport as indicated for the treatment of shock caused by associated trauma or the burn injury.

Electrocardiogram monitoring should be instituted on any patient with a large burn, an electrical injury, or preexisting heart disease. Electrode patches may be a problem to place because the adhesive will not stick to burned skin. If alternate sites for placement cannot be found, an option for monitoring is to insert skin staples such as those used for wound closure and attach the monitor leads to them with alligator clips. This provides a stable monitoring system, particularly for the agitated or restless patient who might displace needle electrodes.[11,43]

A Foley catheter with a urimeter should be placed to accurately monitor urinary output. As with intubation, the catheter should be inserted early, especially for the patient with perineal burns, because edema may make insertion impossible at a later time.[15]

To combat the problem of adynamic[17] ileus, the flight nurse should insert a nasogastric (NG) tube in all burn victims to decompress the stomach. This is especially important for the victim being transported at high altitudes.[15] Initial diagnostic studies should include hematocrit and electrolyte levels, urinalysis, chest x-ray, arterial blood gases with carboxyhemoglobin levels as indicated, and an ECG.[45]

With the exception of escharotomies, open chest wounds, and actively bleeding wounds, wound management in transport consists of simply placing the patient on, and covering him or her with, sterile or clean, dry linen.[25] Wet dressings are contraindicated because of the decreased thermoregulatory capacity of patients sustaining large burns and the possibility of hypothermia. The burn victim should be covered with blankets to avoid hypothermia.[1,2]

Any injections that the flight nurse gives to the burn victim should be given intravenously for at least 72 hours. The generalized edema during this time allows for only sporadic absorption of the medication. As fluid shifts reverse, there can be a "dumping" and a potential overdose of any medications that were given intramuscularly.[15] The exception to this is a tetanus booster, which can be given intramuscularly.

It is essential to have accurate documentation of all treatment provided before and during transport of the burn victim. This information provides the necessary history of the incident and its initial treatment, to allow for consistent and quality planning of patient care at the receiving facility.

Evaluation

Evaluation of the burn victim consists primarily of assessing the effectiveness of problem intervention and the recognition of future potential complications. Not all complications are, however, predictable or correctable.

Circumferential burns to the chest or extremities represent the more easily recognizable complications in burn care. Circumferential burns to the chest wall decrease chest wall compliance, creating respiratory insufficiency and hypoxia, especially in the pediatric population because chest walls are more pliable. This can be further aggravated by generalized edema. The correction for this problem is an escharotomy. This allows the chest to expand fully for more efficient ventilation.

Circumferential burns to the extremities or digits can be equally threatening to the circulatory stability of the affected limb, producing the "5 p's" that represent the signs and symptoms of an arterial injury: pain, pallor, pulselessness, paresthesias, and paralysis. An ultrasonic Doppler device may be helpful in locating pulses in a particularly edematous area.[11,25]

Escharotomies ideally should be performed before

transport and should be performed only under the direction of the receiving physician.[45] There are several principles to remember in performing escharotomies. The procedures should be performed in as sterile an environment as possible to avoid seeding bacteria into already compromised tissue. The incisions should be made carefully and deep enough to penetrate the eschar and decompress the area without causing major bleeding in the zone of stasis because the tissue there is often too friable to maintain sutures. When bleeding does occur, the appropriate treatment is direct pressure to the wound. The incisions should extend slightly beyond the constricted area for maximum effect. (See box below for possible escharotomy sites.) Major vessels, nerves, tendons, ligaments, and joints should be avoided because future range of motion can be adversely affected. Results of the escharotomy should be carefully monitored. In most cases relief of the constriction should be immediate.[11,34,45]

Myoglobinuria that occurs from the release of myoglobin after deep muscle damage can precipitate in the renal tubules and cause acute renal failure. This is especially common after electrical burns, and urine should be monitored for changes, such as a change to a dark tea color, that would indicate the presence of myoglobin. The treatment for myoglobinuria aims to increase fluid administration rates to maintain a urinary output of at least 100 ml/hr until the pigments clear. If this is not successful, the osmotic diuretic mannitol can be added to the intravenous

POSSIBLE ESCHAROTOMY SITES

Chest

Anterior axillary incisions bilaterally joined with a transverse incision along the costal margin (Fig. 16-4)

Extremities

Axially on medial and/or lateral aspect. If a single incision is insufficient to relieve the constriction, then an incision on both sides should be performed

Elbow

Medial aspect anterior to the medial epicondyle

Hand

Axially on the dorsum, between the tendons rather than across them

Fingers

Midlateral axial (Fig. 16-5)

Ankle

Medial aspect anterior to medial malleolus

Foot

Axially on the dorsum between the tendons rather than across them[34,45]

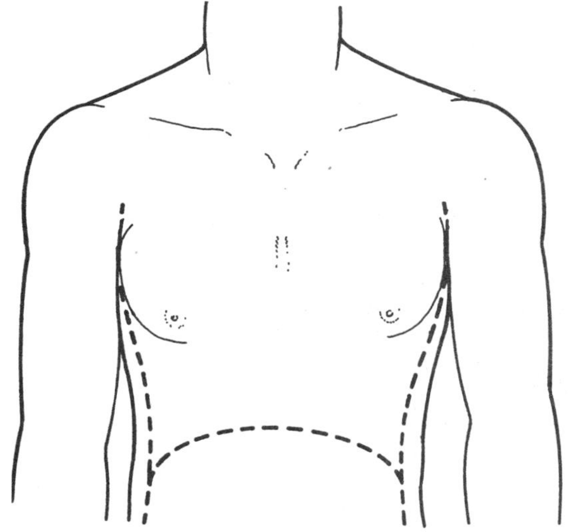

Fig. 16-4. Chest escharotomy sites.

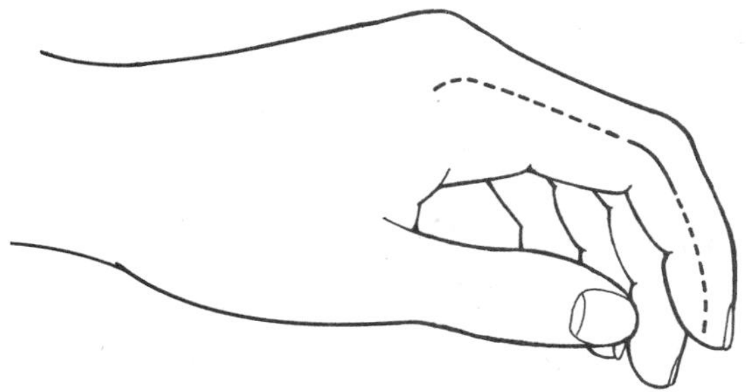

Fig. 16-5. Escharotomy site on the finger.

infusion at the concentration of 12.5 g/L of fluid. Another method of eliminating myoglobin is to alkalinize the urine by administering sodium bicarbonate 1 mEq/kg, because myoglobin is more soluble in an alkaline medium.[43,45]

Pulmonary edema can occur from either overzealous fluid resuscitation or smoke inhalation, and the flight nurse should be careful to monitor respiratory function as fluid administration progresses. The treatment for pulmonary edema is to give inotropic agents and decrease IV infusion rates.

Several acid-base and electrolyte imbalances can occur throughout the course of patient management. Acidosis from the increased lactic acid production can occur, and it can be treated with sodium bicarbonate if increased fluid administration is ineffective. Hyperkalemia from potassium released from the heat-damaged tissues can be reversed in several ways including administration of sodium bicarbonate, glucose and insulin, and/or ion-exchange resins. Hyponatremia from fluid replacement does not reflect a true sodium deficiency and seldom requires any type of treatment. Hypoglycemia is a complication that frequently occurs with infants and young children because of their inability to maintain adequate glycogen stores. Blood glucose should be assessed frequently for pediatric patients. Intravenous fluids can be changed to lactated Ringer's with 5% dextrose if hypoglycemia becomes a problem.[45]

Impact of Transport

For burn victims there are usually two phases of transport. The first is the entry of the burn victim into the EMS system with transport from the scene of the incident to the initial care facility. The second phase is the interfacility transport of the stabilized patient from the initial care facility to a burn center or tertiary care center.[11]

The increasing use of air medical services has had an impact on both phases of burn transport. In early transport, it has made a higher level of medical expertise more rapidly available to a larger service area. This has decreased the amount of time before assessment and resuscitation begins and enables the critically injured patient to reach a definitive care facility quickly. In the second phase of transport, it has markedly decreased the amount of time spent out of a stable environment during transfer to a burn center.[7,33] These have had the combined effect of decreasing the morbidity and mortality of burn victims.[11]

The decision to transport to a burn center is one made based on the condition of the patient, the size of the burn, and, in the case of scene response, the distance to the burn center. Patients who sustain concurrent traumatic injuries should first be evaluated at a trauma center if the traumatic injuries present the greatest immediate risk. If the burn injury is the greater risk to the patient, and initial burn care can be facilitated en route, then transfer to a burn center may be appropriate. The American Burn Association has identified criteria for the transfer of burn victims to a burn center (box).[1,15,45]

CRITERIA FOR TRANSFER OF BURN VICTIMS TO A BURN CENTER

- Second degree burns on more than 25% of body surface area in adults
- Second degree burns on more than 20% of body surface area in children or the elderly
- Third degree burns on more than 10% of body surface area in any age group
- Second and third degree burns that involve and threaten functional or cosmetic impairment of the face, hands, feet, genitalia, perineum, and major joints
- Chemical burns that involve and threaten functional or cosmetic impairment in the face, hands, feet, genitalia, perineum, and major joints
- Electrical burns including lightning injuries
- Any second or third degree burns with concomitant trauma in which the burn injuries pose the greater risk to the patient
- Burns with inhalation injury
- Patients with preexisting medical disorders that could adversely affect patient outcome
- Unavailability of hospitals with qualified personnel or equipment for the care of critically burned children

CHEMICAL BURNS

Chemical burns differ from thermal burns in that the burning process continues until the agent is inactivated by reaction with the tissues, is neutralized, or is diluted with water.[11] The degree of damage by a chemical agent depends on the concentration and quantity of the agent, its mechanism of action, and the duration of contact.[3,45]

Treatment of chemical injuries varies little from that of thermal injuries during the primary survey. After initial life-threatening problems are dealt with, the next priority is to stop the burning process. This requires removal of all saturated clothing and a copious irrigation of the burn wound. In the otherwise stable patient, wound irrigation takes priority over transportation unless the irrigation can continue en route.[11]

Dry chemicals such as lime should be brushed off before irrigation. Water and physiologic saline are the fluids of choice for wound irrigation. The time spent searching for a specific neutralizing agent may be more harmful than simply irrigating with water. The exogenous heat production by neutralization reaction can in itself cause further tissue destruction.[11]

In the treatment of chemical burns, the flight nurse must be aware of the possibility of exposure to the noxious agents and don appropriate protective gear before coming into contact with the patient or the patient's clothing.[45]

RADIATION BURNS

Dealing with radiation burns caused by ionizing radiation is a rare occurrence. The use of air medical transport following a radiation accident will probably be for more critical injuries than for radiation exposure itself.

Radiation burns are treated like other kinds of burns. Any open wounds should be covered with gauze and fastened with an elastic bandage, never with adhesive.[52] The focus beyond the lifesaving measures is to avoid contaminating the flight crew and the aircraft. Gross contamination can be avoided if there is time to plan ahead before liftoff.

Summary

Burn injuries can present a major challenge to flight crew members but an orderly, prioritized approach can greatly simplify their management. A clear understanding of the pathophysiology of burn injuries is essential in providing quality burn care. Not only assessment but also underlying principles of intervention and resuscitation rely on this knowledge base.

Assessment of the burn victim begins with the primary survey. Life-threatening injuries must be treated first, and then, following intervention and control of potentially fatal problems, the priority is to stop the burning process. This activity is followed by appropriate airway control and ventilatory and circulatory support. Special burns such as chemical and electrical injuries have unique consequences that must be observed for early in their management.[43]

To help expedite matters, all ground support should be alerted to stand by to help in air medical transport to avoid keeping the patient out of a stable environment any longer than necessary.[11,45]

ELECTRICAL INJURIES

History and Incidence

A Leyden jar was accidentally discharged by Dutch physicians in 1746, causing the first reported man-made electrical shock.[38] The first recorded death of electrical shock occurred in Lyon, France, in 1879, when a stagehand came in contact with a 250-volt current. The first notable electrical injury in the United States occurred in 1881 when an intoxicated citizen touched a DC generator terminal in Buffalo, New York. Because his death appeared painless and quick, that incident led New Yorkers to suggest that electrocution be used as a means of capital punishment in the United States, and in 1890 the first legal electrocution took place in Auburn, New York.[9]

Over 1000 people die each year of electrical accidents. Contact with electricity accounts for approximately 3% of all burns treated in the United States each year. All ages are affected, the most common victims being those who work with electricity professionally. The age group for which greatest electrical injury rate is noted is infancy to 4 years of age. These injuries are primarily caused by contact with exposed electrical cords and outlets. The second peak appears from ages 20 to 25. Those injuries occur predominately in the male population and are caused by work and industrial accidents.[24]

Physics and Pathophysiology

Because electrical injury is unique in the field of thermal trauma, a flight nurse needs to appreciate the potential widespread anatomic damage to manage these injuries.[8] Significant factors determining severity of electrical injury are (1) voltage and amperage, (2) resistance of internal body structure and tissue, (3) the type and pathway of current, and (4) duration and intensity of contact.[16,24,54]

Ohm's Law

The intensity of the electrical current that passes through victims shows a direct correlation to the tissue damage produce. Ohm's Law supports this correlation.[37]

$$\text{Ohm's Law: Resistance (ohms)} = \frac{\text{Voltage}}{\text{Amperage}}$$

Amperage

Amperage is defined as the number or volume of electrons flowing between two potentials. It cannot be easily measured although it is actually a better indicator of potential tissue damage than voltage is.[54] This is because the skin's resistance changes as it breaks down and blisters from a burn caused by the electrical injury. This is displayed in Joule's Law:

$$\text{Heat} = \text{Amperage}^2 \times \text{Resistance}$$

Voltage

Voltage is defined as the force with which the electrical movement occurs. High-voltage injuries (> 1000 volts) and low-voltage injuries (< 1000 volts) are both common, and either type can cause death. The higher the voltage the more significant the injury. Burns, charring, and extensive blistering commonly occur.[32,42] The type of current, alternating (AC) or direct (DC), can also determine the significance of injury. Alternating current produces a tetanic contraction of muscles that "freezes" the victim to the source. This is not seen with direct current and, therefore, low-voltage AC exposure such as a household current of 110 volts can be more dangerous than a low-voltage direct current. The alternating current also has a greater potential to cause ventricular fibrillation from tetanic chest muscle contractions[22] (Table 16-1).

TABLE 16-1

Effects of amperage by household currents (60 Hz AC)

mAmps	Effect
1-2	Tingling of skin
15-20	Muscle tetany: the "let go" current
50-90	Respiratory arrest (if directed through the medulla)
90-250	Ventricular fibrillation (if the myocardium is transversed)

Resistance

Resistance is described as the degree of hindrance to electron flow. Those tissues containing the most electrolyte media, nerves, blood vessels, and muscles transmit current most easily because they have the least resistance. Tissues, tendons, and fat are most resistant and do not allow conduction, causing burning and surrounding deep muscle damage.[49]

Current Pathway

The current pathway is very critical because it may determine the severity of injury. Current passing through the head and thorax will involve the respiratory center or heart and is likely to produce instant death.[49]

Current passing from hand to foot may not affect the respiratory center but may damage the heart.[22] From the entry point, the electrical current follows the path of least resistance, causing one or more tracks of damage. The energy collects at the grounding point, causing significant tissue necrosis, and subsequently causing an explosive exit through the skin.[8] The mortality of hand-to-hand current passage is reported to be 60%, hand-to-foot current passage is 20%, and foot-to-foot current passage is 5%.[54] It has been noted that direct current tends to leave a discrete exit wound (Fig. 16-6),

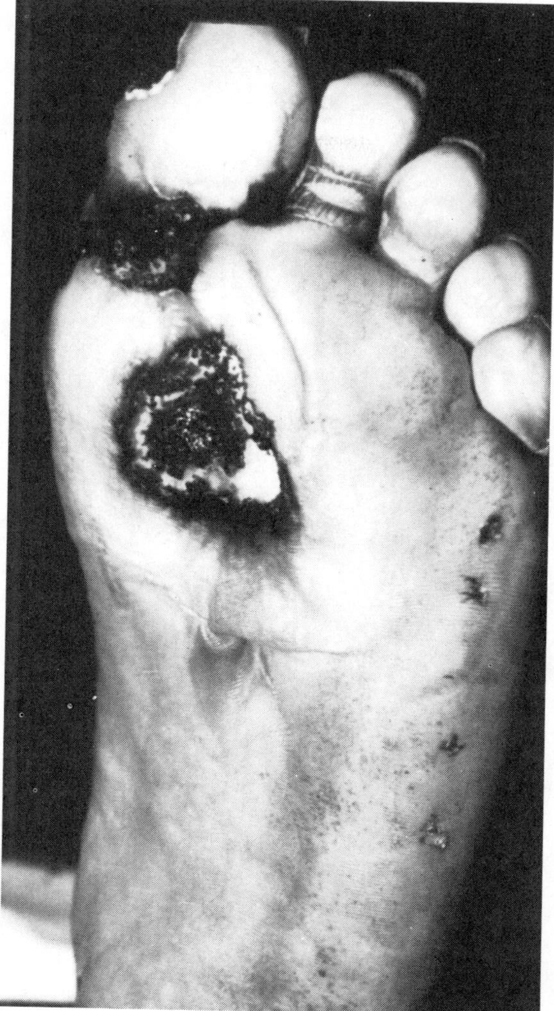

Fig. 16-6. Exit wound from direct current.

whereas alternating current tends to be more explosive[18] (Fig. 16-7).

Direct Contact Burns

The patient actually becomes part of the circuit in the case of direct contact burns. These wounds may appear devastating, and they frequently resemble a crush injury rather than a burn (Fig. 16-8). The most common point of entry is the hand or skull, and the most common exit site is the feet.[18] The sizes of these entrance and exit wounds are no real indicator of the amount of damage done to internal tissue.

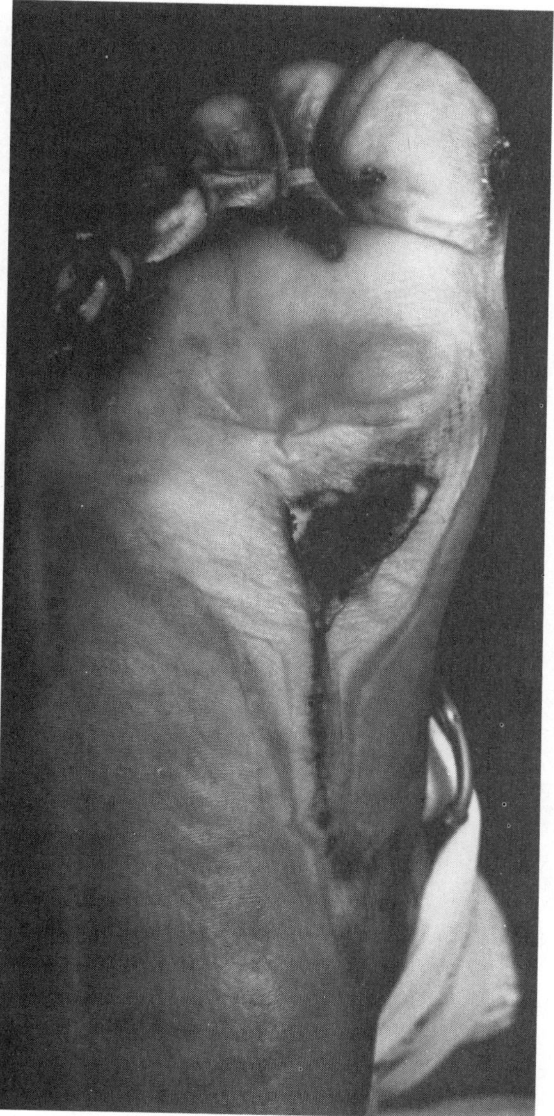

Fig. 16-7. Exit wound from alternating current.

Arc Burns

Arc burns occur when the current leaves the body on its course to the ground. Extremely high energies are produced by the arcing current, ranging from

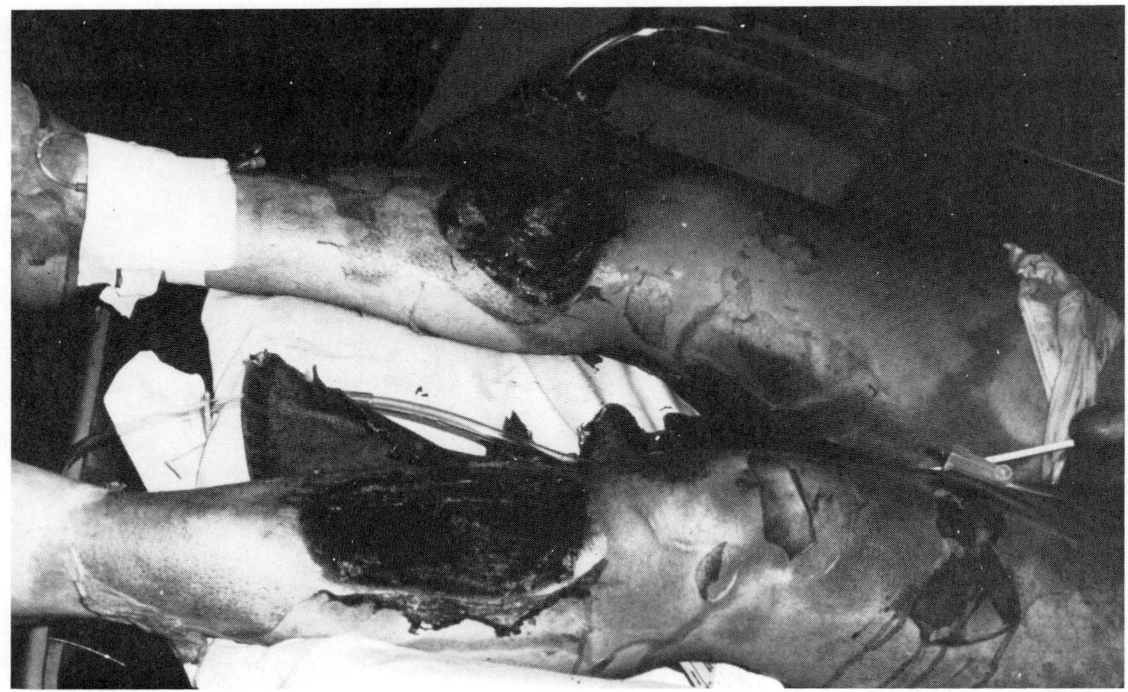

Fig. 16-8. Direct contact burns resembling crush injuries.

3000° to 20,000° C.[8] Wounds are deeper because the heat intensity is closer to the body. Second and third degree thermal burns may be indistinguishable when the heat source is more distant from the body.

Flame Burns

Flame burns occur secondary to the ignition of clothing by the current. These wounds could be severe when the victim is unconscious and has a long exposure to the flame. The ignition of clothing usually occurs with high-voltage injuries that are greater than 350 to 1000 volts.[48] Frequently, high-voltage injuries cause combinations of all types of electrical burns, and it may become difficult to determine the proper course of therapy.

Clinical Manifestations

Cutaneous Injuries

Cutaneous injuries are frequently apparent because the skin is the first point of contact with the electrical current. Dry skin has a greater resistance than wet skin, and thus produces greater generation of heat and subsequently a larger burn.

Flexor crease burns are noted as the hallmark of the true conductive injury.[47] Alternating current produces tetanic contractions of the flexor muscle of the upper extremities, causing the skin layers at the flexed joint to be more closely apposed. As the current path passes through the apposed skin layers, typical arc burns are produced at the wrist, elbow, and antecubital fossa.[48]

Oral commissure burns are commonly seen in children under the age of 2. These burns are typically caused by a child's chewing or sucking on a low-tension (110-V) electrical cord. This type of burn is frequently localized but can cause associated injuries to the tongue, palate, and face (Fig. 16-9).

Cardiac Injuries

As electrical current passes through the body, severe dysrhythmia may occur. Ventricular fibrillation is frequently induced as a 60-cycle alternating current

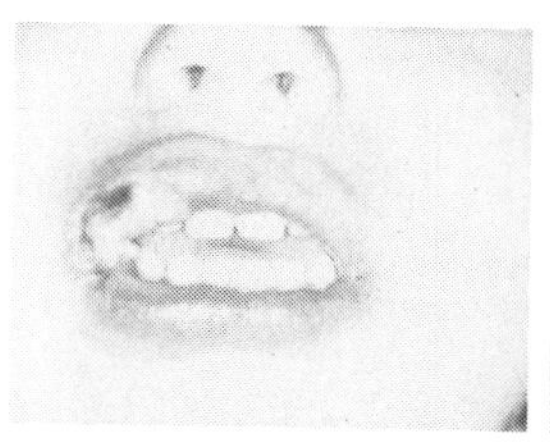
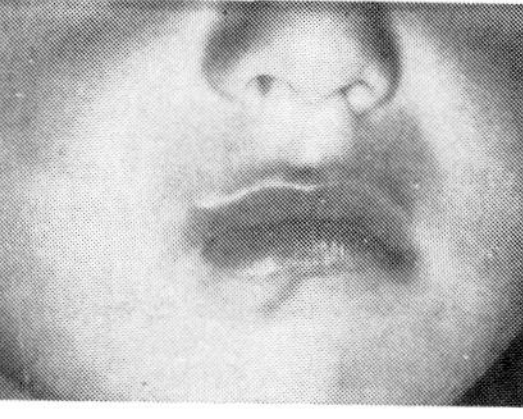

Fig. 16-9. Oral commissure burns in a child under age 2.

passes through the ventricles. Direct current injuries predominantly result in asystole by depolarizing the entire myocardium.[31] In addition to those fatal rhythms, other dysrhythmias such as atrial fibrillation, sinus bradycardia, ventricular and atrial ectopy, supraventricular tachycardia, bundle branch block, and first and second degree block may occur. Coronary artery spasm, coronary endarteritis, and direct myocardial injury are thought to be the cause of these dysrhythmias.[41,48,49] Damage to the myocardium including myocardial rupture is also a result of an electrical injury. These injuries are believed to be caused by the heat generated by the current. Myocardial damage will manifest itself in the same manner as the injury induced by ischemia.[31]

Neurologic Injuries

The skull is a common entry point of electrical current, thus the brainstem is often affected, and can lead to respiratory arrest and potential cerebral hemorrhage or edema. Nervous system tissue is an excellent conductor of electrical current and, therefore, central nervous damage is not uncommon. Effects of electrical injury to the central nervous system are manifested by unconsciousness, seizures, disorientation, or amnesia. Other neurologic complications that have been identified are spinal cord injuries, particularly those associated with electrical current traversing a hand-to-hand or head-to-foot course, and local nerve damage with peripheral neuropathies.[53]

Incomplete spinal cord transection is a common delayed lesion caused by damage to the spinal cord by the heat of the electrical current, or by blunt trauma secondary to falls or severe tetanic contractions of the muscles surrounding the cord.[53] Headaches, cerebellar dysfunctions, optic atrophy, ascending paralysis, and transverse myelitis are neurologic sequelae that are delayed.[13]

Vascular Injuries

Extensive necrosis over vessels may precipitate delayed hemorrhage from large blood vessels.[4] Arterial thrombosis, deep vein thrombosis, and abdominal aortic aneurysms may also result. Progressive venous and arterial thrombosis results in muscle damage that is not apparent on first inspection. A major vessel that has been only partially damaged may cause difficulty with hemostasis in open or newly closed wounds.[4,38,41]

Gastrointestinal Injuries

Intraabdominal injuries involving major organs may be caused by blunt trauma caused by the electrocution or electrical contact points. Life-threatening injuries involving the abdominal organs must be ruled out during the early interventions. Other injuries to the abdominal cavity commonly identified following electrocution are submucosal hemorrhages in the bowel, liver failure, pancreatitis, nausea and vomiting, paralytic ileus, and various forms and degrees of ulcerative disease.[8]

Musculoskeletal Injuries

Long-bone fractures and dislocations and vertebral fractures are caused by the rigorous tetanic muscle contractions that occur. Bilateral scapular fractures have been reported from exposure to a 440-volt, 60-cycle current passing briefly through a man's upper extremities. Bilateral scapula fractures are rare and are usually caused by direct trauma. Because there are multiple muscle attachments that surround the scapula, the severe contractions that occur from the electrical injury lead to stress and subsequent fractures.[10] Amputations have also been the result of severe muscle contractions caused by high-voltage electrical injuries.

Ophthalmologic Injuries

Immediate burns to the eyes, optic atrophy, and the development of cataracts are not uncommon, particularly if the entrance or exit wounds appear on or around the head. Cataracts may develop unilaterally or bilaterally and occur as soon as 4 months or as late as 3 years after the injury.[48]

Pregnancy

Electrical accidents in pregnant women are rare, and only a few have been reported. Lieberman and Mazor[40] studied six pregnant women who survived electrical injuries. All of the exposures were minimal, and there were no cutaneous burns or loss of consciousness. The current pathways were from hand to foot, and the patients did not seek immediate help. Three of the six fetuses were born prematurely and were stillborn. Another showed hemorrhage to the umbilical cord proximal to the fetus. Otherwise the cord and placenta were normal.

The hand-to-foot pathway of current will invariably pass through the fetus. The amniotic fluid and abundant uteroplacental vascularity have a low resistance to current flow, and the fetus becomes an easy victim of electrical injuries. Regardless of how slight the injury may appear, the mother must be transported to the hospital where extensive fetal monitoring can be done.

Renal Injuries

Acute renal failure is a complication resulting from direct damage to the kidney by the electrical current, by blunt trauma to the kidney, or from myoglobinuria.[21] Myoglobin is released as a result of extensive muscle necrosis, and myoglobinuria is proportionate to the amount of muscle damage incurred. The incidence of renal failure may be reduced significantly with aggressive fluid resuscitation.[49]

Management

Prehospital

Because of the rotor wash produced by the helicopter, great caution must be used when landing at a scene where live electrical wires may be hanging freely. Communications with ground personnel regarding the type of scene and landing zone is mandatory before approaching the landing zone.

Removing the victim from the source of current may place rescuers at risk. Wooden poles, rubber gloves, and ropes are not without risk and should be used only by those trained to work with electricity. Extrication is safe only when the power is turned off.[18] It is unfortunate and may even appear cruel not to intervene immediately; however, multiple casualties have occurred when bystanders and rescue workers have attempted to release a victim from electrical current.

Electric lines that have fallen on cars must also be approached with extreme caution. People inside the car are safe as long as they stay inside the car. If victims must be removed immediately because of injury, only trained individuals should attempt to do so. The flight crew must not assume that a downed wire is not dangerous because it is not producing sparks and because the surrounding areas are dark. Wires may become jumbled after they are broken; therefore, telephone cables, fire alarm wires, cable television lines, street lighting wires, and any other attachment to the pole may be carrying the highest voltage available and must be approached with extreme caution. Electrical lines have a tendency to surge, creating a danger of the line jumping and striking someone. Makeshift equipment (tree limbs, wooden ladders, etc.) should not be used to control downed wires, because if the conditions are right they may actually serve as conductors.[18]

Ground current may be produced with downed wires, and the current increases as one gets closer to the wire. Taking long strides may permit current to pass through the legs, therefore, when walking near a live wire, the flight crew should take short shuffling steps to decrease the potential between each foot, thus reducing the risk of injury.[18]

As soon as the scene is secured and the patient is away from the current, the victim's cardiac and respiratory status must be assessed. Arrhythmias must be treated with the same cardiac medications used for any cardiac ischemia, and ACLS protocols should be initiated.

The flight nurse must not allow gross deformities and burns to distract attention from lifesaving interventions. Cervical spine injury is of grave concern because of possible blunt trauma and because of severe tetanic contractions caused by the electrical current. The cervical spine must be protected before moving or attempting to intubate the patient.

Initially, a minimum of two large-bore IVs with normal saline or lactated Ringer's solution should be started. It is difficult to assess the area of surface burns because of the deep injury produced, and multiple liters of fluid may need to be infused. Hemorrhage must be controlled, fractures stabilized, and the patient transported with supplemental oxygen and continuous cardiac monitoring. Patients have been known to recover after long intervals of resuscitation; therefore, prolonged resuscitation efforts are recommended.[21]

Cervical and thoracic spine immobilization must be maintained. Adequate volume replacement, treatment of acidosis, and management of myoglobinuria must also be initiated. It would be incorrect to use one of the burn formulas as the only means of determining fluid requirements for these patients because of the deep tissue damage seen with the apparently mild cutaneous burns.

It is essential to maintain higher rates of urinary output because hemoglobinuria and myoglobinuria are common with electrical injuries. The fluid resuscitation must be based on actual urine flow. A minimum of 50 to 100 ml/hr of urine must be maintained; however, in the presence of urinary hemochromogen, the fluid volume must be of sufficient quantity to maintain a *minimum* output of 100 ml/hr.[32,37]

Lactic acidosis is common because of the significant muscle damage caused by electrical injury. Sodium bicarbonate must be given until an alkaline urine pH is established. Mannitol, 12.5 g, must also be given in the resuscitative phase to increase urinary output and to minimize acute tubular necrosis.[32,37]

Blood transfusion may be necessary only if there is a significant blood loss caused by secondary trauma or in the event that multiple escharotomies or fasciotomies are performed.[32]

Summary

In summary, the patient with electrical injuries may exhibit a wide spectrum of injuries from minor flesh burns to multiple trauma. The quality of treatment that the victim initially receives may determine his or her ultimate level of rehabilitation. Transportation of these patients to an appropriate hospital and early involvement of a burn care specialist is invaluable.

LIGHTNING INJURIES

An estimated 150 to 300 people are killed by lightning each year in the United States. Most lightning injuries occur in the daytime hours of the summer and fall months (Fig. 16-10). The outdoors enthusiast, athlete, camper, farmer, or golfer is more prone to lightning injury because he or she is exposed to the elements more frequently. Lightning injuries pose difficult diagnostic problems. Injuries caused by lightning strikes are dissimilar to those caused by high-voltage contact, and therefore the effects and injuries differ.[16] A lightning bolt may have a voltage up to 1 billion volts and induce currents greater than 200,000 amperes. Although the intensity of lightning is much greater than high-voltage electricity, the duration of exposure is much shorter, ranging from 1/100 to 1/1000 of a second. Because of this, skin burns are less severe than those burns seen with high-voltage injuries (usually first degree and second degree). Many of the injuries associated with tetanic contractions caused by electrical injuries are not of concern in lightning injuries. Blunt trauma may be caused when the victims are hurled to the ground by the current. A victim may suffer a direct strike from a lightning bolt or may experience a splash injury. The splash injury occurs when lightning strikes an object and the stroke jumps to another object that acts as a better conductor. This is the mechanism that causes multiple lightning strikes in people standing in close proximity to an object or to another individual who has been struck.

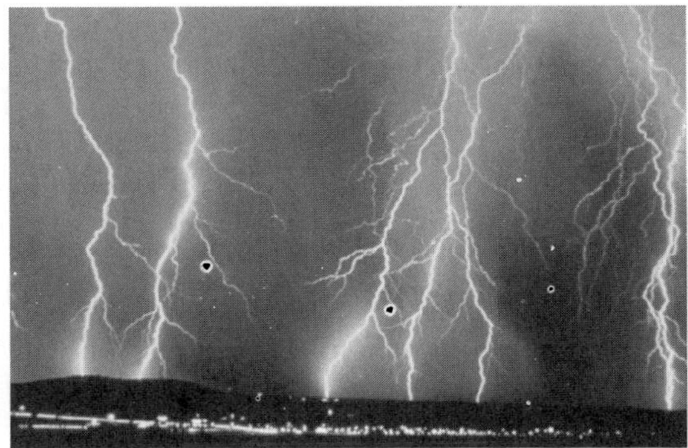

Fig. 16-10. Lightning strike demonstrating the power of lightning.

Types

As stated previously, surface burns are not as severe with lightning injuries because of the short exposure to the current, and third degree burns are rare. Linear and punctate burns are frequently seen with lightning injuries, and feathering burns are pathognomonic to lightning injuries.[5] With a lightning strike, the electrical current turns moisture on the skin to steam and frequently will blow off or shred clothing or shoes[18] (Fig. 16-11).

Minor

Patients with minor injuries usually are conscious; however, they may have lost consciousness transiently and are frequently confused and amnesic. They rarely exhibit burns or any other signs of injury, and vital signs are usually stable.[5]

Moderate

Patients with moderate lightning injuries show more obvious altered mentation and may be combative or comatose. They may have fallen or have been thrown down forcibly from the current, causing fractures and dislocations.

First and second degree burns may be apparent with a moderate lightning strike injury as may tympanic membrane rupture caused by the explosive force of lightning strike. Difficulty palpating peripheral pulses and a mottled appearance of the patient's lower extremities are caused by arteriospasm and are frequently characteristic with a moderate injury. This usually clears in a few hours.[17]

Severe

If lightning current passes through the brain, the direct current or blast effect caused by the strike may damage the brain. The patient will be comatose and may possibly be undergoing a seizure. Closed head injury caused by a fall must also be looked for in these cases.[5]

Cardiac arrest with ventricular fibrillation should be anticipated. The most common cause of death in lightning injuries is cardiopulmonary arrest.[5] Lightning may cause paralysis to the medullary respiratory center, first causing respiratory arrest then cardiac arrest. If immediate ventilation does not occur, a subsequent cardiac arrest will follow, and brain death will occur due to anoxia.[18] Multiple arrhythmias are associated with lightning strikes, including ventricular tachycardia, PVCs, and atrial fibrillation. ST changes associated with ischemia are also common.[36] Many ocular injuries have been reported including detached

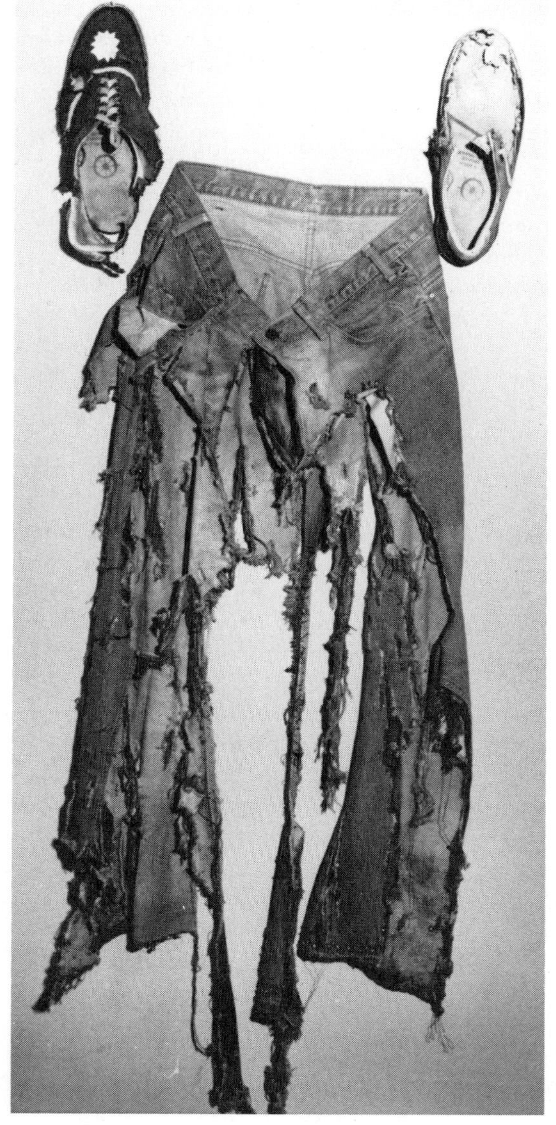

Fig. 16-11. Clothing of a patient struck by lightning.

retina, hyphema, direct thermal burn, corneal lesion, and cataract. As with electrical injuries, cataracts may appear as late as 2 years after the strike, but they are most commonly present in the first few days after the injury.[6]

Patients must be assessed for other signs of trauma caused by the impact of the strike, and life-threatening injuries should be looked for.

Pregnancy

The fetus must be assessed by immediately using fetal heart tones to determine viability. The prognosis of the unborn child is difficult to determine. Half of the pregnancies go on to normal delivery and produce no recognizable abnormality to the child, whereas the other half result in stillbirths.[56]

Prehospital Care

On approaching the scene of a storm, a secured landing site, free from debris and possible downed wires or tree branches must be immediately established. The patient's cardiopulmonary status must be assessed immediately, and CPR and intubation should be initiated on finding the patient in cardiac arrest. As with any unknown injury, the cervical spine must be immobilized before intubation and transport. The patient's cardiac status must be monitored continuously, and arrhythmias should be treated with standard cardiac therapies (ACLS protocols).

Unless significant trauma from a fall or explosive injury is suspected, fluids must be restricted in prevent cerebral edema. Burns seen with lightning injuries are not as extensive as those seen with high-voltage injuries; therefore, massive amounts of fluids are not required unless the patient is in hypovolemic shock. Two IV lines should be established as a "keep open" line and for a medication route. Observation and history taking must be performed with care to treat and transport these victims rapidly.

BURN AND ELECTRICAL INJURIES CASE STUDY #1: ELECTRICAL INJURY

11:15 Life flight ABC is requested to respond to the Boondocks Airport for a 24-year-old male skydiving student who had drifted into high voltage power lines. Ground ambulance was not yet on scene.

11:18 Approval was given from the pilots to accept the flight and preflight safety checks completed.

11:23 Lift off for the 20 minute flight to the scene.

11:28 Ground EMS (BLS Unit) on scene, patient assessment initiated, landing zone being prepared with wires and other hazards communicated to the pilots. En route to the scene the flight nurse and paramedic prepare airway capture and intravenous access supplies.

11:43 Arrival of flight team on scene. Report from EMS Crew Chief: 24-year-old male in contact with high voltage electrical wires near the airfield, fell approximately 10 meters to the ground. Witnesses describe a brief period of unconsciousness but the patient was awake and responding appropriately when EMS arrived, complaining of back and leg pain. During assessment the patient has become gradually less responsive.

11:45 Initial observation reveals that the patient is supine with full spinal immobilization in place, currently responding to painful stimuli only with a Glasgow Coma Scale value of 7. Airway manipulation was hampered by trismus; respiratory rate and effort decreased. The flight nurse elected to perform a rapid sequence induction intubation administering midazolam, lidocaine, and succinylcholine according to program protocol while having the patient's ventilation assisted with a BVM and 100% oxygen.

11:54 The patient was loaded into the aircraft for transport to the regional burn center. Intravenous access was established en route. Total body surface area burned was difficult to determine because the majority of the injury was not visible. Crystalloid fluid was initiated at a wide open rate during transport.

11:57 Report is called to the receiving center where a trauma team is assembled to accept the patient. En route the patient is ventilated to keep CO_2 levels at 28 to 30.

12:15 With no complications arising in flight, the patient is delivered to the trauma receiving team who aggressively treat his head and electrical injuries.

The flight team demonstrated sound knowledge of electrical injury care, recognizing and treating the concomitant trauma and realizing that the extent of an electrical injury cannot be assessed by examination of surface injuries.

BURN AND ELECTRICAL INJURIES CASE STUDY #2: THERMAL INJURY

14:50 The flight team receives a request to respond to an Arctic nursing station for a child with scald injuries from an abusive home situation. The injuries were incurred approximately 1 hour before arrival at the nursing station. The flight nurse relays the request to the pilots so that weather checks can be done while patient information is gathered. The 2-year-old girl is conscious, 12 kg with 40% total body surface area burned superficial and 10% burned deeper. The flight nurse is also informed that the mother is in police custody and an elderly grandmother is in attendance. The flight nurse advises the nursing station nurse to administer oxygen to the child, cover the wounds with clean, dry dressings, keep her warm, initiate intravenous access, and administer sufficient IV fluids to maintain a urine output of 120 ml/hour.

14:58 The pilots report that the flight can be accepted but that the airstrip is across the lake from the nursing station.

15:20 Airborne! The flight nurse takes advantage of the 2-hour flight to make arrangements for a boat to use for transport across the lake and to obtain updates on the patient's condition.

17:30 Arriving at the airstrip, the flight nurses and equipment are transported across the lake by boat where they are met by a truck to take them to the nursing station.

17:50 The flight team arrives at the nursing station where the on-site nurse gives report and introduces them to the patient's grandmother and an aunt who will accompany the child back to the city.

17:57 Flight nurse assessment: quiet, withdrawn child, tolerating oxygen cannula, IV in place with D_5LR infusing at 150 ml/hr. Assessment of injury reveals scald demarcation lines around mid-chest and thighs indicating a forcible submersion. When questioned the patient complains of pain. A narcotic analgesic is administered, a Foley catheter with a urimeter is inserted, and the child is transferred onto the aircraft stretcher and covered with a sleeping bag.

18:20 With careful attention to maintaining warmth, the patient and her aunt are transported across the lake to the waiting aircraft. The child is loaded into the aircraft and given a stuffed toy for comfort during the flight.

18:50 Airborne again, the flight nurses monitor the patient's urine output and adjust fluid administration rates to maintain output of 120 ml/hour. A chemstrip is done to monitor the child's glucose level, and narcotics are administered IV as needed for complaints of pain.

The patient tolerated the flight well and was released to return to her community 2 weeks later with the aunt named as guardian by social services.

REFERENCES

1. American Burn Association: Total care for burn patients: a guide to hospital resources, *Bull Am Coll Surg* 14, 1977.
2. American College of Surgeons: *Advanced trauma life support providers manual,* Chicago, 1993, American College of Surgeons.
3. Archauer B, editor: *Management of the burned patient,* Norwalk, Conn, 1987, Appleton & Lange.
4. Artz CP: Changing concepts of electrical injury, *Am J Surg* 128:600-602, 1974.
5. Auerbach PS, editor: *Wilderness medicine,* ed 3, St Louis, 1995, Mosby.
6. Bartholome CW, Jacoby WD: Cutaneous manifestations of lightning injury, *Arch Dermatol* 1466-1468, 1975.

7. Baxt WG, Moody P: The impact of a rotorcraft aeromedical emergency care service on trauma mortality, *JAMA* 249:3246-3250, 1983.
8. Baxter CR: Present concepts in the management of major electrical injury, *Surg Clin North Am* 50(6):1401-1419, 1970.
9. Bernstein T: Theories of the cause of death from electricity in the late nineteenth century, *Med Instr* 9:267-273, 1975.
10. Beswick DR: Bilateral scapular fractures from low voltage electrical injury, *Ann Emerg Med* 11:676-677, 1982.
11. Boswick JA, editor: *The art and science of burn care,* Rockville, Md, 1987, Aspen Publishers.
12. Carvajal HF: Fluid resuscitation of pediatric burn victims: a critical appraisal, *Pediatr Nephrol* 8(3):357-366, 1994.
13. Christenson JA, Sherman RT: Delayed neurologic injury secondary to high voltage current with recovery, *J Trauma* 20:166-168, 1980.
14. Clark WR: Smoke inhalation, *Burns* 12:163, 1988.
15. Collini FJ, Kealey GP: Burns: a review and update, *Contemp Surg* 34:160-165, 1989.
16. Cooper MA: Electrical and lightning injuries, *Emerg Med Clin North Am* 2(3):489-501, 1984.
17. Cooper MA: Lightning injuries: prognostic signs for death, *Ann Emerg Med* 9:134-138, 1980.
18. Cooper MA: Of volts and bolts, *Emerg Med* 99-121, 1983.
19. Cooper MA, Sherand M: Enhancing recovery from electrical and lightning injuries, *Emerg Med Rep* 8(8):57-63, 1983.
20. Demling RH, Lalonde C: *Burn trauma,* New York, 1989, Thieme Medical.
21. Dixon GF: The evaluation and management of electrical injuries, *Crit Care Med* 11(5):384-387, 1983.
22. Erskine JF: Electrical accidents, *Practitioner* 222:777-781, 1979.
23. Faldmo L, Kravitz M: Management of acute burns and burn shock resuscitation, *AACN Clin Issues Crit Care Nurs* 4(2):351-366, 1993.
24. Gant TD: Electrical injuries, with special reference to the upper extremities: a review of 182 cases, *Am J Surg* 134(1):95-101, 1977.
25. Goldfarb JW: The burn patient, *Air Medical Crew National Standards Curriculum,* Phoenix, 1988, ASHBEAMS.
26. Herndon DN, Rutan RL, Rutan TC: Management of the pediatric patient with burns, *J Burn Care Rehab* 14(1): 3-8, 1993.
27. Hilton JG, Marullo DS: Effects of thermal trauma of cardiac force of contraction, *Burns* 12:173, 1986.
28. Horton JW, White DJ, Hunt JL: Delayed hypertonic saline dextran administration after burn injury, *J Trauma* 38(2):281-286, 1995.
29. Housinger TA: A prospective study of myocardial damage in electrical injuries, *J Trauma* 25(2):122-124, 1985.
30. Huang PP et al: Hypertonic sodium resuscitation is associated with renal failure and death, *Ann Surg* 221(5): 543-554, 1995.
31. Hunt JL: Acute electric burn, *Arch Surg* 115:434-438, 1980.
32. Hurren JS, Dunn KW: Spontaneous pneumothorax in association with a major burn, *Burns* 20(2):178-179, 1994.
33. Judkins KC: Aeromedical transfer of burned patients, *Burns* 14:171, 1987.
34. Kemble JVH, Lamb BE: *Practical burns management,* London, 1987, Hodder and Stoughton.
35. Kinsella J: Smoke inhalation, *Burns* 14:150-155, 1988.
36. Kleiner JP, Welken JH: Cardiac affects of lightning strike, *JAMA* 240:2757-2759, 1978.
37. Kobernick M: Electrical injuries: pathophysiology and emergency management, *Ann Emerg Med,* 11:633-668, 1982.
38. Kouwenhoven WB: Effects of electricity in the human body, *Electrical Engineering* 68:199, 1949.
39. Kumar P, Jagetia GC: A review of triage and management of burn victims following a nuclear disaster, *Burns* 20(5): 397-402, 1994.
40. Lieberman JR, Mazor JR: Electrical accidents during pregnancy, *Obstet Gynecol* 67(6):861-863, 1986.
41. Martyn JAJ: *Acute management of the burned patient,* Philadelphia, 1990, Saunders.
42. Masters FW, Robinson DW: Management of electrical burns. In Lynch JB, Lewis F, editors: *Symposium of the treatment of burns,* vol 5, St Louis, 1977, Mosby.
43. Mikhail J: Acute burn care: an update, *J Emerg Nurs* 14: 14, 20-23, 1988.
44. Miller JG et al: Early cardiorespiratory patterns in patients with major burns and pulmonary insufficiency, *Burns* 20(6):542-546, 1994.
45. Nebraska Burn Institute: *Advanced burn life support provider manual,* Lincoln, Neb, 1987, The Institute.
46. Puffinbarger NK, Tuggle DW, Smith EI: Rapid isotonic fluid resuscitation in pediatric thermal injury, *J Pediatr Surg* 29(2):339-341, 1994.
47. Quimby WC: The use of microscopy as a guide to primary excision of high tension electrical burns, *J Trauma* 18:43, 1978.
48. Rosen P, Baker M: *Emergency medicine: concepts of clinical practice,* St Louis, 1992, Mosby.

49. Salem L, Fisher RP: The natural history of electrical injuries, *J Trauma* 17:487-492, 1977.
50. Shaw A et al: Pathophysiological basis of burn management, *Br J Hosp Med* 52(11):583-587, 1994.
51. Shaw A et al: The early management of large burns, *Br J Hosp Med* 53(6):247-250, 1995.
52. Shleien B: *Preparedness and response in radiation accidents,* Rockville, Md, 1983, US Department of Health and Human Services.
53. Taylor PH: The intriguing electrical burns: a review of 321 electrical burn cases, *J Trauma* 2:309, 1962.
54. Thompson MD, Ashway MD: Electrical injuries in children, Am J Dis Child 137:231-235, 1985.
55. Warden GD: Burn shock resuscitation, *World J Surg* 16(2): 16-23, 1992.
56. Weinstein L: Lightning: a rare cause of intrauterine death with maternal survival, *South Med J* 72:632, 1979.
57. Wilson P: Resolved on burn awareness, *Fire Control Digest* 14:10-15, 1988.

CHAPTER 17

Maxillofacial, Anterior Neck, and Eye Trauma

COMPETENCIES

1. Identify the common mechanisms of injury that result in maxillofacial trauma.
2. Recognize transport considerations for the patient with maxillofacial and eye trauma.
3. Calculate the altitude at which the patient with maxillofacial or eye trauma should be transported.
4. Describe the initial management of the patient with maxillofacial trauma.
5. Provide the appropriate interventions for the patient with an eye injury.

Maxillofacial injuries are rarely life threatening but may result in devastating disfigurement, blindness, and associated psychosocial problems. Anterior neck injuries, conversely, pose a significant threat to the airway and major blood vessels, often causing obstruction and exsanguination. Regardless of the injury, primary assessment and management of all patients remain the same:

1. Clearing and maintaining the airway while taking cervical spine precautions
2. Assuring adequate ventilation and oxygenation
3. Controlling hemorrhage and treating shock

Secondary assessment and management of patients with maxillofacial, anterior neck, and eye trauma require techniques specific to each injury. These techniques are addressed after information regarding the mechanism of injury is provided and basic anatomy and physiology are briefly reviewed. This chapter focuses on the more common maxillofacial injuries in each category.

TRANSPORT CONSIDERATIONS

Whether the flight team is reporting to the scene or is conducting an interfacility transfer, the general principles of emergency medical care still apply. Maintenance of a clear airway while taking cervical spine precautions is always the first consideration. Maintaining a clear airway in a patient with extensive facial or anterior neck trauma may prove challenging because blood, mucus, broken teeth, dislodged dentures, bone fragments, and foreign bodies may all contribute to obstruction of the airway. Obstruction may also be caused by mandibular fractures with posterior displacement of the tongue, nasal and maxillary fractures in obtunded patients, and laryngeal and tracheal injuries.[3] The airway may be cleared either manually or with suction. When manually clearing the airway with a gloved hand, it is necessary to take precautions against inadvertently being bitten by the patient. The cross-finger technique, which is commonly used during endotracheal intubation, works well: The flight nurse uses the thumb and forefinger of one hand to separate the upper and lower teeth or gums and to open the patient's mouth and places gauze padding between the fingers and the teeth to aid in protecting the digits from potentially sharp dental surfaces. Magill forceps can be used to manually remove airway obstructions.

The airway can be suctioned with use of a large catheter tip syringe, bulb syringe, or mechanical device. Suction devices are particularly useful for removing fluids and small particulate matter. Larger foreign bodies usually must be removed manually.

Once the airway has been cleared, it must be maintained to provide adequate ventilation. Patients who have sustained facial and neck injuries often bleed extensively because of the rich blood supply in the area of the face and neck. Once cervical spine injury has been ruled out the patient may be placed in a semi-Fowler's position or higher, which will help gravity to drain secretions and protect the airway. Oral or nasopharyngeal airways are useful for maintaining an open airway but not for protecting it against secretions. Endotracheal or nasotracheal intubation provides maximum protection for the airway when the endotracheal tube is properly positioned at the level of the carina in the trachea and the cuff has been adequately inflated. In the event of maxillary instability, indicating a possible cribriform plate fracture, endotracheal intubation should be attempted orally only under direct laryngoscopic visualization to prevent possible intubation of the brain.

Maxillofacial and neck trauma may be so extensive in some patients that endotracheal or nasotracheal intubation is not possible because of gross deformity of the facial structures or direct trauma to the trachea, with associated laryngeal edema. A cricothyrotomy must be performed when all other forms of airway control are unsuccessful or inappropriate. Because of the sensitive nature of this surgical procedure, it should be performed while on the ground if at all possible and not in flight, where unexpected turbulence may occur. If a situation arises in which it becomes necessary to perform a surgical cricothyrotomy during flight, it is imperative that the pilot keep the aircraft as stable as possible. (See Chapter 8 for a description of airway management.)

If the patient is unable to breathe after the airway has been cleared and maintained, the flight nurse should provide ventilatory assistance; a resuscitation bag (bag-valve mask) or mechanical ventilator is used either to provide breathing assistance to the patient whose respiratory efforts are inadequate or to provide total ventilatory support.

Facial injuries may at first appear to be causing exsanguination because of the extensive bleeding that occurs as a result of the rich vascular supply in the face; however, this is rarely the case. Conversely, anterior neck injuries may cause exsanguination when the carotid and jugular vessels are involved. Shock is usually caused by other associated injuries and must be assessed and treated immediately. For instance, the combination of maxillofacial, anterior neck, and chest trauma occurs frequently, especially in motor vehicle collisions (MVCs). Most bleeding can be controlled with direct pressure applied manually or with pressure dressings. Occasionally, deep and persistent bleeding can be controlled only by direct pressure and subsequent surgical ligation of the external carotid artery.[3]

Facial and eye injuries should be treated only after associated life-threatening injuries have been addressed and the patient has been stabilized. Cervical spine injury should always be suspected in the event of maxillofacial and anterior neck trauma.

Avulsed matter (e.g., eyelids and teeth) should be retrieved when possible and transported with the patient for possible reimplantation. It is also useful to transport objects involved in penetrating trauma for culturing purposes and to aid in determining the source of unidentified foreign bodies. When chemical substances are involved, especially in ocular burns, providing the container to emergency department staff contributes to positive identification and possible use of a more efficacious or specific antidote. For interfacility transports, all medical records, unusual medications, extra blood and body fluid samples, x-ray films, computed tomography (CT) scans, any other diagnostic products, and test results should be transported with the patient.

MAXILLOFACIAL TRAUMA

Mechanism of Injury

The major causes of facial injuries are MVCs, followed by accidents in the home, athletic injuries, animal bites, assaults, and industrial injuries.

Normal Anatomy and Physiology

Facial injuries resulting from MVCs are most often caused when the victim's face strikes the dashboard, windshield, and, in the case of the driver, the steering wheel. Injuries that result from striking the dashboard include fractures of the mid face, nose, zygoma, mandible, and orbital floor. Striking the windshield produces multiple soft tissue injuries, and accidents in cars manufactured before 1966 often produce deep, extensive lacerations, avulsion flap, and complete avulsion injuries. Later model cars have shatterproof windshields made of a chemically tempered inner pane laminated to a plastic inner layer, which causes the windshield to crack but not break into jagged pieces. Facial injuries that occur when persons strike these improved windshields include numerous small superficial lacerations and small triangular avulsion flaps. It has been shown that the proper use of passenger restraint systems, including seat belts, shoulder harnesses, and air bags, can effectively eliminate facial injuries in MVCs because they prevent the victim's face from striking the dashboard, windshield, or steering wheel.

Accidents occurring at home cause a relatively high percentage of facial soft tissue injury and fractures. Mechanisms of injury include explosions, which cause thermal and chemical burns, high-velocity missiles, such as rocks thrown from power lawn mowers, and falls.

Work injuries can be caused by blunt objects or by missiles and are often of a crushing nature. Injuries sustained in heavy construction work can be particularly severe and may result in associated cranial injuries.[6] This type of penetrating trauma may carry a greater threat of tetanus infection from the industrial environment.

Facial Bones

Facial bones are relatively thin and unsupported compared with other bony structures throughout the body. Facial bones function as compressible, energy-absorbing protection for vital organs that lie within and behind them, including the eye, lacrimal apparatus, pharynx, cervical spine, and brain.[6]

Facial Muscles

The muscles of mastication are innervated by branches of the mandibular nerve.[3] Strong contractions of these muscles can cause significant displacement of mandibular fractures. Because of this phenomenon, mandibular fractures are often extremely painful, whereas other types of facial fractures cause relatively minimal discomfort.

Facial Vessels

The face receives its blood supply from branches of the internal and external carotid arteries. The superficial arterial supply comes entirely from the external carotid artery and results in the extensive facial bleeding that occurs with soft tissue injuries of the face. Although bleeding from facial injuries may appear to be exsanguinating, it usually is not, and most bleeding can be controlled by applying simple direct pressure or pressure dressings. It is important that treatment of true life-threatening injuries takes precedence over attention to facial bleeding.[6]

Assessment

Assessment of any patient with facial injuries should begin with the basic ABCs. Facial injuries alone rarely threaten a patient's life, except when they contribute to airway obstruction.

The airway should be assessed for obstructions caused by blood, vomitus, bone fragments, broken teeth, dentures, and damage to the trachea or larynx. Once the airway has been secured and maintained via repositioning of the patient (if not contraindicated) or with use of oral airways, tracheal intubation, or cricothyrotomy, the flight nurse must ensure adequate ventilation. Oxygenation may be improved by the administering oxygen with use of the most appropriate means available, considering the location and extent of the patient's facial injuries. These means may include a nasal cannula, nonrebreather oxygen mask, resuscitation bag, or mechanical ventilator.

Facial injuries should be assessed only after stabilization of the patient's general condition. Assessment of facial injuries requires skill in the areas of observation, palpation, and, when available, radiologic examination.

First, the soft tissues are observed for signs of lacerations, abrasions, avulsions, puncture wounds, hematomas, and any embedded foreign bodies. Facial symmetry is also evaluated by examining the patient for significant structure deformities; it should be kept in mind that few faces are normally perfectly symmetrical.[8,18] The flight nurse can evaluate facial symmetry by viewing the face straight on (face to face) and by viewing it from a position above the supine patient's head while looking toward the feet.

Next, the flight nurse should palpate bony prominences. Although tenderness at the site of facial bone fractures can usually be elicited, severe pain is uncommon,[8,18] with the exception of mandibular fractures, in which muscular contractions cause displacement of the fracture and extreme discomfort results.

The patient must be examined further so that additional signs of injury can be evaluated. Cerebrospinal fluid (CSF) (CSF rhinorrhea and CSF otorrhea) is usually associated with fractures of the cribriform plate or anterior cranial fossa. Early detection of CSF is difficult in the presence of facial bleeding, and positive identification requires laboratory analysis for protein, sugar, and mucin.[3] The patient should also be evaluated for abnormal extraocular movements (EOMs), pain or deviation of the mandible on opening, trismus (limitation of movement as a result of pain), mobility of the teeth, lengthening of the face, paresthesia, medial canthal deformity, subconjunctival ecchymosis, and pupil height, equality, and reaction to light.

Injuries to the face may involve the third, fourth, fifth, and seventh cranial nerves (Table 17-1). The third nerve, the oculomotor nerve, supplies the majority of the ocular muscles to provide ocular movement, elevation of the upper eyelid, and pupil constriction. Injury to the third nerve may be evaluated by testing pupil response to light and the ability of the patient to perform EOMs. The fourth cranial nerve, the trochlear nerve, enables downward and inward movement of the eye. It is evaluated by assessing the patient's ability to feel objects touched to the face or to feel pain, numbness, tingling, and hot or cold sensations. Movement of the jaw may be assessed by asking the patient to bite down and by opening the patient's mouth against resistance. The facial nerve, the seventh cranial nerve, is responsible for facial expression, closing the eyelids, secretions of the glands of the mouth and eyes, and taste from the anterior two-thirds of the tongue. This nerve divides into several branches, including the temporal, zygomatic, and buccal branches. The temporal branch can be evaluated by having the patient raise his or her eyebrows and wrinkle the forehead. Integrity of the zygomatic branch is tested by having the patient close both eyes tightly. The buccal branch is assessed by having the patient purse his or her lips and wrinkle the nose.

X-ray films are often available for patients being transported from a facility, and the flight nurse will usually have time to evaluate them. CT films may also be available and are particularly valuable for diagnosing fractures of the middle third of the face, especially blow-out fractures of the orbital floor.[3]

TABLE 17-1

Cranial nerve damage associated with facial trauma

Cranial nerve	Name	Effect	Test
III	Oculomotor	Ocular movement Pupil constriction Upper eyelid elevation	Pupil response EOMs
IV	Trochlear	Downward/inward ocular movement	EOMs
V	Trigeminal	Facial sensation Jaw movement	Touch face Open mouth against resistance
VII	Facial	Facial expression Eyelid closure Taste from anterior two-thirds of tongue Secretions of mouth and eye glands	Temporal branch: Raise eyebrows, wrinkle forehead Zygomatic branch: Close eyes tightly Buccal branch: Purse lips, wrinkle nose

Pathophysiology and Treatment

Soft Tissue Injuries

Contusion/Hematoma. Contusions, which result from blunt trauma, do not generally cause problems unless they are associated with an underlying hematoma. Some hematomas spontaneously reabsorb, whereas those that become encapsulated must be evacuated. In the early stages of formation a hematoma can be evacuated through a small incision to release the "jellylike" substance contained within.

Abrasions. Abrasions usually only require cleansing with a mild soap. They are either left uncovered or, in more painful cases, are protected from air by a thin layer of antibacterial ointment and a serum-absorbent dressing. Large third-degree abrasions are often treated as burns and sometimes require skin grafts. Small particles embedded in the dermal layer, often as a result of contact with asphalt or gravel, will become fixed in the tissue and cause permanent tattooing of the skin if not removed within 12 hours. A sterile surgical scrub brush and mild soap are usually adequate for removal of the particles under local or general anesthesia. Once the particles are fixed in the tissues, mechanical dermabrasion becomes necessary. Grease or oil around the wound may be removed with small amounts of ether or acetone.

Lacerations. Lacerations are the most common facial injury.[3,8,16] When facial lacerations are evaluated, consideration is given to possible associated damage to deeper structures, including the parotid duct, facial nerves, vascular structures, and facial skeleton. With the exception of animal bites and accidental tattooing, most soft tissue wounds of the face can be repaired up to 24 hours after the injury without serious risk of infection or of jeopardizing the final aesthetic result, providing proper cleansing and dressing have been accomplished.[3,6]

Lacerations of the cheek require special attention because of the importance of the underlying structures, including branches of the facial nerve, the parotid gland, Stensen's duct, and the muscles of mastication. Pressure dressings are often used for extensive facial laceration repair to support the tissues and maintain close approximation of the wound edges, eliminate dead space, restrict venous and lymph accumulation, reduce fibrin deposition and excess scar formation, minimize tension on the sutures, and prevent wound contamination. They are normally left in place for a minimum of 48 to 72 hours. Dressings that become saturated with secretions should be reinforced and should not be replaced in flight. Exposure of an open wound to the contaminated aircraft environment could result in serious infection. All wounds should be appropriately cleansed and the patient's tetanus status evaluated.

Nerve Injury

The cranial nerves associated with facial trauma are the oculomotor, trochlear, trigeminal, and facial nerves. Damage to the oculomotor nerve results in decreased ocular movement, inability to raise the eyelid, and a delayed or absent pupillary response. Trochlear nerve damage results in the absence or limitation of downward and inward movement of the eye. The absence of facial sensation and limitation of jaw movement are caused by damage to the trigeminal nerve.

Major branches of the facial nerve are located deep in the cheek area, are well protected by overlying tissue, and are seldom injured by accidental trauma.[3] Although injury to this nerve can cause facial drooping on the affected side, the most severe functional deficit results from damage to the temporal branch of the facial nerve, which causes paralysis of the eyelid and subsequent exposure of the cornea.[3] Care of these patients during transport includes instillation of artificial tears and taping of the eyelids to prevent dehydrated corneal tissue, which can lead to corneal abrasion and ulcers. This treatment is particularly significant during extended flights at higher altitudes where the humidity may decrease from 1% to 3%.[34]

Parotid Gland and Stensen's Duct

Because the parotid gland and Stensen's duct are more superficial than the facial nerve branches, they are more susceptible to injury. Any deep lacerations in the area of the parotid (Stensen's) duct (from the lower border of the acoustic meatus to a point midway between the nose and upper border of the lip) need to be assessed for parotid duct injury. Leakage of clear fluid in this area is indicative of damage. Because the buccal branch of the facial nerve runs parallel to and sometimes across the parotid duct, it may be simultaneously damaged, resulting in drooping of the affected half of the upper lip. This phenomenon serves as an additional indicator of parotid damage.

Fractures

Orbital Fractures. Fractures of the orbit include orbital blow-out fractures and supraorbital fractures. A "pure" orbital blow-out fracture specifically involves only the orbital floor and not the surrounding orbital rim structures. An "impure" blow-out fracture occurs with injury to the rim of the orbit and is often associated with nasoorbital fractures, Le Fort's fractures, frontal sinus fractures, and malar fractures. The orbital floor is particularly susceptible to fractures because of the relatively thin nature of the bony structure. An orbital blow-out fracture occurs when an object of greater diameter than that of the bony orbital rim strikes the globe and the surrounding soft tissues. The force of impact on the globe pushes it into the orbit, thereby causing compression of the orbital contents. The sudden increase in intraocular pressure is transmitted to the weakest part of the structure, the orbital floor, resulting in its fracture and herniation of the orbital contents into the maxillary sinuses. When the traumatic force dissipates, the bony structures of the orbital floor attempt to return to their normal position, entrapping the prolapsed orbital contents. Objects commonly responsible for these types of fractures include baseballs, tennis balls, hockey pucks, fists, and elbows. Smaller objects, such as squash balls or racquet balls, usually cause rupture of the globe without fracture.

Clinical signs and symptoms of orbital blow-out fractures include periorbital edema, periorbital and subconjunctival ecchymosis, diplopia, enophthalmos (recessed globe) resulting in unequal pupil height, unilateral epistaxis, air-fluid levels in the maxillary sinus, infraorbital nerve paresthesia of the anterior cheek, and decreased extraocular movement. These signs are also indicative of zygomatic fractures, which can be ruled out by a Waters view x-ray, which includes the orbital roof and floor, the zygomatic bone, and the temporal arch. CT and MRI scans and ultrasound procedures may also prove useful.

A complete ophthalmic examination is necessary to rule out other ocular injuries, including injury to the globe and optic nerve and lacerations of the eyelids and lacrimal system. All patients require evaluation and documentation of pupil reactivity. If time permits, an ophthalmoscopic examination can be performed to assess any retinal damage. Visual acuity and extraocular movement should be assessed in the conscious patient. A crude evaluation of visual acuity can be performed in the field by having the patient read the printed words on an intravenous bag or on the patient consent form.

Initial treatment for orbital blow-out fractures consists of loose binocular bandaging (covering both eyes) to reduce movement of either eye. Because the patient will not be able to see, the flight nurse should inform the patient of any procedure or activity that is about to occur, including loading the patient into the aircraft, takeoff, and landing, to relieve the patient's anxiety and reduce intraocular pressure that could lead to further damage. The patient should be transported in a supine position with the head immobilized and the flight nurse should administer low-flow oxygen to prevent problems of hypoxia, particularly because the eye is such an oxygen-sensitive organ. Patients should be transported at lower altitudes because the fracture creates a communication with the maxillary sinus and air from the sinus may expand and apply increased pressure to the entrapped orbital contents. The flight nurse should request an altitude restriction no greater than the destination altitude.

Nasal Fractures. The nose is the most frequently fractured facial structure. Nasal fractures and nasal-orbital-ethmoid fractures are included in this category.

Nasal fractures may involve the bony nasal complex and nasal septum. Clinical signs and symptoms of nasal fractures include airway obstruction (caused by displaced bone fragments, blood, and edema); facial asymmetry, deformity, or angulation; crepitus; periorbital ecchymosis; edema; tenderness; and unilateral or bilateral epistaxis. CSF leak, subconjunctival ecchymosis, and nasal septal deformity may also be seen. The nasal bones may be deviated to one side or depressed, and bony irregularities ("step-offs") may be palpated at the fracture site. Edema surrounding the injured area may render it difficult to determine the presence or extent of nasal fracture or deformity.

Initial treatment involves clearing and maintaining the airway and controlling epistaxis. The airway should be cleared with suctioning and maintained by the most appropriate means available. Epistaxis can usually be controlled by external direct pressure (compression of the anterior nares). Persistent bleeding may require the use of a topical vasoconstrictor, such as 0.5% phenylephrine hydrochloride (Neo-synephrine). Profuse epistaxis rarely occurs and can be treated by nasal packing. The patient should be transported in a semi-Fowler's position or higher, if not contraindicated, to facilitate gravitational drainage of blood and other secretions.

Septal hematomas, which are often associated with nasal fractures, are a unilateral or bilateral accumulation of blood between the septal cartilage and the overlying mucoperichondrium. These hematomas should be treated promptly by incision and evacuation of the clot to prevent a permanent "saddlenose" deformity caused by necrosis of the septal cartilage and abscess formation.

Zygomatic Fractures. Because of its prominent position and contour, the zygoma (also called the *malar eminence*) is highly susceptible to injury; however, because of its sturdy construction, the body of the zygoma is rarely fractured. The two most common types of zygomatic fractures are zygomatic complex fractures and zygomatic arch fractures. The usual causes of these fractures are physical assault and MVCs. Orbital floor fractures are frequently associated with zygomatic fractures and manifest similar clinical signs. Differentiation is made with x-ray films.

Clinical findings associated with zygomatic fractures include periorbital and subconjunctival ecchymosis and edema, crepitus, and paresthesia of the anterior cheek from injury of the infraorbital nerve or zygomaticotemporal branch of the fifth cranial (trigeminal) nerve. Flattening of the cheek may also occur from displacement of the zygoma. One or more of the following signs and symptoms may also appear: facial asymmetry with unilateral depression when comparing zygomatic height, decreased extraocular movement, diplopia, strabismus (deviation of the eye), enophthalmos, unilateral epistaxis, depression of the infraorbital rim, mechanical limitation of mandibular movement, trismus (limitation of movement as a result of pain), palpable "step-offs" at fracture sites, and unequal pupil height. The flight nurse must also examine the orbit to rule out injury to the globe. It is important to realize that traumatic forces sufficient to cause zygomatic, orbital, and maxillary fractures may also cause potentially fatal intracranial injury; therefore, neurologic examinations are necessary. Edema and hematomas at the site of injury may mask some clinical signs; x-ray films can confirm the presence of fractures.

Early treatment of this injury is similar to that of an orbital blow-out fracture. Preparation of the patient for transport should include loose binocular bandaging to reduce eye movement in the event of orbital soft tissue involvement, immobilization of the head, and an altitude restriction to reduce the effects of decreased barometric pressure and air expansion in damaged sinuses, which could contribute to increased intraocular pressure. Constant communication with a patient whose eyes are bandaged is imperative to alleviate anxiety and reduce intraocular pressure.

Considerable force is required to fracture the zygomatic arch. The most remarkable clinical manifestations of this injury are flattening of the lateral cheek area and the inability of the patient to open his or her mouth.[3] Additional signs and symptoms are facial asymmetry, crepitus, unilateral orbital ecchymosis, edema, and tenderness over the affected area.

Treatment during transport should focus on immobilization of the head and protection of the cervical spine because of the amount of force required to produce a zygomatic arch fracture.

Maxillary Fractures. Fractures of the maxilla may occur as isolated injuries or in combination with fractures of adjoining structures. Fractures of the middle third of the face are usually the result of a violent blunt force to the face.[6] The most common maxillary fracture involves the maxillary alveolar arch; this is a fracture of the maxillary bone (usually the anterior segment) that directly supports the teeth. Signs and symptoms include ecchymosis, dental malocclusion, and mobility of the teeth.[24]

Treatment before transport should include ensuring that the airway is cleared and removal of broken teeth, bone fragments, and blood, if present. The patient should then be transported, preferably to a facility with oral surgery capabilities, with the head immobilized to reduce motion of the fracture site and resultant pain. If oral bleeding persists and threatens to interfere with the airway, the patient should be placed in a semi-Fowler's position or higher to assist in gravitational drainage, unless this is contraindicated for another reason. Avulsed teeth should be transported with the patient for possible reimplantation.

Maxillary fractures should be reduced and stabilized as soon as possible. Endodontic consultation and intervention may also be required to preserve any teeth to which blood supply has been jeopardized. Antibiotic therapy is instituted for all alveolar fractures.

Le Fort fractures involve the middle one third of the face, which is composed of the maxillary, zygomatic, nasal, lacrimal, ethmoid, and sphenoid bones and the bony nasal septum. Specific structural weaknesses of these bones dictate the location of these fractures. Le Fort fractures are divided into three categories: Le Fort I, or transverse maxillary fractures; Le Fort II, or pyramidal fractures; and Le Fort III, or complete craniofacial disjunction. An isolated or "pure" Le Fort fracture is rare, because forces severe enough to cause Le Fort injuries usually result in multiple fractures of the midfacial bones.[6] Determination of the appropriate Le Fort fracture through correlation of historical, clinical, and radiographic data is important because proper treatment is specific to each type. Le Fort fractures may occur in combinations of any two or all three fracture types. When this occurs, treatment becomes extremely complex because of the lack of existing stable bony structures to which fractured segments are transfixed to provide stabilization and support for reduced fractures. It is recommended that antibiotics be administered to patients with any type of Le Fort fracture because of the communication between the sinus and the fracture lines.

The Le Fort I fracture is described as a horizontal fracture extending through the maxilla between the floor of the maxillary sinus and the orbital floor[3,8] (Fig. 17-1). Signs and symptoms include crepitus, ecchymosis, bilateral epistaxis, dental malocclusion, and mobility of the maxilla that can be determined by grasping the upper dental arch and attempting to manipulate it. In addition, lengthening of the face, nasal septal deformity, and paresthesia of the anterior cheek from infraorbital nerve involvement may be present.

A Le Fort II fracture is defined as a subzygomatic midfacial fracture with a floating fragment that is shaped like a pyramid and separated from the cranium and lateral aspects of the face[3] (Fig. 17-2). Consistent signs and symptoms include crepitus, ecchymosis (periorbital and subconjunctival), bilateral epistaxis, infraorbital rim defect, lengthening of the face, dental malocclusion, and paresthesia of the anterior cheek. CSF leak as a result of a cribriform plate fracture, decreased extraocular movement, diplopia, enophthalmos, limited mandibular movement, medial canthal deformity, nasal septal deformity, and unequal pupil height may also be associated with this type of fracture.

A Le Fort III fracture is a bilateral suprazygomatic fracture resulting in a floating fragment of the midfacial bones, which are totally separated from the cranial base[3] (Fig. 17-3). The clinical signs and symptoms are similar to those associated with Le Fort II fractures with the deletion of the infraorbital defect and the addition of the lateral orbital rim defect.

Because of the considerable force required to produce a fracture of this magnitude, substantial soft tissue injury is frequently associated with the Le Fort III fracture, including severe intrafacial hemorrhage that requires immediate surgical intervention. Stabilization of these fractures involves open reduction; intermaxillary fixation is sometimes used when concomitant mandibular fractures eliminate the ability to secure the maxilla to the mandible for stabilization during the healing process.

Initial treatment of the patient with Le Fort fractures includes clearing the airway of teeth, bone fragments, blood, and mucus. The airway may also be compromised by the displacement of the edematous soft palate into a traumatized oropharynx.[3,6,8] Correction of this situation requires endotracheal intubation or surgical cricothyrotomy to secure and protect the airway, because it is unlikely that an oropharyngeal or nasopharyngeal airway would be

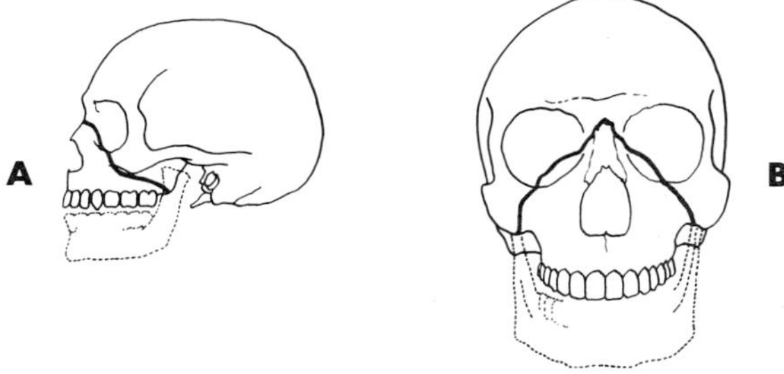

Figure 17-2. Le Fort II fracture. **A,** Lateral view. **B,** Frontal view. (From Sheehy SB: *Emergency nursing: principles and practice,* ed 3, St Louis, 1992, Mosby.)

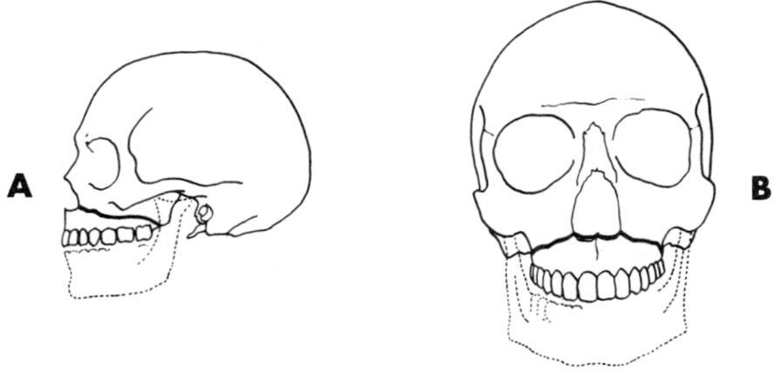

Figure 17-1. Le Fort I facial fracture. **A,** Lateral view. **B,** Frontal view. (From Sheehy SB: *Emergency nursing: principles and practice,* ed 3, St Louis, 1992, Mosby.)

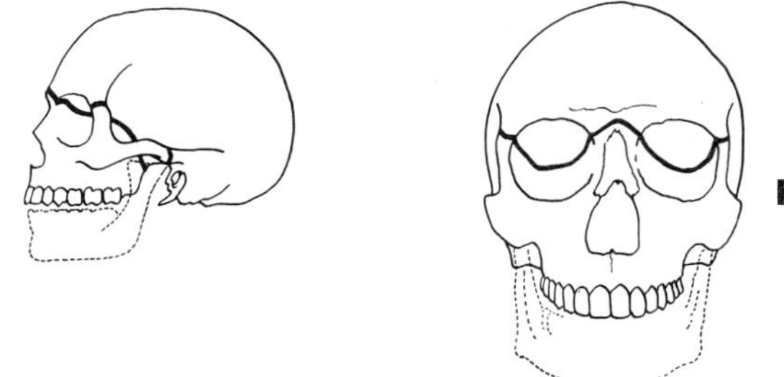

Figure 17-3. Le Fort III fracture. **A,** Lateral view. **B,** Frontal view. (From Sheehy SB: *Emergency nursing: principles and practice,* ed 3, St Louis, 1992, Mosby.)

sufficiently long to bypass the affected area. Endotracheal intubation should be performed via the oral route and should be attempted only with direct laryngoscopic visualization to prevent accidental intubation of the brain through a cribriform plate fracture. An orogastric tube may also be placed with use of direct visualization. Nasotracheal intubation and nasogastric tube placement should not be attempted. In addition, assisted ventilation may be required, and the flight nurse should administer oxygen for all traumatic injuries of this severity.

Immobilization of the head and cervical spine are imperative, because the magnitude of force required to create Le Fort fractures can also produce associated cervical injuries. Hemorrhage within the facial structures may occur, particularly with Le Fort III fractures that result in complete craniofacial disjunction. Fluid replacement with a crystalloid solution is initiated to assist in the prevention of shock. When possible, and if time permits, missing teeth should be transported with the patient for possible replantation.

During interfacility transports with patients who have had their fractures stabilized with wires or rubber bands attaching the maxilla to the mandible, it is essential that the flight nurse know how to immediately release the devices in the event the patient begins to vomit. Wires either have a quick release mechanism or need to be severed with wirecutters. Rubber bands can usually be cut with scissors. If unfamiliar stabilization devices are encountered, it is imperative that the flight nurse consult with the referral center nursing or medical staff before departing from the facility. If wirecutters are required, the flight nurse should ensure that they are available in the aircraft or packs.

Mandibular Fracture and Dislocation. The prominence and vulnerable location of the mandible make it highly susceptible to injury. Lower jaw fractures are twice as common as mid face fractures. Physical assault, MVCs, and sports-related activities account for most injuries to the mandible. In addition, significant associated injuries, such as closed head injury, fractures of facial and other bones, and major lacerations of the face, tongue, and scalp, have been present in approximately 40% of patients with fractures of the mandible.[6] Initial management of the patient requires particular attention to associated airway and cervical spine disorders. A compromised airway may result from grossly displaced fractures, prolapse of the tongue as a result of mandibular arch instability, and the presence of blood, mucus, and avulsed or broken teeth. Cervical spine injury should always be suspected in the presence of serious head and facial trauma.

Patients with mandibular fractures may manifest any combination of the following clinical signs and symptoms, depending on the type of fractures incurred. The most consistent physical finding is dental malocclusion with a lateral crossbite.[8] Additional findings may include facial asymmetry, preauricular edema on the fractured side, deviation of the mandible toward the fractured side with opening of the mouth, limitation of mandibular movement caused by structural defects and/or pain, ecchymosis over the fracture site, crepitus over the fracture site, lengthening of the face with a bilateral fracture, paresthesia of the lower lip and chin from inferior alveolar nerve damage, abnormal mobility of the teeth, and tenderness on palpation of affected areas. Intraoral damage may also occur with ecchymosis, mucosal disruption, a hematoma on the floor of the mouth, fractured or displaced teeth, and bleeding from the mouth. Forceful muscular contractions of the anterior depressor (retractor) group and posterior elevator group can cause significant displacement of the bone fragments with resultant severe pain.

Dislocation of the mandible occurs when the mandibular condyles are unilaterally or bilaterally forced to a position anterior to the articular eminence of the temporal bone. Severe spasm in the muscles of mastication causes extreme pain and the familiar open-bite deformity common to this injury. Dental malocclusion and limitation of mandibular movements from structural defect and pain also occur. In unilateral dislocation injuries, the chin tends to deviate to the side opposite the dislocation, whereas bilateral dislocation causes lengthening of the face.

Initial management of the patient with mandibular injuries should focus on clearing the airway and maintaining cervical alignment immobilization. After assessment, treatment, and stabilization of other associated injuries, the mandible may be immobilized with use of a circumferential head dressing (Barton's bandage) to support the damaged structures, restrict jaw movement, and minimize pain. The flight nurse must be able to quickly loosen this dressing to provide access to the airway in the event that the patient vomits.

Any device used to cause fixation of the mandible to the maxilla and close the mouth must have a quick release method to permit access to the airway in the event that the patient vomits. This may be in the form of a quick-release mechanism, wirecutters, or scissors, and the flight nurse must ensure that equipment is available on the aircraft for this purpose. Antibiotic therapy with penicillin or ampicillin is routinely administered to patients with fractures that are open to the oral cavity, communicate through the skin, or involve the region of the dental roots. Mandibular dislocations are manually repositioned as soon as possible with use of a muscle relaxant, sedative, or occasionally a general anesthetic.

ANTERIOR NECK TRAUMA

Mechanism of Injury

Anterior neck injuries are caused by either blunt or penetrating trauma. Blunt trauma, in the form of externally applied anterior-posterior forces, can compress the larynx and trachea against the cervical vertebrae, causing fracture and dislocation of the cartilages, avulsion of the epiglottis, vocal cords, and ligaments, and injury to the vessels and nerves, with resultant airway deficiencies. The most common cause of injury in blunt neck trauma is an MVC. When seat belts are not worn, motor vehicle occupants risk striking their necks on the dashboard and, in the case of the driver, the steering wheel. The use of two-point lap belts (without the shoulder harness) reduces fatalities but allows the neck to be thrown forward, resulting in hyperextension injuries.

Normal Anatomy and Physiology

Sports and recreational activities also contribute significantly to blunt injuries of the anterior neck. Contact sports such as boxing, wrestling, karate, basketball, football, and hockey encourage sudden, unexpected neck blows. Recreational pursuits, including riding motorcycles and all-terrain vehicles, jet skiing, waterskiing, horseback riding, snowmobiling, and snow skiing, can lead to "clotheslining" injuries of the neck from running into wires, ropes, and fences.[5] A "clothesline" injury often results in complete separation of the larynx and trachea.

The industrial environment can be the setting for strangulation-type injuries caused by clothing (e.g., a scarf or tie), jewelry, or equipment (e.g., a rope or cords) that is worn around the neck being caught in machinery. Air medical crew members themselves are at risk for this type of injury when they wear stethoscopes and other paraphernalia around their necks in the presence of violent, incoherent patients.

Penetrating injuries to the anterior neck are most frequently caused by violent altercations. Stab wounds from knives, screwdrivers, ice picks, scissors, and a host of other conceivable weapons are common. Penetrating wounds also result from flying missiles, especially bullets. The energy transmitted by a bullet allows wide dissipation and severe destruction of tissue within and outside its path. Large portions of soft tissue and cartilaginous support structures can frequently be completely displaced by the explosive effect.[5]

Skeletal Structures

Of foremost importance among skeletal structures is the larynx, which is primarily responsible for ensuring a passageway for respiration through a system of cartilaginous and valvular structures that allow air into the pulmonary tree while preventing other substances from being aspirated. The larynx is located below the root of the tongue and hyoid bone and at the uppermost section of the trachea. The thyroid cartilage is the most prominent in the larynx and serves as an anatomic landmark in performing cricothyrotomies. It also provides support to the epiglottis and vocal cords. The cricoid cartilage, which articulates with the thyroid cartilage inferiorly, differs from the other laryngeal and tracheal cartilages in that it is the only completely intact ring.[21] The arytenoid cartilage forms true joints with the cricoid cartilage. They are susceptible to traumatic dislocation from anterior-posterior forces to the larynx.

This type of injury causes narrowing of the glottic airway, resulting in obstruction and decreased mobility of the vocal cords.[5]

The larynx is somewhat protected from injury by the forward position of the mandible, the sternum, and the clavicles. Most of the time the head instinctively drops forward to cover the anterior neck with the mandible and it receives the major impact. In addition, intercartilaginous ligaments render the laryngeal and tracheal cartilages relatively mobile and serve to dissipate external sudden forces.[5,16,17]

The trachea lies anterior to the esophagus and is the connecting structure between the larynx and the main bronchi. It consists of a series of C-shaped cartilages that do not communicate posteriorly. The trachea is lined with mucous membrane and cilia (small hairlike structures) that assist in keeping the airway free of foreign substances. Posterior to the trachea lies the esophagus. This hollow organ extends from the pharynx to the stomach and is an integral part of the digestive system. It consists of an outer fibrous tissue, a muscular layer, a submucous layer, and an inner mucous membrane. The esophagus and larynx communicate at the laryngeal/pharyngeal aspect of the throat. The soft palate and epiglottis close to form a seal over the larynx to protect it from aspiration during swallowing.

The thyroid gland is positioned just below the thyroid cartilage and anterior and lateral to the trachea. It is the largest of the endocrine glands and produces hormones, including thyroxine and triiodothyronine, that serve to promote normal growth and metabolism. The thyroid gland also stores iodine.

Muscles

The muscles of the neck provide support and some lateral protection of vital structures, such as the internal jugular and carotids, from injury. The anterior larynx and trachea are not covered by muscular tissue and are therefore more vulnerable to the effects of impacting forces.

Vascular Structures

The common carotid arteries lie lateral and somewhat posterior to the larynx and trachea. Further down the trachea, the subclavian artery emerges. The subclavian vein passes in front of the lower trachea and branches into the internal and external jugular veins that are located in the lateral aspect of the neck. In addition, the thyroid vein (a bifurcation of the subclavian vein) and the thyroid artery serve to vascularize the thyroid gland. The larynx is supplied with blood by the superior and inferior laryngeal arterial branches of the thyroid arteries and their accompanying veins. Disruption of the major vessels in the neck could cause severe hemorrhage and shock and contribute to airway obstruction in the form of aspiration of blood and hematomas applying pressure to the airway structures.

Nerves

The superior laryngeal nerve, which lies in the supraglottic/glottic area, is responsible for pharyngeal sensation and the ability to handle secretions. Immediately lateral to the cricothyroid joint are the recurrent laryngeal nerves, which contribute to vocal cord function and the ability to speak (phonation).

Assessment

All patients with major head or chest trauma should be evaluated for neck injuries. Because injury to the anterior neck could have devastating effects on the airway, it must be checked immediately for any obstruction from loss of structural integrity of the laryngeal or tracheal cartilages, soft tissue edema causing pressure on or within the airway, or foreign substances such as blood, vomitus, and bone or cartilage fragments. The airway may also be compromised by a penetrating wound that communicates to the outside, thus creating a leak in the respiratory system. Symptoms of respiratory distress may include dyspnea, inspiratory stridor, cyanosis, and changes in voice quality. Any indications of respiratory distress require prompt treatment with suctioning, oxygen and, if warranted, invasive support by nasal or endotracheal intubation or surgical cricothyrotomy. The flight nurse must also suspect cervical spine injury and maintain anatomic alignment and immobility until C-spine injury is ruled out.

External evaluation consists of visually examining the neck for any signs of trauma. The skin is checked for lacerations, abrasions, and puncture wounds. Any soft tissue edema and hematomas should be noted and evaluated for potential airway compromise. Evidence of strangulation, such as bruising, should also be noted. Subcutaneous emphysema and crepitus may be present and indicative of a tear in the pharynx, esophagus, or trachea that can extend from the face to the groin.[5,8,13] The flight nurse should palpate the trachea to determine stability of the laryngeal and tracheal cartilages and to check for midline position. Flattening of the cricothyroid prominence indicates probable laryngeal collapse. The trachea should also be auscultated to ensure the presence of airflow. The flight nurse should then palpate and auscultate the carotid arteries to determine the presence of adequate circulation. If conscious, the patient can be asked to respond verbally so that vocalization ability can be evaluated. Vocalization ability can range from mild hoarseness to complete aphonia, the latter indicating possible vocal cord involvement.

Internal evaluation of the neck consists of a laryngoscopic examination, which should be performed very carefully and gently to prevent further damage. The posterior pharynx should be evaluated for any potential obstructive substances, lacerations, and soft tissue edema. The flight nurse should evaluate the epiglottis for proper position and functioning and should look primarily for avulsion, a major contributor to aspiration problems. Any edema of the epiglottis should be noted because it can obstruct the airway. Extreme caution is warranted when performing laryngoscopic examination under these circumstances because of potential irritation of the epiglottis by the laryngoscope blade, causing further edema. The flight nurse should also examine the larynx for evidence of aspiration, structural integrity of the surrounding cartilage, and appearance of the vocal cords, and should check at that time for lacerations, avulsion, and edema.

Pathophysiology and Treatment

Airway management and ventilation are particularly significant in the case of anterior neck trauma, considering the vulnerability of the larynx and trachea. Patients with no symptoms or minimal symptoms may subsequently experience rapid progression of edema with loss of airway and should be monitored closely. The flight nurse should also control hemorrhage and shock. Any trauma involving the major vessels of the neck requires immediate intervention to prevent exsanguination. Supportive therapy for all patients with anterior neck injuries includes immobilization, elevation of the head and neck (if not contraindicated), oxygen with cool mist humidification, continuous neurologic examinations, and tetanus toxoid for any wounds.

Blunt trauma to the anterior aspect of the neck may cause injury to soft tissue (abrasions, contusions, and hematomas), laryngeal nerves, the thyroid gland, the epiglottis, and vocal cords, as well as fracture-dislocation of the laryngeal and tracheal cartilages. Penetrating trauma can produce these injuries plus lacerations, puncture wounds, and injury to the major vessels in the neck. It is common for both blunt and penetrating trauma to be involved.[7,16,17,26]

Soft Tissue Injuries

Hematoma and Edema

Hematomas of the anterior neck may cause sufficient pressure on the airway as to result in respiratory distress. Because evacuation of hematomas in the field is not recommended, the airway should be protected from constriction by use of an endo- or nasotracheal tube. Oxygen administered via cool humidification may assist in retarding further swelling. If not contraindicated by other injuries, elevating the patient's head and neck in a semi-Fowler's (or higher) sitting position will prevent additional pooling of blood and assist drainage of the area.

Edema of the pharynx, larynx, trachea, epiglottis, and vocal cords causes respiratory distress and may result in complete airway obstruction. Endotracheal intubation under direct laryngoscopy should be performed at the first sign of respiratory dysfunction. Once an edematous airway is obstructed, surgical cricothyrotomy becomes necessary to establish an open airway. Laryngoscopy, in the presence of edema, should be performed extremely carefully and gently because any irritation of the tissue by the laryngoscope blade or endotracheal tube could exacerbate the problem to the point that the flight nurse may not be able to pass the tube at all. For this reason, blind intubating should be performed rarely or avoided if possible. When edema is present, use of a smaller endotracheal tube may be necessary to ensure passage through the swollen airway. Cool humidified oxygen and elevation of the head and neck (if not contraindicated) may provide additional benefits to managing airway edema.

Lacerations and Puncture Wounds

Lacerations and puncture wounds, which are usually the result of penetrating trauma, can have devastating effects on the vital structures in the neck.[33] Superficial lacerations and puncture wounds need only be cleansed and covered with a clean dressing. For oozing wounds, the flight nurse must reinforce the dressing as it becomes soiled with drainage instead of changing it. Opening the wound to the aircraft environment can increase the chance of infection. The flight nurse should also ascertain when the patient last had a tetanus shot.

When a patient has deep, penetrating wounds, bleeding must be controlled by direct pressure. Suctioning will be necessary if blood accumulates in the airway. The flight nurse must determine the presence of any associated underlying injuries, including damage to the major blood vessels, nerves, thyroid gland, or laryngeal/tracheal structures, and treat the patient accordingly. Deep or extensive lacerations and puncture wounds require subsequent exploration, debridement, and antibiotic therapy.

The location of the carotid arteries and internal jugular veins in the neck renders them extremely vulnerable to injury. Laceration of these major vessels can result in rapid exsanguination if bleeding is not controlled. In addition, the major vascular supply to the larynx is from the superior and inferior laryngeal arterial branches of the superior and inferior thyroid arteries and their accompanying veins. Disruption of these vessels can cause severe hemorrhage. Controlling hemorrhage by means of constant direct pressure is imperative. If the flight nurse is unable to control the bleeding in this manner, the vessels can be clamped as a last resort with use of sterile clamps or even the flight nurse's fingers. Fluid replacement should be aggressive with use of whole blood, when available, or plasma expanders or crystalloid solution to control shock. The flight nurse should apply pressure only to the affected vessels; for instance, obstructing both carotid arteries when only one side is affected will obstruct blood flow to the brain. As with all trauma patients, oxygen should be administered. If the vessels are hemorrhaging internally, blood may accumulate in the airway, causing obstruction and aspiration. In this case, suctioning along with endotracheal intubation will be necessary to maintain a clear patient airway. Definitive therapy includes surgical repair and administration of antibiotics.

Nerve Injury

Damage to the recurrent laryngeal nerve will result in dysfunction of the vocal cords. Paralysis of this nerve will cause a weak, breathy voice and cough and the potential for aspiration. Atrophy of the vocal cords usually develops over the course of a few weeks and may not be immediately apparent. Trauma to this nerve can occur with a cricoid injury, laryngotracheal separation, or compression of the cricoid and arytenoid articulation. After the initial assessment is completed, the flight nurse should immobilize the patient's head and neck region and instruct the patient not to speak or cough to prevent further damage; he or she should also monitor the patient closely for evidence of aspiration and protect the airway as necessary.

Injury to the superior laryngeal nerve is common in supraglottic and glottic trauma. Damage caused by contusion, stretching, or division of this nerve results in loss of pharyngeal sensation and the ability to manage secretions. Thus the patient will not be able to feel foreign substances in the throat and will need to be carefully observed for respiratory distress as a result of airway obstruction. Assistance with managing secretions is also necessary to prevent aspiration.

Surgical repair and anastomosis of injured nerves, when attempted after edema has subsided, have reportedly met with limited success. Spontaneous recovery, if it occurs, will usually take place in 6 to 12 months.

Thyroid Gland Injury

The location of the thyroid gland on either side of the upper trachea and anterior to the larynx makes it a prime target for injury associated with anterior neck trauma. Because this organ is highly vascular in nature (the thyroid gland has one of the highest rates of blood flow of all the organs in the body), hemorrhage becomes the primary concern in case of injury. Bleeding should be controlled by direct pressure while the patient is closely evaluated for airway obstruction and shock. Suctioning, airway management, fluid replacement, oxygen administration, and immobilization of the head and neck are integral to treatment of the patient with a thyroid gland injury. Surgical intervention will usually include repair or cauterization of vessels or, depending on the severity of the injury, removal of the damaged tissue. Long-term effects of thyroid gland damage may necessitate supplemental thyroid hormone therapy.

Laryngeal and Tracheal Injury

Fracture or dislocation of the laryngeal and tracheal cartilages can present grave consequences to the respiratory system through loss of structural integrity and the presence of bone fragments and blood in the airway. It is important to note that calcification and ossification of the larynx and trachea occur around the age of 20 years. Before that age, the cartilages are flexible and will usually rebound instead of sustaining true fractures. Blunt trauma in patients under age 20 years usually manifests in nerve and joint damage.

A hyoid bone fracture often occurs as an isolated sports injury. Depending on the severity of the force causing the fracture, laceration and distortion of the epiglottis may result. Intense pain, dysphagia, and crepitus are common with this type of injury. Airway obstruction may also occur as a result of partial severance of the epiglottis.

Separation of the hyoid and thyroid cartilages may also produce dislocation of the epiglottis, leading to problems with aspiration. Severance of the thyrohyoid membrane may also occur, resulting in an air leak and subcutaneous emphysema.

Fractures of the thyroid cartilage complex may be either linear or comminuted with varying degrees of internal derangement. Associated damage may include avulsion of the epiglottis and vocal cords, laceration of the mucous membranes, and dislocation of the arytenoids. Blood and bone fragments are likely to exist in the larynx, causing obstruction to the airway.

Cricothyroid dislocation can be a serious and subtle injury and is often seen in "clothesline" accidents in which a person runs into a stretched wire or cord that strikes between the cricoid and thyroid cartilages, forcing them apart and dislocating the cricoarytenoid joints. Patients recovering from this injury face significant risk of manifesting ankylosis, laryngeal stenosis, and "end stage" laryngeal disease.[6]

A cricoid fracture is often found in association with a thyroid cartilage fracture. Laryngeal nerve paralysis is common in cricoid fractures and laryngotracheal avulsion injuries.

Tracheal fracture occurs either between the tracheal rings or at the cricotracheal junction. Avulsion of the trachea from the larynx occurs from tearing of the cricotracheal membrane. This injury often results in immediate death from severe respiratory obstruction and leakage of air into subcutaneous tissues. When a patient sustains this injury, the trachea should be clamped or occluded with Vaseline gauze and taped for external stability. Immediate intubation should be performed for internal stability and airway control. Bilateral transection of the recurrent laryngeal nerves commonly occurs in this type of injury. In addition, esophageal tears may also occur.

Patients with any type of laryngeal and tracheal injuries require immediate evaluation for respiratory distress and subsequent airway management. Suctioning is necessary to remove blood and bone fragments lodged in the airway. Intubation provides internal stability to damaged areas, protection of the airway, and a means for ventilation. Humidified oxygen should be administered, fluids should be replaced, and the head and neck should be immobilized, and the patient should be transported immediately to the nearest appropriate facility.

Esophageal Injury

Because of its position posterior to the trachea, the esophagus is somewhat protected from external forces. However, esophageal injury may be associated with tracheal fractures, penetrating trauma from stab wounds or gunshot wounds, or ingestion of caustic substances. Blood draining into the stomach from esophageal tears can cause regurgitation, which is particularly dangerous when the airway is already compromised by other injuries resulting in, for example, dysfunction of the epiglottis.

Esophageal rupture results in a high mortality rate. Serious complications manifest when gastric contents spill into the chest cavity, causing mediastinitis. The patient may experience pain on swallowing, dyspnea, subcutaneous emphysema, pneumothorax, and gastric contents in the chest tube. A pleural effusion or air in the mediastinum may be seen on x-ray films. Surgical intervention is required to repair the injury.[1,20,27,29,30,32]

Placement of a nasogastric tube in the presence of esophageal injury should be accomplished very carefully to prevent further tissue damage or inadvertent intubation of the mediastinum. A nasogastic tube provides drainage of gastric contents, minimizes the chance of vomiting, and reduces further contamination of the mediastinum. When placing a nasogastric tube, the flight nurse can minimize the risk of aggravating esophageal injuries by advancing the tube gently and slowly without forcing it past obstructions and may use a tube with a smaller diameter for less traumatic placement. For active esophageal bleeding, iced saline solution flushes may be used. A Sengstaken-Blakemore tube, which is often used for treatment of esophageal varices, may prove beneficial in controlling bleeding by asserting direct pressure within the esophagus. In addition, the patient should receive oxygen and fluid replacement. Placing the patient in a semi-Fowler's or Fowler's position (if not contraindicated) will assist in preventing reflux of gastric contents and further irritation of the esophagus.

EYE TRAUMA

Mechanism of Injury

Severe injury to the eye can result in a reduction of visual acuity, cosmetic deformities of the face, and, most tragically, blindness. Traumatic forces to the face and head can cause direct or indirect injury to the globe of the eye, the eyelids, optic nerve, optic blood vessels, lacrimal apparatus, and bony orbital structures. The globe and optic nerve may be damaged by penetrating displaced bone fragments. The optic nerve is more likely to be affected by compression of the optic foramen or shearing at the optic chiasm (the junction in the forebrain where nerve fibers from the medial side of the retina cross over to join fibers of the opposite retina). Motor vehicle accidents, accidents resulting from sports and recreational activities, violent altercations, and household and industrial accidents are responsible for the vast majority of blunt and penetrating injuries to the eye.[2,19,22]

Unrestrained car occupants frequently sustain severe facial and eye trauma in MVCs. Drivers not wearing seat belts with shoulder harnesses often strike their faces on the steering wheel and, along with unrestrained front seat passengers, the dashboard and windshield. These accidents usually cause damage to the bony orbital structures with potential involvement of the globe, eye muscles, and optic nerve. Motorcyclists who do not wear helmets with protective face shields or goggles often have foreign bodies in the form of bugs, rocks, dirt, and sand embedded in their eye(s). These riders are at significant risk for severe facial and ocular injuries, especially when their faces strike asphalt, trees, or other vehicles.

Sports injuries to the eye result when persons are hit by tennis balls, racquet balls, squash balls, handballs, hockey pucks and sticks, and baseballs. Larger objects (baseballs) tend to cause orbital blow-out fractures, whereas objects smaller than the orbital rim (handballs) cause direct injury to the globe. Blows to the head and eye area can have a contrecoup effect resulting in rupture of the globe and retinal detachment opposite the impact site. Swimming in improperly treated pools can cause chemical burns to the eye. Ultraviolet corneal burns from overexposure to the sun reflecting off snow can result when snow skiing. Most ocular sports injuries can be prevented with use of helmets and protective eyewear or goggles specifically designed for the sport activity.

Darts, BB guns, and pellet guns have all been responsible for penetrating eye injuries. Various forms of fireworks such as flares and sparklers cause serious eye trauma every year, especially during holiday periods.[23]

Violent altercations often result in severe injury to the eye. Fists, rocks, guns, knives, ice picks, and screwdrivers all make formidable weapons. Mace and tear gas usually cause significant but only temporary discomfort without permanent damage.

Household and industrial accidents account for the greatest number of burns to and foreign bodies in the eyes. Chemical burns can be caused by most household and industrial cleaning products when they are splashed or sprayed into the eyes. Chemical burns are caused by alkalis or acids. Alkali burns caused by lye (NaOH or KOH), fresh lime (CaO), and ammonia are the most frequent in the United States.[2] Alkali burns usually cause more damage to the eye than do acid burns, with the exception of extremely strong acids (such as hydrofluoric acid) and acids that contain heavy metals. Thermal burns to the eye are caused by flames, steam, explosions, flying ashes, or molten metal. Glassblowers, welders, and metal-furnace stokers are susceptible to infrared flash burns. Radiation burns result from atomic blasts and accidents, which mostly occur at nuclear power facilities. Ocular sequelae may also develop in patients receiving radiation treatment for head and neck cancer. Industrial laser accidents are becoming more common and result in macular burns. Accidentally gazing into a laser beam can have sudden and tragic consequences.[2,12,15,28]

Intraocular foreign bodies frequently become embedded when a person neglects to wear safety goggles. Hammering, chiseling, and drilling often create minute chips that can become embedded in the eyes. Blast injuries cause multiple foreign bodies of glass, metal, and wood to become embedded in the eyes. Foreign bodies are often contaminated with dirt, oil, and grease, which can further complicate the injury. Objects thrown from lawn mowers and mixers and high-pressure hoses and sandblasters can cause severe ocular trauma. Domestic and wild animal bites are also responsible for eye injuries, especially in small children who unintentionally aggravate an animal.

Normal Anatomy and Physiology

The eye is a delicate organ that is partially protected from injury by the bony orbital rim and malar eminences (cheekbones) of the face. These structures protrude slightly past the globe of the eye and receive the brunt of the impact when the offending object is larger than the eyeball. The eyelid protects the eye from becoming dehydrated and from contamination by foreign substances. The outer section of the eye consists of the cornea, sclera, and Tenon's capsule. The cornea is the clear, transparent structure covering the anterior aspect of the eye. Light passes through the cornea en route to the retina to produce vision. The sclera is the opaque, tough, fibrous layer that covers approximately five sixths of the eye from where it meets the cornea (posteriorly to the optic nerve). The sclera is white but may turn yellow in the presence of jaundice or orange with use of the drug rifampin. Tenon's capsule is a loose connective tissue that covers the sclera and becomes continuous with the dura (external sheath) of the optic nerve and mucosal lining of the sinuses surrounding the orbit.[10]

The middle area of the eye, called the uveal tract, consists of the iris, ciliary body, and choroid. The iris is located behind the cornea and functions as a diaphragm to control the amount of light that passes through the pupil and the retina. Muscle fibers, innervated by the third cranial nerve, allow the pupil to dilate and contract in response to available light.

The ciliary body connects the iris to the choroid and is composed of ciliary muscle and ciliary processes. The ciliary muscle is responsible for accommodation of the lens, affecting the degree of visual acuity from myopia (nearsightedness) to hyperopia (farsightedness). The ciliary body also produces aqueous humor, a free-flowing clear fluid that occupies the space anterior and lateral to the lens. Aqueous humor is continuously formed and reabsorbed through Schlemm's canal. The balance between the formation and reabsorption of this substance determines intraocular pressure.

The choroid is a highly vascular layer of the eye underlying the sclera and adhering to the retina. Whereas the retina has its own blood supply from the central retinal artery, the outer layers containing the rods and cones are dependent on the supply of blood from the choroid, as is the entire macular area.

The retina is the light-sensitive portion of the eye that surrounds the vitreous body. The rods and cones located within the retina detect light and color. The macula, which is in the center of the retina, is about I square millimeter in size and is composed entirely of cones, making it especially capable of acute and detailed vision. The central portion of the macula is called the fovea, which is the area of clearest vision because of the retinal layers being displaced to one side, which allows light to fall directly on the cones. The point at which the optic nerve leaves the eye has no rods or cones and is therefore called the blind spot.

The three chambers of the eye are the anterior chamber, posterior chamber, and vitreous cavity. The anterior chamber is the area posterior to the cornea and anterior to the iris. The posterior chamber occupies the space between the iris and the lens. Both anterior and posterior chambers contain aqueous humor. The largest area within the eye is the vitreous cavity, which lies posterior to the lens and is surrounded by the retina. The chamber contains vitreous humor, a clear gelatinous mass held together by a network of fine fibers. The vitreous humor acts to diffuse light to the retina and gives structure to the posterior globe of the eye.

Ocular Nerves and Muscles

Cranial nerves II, III, IV, and VI are primarily involved with ocular functions. The rods and cones in the retina contain biochemicals that decompose on exposure to light, thereby exciting the optic nerve (cranial nerve II) fibers. The neural impulse travels from the optic nerve to the optic chiasm and on through the optic tracts, which lead to the visual cortex in the occipital lobe of the brain where visual images are recognized and interpreted. Cranial nerves III, IV, and VI are related to ocular movements. These three nerves are responsible for controlling the ocular muscles to ensure that both eyes function in concert and remain parallel through all movements. The oculomotor nerve also functions to constrict the pupil and elevate the upper eyelid.

Assessment

Assessment of the eye involves evaluation of the external structures, visual acuity, EOMs, and, if time permits and an ophthalmoscope is available, internal structures as well.[4] Examination should be performed very carefully and gently with no pressure applied to the orbital rims or globe that could cause further injury. It is also essential that the flight nurse obtain a historical account of the traumatic event to fully evaluate the injury.

The bony orbital rims are gently palpated to determine stability, depressions, and crepitus. The eyelids are examined for lacerations, avulsions, edema, contusion, and foreign bodies. Cranial nerve III (oculomotor) is assessed by having the patient elevate his or her upper eyelids, and cranial nerve VIII (facial) is assessed by having the patient close the eyes. Inability to close the eyes could result in severe dehydration of the corneas. If the eyelids are swollen shut and the patient cannot voluntarily open them, the flight nurse should not attempt to force them open because that could lead to further injury. The remainder of the evaluation would have to be deferred and should be charted as such.

If the patient is able to open his or her eyes, the flight nurse should next evaluate visual acuity. A pocket-sized visual acuity chart is used, if available. Otherwise, anything with printing on it, including transport forms, equipment packaging, and intravenous bags, can serve. The flight nurse must remember to document the distance the object was held from the face. The patient should be asked to read the print with one eye at a time; the other eye should be covered with anything that will occlude vision without applying any pressure. The injured eye is tested first and the resulting data are interpreted by determining the patient's normal visual acuity and comparing the results of the injured eye to the unaffected eye. Diminished visual acuity in the injured eye may indicate a partial dislocation of the lens. The flight nurse should also note whether the patient normally wears glasses or contacts and should check vision with corrective lenses first, if they are already being worn, and then without them. The patient must be able to read to participate in this exercise; illiteracy or foreign language limitations will require alternate methods of evaluation. If the patient is unable to read or see the print, the flight nurse can test for the ability to count fingers at a distance.

Extraocular movements are evaluated by having the patient follow the flight nurse's finger through the six cardinal positions of gaze while keeping his or her head still and facing forward. The flight nurse can observe for nystagmus by having the patient hold the lateral and upward gaze for a few moments. EOMs test for functioning of cranial nerves III, IV, and VI, as well as ocular muscles.

The flight nurse should observe the conjunctiva for hemorrhage and foreign bodies. Localized subconjunctival hemorrhage may indicate perforation of the globe.[8] Conjunctival crepitus results from fractures of the paranasal sinuses and appears as tiny bubbles in subconjunctiva. If the flight nurse suspects a chemical burn, he or she should search for any particulate matter in the conjunctival folds and remove it with a cotton swab. The flight nurse should examine the conjunctiva of the upper lid by everting the lid over the stick end of a cotton applicator.

The sclera is evaluated for any change in color and for the presence of blood. Lacerations and abrasions of the cornea are difficult to detect without fluorescein staining and an ultraviolet light. Foreign bodies and the presence of corneal opacity should also be noted. The flight nurse should also check for the presence of contact lenses (hard or soft) and evidence of an ocular prosthesis.

The flight nurse should observe the anterior chamber for depression or shallowing that may indicate choroidal hemorrhage or detachment, or leakage from a penetrating wound, and should note any presence of hyphema (blood in the anterior chamber), estimating the size in millimeters.[8] Exophthalmos (protrusion) or enophthalmos (posterior displacement) of the globe should be noted and may indicate orbital fractures or hemorrhage.

A thorough examination of the pupils is critical to assessing ocular trauma and intracranial injuries. Intracranial injury should always be suspected after severe trauma to the eye. The flight nurse should evaluate the pupils for size, shape, equality, and direct and consensual reaction to light and should shine a light directly into the eye to test for a direct light response. Shining the light into one pupil and checking the response in the other determines consensual light response. A fixed and dilated pupil may indicate direct injury to the globe, increased intracranial pressure, direct injury to the third cranial nerve, or a previously instilled mydriatic drug. In the case of oculomotor (cranial nerve III) nerve damage, pupillary dilation is often associated with other manifestations such as ptosis (drooping eyelid) and extraocular muscle function. An ocular prosthesis will also give false data.

If time and circumstances permit, performing an ophthalmoscopic examination can provide essential information regarding the internal structures of the eye. The flight nurse may shine the ophthalmoscope light initially on the pupil to observe for any opacity of the lens and, looking beyond, see the optic disc come into view and appear red-orange in color, smooth, and round or vertically oval. The flight nurse can also observe the optic disc for any signs of papilledema, which is edema and hyperemia (excess blood), an indication of increased intracranial pressure. Blood vessels should be followed from the disc to the margin of the fundus while observing for abnormalities, including nicking. Veins are normally larger and darker and they pulsate, whereas arterioles are smaller, brighter, and do not pulsate.[10] The flight nurse can also examine the patient for hemorrhages, exudate, retinal edema, foreign bodies, and posterior perforation of the globe. If possible, the flight nurse can have the patient look directly into the light so the macula and fovea can be examined.

X-rays are used to detect orbital fractures and foreign bodies within the eye. CT is valuable for finding foreign material within the eye that is not visible by other radiographic techniques. Wood, plastic, glass, and metals of low density are all clearly visible in the CT scan.[2]

Pathophysiology and Treatment

Although eye injuries are not life threatening in themselves, they can have devastating consequences, including blindness. Eye injuries should be evaluated and treated only after life-threatening problems have been addressed and the patient is stabilized. Eye injury should always be suspected in the presence of maxillofacial and intracranial injuries.

Eyelid Lacerations

Eyelid lacerations may be superficial or full-thickness in nature. Initial treatment consists of controlling bleeding, irrigating the area with saline solution, and applying a sterile dressing. Careful examination of the eye is required to determine any associated injuries to the globe. Definitive therapy requires debridement, a search for foreign bodies, and layer-by-layer closure of the tissue with fine-suture material.

In the event of partially or completely avulsed eyelids, priority must be given to protecting the globe from severe dehydration and foreign bodies. A piece of plastic can be placed over the eye during transport to maintain moisture and prevent contamination by foreign substances. The flight nurse should seal the edges of the plastic to the skin surrounding the eye with use of ointment or tape. Because eyelid tissue can be grafted, the scene of the accident should be searched for any avulsed pieces to transport with the patient for reimplantation.

Corneal Abrasions, Scratches, and Lacerations

Disruption of the corneal tissue can be caused by any foreign body in the eye. Contact lenses are the most prevalent cause of corneal abrasions as a result of overuse and the presence of foreign substances between the lens and cornea. Any erosion of the corneal epithelial cells causes sudden onset of pain, lacrimation, photophobia, blepharospasm, and the sensation of the presence of a foreign body. Blinking and extraocular movements are instinctive but only aggravate the problem.[25] Initial treatment involves examining the eye for the presence of foreign bodies, irrigation with saline solution, and loose binocular bandaging to reduce eye movements. It may be extremely difficult for the patient with painful corneal trauma to keep his or her eyes open long enough for examination or irrigation. An ophthalmic analgesic (e.g., proparacaine hydrochloride [Ophthaine]) may be necessary for the patient to tolerate such procedures. Definitive therapy includes evaluation with fluorescein staining and fluorescent light to determine the extent and location of epithelial damage and application of a semi-pressure eye patch. When applying the eye patch, the flight nurse should ensure that the eyelids are completely closed and that the dressing is sufficiently firm to prevent the lids from opening and closing beneath it. Corneal abrasions and scratches usually resolve in 24 to 48 hours. Superficial corneal lacerations rarely need suturing unless there is loss of substance or a gaping wound.[8] Whenever the eye has been lacerated, the flight nurse must be careful to avoid any pressure on the globe to prevent extrusion of intraocular contents. X-rays of any corneal lacerations should be taken to rule out the presence of foreign bodies.[8]

Foreign Bodies

Foreign bodies are classified as conjunctival, corneal, and intraocular. Conjunctival foreign bodies are located by everting the eyelids. Once located, the object is removed with irrigation or a sterile cotton swab. Corneal foreign bodies may or may not be visible on initial examination. Corneal foreign bodies not successfully removed by irrigation or gentle swabbing should be further evaluated with use of a slit lamp. Deeply embedded foreign bodies and resultant rust rings must ultimately be removed with an ocular spud or 25-gauge needle. The eye is then bandaged. Whenever periorbital or ocular tissues are lacerated or punctured, a retained intraorbital or intraocular foreign body should be suspected. The presence of multiple foreign bodies is common with explosions and shotgun or other blast injuries.

Protruding intraocular foreign bodies must be stabilized and covered with a protective cup or cone device secured with tape during transport to prevent further damage. The unaffected eye should also be bandaged to minimize binocular eye movements. The flight nurse should make no attempt to remove the object. An intravenous line and oxygen can be initiated while in flight to the nearest facility that has ophthalmology services available.

"Metal on metal" injuries occur when a person beats on a piece of metal with a metal hammer or chisel. The objects involved should be transported with the patient so their composition can be determined and for culturing purposes. Copper and brass are particularly destructive to the vitreous and retina and can cause tragic results. The flight nurse should also note whether the instrument that produced the damage was contaminated with oil, grease, or dirt.[2]

Because glass varies in radiodensity, any available fragment should be transported to the medical facility to be examined by x-ray for radiopacity. If it is determined not to be radiopaque, CT will be necessary to locate retained fragments. The location, size, shape, and composition of the foreign body will determine whether it ultimately can be surgically removed or must be left in place.

Burns

Burns of the eye are caused by chemicals, heat, radiation, lasers, infrared rays, and ultraviolet light. A true ocular emergency exists when burns are caused by acid or alkali. Alkaline substances pose a greater threat because of their capacity for more rapid absorption into the cornea and anterior chamber. Alkalis combine with the lipids of cellular membranes, causing total cell disruption with softening of the tissue.[8] Further penetration by additional alkaline material follows, thus creating a cycle that may persist for days or until the alkaline supply has been exhausted. Damage includes immediate corneal opacification with subsequent ischemia, coagulation necrosis of the conjunctiva and sclera, and possible perforation of the globe through the conjunctiva, sclera, choroid, and retina. Further sequelae include late glaucoma, cataracts, and dry-eye syndrome caused by destruction of the lacrimal system. An initial rise in intraocular pressure occurs from shrinkage of the outer tissues of the eye, and a rise later occurs that is attributed to scarring and sclerosis of outflow channels (Schlemm's canal).

Acidic substances cause damage within the first few hours of exposure. Acids tend to neutralize themselves by quickly precipitating tissue proteins, thereby creating a physical barrier against further penetration. Because of the buffering effect of tissue proteins, the damage tends to be localized to the area of contact. However, strong acids (such as hydrofluoric acid) and acids that contain heavy metals rapidly penetrate the cornea, causing severe marbling opacification.

Treatment of chemical burns requires immediate irrigation with copious amounts of water or saline solution. An intravenous bag of saline solution connected to intravenous tubing works well as an irrigation system. Specific devices such as the Morgan lens can help make irrigation easier. Irrigation, with use of at least 1 L per eye, should continue for a minimum of 30 minutes and be repeated for more serious burns. Ocular burns cause severe pain and orbicularis spasm, making it difficult for the patient to cooperate in the treatment process. A topical ophthalmic anesthetic (Ophthaine) provides pain relief and makes irrigation easier. After thorough irrigation, the flight nurse should examine the eyes for any particulate matter in the conjunctival folds and fornices. Double eversion of the upper lid is necessary to accomplish this examination. Any remaining particles can be removed with use of sterile cotton swabs. If the chemical container is available (and of reasonable size), transporting it with the patient permits precise identification of the agent involved.

The extent of permanent injury is a function of the nature and concentration of the chemical and the amount of elapsed time between exposure and decontamination. The extent of damage from chemical burns is often evaluated by the severity of corneal opacification, as measured by the ability to see details of the anterior chamber and iris.[2] Riot-control agents (such as Mace and tear gas) result in temporary discomfort but rarely cause permanent damage to the eyes. In cases of exposure to these agents, irrigation and complete examination are usually sufficient intervention.

Thermal burns of the eyes result from flash fires, flying cinders and ash, hot glass, and molten metals. Resultant damage may include partial and full-thickness burns of the eyelids, keratitis (inflammation of the cornea), corneal ulceration or perforation, and subsequent infection. Airway involvement must always be suspected with any facial burns. Subsequent to airway management, the flight nurse should undertake prevention of shock by administering intravenous fluids and oxygen. Protection of the cornea is imperative and may be accomplished with use of moist dressings or plastic wrap over the eye. Corneal burns are ultimately treated with topical cycloplegics (atropine and its relatives) and antibiotics; if severe scarring occurs, corneal grafts may be necessary.

Radiation burns can ultimately cause cataracts, infrared light produces heat cataracts with prolonged exposure, and ultraviolet light causes keratitis. Preliminary symptoms of ultraviolet burns usually appear 6 to 10 hours after exposure and include severe pain, photophobia, and blepharospasm. Laser beams cause macular burns with an immediate decrease in visual acuity. Because no effective emergency or long-term treatment exists for these types of burns, prophylaxis is imperative. Wearing proper eye protection and avoiding exposure are the key elements to prevention of these injuries.

Hyphema

Blood in the anterior chamber of the eye is known as a *hyphema* and is caused by a direct blow to the globe. Traumatic hyphemas are often associated with other injuries such as orbital blow-out fractures, vitreous hemorrhage, dislocation of the lens, retinal detachment, and scleral rupture. Prognosis, in the case of hyphema, is directly related to the amount of blood in the anterior chamber.[8] Small hemorrhages (4 mm in height or less) usually reabsorb in a few days with a low rate of complications. Large hyphemas are more likely to rebleed with subsequent poor prognosis. Secondary hemorrhages develop in approximately 20% of all hyphemas[2] and appear 2 to 7 days after the injury.

For unknown reasons, the presence of blood in the anterior chamber produces drowsiness. Neurologic causes should be ruled out, especially if there is any suspicion of associated head injury. Preparation for transport consists of immobilizing the patient, binocular bandaging, and elevating the head to 40 degrees. The patient should be protected from doing anything that increases intraocular pressure (e.g., straining, coughing, vomiting, or enduring a Valsalva maneuver), which would exacerbate the bleeding. Controversy regarding the most effective continued treatment of hyphemas ranges from total bed rest, sedation, and binocular bandaging to ambulation, no sedation, and bandaging of the affected eye only. The flight nurse should instill atropine in the eye for cycloplegic and mydriatic purposes. Hospitalization is necessary for daily observation of intraocular pressure, hyphema blood level, evidence of rebleeding, and corneal blood staining. If the blood does not reabsorb promptly, blood pigment enters the corneal tissue, producing blood staining in the presence of a total hyphema and elevated intraocular pressure. This opacity may persist for several years. Glaucoma is a frequent complication with hyphemas and is the result of traumatic recession of the anterior chamber angle, with subsequent impairment of aqueous flow. Chronic glaucoma may take years to develop, thereby requiring continued regular evaluations. Surgical intervention becomes necessary when intraocular pressure cannot be medically controlled or if the hyphema is large and black, indicating a clot.

Lens Dislocation and Subluxation

Direct trauma to the globe can cause the zonular fibers encircling the iris to break. These structures are responsible for suspending the lens in the pupillary space by anchoring to the ciliary body. The lens becomes subluxated when 25% or more of the fibers are affected.[9]

When all of the fibers are broken, the lens becomes dislocated and may fall into the vitreous cavity, pupillary space, or anterior chamber. Symptoms include trembling of the iris with quick movements (iridonesis), decreased visual acuity, distortion, and diplopia. Slit-lamp examination is likely to demonstrate irregular depth of the anterior chamber and the presence of vitreous in the anterior chamber. When the lens ends up in the anterior chamber, it often blocks the outflow channels, resulting in a buildup of aqueous fluid and increased intraocular pressure. The lens may also block the pupil, contributing further to glaucoma. Emergency surgical intervention becomes necessary when these conditions exist, although the high potential for vitreous extrusion renders surgery hazardous.

Initial preparations for transport of patients with these injuries include immobilization of the patient (especially the head), elevation of the head, loose binocular bandaging to reduce eye movements, and prevention of any Valsalva-like maneuvers that could cause increased intraocular pressure. Patients with lens dislocation into the vitreous are not at risk for glaucoma and are usually given a contact lens to wear after inflammation has subsided.

Retinal Detachment

Retinal detachment may be caused by either blunt or penetrating trauma and usually occurs months or years after the original injury was sustained. Disruption of the retina occurs at the time of injury. The size and location of detachment dictates the degree of visual impairment. If the macular area is involved, severe loss of vision can be expected. Detachment in other areas results in peripheral field defects or blurred vision in the quadrant opposite the location of disruption.

Symptoms of retinal detachment include a history of light flashes, the presence of floating black specks, and curtainlike narrowing of the peripheral vision. Vitreous hemorrhage will also be evident on ophthalmologic examination. Immediate intervention includes immobilization of the head and use of binocular patches.

Vitreous Hemorrhage

Retinal tears are the most common cause of vitreous hemorrhage. Other causes include rupture of the sclera, damage to the ciliary body, or a choroidal tear. Persons with diabetes, sickle-cell anemia, and retinal neovascularization disorder are particularly vulnerable to vitreous hemorrhage. Blood from the choroid and retina flows into the vitreous, causing the patient to see "floaters." Severe vitreous hemorrhage can result in sudden and profound loss of vision.

The head of a patient with vitreous hemorrhaging should be immobilized and elevated to reduce pressure within the intraocular vessels and allow gravitational settling of intravitreal blood. Binocular bandages minimize movement of the eyes. The flight nurse should ensure that the patient does not attempt any Valsalva maneuvers that would lead to increased intraocular pressure. Most vitreous hemorrhages eventually reabsorb spontaneously within weeks or months. Persistent hemorrhages are surgically treated by vitrectomy 6 or more months after the injury to allow for possible spontaneous reabsorption.

Global and Scleral Rupture

Because not all ruptures are visible, the flight nurse must be alert to specific signs and symptoms, including hypotonus (soft) eye, a deep anterior chamber, conjunctival hemorrhage, loss of vision, and presence of pain. Uveal or retinal tissue prolapse and loss of intraocular contents may also occur.

Immediate management of patients with global or scleral ruptures involves immobilizing the head and placing a protective shield or cup over the affected eye, taking care to avoid application of any pressure. Rapid transport of the patient to a facility with ophthalmic surgical capabilities is imperative.

Optic Nerve Injury

Contusion, transection, or avulsion of the optic nerve may result from severe trauma to the head. Any patient with suspected intracranial hemorrhage should be evaluated for optic nerve involvement. Contusion of the optic nerve is usually caused by blunt trauma over the anterior aspect of the skull in the superior-lateral brow area of the affected eye. Compression of the nerve by contusion, hematoma, or depressed fracture can cause varying degrees of vision loss. Pupillary abnormality may be the only initial evidence of damage to the visual pathway, with optic disc pallor manifesting in 2 to 3 weeks.[10,14] Treatment includes surgical intervention in cases in which nerve sheath hemorrhage or fracture of the optic canal is present. Administration of high-dose corticosteroids is recommended to decrease any further injury to the nerve. The dosage, which is 30 mg/kg administered intravenously during a 20 to 30 minute period followed by an infusion of 5.4 mg/kg for 23 hours, is the same for patients with spinal cord injuries as well.[10]

Stabbing injuries are the most common cause of optic nerve transection. Small puncture wounds around the orbit may not always be apparent and should be carefully evaluated. The optic nerve may also be lacerated by displaced bone fragments from a depressed cranial fracture. Sudden vision loss and afferent pupillary defect are indicative of a transected optic nerve.

Avulsion of the optic nerve can result from severe temporal trauma. The damage occurs when forces cause the globe to suddenly move forward while the optic nerve remains tethered in place at the point where it leaves the eyes. Intracranial optic nerve damage can occur when a blow to the back of the head or the impact of a fall causes the brain to shift backward. With the optic nerve anchored within the optic canal, this sudden motion causes shearing of the nerve just posterior to its entrance into the cranium.

The result is sudden, permanent, and usually complete loss of vision.

Any patient suspected to have optic nerve injury should be immobilized for transport with binocular bandaging applied to reduce eye movement.

Extrusion

Severe trauma sometimes results in extrusion of the eyeball. No attempt should be made to place the eye back into the socket. Moist saline solution dressings and a protective covering over the affected eye are necessary for transport.[31] Several pieces of gauze with a hole cut in the center can be placed over the extruded eye to stabilize it, and a cup or cone should be taped in place over the eye to protect it from further injury. The flight nurse should also bandage the unaffected eye to prevent any ocular movement. The patient should be transported with his or her head immobilized and in a supine position to the nearest facility with an available ophthalmologist.

SUMMARY

Maxillofacial, anterior neck, and eye injuries frequently occur simultaneously as a result of severe traumatic forces to the head and neck. These injuries, which rarely occur in isolation, often include fractures and injuries to the soft tissues, nerves, vessels, and glands. Traumatic facial injuries can appear devastating and even life threatening at first. However, despite initial appearances, the flight nurse should focus attention on ensuring a clear airway, breathing, and control of hemorrhage. Injuries to the maxillofacial and anterior aspect of the neck can compromise the airway because of the presence of blood, mucus, broken teeth, displaced dentures, bone fragments, a prolapsed tongue, and pharyngeal edema or hematoma. Airway obstruction is the primary concern in patients with this type of trauma.

Only after the patient has been stabilized through proper recognition and treatment of associated life-threatening disorders should treatment of maxillofacial, anterior neck, and eye injuries occur. For most types of injuries this includes immobilization of the head, stabilization of fractures and other damaged structures, and dressing of open wounds. On interfacility flights, inquiry should be made about the patient's tetanus protection status, possible allergies to antibiotics, and any additional medication regimens. The evaluation of x-ray films and CT and MRI scans is also useful, if time permits.

If at all possible, patients with severe maxillofacial, anterior neck, and eye injuries should be transported to facilities that can provide appropriate tertiary care, including maxillofacial surgery, oral surgery, emergency dental care, eye, nose, and throat surgery, ophthalmology services, plastic surgery, and oculoplastic surgery. With proper initial and definitive treatment, patients with injuries to the face and neck often recover without significant functional or cosmetic deficiencies.

MAXILLOFACIAL TRAUMA AND EYE INJURY CASE STUDY

A flight team was dispatched to the scene of a motorcycle crash. An 18-year-old male who was not wearing a helmet was riding his motorcycle at speeds exceeding 100 miles per hour and "hopping over hills" when he lost control of the bike and was thrown onto the pavement. His body motion was stopped by his head. The basic life support rescue crew at the scene described an unconscious patient with multiple facial abrasions and lacerations, and an enucleated left eye.

When the flight team arrived, they found a young white male patient whose ventilations were being assisted with a bag-valve mask. His Glasgow Coma Scale score was 6 (eye opening, 1; verbal response, 1; motor response, 4). The patient had extensive facial injuries and was unstable. His left eye was enucleated and lying on his cheek, covered with a metal dressing. His right eye was not visible in its socket. Blood was coming from his mouth. He was making some respiratory effort and his chest expansion was equal with ventilation. He had a palpable radial pulse of 120.

An intravenous line was inserted, the patient was hooked up to a heart monitor and was given fentanyl for sedation, and an RSI was performed for orotracheal intubation. Despite the patient's facial instability, a tube was easily inserted on the first attempt once relaxation occurred. The patient had a blood pressure of 110/68, a pulse rate of 120, and a respiratory rate of 16.

A rapid secondary assessment was performed. Both lower extremities were deformed, but no open fractures were found. Each extremity was placed in a pneumatic splint. The patient's cervical spine was immobilized and the patient was placed on a backboard and loaded in the aircraft.

During transport, the patient continued to bleed profusely from his mouth and nose. Continuous suctioning was required. The flight team was unable to evaluate his right eye, and the left eye remained covered on his left cheek. The patient was transported to a trauma center.

A CT scan of the patient's head revealed multiple skull fractures, a Le Fort III facial fracture, and a diffuse axonal injury. The CT scan also showed that the patient's right eye had fallen to the back of its socket. The left eye was surgically removed. No other significant injuries were identified except for femur fractures; his legs were placed in traction.

The patient was admitted to the surgical intensive care unit. His condition continued to deteriorate despite aggressive neurologic management and he was declared brain dead 72 hours after injury. His family consented to organ donation.

Discussion

The most important concern when caring for a patient with maxillofacial trauma is establishing an airway. Choosing the most appropriate method to manage the airway can be a challenge in patients with this type of injury. Although the patient had extensive facial trauma, he was clenching his teeth. The flight team elected to use RSI and were successful with this procedure. Others may have chosen to perform a surgical cricothyroidotomy. Whatever method the flight team chooses, they need to have the necessary skills to perform the procedure.

Because of the unusual nature of the eye injury, the flight nurse had to ensure that the eye was protected to prevent further injury in case there was a chance of saving the eye. This case illustrates another example of the need for motorcyclists to wear helmets.

REFERENCES

1. Beal SL, Pottmeyer EW, Spisso JM: Esophageal perforation following external blunt trauma, *J Trauma* 28(10): 1425, 1988.
2. Bedrossian EH Jr: Evaluation of orbital injuries, *Adv Ophthalmic Plast Reconstruct Surg* 6:37, 1987.
3. Boroer TC: Maxillofacial and soft tissue injuries. In Cardon V et al, editors: *Trauma nursing,* Philadelphia, 1994, WB Saunders.
4. Boyar C: Ocular examination, *Emerg Med Clin Am* 6(1): 111, 1988.
5. Cogbill TH et al: The spectrum of blunt injury to the carotid artery: a multicenter perspective, *J Trauma* 37(3): 473–479, 1994.
6. Henneman E, Henneman P, Oman K: Ventilation and gas transport: pulmonary, thoracic and facial injuries. In Neff J, Kidd P, editors: *Trauma nursing: the art & science,* St Louis, 1993, Mosby.
7. Hermon A et al: Complete cricotracheal separation following blunt trauma to the neck, *J Trauma* 154(6):619, 1987.
8. Jacobs B, Baker P: *Trauma nursing core course,* Park Ridge, Ill, 1995, Emergency Nurses Association.
9. Joondeph BC: Blunt ocular trauma, *Emerg Med Clin North Am* 6(1):147, 1988.
10. Karesh J, Keyes B: Ocular trauma. In Cardon V et al, editors: *Trauma nursing,* Philadelphia, 1994, Saunders.
11. Kersten RC: Blowout fracture of the orbital floor with entrapment caused by isolated trauma to the orbital rim, *Am J Ophthalmol* 103(2):215, 1987.
12. Liu HF et al: Ocular injuries from accidental laser exposure, *Health Physics* 56(5):711, 1989.
13. Meyer P et al: Esophageal perforation: the need for early diagnosis, *Chest* 94(4):893, 1988.
14. Middleton TH III, Smith RR: Optic nerve avulsion secondary to traumatic enucleation, *Neurosurgery* 21(1):89, 1987.
15. Morgan SJ: Chemical burns of the eye: causes and management, *Br J Ophthalmol* 71(11):854, 1987.
16. Eyers EM, Iko BO: The management of acute laryngeal trauma, *J Trauma* 27(4):448, 1987.
17. Ordog GJ: Penetrating neck trauma, *J Trauma* 27(5):543, 1987.
18. O'Toole M: Facial emergencies. In Semonin-Holleran R, editor: *Emergency nursing review,* St Louis, 1996, Mosby.
19. Patel BC: Penetrating eye injuries, *Arch Dis Childhood* 64(3):317, 1989.
20. Pillay SP et al: Oesophageal ruptures and perforations: a review, *Med J Australia* 150(5):246, 1989.
21. Rohen JW, Yokochi C: *The color atlas of anatomy,* New York, 1984, Igaku-Shoin Medical Publishers.
22. Rosenberg PN, Stasior OB: Optic nerve avulsion and transection, *Adv Ophthalmic Plast Reconstruct Surg* 6:63, 1987.
23. Rosenthal AR, Oakley G: Firework related ocular injury, *J Roy Soc Med* 81(10):559, 1988.

24. Rowe NL, Williams JL: *Maxillofacial injuries,* vol I and II, Edinburgh, 1985, Churchill Livingstone.
25. Searl SS: Minor trauma, disastrous results, *Surv Ophthalmol* 31(5):337, 1987.
26. Shotton JC: Stab wounds of the neck: observations on management, *Clin Otolaryngol* 13(5):335, 1988.
27. Taylor RB: Esophageal foreign bodies, *Emerg Med Clin North Am* 5(2):301, 1987.
28. Vernon SA: Fireworks and the eye, *J Roy Soc Med* 81(10): 569, 1988.
29. Weigelt JA et al: Diagnosis of penetrating cervical-esophageal injuries, *Am J Surg* 154(6):619, 1987.
30. Weiman DS et al: Combined tracheal and esophageal transection from blunt trauma to the neck, *J South Carolina Med Assoc* 84(3):111, 1988.
31. Wesley RE et al: Management of orbital-cranial trauma, *Adv Ophthalmic Plast Reconstruct Surg* 7:3, 1987.
32. Wilde PH, Mullany CJ: Esophageal perforation: a review of 37 cases, *Australian New Zealand J Surg* 57(10):743, 1987.
33. Wood J, Fabian TC, Mangiante EC: Penetrating neck injuries: recommendations for selective treatment, *J Trauma* 29(5):602, 1989.
34. Wraa C: Transport considerations for the trauma patient. In Semonin-Holleran R, editor: *Prehospital nursing: a collaborative approach,* St Louis, 1994, Mosby.

CHAPTER 18

Pediatric Trauma

COMPETENCIES

1. Evaluate and perform primary airway interventions for the pediatric patient.
2. Correctly calculate doses and assemble equipment for rapid sequence induction (RSI) for the pediatric patient.
3. Perform appropriate pediatric spinal immobilization.
4. Correctly calculate colloid and blood replacement for fluid resuscitation for the pediatric patient.
5. Perform specific interventions related to pediatric traumatic injuries.

About 25,000 children die each year as a result of accidents. For every death four more children are permanently disabled and 100 temporarily disabled. The cost in dollars is in the billions.[21] The cost in emotional impact on children, families, health care professionals, and communities is immeasurable.

Two of three victims of pediatric trauma are boys. Of all child victims, 37% are of preschool age (0 to 5 years old) and 63% are school aged (6 to 20 years old). Blunt trauma accounts for approximately 85% of all injuries. As a rule, multiple organs are injured.[8,24] The solid organs are injured most often; in decreasing order of frequency they include the brain, lung, liver-spleen, pancreas, and kidney.[20] Physical findings may be subtle despite serious injury, making evaluation and rapid, correct treatment difficult. The most frequent injuries to hollow organs include perforations of the proximal jejunum, duodenum, and bladder. Fractures of the long bones occur in 23% of these children. Penetrating trauma accounts for about 12% of injuries.[20] Although diagnosis is relatively easy in these cases, massive bleeding is a major factor and makes the mortality rate high.[26]

Mechanism of injury varies greatly from one area of the country to another, but the single largest cause of traumatic deaths is motor-vehicle–related accidents.[20,21] Other major causes of injury include falls, gunshot/stab wounds, child abuse, drowning, and fire.

Of traumatic deaths, 50% occur in the hour after injury.[25] Injuries that cause death in this period include major damage to the brain, brainstem, spinal cord, heart, and aorta. If the site where the trauma occurred is very close to a major trauma center with a sophisticated transport system available, some of these patients may be salvaged, but the percentage will be small. The area in which prehospital care providers have the potential to make the biggest difference is with those children who die within 1 to 3 hours of injury. About 30% of traumatic deaths occur in this period as a result of accidents resulting in brain trauma and bleeding from multiple sites (epidural/subdural hematomas, hemopneumothorax, abdominal injuries, and pelvic and long-bone fractures).[25] The injuries result in loss of consciousness, respiratory insufficiency, and major (but usually reversible) blood loss. Injury recognition, short response time, limited but appropriate intervention in the field, sophisticated and knowledgeable transport, short transport time, and the immediate availability of comprehensive pediatric trauma services can save the lives of thousands of children annually.[1]

AIRWAY

Assessment, Intervention, and Complications

Securing and maintaining the child's airway is always the first priority. This seems obvious, but many children still die each year of hypoxia associated with otherwise nonfatal injuries. When managing the child's airway, flight nurses need to consider what pitfalls can be encountered because of anatomic structure. A child's trachea is narrow and anterior, and the soft cartilaginous rings provide minimal support. The trachea can be partially or totally obstructed by a moderate amount of bleeding, vomitus, mucus, or swelling or by incorrect positioning. A child's tongue is large in relation to the oral cavity and may easily obstruct the narrow airway passage, particularly if the child is unconscious. Because their intercostal muscles are relatively weak, children are primarily diaphragmatic breathers. Any compromise of the diaphragm such as gastric distention, diaphragmatic rupture, or abdominal bleeding may cause respiratory distress.

Injury to the cervical spine must be suspected in all pediatric trauma patients, particularly those with any injury above the clavicles, those who are unconscious, and those who are too young to effectively communicate type and location of pain and sensory deficit. The cervical spine must be immobilized in conjunction with any procedures that open and maintain the airway. Rigid cervical collars and head immobilizers are now available in pediatric sizes. Very young children and infants may be too small to fit even pediatric-size immobilization devices, so improvisation becomes a real art. If even the smallest rigid cervical collar is too large, the young child or infant's head and cervical spine can be immobilized by placing the child on a backboard (maintaining manual axial immobilization) and placing rolled-up towels or foam blocks on either side of the head.[9,22] Tape can then be used to secure the child's head to the backboard. The flight nurse must be careful when placing tape under the chin portion of the cervical collar because the tape may compromise the ability to clear and maintain the airway. A traumatized child commonly vomits, so the child must be secured in such a way that log rolling is easily performed while good alignment of the cervical spine is maintained (box). Infant or child car seats are not appropriate or adequate for spinal immobilization.[19]

A common mistake in airway management is to reach immediately for the laryngoscope and endotracheal tube, bypassing the simple, noninvasive, lifesaving procedures. Tracheal intubation is difficult to perform on children, particularly injured children, and it requires skill and continuing experience. A chin lift and jaw thrust are appropriate interventions for basic airway control.[2] Proper positioning may be the only treatment necessary to maintain an open airway.

The next step is removal of any foreign matter from the mouth and nose. Blood, mucus, vomitus, food, and broken teeth should be promptly suctioned

PEDIATRIC SPINAL IMMOBILIZATION

In the pediatric trauma patient, airway and cervical spine control are essentially performed simultaneously. After the airway and cervical spine have been assessed and appropriate interventions accomplished, pediatric spinal immobilization must be completed. Summarized here are new developments in the emergency medical services industry regarding pediatric spinal immobilization.

Spinal Boards

Boards are extrication devices, not immobilization devices.
Board securely wraps entire patient.
Head, even without padding, is in a flexed position.
Boards are used when access to the patient is limited.

Infant Seats

Infant seats are not immobilization devices.
When child is left in seat and padded, head is in a flexed position.
Infant seats are used when head cannot be placed in neutral position.
Infant seats are used when airway cannot be maintained.
Infant seats are used when access to patient is limited.

Neutral Positioning in the Pediatric Trauma Patient

The child is normally in a flexed position.
Cervical collars are often not sized correctly.
Infant seats frequently accentuate flexion.
Ideal position is neutral.
Neutral positioning is usually used on children ages 0 to 8 years.
Two accepted standards:

1. Measure the angle from supraorbital ridge to maxilla in sagittal plane bisecting the eye.[22]
2. Draw a horizontal line from external auditory canal to axilla.[9]

The child should appear to be looking straight ahead while on a flat backboard.

Padding the Board[9,22]

Position of padding:
Place padding from the shoulders to the heels, and elevate body rather than recess head.
Padding types:

1. Commercially available pieces of rectangular Styrofoam are used.
2. Blankets, bedspreads, bath blankets, and/or sheets are piled to place the head in neutral position.
3. Height of padding needed to place the head in neutral position is approximated.

out, and suctioning should be repeated often enough to keep the airway clear. Rapid, frequent suctioning is preferable to prolonged suctioning because suctioning stimulates the vagus nerve and may cause bradycardia.[4,5]

Even if color and perfusion appear adequate, the flight nurse should administer supplemental oxygen. Pulse oximetry can be helpful in monitoring oxygenation. The increase in use of pulse oximetry during transport has demonstrated that most patients have improved oxygen saturation, even though they do not physically appear to need it. Most young children who are awake enough to protest an oxygen mask will do so. They may better tolerate a nasal cannula with the prongs cut off or a mask held close to the face with the flow turned up.

An oral airway can be a useful adjunct in an unconscious child. The flight nurse can choose the appropriate size by finding an airway that is equal to the distance from the child's front teeth to the ear. The flight nurse should take care when inserting the airway because the tissues of the palate and tongue bleed easily. Inserting the airway in anatomic position without rotation is preferable. A tongue depressor should be used to facilitate insertion.

With correct positioning and high-flow oxygen, the child can usually be adequately ventilated with a bag and mask. Effective bag-valve mask ventilation also depends on the proper size mask and type of bag. The mask must fit the configuration of the child's face well, or obtaining a good seal will be difficult. The mask should be transparent to permit observation of the child's lip color and quick recognition of vomiting. Bags that allow the delivery of high pressures without a "pop-off" valve are especially helpful for children who are difficult to ventilate. This type of bag also makes changes in lung compliance more obvious to the person doing the ventilating. Gastric dilation can be minimized by use of the Sellick maneuver during assisted bag-valve mask ventilation of unconscious infants and children. In this maneuver, gentle manual pressure is applied to the cricoid cartilage, compressing the esophagus between the cricoid ring and the cervical spine. The flight nurse must be careful not to compress the trachea and obstruct the airway, especially in infants. A nasogastric or an orogastric tube should be inserted before transport to decrease gastric distention. Oxygen-powered breathing devices are contraindicated for pediatric use because the tidal volume is difficult to control and high airway pressure can produce gastric distention or a tension pneumothorax.[2]

Endotracheal Intubation

If ventilation remains inadequate or transport time is prolonged, endotracheal intubation becomes necessary. Endotracheal intubation presents unique challenges in small children.[7] When choosing the appropriate size of endotracheal tube, the flight nurse must consider that the narrowest portion of the child's trachea is at the cricoid cartilage, below the vocal cords, and approximates the size of the child's little finger or external nares. Therefore a tube about the size of the child's little finger or one that will fit easily into the external nares is usually the right size. Preselection of tubes one size larger and one size smaller will save some time if the tube chosen for the intubation proves to be the wrong size. The vocal cords themselves are delicate and easily injured, as is the tracheal mucosa. The single passage of a too-large tube may strip the tracheal mucosa, causing airway damage. A properly fitted tube should develop an air leak at 15 to 20 cm H_2O inspiratory pressure. No air leakage means that the tube is too big. Uncuffed tubes are used for children younger than 8 years because inflation of a cuffed tube in a young child may result in subglottic stenosis or laceration of the membranous portion of the trachea with subsequent pneumomediastinum, pneumopericardium, or tension pneumothorax. The box lists guidelines for selecting laryngoscope blades and endotracheal tubes.[18]

Before intubation, the child should be preoxygenated with 100% oxygen and a bag-valve mask. Oral intubation is recommended for children younger than

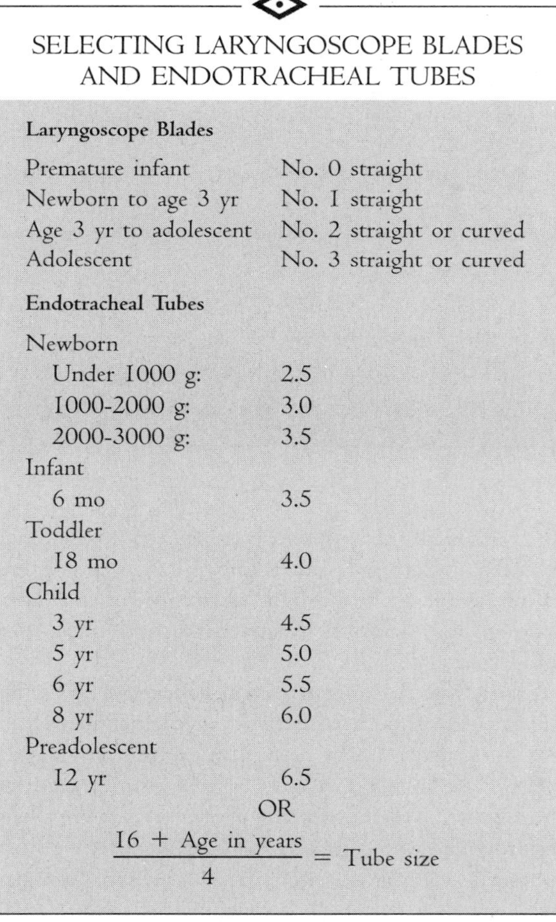

SELECTING LARYNGOSCOPE BLADES AND ENDOTRACHEAL TUBES

Laryngoscope Blades

Premature infant	No. 0 straight
Newborn to age 3 yr	No. 1 straight
Age 3 yr to adolescent	No. 2 straight or curved
Adolescent	No. 3 straight or curved

Endotracheal Tubes

Newborn	
Under 1000 g:	2.5
1000-2000 g:	3.0
2000-3000 g:	3.5
Infant	
6 mo	3.5
Toddler	
18 mo	4.0
Child	
3 yr	4.5
5 yr	5.0
6 yr	5.5
8 yr	6.0
Preadolescent	
12 yr	6.5

OR

$$\frac{16 + \text{Age in years}}{4} = \text{Tube size}$$

8 years. Nasal intubation is preferred for older children, especially if some spontaneous respiration is present. Nasal intubation should not be attempted if the child has a basilar skull fracture through the cribriform plate.

Rapid Sequence Induction

Management of the airway and oxygenation are performed at the beginning of the primary assessment of airway, breathing, and circulation (the ABCs). Emergency control of the airway may be necessary and one of the best techniques can be accomplished by rapid sequence induction (RSI) intubation.

RSI has been described in emergency, surgical, pediatric, anesthesia, and nursing journals. Many protocols have been published for the step-by-step process and all the different drugs used at different institutions. The protocol contained in the box is used by a level I trauma center and is from the University of Michigan Section of Emergency Medicine. This protocol can be used as a guide or starting point from which a program can develop a tailored protocol.

Hypoxia is a common complication of intubation of the pediatric trauma patient. It most often occurs with prolonged attempts at intubation. Pulse oximetry is helpful at this time.

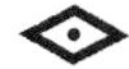

UNIVERSITY OF MICHIGAN SECTION OF EMERGENCY MEDICINE
RSI INTUBATION PROTOCOL FOR TRAUMA PATIENTS

Suspected Traumatic Brain Injury

Preoxygenate:
100% oxygen by nonrebreather mask or four vital capacity breaths
Pretreatment:
Lidocaine (1.5 mg/kg IV)
Fentanyl (3-5 μg/kg IV)
Atropine (0.02 mg/kg)
Induction:
Etomidate (0.2-0.3 mg/kg IV)
Paralysis:
Succinylcholine (1.5 mg/kg IV)

Intubation with cervical spine immobilization

Checking of tube position by:
Presence of chest rise
Bilateral breath sounds
Positive finding on end tidal CO_2 detector
Chest radiography

Consideration of additional sedation and long-term neuromuscular blockade if necessary

No Suspicion of Traumatic Brain Injury

Preoxygenate:
100% oxygen by nonrebreather mask or four vital capacity breaths
Pretreatment:
Atropine (0.02 mg/kg) for children receiving succinylcholine

Inaction for 2-3 minutes if possible

Induction:
Etomidate (0.2 to 0.3 mg/kg IV)
Paralysis:
Succinylcholine (1.5 mg/kg IV)

Intubation with cervical spine immobilization

Checking of tube position by:
Presence of chest rise
Bilateral breath sounds
Positive finding on end tidal CO_2 detector
Chest radiography

Consideration of additional sedation and long-term neuromuscular blockade if necessary

Unlikely Successful Intubation

Consideration of:
Fiberoptic intubation
Cricothyrotomy
Retrograde intubation
Needle cricothyrotomy/transtracheal jet ventilation

The distance from the vocal cords to the bifurcation of the trachea varies from 4 to 5 cm in an infant to approximately 11 cm in an older child. Endotracheal tube placement must therefore be precise, not only in terms of placement through the vocal cords but in the distance the tube is passed after going through the cords. A tube passed too far will result in a mainstem bronchus intubation. A tube not passed far enough through the cords may be dislodged if the child coughs, gags, flexes, or extends the neck or is moved. In an infant, the tip of the tube can move as much as 2 cm during flexion or extension of the head. Therefore the child's ventilatory status and, if necessary, tube position should be rechecked every time the child is moved. Good tube placement is evaluated by auscultation of all lung fields and the gastric area and by observation of chest rise. Effective ventilation is assessed by ongoing monitoring of the child's heart rate, color, end-tidal carbon dioxide ($ETCO_2$) monitoring, capillary refill, and pulse oximetry, if available. If the child is intubated orally, an oral airway may be placed to prevent the child from biting down on the tube and occluding it. Care should also be taken to prevent kinking of smaller endotracheal tubes caused by the weight and position of the resuscitation bag.

Insertion of an oral or a nasogastric tube is part of airway management. When the child is intubated, the normal mechanism for protecting the airway is bypassed. If the tube fits properly, an air leak exists that protects the trachea from ischemic damage by the tube. There is also easy access to the lungs for any aspirated material. If the child has been ventilated by bag-valve mask for any length of time, air will be present in the child's stomach.

Normally, a nasogastric or an orogastric tube is placed after successful intubation; placement intubation allows the cardiac sphincter to be incompetent, leading to an increase in aspiration. Before intubation, cricothyroid pressure is used to control gastric contents. If preoxygenation with a bag-valve mask happens to lead to acute gastric distention with resulting cyanosis, bradycardia, and difficulty in ventilation, an orogastric tube should be placed for decompression first. Decompressing the stomach is also necessary if peritoneal lavage will be performed. Nasal insertion of the gastric tube, as with the tracheal tube, should be avoided if the possibility exists that the tube will pass into the brain.

Cricothyrotomy is rarely necessary for the pediatric patient. Indications for the procedure include complete or nearly complete airway obstruction. This may occur with a fractured larynx, severe maxillofacial trauma, or laryngeal foreign body. Surgical cricothyrotomy is typically performed for children older than 8 years.

Needle cricothyrotomy is usually performed for children younger than 8 years.[19] In this procedure, a 12- or 14-gauge angiocatheter with a syringe attached to the hub is inserted. After the cricothyroid membrane is located, the skin covering is cleaned with povidone-iodine (Betadine) or alcohol and tightened across the membrane. The needle is placed directly in the midline and advanced at a 45-degree angle toward the feet while suction is kept on the syringe during insertion until air is aspirated. Because the membrane is soft, cannulation of the esophagus must be avoided by exerting excessive pressure. After the plastic catheter is advanced, the stylet is removed. An intermittent jet of oxygen is delivered to the catheter hub through oxygen tubing attached to the Y connector or a 3-mm pediatric endotracheal tube adapter attached to a ventilating bag.[12] An oxygen source delivering 50 psi or more is needed for adequate ventilation. The chest should rise when oxygen is delivered, but exhalation occurs passively. With the Y-connector setup, the connector is occluded for 1 to 2 seconds or until the chest rises and then released for 3 to 4 seconds to allow for exhalation. Manual compression of the chest may be used to assist the exhalation process. Commercial insufflation devices that allow psi to be calibrated for delivery of weight-appropriate tidal volumes are now available.

Regardless of whether any type of airway adjunct has been used, the effectiveness of ventilation must be assessed frequently. Both sides of the chest must be expanding equally, and bilateral breath sounds must be auscultated. Color, perfusion, and physiologic parameters should be improving or be within normal limits. The use of portable pulse oximeters, $ETCO_2$ monitors, and other noninvasive monitors for air transport has greatly improved the ability to monitor ventilation and oxygenation in an environment in which poor lighting, vibration, and noise make physical assessment difficult.

THORACIC INJURIES

Assessment, Intervention, and Complications

Injuries to the thorax may dramatically affect ventilation. A child's chest wall is thin; the thorax is small and round. As a result, sounds in the chest cavity reverberate easily and can be misinterpreted. Breath sounds, referred from one or another area of the chest, may be heard over an area of pneumothorax or atelectasis, masking a potentially lethal problem.

Tension Pneumothorax

Although uncommon, a tension pneumothorax may be life threatening. Indications include diminished or absent breath sounds on the side of the collapsed lung, distended neck veins, shock from the compression of the vena cava, and decreased venous return. Diagnosis is made clinically on the basis of the mechanism of injury and the symptoms listed, as well as difficulty in ventilation through an endotracheal tube (once it has been shown the endotracheal tube is not occluded and in the proper position). A diagnosis should not be made on the basis of chest radiography.[19] If the child receives oxygen under pressure (bag-valve mask or endotracheal tube bag), the tension inside the chest increases. As tension increases, the heart's ability to fill effectively diminishes and cardiac arrest is imminent. A rapid needle thoracentesis converts the tension pneumothorax to a simple pneumothorax. A 14- or 16-gauge angiocatheter is inserted in the second intercostal space midclavicular line, and the patient is reassessed. Needle thoracostomy may be repeated if symptoms recur. The needle is inserted over the top of the rib (blood vessels and nerves being located at the bottom of the rib) and aimed in a posterior direction. Needle thoracostomy is only a temporizing measure, and a chest tube must be placed for definitive management.[19] If the child has multiple injuries, continued severe respiratory symptoms, or a pneumothorax of 15% or greater, consideration must be given to insertion of a chest tube before transport.

Pneumothorax and Hemopneumothorax

Simple pneumothorax and hemopneumothorax are the most common types of chest injuries in children. A suspected large hemothorax (unilateral dullness on percussion of the chest, unilateral diminished breath sounds, and signs and symptoms of shock with known or suspected chest injury) is treated with aggressive fluid therapy with large-bore intravenous (IV) lines and blood, if available. Monitoring of chest tube output from hemothoraxes with aggressive fluid resuscitation is an important aspect in the management of children with this injury. Open pneumothorax is treated by the insertion of a chest tube through an alternate site and placement of an occlusive dressing over the open wound. If time and circumstances do not permit a chest tube, a dressing taped on three sides, creating a flutter valve, may be applied. The definitive management of these injuries is chest tube insertion.[19]

Rib Fractures

The cartilage in a young child's ribs is so flexible that it generally takes significant force to fracture a rib. Rib fractures in children younger than 8 years are uncommon and indicate that the child has sustained major chest-wall trauma. For this reason, flail chest is not common in children. When flail chest occurs, it is usually accompanied by severe pulmonary contusion. Cardiac contusion, pneumothorax, and hemothorax are also possible. Flail chest may be managed initially with manual stabilization of the flail segment or the taping of a bulky dressing over the defect. If the child remains in severe respiratory distress, intubation and assisted ventilation become necessary.

Cardiac Injuries

The incidence of heart injuries resulting from blunt trauma in children is relatively low. The child's chest wall has more elastic properties than an adult's. The flight nurse may overlook cardiac injuries in the absence of rib fractures. Cardiac monitoring should be performed routinely in all pediatric trauma patients. A high index of suspicion for cardiac and great vessel damage should be included in the assessment of children with blunt chest trauma.

CIRCULATION, SHOCK, AND VASCULAR ACCESS

Assessment, Intervention, and Complications

A common error in the management of pediatric trauma is failure to recognize that the child is seriously injured. Early detection of impending shock in the pediatric trauma patient must be given meticulous attention. A child often appears clinically very stable one minute and "crashes" the next when cardiovascular collapse occurs. Familiarity with normal physiologic parameters in children aids early detection of shock. (The box depicts the physiologic parameters in children.)

Pediatric patients generally tolerate blood loss of up to 15% of total estimated blood volume without much change in normal physiologic parameters. They may experience tachycardia from fear, pain, or crying, but a safer assumption is that the tachycardia is the first sign of shock. IV access should be obtained immediately and a fluid challenge given. A bolus of 20 ml/kg of Ringer's lactate should be tolerated well by any child in whom mild shock is suspected.

Once the child has lost between 15% and 25% of estimated blood volume, capillary refill time becomes slightly prolonged (longer than 2 seconds), the skin begins to cool and become pale or mottled, and the child may become tachypneic. The anxiety that is seen is often attributed to fear or pain, but it may be the initial stage of decreased level of consciousness. The patient remains tachycardic, and the blood pressure begins to change. At this mild stage of shock, the systolic pressure often remains within normal limits, but the diastolic pressure increases and the pulse pressure is narrowed. In many emergency settings, systolic pressure is the only pressure parameter measured, and the narrowing pulse pressure is not appreciated. The diastolic pressure is generally two thirds of the systolic pressure. A pressure of 90/60 mm Hg is within normal limits, but a pressure of 90/70 mm Hg suggests mild hypovolemia. An accurate blood pressure reading is sometimes difficult to obtain in pediatric patients. Blood pressure may not become abnormal until shock has become severe. Measurement of other parameters (heart rate, capillary refill, and urine output) becomes instrumental in diagnosing shock in the pediatric patient.[19]

GUIDELINES FOR PHYSIOLOGIC PARAMETERS IN CHILDREN

Heart Rate

Infant: 120-160 beats/min
Preschool age: 100-120 beats/min
School age: 80-100 beats/min

Respiratory Rate

Infant: 40-60 breaths/min
Preschool age: 30-40 breaths/min
School age: 20-30 breaths/min

Blood Pressure

Systolic pressure = (Age in years × 2) + 80
Diastolic pressure = ⅔ systolic pressure

Estimated Blood Volume

80 ml/kg

Urine Output

Infant: 2 ml/kg/hr
Child over 2 yr: 1 ml/kg/hr

Average Weight for Age

Premature infant: 1 kg
Term infant: 3 kg
6 mo: 6 kg
12 mo: 8 kg
18 mo: 12 kg
2 yr: 14 kg
5 yr: 20 kg
10 yr: 35 kg

Many children compensate for blood loss of up to 50% of total blood volume before showing obvious signs of shock. At that point, things often seem to fall apart all at once—capillary refill time is prolonged, blood pressure decreases dramatically, skin is cold and mottled, and urine output is decreased. A child in severe shock and very unstable hemodynamically is often still conscious and responsive.

Hypovolemic shock must be recognized early and treated aggressively. Large volumes of lactated Ringer's solution must be administered as quickly as possible (within minutes), so two well-functioning, large-bore IV lines are a necessity. Drawing lactated Ringer's solution into a syringe and manually infusing it through an IV line is a rapid method of delivering boluses. Venous access is often difficult in relatively healthy children and much more so in children who are in shock, who are peripherally vasoconstricted, hypothermic, and uncooperative. Percutaneous peripheral IV lines are perhaps the simplest and most complication-free lines to insert in children and will often accept a size-larger catheter than cursory evaluation would indicate.

Research using a wide variety of catheters, fluids, and delivery techniques has shown that a larger-diameter catheter results in increased flow rates and that the greater length of the same-gauge catheters results in decreased flow rates. The recommendation is that the choice of IV catheter should be the largest gauge and shortest length reasonable for the child's size.[11]

Peripheral IV Line Placement

When a peripheral IV line is being placed, an over-the-needle catheter should be used because butterfly needles tend to be infiltrated easily. Common sites of peripheral IV line insertion are the cephalic, basilic, and median cubital veins in the arm and the saphenous vein and veins in the dorsal arch in the leg. The external jugular vein is often prominent in children and is an acceptable site for IV cannulation as long as cervical spine stability is maintained. Scalp veins are helpful in administering medications but are rarely helpful in fluid resuscitation.[2] Before insertion, the catheter may be flushed with saline solution. This generally allows the flashback to be seen more quickly, and advancement of the catheter can be halted before the back side of the vein is punctured. Attachment of a T connector to the hub of the catheter after insertion helps prevent the catheter from being dislodged and makes it easier to change IV tubing when necessary. If the IV line is in an extremity, the extremity should be restrained in as natural a position as possible and any bony prominences padded. IV lines should not be placed in injured extremities or an extremity in which trauma proximal to it is obvious or suspected. The external IV catheter should be well protected without the site being obscured because resuscitation with large fluid volumes and caustic medications can cause IV lines to be infiltrated readily.

Central venous access is difficult to establish in children younger than 8 years and is associated with significant complications.[14] Central venous access (by way of the femoral, internal jugular, or subclavian vein) may be necessary during resuscitation if peripheral cannulation or intraosseous needle placement is unsuccessful or contraindicated.[19] Central venous access is not recommended as the main vascular access during resuscitation.

Intraosseous Infusion

Intraosseous infusion has been suggested as an easy, safe, reliable, rapid, and relatively complication-free method of gaining circulatory access. Insertion is indicated in children 6 years or younger who require acute critical care and in whom peripheral IV access is not rapidly obtained.[13] Placement of an intraosseous needle for resuscitation should be considered if peripheral cannulation is not accomplished in 90 seconds or after three attempts, whichever comes first.[2] Equipment is minimal: 16- to 20-gauge short bone marrow or spinal needle, povidone-iodine (Betadine), a flush-filled syringe, and a T connector. The insertion site is the anterior medial surface of the tibia, 2 to 3 cm below the proximal tibial tuberosity. Insertion at this location avoids the epiphyseal growth plate. The needle is inserted perpendicular to the tibial surface and advanced in a twisting, boring fashion. Generally, a soft pop is felt as the needle enters the bone marrow cavity. The needle should be stable and stand upright by itself. Blood and bone marrow may be aspirated, but failure to do so does not necessarily indicate improper placement. Fluid should flow freely without signs of subcutaneous infiltration. IV fluid, blood, blood products, and medications may be given by this route. The intraosseous route is considered temporary and should be discontinued as soon as other reliable large-bore lines are in place.[23] Among the reported infrequent complications are osteomyelitis and subcutaneous abscess.[10] Contraindications to placement include fracture of the bone or failed intraosseous needle placement at the intended site. Alternate sites for placement include the distal femur, the proximal humerus, and rarely, the sternum.[19]

Pneumatic antishock garments (PASGs) are somewhat controversial as an adjunct in the treatment of shock, but some indications for their use exist. The garment may be useful in stabilizing underlying fractures and controlling soft-tissue bleeding. The garments are now available in toddler (18 months to 4 years) and pediatric (4 to 10 years) sizes.

Once circulatory access is gained, fluid administration should be initiated immediately and aggressively. Lactated Ringer's solution is administered as a bolus of 20 ml/kg of body weight. Children (including infants) in shock often need large amounts of fluid as quickly as it can be given. Children in severe hypovolemic shock often require 40 to 60 ml/kg of resuscitation in the first hour. In some cases with ongoing fluid loss, 200 ml/kg may be necessary in the first few hours of resuscitation. Children in septic shock often require 60 to 80 ml/kg in the first hour of resuscitation.[2] A lactated Ringer's bolus can be repeated once. If after a 40 ml/kg bolus the child continues to show symptoms of shock, an infusion of O-negative blood, 10 ml/kg, should be administered. Typed and cross-matched blood is certainly preferable but is rarely available in emergency situations.[2] Many trauma centers have O-negative blood immediately available from the blood bank for the flight team to take with them if necessary. On a longer flight, a referring hospital may have time to type and cross-match blood. Type-specific blood is acceptable if time does not permit cross-matching. The blood should be transfused in 10 ml/kg boluses. IV fluids should be warmed as soon as possible; room-temperature fluids are colder than severely hypothermic patients. Infusion of boluses of cold fluid, especially into infants and small children, can lower body temperature significantly. If IV access is obtained in a leg where a PASG is being used, the fluid must be infused under pressure (with the use of an infusion pump or a pressure bag). Pressure bags may be necessary to provide fluid infusion through an intraosseous needle during transport.

NEUROLOGIC INJURY

Assessment, Intervention, and Complications

A small child's head is one fourth to one third of total body size and has a large circulating blood volume. Injuries to the face and scalp, which may appear relatively minor, can result in blood loss severe enough to cause shock. The cranial bones are normally not fused until the child is approximately 16 to 18 months old. Before that, enough blood loss to cause shock can accumulate intracranially as a result of a closed-head injury. Cranial enlargement may initially allow for the increase in intracranial volume without significant increase in intracranial pressure (ICP). In children older than 2 years, closed-head injuries generally do not allow for enough volume loss to cause shock. If in shock, the child must be evaluated for other significant injury as the cause. Also of significance in children is their hyperemic response to head trauma. After a severe blow to the child's head, cerebral autoregulation is lost, an influx of blood engorges the cerebral vasculature, extracellular and intracellular edema develops, and ICP increases.

Increased ICP contributes to death in many patients with head injury. The most effective treatment of hyperemia is intubation and controlled hyperventilation with 100% oxygen. As the PCO_2 is lowered, cerebral blood vessels constrict, thereby decreasing ICP. Increasing cerebral oxygenation helps decrease brain injury. Elevation of the head 15 to 30 degrees in a midline position facilitates cerebral venous drainage and decreased ICP.[19] With full cervical spine immobilization the head of the backboard may be raised to achieve the same result.

A rapid neurologic examination in which level of consciousness, pupillary response to light, extraocular movements, and motor function are evaluated is necessary to establish the child's postinjury baseline. If possible, the child's preinjury baseline should also be determined, including any preexisting deficits.

Level of Consciousness

Level of consciousness may be described by a multitude of terminologies, scales, and scores, all of which are adaptable to pediatrics to a certain degree. However, it may be more helpful and accurate to give a brief description of what the child is or is not responding to and what the response is. Children of different cultures often respond differently to stimuli. Some understanding of the child's cultural background is helpful in determining the appropriateness of their response. Glasgow Coma Scale (GCS) grading should be performed initially, during transport, and at the receiving institution. Table 18-1 illustrates the GCS, which compares infants with adults and children.[17]

Pupillary Assessment

Both pupils should be checked for size in millimeters, equality, and both direct and consensual response to light. Some children have anisocoria, a normal discrepancy in pupil size. Trauma to the eye itself or to the orbit, muscles, and nerves may cause a variation in pupil size not necessarily associated with brain injury. When one pupil becomes progressively larger and less reactive or is first seen as dilated and nonreactive, a progressive herniation of the uncus of the temporal lobe of the brain through the tentorial notch may be occurring. As the uncus moves downward, it compresses the third cranial nerve. Parasympathetic fibers on the outside of the third nerve are compressed, allowing the sympathetics to take over and dilate the pupil. As the nerve is further compressed, fibers inside the nerve that controls extraocular movements are deactivated, causing a downward, outward deviation of the eye. Ultimately, the midbrain is compressed; a vegetative state or death can ensue. Compression of the brain stem is generally caused by a focal insult such as an epidural hematoma or localized edema. The lesion will be on the same side as the affected pupil. A hemiparesis may develop on the contralateral side as the cerebral peduncle carrying the motor fibers is compressed. Atropine, administered locally or systemically, causes the pupil to dilate and become unresponsive to light. If the child has been resuscitated with atropine, the pupils may be fixed and dilated as a result.

Diencephalic or small, reactive pupils occur when impairment takes place at the level of sympathetic involvement. This reaction would be typical for a child exposed to narcotic agents such as phenobarbital and diazepam. It is also common during sleep when the sympathetic system is not active.

TABLE 18-1

Glasgow Coma Scale

Response	Adults and Children	Infants	Points
Eye-opening	No response	No response	1
	To pain	To pain	2
	To voice	To voice	3
	Spontaneous	Spontaneous	4
Verbal	No response	No response	1
	Incomprehensible	Moans at pain	2
	Inappropriate words	Cries at pain	3
	Disoriented	Irritable	4
	Conversation	Coos, babbles	5
Motor	No response	No response	1
	Decerebrate posturing	Decerebrate posturing	2
	Decorticate posturing	Decorticate posturing	3
	Withdraws from pain	Withdraws from pain	4
	Localizes pain	Withdraws from touch	5
	Obeys commands	Normal spontaneous movement	6

Midpositioned, fixed pupils occur when a diffuse pressure forces the brainstem through the tentorial notch and it becomes kinked and compressed. Such pressure may result from cerebral edema due to hypoxia, massive fluid overload, or head injury–induced hyperemia. The parasympathetics are affected first, and both pupils dilate and react only sluggishly. As the impaction increases, the sympathetics are also damaged. This damage leaves the pupils at midposition because both regulatory systems have been damaged.

Extraocular Eye Movement

Extraocular eye movement is controlled by the four rectus and two oblique muscles and the third, fourth, and sixth cranial nerves. The eyes may be evaluated for movement by having the child follow a bright light or toy upward, downward, and to the left and right. Each eye should be observed for individual movement, as well as whether the eyes move together in a conjugate gaze.

In an awake, alert child, turning the head quickly to one side causes a conjugate deviation of the eyes toward the side the head is turned to. In the unconscious child, turning the head quickly to one side should produce a conjugate deviation of the eyes toward the opposite side. This is called *doll's eyes,* or the *oculocephalic reflex.* Infants normally have doll's eyes until they are old enough to track well with their eyes. The oculocephalic reflex is not resilient and may be knocked out by pancuronium bromide, trauma, or hypoxia. This reflex should never be evaluated in a traumatized child until a cervical spine injury has been ruled out.

Damage to the eye or its surrounding structures may cause trapping or compression of muscles and nerves that control pupillary response to light or eye movement. It is important to distinguish between this type of damage and damage caused by brain injury so that the correct problem can be expeditiously treated. A blowout fracture of the orbit of the eye can entrap the inferior rectus, inferior oblique muscle, or both and result in restriction of extraocular movement.

Palsies of the cranial nerves that control eye movement may result in varied findings. Although palsies of the third cranial nerve are uncommon in children, they can result from trauma and increased ICP. Such a palsy is evident in the previously discussed case in which the uncus of the temporal lobe of the brain herniates downward through the tentorial notch. Manifestations of such a palsy include drooping of the upper eyelid, a larger pupil on the affected side, and poor ability to move the eye up, down, or in. Sixth-nerve palsies are common in children. Meningitis, increased ICP, skull fractures, intracranial tumors, middle-ear infections, and mastoiditis may cause the characteristic inability to turn the eye out past the midline, diplopia, and head turning toward the side of the palsy.

Motor Function

Evaluation of the child's motor function should be begun while initial assessment and stabilization procedures are underway. Spontaneous and elicited movement in all extremities and impairment, if any, should be observed. If time permits, each extremity should be checked for the "five p's": pain, pallor, pulselessness, paresis, and paralysis. If possible, the degree of weakness and side or specific body part that is weaker should be indicated. If spinal cord injury is a possibility, the level of the body at which sensory and motor impairment begins should be indicated.

Decorticate posturing is manifested by adduction and flexion of the arms on the chest, flexion of the wrists and elbows, extension and internal rotation of the legs, and plantar flexion at the ankle. It is indicative of a lesion or insult anywhere down to the upper third of the midbrain. It is an early indication of the massive diffuse pressure that eventually causes pupils to become midpositioned and fixed.

Decerebrate posturing is manifested by adduction, extension, and internal rotation of the arms; flexion of the wrists; extension and internal rotation of the legs; and plantar flexion at the ankles. It is indicative of a lesion or insult extending down through the midbrain to the pons. It may be accompanied by dilated or midposition pupils that are nonreactive.

Temperature, respirations, pulse, and blood pressure are an integral part of the neurologic examination and may give valuable clues to the location and severity of the neurologic insult. Increased temperature may be indicative of shock or loss of the body's usual thermoregulatory system for some other reason. Increased body temperature increases cerebral blood flow and therefore increases ICP.[15]

Hypothermia can be equally devastating. Children have a large body surface area in proportion to weight and have less subcutaneous fat. These factors contribute significantly to problems with thermoregulation. Even limited exposure, such as that occurring with undressing the child for evaluation and treatment in a protected environment, can cause the child to become hypothermic within minutes. Because the child's head is such a large part of the total body surface area, simply covering the head can greatly aid in preventing hypothermia.

Mild hypothermia (body temperature of 35° to 31° C) produces ataxia, difficulty in speaking (dysarthria), and tachycardia. Moderate hypothermia (body temperature of 31° to 35° C) produces delirium, acidosis, reduced metabolic rate, bradycardia, electrocardiographic changes, and stupor. Severe hypothermia (body temperature of 25° to 20° C) produces hypoventilation, coma, no spontaneous movement, no reflexes or pupillary response to light, apnea, and death. Hypothermia may have a protective effect on neurologic function in some cases. The metabolic demands of the brain are reduced, and the tolerance for hypoxia and ischemia increases.

Respiratory rate and pattern should be recorded and changes noted. Different patterns may point to specific areas of neurologic insult. Cheyne-Stokes respiration consists of a crescendo and decrescendo pattern with a brief period of apnea between patterns. It indicates diffuse diencephalic or upper midbrain involvement. Central neurogenic hyperventilation consists of deep repetitive breaths and is generally unresponsive to oxygen therapy. It indicates injury to the brainstem at the level of the pons.

A decreased pulse, a widening pressure, and decreased level of consciousness (the Cushing response) may indicate increasing ICP. Because this is generally a late sign of high ICP, it should not be used as an early indicator of trouble.

ABDOMINAL INJURY

Assessment, Intervention, and Complications

Blunt trauma accounts for 80% to 90% of abdominal injuries in children.[16,20] Injury results from compression of an organ against the spine, direct transfer of energy to an organ, or rapid deceleration with subsequent tearing of tissue. Solid organs are injured more frequently than hollow viscera. Physical findings may be minimal despite serious injury, delaying diagnosis and prompt, appropriate intervention. Critical findings on examination include hemodynamic instability, an enlarging abdomen with no other site of intravascular volume loss, peritoneal irritation with involuntary guarding, and abdominal-wall rigidity. A child with major trauma often has a head injury that may mask lethal abdominal trauma. Respiratory rate and pattern and response to pain, indicators that tell about the child's abdomen, may be dramatically affected by head injury.

The abdomen, chest, pelvis, and perineum should be inspected for contusions, abrasions, lacerations, and penetrating wounds. Respiratory rate and pattern must be carefully and serially observed. Children are normally abdominal (diaphragmatic) breathers. Peritoneal irritation from blood or intestinal contents changes the breathing pattern. The child now uses the chest to breathe, avoiding deep inspiration and expiration (including crying) because these actions cause severe pain. Respirations are rapid and shallow as the child "splints" with each breath.

Serial measurements of abdominal girth at the level of the umbilicus are another helpful evaluation tool, one not altered by decreased level of consciousness. The abdomen may distend as a result of an accumulation of gas (swallowed air or an ileus), liquid (blood, intestinal contents, urine, bile, and pancreatic juices), or both. Marking the area measured with a pen will allow consistent, accurate measurements of abdominal girth. Absent or decreased bowel sounds may be normal or indicate an ileus. A bruit may indicate significant arterial injury. Abdominal auscultation should be performed before palpation.

The entire abdomen is palpated for masses, guarding, tenderness, and rebound pain. If the child is old enough, cooperative, and awake and alert, testing for rebound pain can be accomplished by asking the child to cough rather than by the usual rapid release of manual pressure.

The pelvis is evaluated by the compression of the wings of the ilium and symphysis pubis. If pain is elicited with these maneuvers or with adduction of the legs, a pelvic fracture is to be suspected. Applying and inflating a PASG is helpful in decreasing bleeding from pelvic fractures and may stabilize the fracture.[19]

The most common specific abdominal injury in children is laceration of the spleen. It generally results from a blow to the left upper quadrant, such as contact with bicycle handlebars, and may not have associated rib fractures. Signs and symptoms may include respiratory distress, tachycardia, pallor, hypotension, pain in the left upper quadrant, pain in the left chest with inspiration, Kehr's sign (compression of the left upper quadrant producing left shoulder pain), nausea, and vomiting.

The major cause of death from abdominal trauma, accounting for as many as 40% of the deaths,[6] is trauma to the liver. Associated injury of the inferior vena cava is a major contributor to the high mortality rate. More than 90% of liver injuries are the result of blunt trauma,[6] and associated rib fractures are relatively common. Blood loss will cause shock, including hypotension, if the loss is more than 25% of circulating blood volume. In addition, the child may have right shoulder pain, right upper quadrant tenderness, and demonstrate guarding.

Pancreatic injury is indicated by diffuse abdominal tenderness, abdominal pain, and vomiting. The child may be hemodynamically unstable because of massive retroperitoneal bleeding or sequestration of third-space fluids. The child initially seen with hypovolemic shock due to an isolated injury to the pancreas is rare and more commonly has associated injuries to adjacent major blood vessels.

Injury to the kidney is common in children. The ribs are softer and abdominal muscles less developed than an adult's, providing less protection from blunt trauma. Signs and symptoms include hematuria, flank pain, flank tenderness, peritoneal signs, shock, and infrequently, a palpable mass. Hematuria is not always present, even in severe renal injuries. A high index of suspicion for these injuries based on mechanism of injury is necessary. Placement of a Foley catheter in suspected renal injury allows for accurate measurement of urine output and evaluation of fluid resuscitation.

Treatment of abdominal trauma in the pretertiary care facility setting should focus on aggressive and scrupulous management of the airway and ventilation and restoration and maintenance of hemodynamic stability, as described earlier. If major injuries to the pelvis or retroperitoneum have occurred, fluid boluses administered in the legs may not reach the central circulation. A gastric tube and urinary catheter should be placed.

ORTHOPEDIC INJURY

Assessment, Intervention, and Complications

The goals of managing pediatric extremity trauma are to promote healing of the fracture without deformity, prevent loss of motion in any involved joints, and allow normal growth. The child has differences in the skeletal structure that create additional concerns in the correct initial treatment of bony injuries. The long bones of infants and young children have wide epiphyseal growth plates. Fractures involving the growth plate may heal rapidly without permanent sequelae but may also cause partial or complete growth disturbance and subsequent shortening and angular deformity of the extremity. Thick periosteal "sleeves" link and support the proximal and distal ends of the bone. The periosteum—along with the porous, bendable nature of the bone—can cause fractures of the diaphyseal portion of the bone to snap back into relatively normal alignment with little displacement and little evidence of fracture. The ligaments of the child's joints are extremely strong and well attached, making joint dislocations rare.

Examination of the extremities begins with observation for abrasions, contusions, lacerations, swelling, and obvious deformities that would indicate possible damage to an underlying bone or joint. The neurovascular status of each extremity is documented by evaluation of peripheral pulses, capillary refill, color, warmth, movement, and sensation.

Suspected fractures are splinted to prevent further soft-tissue damage and reduce pain. Extremities are splinted in the position in which they were found, immobilizing the bone and joint both proximal and distal to the injury. Alignment of deformities should be attempted only if significant compromise in the neurovascular status has already occurred or the deformity interferes with proper spinal immobilization or patient assessment. Many pediatric splinting and immobilizing devices are available. Several allow immobilization of the head, cervical spine, back, and all four extremities at once.

Children, like adults, can sustain significant blood loss from both open and closed fractures. Bleeding should be controlled with local pressure when possible. Fluid resuscitation should take into account the obvious or hidden losses that are estimated to have occurred from the fracture.

URINARY CATHETER

Measurement of urine output is critically important during the initial phases of shock resuscitation. Insertion of a urinary catheter is helpful for measuring the effectiveness of fluid resuscitation in pediatric burn and trauma patients. It is also beneficial in head-injury cases, especially when diuretics have been administered. The bladders in such children may overdistend and rupture if not drained. Urinary catheter placement is contraindicated if passage of the catheter meets with resistance or a urethral injury is suspected.

CHILD ABUSE AND NONACCIDENTAL TRAUMA

In the care of any traumatized child whose mechanism of injury is not clearly documented, abuse or nonaccidental trauma must be part of the differential diagnosis.

Time and circumstances do not always permit extensive history taking, but "red flags" that may arise in even a brief history should make the examiner suspicious. Was the time between when the accident/injury occurred and medical attention began reasonable or prolonged? Is the described mechanism of injury consistent with the actual injury seen? If more than one caregiver is giving the history, does each describe similar circumstances, or do significant parts of the story differ? Is the accident consistent with the developmental level of the child? For example, is it reasonable that a 1-month-old infant could sustain multiple skull fractures by "rolling over" off the couch? Are the caregiver's expectations of the child's behavior and abilities reasonable for the child's developmental level? Do the caregivers or the child's medical record indicate a history of multiple injuries over a period of time? Is the child in a high-risk group for abuse (chronically or frequently physically ill, mentally impaired, or described as being particularly "difficult" or "accident prone")? Are there obvious problems with family dynamics?

As previously discussed, the signs of impending respiratory and cardiovascular collapse in children may be subtle. If the mechanism of injury is unclear or suspicious, as is often the case in abuse, excellent physical examination skills are needed to thoroughly and quickly assess immediate needs and begin intervention.

The most commonly injured organ in abuse is the skin. Although bruises and contusions are seen in virtually all children, the distribution and appearance differ with abuse. Most healthy and active children sustain bruises regularly over bony prominences on the extremities and face. Nonaccidental bruising tends to be central, present on soft-tissue surfaces, and more extensive. Multiple bruises in various stages of healing may be seen. Bruising may appear in the specific configuration of the object or method used to inflict the trauma, such as a handprint on the side of the face, circumferential rope burns around wrists or ankles, belt marks (either the strap or buckle imprint), or bite marks. Splash, immersion, or "branding" burns may be seen. Traumatic alopecia and even cephalhematoma may be seen in a child who has been violently pulled by the hair.

Some suspicious outward physical signs may mimic abuse but are not the result of intentionally inflicted injury. Babies who are victims of sudden infant death syndrome (SIDS) may have significant postmortem pooling of the circulation that appears as bruising. Mongolian spots, hyperpigmented areas of skin most commonly seen in dark-skinned racial groups, may be confused with unexplained bruises. The spots are present at birth and fade between a few months and 3 or 4 years of age. The results of "coining," an Asian cold medicine ritual, are seen when Asian immigrants have treated their children for fever. Warm oil is placed on the skin and the edge of a coin repeatedly rubbed across it. The resulting capillary dilation and friction produce bruising. This is reportedly not painful to the child and may be likened to a massage.

The most common mechanism of abuse-caused death is injury to the head, central nervous system, or both. Commonly seen injuries include skull fractures, intracranial injuries (cerebral edema, subdural and epidural hematomas), intracerebral injuries (hematomas, contusions, and lacerations), and shaking injuries. Bruising of the ears and periorbital area and hemotympanum may be seen.

Shaking injuries can cause lethal damage without significant external evidence or skull fracture. Bleeding and contusion of the brain can result in decreased levels of consciousness ranging from lethargy to coma, seizures, and even respiratory or cardiac arrest. Bruising on the upper arms or shoulders may be evident when the child has been firmly held and shaken. Retinal hemorrhages may be seen on funduscopic examination.

Skeletal trauma is a common finding in physical abuse. On radiography, multiple old fractures may be seen in a child with one or more obvious new fractures. The location and type of fracture may be suggestive of abuse, unless significant trauma such as an automobile accident or accidental fall can be documented. Fractures of the femur or ribs in a young child are unusual because of the type and amount of force required to produce them. Other unusual fractures are those of the pelvis, sternum, scapulae, and vertebrae.

Gastrointestinal trauma accounts for a large number of fatal abuse injuries. Blunt trauma to abdominal organs can result in severe shock and rapid death. Mouth trauma of the frenulum and teeth can result from forced feeding. Even though oral trauma is seldom life threatening, it should be considered a red flag that raises suspicion other injuries may be present.

Genitourinary injury from abuse may be seen in the form of direct trauma or sexually transmitted infections. Sexual abuse may leave signs of physical damage to both the gastrointestinal and genitourinary systems. It may also be evidenced by signs of emotional damage.

Cardiopulmonary trauma is rare in abuse, but reported injuries include pulmonary or myocardial contusion, pneumothorax, hemothorax, and cardiac tamponade. The story given to explain this type of injury should reconcile with the type and significant amount of force necessary to cause such potentially lethal damage.

Other types of abuse are not traumatic per se but may contribute to the child's lack of well-being and may be seen in conjunction with nonaccidental trauma. They include forced ingestion of drugs, alcohol, and household cleaners and electrolyte disturbances caused by starvation or inappropriate diet.

It is the responsibility of every health care professional to know the legal requirements for reporting abuse in their area and to follow through with reporting suspected abuse to the appropriate social service or police agency. Documentation in the child's patient record forms the basis on which protective services and the courts can act and should therefore be thorough and objective.

SUMMARY

Children lack the skill and understanding to communicate their needs effectively. Learning to look for and interpret signs and symptoms is a unique challenge in dealing with the pediatric population.

PEDIATRIC TRAUMA CASE STUDY

The air medical communication center dispatched their rotor-wing aircraft to a small rural hospital 60 miles away with the following information: An 8-year-old, 30-kg girl was the unrestrained front-seat passenger in a pickup truck that struck a utility pole at a high rate of speed. The driver of the truck was pronounced dead at the scene. The patient was ejected through the windshield and was unconscious, according to bystanders, for 5 minutes. She was placed in full cervical spine immobilization and rapidly transported to the nearest hospital. The physician at the referring hospital stated that the patient exhibited decorticate posturing to painful stimuli but was otherwise unresponsive. Her initial vital signs were blood pressure, 70/50; heart rate, 185; respiratory rate, 48;

and temperature, 37.2° C. They were attempting to intubate and establish venous access at the time of communication.

On the patient's arrival at the referring facility the flight nurse's examination revealed an 8-year-old girl in full cervical spine immobilization with a respiratory rate of 52. Her airway was open and clear on initial evaluation. The patient was on a nonrebreather mask with 100% oxygen. The referring physician stated that he had been unable to intubate this patient even after making several unsuccessful oral attempts. No radiographs or laboratory tests had been performed.

At this point, RSI for intubation was undertaken by the flight crew with the assistance of the referring facility's staff. Atropine sulfate 0.3 mg and fentanyl citrate 30 μg/kg were administered intravenously, followed by 60 mg of IV succinylcholine. Cricoid pressure was applied and continued throughout the intubation procedure. Hyperventilation with 100% oxygen by bag-valve mask was provided, yielding a pulse oximetry reading of 100%. After manual in-line stabilization of the cervical spine, the front of the cervical collar was removed. Once full paralysis was obtained and after further hyperventilation, the patient was successfully orally intubated with a 5.5-mm endotracheal tube, which was taped at 17 cm at the lip. Correct placement was verified by means of auscultation, and the presence of CO_2 was measured by use of an $ETCO_2$ monitor. The cervical collar and lateral immobilization device were replaced after successful intubation.

The remainder of the primary survey revealed clear breath sounds bilaterally without obvious external signs of thoracic trauma. No crepitance or flail segments were palpated. The respiratory rate after intubation was 36, and the patient's respiratory effort was assisted with 100% oxygen by bag-valve mask (BVM).

The child's skin was pale, cool, and mottled, with a capillary refill time of 6 seconds. Her radial pulse was 188 and weak. Electrocardiography revealed sinus tachycardia without ectopic beats. A 24-gauge butterfly needle had been placed in the left hand, and a solution of D5.45NS was infused at 25 ml/hr. This solution was changed to lactated Ringer's solution by the flight nurse, but the flow rate could not be increased at this IV site.

After three unsuccessful attempts at placing a larger peripheral IV catheter, an intraosseous needle was placed in the right proximal tibia. Two 600-ml boluses of lactated Ringer's solution were infused, with no change in this patient's hemodynamic status. Her heart rate remained 190, with a capillary refill time of 7 seconds. A 300-ml bolus of O-negative blood was given by the flight nurse; at this point the patient's heart rate decreased to 120 and the capillary refill time decreased to 3 seconds.

The patient remained unconscious, with decorticate posturing to painful stimuli. Pupil size was noted to be 4 mm, and both pupils were sluggishly reactive to light. Movement of all extremities was noted. Full cervical spine precautions with backboard and straps were continued.

A brief secondary survey revealed an 8-cm temporal laceration, without active bleeding, and multiple facial abrasions. No drainage was noted from the ears or nose, and the face and mandible were stable to palpation. The patient's clavicles were uninjured, and the thoracic examination findings were unchanged.

The abdomen was found to be distended and firm, without audible bowel sounds. Decorticate posturing was noted on palpation of the abdomen. The pelvis was grossly unstable to palpation, and large areas of ecchymosis were present in the perineal region.

No obvious upper- or lower-extremity injury was found on palpation, and peripheral pulses were present in all extremities. An orogastric tube was placed; it returned a small amount of undigested food. A rectal examination by the referring physician revealed good sphincter tone and no occult bleeding. No apparent external urethral trauma was seen. A Foley catheter was placed; frank hematuria was evident.

A PASG was applied and all compartments inflated to stabilize the suspected pelvic fracture. At this time the patient's backboard was secured to the helicopter stretcher and transport to the tertiary facility initiated. Vital signs before departure were blood pressure, 110/60 mm Hg; heart rate, 106; respiratory rate, 32; rectal temperature, 36.8° C; and pulse oximetry saturation, 100%.

Assisted ventilation with 100% oxygen and an $ETCO_2$ monitor was continued in transport. An 18-gauge IV catheter was successfully placed in the right antecubital fossa, and lactated Ringer's solution was infused at 100 ml/hr.

Approximately 10 minutes from the tertiary hospital the patient's systolic blood pressure dropped to 68 mm Hg on palpation, with a heart rate of 190. The patient was easily ventilated, and the pulse oximetry reading remained 100%. A second 300-ml bolus of O-negative blood was infused; it increased the blood pressure to 108/68 mm Hg and decreased the heart rate to 104. The patient produced 80 ml of blood-tinged urine during the transport.

The remainder of the patient's assessment was unchanged through the 25-minute transport, and she was admitted to the emergency department of the level I tertiary hospital 1 hour and 40 minutes after injury.

Emergency computed tomography scan of the head revealed cerebral edema but no focal intracranial lesion. Cervical spine and chest films were negative for injury, but numerous pelvic fractures were found on radiography.

After another episode of hypotension requiring transfusion therapy, the patient was taken to the operating room, where a large liver laceration was found and repaired during laparotomy. No additional intraabdominal injuries were noted. Her pelvic fractures were surgically stabilized, and she was admitted to the pediatric intensive care unit.

The patient was successfully extubated on her third postoperative day and placed in the trauma stepdown unit 5 days after injury. After 2 weeks on the rehabilitative service, she was discharged home to continue physical therapy on an outpatient basis. Approximately 6 months after injury, she had made a full recovery and was functioning at an age-appropriate level in all cognitive tests.

DISCUSSION

Management of complications found in the primary survey is critical to the successful management of the traumatically injured child.

Airway control (in conjunction with stabilization of the cervical spine) was promptly and effectively managed by the flight nurse in this case study. By intubating this patient, the flight nurse was able to ventilate this patient adequately, as well as assist in airway protection from aspiration. Knowledge of weight-appropriate drug dosages for rapid sequence intubation allowed management of the airway in conjunction with the clinical benefits offered by these medications. After securing the airway and assisting ventilation, the flight nurse quickly focused on this patient's circulatory compromise.

The identification of shock and the aggressive management with both the intraosseous needle and fluid resuscitation was instrumental in the stabilization of the patient described here. Again, acute awareness of the fluid needs of pediatric patients based on their kilogram weight made it possible for the flight nurse to control what in all likelihood would have developed into a lethal complication for this child.

A neurologic examination served as a baseline for serial examinations but showed no necessity for acute intervention. Diuresis may be considered in the hemodynamically stable patient with focal findings, but it was not indicated in the early management of this patient.

After completing the interventions necessary in the primary survey, the nurse noted during a rapid secondary survey the probable cause of the patient's hypovolemia (intraabdominal bleeding and pelvic fractures) and guided interventions to further stabilize the patient.

The placement of the PASG, orogastric tube, and Foley catheter prevented further patient complications and, in the case of the Foley catheter, assisted in the measurement of fluid needs and circulatory status.

Reassessment, as in all trauma patients, was extremely beneficial. The flight nurse was able to document that initial interventions had improved the patient's clinical examination and had produced no deleterious side effects such as hypothermia. Reassessing the patient in transport also identified the second hypotensive episode, which was correctly treated with transfusion therapy.

The coordination in care of the referring hospital, the transport team, and the receiving hospital provided this child with all the resources necessary for her eventual positive outcome.

REFERENCES

1. American Academy of Pediatrics Committee on Hospital Care: Guidelines for air and ground transportation of pediatric patients, *Pediatrics* 78:5, 1986.
2. American Heart Association, American Academy of Pediatrics: *Textbook of pediatric advanced life support,* ed 2, Dallas, 1994.
3. Cook G: Starting IVs with the four tourniquet technique, *J Emerg Nurs* 12(4):200, 1987.

4. Eichelberger MR, Pratasch GL: *Pediatric trauma care,* Rockville, Md, 1988, Aspen.
5. Emergency Nurses Association: *Trauma nursing core course,* 1995, Park Ridge, Ill, The Association.
6. Fleischer GW , Ludwig S, editors: *Textbook of pediatric emergency medicine,* ed 2, Baltimore, 1988, Williams & Wilkins.
7. Harris BH et al: The crucial hour, *Pediatr Ann* 16:301, 1987.
8. Haller JA: Pediatric trauma: the no. 1 killer of children, *JAMA* 249:47, 1983.
9. Herzenberg JE et al: Emergency transport and positioning of young children who have an injury of the cervical spine: the standard backboard may be dangerous, *J Bone Joint Surg* 71-A:1, 1989.
10. Hodge D: Intraosseous infusions: a review, *Pediatr Emerg Care* 1(4):215, 1985.
11. Hodge D, Fleischer G: Pediatric catheter flow rates, *Am J Emerg Med* 2(5):403, 1985.
12. Katz J, Steward DJ: *Anesthesia and uncommon pediatric airway diseases,* Philadelphia, 1987, Saunders.
13. Manley L, Haley K, Dick M: Intraosseous infusion: rapid vascular access for critically ill or injured infants and children, *JEN* 14:2, 1988.
14. Matlak M: *Current problems in the management of pediatric trauma,* Ninety-seventh annual Ross Conference, Phoenix, May 1988.
15. Mayer T, Walker ML: Emergency intracranial pressure monitoring in pediatrics, *Clin Pediatr* 1:7, 1982.
16. Mayer T et al: *Emergency management of pediatric trauma,* Philadelphia, 1985, Saunders.
17. Moore P: When you have to think small for a neurological exam, *RN,* p 8, June 1988.
18. Morrow JC: Simplifying nursing management of pediatric airways and intravenous infusions, *JEN* 14:2, 1988.
19. National Flight Nurses Association: *Textbook of flight nurse advanced trauma course,* Park Ridge, Ill, 1994, The Association.
20. National Institute of Disability and Rehabilitation Research: *Pediatric trauma registry, summary report,* 1988, The Institute.
21. National Safety Council: *Accidents facts,* 1987 edition, The Council.
22. Nypaver M, Treloar D: Neutral cervical spine positioning in children, *Ann Emerg Med* 23:208, 1994.
23. Rosetti VA et al: Intraosseous infusion: an alternative route of pediatric vascular access, *Ann Emerg Med* 14:9, 1985.
24. Trunkey D: Trauma, *Sci Am* 249:28, 1983.
25. Tsai A et al: Epidemiology of pediatric prehospital care, *Ann Emerg Med* 16:12, 1987.
26. US Department of Health and Human Services and US Department of Transportation: *Pediatric emergency medical services training program,* ed 4, Washington, DC, 1987 GPO.

CHAPTER 19

Neurologic Medical Emergencies

COMPETENCIES

1. Provide respiratory support, airway management, cardiovascular support and neurologic support to the comatose patient.
2. Realize the importance of serial examinations in the care of the comatose patient.
3. Emphasize safety of the patient and crew during transport of the patient with seizures.
4. Provide life-sustaining and supportive care with appropriate and aggressive interventions to patients with cerebrovascular episodes to achieve maximum potential for recovery.
5. Review need for universal precautions in patient transport.
6. Review need for effective communication.

Several nontraumatic neurologic emergencies require rapid assessment, stabilization, diagnosis, and transfer to definitive care. The flight nurse plays an important role in the outcome of these patients; therefore a thorough understanding of the pathophysiology, etiology, and management of these emergencies is crucial.

Neurologic medical emergencies may present individually or concurrently. Their causes differ, depending on the disorder, but emergency treatment is aimed at controlling the airway, stabilizing and supporting the cardiovascular system, minimizing additional cerebral insult, and protecting the patient from physical harm during expeditious transfer to definitive care.[1]

NEUROLOGIC PATHOPHYSIOLOGY

Alteration in the intracranial pressure (ICP) is directly or indirectly of prime concern in the care of patients with neurologic emergencies.[14,18,27] Following is a discussion of how normal ICP is maintained, how it is altered, and how changes in it should be managed.

Pressure-Volume Relationships

In understanding the diagnosis and management of ICP problems, it is helpful to think of the intracranial contents as having three components: cerebrospinal fluid (CSF), blood volume, and brain. In the average situation, approximately 100 ml of CSF is accompanied by 150 ml of blood and 1250 ml (or grams) of brain. In the normal course of events, brain volume is not altered. However, the average volume of fluid in the CSF and in the blood is rather dynamic, and throughout the day the volumes of these two compartments may vary considerably. These variations occur in response to alterations in ICP.[16,25,27]

The way relationships among the volume of CSF, the volume of blood, and the volume of brain maintain a relatively constant ICP is described in the modified Monroe-Kellie hypothesis, which states that increases and decreases in the volume of one or more compartments will be offset by appropriate reductions or increases in the volume of the other compartment or compartments to maintain a constant ICP (Fig. 19-1). Because brain volume changes little (and when it does, it involves mainly interstitial water), most normal variations occur in the volumes of CSF and blood.[16,25,27]

Should an intracranial mass or cerebral edema begin to develop, this volume relationship is extremely important early in the insult to compensate for the increase in mass. In the skull, particularly after childhood, when the sutures begin to fuse, the intracranial contents are housed in a nondistensible structure. As a mass or cerebral edema begins to develop, there must be an immediate reduction in the volumes of one or more compartments for ICP not to begin to increase immediately because the contents themselves are largely water and are relatively noncompressible.[27] The viscoelastic properties of the brain are such that if a mass, such as a growing tumor, exerts slowly increasing pressure, the brain may compensate through the slow loss of water or cellular elements through atrophy. However, with acute changes in the size of a mass, such as in an acute epidural hematoma, the brain is relatively noncompressible.

To understand the ability of the intracranial components to compensate for the development of a mass (it is helpful to think of the combined volume of cerebral edema as mass), it is useful to look at the pressure-volume curve.[16,27,33] (See Fig. 19-2.) It can be seen that at first, as a change in volume of mass occurs, there is no change in ICP. This phenomenon is the result of compliance and is accomplished by reduction in volume of CSF and blood. At some point, however, compliance is lost, and additional changes in volume result in great increases in ICP. In the acute state of cerebral edema, or a rapidly developing intracranial hematoma, the total shifts in volume amount to approximately 50 to 75 ml.[16,24,27,34]

$$K \sim V_{CSF} + V_{Blood} + V_{Brain}$$

Fig. 19-1. Modified Monroe-Kellie hypothesis.

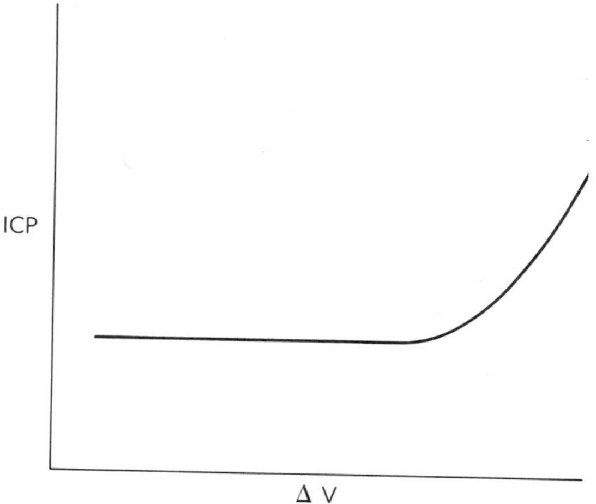

Fig. 19-2. Pressure-volume curve.

Cerebrospinal Fluid Volume

The volume of CSF is controlled by the rate of production and the rate of absorption of CSF. Production, except in the presence of very high ICP, remains relatively constant in the adult at about 0.35 ml/min. It is a secretory process in which CSF is actively secreted by the choroid plexus in the lateral, third, and fourth ventricles. The fluid leaves the ventricular system and then circulates throughout the subarachnoid space, finally reaching the subarachnoid space overlying the cerebral convexities, where it is absorbed passively by way of the arachnoid granulations located parasagittally along the sagittal sinus. The fluid passes through the structures of the granulation into the cerebral venous system and is carried away with venous blood.[24,27]

Absorption is pressure driven, with the rate of CSF absorption proportional to the ICP. CSF volume is pathologically increased by an interference with absorption.[8,21,27] This increase can be caused by a mass or stricture in the ventricular system that prevents the CSF from exiting into the subarachnoid space. This accumulation of CSF is termed *obstructive* or *noncommunicating hydrocephalus*.[8,27]

Alternatively, after the CSF leaves the ventricular system, its circulation may be disturbed so that the fluid cannot reach the arachnoid granulation, resulting in communicating or nonobstructive hydrocephalus. Because the subarachnoid space is quite large, a focal lesion such as a tumor ordinarily will not produce this type of obstruction. Instead, a widespread disorder such as inflammation of the meninges or increased CSF protein will result in such obstruction.[26]

The management of hydrocephalus, whether acute or chronic, requires the diversion of the CSF around the site of blockage.[3,21,33] In general, this requires a procedure in which the neurosurgeon places a tube in a lateral ventricle by way of a surgically created defect in the skull, through a burr hole made with a small twist-drill trephine. The tube may be left in temporarily if the condition is transient, as in meningitis or if an obstructing tumor is soon to be removed. However, the tube may be made internal, in the form of a ventriculoperitoneal diversion shunt, if the condition is permanent, as in the presence of congenital stenosis of the aqueduct of Sylvius, the small CSF pathway connecting the third ventricle with the fourth ventricle.[3,27]

Cerebral Blood Volume

Cerebral blood volume comprises two relatively independent components, the arterial blood volume and the venous blood volume. Arterial blood volume accounts for approximately 25% of the total cerebral blood volume; venous blood volume accounts for the other 75%.[23,24]

Arterial cerebral blood flow (and volume) under normal circumstances remains relatively independent of systemic mean arterial blood volume and pressure through a process called *autoregulation.* Autoregulation is influenced by pressure and biochemical parameters.[2,3,27]

As mean systemic arterial pressure increases cerebral arterial blood vessels constrict, preventing the increase in blood volume and flow that would normally occur. If the mean systemic arterial blood pressure decreases, the cerebral arteries dilate, increasing cerebral blood flow. Thus between a mean systemic arterial pressure of approximately 60 and 140 mm Hg, cerebral blood flow may be maintained in a constant state (Fig. 19-3, *A*).[23,27]

Arterial blood volume is also influenced by complex biochemical or metabolic action that can be summarized by the association of $PaCO_2$ and blood flow (Fig. 19-3, *B*).[22,26,33] Increased $PaCO_2$ or decreased PaO_2 results in dilation of the blood vessel, presumably in response to greater cerebral metabolic

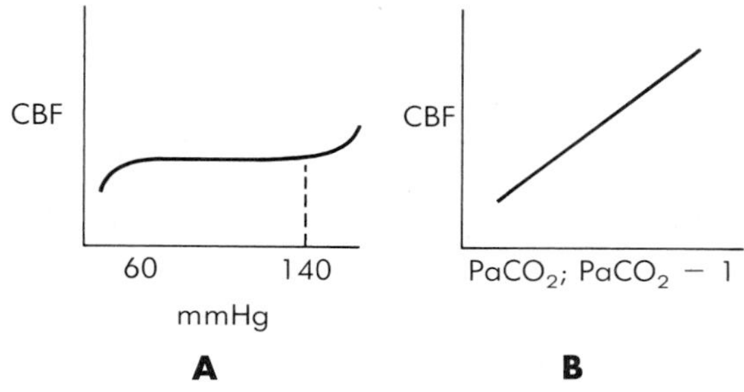

Fig. 19-3. A, Autoregulation maintains constant cerebral blood flow. **B,** Cerebral blood flow increases with increased $PaCO_2$.

needs.[23,27,34] As $PaCO_2$ decreases, blood volume and flow will be reduced. Thus it can be seen that this component of autoregulation may be influenced by respiratory control, with hyperventilation resulting in decreased cerebral blood flow and hypoventilation resulting in increased cerebral blood flow.[1,2,27,34]

Venous blood volume is passively influenced by the delivery of blood from the arterial side and the ability of the cerebral venous system to drain from the head. This drainage depends on two influences: hydrostatic pressure and central venous pressure. Elevation of the head increases hydrostatic pressure on the venous side, permitting more rapid drainage from the cerebral venous system, mainly through the internal jugular veins bilaterally. Increased central venous pressure, whether caused by increased intrathoracic pressure or by right heart failure, decreases cerebral venous return.[2,27,34]

Respiratory management can greatly influence the volume of cerebral venous blood. If intrathoracic pressure is increasing because, for example, the patient is straining on an endotracheal tube, a decrease in cerebral venous drainage (and thus an increase in cerebral venous blood volume) will occur.[16,34]

Brain Volume Cerebral Edema

Brain volume, except for a relatively insignificant alteration in interstitial water, does not change under ordinary circumstances. However, with injury, cerebral brain water may accumulate in the form of cerebral edema. This brain water may be found mainly in the cells, where it is called *cytotoxic edema,* or in the interstitial spaces, called *vasogenic edema.*[3,29]

Cytotoxic edema is produced by injury to cells, as occurs in hypoxia and certain metabolic diseases. Under these circumstances, cell membranes are damaged and certain intracellular metabolic processes become deranged. The normal metabolic pumps (e.g., sodium, potassium, calcium) do not function properly, and water, moving along osmotic gradients, accumulates intracellularly.[24,27]

Vasogenic edema is produced mainly by a disruption in the blood-brain barrier, which allows larger molecules than normal to cross from the blood along concentration gradients into the interstitial spaces. This movement of ions and protein alters interstitial osmotic pressure, permitting water to pass into the interstitial spaces of the brain.[24,27]

COMA

All neurologic emergencies discussed in this chapter can lead to coma. (The pathophysiology of coma is discussed in Chapter 12.) Following is a discussion of the precipitating causes, diagnosis, and patient care interventions for the broad categories of coma.

Assessment

The flight nurse relies on thorough assessment and objective data in examining the comatose patient because subjective data cannot be obtained. A thorough history including the events preceding coma, medical history, and therapy instituted are of prime concern and should be obtained from family and transferring medical personnel. The flight nurse assessment of the comatose patient is crucial in differentiating potential causes of the comatose state and determining the proper treatment protocol.[6]

During the assessment, it is useful to use a system approach in evaluating the comatose patient (see Chapter 12) and establishing a differential diagnosis.

Differential Diagnosis of the Comatose Patient: UNCONSCIOUS

On the basis of the differential diagnosis, certain actions may be instituted by the flight nurse in terms of therapy or diagnosis. The components of a reasonable differential diagnosis of the comatose patient may be recalled by remembering the items, the initial letters of which spell the word "unconscious" (box).

U = **Units of Insulin.** Units of insulin relates to the presence of both hyperglycemia and hypoglycemia, regardless of whether the patient is diabetic. The flight nurse, in considering the possibility of either one, would want to give the patient with coma of unknown cause IV glucose, up to 50 ml of 50% concentration ($D_{50}W$). If the patient appears malnourished and has a known history of alcohol abuse, thiamine (100 mg) may be added to the maintenance IV fluid.

N = **Narcotics.** The word "narcotics" should prompt the flight nurse to consider any and all drugs, not only narcotics, including street drugs, but pre-

MNEMONIC FOR THE DIFFERENTIAL DIAGNOSIS OF COMA

U Units of insulin
N Narcotics
C Convulsions
O Oxygen
N Nonorganic
S Stroke
C Cocktail
I ICP
O Organism
U Urea
S Shock

scription and nonprescription drugs. Naloxone may be useful in the diagnosis of opiate overdose; however, the appropriate management is control of the airway. Appropriate diagnostic studies include blood and urine drug screens.

C = **Convulsions.** Seizures of both idiopathic origin and those associated with structural lesions such as stroke, trauma, brain tumor, and arteriovenous malformation should be considered.

O = **Oxygen.** Hypoxia and carbon monoxide poisoning should be considered.

N = **Nonorganic.** Very rarely, apparent coma will be of psychogenic origin.

S = **Stroke.** Ischemic stroke may be the result of thrombi or emboli of cerebrovascular or cardiovascular origin. Assessment of cardiac status in search of arrhythmias and appropriate intervention is important.

C = **Cocktail.** The cocktail image should suggest alcohol and its various syndromes to include a postictal state, Wernicke's encephalopathy, and overdose.

I = **Intracranial Pressure.** Increase in ICP should be considered.

O = **Organism.** Organisms result in infections and manifest bacterial, fungal, and viral causes. They mainly infect the central nervous system or result from systemic sepsis.

U = **Urea.** The miscellaneous metabolic causes of coma such as diabetes, liver disease, and kidney failure should be considered. Generally available laboratory examinations that survey blood and urine chemistries are helpful in excluding this category.

S = **Shock.** Of primary concern in suspected shock is hypovolemic shock resulting from trauma or from spontaneous vascular rupture such as dissecting aortic aneurysm. The possibility of trauma should engender the thought of an accompanying head injury. The appropriate diagnostic procedure in such a case is computed tomography (CT). Shock may also be cardiogenic or septic in nature, and the appropriate examinations to include electrocardiography, central venous pressure, and blood cultures will be useful.

Plan and Implementation

In developing a plan of care for the comatose patient during air medical transport, the cause of the comatose state must be considered and care implemented accordingly. A systematic approach should be used in the evaluation and care of the comatose patient, as with any seriously ill or injured patient. Universal precautions should be initiated before contact with any patient. Gloves, goggles, and a protective barrier (or spare uniform, if available) should be worn if the possibility of contact with a patient's body fluids exists.

In the comatose patient the airway should be secured first; then an IV line should be established. If the cause of the coma is truly unknown, samples for blood work to include blood gases, chemistry studies, drug screens, and toxicology should be drawn while the IV line is being secured.[1,23] This should be immediately followed by IV glucose and, if appropriate, thiamine.[1,23] The maintenance fluids depend on the vital signs and the suspected cause of coma. If hypovolemia or a head injury is suspected, then a balanced salt solution (such as normal saline or Ringer's lactate) is indicated. Otherwise, maintenance infusions of 5% dextrose and water to keep the line functional are appropriate. CT is the diagnostic procedure of choice for the unconscious patient to rule out a mass lesion, stroke, and hydrocephalus.[24] It may also be useful in the diagnosis of certain forms of encephalitis, particularly that of herpes simplex, which tends to localize in the temporal lobe.[12]

Approximately 60% of patients in coma will have some diffuse or systemic problem such as metabolic coma, encephalitis, sepsis, or AIDS. Neurologic symptoms develop in at least 39% of all patients with AIDS; the most common is AIDS encephalopathy.[15] The comatose state indicates a secondary involvement of the brain. The main problem is identification of the underlying systemic or diffuse cause of the patient's illness. Another 25% of patients in coma present as stroke victims; such presentations include not only embolic and ischemic conditions but subarachnoid hemorrhage and hypertensive hemorrhage into the brainstem. Patients with such disorders require maintenance of the airway and fluids until the definitive diagnosis can be established. The remainder of patients, approximately 15%, have a mass lesion as the underlying cause of coma. Examples of lesions include brain tumors, hematomas, and brain abscesses.[4,5,12,24]

Practical Considerations in the Examination of the Comatose Patient

In all comatose patients, rapid assessment and diagnosis of the problem are critical to the success of treatment because significant delay will result in major morbidity and mortality.[24,26] Thus it is critical that after examination the unconscious patient be classified in one of the three categories described. This classification requires reevaluation of the patient. Table 19-1 demonstrates a correlation between the anatomic level of the lesion and the physiologic disturbance produced by the lesion, as demonstrated in the neurologic examination.

If repeated examinations demonstrate deterioration of the patient's condition with progressive loss of anatomic and physiologic function, the presence of a dynamic lesion may be assumed; a mass lesion must be immediately excluded.

If reevaluation reveals a stable, unchanging situation, it may be assumed that a static lesion is present, most likely a stroke. For example, pontine hemorrhage is manifested by small, equal pupils and abnormal oculocephalic or oculovestibular reflex examination findings, flaccid motor response, and unconsciousness.[5,6,22]

If the repeated examinations reveal a diffusely distributed neurologic picture and, especially, if that picture seems to wax and wane in severity, then a diffuse systemic cause is most likely to blame.[7] For example, a patient with drug intoxication may be lightly stuporous but exhibit pinpoint pupils and near-apnea in the absence of significant painful stimulation.

Summary

The comatose patient presents a challenge. The patient cannot provide a direct history or a chief complaint. Therefore a history from family members or bystanders, in addition to clinical data, are necessary for a working diagnosis. All comatose patients require supportive care directed at prevention of complications.[1,6,16] Not infrequently, the comatose patient will require intervention for respiratory support, airway management (and consideration of hyperventilation), cardiovascular support (to maintain fluid balance and possible dysrhythmia control), and neurologic support (for control of seizures and ICP maintenance).[1,6,16,23]

Serial examinations are vital in the care of a comatose patient. As with all acutely critically ill or injured patients, the neurologically impaired (comatose) patient is not in a static condition. Repeated examination is essential if appropriate and timely interventions are to be instituted.

On the basis of examination findings communicated to the emergency center, CT can be performed on the patient's arrival at the receiving facility. This may require an alteration in the schedule of the CT scan equipment; hence it is important that the patient's needs be prioritized as assessed during the transfer phase.

SEIZURES

Patients with seizures are often transported by air. Of primary concern in the aircraft is the safety of the patient and crew, with particular attention to techniques to protect and restrain the patient prone to or exhibiting seizure activity.

The annual incidence of seizure is estimated to be approximately 0.5% of the population (48 per 100,000) in the United States. Incidence is greater among males, particularly after the age of 20.[3,14,30]

TABLE 19-1

Physiologic disturbance correlated with anatomic level of lesion

Parameters	Cerebral cortex	Diencephalon (thalamus)		Midbrain	Pons	Medulla
Mental status	Awake, alert, lethargic, obtunded	Light stupor	Deep stupor	Coma	Coma	Coma
Motor response	Appropriate	Focal response to pain	General response to pain	Decerebrate posturing, decorticate posturing	Flaccid	Flaccid
Pupil response	Normal size and reactivity	Small	Small	Mid-position	Small	Small
Oculocephalic, oculovestibular reflex	Not testable	Normal response	Normal response	Abnormal	Abnormal	Abnormal*
Respiratory status	Variable	Variable	Cheyne-Stokes	Central neurogenic hyperventilation	Apneustic pattern	Apnea

*May be normal with isolated medullary injury.

This may be due to a higher incidence of head injury with subsequent seizure activity. The highest incidence, however, is among children younger than 5 years (152 per 100,000 population annually). Overall, 650 per 100,000 population are affected by seizure activity in the United States. The prevalence is relatively constant between the ages of 10 and 60 years.[3,14]

Early, aggressive management of the patient with seizures is important; rapid transport with appropriate intervention for control of the seizure, management of the airway and cardiovascular system, and treatment of any associated condition clearly reduce morbidity and mortality.

Pathophysiology

The onset of epileptic seizures is associated with several types of generalized and focal brain lesions. The underlying neuropathophysiologic disturbances, however, are poorly understood. Although it is reasonable to believe that an alteration exists in the neuronal pool or in the extracellular environment (both general theories having their advocates), neither laboratory investigations nor clinical experience with specific antiepileptic drugs has yielded a common therapy.[3,18]

It is known, however, that similar-appearing epileptic syndromes may occur, caused by focal lesions such as brain tumors, arteriovenous malformations, stroke, and generalized states such as head trauma and viral or metabolic encephalopathies. Additionally, in some idiopathic epilepsy syndromes no obvious underlying cause is apparent. With more sophisticated recording techniques, several idiopathic epileptic syndromes are being associated with the presence of focal lesions such as occult infarcts or sclerosis following birth trauma.[16,18]

Some patients present with status epilepticus syndrome. These patients are to be considered true neurologic emergencies; ischemic changes at the neuronal level, similar to those seen in patients with severe hypoglycemia and cerebral hypoxia, develop.[3,30]

Neuronal ischemic changes were once thought to be caused by decreased respiratory effort. They are theorized to occur in combination with ictal events including marked increase in metabolic rate and membrane changes affecting the transport of small ions at the neuronal level.[16,30]

Assessment

Several classification schemes for epilepsy have been proposed. The one with the most current widespread acceptance is from the International League Against Epilepsy,[3,30] which characterizes the syndromes as (1) partial seizures that begin locally and may or may not spread generally, (2) generalized seizures that begin bilaterally and are symmetrical, (3) a large group of unclassified, poorly understood syndromes, and (4) status epilepticus.

The same assessment criteria should be used regardless of the classification of seizure activity exhibited. The assessment criteria should include a thorough history, physical examination, and neurologic evaluation. The onset and type and duration of seizure activity should be determined from the history. Additional pertinent information includes allergies, medications, and any recent illness or injury.

In the physical examination the airway is always of primary importance. The examiner must be alert to signs of trauma that may have occurred before or concurrent with the seizure activity. The physical assessment should then include motor, sensory, and psychomotor evaluation. The degree of involvement of these areas will depend on the individual patient presentation. Involvement may range from isolated focal activity to generalized status involvement.[3,6,30]

Regardless of the level of involvement, motor activity is involuntary. It begins with the tonic phase, a continuous tense muscular state. This is followed by a hypertonic phase with hypertension and muscle rigidity. The clonic phase is characterized by rapidly alternating muscle rigidity and relaxation. During the clonic phase sphincter control is lost, and the patient may be incontinent. Tachycardia, hyperventilation, and salivation result from autonomic discharge during seizure activity. Sensory assessment is subjective because the patient's complaints may include visual, auditory, or proprioceptive phenomena. Psychomotor assessment is the determination of the level of consciousness, which may vary widely depending on the type of seizure activity and the time of evaluation.

Other psychomotor observations include amnesia and repetitive behavioral patterns.[10,18,30]

Plan and Implementation

A plan of care for the seizure patient requiring air medical transport includes a rapid, thorough assessment; aggressive intervention; and safe transfer to tertiary care.

Implementation of the plan involves management of the airway for prevention of hypoxia, support of the cardiovascular system, control of the seizure activity, and protection of the patient from physical injuries and additional complications associated with the seizure activity. Management of the underlying illness or injury that predisposed the patient to seizures may also be necessary.

Several drugs are effective in the control of various seizures. The most commonly used specific antiepileptic drugs include phenytoin, carbamazepine, and valproate sodium. The most widely used nonspecific antiepileptic drugs include the barbiturates and the benzodiazepines, most commonly diazepam.[6,30] Because in air medical transport the seizure patient is generally monitored for only a short period, often without benefit of any detailed previous medical history, two decisions must be made: Should treatment be instituted? What drug therapy should be used?

All patients with a generalized presentation of seizures characterized by bilateral tonic-clonic activity, altered level of consciousness, and, possibly, urinary or fecal incontinence should be treated aggressively. These patients quickly become relatively hypoxic as a result of the seizure activity. Hypoxia tends to aggravate the seizure disorder and make it more difficult to treat. The hypoxia occurs at two levels: generalized tissue hypoxia and cellular hypoxia. General tissue hypoxia occurs because the intense motor activity of the seizure interferes with adequate respiration. This aspect of the seizure disorder can be managed with the use of paralytic agents in association with proper airway management. However, the intense neuronal activity characterized by sustained or rapidly intermittent bursts of neuronal discharge produces additional hypoxia at the cellular level. This hypoxia can result in a more long-term neuronal injury and is the reason for the aggressive use of an antiepileptic drug. The patient with a focal seizure (or partial seizure) characterized, for example, by facial twitching or motor activity limited to one extremity with no alteration of consciousness need not be managed aggressively for short periods of time if attention must be paid to a more serious medical problem. However, it should be recognized that a focal epileptic syndrome can become generalized fairly rapidly, so such progression should be anticipated.[3,10]

Status epilepticus is the most dangerous syndrome. It is the most refractory to treatment, and the stress of the intense motor activity can cause not only respiratory insufficiency but, in the elderly, myocardial strain leading to myocardial injury.[30] Intense hypertension may also occur during status seizures, resulting in expected complications such as intracerebral hemorrhage.

Practically speaking, the acute management of a generalized seizure syndrome is simple and straightforward. An IV line must be placed for administration of the appropriate medication. Attention to the airway is most important, and intubation should be considered for all patients with generalized seizure activity, especially if a significant alteration in level of consciousness is present. A person in the generalized tonic-clonic seizures often referred to as grand mal epilepsy may have such trismus that oral intubation is impossible. Nasal intubation should definitely be attempted. The trismus may be broken if the seizure is stopped with IV antiepileptic medication or with the careful use of paralytic agents.

Generalized epilepsy leading to status epilepticus is most often seen in the acute state in one of two situations: (1) with generalized encephalopathy, including that immediately following trauma; and (2) in patients who are known epileptics, who have reduced drug intake, and whose blood levels have fallen below therapeutic concentrations.[18,30]

The initial drug of choice for the patient with an acute seizure is IV diazepam, 5 to 10 mg over 1 to 2 minutes. This dose can be repeated every 2 to 5 minutes as necessary. Rarely will more than two to three separate administrations of these doses be necessary. Patients with a long history of epilepsy and nontherapeutic drug levels may be quite refractory to IV diazepam. Lorazepam 2 to 4 mg IV may be considered.[10,17,30]

Patients with recurrent seizures, whether they are experiencing seizures for the first time or have chronic epilepsy, may be given phenytoin in a relatively rapid loading dose of 18 mg/kg IV (in normal saline solution) at a rate of 50 mg/min. Because this dose can precipitate supraventricular and ventricular arrhythmias, it is wise to observe the patient with a heart monitor. If arrhythmias are noted, administration of the drug should cease. If the cardiac rhythm returns to normal, especially if seizures continue, resumption of the administration of the phenytoin is appropriate at half the previously noted rate of administration.[10,30]

Evaluation

Obviously, patient outcome depends not only on the intervention but also on precipitating factors and any complications the patient might experience. The optimal goal in caring for the patient with seizures is prompt control of the seizure activity to minimize cerebral insult and prevent complications.

Evaluation data might include arterial blood gas values, chest radiographs, laboratory results including medication blood levels, and, possibly, CT to rule out cerebral pathology on the patient's admission to the receiving facility. In the trauma patient exhibiting seizure activity, radiographs of the skull and cervical spine would also be evaluated.

Summary

Patients who present with seizure activity or in whom it develops pose special problems. Most obvious is the safety of the uncontrolled seizure patient during air medical transport. The patient, crew, and aircraft must be protected from the danger associated with the unpredictable motor responses of the seizure patient. Extra care should be taken in the application of protective patient restraints, and aggressive pharmacologic therapy should be instituted for all seizure patients.

Of particular note are visually induced seizures. The photosensitivity type is most prevalent. These seizures are induced by light flashes[10,14]; patients prone to these seizures may experience them in flight as a result of the strobe effect of aircraft lights. Pattern-induced seizures may occur in response to the light-dark pattern caused by a slowly rotating main rotor during start-up and shutdown.

CEREBROVASCULAR DISEASE

Cerebrovascular disease frequently results in interference with cerebral blood flow, causing ischemia of brain tissue. The challenge is to recognize when this condition exists and to protect the patient from further decrease in blood flow and poor delivery of oxygen, glucose, and other substrates essential to brain tissue.

Stroke, as it was called in the past, is now termed *brain attack.* This new terminology is purposely used to resemble the term "heart attack" and to underscore the fact that it is a medical emergency.[19]

Atherosclerosis and hypertension lead to approximately half a million strokes annually; of that number, approximately 150,000 victims survive. According to the American Heart Association, stroke is the leading cause of permanent disability in adults. Of the three major categories of stroke, thromboembolism accounts for most, with an approximate 70% incidence. Hemorrhagic stroke is responsible for an estimated 20% incidence (subarachnoid hemorrhage, 8%; intracerebral hemorrhage, 12%). The remaining 10% are unclassified.[11,19,23,25] The need to view stroke as a medical emergency is imperative to improving the outcome of stroke victims. The flight service is essential for providing rapid transport of the stroke patient to a tertiary care center where screening procedures such as CT, angiography, endovascular techniques, and intraarterial thrombolytic therapy are available as deemed necessary.[11,19]

Regardless of the underlying cause, a cerebrovascular episode requiring air medical transport is frequently abrupt in onset and dynamic in progression. Treatment is directed at life-sustaining intervention, with emphasis on prevention of extension of injury. Prognosis varies depending on the extent of involvement and the affected area of the brain. Recovery may be maximized by the prevention of additional cerebral insult through aggressive airway and cardiovascular support.[17,23,25]

Pathophysiology

A knowledge of normal cerebral circulation aids in the understanding of the pathophysiology of cerebrovascular disease. The importance of avoiding hypoxia has been discussed. Because the brain cannot store glucose, this substance must be constantly supplied in the blood flow. Critical reductions in glucose resulting from hypoglycemia or decreased perfusion can cause irreversible cellular damage.

The brain receives its blood from two sets of vessels. Two common carotid arteries in the anterior neck bifurcate, each into an external carotid artery that supplies primarily facial tissue; and the internal carotid arteries that provide most of the blood supply to the brain through its major subdivisions, the anterior cerebral and the middle cerebral arteries. In the posterior aspect of the neck on either side lie the vertebral arteries. These combine shortly after they pass through the foramen magnum into the single basilar artery, which mainly supplies the brainstem. The posterior cerebral arteries from the vertebral basilar system communicate through two posterior communicating arteries with the internal carotid arteries. A small anterior artery permits communication between the two anterior cerebral arteries. Thus at the base of the brain a significant collateral circulation called the *circle of Willis* is formed where blood can flow as needed from one internal carotid system to the opposite internal carotid system, or to the vertebral basilar system, or to any combination of connections between the internal carotid systems and the vertebral basilar system.[2,16,25]

In addition, extensive collateral vessels may develop between the external carotid system and the internal carotid system. These collaterals are supplied mainly through facial anastomoses by way of the ophthalamic artery and through anastomoses between scalp vessels and vessels of the dura and arachnoid, called *leptomeningeal vessels.* Beyond this, however, in the depths of the brain, no collaterals assist deficient circulation. Therefore occlusion of smaller vessels from the surface of the brain inward will result in ischemia and infarction.[2]

The main features governing blood flow are summarized only briefly here. In the range of a mean systematic arterial pressure of 60 to 140 mm Hg, cerebral blood remains relatively constant through autoregulation (Fig. 19-3, *A*). The cerebral blood vessels, especially those of capacitance (in the substance of the brain), constrict or dilate depending on the pressure of blood flow to maintain the constant flow. This system is also governed by metabolic considerations, with increased blood flow occurring with increased $PaCO_2$ (Fig. 19-3, *B*). In the face of increased $PaCO_2$, and if cerebral blood flow is impaired, a decrease in PaO_2 will occur and is significant. In a severe hypoxic state, the blood vessels react not mainly on the basis of $PaCO_2$ but on the basis of PaO_2 with increased dilation seen as hypoxia worsens.[23,25]

Cerebral Ischemia

Cerebral ischemia is the term applied to brain tissue injury resulting from decreased cerebral blood flow.[2] The decrease in blood flow may be caused by systemic problems such as severe hypovolemia and myocardial failure. Because these issues are discussed in other chapters, they will not be discussed here. The primary concern is decreased regional or local cerebral blood flow resulting from vascular occlusion. The occlusion may be the result of an intraluminal process—that is, the development of a thrombosis or the arrival of an embolus—or it may be the result of extrinsic pressure from a mass in the brain tissue itself.[2,23]

The most common cause of vascular occlusion, resulting in the classic appearance of a stroke, is an embolus from some other part of the vascular system. Approximately one third of these emboli (especially in older persons) come from disease in the heart. Previous myocardial infarctions or valvular diseases may result in the development of mural thrombi, which are the source of emboli. In the great vessels a common location for thrombi formation is the bifurcation of the common carotid into the internal and external carotid. Disease at this location can often be detected by the auscultation of a bruit over the carotid bifurcation at the border of the involved sternocleidomastoid muscle just at the level of the angle of the mandible.[25] Auscultation must be performed carefully to prevent the dislodging of thrombi in the underlying vessel.

The next most common cause of cerebral ischemia is spontaneous intracerebral hemorrhage from cerebral aneurysms or arteriovenous malformations; that of accompanying hypertension is the most prevalent. As a result of this hemorrhage, the first vascular response is to contract and constrict to control hemorrhage in the region of the vascular injury. Second, as the hematoma develops in the brain tissue, the mass effect can place significant pressure on the distal arterioles, and capillary blood pressure becomes relatively low. Approximately 85% of hemorrhagic cases involve the cerebral hemispheres, and only a relatively small number occur in the cerebellum and brainstem as a result of involvement of the vertebral basilar system. In the case of hemorrhage in the cerebellum, the fourth ventricle may be acutely obstructed by the hematoma, resulting in sudden increase in ICP caused by impeded CSF flow. This increase will be managed by the neurosurgeon with ventriculostomy drainage.[4,23,25]

In the extremely rare instance when such a patient is transferred, the neurosurgeon should be consulted on a case-by-case basis with regard to the care of the ventriculostomy or any other implanted device to monitor ICP before transport.

A small subset of hemorrhagic cases involve the rupture of intracranial aneurysms into the subarachnoid space. This subarachnoid hemorrhage, besides causing primary brain injury, may result in cerebral ischemia caused by cerebral vasospasm. There is little to distinguish this condition from other strokes except the complaint of the patient of severe, often focal, headache just before the hemorrhage.[5,9,32]

The use of crack cocaine has not only been implicated as a cause of intracranial hemorrhage but has been associated with acute intracranial arterial occlusive disease.[16]

The development of intracerebral thrombi as a cause of cerebral ischemia is relatively uncommon. Such development is most likely when there exists a primary disease of the blood vessels such as occurs with meningitis or with some of the vasculitides that accompany more widespread immunologic conditions such as rheumatoid arthritis, dermatomyositis, and the polyangiopathies. A small group of patients with primary myopathies may exhibit cerebral symptoms of ischemia. The pathophysiology is not clear, but it may be a combination of cerebrovasospasm and primary thrombosis.[4,25]

The signs and symptoms the patient presents with will depend on the portion of the cerebral circulation involved and the cause. The classic presentation of the embolic state is that of the transient ischemic attack. In this condition, the embolus lodges at the bifurcation of a cerebral blood vessel, temporarily producing decreasing blood flow and symptoms appropriate to the involvement of that part of the brain such as a contralateral hemiparesis or numbness in the face. After a few minutes or hours the embolus breaks up, and the material passes more distally, restoring blood flow. Within 24 hours the patient has recovered. If this clearing of the blood flow avenue does not occur, significant injury of the tissue may result, including tissue death; a frank stroke has then occurred. If a small vessel supplying the internal capsule is involved, a dense hemiplegia may develop. Should the embolus lodge in a major branch of the internal carotid artery, such as the anterior cerebral or middle cerebral arteries, the posterior cerebral artery, or the internal carotid itself, major destruction of the hemisphere will occur, and the patient may have an accompanying severe depression of level of consciousness, including coma. If the embolus involves the vertebral basilar system, various combinations of cranial nerve and cerebellar findings may be apparent, but the hallmark of vertebral basilar stroke is sudden coma.[2,25,29]

Plan and Implementation

As mentioned previously, care of the patient with a cerebrovascular episode is directed toward prevention of additional cerebral insult. Every attempt must be made to maximize cerebral blood flow, to control increased ICP, and to manage associated conditions such as cardiac dysrhythmias and seizures.

Thrombolytic therapy was recently shown to be beneficial in acute ischemic stroke. Timing is crucial in these patients because evidence suggests that ischemic brain injury occurs when arterial occlusion continues longer than 2 or 3 hours and an increasing amount of brain is infarcted if occlusion persists beyond this time. Local thrombolytic therapy should be started within 6 hours of the time of neurologic deterioration.[19]

Once again, airway support is paramount, often requiring intubation and ventilatory support. The use of mechanical ventilation and arterial oxygen-saturation and end-tidal CO_2 ($ETCO_2$) monitoring during flight has proved effective in managing the patient with a neurologic medical emergency. IV access is necessary for fluid maintenance and medication administration. As with all neurologic emergencies, protection of the patient from physical harm is necessary, with particular attention to safety restraints.

Summary

Cerebrovascular disease is common in the adult population of the United States. Morbidity and mortality vary, depending on the type and extent of lesion and associated conditions or complications. Patients experiencing cerebrovascular episodes are frequently transferred to tertiary care facilities for further diagnostic studies and intervention. The initiation of life-sustaining care and supportive care throughout the transfer are valuable links in the transfer process. The overall mortality rate for cerebrovascular episodes can be generally divided into the three causes: cerebral hemorrhage, 80%; subarachnoid hemorrhage, 20% to 30%; and embolic occlusion, 25% to 30%. With appropriate and aggressive intervention, the maximal potential for recovery and subsequent rehabilitation can be ensured in the patient who has sustained a cerebrovascular episode.[25]

NEUROLOGIC MEDICAL EMERGENCIES CASE STUDY

The flight crew was dispatched to a scene where a 46-year-old woman, who had earlier called 911 complaining of a severe headache and neck pain, was found unresponsive by basic life support unit personnel.

Flight Crew Examination

On the arrival of the flight crew, the patient appeared to be having a seizure. An oxygen mask had been applied to the patient by the emergency medical technician. A neighbor stated that she did not know whether the patient was allergic to any medications or whether she took any medications. Assessment revealed bilateral breath sounds to be present and clear. An IV line of lactated Ringer's solution was started and 5 mg IV diazepam given. The seizure activity stopped after 15 seconds. The patient remained unresponsive to verbal or painful stimuli. The patient had spontaneous respiration. An attempt at nasal endotracheal intubation was unsuccessful. The patient was clenching her teeth very hard, so the decision to intubate orally with the use of succinylcholine was made. The Propaq monitor was applied to the patient. Blood pressure was 204/110 mm Hg, heart rate 103, and oxygen saturation 90%. The patient had shallow respirations of 12 breaths/min. Her pupils were equal at 7 mm but nonreactive to light. A rapid sequence intubation protocol was followed in which the patient was initially given 2 mg IV midazolam, 60 mg IV lidocaine (suspected head injury), and 1 mg IV vecuronium. A bag-valve mask and suction were ready. With an estimated patient weight of 60 kg, 60 mg IV succinylcholine was given. The patient was ventilated with a bag-valve mask; once paralyzed, she was intubated orally with a 7.5 endotracheal tube, with cricoid pressure. With endotracheal tube placement confirmed with detection of bilateral breath sounds and $ETCO_2$ monitoring, the patient was prepared for transport to the nearest facility with CT and neurology consultation capabilities. An 18Fr nasogastric tube was placed before liftoff.

In Flight Care

Mechanical ventilation was started en route, with the $ETCO_2$ adapter in place. Ventilation settings were FIO_2, 100%; TV, 600; AC, 20. Oxygen saturation was 100%. $ETCO_2$ was 25 mm Hg. The patient's head was elevated 45 degrees. Heart rate remained 90 with normal sinus rhythm, blood pressure 196/117 mm Hg. Medical control issued an order to give 60 GM IV mannitol 20%. A second IV line of lactated Ringer's solution was started at a keep-vein-open rate. The nasogastric tube was adjusted for low continuous suction, with 100 ml of gastric contents returned. Frequent neurologic checks revealed unchanged pupils. The patient did not respond to verbal or painful stimuli. No seizure activity was noted. Additional assessment revealed warm, dry skin with 2-second capillary refill. The patient's abdomen was soft, and her extremities appeared normal. The need for an immediate CT of the head was included in the radio report. The patient was seen in the emergency department after the 15-minute flight.

Interventions

In the ER a Nipride drip was started to keep the BP less than 200/100 mm Hg. A Foley catheter was placed and blood specimens for laboratory work drawn. Emergency CT of the head was then performed.

Outcome

CT showed diffuse subarachnoid hemorrhage. Cerebral angiography revealed a complex anterior communicating artery aneurysm and no spasm. Craniotomy for aneurysm clipping was then performed. The next day the patient opened her eyes and moved all extremities on command. The patient's intensive care unit stay included an arterial line, central venous pressure line, tube feedings, antibiotics, and phenytoin. Extubation was performed 7 days after surgery, and the patient was transferred to the rehabilitation unit 10 days later. Her rehabilitation included consultations from occupational therapy, physical therapy, and speech pathology. On discharge, 50 days from the date of injury, the patient was walking on her own, and was eating a regular diet. The patient did sustain visual impairment in her left eye (Terson's syndrome).

Discussion

On the basis of this patient's history of severe headache and neck pain, the seizure activity, and the quick and thorough assessment and the appropriate interventions during air medical transport, this patient had a positive outcome. On the initial assessment and suspect of a head injury, care was implemented accordingly. Airway management was the priority. By hyperventilating the patient PCO_2 was decreased, which in turn decreased blood volume and flow. When the patient's head was elevated, the cerebral venous return increased, allowing for rapid drainage by way of the internal jugular veins. Mannitol, an osmotic diuretic, was given to decrease cerebral edema. Because the patient's need for emergency CT was noted in the radio report, hospital personnel were prepared to care for this patient.

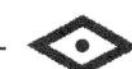

CURRENT RESEARCH AREAS IN NEUROLOGIC MEDICAL EMERGENCIES

Researchers continue to seek answers in areas that may enhance care and improve outcome of the patient with a neurologic medical illness. Current research should be applied whenever possible. Listed below are some areas of current research.

Rationale for Treatment of Stroke as a Medical Emergency

Camarata PJ, Heros RC, Latchaw RE: Brain attack: the rationale for treating stroke as a medical emergency, *Neurosurgery* 34(1):144-158, 1994.

McDowell RH, et al: Stroke: the first six hours, *J Stroke Cerebrovasc Dis* 4(1):133-144, 1993.

Thrombolytic Therapy

Bowes MP et al: Monoclonal antibodies preventing leukocyte activation reduce experimental neurologic injury and enhance efficacy of thrombolytic therapy, *Neurology* 45(5):815-819, 1995.

Oman KS: Commentary on TPA in acute stroke: risk or reprieve? *ENA Nurs Scan Emerg Care* 3(6): 5, 1993.

Transcranial Doppler Ultrasonography

Martin NA, Thomas KM, Caron M: Transcranial doppler: techniques, applications and instrumentation, *Neurosurgery* 3:761, 1993.

Sheinberg M et al: Continuous monitoring of jugular venous oxygen saturation on head-injured patients, *J Neurosurg* 76:212-217, 1992.

Neurogenic Pulmonary Edema

Hickey JV: *Neurogenic pulmonary edema: the clinical practice of neurological and neurosurgical nursing*, ed 3, Philadelphia, 1992, Lippincott.

Mannitol Use in Intracranial Bleeds

Gigliuto CM, Stone KE, Algus M: The use of mannitol in intracerebral bleeds in the medical ICU, *N J Med* 88(1):48-51, 1991.

REFERENCES

1. Albin MS, Babinski M: *Intensive life support of the neurosurgical patient: critical care of neurological and neurosurgical emergencies,* New York, 1980, Raven Press.
2. Bannister SR: *Brain's clinical neurology,* London, 1985, Oxford University Press.
3. Barker E: *Neuroscience nursing,* St Louis, 1994, Mosby.
4. Barnett HJM et al, editors: *Stroke: pathophysiology, diagnosis and management,* New York, 1986, Churchill Livingstone.
5. Biller J et al: Spontaneous subarachnoid hemorrhage in young adults, *Neurosurgery* 21:664-667, 1987.
6. Bubb DI: Neurological problems. In *RN neurological problems: nursing assessment,* series 3, Oradell, NJ, 1984, Medical Economics Books.
7. Clifford DB: The somatosensory system and pain. In Pearlman AL, Collins RC, editors: *Neurological pathophysiology,* ed 3, New York, 1984, Oxford University Press.
8. Daube JR et al: *Medical neurosciences: an approach to anatomy, pathology, and physiology by systems and levels,* ed 2, Boston, 1986, Little, Brown.
9. Doczi T et al: Blood-brain barrier damage during the acute stage of subarachnoid hemorrhage as exemplified by a new animal model, *Neurosurgery* 18:733-739, 1986.
10. Forster FM, Booker HE: The epilepsies and convulsive disorders. In Baker AB, editor: *Clinical neurology,* vol 3, Philadelphia, 1984.
11. Garza M: Brain attack, *JEMS* 18(4):60-62, 1993.
12. Gelb LD: Infections. In Pearlman AL, Collins RC, editors: *Neurological pathophysiology,* ed 3, New York, 1984, Oxford University Press.
13. Gilroy J: *Basic neurology,* ed 2, New York, 1990, Pergamon Press.
14. Glaser GH: Convulsive disorders (epilepsy). In Merritt H, editor: *A textbook of neurology,* ed 6, Philadelphia, 1979, Lea & Febiger.
15. Greenberg M: Neurologic manifestations of AIDS. In Greenburg M, editor: *Handbook of neurosurgery,* ed 3, Lakeland, Fla, 1994, Greenberg Graphics.
16. Guberman A: *Clinical neurology,* Boston, 1994, Little, Brown.
17. Holleran RS: *Prehospital nursing: a collaborative approach,* St Louis, 1994, Mosby.
18. Lothman EW, Collins RC: Seizures. In Pearlman AL, Collins RC, editors: *Neurological pathophysiology,* ed 3, New York, 1984, Oxford University Press.
19. Macabasco AC, Hickman JL: Thrombolytic therapy for brain attack, *J Neurosci Nurs* 27:138-148, 1995.
20. Merritt H, Houston H: *A textbook of neurology,* ed 6, Philadelphia, 1979, Lea & Febiger.
21. Miller JD, Garabi J, Pichard JD: Induced changes of cerebrospinal fluid volume: effects during continuous monitoring of ventricular fluid pressure, *Arch Neurol* 28: 265-269, 1973.
22. Millikan CH, McDowell F, Easton JD: *Stroke,* Philadelphia, 1987, Lea & Febiger.
23. McHenry Jr LC: *Cerebral circulation and strokes,* St Louis, 1978, Warren H Green.
24. Plum F, Posner JB: *Diagnosis of stupor and coma,* ed 3, Philadelphia, 1983, FA Davis.
25. Powers WJ, Raichle ME: Stroke. In Pearlman AL, Collins RC, editors: *Neurological pathophysiology,* ed 3, New York, 1984, Oxford University Press.
26. Saper CB: Hypothalamus and brainstem. In Pearlman AL, Collins RC, editors: *Neurological pathophysiology,* ed 3, New York, 1984, Oxford University Press.
27. Schmidley JW: Cerebrospinal fluid, blood-brain barrier, and brain edema. In Pearlman AL, Collins RC, editors: *Neurological pathophysiology,* ed 3, New York, 1984, Oxford University Press.
28. Skinhoj E, Standgoard S: Pathogenesis of hypertensive encephalopathy, *Lancet* 1:461, 1973.
29. Toole JF: Vascular diseases of brain and spinal cord. In Merrit H, editor: *A textbook of neurology,* ed 6, Philadelphia, 1979, Lea & Febiger.
30. Treiman DM, Delgado-Escueta AV: Status epilepticus. In Thompson RA, Green JR, editors: *Critical care of neurological and neurosurgical emergencies,* New York, 1980, Raven Press.
31. Tsemetzis SA: Surgical management of intracerebral hematomas, *Neurosurgery* 16:562-572, 1985.
32. Overbeeke JJ et al: Higher cortical disorders: an unusual presentation of an arteriovenous malformation, *Neurosurgery* 21:839-842, 1987.
33. vanEifndhoven JHM, Avezaat CJJ: Cerebrospinal fluid pulse pressure and the pulsatile variation in cerebral blood volume: an experimental study in dogs, *Neurosurgery* 19:507-522, 1986.
34. Williams FC, Spetzler RF: Hemodynamic management in the neurosurgical intensive care unit. In *Clinical neurosurgery,* 35:101-163, Baltimore, 1987, Williams & Wilkins.

CHAPTER 20

Cardiovascular Emergencies

COMPETENCIES

1. Perform a cardiovascular assessment before and during transport.
2. Identify and treat lethal arrhythmias.
3. Identify a patient having an acute myocardial infarction.
4. Provide treatment for the patient with hypertension.
5. Perform invasive monitoring during transport.

For the flight nurse, one of the most challenging aspects of caring for critically ill patients involves the air medical transport of patients with acute cardiovascular diseases. The demand for air medical transport of patients dependent on invasive devices and sophisticated technology continues to increase. This chapter describes advances in clinical flight nursing for patients with acute myocardial infarction (AMI), congestive heart failure (CHF), aortic dissection, and other manifestations of cardiovascular disease, with a focus on assessment and management of these patients relative to the air medical environment.

INCIDENCE

The magnitude of cardiovascular disease as a national problem is evidenced by the fact that coronary heart disease continues to be one of the most predominant health problems in the United States. There are more than 65 million Americans with cardiovascular disease, including hypertension, coronary artery disease (CAD), rheumatic heart disease, and stroke. Approximately 45% of all deaths in the United States are caused by cardiovascular disease, and nearly half of these deaths are in patients younger than age 65.[43] People who experience MI, congestive heart failure (CHF), aortic dissection, and other manifestations of cardiovascular disease in small or isolated community hospitals often require rapid skilled transfer to a tertiary care facility to benefit from further evaluation and emergency thrombolytic therapy, angioplasty, surgery, or another intervention. Topol et al.[85] demonstrated the safety of interhospital air medical transport of patients with evolving MI and IV fibrinolytic therapy infusing during flight. Other studies have been done addressing the overall safety of interhospital air medical transport of these critical patients.[15,48,85] These studies help verify the safety of transporting critically ill patients with AMI in well-equipped aircraft with highly trained medical personnel. However, continued research is necessary to establish the safety and efficacy of air medical transport of cardiovascular patients dependent on sophisticated technology such as the intraaortic balloon pump (IABP), extracorporeal membrane oxygenation (ECMO), and ventricular assist devices, as well as those experiencing aortic dissection and other manifestations of cardiovascular disease.[60,71]

Transporting critically ill cardiovascular patients by air involves a number of issues unique to the air medical environment. These issues include the effect of altitude on the cardiovascular system, performance of cardiopulmonary resuscitation during transport, and defibrillation during flight.

ALTERATIONS OF CARDIOVASCULAR PHYSIOLOGY AT ALTITUDE

Hypoxia poses one of the greatest threats to a patient with coronary artery disease. Decompensation of patients with acute cardiovascular disease being transported at altitude is generally caused by hypoxic hypoxia, which is defined as an oxygen deficiency in the body tissue sufficient to cause impaired function.[18] Individual tolerances vary, but generally the patient with cardiovascular disease is at risk above 6000 feet. Physiologic changes occur as barometric pressure at altitude decreases, causing a reduction in the alveolar partial pressure of oxygen. This reduction in the amount of oxygen in the blood decreases available oxygen to the tissues. Compensatory changes that occur to maintain an adequate oxygen supply to the body tissues include increased respiratory rate, heart rate, and cardiac output. This increased demand on the heart also necessitates increased blood flow to the heart muscle.[22] In healthy people, cardiac reserve allows the body to compensate and meet the demand for increased blood flow to the tissues by altering heart rate, stroke volume, or both, and to increase blood flow to the heart muscle by dilating the coronary arteries. Cardiovascular heart disease may limit this ability to increase cardiac output in response to increased demand. Patients with CAD who are unable to compensate for the increased workload imposed on the heart by the decreased oxygen tension of high altitude may experience chest pain, congestive heart failure with pulmonary edema, cardiac arrhythmia, or cardiac arrest.[18] Decisions regarding altitude limitations must be based on the history and assessment of individual patients and close in-flight observations. All patients with cardiovascular disease should receive supplemental oxygen when transported by air; the effects of altitude can be compensated for if the aircraft is pressurized at high altitudes and supplemental oxygen is used. Controversy exists over altitude limitations for patients with cardiovascular compromise. The American College of Chest Physicians has recommended altitude limits for patients with known cardiorespiratory disease when supplemental oxygen is not available. In the fixed-wing population, limiting cabin altitude to a maximum of 6000 feet has been shown to eliminate problems for people with cardiovascular disease who may be unable to maintain full oxygenation of tissues.[28]

SPECIAL CONSIDERATIONS FOR CARDIOPULMONARY RESUSCITATION IN THE AIR MEDICAL ENVIRONMENT

Cardiac arrest is of special concern to nurses involved in the air medical transport of critical patients because the performance of cardiopulmonary resuscitation (CPR) in the confined space of an aircraft is often difficult and challenging. The American Heart Association revised its guidelines for CPR in 1986.[2,3] Flight nurses are expected to have current certification in Advanced Cardiac Life Support (ACLS) through the American Heart Association to practice independent patient care in the air medical environment.[65] The ACLS guidelines are the standard of practice for resuscitation of the patient in cardiac arrest and should be used as guidelines in the event of cardiac arrest in the air medical environment.[3] Thorough preflight assessment, planning, and intervention; prompt correction of arrhythmias; and continuous maintenance of adequate oxygenation may help prevent the need for CPR. However, flight nurses should prepare in advance for in-flight emergencies such as cardiac arrest. Preparation includes ensuring that resuscitation equipment is easily accessible, oxygen is readily available, and ACLS drugs are well labeled and within easy reach. Generally, the number of crew members available to perform basic and advanced life resuscitation is limited to only two medically trained personnel. To respond effectively and rapidly in the event of an emergency, these team members must establish well-defined roles and responsibilities.

Special consideration should be given to aircraft configuration when anticipating the potential need for CPR in flight. The position and height of the stretcher off the floor in relation to seating of the medical crew is important to facilitate proper hand and arm positioning when providing chest compressions. In addition, a well-planned configuration will minimize the need for crew members to extend or release their seatbelts when administering CPR and other therapeutic interventions.[65] More detailed studies are necessary to ascertain the efficacy of CPR in medically configured helicopter and fixed-wing aircraft.

Airborne Defibrillation

Cardiac arrest results from a variety of arrhythmias amenable to defibrillation, including ventricular fibrillation and ventricular tachycardia. The most critical factor in determining the success of resuscitation is the time to successfully restore an effective spontaneous circulation, which is dependent on the use of advanced techniques such as defibrillation.[45] Current American Heart Association ACLS standards[2,3] recommend that defibrillation be immediate in the treatment of confirmed ventricular fibrillation and unstable ventricular tachycardia. The close quarters, metallic environment, and proximity of vital electronic equipment in the helicopter environment had generated concern among flight personnel carrying out defibrillation in the air. One study addressed the potential risks of airborne defibrillation. The results demonstrated that defibrillation with current equipment in a medically equipped twin-engine helicopter is safe and would be expected to be safe in all types of rotary aircraft used for emergency medical transport.[21] Despite cramped quarters and sensitive electrical equipment, defibrillation can be carried out without hesitation whether the aircraft is on the ground or in flight, providing that standard defibrillation precautions are observed. Standard defibrillation precautions in the air medical environment include following ACLS defibrillation standards for selecting energy levels and placement of self-adhesive monitor/defibrillation pad or handheld paddles. Stults et al.[82] demonstrated that self-adhesive monitor/defibrillator pads are superior to standard monitoring leads and handheld electrode paddles in the management of prehospital ventricular defibrillation (Fig. 20-1). Many transport cardiac monitors permit remote defibrillation. When defibrillation pads are appropriately placed and equipment is ready before transport, defibrillation can be quicker and safety enhanced. In addition to proper energy levels and pad placement, it is also essential to inform the pilot before defibrillation and to maintain clearance

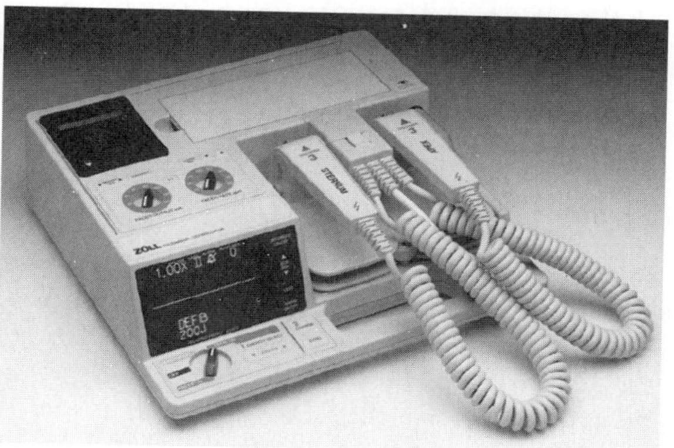

Fig. 20-1. Integrated cardiac resuscitation system that utilizes a single pair of electrodes to monitor, defibrillate, and pace. (Courtesy ZOLL Medical Corporation, Burlington, Mass.)

from the patient and stretcher when discharging the current.

CORONARY ARTERY DISEASE

Definition

Coronary artery disease, one of the most common health problems today, is characterized by a progressive narrowing of the lumen of coronary arteries called *atherosclerosis.* Atherosclerosis is a disease process that results in the development of thick, hard atherosclerotic plaques referred to as *atheromas* or *lesions* that obstruct the lumen in coronary arteries.[50] These lesions propagate in areas with turbulent blood flow such as vessel bifurcation or vessels with decreased lumen diameter. A brief review of coronary anatomy will facilitate understanding of the pathophysiology of coronary artery disease.

The coronary circulation consists of the right and left coronary arteries that arise from the coronary ostia in the aortic root. The left main coronary artery divides into the left anterior descending (LAD) and left circumflex (LCX) arteries. The branches of the main vessel take a diagonal route over the left ventricle and are located between the anterior descending and circumflex arteries. These diagonal left ventricular branches are commonly referred to as *diags.* The LAD artery supplies the left ventricle, the septum, and parts of the right ventricle. It also supplies the anterior portion of the apex and sometimes portions of the inferior and posterior apex. The LCX travels through the lateral left ventricle and the apex, and branches from the LCX supply the posterior and lateral walls of the left ventricle.

The right coronary artery (RCA) is located in the right atrioventricular (AV) sulcus. It crosses the crux of the heart and becomes the posterior descending artery (PDA). The RCA predominately supplies the right atrium and right ventricle and forms branches supplying the inferior surface of the left ventricle. In some cases the LCX crosses the crux to become the PDA. The heart is said to have left coronary dominance if the LCX becomes the PDA and is considered right dominant if the RCA becomes the PDA.

Interarterial vessels interconnect with each other, providing the shunting of arterial flow to areas of increased need. These vessels are responsible for forming collateral vessels that develop after ischemia and infarction and are found throughout the layers of the myocardium. There are a variable number of collaterals, depending on the degree of atherosclerotic heart disease, hypoxemia, and chronic anemia. A schematic representation of the coronary anatomy is illustrated in Fig. 20-2.

The cardiac venous system contains two major areas for venous return to the right side of the heart. The anterior veins empty into the right atrium directly and consist of vessels covering the anterior right ventricular wall. They drain in a direction toward the AV sulcus (groove on the external surface of the heart marking the joining of atria and ventricles). The great cardiac vein drains the left ventricular myocardium and the interventricular septum. The great cardiac vein terminates in the coronary sinus, which opens into the right atrium. A small endothelial flap covers the opening of the sinus, preventing backflow during atrial contraction.[53]

Pathophysiology

Atherosclerotic lesions can partially or totally obstruct one or several of the coronary arteries. The severity of clinical symptoms is determined by the location and extent of the culprit lesion or lesions. The lesions themselves are formed by a complex process that is not well understood.

Four theories have been proposed regarding the pathogenesis of atherosclerosis. These include the lipogenic, thrombogenic, monoclonal, and the response-to-injury theories.[14] The response-to-injury theory currently has the most support. According to this theory, the endothelial cell is injured mechanically or chemically, which promotes platelet adhesion and aggregation and proliferation of smooth muscle cells into the intima, forming the atheroma.[74] The injured endothelial cell secretes a growth factor for smooth muscle cells and promotes attachment of monocytes to its surface, thus leading to the development of the fatty streak of atherosclerosis.

The lesions begin to form within the intimal layer of the artery but extend into the media as the plaque enlarges. They progress over the years and result in significant or total blockage of the coronary arteries.

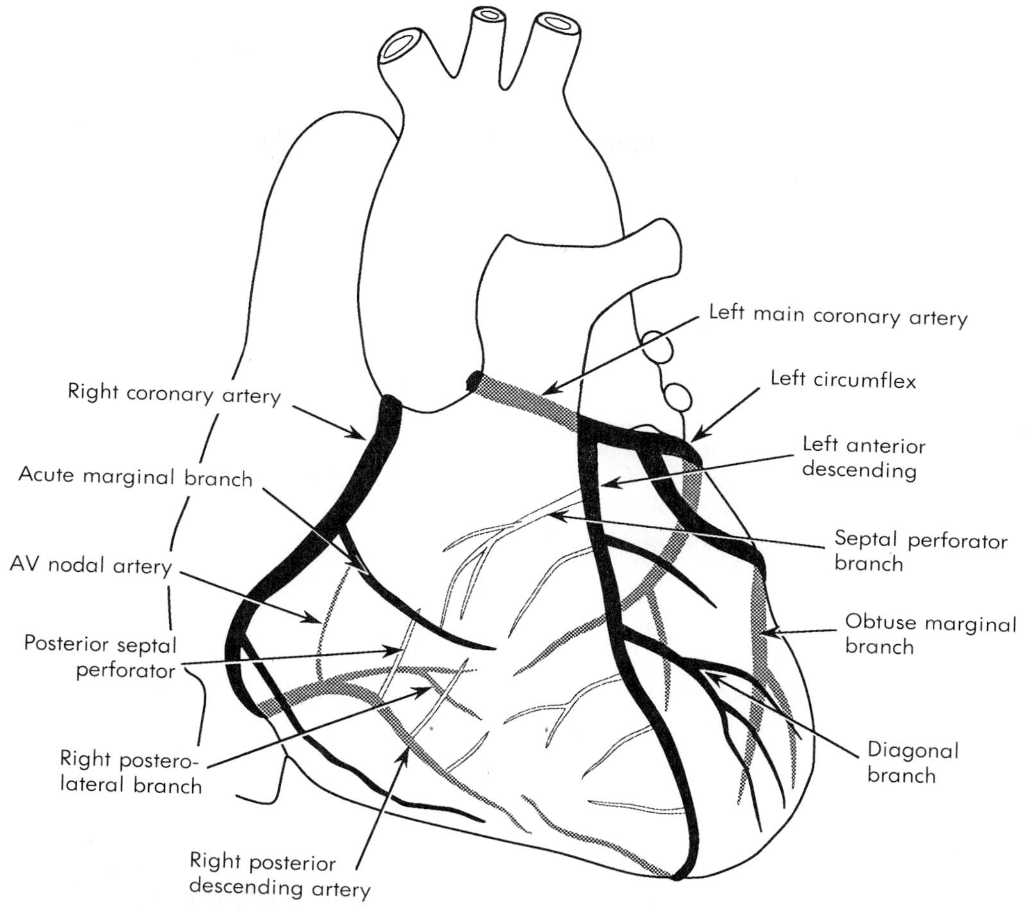

Fig. 20-2. Coronary anatomy. (Courtesy Darrell Debowey, Ann Arbor, Mich.)

Fortunately, research has shown that plaque formation is not only preventable but also reversible.[63]

Coronary artery disease manifests itself in a variety of cardiovascular disorders including silent ischemia, stable and unstable angina, and AMI.

Angina

Angina pectoris or *angina* is a symptom of myocardial ischemia that literally means "choking of the chest." It is caused by an imbalance between myocardial oxygen supply and demand. This impairment of oxygen delivery can be caused by a temporary occlusion of a coronary artery because of spasm, coronary artery stenosis, thrombus, or any combination of these. Other causes of decreased blood supply to the coronary arteries include low blood pressure, low blood volume, and drug effects. Angina can also be precipitated by factors that increase myocardial oxygen demand such as exercise, emotional stress, cold, smoking, sexual intercourse, or a heavy meal.[62] One or several of these factors may disrupt the balance of supply and demand resulting in the inability of the diseased artery to meet the oxygen needs for that area of myocardium. The end result is a buildup of metabolites in the ischemic tissue that activates the nerve endings, and anginal pain occurs.[62]

Categories

Angina can be divided into several categories depending on the onset, severity, duration, and alleviation of symptoms. These categories include classic or stable angina, crescendo or unstable angina, coronary spasm or variant angina, mixed angina, and silent angina or, more commonly termed, *silent ischemia.*

Stable angina is usually precipitated by physical exertion or emotional stress. The pain typically lasts 1 to 5 minutes, is relieved by rest, and is noted to be unchanged over several months. The anginal attacks are similar and are relieved by the same mode of therapy.

Unstable angina is a phrase denoting stable angina that has changed in the timing, frequency, intensity, duration, and quality. It is provoked by lower exercise workloads than is stable angina. There is also an increased severity of pain associated with unstable angina that lasts longer than 10 minutes despite rest and the use of sublingual nitroglycerin. The symptoms of unstable angina typically mimic the symptoms of AMI, making diagnosis and treatment much more difficult. Pharmacologic management of this type of angina is also more complex. These patients are at an increased risk for experiencing sudden death or AMI.[50]

The terms *variant angina* and *coronary artery spasm* are often used interchangeably, although this may not be accurate. Coronary artery spasm has been defined as a transient total or subtotal narrowing of a coronary artery sufficient to cause ischemia. Variant angina is characterized by spontaneous episodes of chest pain related to a decrease in coronary blood supply frequently noted at rest or on early rising. This type of angina may have a circadian pattern and is almost always relieved by nitroglycerin. The most common cause of variant angina is coronary artery spasm; however, the cause cannot be assumed.[70] The same signs and symptoms may also be present in patients with severe atherosclerotic obstruction with only slight changes in coronary artery tone or with platelet or thrombus occlusion.

Mixed angina has been described by some clinicians as a combination of stable angina and coronary spasm.[50] These patients usually have a fixed obstruction with concomitant spasm that precipitates ischemia with or without increased oxygen demand.

The term *silent ischemia* has been used to describe objective evidence of ischemia in asymptomatic patients with or without documented CAD. Objective evidence includes electrocardiographic (ECG), exercise test, or radionuclide findings suggestive of coronary ischemia. There are several explanations for the absence of angina or anginal symptoms in patients with silent ischemia including the observation that patients with this "silent" angina exhibit less sensitivity to pain in general than do patients with reproducible angina.[76] Another postulated explanation is that this syndrome may be related to a reduction in myocardial oxygen supply secondary to spasm in contrast to an increase in myocardial oxygen demand as noted in stable angina.[53]

Pathophysiology

During normal myocardial metabolism, an aerobic process, the heart extracts about 70% of available oxygen supplied in the coronary artery blood. Increases in myocardial oxygen demand are normally met by increases in blood flow. Coronary arteries that have an obstruction to flow, as in atherosclerosis, are unable to compensate by increasing blood flow in response to an increase in demand. Therefore therapy is aimed at decreasing the myocardial oxygen need. The major determinants of myocardial oxygen demand are heart rate, contractility, and wall stress.[70]

Blood flow in the coronary arteries is also determined by the size of the coronary arteries and their collateral vessels. The factors that influence flow are diastolic pressure in the aorta, diastolic time (the major portion of coronary artery perfusion occurs during diastole), and coronary resistance. If diastolic time or left ventricular filling time is shortened, as occurs with rapid heart rates, filling is inadequate. Coronary artery resistance is controlled mostly by the intramyocardial arterioles, and spasm results in an abrupt decrease in blood flow.[70] Another potential cause of unstable angina is the presence of an intracoronary thrombus. This was recently visualized via coronary angioscopy during coronary artery bypass surgery in patients with unstable angina.[77]

Assessment and Diagnosis

Classic angina is usually described as substernal chest discomfort or pain with a sensation of pressure or heaviness that occurs with activity and is relieved by rest. The chest discomfort may be associated with burning or itching in the chest that gradually increases in intensity and is followed by a gradual fading away. In rare cases a patient may report dyspnea, or back or jaw pain without associated chest pain. The location of the chest pain is most commonly in the middle or lower sternum or over the left precordium. Patients may also note left shoulder pain or upper arm pain. The pain sometimes extends down the arm and involves the fourth and fifth fingers. Patients may also have associated symptoms including nausea, vomiting, diaphoresis, dyspnea, and exhaustion.

Physical examination usually reveals a patient whose cool and clammy skin appears pale or dusky-colored, and who shows signs of labored breathing. Cardiac dysrhythmias may occur related to transient ischemia of heart tissue. Patients may also experience an increase in heart rate and blood pressure.

In stable angina, the ECG has limited diagnostic value. Transient ST depression of 1 mm or greater has been recorded in some patients during an episode of angina and has also been observed in patients experiencing silent ischemia but no pain. This ST segment depression is characteristic of myocardial ischemia but is unfortunately only detected by ECG during an anginal episode. In variant angina, the ECG is more diagnostically valuable. The ECG will display transient ST segment elevations in the leads corresponding to the ischemic areas, and some cases of ST depression have been reported as well. Dysrhythmias may also occur with variant angina and spasm.

Management

Management of the patient with angina includes admission to a coronary care or critical care unit for continuous ECG monitoring and treatment of symptoms, which may require air medical transport to a definitive care hospital. Many of these patients are admitted to rule out an MI. The goal of treatment is to either increase the coronary blood supply or decrease the myocardial oxygen demand, or both. This may be accomplished through pharmacologic, mechanical, or surgical interventions.

Pharmacologic Therapy. Pharmacologic therapy includes three classes of agents used for patients with CAD or spasm. These three classes are nitrates, beta-adrenergic blocking agents, and calcium channel antagonists. Thrombolytic therapy is also being investigated as an alternative treatment for unstable angina.

Nitrates are widely accepted and are usually used as the first-line agents for both angina and coronary spasm. They are classified as short-acting nitrates and longer acting nitrates. Nitroglycerin (NTG) is used sublingually for acute anginal attacks or coronary spasm because of its rapid onset of action. It is also used as prophylaxis before an activity that is known to precipitate an attack. Intravenous NTG is also used in acute anginal episodes because the dose can be easily regulated, and consistent drug levels can be maintained.[62] The longer acting nitrates such as isosorbide dinitrate and isosorbide 5-mononitrate are used to increase exercise tolerance and prevent further anginal episodes or spasm attacks.

Nitrates act by improving coronary blood flow primarily by direct smooth muscle relaxation. Blood return to the heart is decreased because of venous pooling from general vasodilation. Decreased venous return causes a decline in cardiac output and lowers systemic arterial pressure. This reduces ventricular wall tension and oxygen consumption, relieving anginal pain.

Whereas NTG increases myocardial oxygen supply, beta blockers decrease oxygen demand. Beta-blocker agents interrupt sympathetic impulses by competing with the neurotransmitter norepinephrine at the beta-sympathetic nerve endings. Beta-receptor inhibition results in decreased heart rate and contractility and slowed impulse transmission through the cardiac conduction system. These effects, coupled with a decreased renin production, lead to a decrease in systemic blood pressure.[62] Most of the beta blockers have been found to increase exercise capacity in CAD and to increase diastolic filling time, thereby increasing coronary perfusion. Propranolol has been shown to be useful for prophylaxis of stable angina.

Calcium channel antagonists have been widely used recently for the management of angina. The mechanism of action is inhibition of the movement of calcium ions across myocardial and vascular smooth muscle. This action produces vasodilation of the coronary arteries and collateral vessels, a decrease in myocardial contractility (decrease in myocardial oxygen demand), vasodilation of the peripheral arteries (decrease in systemic blood pressure), and a decrease in cardiac conduction.[50] Calcium channel antagonists have a slower onset of action compared with nitrates but are much longer acting. Patients with unstable angina in which medical management is difficult may require a combination of long-acting nitrates, a beta blocker, and a calcium channel antagonist. Table 20-1 on pp. 384-385 lists the various classes of antianginal agents and describes their actions, route of administration, and adverse effects.

Angiotensin-converting enzyme (ACE) inhibitors can reduce mortality in patients recovering from an MI. They act by reducing ventricular dilatation after infarction. ACE inhibitors may also reduce the rate of reinfarction and improve the prognosis of chronic heart failure.[16,54]

Thrombolytic therapy is an important tool in treatment of AMI. Randomized trials have shown beneficial effects in both long- and short-term mortality with presentation of left ventricular function.[51] In patients with unstable angina, intracoronary thrombosis has been detected in several studies.[24] The thrombus was not observed in patients with stable angina. Therefore in patients with unstable angina, administration of a thrombolytic agent may be effective for dissolving intracoronary thrombi, thus alleviating anginal symptoms.[33] A complete discussion of thrombolytic therapy is presented in the AMI section of this chapter.[5]

Mechanical and Surgical Intervention. Mechanical intervention for patients with angina and for patients after infarction continues to receive much attention worldwide. Since 1977 the standard mechanical means of treating severe CAD has been percutaneous transluminal coronary angioplasty (PTCA). Beginning in the mid-1980s, alternative methods of mechanical interventions have been explored, including the atherectomy catheters, rotational catheters, laser angioplasty, and intracoronary stents.

PTCA is a procedure used to dilate occluded or partially occluded coronary arteries. This is accomplished by insertion of a guiding catheter via the femoral or brachial artery, which is then advanced retrograde into the ascending aorta. Angiography is performed during the guide-wire insertion to identify the lesion and to provide a view for passing the catheter. A dilation catheter with a deflated balloon attached is advanced through the guiding catheter into the stenotic area of the artery. The balloon is then inflated in a stepwise fashion until the desired residual pressure gradient is obtained. The balloon actually induces a "controlled injury" when exerting lateral force against the arterial wall. These changes include compression, splitting, or redistribution of the plaque and stretching of the wall. The fibrous cap is disrupted, and the resulting exposed debris is removed by phagocytosis. The result is an increased diameter with improved blood flow through the previously stenotic segment.

Although PTCA has been used extensively in the past decade, several limitations have been identified, prompting researchers to develop alternative means of removing atherosclerotic plaque from the coronary arteries. These limitations include a 5% to 15% incidence of unsuccessful PTCA, a 5% incidence of acute occlusive complications, and a restenosis rate as high as 20% to 35% within 6 months of the PTCA procedure.[7]

Coronary artery bypass surgery has been and will continue to be a coronary artery revascularization procedure appropriate for patients with severe CAD, left main artery disease, and in patients in whom other revascularization procedures have failed.[19]

Myocardial Infarction

Myocardial infarction is one of the most serious complications of CAD and remains the leading cause of death in the United States. An AMI results in total cessation of blood supply in the affected coronary artery, resulting in diminished or absence of oxygen supply to the heart, in turn causing ischemia, injury, and necrosis to the area of myocardium supplied by the affected coronary artery.

The process is dynamic and complex, beginning with the establishment of an atherosclerotic plaque on the intimal layer of the coronary artery and culminating with a thrombus formation on the plaque surface. The infarction process starts within minutes of total coronary occlusion and continues for several hours. In addition to thrombus formation, coronary spasm and platelet aggregation also have been suggested as factors responsible for precipitating an AMI.

Pathophysiology

An acute thrombotic occlusion is currently accepted as the precipitating event in MI. The events that incite thrombus formation appear to be rupture or cracking of the thin fibrous cap and release of the plaque constituents into the coronary lumen. The mechanisms through which this occurs include contact of platelets with denuded collagen, which leads to thrombocyte adherence and the accumulation of a platelet plug; release of tissue thromboplastin from the plaque contents, initiating the clotting cascade; and mechanical obstruction of the artery by plaque components.[50] Fig. 20-3 illustrates the process of thrombogenesis.

Coronary spasm can cause an infarct by predisposing the formation of thrombi or platelet aggregation, which may lead to prolonged total obstruction and infarction. Platelet aggregation has also been cited as the cause of an MI because turbulent blood flow at the site of a stenotic area creates favorable conditions for platelet adhesion and aggregation.[14]

Infarction of the myocardium usually develops distal to the occluded artery and is determined by the amount of blood that is able to flow into the ischemic artery and by the duration of time required for flow to be reestablished. Blood flow can be resumed via collateral circulation, clot lysis, retraction of the vessel wall that has been in spasm, or through mechanical means such as PTCA or coronary bypass surgery. Reimer and Jennings[73] demonstrated that prolonged ischemia results in myocardial necrosis up to 6 hours after total occlusion of the coronary artery. Interventions are therefore aimed at reperfusing the ischemic myocardium as quickly as possible after symptom onset. Myocardial cellular death is also dependent on (1) the rate of development of the obstruction, (2) the coronary artery that is occluded, (3) the quantity of myocardium supplied by that artery, (4) the quantity of collateral flow, and (5) the presence, site, and severity of any coronary artery spasm.[1]

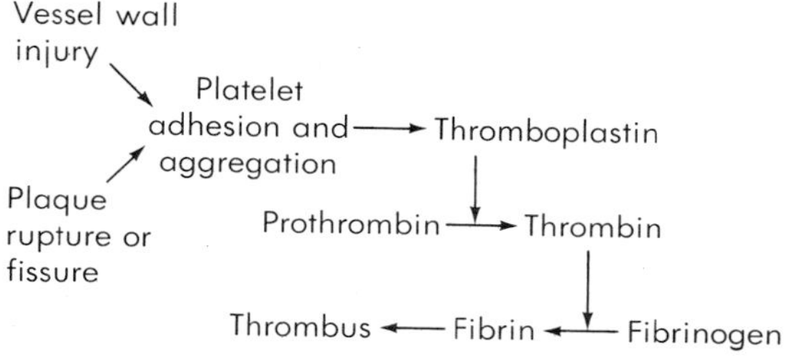

Fig. 20-3. Thrombogenesis.

Types and Location of Infarcts

Infarcts can be divided into transmural and nontransmural, or subendocardial, infarcts. A transmural infarct extends through the full thickness of the myocardium including the endocardium and epicardium. In a subendocardial infarct the necrosis is limited to the subendocardial surface. Patients who have a transmural infarct are at much greater risk of losing functional myocardium and developing complications associated with MI. The majority of infarcts occur in the left ventricle and interventricular septum, although some patients sustain damage to the right ventricle.

An anterior wall MI is caused by obstruction of the LAD artery. An LAD occlusion also causes infarction of the apical region of the left ventricle, portions of the septum, anterolateral wall, papillary muscles, and inferoapical wall of the left ventricle (Fig. 20-4).

A lateral wall or posterior infarct is caused by obstruction of the LCX artery, and an RCA occlusion results in an inferior infarct (inferoposterior wall of the left ventricle) as well as the inferior portions of the septum and the posteromedial papillary muscle[1] (Fig. 20-5). The size and location of an infarct depend on the distribution of the obstructed vessels.

TABLE 20-1

Medications used in treatment of angina

Class	Drug	Route	Actions	Adverse effects
Nitrates	Nitroglycerin	Intravenous Sublingual Ointment	IV route preferred in acute episodes Direct smooth muscle relaxation leads to general vasodilation and reduces venous return to heart. Decrease in cardiac output lowers arterial pressure, which causes a reduction in ventricular wall tension and oxygen consumption	Reduced coronary perfusion pressure leads to decreased cardiac output. The following side effects can result: hypotension, syncope, headache, flushing, dizziness, methemoglobinemia; occasionally hypoxemia tolerance may develop
	Isosorbide dinitrate	Oral Sublingual Sustained release		
Beta blockers	Propranolol	Intravenous Oral	Decreases oxygen demand Decreases heart rate and contractility and slows atrioventricular conduction caused by interference with sympathetic nerve endings. Decreases renin production Affects bronchioles and systemic vessels as well	Severe myocardial depression can lead to heart failure Airway constriction of concern in patients with respiratory disease Other side effects: fatigue, weakness, mental depression Unopposed alpha stimulation can lead to coronary vasoconstriction and exacerbate variant angina or peripheral vascular disease
	Nadolol	Oral	Same as propranolol	
	Pindolol		Has some intrinsic sympathomimetic activity	
	Esmolol	Intravenous	Short-acting preparation Same as propranolol	

Selective	Atenolol	Oral	Similar to nonselective agents with respect to cardiac actions. Selective only at low doses	
Calcium ion antagonists	Nifedipine	Oral, subcutaneous, intravenous	Coronary vasodilation, reduced myocardial contractility, and lowered systemic vascular resistance caused by slowed calcium transport into cells	Most common side effects: hypotension, peripheral edema Initial administration can lead to increased attacks
	Verapamil Diltiazem	Oral, intraveous Oral	Slow channels in cardiac cells and smooth muscle affected Nifedipine reduces oxygen extraction in coronary arteries, decreases blood pressure, and relieves coronary spasm	Headaches and peripheral edema most common with nifedipine Elevated digoxin levels Headaches, palpitations, flushing, nausea, and nervousness can occur with any agent Diltiazem and verapamil can pro'duce heart block
Combination therapy	Nifedipine and propranolol or Diltiazem and propranolol		Nifedipine prevents ischemia by vasodilation, and propranolol prevents a reflex increase in heart rate Increased exercise capacity	Monitor for bradycardia, hypotension, dysrhythmias, congestive heart failure These combinations under investigation

From Miller CL: Cardiac medications *Focus Crit Care* 15(4)23-29, 1988; and Stine R, Chudnofsky C: *A practical approach to emergency medicine,* ed 2, Boston, 1994, Little, Brown, p 113.

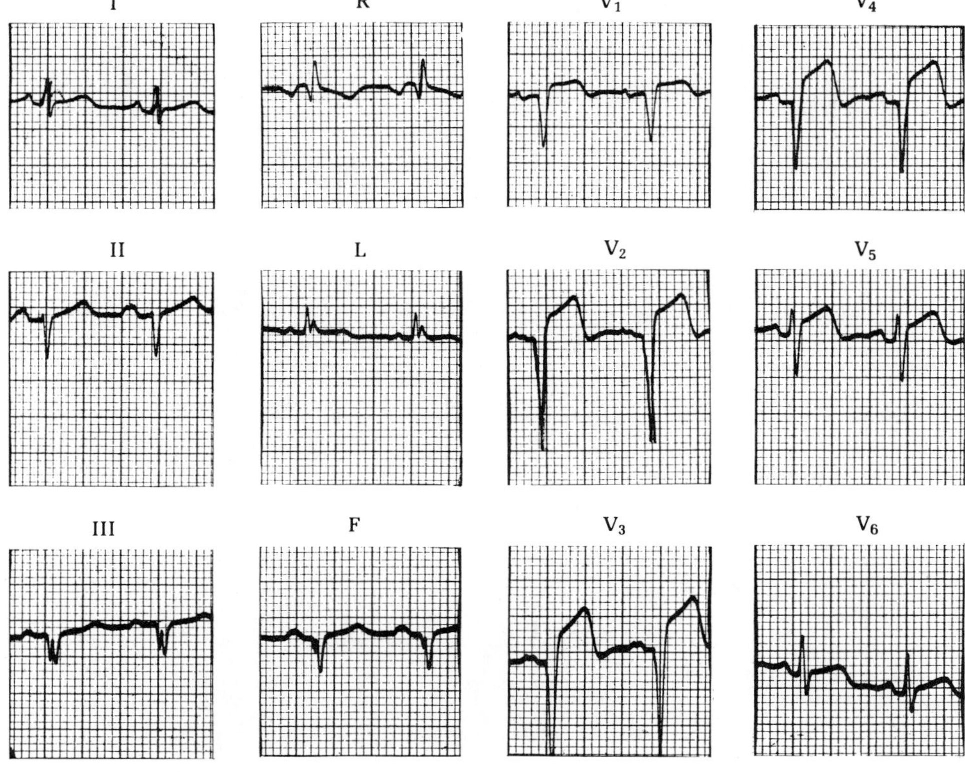

Fig. 20-4. Anterior MI shown on ECG. (From Conover C: *Understanding electrocardiography,* ed 5, St Louis, 1994, Mosby.)

Assessment and Diagnosis

Mild to severe pain is almost always present during an AMI and is usually substernal in origin, radiating across the precordium to the back, arms, neck, or jaw. When describing the pain, some patients report radiation or localization to neck, jaw, back, shoulder, left arm, or near the epigastric area. The epigastric area pain is often confused with indigestion. The onset of symptoms is often abrupt and without provocation and will last for at least 30 minutes. The pain is unrelieved with NTG and is usually accompanied by reports of nausea, vomiting, diaphoresis, and shortness of breath.[80]

On physical examination, patients look acutely ill and are in severe discomfort, with facial grimaces indicating pain. They may clutch their chests, sit forward, and may appear diaphoretic, pale, and restless. The patients with evolving MI may also have nausea. Their skin color may be either normal or have a gray, ashen appearance, and the skin may be moist, warm, or cool.

Excessive sympathetic stimulation via the autonomic nervous system may affect the vital signs by elevating the blood pressure (BP) and increasing the heart rate. Parasympathetic overactivity, the result of activation of the vagal reflex, may result in bradycardia with concomitant hypotension. This is most often seen in patients with inferior infarcts and is reversible with administration of fluids and atropine. The respiratory rate is usually elevated as a result of the pain and anxiety but should return to normal once the pain and stress are alleviated.

Heart sounds are often difficult to hear but the presence of an S_4 usually indicates ischemic heart

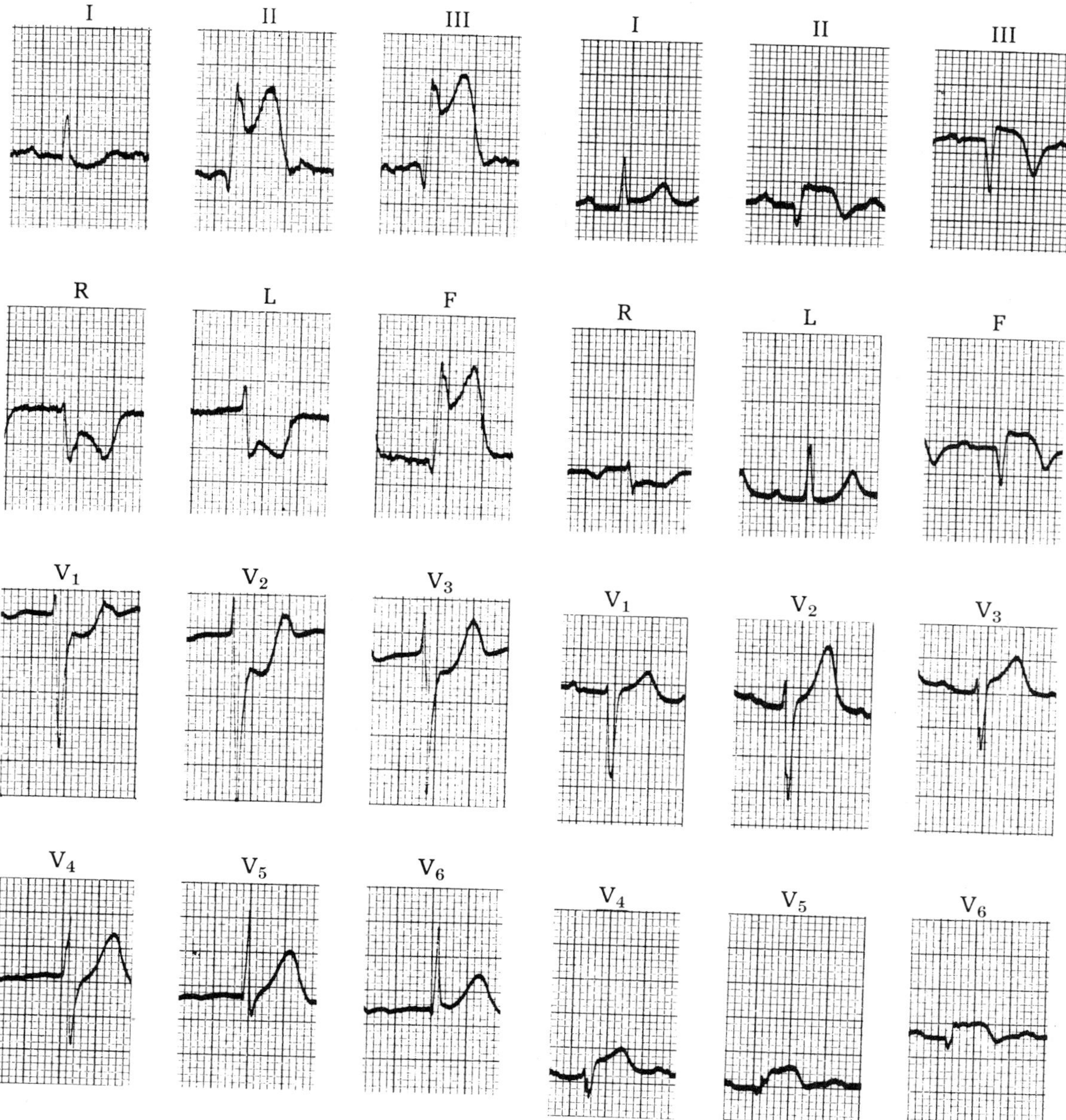

Fig. 20-5. Inferior MI ECG changes. (From Conover C: *Understanding electrocardiography,* ed 5, St Louis, 1994, Mosby.)

disease. Patients with extensive infarctions may have an S_3, which reflects severe left ventricular dysfunction. It is not uncommon in patients with transmural anterior infarctions. In the presence of papillary muscle dysfunction, there may be systolic murmurs as a result of acute mitral regurgitation. A pericardial friction rub may also be auscultated. Moist bibasilar rales may be present in patients with left ventricular failure postinfarction.

In right ventricular infarcts the jugular veins are distended. The jugular venous pressure is also elevated in cardiogenic shock and reduced with hypotension or hypoperfusion.

A 12-lead ECG is necessary to confirm the diagnosis of AMI. The ECG finding most frequently seen and most indicative of an AMI is ST segment elevation of > 0.1 mV in at least two contiguous ECG leads corresponding to the involved coronary artery. Reciprocal ST segment depression may be evident in the opposite leads reinforcing the acuity of the ST segment elevation over the area of infarction.[67] ST segment depression in leads V_1 and V_2 is also indicative of a true posterior MI, making this a difficult infarction to diagnose, because ST segment depression usually indicates ischemia and not infarction. In coronary spasm, ST segment elevation may also be seen but will resolve with NTG, thus differentiating it from an AMI. Table 20-2 illustrates the location of various infarcts and associated ECG changes.[81]

Management

Management of the AMI patient has changed dramatically in the past decade with improvements in hemodynamic monitoring, pharmacologic support, mechanical and surgical therapy, and the development of temporary ventricular assist devices. Current interventions, specifically thrombolytic therapy, PTCA, and bypass surgery, are aimed at reperfusing the ischemic myocardium, thus preserving left ventricular function and ultimately decreasing the morbidity and mortality associated with an AMI.[11]

Pharmacologic Therapy. The reduction of pain is a critical factor in the care of patients with AMI. Intravenous morphine sulfate still remains the drug of choice for pain control. It combines a potent analgesic effect with hemodynamic actions that reduce myocardial oxygen demand. Morphine has a vasodilator effect that reduces preload and afterload and sympathetic tone, causing a decrease in heart rate and therefore reducing oxygen demand. Morphine may be administered liberally in the setting of an AMI in doses of 2 to 4 mg at 5- to 15-minute intervals. The patient should be observed for side effects, which may include hypotension, bradycardia, decreased respirations, and change in mentation.[86]

TABLE 20-2

Location of MI and associated ST segment changes

Location of infarct	Leads with ST segment elevation	Leads with ST segment depression and/or reciprocal changes
Inferior	2, 3, aVF	I, aVL, V_1-V_4
Anterior (extensive)	I, aVL, V_1-V_6	2, 3, aVF, aVR
Anteroseptal	V_1-V_4	
Anterolateral	I, aVL, V_3-V_6	
Lateral	I, aVL, V_5-V_6	2, 3, aVF
High anterolateral	I, aVL	
Posterior	V_6	V_1-V_2

Nitrates are also commonly used to treat acute infarct patients. They are beneficial because of their ability to decrease oxygen demand. Vasodilation of the coronary arteries explains their effectiveness in decreasing chest pain. An IV NTG infusion is usually begun at a dosage of 1 to 10 μg/min and titrated to relief of chest pain while maintaining the systolic BP at greater than 90 mm Hg. Nitrates should be used concomitantly with morphine to alleviate chest pain.

Beta-blockers and calcium channel blockers are also used to treat MI, though not usually during the initial presentation. Antiarrhythmics are used for the prophylaxis and treatment of dysrhythmias associated with AMI and are discussed in a following section.

Thrombolytic Intervention. Once it was established that coronary thrombus was the precipitating event in an AMI, interest in thrombolytic therapy escalated. The goal of thrombolytic therapy was to lyse coronary thrombi and restore blood flow to prevent the ischemic area from evolving into a completed infarct, thus reducing mortality. Multiple clinical trials have shown that administration of a thrombolytic agent within 6 hours after the onset of symptoms during an AMI dramatically reduces mortality.[31] Since the late 1970s and early 1980s, several agents have been used. Two commonly used thrombolytic agents are streptokinase and recombinant tissue plasminogen activator (TPA). In the years to come, research may produce even more agents. These agents work by dissolving the coronary thrombi through activation of the plasma protein plasminogen. Plasminogen is then converted to plasmin, which degrades fibrin, the basic component of a thrombus.[68,84]

Each thrombolytic agent differs slightly in its mechanism of action, plasma half-life, effect on fibrinogen, and adverse effects.

No agent of choice has been identified with regard to thrombolytic therapy. Each individual cardiologist chooses an agent based on the patient's history, clinical presentation, and any unusual circumstances associated with that patient's care. It is therefore imperative that the flight nurse be familiar with the various agents, methods of dosing, and care of patients receiving thrombolytic therapy, to ensure accurate and safe treatment. Close in-flight monitoring of these agents is essential. Infusion devices must be checked for accuracy and reliability to ensure accurate dosing.

One of the most severe complications associated with thrombolytic therapy is intracranial hemorrhage. Because thrombolytic agents have the potential to lyse beneficial hemostatic thrombi as well as pathologic thrombi, proper screening and patient selection are essential. Thrombolytic therapy is absolutely contraindicated in patients who are at a high risk of intracranial or internal hemorrhage, and every effort should be made to exclude these patients from receiving lytic therapy (see box).

A patient receiving thrombolytic therapy is at high risk of bleeding complications. To minimize these, all invasive procedures and venipunctures should be avoided if at all possible, and compression dressings should be applied over puncture sites to decrease the amount of oozing. The sites should be carefully observed throughout the transport process, and dressings should remain in place until hemostasis is attained. If pacing is required, an external pacemaker is recommended for patients receiving thrombolytic therapy.

Mechanical and Surgical Intervention. Both mechanical and surgical techniques are used in the management of the AMI patient. Since 1982, PTCA has been investigated as an alternative treatment for AMI.[78] This procedure has been used both as a primary

ABSOLUTE CONTRAINDICATIONS FOR THROMBOLYTIC THERAPY

- History of intracranial bleeding or cerebrovascular accident
- High risk of internal hemorrhage or active internal hemorrhage
- Uncontrolled hypertension
- Recent intracranial or intraspinal surgery
- Intracranial tumor
- Arteriovenous malformation and aneurysm
- History of known bleeding diathesis

intervention and as an emergency procedure after failed thrombolytic therapy in an attempt to limit infarct size. The advantages of the immediate interventional use of PTCA include improvement of global and regional left ventricular function, decrease in the underlying stenosis of the affected coronary artery, recanalization of the infarct artery in patients in whom lytic therapy has failed, and as an alternative treatment in patients who are excluded from lytic therapy.[12] The greatest disadvantage of immediate PTCA in AMI is the time delay involved in getting the patient to an interventional catheter laboratory and the requirement for trained personnel and sophisticated equipment. Complications may also occur as a consequence of the PTCA procedure. These include coronary dissection, reocclusion, coronary spasm, dysrhythmias, hemorrhage, and circulation impairment to the affected extremity.

Surgical intervention or coronary artery bypass graft (CABG) surgery is performed to improve the myocardial blood supply for patients with CAD and has recently been used as an intervention for AMI. The indications for emergency CABG surgery include unstable angina unresponsive to medical therapy, evolving AMI with multivessel disease, and evolving MI when thrombolytic therapy or PTCA, or both, are unsuccessful.[57] The timing of CABG surgery is an important factor in determining the success of the procedure. Early reperfusion, within 6 hours, improves both short- and long-term survival rates. CABG surgery after thrombolytic therapy has also been performed successfully; however, the potential for bleeding is a significant concern for these particular patients. The advantages of the use of primary CABG surgery as an intervention for MI include better treatment of global ischemia, a more complete revascularization, and easier accessibility to reperfusing distal obstructions.[47] The disadvantages include the need for highly sophisticated facilities and personnel and the protracted time delay.

Several complications may also occur as a result of CABG surgery in AMI. These are graft closure, dysrhythmias, low cardiac output, hemorrhage, cardiac tamponade, fluid and electrolyte imbalance, hypertension or hypotension, pulmonary embolism, cerebrovascular accident, and renal failure.

DYSRHYTHMIAS

Variations in the rate and rhythm of the heart are classified as dysrhythmias. They are caused by a variation in the rate of discharge of the sinoatrial (SA) node, ectopic impulses that compete with the SA node, or abnormal conduction of impulses from the SA node through the heart. Dysrhythmias can be categorized as tachydysrhythmias, which include sinus tachycardia, supraventricular dysrhythmias, and ventricular dysrhythmias, and bradydysrhythmias, including sinus bradycardia and conduction disturbances.

Pathophysiology

The cells that conduct the electrical current through the heart are known as the *pacemaker* or *automatic* cells. The pacemaker of the heart, the SA node, is located at the junction of the superior vena cava and the right atrium. An electric impulse is initiated at this node, and it travels through the internodal pathways to the AV. The AV node is located in the right atrium, directly above the tricuspid valve and anterior to the coronary sinus. The electrical impulse travels through the AV node, then moves through a common bundle of His, which divides almost immediately into the right and left bundles. The left bundle divides further to form two direct pathways to the anterior and posterior papillary muscle. The electrical impulse then permeates the many small fibers of the Purkinje network, beginning at the endocardium, and ending within the ventricular myocardium.[50]

Dysrhythmias are the result of an irritable focus or foci within the electrical conduction system. There are several contributing mechanisms to the development of dysrhythmias. The ischemic process and postnecrotic entities and underlying cardiac disease may enhance myocardial electrical instability. In addition, the development and treatment of myocardial failure result in mechanical dysfunction, metabolic changes, and electrolyte shifts, which contribute to the rhythm disturbances. Invasive cardiac instrumentation or pharmacologic therapy also have the potential to provoke serious dysrhythmias.

Assessment, Diagnosis, and Treatment

Ventricular Dysrhythmias

Ventricular ectopic activity is a very common phenomenon in AMI, and ventricular tachydysrhythmias are the most preventable cause of death occurring in MI. Ventricular dysrhythmias represent electrical instability of the ventricle as a result of the necrotic process.[60] The reader is referred to the American Heart Association's ACLS guidelines for specific algorithms to treat arrhythmias.

Ventricular Premature Beats (VPBs). Ventricular premature beats represent early ventricular depolarizations that occur before the next sinus beat. A wide, bizarre configuration represents abnormal impulse conduction. VPBs are fairly benign and are usually left untreated. They may, however, escalate to ventricular tachycardia or fibrillation, requiring careful observation of these patients.

Ventricular Tachycardia (VT). Ventricular tachycardia is three or more beats at an accelerated rate, usually greater than 100 beats/min. The rhythm may be well tolerated or associated with hemodynamic compromise. If the patient is conscious, treatment may include a precordial thump followed by antiarrhythmic therapy, or antiarrhythmic therapy alone may be sufficient. In an unconscious patient, asynchronous cardioversion is the best treatment. Some patients tolerate this form of dysrhythmia well and can be managed by antiarrhythmic therapy alone. Antiarrhythmic therapy includes using lidocaine (1 mg to 1.5 mg/kg bolus followed in 5 to 10 minutes by 0.5 to 0.75 mg/kg bolus to maximum total of 3 mg/kg bolus). Lidocaine can be followed with procainamide (20 to 30 mg/kg to a maximum of 17 mg/kg) if needed. Intravenous bretylium may be used if the VT is refractory to other pharmacologic therapy.[37]

Ventricular Fibrillation (VF). Ventricular fibrillation is chaotic depolarization from multiple areas of the ventricle; no effective contraction occurs resulting in severe hemodynamic compromise. VF is the most common mechanism of cardiac arrest from myocardial ischemia or infarction and leads to sudden death if it is not converted to a more normal rhythm. The best treatment for VF is defibrillation. CPR should be initiated until defibrillation occurs. If defibrillation fails, adjunctive pharmacologic therapy should be initiated. Epinephrine makes VF more susceptible to defibrillation. Lidocaine hydrochloride or bretylium tosylate can also be used adjunctively to defibrillation because they increase the ventricular fibrillation threshold.

Prophylactic administration of antiarrhythmic agents in the AMI patient is accepted by most clinicians. Lidocaine is the drug of choice because it improves conduction in the ischemic zone of myocardium. Procainamide hydrochloride is the second line of therapy.

Accelerated Idioventricular Rhythm (AIVR). Accelerated idioventricular rhythm is defined as a ventricular rhythm with a rate of 60 to 110 beats/min. Most episodes are of short duration and will terminate abruptly, slow gradually before stopping, or be overdriven by the basic cardiac rhythm. This rhythm is usually not treated but must be observed closely because of its propensity to degenerate into ventricular tachycardia or fibrillation.

Bradydysrhythmias

Sinus Bradycardia. Sinus bradycardia is manifested by a heart rate less than 60 beats/min. It is a result of slowing of impulse formation by the sinus node and is most often associated with an inferior or posterior wall MI. It may also result from ischemic effects on the sinus node. The treatment of choice for sinus bradycardia is atropine (0.5 to 1.0 mg every 2 minutes to a total dose of 0.03 to 0.04 mg/kg), which enhances sinus node automaticity and AV conduction. Atropine should be initiated when the patient becomes symptomatic, exhibiting signs of CHF, hypotension, or refractory ventricular ectopic activity. If symptomatic bradycardia persists, temporary pacing may be required. This can be accomplished by application of an external pacemaker (which is preferred in the patient being considered for or receiving thrombolytic therapy) or by insertion of a transvenous pacemaker.

External Pacing. An external pacemaker or noninvasive temporary pacemaker (NTP) provides immediate pacing in an emergency without the risk of complications related to an invasive procedure. Pacing is accomplished by using large electrodes that are placed over the precordium and on the posterior left side of the chest beneath the scapula. Standard electrodes provide the ECG tracing and allow demand-mode operation. The NTP will operate asynchronously if the sensing electrodes are not in place. The pacing rate may be varied from 30 to 180 per minute and output from 0 to 140 mA.[26]

Temporary Pacing. Temporary pacing is indicated for patients experiencing acute symptomatic bradycardias or other life-threatening conduction disturbances that could be corrected with temporary cardiac pacing. Although the cause and reversibility of the bradydysrhythmia may not be known, prompt institution of backup pacing may be crucial to maintain hemodynamic stability. During transport an external pacemaker may be used until a transvenous pacemaker can be inserted. External pacing is performed according to ACLS protocols. Ventricular pacing is used in most clinical situations, although atrial or AV sequential pacing may be indicated. The percutaneous transvenous routes for electrode catheter insertion are the antecubital, internal jugular, subclavian, and femoral veins.[37,42] The catheters are inserted using aseptic technique, and the position of the electrode is validated by fluoroscopy.

Some of the complications encountered with temporary cardiac pacing that may occur during air medical transport include sensing problems, failure to capture, myocardial penetration, and cardiac tamponade. Undersensing or "failure to sense" may be caused by malposition of the catheter, poor intracardiac signal quality, or generator malfunction. Undersensing is managed by turning the sensitivity setting of the pulse generator to full-demand position.[37]

Oversensing, which results in pauses in paced rhythm, can result from sensing of atrial electrical activity if the pacing lead is positioned near the tricuspid valve, from sensing of T waves, or from sensing voltage transients that are the result of lead wire fracture, environmental influences, or signals from the generator. The problem of oversensing can be resolved by turning the sensitivity setting toward the asynchronous position until the unwanted signals are no longer sensed.[37]

Failure to capture can be related to malposition of the lead or to an increase in the myocardial stimulation threshold. To resolve this the current output should be increased until consistent capture occurs. If the underlying problem is electrolyte imbalance, that should be corrected. The position of the lead should be checked and repositioned if necessary.

Myocardial penetration or perforation into the pericardial space is usually accompanied by a pericardial friction rub and often by a squeaking systolic sound or murmur. If the pacing has migrated, it should be repositioned. If cardiac tamponade occurs in association with perforation, immediate pericardiocentesis should be performed.

First-Degree AV Block. First-degree AV block is characterized by prolongation of the PR interval beyond 0.20. The usual range for the prolonged PR interval is 0.21 to 0.40, but the interval may extend to as long as 0.80. In this form of AV block, each atrial impulse is conducted to the ventricles. First-degree AV block is rarely treated, but the cause should be determined and corrected.

Second-Degree AV Block. Mobitz type I (Wenckebach AV block) is characterized by the progressive prolongation of the PR intervals until a single P wave is not followed by a QRS. The RR intervals become progressively shorter until the P wave is blocked. This type of dysrhythmia has little clinical significance and is not treated. It is generally thought to be related to hyperactive vagal tone.

Mobitz type II is recognized when the P waves are periodically blocked from conduction to the ventricles without a progressive prolongation of the PR interval or a progressive shortening of the RR interval. In this type of block, the PR interval of all conducted beats is constant. Because Mobitz type II is usually a precursor of complete AV block and is generally irreversible, a permanent pacemaker is usually required.

Third-Degree AV Block or Complete Heart Block. This potentially lethal conduction abnormality is characterized by separate and independent atrial and ventricular activity. The atria are controlled by either sinus or ectopic atrial pacemakers, and the ventricles are controlled by a pacemaker that is distal to the AV block. The heart rate can go as low as 20 to 40 beats/min with this type of block. Treatment almost always involves the use of an external pacemaker or transvenous pacemaker. Pharmacologic therapy with atropine, epinephrine, or isoproterenol may be tried, and CPR may be necessary until a pacemaker can be placed.[44]

Supraventricular Dysrhythmias

Supraventricular dysrhythmias originate above the ventricle and reflect atrial irritability. These arrhythmias include premature atrial contractions, atrial tachycardia, atrial flutter, and atrial fibrillation.

Premature Atrial Contractions. Premature atrial contractions are an early atrial depolarization. They are predictors of impending supraventricular dysrhythmias and do not require intervention.

Atrial Tachycardia. Atrial tachycardias possess a regular rhythm, although variable AV conduction may be present. The heart rates vary from 140 to 240 beats/min. The P waves are usually obscured because of the rapid heart rate, and the QRS complexes tend to be narrow.

Atrial Flutter. Atrial flutter presents as a series of rapid regular flutter waves with a rate from 220 to 350 beats/min. Conduction through the AV node delays impulses, thus preventing rapid ventricular rates. Therapy of choice in sustained atrial flutter is DC cardioversion at low energy levels (25 to 50 J). Pharmacologic conversion may be accomplished by administering digitalis (1.0 to 1.5 mg IV over 12 hours).[37]

Atrial Fibrillation. Atrial fibrillation represents chaotic atrial activity with the atrial rate ranging from 300 to 700 beats/min. Impulses are randomly conducted through the AV node to the ventricles, resulting in a typically irregular ventricular response. Atrial fibrillation results in loss of effective atrial contraction, which reduces cardiac output and promotes mural thrombus development.

Treatment for patients in stable condition with atrial dysrhythmias includes pharmacologic management with IV digitalis, verapamil, quinidine, procainamide, or beta blockade. If the patient's condition becomes unstable or if drug-induced conversion is unsuccessful, cardioversion may be necessary.[49]

Sinus Tachycardia. Sinus tachycardia initiates in the sinus node and is characterized by a heart rate greater than 100 beats/min. It is a physiologic response to a demand for a higher cardiac output, and treatment is directed toward correcting the physiologic demand, as opposed to correcting the rapid heart rate. IV or oral beta blockers may be used when the tachycardia is detrimental.

CARDIOGENIC SHOCK

Cardiogenic shock is one of the most severe complications of AMI. It is the result of extensive damage to approximately 40% or more of the left ventricle, with the mortality rate in medically treated patients approaching 70% and higher. During the past two decades, the primary goal of therapy for the AMI patient has been to manage or prevent pump failure. Because the amount of ventricular failure is directly related to the extent of infarction, therapies aimed at limiting MI size, such as thrombolytic therapy, have significantly reduced the incidence and extent of pump failure. However, the most extreme form of pump failure after an AMI remains cardiogenic shock.

Extreme cardiac pump failure results in the inability of the heart to perfuse the vital organs. Clinical evidence of hypoperfusion to the vital organs along with significant systemic hypotension are the classic signs of cardiogenic shock.

Pathophysiology

The inadequate cardiac pumping that is present in cardiogenic shock results in a decreased cardiac output, hypotension, and inadequate tissue perfusion. This leads to blood pooling in the left ventricle and ultimately pulmonary congestion, as the blood begins to retrogress in the cardiopulmonary circulation. The hemodynamic changes evident include a decrease in stroke volume (SV), resulting in elevations in left ventricular end-diastolic pressure, left atrial pressure, and pulmonary capillary wedge pressure (PCWP). The concomitant hypotension causes a decrease in coronary artery perfusion, further contributing to myocardial depression.[10,56]

Assessment and Diagnosis

Patients in cardiogenic shock appear acutely ill. They often have an ashen appearance, and their skin is cool and clammy. Most patients have a depressed sensorium as a result of hypoxemia.

Physical examination often reveals profound hypotension, signs of peripheral hypoperfusion, hypoxemia, acidosis, rales, and oliguria. Hemodynamically, patients in cardiogenic shock manifest marked hypotension with systolic BP less than 80 mm Hg, low cardiac index less than 1.8 L/min/m^2, decreased urinary output (UO), elevated heart rates, and a pulmonary artery wedge pressure greater than 18 mm Hg. They also exhibit pulmonary congestion and arterial hypoxemia. Arrhythmias may occur as a result of hypoxemia, and a chest x-ray film reveals pulmonary vascular congestion.

Management

Patients in cardiogenic shock require frequent assessment of hemodynamic parameters including BP, heart rate, and pulmonary artery pressures (if a Swan-Ganz line is present). These patients should be kept in a supine position to improve cerebral blood flow and blood flow to the heart. They should be frequently assessed for peripheral perfusion, presence of edema, and color and warmth of skin. Oxygen should be administered, and most patients will require intubation with positive-end expiratory pressure (PEEP) if pulmonary congestion is severe. Intake and output should be monitored carefully, as well as blood gases, hemoglobin, and hematocrit to assess oxygen-carrying capacity and function.

Pharmacologic Therapy

Pharmacologic management includes the use of inotopic agents such as dopamine, Dobutamine, and Inocor to improve cardiac output by increasing contractility. Vasodilators are also used to increase forward flow by reducing afterload; these drugs include nitroprusside and NTG. Vasoconstrictors like Levophed, a norepinephrine bitartrate, may be used if profound hypotension persists.[49]

Intraaortic Balloon Counterpulsation (IABC)

When pharmacologic support and adjunctive therapies fail to improve low cardiac output and poor perfusion associated with cardiogenic shock, alternative devices are often employed, such as the use of the intraaortic balloon pump (IABP) and left ventricular assist device (LVAD).[6]

Balloon-pump counterpulsation can augment the cardiac output by as much as 10% to 20%.[72] It accomplishes this by raising the intraaortic pressure during diastole and lowering intraortic pressure during systole. The insertion procedure involves placing a distensible, nonthrombogenic balloon into the femoral artery percutaneously and advancing it until the balloon lies in the thoracic aorta with the tip 2 cm distal to the aortic arch. The balloon is then inflated and deflated in synchrony with the cardiac cycle. During diastole, when the balloon is inflated, blood is displaced both proximally and distally. Proximal displacement enhances coronary artery perfusion and cerebral perfusion; distal displacement improves systemic perfusion. The physiologic changes that occur as a result of the IABP include an increase in UO and improved capillary refill.

Several complications associated with the use of the IABP include emboli, thrombosis, thrombocytopenia, infection, rupture of the aorta, rupture of the balloon, impaired circulation, bleeding, and inability to wean. Because the IABP is dependent on partial intrinsic ventricular function, patients who have extremely limited or no intrinsic ventricular function may require more aggressive therapy with an LVAD.[10]

Air Medical Transport of Patients with an IABP or LVAD. Management of the patient in severe cardiogenic shock is challenging and complex. The challenge is further intensified when the patient requires transport to definitive care. The cost and complexity of specialized equipment, the space required for additional staff and equipment, and the need for highly trained personnel all suggest that the air medical transport of patients requiring IABP or LVAD intervention be undertaken only by teams proficient in the use of these therapies in the air medical environment. Organizing a smooth transition from the critical care area to the air medical environment requires a team effort to ensure that the hemodynamic stability of the patient is not interrupted. This can be accomplished by organizing the transport team and efficiently using space aboard the aircraft to accommodate equipment and allow the crew to adequately visualize the patient, monitors, and vasoactive medications (Fig. 20-6). It is also imperative that adequate

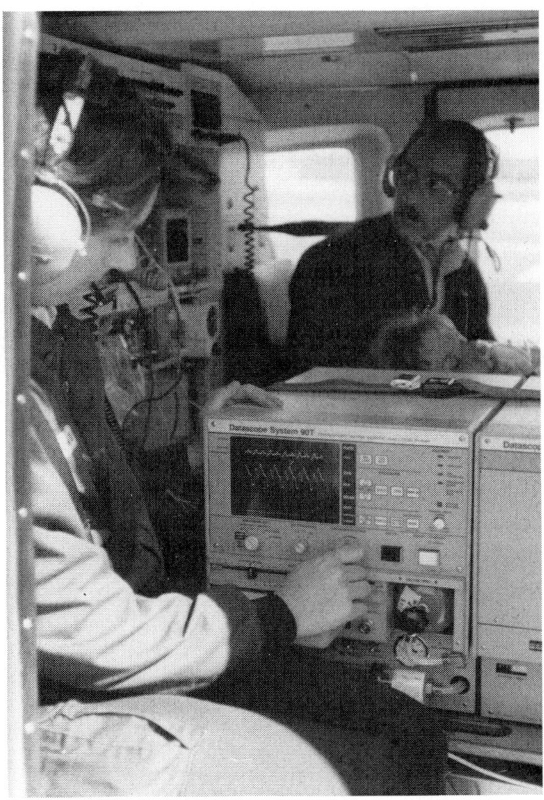

Fig. 20-6. Helicopter transport of intraaortic balloon pump (IABP)-dependent patient. (Courtesy of Life Link III, St. Paul, Minn.)

oxygen and electrical power are available during all facets of the transport process. To avoid catastrophic inadvertent disconnection of the device during transport, all equipment must be well secured, and the patient may require sedation.[89]

An additional special consideration is the effect of the hypobaric environment during flight. Boyle's law suggests that as altitude increases, volume within the intraaortic balloon will decrease, possibly resulting in incomplete inflation and less-than-optimal augmentation. A limited number of studies address this issue; however, it has been recommended that precautions be taken when dealing with any enclosed gas at altitude and that the IABP be reprimed during ascent, at cruising, altitude, and during descent.[61,89] Further and more detailed studies are necessary to examine the exact status of the IABP at altitude.[58]

Ventricular Assist Devices

The use of a ventricular assist device (VAD) is indicated when maximal conventional therapy has failed and profound cardiogenic shock develops.[10] Three groups of patients may benefit from the use of a VAD: (1) patients with AMI in cardiogenic shock, (2) patients with postcardiotomy ventricular failure who cannot be weaned from cardiopulmonary bypass, and (3) candidates for cardiac transplantation whose conditions deteriorate before a donor can be found.[75] The general principle behind the use of VADs is the same, and that is based on the "stunned myocardium" theory. Severe myocardial ischemia may produce stunned myocardium that is reversible. The myocardium that has minimal or no intrinsic function may be able to regain function if allowed to recover. A VAD allows the myocardium to rest by diverting blood from the natural ventricle to an artificial pump that maintains the circulation. Several types of assist devices are available including VADs that are surgically implanted and those that are inserted percutaneously.

VADs that can be inserted percutaneously have received much attention recently because they can be inserted quickly and do not require surgical opening of the chest. Insertion involves a simple cutdown procedure of the femoral artery through which a cannula is inserted. Bypass can then be initiated without mobilization of the surgical team.

Another percutaneously inserted VAD is the cardiopulmonary support system (CPS). This system is designed to provide rapid and portable total cardiopulmonary bypass. The system is preassembled and can be primed in 5 minutes. Both the femoral artery and femoral vein are cannulated, and the bypass is initiated. A vortex pump is used without a cardiotomy reservoir, which allows suction rather than gravity venous return. This provides marked cardiac decompression during bypass. The advantage of the CPS is that it can be instituted very quickly in the cardiac catheterization laboratory, the intensive care unit, or even the patient's room. It has been used for patients with cardiac arrest or cardiogenic shock, postbypass cardiovascular collapse, pulmonary embolism, cardiomyopathy, left ventricular rupture, and for patients undergoing left main coronary angioplasty.

Another percutaneously inserted VAD is the extracorporeal membrane oxygenator. ECMO uses a membrane oxygenator system connected to a heat exchanger and a roller pump system. Venovenous or venoarterial cannulation is used for blood outflow and inflow. Adult ECMO is only indicated in a select group of patients with such severe respiratory or cardiac compromise that they have not improved with conventional therapy. It is most commonly used with respiratory failure due to adult respiratory distress syndrome (ARDS), pneumonia, severe asthma, cardiac failure, or trauma. These patients have generally exhausted vigorous respiratory care and are acutely ill with a mortality risk as high as 90%.[4]

Surgically implanted VADs require surgical implantation of a cannula by means of a median sternotomy or thoracotomy incision. They are used for patients in cardiogenic shock requiring open heart surgical intervention and those undergoing open heart procedures who experience an AMI during or immediately after the procedure. There are two types of VADs, the right ventricular assist devices (RVADs), which divert blood around the right ventricle, and the LVADs, which divert blood around the left ventricle. The RVAD uses a cannula placed in the right atrium for the outflow of blood and a cannula placed in the pulmonary artery for the return of blood. With the LVAD, blood is removed from the left atrium and returned to the systemic circulation by means of the aorta.[10]

There are several different types of surgically implanted VADs. These include (1) roller pumps that propel blood forward by compressing the blood at a manually set point, creating a nonpulsatile flow,[64] (2) centrifugal devices that circulate high volumes of blood under relatively low pressure, and (3) pneumatic devices that provide pulsatile flow by using jets of compressed air to drive or eject blood.

Complications associated with all of the VADs are thromboembolism, hemolysis, mechanical failure, and infection.

CONGESTIVE HEART FAILURE

Definition

Heart failure or CHF is a condition in which the heart cannot pump sufficient blood to meet the metabolic needs of the body. It is characterized by a syndrome in which cardiac dysfunction is associated with reduced exercise tolerance, a high incidence of ventricular arrhythmias, and a shortened life expectancy.[17] Sudden death occurs in patients with existing ventricular dysfunction, most of whom are in heart failure. However, some patients with ventricular dysfunction have a normal exercise tolerance; thus therapy includes not only treatment for symptomatic patients but preventive treatment for asymptomatic patients as well. The three most common causes of heart failure are left ventricular aneurysm, mitral regurgitation caused by papillary muscle dysfunction, and an inadequate quantity of normally contracting myocardium.

Pathophysiology

Heart failure results in a reduction in stroke volume that initiates several mechanisms that act to restore stroke volume. These compensatory mechanisms are sympathetic stimulation (tachycardia and vasoconstriction) and activation of the renin-angiotensin-aldosterone system. Unfortunately, these mechanisms increase myocardial oxygen demand and thus are potentially detrimental to myocardial function.

Assessment and Diagnosis

A careful history usually reveals the cause of heart failure, such as MI, hypertension, or alcoholism. The patient will experience shortness of breath, which begins initially with exertion and progresses to shortness of breath at rest. In severe heart failure, the patient cannot tolerate the supine position and must sit upright or lean over a table to breathe.

Physical examination reveals elevated central venous pressure, pulsus alternans, or a dicrotic pulse, and pulmonary rales that may extend to the lung apices. In right ventricular failure, an S_3 is often heard, as well as a holosystolic murmur of tricuspid regurgitation. Hepatomegaly is felt, and peripheral pitting edema is seen, along with sacral edema if the patient has been on bed rest. In left ventricular failure the apical impulse is usually displaced laterally and downward, and S_1 is diminished. The S_2 is sometimes paradoxically split, and an S_3 gallop is present. A systolic murmur of mitral regurgitation is often heard.[36]

The ECG may assist in determining the cause of the heart failure. Laboratory data are nonspecific, although arterial hypoxemia and metabolic acidosis are common, and respiratory alkalosis may be present with significant tachypnea. Chest x-ray films reveal cardiomegaly and pulmonary congestion or frank pulmonary edema.[36] Invasive monitoring reveals an elevated pulmonary artery wedge pressure, elevated systemic vascular resistance, and low cardiac output.

Management

The two goals of therapy for heart failure patients are (1) to relieve symptoms, thus improving the quality of life, and (2) to prolong life. Management of acute heart failure focuses on the reduction of preload for relief of pulmonary edema, reduction of afterload with vasodilators to enhance stroke volume, and enhancement of contractile function. Intravenous diuretics and nitrates are used for preload reduction. The calcium blocking agent nifedipine has also been used in select cases as a preload reducing agent. Orally administered afterload reducing agents and angiotensin-converting enzyme inhibitors are used in the chronic, as opposed to the acute, setting. Inotropic agents are rarely used to enhance contractility because of the increase in myocardial oxygen demand, unless shock is present.[36] Continuous ECG monitoring is required (potential ventricular dysrhythmias caused by electrolyte imbalances), and strict intake and output measurements must be maintained.

CARDIOMYOPATHY

Cardiomyopathy is a general term used to describe disease involving the muscle itself. The cardiomyopathies are unique because they are not the result of ischemic, hypertensive, congenital, valvular, or pericardial diseases.

Cardiomyopathies can be functionally classified into three categories: (1) dilated or congestive cardiomyopathy, which is characterized by ventricular dilatation, contractile dysfunction, and symptoms of heart failure; (2) hypertrophic cardiomyopathy, which is marked by inappropriate left ventricular hypertrophy with preserved or enhanced contractile function; and (3) restrictive cardiomyopathy, characterized by endocardial scarring of the ventricle with impairment of diastolic filling.

The cardiomyopathies are further classified as either primary or secondary. For primary cardiomyopathy, the basic pathologic process involves the myocardium rather than other cardiac structures, and the cause of heart disease is unknown. For secondary cardiomyopathy, the cause of the myocardial abnormality is known, and the cardiomyopathy is one manifestation of the disease process.[12]

Dilated Cardiomyopathy

Dilated cardiomyopathy is characterized by cardiac enlargement and, in the majority of cases, heart failure as a result of impairment of systolic pump function. All four heart chambers are dilated, resulting in marked cardiomegaly; the ventricles are usually more dilated then the atria. Dilated cardiomyopathy is the end result of myocardial damage produced by a variety of toxic, metabolic, or infectious agents.[12] Some examples of these secondary causes that may precipitate dilated cardiomyopathy include alcohol, hypertension, pregnancy, viruses, and hyperthyroidism.[88]

Pathophysiology

Ventricular function is impaired as the disease of dilated cardiomyopathy progresses, resulting in an elevated end-systolic volume and a reduction in stroke volume and ejection fraction. As a compensatory response, cardiac output initially rises but will eventually decline in exercise or stress. Thrombus formation is enhanced because of the retention of blood in the cardiac chambers. The coronary arteries are usually normal. At the end stage of dilated cardiomyopathy, cardiac output declines and right-sided heart failure occurs, causing biventricular failure.

Assessment and Diagnosis

As end-systolic volume increases, pulmonary symptoms are manifested. Dyspnea on exertion progresses to orthopnea, then to paroxysmal nocturnal dyspnea

(PND), and dyspnea at rest. Fatigue and weakness usually accompany these symptoms. Right-sided heart failure causes increased jugular venous distention (JVD), hepatomegaly, splenomegaly, ascites, and peripheral edema. Patients may also have abdominal pain, which is a reflection of liver congestion.

On physical examination the patient is breathless at rest or on exertion. The skin may be cool, pale, or cyanotic with peripheral edema. Palpation may reveal ascites, JVD, and pulsatile liver engorgement. An S_3 and an S_4 heart sound are often auscultated as a summation gallop in patients with rapid heart rates. There may be a reduction in pulse pressure and the presence of systolic murmurs.

Management

Treatment of dilated cardiomyopathy includes measures to improve the symptoms of heart failure and increase stroke volume. Cardiac glycosides and other inotropic agents such as amrinone, dopamine, and dobutamine are used for their positive inotropic effects. Diuretics decrease blood volume in heart failure patients, and anticoagulation prevents systemic and pulmonary emboli. Beta-blocking agents may be used in patients with tachycardia at rest. Vasodilator therapy is used to lessen the symptoms of failure and increase exercise tolerance; venodilators are used to decrease preload. Nitrates are most commonly used for this purpose. Unfortunately, all forms of medical treatment are palliative rather than curative in the treatment of dilated cardiomyopathy.

Hypertrophic Cardiomyopathy

Hypertrophic cardiomyopathy is a disease of unknown cause that has a hypertrophic, nondilated ventricle, in the absence of a cardiac or systemic disease that could produce left ventricular hypertrophy.[50] Although the cause is unclear, heredity, specifically an autosomal dominant trait, has been linked to hypertrophic cardiomyopathy. This type of cardiomyopathy had been known until recently as idiopathic hypertrophic subaortic stenosis (IHSS).

Pathophysiology

Hypertrophic cardiomyopathy is identified by thickening of the ventricular septum greater than the left ventricular free wall. It is further characterized by disorganization of the myocardial fibers within the ventricular septum. Other secondary characteristics include a fibrous plaque on the mural endocardium of the septum, a decrease in ventricular cavity size, anterior and posterior mitral valve thickening, and left atrial dilation in adults in response to the increased ventricular filling pressure.

A variety of patterns of hypertrophy occurs within the ventricular septum. The most common form of hypertrophy encompasses a large portion of the ventricular septum and anterolateral portion of the left ventricular free wall. Other areas of hypertrophy include the anterior portion of the septum and all areas of the left ventricle except the basal anterior ventricular septum. Many patients have some mitral regurgitation related to the abnormal bending and pulling of the papillary muscles from hypertrophy. The asymmetric hypertrophy in the left ventricle and the abnormal myofibrils produce hemodynamic changes in the left ventricle. These changes include a decrease in ventricular compliance, a decrease in diastolic filling volume, an elevated pressure gradient across the outflow tract, and a very rapid initial systolic contraction.

Assessment and Diagnosis

Patients with hypertrophic cardiomyopathy are usually young (in their second or third decade of life), active, and athletic. They typically are initially seen with a systolic murmur of late onset heard at the left sternal border and apex that radiates to the axilla. The murmur is increased by standing or during the Valsalva maneuver. The arterial pulse is abrupt and has a jerky quality.

The most common symptom is dyspnea; other symptoms include angina, fatigue, syncope, palpitations, PND, heart failure, and vertigo. Most of the symptoms are worsened with exertion. The ECG in hypertrophic cardiomyopathy reflects hypertrophy and atrial abnormality. Approximately 20% of these patients have atrial fibrillation.

Management

Management of patients with hypertrophic cardiomyopathy consists of symptom relief and prevention of complications. Pharmacologic interventions that increase or maintain left ventricular end-diastolic volume and reduce ventricular contractility are usually used. Propranolol is most commonly used because it inhibits inotropic and chronotropic actions, prolongs cardiac diastole, decreases myocardial oxygen consumption, improves the distensibility of the left ventricle, and increases diastolic filling time.[50] For long-term management, calcium channel blocking agents are used. The antiarrhythmic agent amiodarone is used for those patients with frequent ventricular ectopy or ventricular tachycardia. Prophylactic antibiotic therapy is indicated both before and after surgical procedures for protection from infective endocarditis.

Restrictive Cardiomyopathy

Restrictive cardiomyopathy is the least common of the cardiomyopathies in Western countries. It resembles constrictive pericarditis clinically and is characterized by abnormal diastolic function as a result of abnormal cardiac stiffness.

Pathophysiology

There is usually mild cardiac enlargement with restrictive cardiomyopathy without significant ventricular dilatation. The walls of both ventricles are firm, noncompliant, and thickened. The cause is usually unknown, but many specific pathologic processes may develop into restrictive cardiomyopathy, including myocardial fibrosis, hypertrophy, or infiltration.

Assessment and Diagnosis

Most patients have chest pain, dyspnea on exertion, and fatigue. Because of the heart's inability to increase cardiac output, exercise tolerance is limited. JVD, peripheral edema, ascites, anasarca, and hepatomegaly may be noted. Mitral and tricuspid murmurs and S_3 or S_4 heart sounds are usually present. The ECG commonly reveals sinus tachycardia and atrial fibrillation with biventricular hypertrophy and decreased voltage.

Management

Medical management of restrictive cardiomyopathy is similar to that for heart failure in that it is symptom limiting. The treatment focuses on fluid restriction, diuretic therapy, anticoagulation, and administration of digitalis if atrial fibrillation is present.

Surgical treatment consists of resection of thickened endocardial tissue. Valve replacement surgery is also done when necessary.

VALVULAR DYSFUNCTION

Definition

Valvular dysfunction can result from either congenital or acquired causes that expose the valve to hemodynamic stress and may accelerate the degenerative changes that cause dysfunction. Changes that cause narrowing of the valve orifice are classified as stenosis. Changes leading to valvular insufficiency because of improper closing of valves are classified as regurgitation.[50]

Mitral Stenosis

Pathophysiology

Mitral stenosis is a narrowing of the mitral orifice and is usually caused by rheumatic fever. The pathologic changes that occur in mitral stenosis are fusion of the commissures, fibrosis and thickening of the leaflets, shortening and fusion of the chordae and papillary muscles, or both, and calcification of the leaflets. As the valve area is reduced, the gradient across the valve increases. Critical mitral stenosis occurs when the mitral valve opening is reduced to 1 cm^2; the normal mitral valve has an area of 4 to 6 cm^2. The stenosis leads to elevations in left atrial pressure that cause increased pulmonary venous and pulmonary artery wedge pressure.

Assessment and Diagnosis

The principal symptom of severe mitral stenosis is dyspnea with minimal exertion and episodes of orthopnea, PND, or pulmonary edema. Fatigue is also common, as are palpitations if atrial fibrillation has developed. Systemic venous hypertension with increased JVD, hepatomegaly, ascites, splenomegaly, and peripheral edema develop when severe mitral stenosis leads to pulmonary vascular resistance and right-sided heart failure.[50] Thromboembolism may be a presenting symptom because most of these patients are in atrial fibrillation.

Physical examination reveals a dyspneic patient (the degree of dyspnea depends on the severity of the stenosis) with pinkish-purple patches on his or her cheeks. The point of maximal impulse (PMI) is usually normal.

Management

Medical management of mitral stenosis includes preventing complications such as systemic embolism or bacterial endocarditis and treating atrial fibrillation. Symptomatic patients are treated with oral diuretics and sodium restriction.

Surgical management of mitral stenosis includes closed mitral commissurotomy, open mitral commissurotomy, and mitral valve replacement. Nonsurgical treatment with mitral valvuloplasty may be appropriate for some patients.

Mitral Regurgitation

Pathophysiology

Acute mitral regurgitation (MR) is a potentially fatal occurrence and is the result of rupture of the mitral valve. This valve disruption is caused by rupture of the base of a papillary muscle, usually caused by ischemic necrosis. Rupture of both valve leaflets is incompatible with life; however, if only one leaflet ruptures, resulting in an incompetent valve, prognosis is much better. From acute severe MR, pulmonary edema, left ventricular volume overload, and passive pulmonary hypertension develop. The pulmonary edema and hypertension are a result of left atrial hypertension from acute volume overload in a chamber of normal size and compliance.[40]

Assessment and Diagnosis

The primary symptom of MR is dyspnea with auscultation of both S_3 and S_4 gallop sounds. The MR murmur is of variable intensity; it is sometimes not holosystolic and may be crescendo-decrescendo in contour. If both leaflets are involved, the murmur is very loud and widespread.

The ECG may be normal or show evidence of an AMI. The rhythm is usually sinus rhythm; atrial fibrillation is indicative of chronic MR. Invasive monitoring discloses a prominent systolic regurgitant wave in the pulmonary artery wedge pressure tracing.

Management

Medical management is used to stabilize the patient's condition before surgical treatment. Diuretics are used to treat the pulmonary edema, and afterload-reducing agents (nitroprusside) are given intravenously to lower systemic vascular resistance and enhance stroke volume. Digitalis may be used in the non-AMI patient. Hypotension is usually treated with dopamine, and hemodynamic support with the IABP may be necessary.

Aortic Stenosis

Pathophysiology

Aortic stenosis (AS) usually results from a congenital or degenerative origin. The reduction in the valve orifice causes obstruction to the flow of blood from the left ventricle into the aorta during ventricular systole resulting in ventricular wall thickening. Left ventricular hypertrophy occurs as a compensatory mechanism, and ultimately the left ventricle may fail completely, leading to a critically low cardiac output.[50]

Assessment and Diagnosis

The classic clinical manifestation of severe AS is chest pain, syncope, and heart failure. Physical examination reveals a harsh crescendo-decrescendo systolic ejection murmur that begins after the S_I sound. A widened pulse pressure with a normal diastolic pressure is common in compensated AS, and a narrowed pulse pressure is common in noncompensated AS. Left ventricular hypertrophy produces a sustained thrust or heave of the apical impulse with displacement of the impulse downward and to the left when ventricular failure develops.

In decompensated severe AS, the ECG may reveal left atrial hypertrophy. Conduction abnormalities are also common in patients with AS.

Management

Patients with severe AS with associated left ventricular dysfunction and myocardial ischemia respond well to careful administration of nitroprusside.[50] These patients also benefit from use of the IABP. Diuretics and beta-blocking agents should be used cautiously. Surgical intervention includes aortic valve replacement, and nonsurgical intervention with aortic valvuloplasty may be indicated.

Aortic Regurgitation

Pathophysiology

Acute aortic regurgitation (AR) results in a large volume overload at high pressure to the left ventricle, which cannot adapt acutely. Acute AR causes an early impairment in ejection, resulting in low forward stroke output, left atrial hypertension, and pulmonary edema. Causes include infective endocarditis, aortic dissection, and nonpenetrating chest or upper abdominal trauma.[40]

Assessment and Diagnosis

The patient with acute AR is acutely ill with tachycardia, peripheral hypoperfusion, and congestive heart failure. Physical examination reveals a widened pulse pressure. S_1 is diminished, and there is no S_4. The diastolic murmur may be of variable intensity. The ECG may be normal or show left ventricular hypertrophy if aortic dissection is present.

Management

Medical management for patients with AR is a temporary measure until surgery can be performed. Pulmonary edema should be treated with diuretics, and afterload-reducing agents are used to lower systemic vascular resistance. This increases forward stroke volume and reduces regurgitant volume. Use of the IABP is contraindicated because it increases aortic regurgitation.[40]

ACUTE PERICARDITIS

Pericarditis refers to inflammation of the pericardium and can have a number of causes. The most common conditions associated with the development of pericarditis include MI, infection, collagen vascular diseases, uremia, malignancy, drug therapy, and trauma.

The pericardium is a closed fibrous sac that envelops the heart. It consists of an inner serous membrane, the visceral pericardium that is closely adherent to the superficial myocardium and coronary vessels. The fibrous outer layer that surrounds the heart is the parietal pericardium. The space between the visceral and parietal layers normally contains between 10 to 20 ml of pericardial fluid that acts as a lubricant between the contracting surfaces. The exact role of the pericardium is not clear. However, it is believed to serve as a lubrication system, ensuring that cardiac motion is unimpaired by surrounding mediastinal structures. Because the pericardium resists stretching, it functions as a protective mechanism to prevent sudden dilation of the heart. The pericardium may also protect the heart from infection.[69]

The pathologic changes and clinical features associated with the inflammation of acute pericarditis depend on their cause. For example, pericarditis is a common sequela of transmural MI. The epicardial layer in contact with the pericardium may become roughened, irritating the pericardial surface and creating an inflammatory reaction.[60]

Assessment and Diagnosis

The presentation of pericardial heart disease depends on the pericardium's response to injury and subsequent effect on cardiac function. Diagnosis and recognition of acute pericarditis in the emergent situation are largely dependent on patient history of pleuritic chest pain. The physical examination may reveal a pericardial friction rub and, possibly, ECG demonstration of ST elevation (associated with subepicardial inflammation or injury) of 1 to 3 mm, involving the precordial leads. Sequential ECGs over a number of days demonstrate the evolution of pericarditis and therefore are limited as a diagnostic tool in the emergent situation.[66]

In acute pericarditis the most common symptom is precordial or retrosternal chest pain, which is frequently described as stabbing or sharp in nature. The pain may occur gradually or begin suddenly, radiating to the shoulders, arms, or back. A classic symptom is pain radiating to the trapezius ridges from inflammation of the adjoining diaphragmatic pleura.[55] Chest pain caused by acute pericarditis may be aggravated by inspiration, coughing, or movement and may be relieved when the patient sits up and leans forward. Associated signs and symptoms include (1) fever and leukocytosis, (2) dyspnea related to increased pain with inspiration, (3) dysphagia related to irritation of the esophagus by the posterior pericardium, and (4) sinus tachycardia.

Physical examination reveals a pericardial friction rub that may be heard at various times and in various locations during the patient's course. The friction rub resembles a high-pitched grating or scratching sound. It is best heard with the diaphragm of the stethoscope placed at the lower left sternal border or apex with the patient sitting and leaning forward during held expiration. The presence of a friction rub does not exclude the presence of a large pericardial effusion or tamponade.[34,66] A normal BP should be present without paradoxical pulse or venous distention. If the flight nurse observes signs of restriction to ventricular filling, he or she should consider the presence of pericardial tamponade or effusion.

Management

Evaluation and monitoring of acute pericarditis are important in the emergency setting to establish whether the pericarditis is associated with an underlying problem, such as MI or pericardial effusion, requiring specific therapy. The flight nurse should monitor for complications of pericarditis such as signs of pericardial effusion that may accumulate rapidly and cause cardiac tamponade.

The chest pain of pericarditis may be managed by analgesics and antiinflammatory agents such as aspirin, indomethacin, and nonsteroidal antiinflammatory drugs such as ibuprofen. Steroids may also be indicated.[87] The patient should be observed for atrial arrhythmias, such as beats and bursts of atrial tachycardia, which often accompany acute pericarditis. Unless these arrhythmias progress to sustained atrial tachydysrhythmias, treatment may not be recommended.[34]

CARDIAC EFFUSION AND TAMPONADE

Pericardial effusion refers to the development of fluid within the pericardial sac as a response to injury of the parietal pericardium or with all causes of acute pericarditis. Cardiac tamponade occurs when the accumulation of fluid occurs to such an extent that cardiac output is significantly compromised.[55] For emergency practitioners, cardiac tamponade is one of the most dramatic emergencies.

Pathophysiology

The hemodynamic effects of effusion are related to the speed of accumulation of the fluid. Rapid accumulation of 150 to 200 ml may produce acute cardiac tamponade; in contrast, the slow accumulation of 1000 ml of fluid may be well tolerated.[52] Under normal conditions, between 15 and 50 ml of fluid may be present in the pericardial space. The development of a larger volume of fluid may result from pericardial inflammation of any cause, heart failure or traumatic injury to the heart, aortic dissection, or neoplasm. The presence of additional fluid causes the intrapericardial pressure to increase. When intrapericardial pressure is increased, diastolic filling of the ventricles is impeded, resulting in a rise of ventricular pressure and decreased cardiac output. As the increased intrapericardial pressure reaches a critical level, a precipitous decrease in arterial pressure occurs.[52]

Assessment and Diagnosis

Mild to moderate percardial effusion may not produce symptoms. If the fluid accumulates slowly, the fairly noncompliant pericardium stretches to accommodate the increasing volume with little or no rise in intrapericardial pressure, until it reaches a size where it can no longer stretch. However, if the fluid accumulates rapidly, a small volume can be life threatening. Clinical symptoms of cardiac tamponade are related to systemic venous congestion, a reduction in cardiac stroke volume, and respiratory effects of impaired ventricular filling. The classic signs, described as Beck's triad, include distended neck veins resulting from elevated CVP, decreased BP, and distant heart sounds.[55] Other signs of acute tamponade include early sinus tachycardia with reactive vasoconstriction and pulsus paradoxus (abnormal fall in systolic pressure during inspiration caused by differential filling of the ventricles). If early signs of cardiac tamponade are not treated, rapid development of severe hypotension, profound circulatory failure, and shock result.[69] Chest x-ray films may demonstrate a widening cardiac silhouette.

Paradoxical Pulse

A finding of paradoxical pulse is elicited by measuring BP during quiet respiration. The technique involves pumping the blood pressure cuff above the systolic sounds and slowly deflating the cuff until the first systolic sound is heard. Normally, on inspiration, the systolic sound should disappear. The flight nurse should continue to deflate the cuff until all systolic sounds can be heard on inspiration and expiration. The paradox is the difference in millimeters of mercury between the pressure where the systolic sound disappears and the pressure at which *all* systolic sounds are heard. A paradox of less than 10 mm Hg is a normal reflection of the inspiratory fall of aortic systolic pressure; however, it is exaggerated in the presence of cardiac tamponade. An inspiratory fall in systolic BP exceeding 10 mm Hg indicates the presence of a paradoxical pulse.[55]

Management

Emergent evacuation of the pericardial fluid is definitive therapy in the presence of acute cardiac tamponade. Hemodynamic support during preparation of the patient for pericardiocentesis includes administration of IV fluid, blood, plasma, or saline, and ECG monitoring. Pericardiocentesis is accomplished by needle aspiration of pericardial fluid. Positive-pressure ventilation should be avoided if possible, because it has been demonstrated to further depress cardiac output in patients with cardiac tamponade.[55]

NONTRAUMATIC AORTIC DISSECTION

One of the most commonly seen life-threatening disorders of the aorta is dissection. Aortic dissection occurs when an intimal tear develops in the aorta, resulting in hematoma formation in its medial layer and subsequent longitudinal separation of the layers of the aorta. Dissections can originate anywhere along the length of the aorta, but the most common point of origin is in the ascending aorta (proximal dissection) within a few centimeters above the aortic valve.[23] Conditions associated with aortic dissection include atherosclerosis, hypertension, Marfan's syndrome (a nonatherosclerotic disorder of connective tissue involving massive degeneration of elastic fibers in the aortic media), syphilis, and autoimmune diseases.[25] Half of the dissections occurring in young female patients occur during pregnancy.[30]

Classification of aortic dissection is based on the extent of the dissecting process and its anatomic location. A type I dissection occurs in the ascending aorta and extends distally, beyond the aortic arch. In type II, the dissecting process is limited to the ascending aorta and is most often associated with aortic valvular incompetence and with Marfan's syndrome. Type III dissection in most patients occurs just distal to the origin of the left subclavian artery and extends distally, possibly involving the abdominal aorta.[20] Patients with distal dissection are usually managed medically unless the dissection is complicated by rupture of the aorta or compromise of the blood supply to a vital organ. Surgery, emergent if necessary, is indicated for most patients with proximal dissection.[79]

Assessment and Diagnosis

Patients with aortic dissections have sudden, severe pain that is more intense than they have ever experienced. The pain may be described as ripping, cutting, and tearing, often originating in the back or substernal area, possibly extending down into the legs. The pain may change in location as the dissection proceeds. Other signs result from obstruction of major vessels originating from the aorta. Depending on the location of the dissection and the compromised vessels involved, MI, cerebral insufficiency, cerebral vascular accident, hemiplegia or paraplegia, renal failure, and intestinal infarction may result.

The patient with acute dissection is in severe distress and is "shocky" with pallor, sweating, peripheral cyanosis, and restlessness. However, the BP may be normal or elevated, often as high as 200 mm Hg systolic, with a significant difference between both arms. Differential BP and pulses may indicate compromise of blood flow to one or both subclavian arteries. Absence of femoral pulses may indicate extension of the dissection into the aortic bifurcation, compromising circulation to one or both legs. If the patient is hypotensive, cardiac tamponade or aortic rupture should be suspected.[35]

Diagnosis of aortic dissection can often be made by physical examination alone. Transport of the acute patient should not be delayed to obtain a chest x-ray. However, if a chest film is available on arrival of the transport team, it may be a useful in conjunction with other diagnostic signs. X-ray findings suggestive of an acute aortic dissection are (1) mediastinal widening, (2) extension of the aortic shadow beyond a calcified aortic wall, (3) a localized bulge on the aortic arch, and (4) tracheal deviation, or (5) a left pleural effusion.[79]

Management

Prompt initiation of therapy and transport of patients with acute aortic dissection remains a challenge for flight nurses who are often caring for these patients during the brief interval between the onset of symptoms and the occurrence of life-threatening complications. Interventions are aimed at halting the progression of the dissecting force by lowering the BP and diminishing left ventricular contractility. Left ventricular contractility determines the rate of acceleration of blood in the aorta and is a major factor in the generation of shearing forces on the aortic wall.[27] Expert care and transport to definitive care requires pain relief and continuous ECG and BP monitoring. Blood pressure should be aggressively lowered, usually 100 to 110 mm Hg, with sodium nitroprusside, using caution not to compromise renal or cerebral circulation.[79] Because of its rapid onset and short duration of action, nitroprusside infusions should be placed on the most accurate delivery pump available for transport. The dose should be titrated to BP response. For patients without significant bradycardia, AV block, congestive heart failure, or bronchospasm, beta-adrenergic blockade and its subsequent negative inotropic effect help reduce the pulsatility of aortic flow and the pulse rate.[27] Pain may be managed with IV narcotic analgesia while the flight nurse constantly observes for signs of respiratory compromise.

Flight personnel should also be prepared to initiate intubation and assisted ventilation in the event that the patient's condition deteriorates. At least two large-bore IV access sites should be established for transport. Fluids should be kept to a minimum unless severe hypotension or rupture of the aorta occurs in flight. Blood should be available for transfusion during the flight if cardiac output becomes compromised. Inadequate pain or BP control and evidence of progressive dissection indicate an urgent need for surgical intervention. The flight team should not delay transfer to wait for laboratory results, blood products, or x-rays. Coordination of efforts among air medical transport personnel and the referring and receiving hospitals will expedite admission to the surgical department for prompt intervention.

HYPERTENSIVE CRISIS

A hypertensive crisis is a very rapid, progressive rise in BP sufficient to cause potential irreversible damage to vital organs. The major organs at risk are the brain, heart, and kidneys. Hypertensive crisis may occur in the clinical course of any patient with a persistent BP elevation, or it may occur as the initial presentation of a hypertensive patient. There are no predetermined criteria for the level of BP necessary to produce a hypertensive emergency; the level of BP usually associated with hypertensive crisis is 130 mm Hg diastolic. The evidence of organ dysfunction is the basis for diagnosis. Patients without prior hypertension may not tolerate BP levels as high as can those patients with chronic hypertension.[59]

Assessment and Diagnosis

The underlying pathologic process in accelerated hypertension and subsequent hypertensive crisis is a progressive arteriolopathy with inflammation and necrosis of arterioles.[8] The effects of these changes within the small arterioles are directly visible in the retina. The pathophysiology underlying specific target organ damage varies.[39] However, the important clinical features of accelerated hypertension include signs and symptoms of hypertensive encephalopathy, renal damage, and cardiac failure.

The most devastating complication of hypertension is hypertensive encephalopathy. This condition is generally thought to result from an abrupt sustained rise of BP exceeding the limits of autoregulation of the cerebral circulation.[8] Hypertensive encephalopathy may be characterized by the presence of progressive central nervous systems signs and symptoms including severe headache, nausea, vomiting, and visual difficulties. Focal neurologic findings can include blindness, seizures, aphasia, and hemiparesis. If left untreated, symptoms may progress to convulsions, stupor, coma, and death. This condition is a true emergency, and the goal of therapy is to lower the mean arterial pressure over a 30- to 60-minute time interval to normalize cerebral blood flow.[45]

Alterations in left ventricular performance secondary to increased afterload are the primary mechanism by which an acute rise in pressure affects the cardiovascular system.[45] Left ventricular failure, myocardial ischemia, or both, can occur as a result of accelerated hypertension. These conditions may progress to pulmonary edema or AMI as a consequence of increased myocardial oxygen demand. Signs and symptoms of left ventricular failure include chest pain, dyspnea, production of pink frothy sputum, rales, and bronchospasm.

Management

The goal of therapy for patients demonstrating signs of hypertensive encephalopathy, acute renal failure, or cardiac decompensation is to lower the BP in a controlled manner within 30 to 60 minutes to what is "normal" for that patient. For the flight nurse, the resolution of signs and symptoms should be used as a primary guide in the control of the pressure, in addition to the level of BP, because it may be difficult to obtain frequent accurate BP in flight. Monitoring the patient's cardiac rhythm and BP (by the most accurate means possible), observing the patient's level of consciousness, and assessing for signs of impending pulmonary edema or cardiac failure helps the flight nurse evaluate whether the antihypertensive agents are effective. Either nitroprusside or diazoxide may be used when immediate antihypertensive therapy is required.

Sodium nitroprusside acts by direct peripheral vasodilation with balanced effects on arterial and venous blood vessels. The antihypertensive effect of IV sodium nitroprusside is apparent within seconds and is dose dependent. Once the drug is discontinued, the pressure rises rapidly to the previous level within 1 to 10 minutes. Infusion rates must be closely monitored to avoid sudden fluctuations in BP. Diazoxide exerts its hypotensive effect by reducing arteriolar vascular resistance through direct relaxation of arteriolar smooth muscle. When the drug decreases arterial pressure, baroreceptor reflexes are activated, leading to cardiac stimulation with increased heart rate, stroke volume, and cardiac output, resulting in mechanical stress on the aorta. For this reason diazoxide should not be used for patients with dissection of the aorta and for patients with known CAD.[8] Once the BP is controlled, the BP remains low and returns only gradually over 4 to 12 hours, giving it an advantage over nitroprusside in clinical situations where it is difficult to monitor the patient's condition closely for a long period of time.[59] Other antihypertensive agents useful in the emergent situation are summarized in Table 20-3.

HEMODYNAMIC MONITORING IN CARDIOVASCULAR ASSESSMENT

Accurate hemodynamic assessment is essential during the transport of the patient with cardiovascular compromise. Space limitations, noise levels, and vibration in the air medical environment often preclude the use of sophisticated invasive hemodynamic monitoring equipment during transport. However, the proficient flight nurse will develop and refine the use of visual and tactile assessment skills to clinically evaluate the patient. Especially valuable are frequent examinations of mental status, skin color and temperature, pulse rate and quality, and UO.

Cardiac Output

The ultimate goal of monitoring and manipulation of hemodynamic parameters is to provide adequate perfusion of the body. This can be accomplished by directing and maintaining adequate cardiac output. Assessing the cardiac output provides a useful measure of the pumping ability of the heart. *Cardiac output* is defined as the product of the heart rate and stroke volume, which is the amount of blood ejected from the left ventricle with each contraction. Changes in cardiac output result from altering the rate of the heartbeat or the stroke volume. The major factors that influence stroke volume are contractility, preload (venous return or diastolic filling), and afterload (re-

TABLE 20-3

Drugs commonly used in hypertensive emergencies

Drug	Usual Dose	Mechanism and onset of action	Duration of action	Side effects
Sodium nitroprusside (Nipride)	Prepare 50-100 mg/500 ml D5W; administer at rate of 0.05-020 mg/min	Arterial and venous vasodilator, immediate onset of action	3-5 min	Severe hypotension, nausea, restlessness, thiocyanate toxicity, methemoglobinemia
Labetalol (Normodyne)	5-50 mg IV every 10 minutes as needed; may be administered as a continuous IV infusion (2 mg/min) thereafter to maximum dose of 300 mg	Alpha- and beta-blocking agent, onset immediate; decrease blood pressure without changing heart rate	2-4 hr	Bradycardia, bronchospasm, profound hypotension
Furosemide (Lasix)	40-80 mg IV over 1-2 min	Diuretic, venous vasodilator, onset 1-5 min	1-12 hr	Electrolyte imbalance

From Keen J, Baird M, Allen J: *Critical care and emergency drug reference,* St Louis, 1994, Mosby.

sistance imposed by normal aortic impedance)[87] (see Fig. 20-7).

Noninvasive Hemodynamic Monitoring

Noninvasive methods used to assess the hemodynamic status of the patient include the monitoring of the patient's capillary refill, pulse rate and quality, BP, mentation, UO, and skin temperature. Mental status changes are important in determining the patient's overall condition. Significant changes in mentation occur in late shock when flow is compromised to the vital organs. Skin temperature and color, capillary refill, and UO in the absence of renal disease reflect tissue perfusion as it relates to cardiac output and intravascular volume. Thomas and Clemmer[83] suggest using a combination of noninvasive methods to create a picture of the adequacy of cardiac output during aeromedical transport of critical patients.

Assessing the patient's capillary refill provides information about the ability to perfuse all body organs. When cardiac output falls, the body prioritizes tissue perfusion by increasing peripheral resistance and shunting blood away from the peripheral areas toward the body central core to preserve heart, brain,

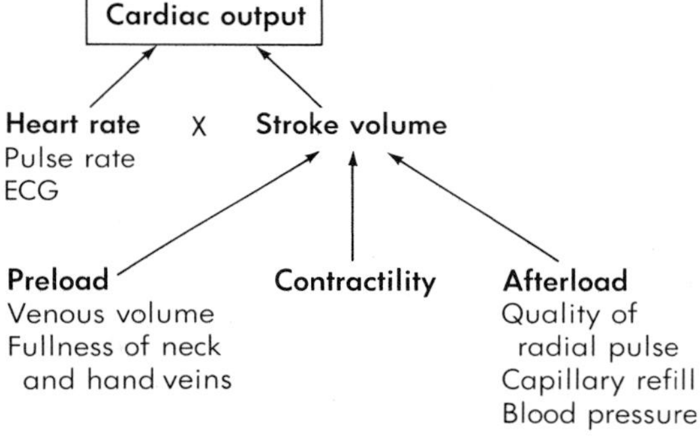

Fig. 20-7. Noninvasive assessment of cardiac output.

and kidney function. A capillary refill time in the distal extremities of 2 seconds or longer is considered a delayed response and an indication of vasoconstriction. A normal capillary refill time of less than 2 seconds is one indication of adequate cardiac output.[83]

The heart rate and quality of the pulse are easily obtained parameters in the air medical environment and provide vital information about the patient's ability to adequately perfuse vital organs. Alteration in heart rate is controlled by both the parasympathetic and sympathetic nervous systems. Changes in heart rate resulting from neural control directly affect cardiac output by altering ventricular filling time and, subsequently, stroke volume. Simply stated, if stroke volume decreases as a result of hypovolemia (decreased preload filling), decreased contractility, or an increased peripheral vascular resistance (afterload), cardiac output can be temporarily stabilized by increasing the heart rate. Indeed, tachycardia in early shock states is a compensatory mechanism to stabilize cardiac output. If appropriate resuscitation is initiated, heart rate slows, and the period of relaxation between heartbeats is longer, increasing ventricular filling time and stroke volume.[32] Heart rate is best interpreted relative to stroke volume, venous pressure, and peripheral resistance.

The quality of the pulse, or pulse contour, allows the flight nurse to estimate the stroke volume and the heart's capacity to pump blood to peripheral tissue.[83] A forceful, bounding pulse correlates with high stroke volume and reduced peripheral vascular resistance.[32] A consistently weak and thready radial pulse may indicate a low stroke volume or increased peripheral vascular resistance. Poor radial pulse contour may be an early sign of peripheral vasoconstriction. If it is associated with a slow pulse, poor pulse contour may also suggest that normal compensatory mechanisms are failing, as in profound shock.

Hypotension is best evaluated in terms of peripheral perfusion. Early signs of inadequate peripheral perfusion would be a decreased UO; cold, clammy skin; reduced capillary refill; and poor radial pulse contour. Measuring the blood pressure lets the flight nurse estimate the extent of hypotension. A low BP in the face of other signs of poor tissue perfusion is a late and threatening sign of impending circulatory collapse, requiring aggressive intervention.[83] Blood pressure can be obtained noninvasively in the air medical environment by the use of mechanical Doppler augmentation, automated BP devices, or palpation of the radial pulse with a sphygmomanometer and cuff. The cuff pressure measurements are usually adequate for a hemodynamically stable patient; however, for the unstable patient, the accuracy is questionable in the presence of hypertension, hypothermia, and shock.[46] A recent preliminary study demonstrated the difficulty of obtaining reliable BP in the air medical environment.[9] All of the instruments tested were susceptible to problems frequently encountered in the air medical environment, including noise levels, vibrations, sudden movement, and limited access to the patient. Although BP measuring devices can be useful to monitor trends in the patient's hemodynamic status, the results of this study and the experience of air medical practitioners emphasize the need to evaluate the patient's hemodynamic status by multiple methods rather than relying on one specific parameter such as BP.

Percutaneous Devices for Assessment of Oxygenation Status

The effects of altitude on the cardiovascular system are numerous. Adequate tissue oxygenation remains the highest priority in critically ill patients. The assessment of a patient's oxygenation and hemodynamic status can be augmented by various noninvasive transcutaneous devices that respond to physiological changes in oxygenation and perfusion. Many monitors are available to monitor pulse oximetry during transport.

Invasive Hemodynamic Monitoring

When transporting a patient who has been admitted to a coronary care unit, the goal of transport is to provide a high level of care equal to that in the intensive care unit. Often the patient has invasive intravascular catheters in place. Hemodynamic monitoring in a critically ill patient by means of intravascular catheters provides a reliable means of verifying diagnosis and obtaining continuous information to guide therapy and monitor clinical changes.[38] For example, intraarterial pressure is more accurate than noninvasive sphygmomanometry in patients who are obese, hypotensive, peripherally vasoconstricted, or severely hypertensive. Pulmonary artery wedge pressure may be a valuable aid in assessing patients who require specific interventions such as volume loading, afterload reducing, or inotropic agents, or for patients on IABC. These parameters can help the flight nurse guide therapy. However, caution should be used not to concentrate on one cardiodynamic variable without a full evaluation of all physiologic information available, such as heart rate, capillary refill, pulse contour, BP, and UO.

Before transport, interpretation of intravascular hemodynamic parameters and trends provide the flight nurse with valuable information regarding the cardiovascular status of the patient. To practice safely, flight nurses caring for patients who require invasive hemodynamic monitoring must have knowledge of normal hemodynamic values, understand the significance of changes in these values over time, and demonstrate competency when using hemodynamic equipment. Table 20-4 summarizes the definition, application, and normal values of some of the more commonly seen invasive monitoring devices. Fig. 20-8 gives an example of such a device.

Preparation for transport of patients with existing intravascular monitoring lines varies from program to program; however, attention to detail and careful handling of the intravascular line are essential to avoid potential complications. When preparing a patient with intravascular monitoring lines for transport, the flight nurse must label all lines clearly, secure all connections, place sterile caps over all exposed ports, and maintain a heparin flush system during transport. Little research has been done in the air medical environment to substantiate the accuracy of these invasive measures of hemodynamic status during air medical transport. This emphasizes the need for the flight nurse to use a combination of invasive and noninvasive assessment methods to evaluate a patient's status throughout the transfer process.

THE NURSING PROCESS AND AIR MEDICAL TRANSPORT OF THE CARDIOVASCULAR PATIENT

To efficiently organize the care and transport of critically ill patients, the flight nurse's performance must be consistent with a cognitive knowledge of the nursing process as it relates to the unique air medical environment.[65] The nursing process helps the flight nurse formulate goals and a plan of action for the complex patients under his or her care. The nursing process—assessment, planning, intervention, and evaluation—is here related to air medical transport.

Assessment

Assessment of the cardiovascular patient begins with the initial information elicited from the referring agency by dispatch personnel. This information can be invaluable when selecting appropriate equipment for the flight (especially when flying in an aircraft with limited space and weight restrictions), anticipating in-flight emergencies, and preparing the receiving agency for the patient. Time en route to the referring agency can be spent developing a preliminary database and plan of care based on initial information obtained from dispatch and the referring agency.

For the cardiovascular patient, assessment and preparation for transport are directed toward recognition, prevention, and correction of hypoxia, and maintenance of adequate tissue perfusion and cardiac output. The amount of time spent on assessment of the cardiovascular patient depends on the severity of the illness and the need for rapid intervention. The flight nurse should ascertain as much information in the most efficient way possible to provide safe and efficient transport to a definitive care institution.

A brief history of the event may be elicited from the patient, family members, or referring agency personnel. A general appraisal of the cardiovascular patient can be made while approaching the bedside, observing, at that time, skin color, diaphoresis, activity (AMI patients characteristically move about trying to find a comfortable position), and respiratory distress. The flight nurse can also note whether IV infusions have been initiated, whether they are running wide open, vasoactive drugs are infusing, oxygen is being delivered, and what rhythm is on the cardiac monitor. An initial perception of the situation helps to organize and direct management of the patient for efficient and safe transport.[41]

Physical examination is often abbreviated to the situation using skill and judgment to determine what is vital and appropriate to evaluate under the circumstances. Hands-on assessment of the cardiovascular patient includes confirmation of vital signs and the identification of implications for continued emer-

TABLE 20-4

Summary of frequently used hemodynamic parameters

Hemodynamic pressure	Definition and clinical application	Normal range
Mean arterial pressure (MAP)	Average perfusion pressure throughout the complete cardiac cycle, which is ⅓ systole and ⅔ diastole. Average pressure responsible for the arterial to venous pressure gradient, which is an important influence on tissue flow.	65-100 mm Hg
Central venous pressure (CVP)	Reflects filling pressure of the right ventricle when the tricuspid valve is open. Reflects venous return to the right atrium; thus conditions that reduce venous return result in a decreasee in CVP. Clinically used as a guide to overall fluid balance.	2-6 mm Hg 2.7-12 cm H_2O
Pulmonary artery pressure (PAP) systolic, diastolic, mean	Pulsatile pressure in the pulmonary artery. Pulmonary artery end-diastolic pressure (PAEDP) reflects filling pressure to the left ventricle.	PA Systolic = 20-30 mm Hg PA Diastolic = 5-10 mm Hg
Mixed venous oxygen saturation (SvO_2)	Fiberoptic catheter available on newer generation pulmonary artery catheters. Reflects overall tissue utilization of oxygen as a net result of cardiorespiratory function and tissue perfusion.	60%-80%
Pulmonary capillary wedge pressure (PCWP)	Reflection of the left ventricular filling presure when the mitral valve is open and the balloon-tipped distal end of the catheter is "wedged" into a small capillary arteriole. Clincally useful as a marker for fluid administration or restriction.	5-12 mm Hg
Cardiac output (CO)	Blood ejected from the heart into systemic circulation per minute. Clinically measured with a pulmonary artery catheter using the thermodilution cardiac output method. Decreased CO may be a result of decreased preload (massive vasodilation, diuresis, fluid shifts, arrhythmias), decreased contractility (MI, ischemia), increased afterload, or systemic vascular resistance.	Heart rate × Stroke volume 4-8 L/min

Continued

TABLE 20-4

Summary of frequently used hemodynamic parameters—cont'd

Hemodynamic pressure	Definition and clinical application	Normal range
Cardiac index (CI)	Cardiac output calculated to individual body size. Clinically more precise than cardiac output because it is individualized to height and weight.	2.4-4.0 L/min
Systemic vascular resistance (SVR)	Resistance to left ventricular ejection created by the systemic arteries and arterioles. Clinically, as SVR rises, cardiac output falls.	800-1200 dynes/sec/cm^{-5}
Pulmonary vascular resistance (PVR)	Resistance to right ventricular ejection created by the pulmonary arteries and arterioles. Clinically, as PVR rises, the output from the right ventricle falls.	40-100 dynes/sec/cm^{-5}
Left atrial pressure (LAP)	Reflects filling pressure in the left ventricle when the mitral valve is open. Clinically, the distal end of the LA line is inserted into the left atrial appendage after cardiac surgery. It is used to determine how efficiently the left ventricle is ejecting its volume (higher LAP, the lower ejection fraction from the left ventricle).	4-12 mm Hg

Adapted from Kinney M, Packa DR, Dunbar S: *AACN's clinical reference for critical care nursing,* ed 2, New York, 1988, McGraw-Hill; and Lough ME: Introduction to hemodynamic monitoring, *Nurs Clin North Am* 22(1)89-110, 1987.

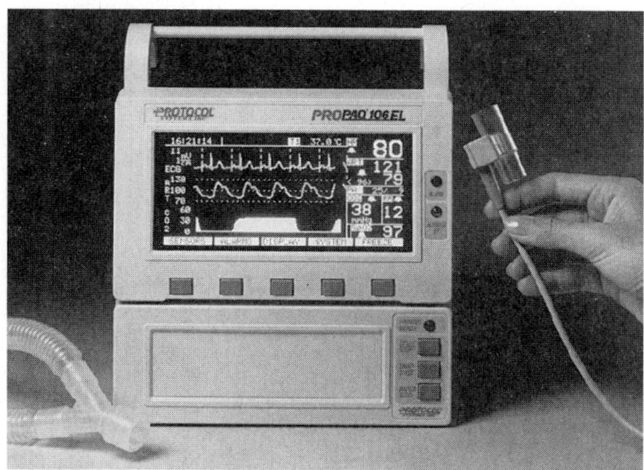

Fig. 20-8. The Protocol monitor serves as an example of a multiuse monitor. It not only monitors the patient's ECG, but can provide noninvasive blood pressure monitoring, pulse oximetry, and monitoring for invasive lines such as arterial and pulmonary lines. (Courtesy Protocol Systems, Inc, Beaverton, Ore.)

gency care. Initial evaluation of airway, breathing, and circulation is done in accordance with basic cardiac life support guidelines. If the cardiovascular patient is not in immediate need of cardiopulmonary resuscitation, the overall cardiovascular status should be evaluated.

Planning and Intervention

The National Flight Nurses Association (NFNA) practice standards state that "the flight nurse derives a valid plan prioritizing the patient's needs based on actual or potential threats."[65] Adequate management and preparation of the patient for air medical transport can greatly reduce the need for resuscitative measure in flight. Planning care for transport of the critical cardiovascular patient includes anticipating complications that may occur as a result of the disease process and preventing predictable emergencies; for example, ventricular ectopic activity is a universal phenomenon in AMI and the most preventable cause of death occurring during AMI.[60] The flight nurse transporting a patient with AMI anticipates this potential emergency and ensures that the patient has adequate IV access. He or she also has defibrillation equipment and a lidocaine bolus readily accessible in the event that a ventricular arrhythmia with subsequent hemodynamic compromise occurs.

Evaluation

Throughout the transport process, the flight nurse systematically evaluates the patient's progress, analyzes data, and modifies the plan of care based on the patient's response to therapy.[65] In the air medical environment, continual assessment and monitoring of the patient provide data regarding the success or failure of each intervention. The following case study illustrates the nursing process relative to the air medical transport of a patient with an evolving MI.

CARDIOVASCULAR EMERGENCIES CASE STUDY

History

An air medical transport team was called to handle a 50-year-old male accountant with no previous history of cardiac disease. He was transferred from a local community hospital to a major university health center by rotor wing transport for evaluation and treatment of inferior wall MI. Risk factors for CAD included smoking one pack of cigarettes a day and occupation-related stress.

The patient had severe precordial chest pain radiating to the left arm and associated with intense diaphoresis 2 hours before his admission to the community hospital emergency services. The initial 12-lead ECG was consistent with inferior wall MI. Chest pain was unrelieved with sublingual NTG, and IV morphine was administered to a total dose of 12 mg with moderate relief of pain. An NTG infusion was also initiated at 30 μg/min. He experienced a bigeminal rhythm, which was treated with a 75 mg lidocaine bolus and subsequent 2/mg/min IV infusion. The air medical transport team was requested by the emergency services physician. The flight nurses were notified of the patient's history, ECG findings, vital signs, weight, and current status before leaving the base agency for the 40-minute flight.

Air Medical Transport

En route to the community hospital, it was determined that the patient was to receive TPA, a drug that was unavailable at the community hospital where he had been admitted. The TPA infusion and loading bolus were of thrombolytic therapy. Immediately on arrival at the community hospital, the flight nurses elicited a history, assessed the patient, and then reviewed the diagnostic ECG. Physical examination revealed a pale, alert, oriented man. Blood pressure was 110/80 mm Hg, capillary refill was within 2 seconds, apical pulse was 72 with normal sinus rhythm, and radial pulse was strong and regular. There was no abnormal neck vein distention, and his lungs were clear on auscultation. The respiratory rate was 18 breaths per minute with 6 L/min oxygen delivered by nasal cannula. Results of cardiac examination were normal and without evidence of abnormal heart sounds, rubs, or murmurs. The 12-lead ECG demonstrated 7 to 8 mm ST segment elevation in CCAOs II, III, and aVF. These changes were significant for inferior MI. The patient denied risk factors associated with contraindications for thrombolytic therapy. An additional IV line was initiated for the thrombolytic drug. Samples for the baseline laboratory data had been drawn by the emergency department staff; however, results were unavailable. The patient was given a 15 mg bolus of TPA followed by an infusion of 50 mg TPA (0.75 mg/kg) over 30 minutes followed by 35 mg TPA (0.50 mg/kg) over 60 minutes. In addition, the patient was given a 5000 mg bolus of heparin followed by 1000 U/hr infusion. The patient was given 325 mg of aspirin by mouth. To prepare the patient for the flight, the self-adhesive monitor/defibrillator electrodes were placed on the chest for optimum ECG monitoring and rapid countershock if ventricular fibrillation occurred. The lidocaine, TPA, and NTG infusions were placed on portable infusion pumps. The third IV site was easily accessible in the event that further pharmacologic intervention or fluid therapy was necessary during the 40-minute flight. In addition, the flight team introduced themselves to the family, briefly described the transport process, and explained what they should expect when they arrived at the hospital.

During the flight, the patient initially experienced increased chest pain. The BP remained above 90 mm Hg, systolic, and the NTG infusion was increased to provide pain relief. At approximately 45 minutes after the initiation of TPA and 10 minutes into the flight, the patient became diaphoretic and complained of nausea. He also experienced a run of self-limiting ventricular tachycardia without evidence of hemodynamic compromise. A second lidocaine bolus was given, and the infusion was increased to 4 mg/min with no further arrhythmias. Fifteen minutes into the flight the patient stated that his pain had resolved. Blood pressure was 110 mm Hg systolic per Doppler; pulse rate 78 beats/min, strong and regular; cardiac rhythm was normal sinus on lead II. He was taken directly to the cardiac catheterization lab on arrival at the University Medical Center.

Outcome

Emergent catheterization 60 minutes after initiation of TPA revealed a TIMI grade 3 flow (normal flow) of the right coronary artery with a 90% proximal lesion. He underwent PTCA with the proximal lesion reduced in gradient from 60 mm to less than 5 mm. It was believed that reperfusion occurred during aeromedical transport at approximately 45 minutes after the initiation of the TPA infusion.

The patient experienced some periinfarct arrhythmias, including nonsustained ventricular tachycardia and premature beats. These arrhythmias responded to antiarrhythmic therapy. There were no significant bleeding problems; however, several hours after catheterization, bleeding from the right groin catheter site required manual pressure for 15 minutes. TCT was 75.9 and the routine heparin infusion was discontinued for several hours. CPK peaked at 600 (with positive MB fraction).

Summary and Discussion

This 50-year-old man experienced his first symptoms of CAD as inferior wall MI. He was admitted to the community hospital 2 hours after the onset of pain. En route to the referring institution, the flight nurses began to devise their strategy and plan of care for the patient based on preliminary data. On arrival, the essential history and physical were performed to verify the diagnosis and to plan interventions. Infusion of TPA was initiated without delay and within 3 hours of the onset of pain. The patient probably experienced reperfusion in flight, approximately 45 to 60 minutes after initiation of TPA therapy. Clinical reperfusion was evidenced by the simultaneous occurrence of a ventricular dysrhythmia, relief of chest pain, and normalization of ST segment elevation.[2] The flight team had prepared for these predictable emergencies and intervened with appropriate therapy to avoid further complications. The flight nurses also evaluated and documented the outcome of their interventions (pain relief and absence of further arrhythmias). The patient was safely and expeditiously transported to a university health center cardiac catheterization laboratory, where the admission ECG revealed resolution of ST segment elevation. The patient received emergent and successful PTCA with only minor postprocedure bleeding problems. After returning home, he gradually mobilized to the point of returning to his usual baseline level of activity.

REFERENCES

1. Alpert JS, Braunwald E: Acute myocardial infarction: pathological, pathophysiological, and clinical manifestations. In Braunwald E, editor: *Heart disease*, Philadelphia, 1984, Saunders.
2. American Heart Association: Standards and guidelines for cardiopulmonary resuscitation and emergency cardiac care, *JAMA* 255(21):2841-3044, 1986.
3. American Heart Association: *Textbook of advance cardiac life support*, Dallas, 1994, The Association.
4. Anderson H et al: Cardiopulmonary bypass, *Surgery* 114(2):161-173, 1993.
5. Anderson JL: Streptokinase and acylated streptokinase: biochemical properties and clinical effects. In Topol EJ, editor: *Acute coronary intervention*, New York, 1988, Alan R Liss.
6. Bartlett RH: *Extra corporeal life support manual*, Ann Arbor, Mich, 1991.
7. Bates ER, O'Neill WW, Topol EJ: Percutaneous atherectomy catheters, *Cardiol Clin* 6(3):373-382, 1988.
8. Becker CE, Benowitz NL: Hypertensive emergencies, *Med Clin North Am* 63(1):127-140, 1979.
9. Benson NH et al: Blood pressure measurement: comparison of multiple methods in an aeromedical environment, *Aeromed J* 3(5):90-94, 1988.
10. Berron K: Role of the ventricular assist device in acute myocardial infarction, *Crit Care Nur Q* 12(2):25-37, 1989.
11. Braunwald E: The aggressive treatment of acute myocardial infarction, *Circulation* 71:1087-1092, 1985.
12. Braunwald E: *Heart disease: a textbook of cardiovascular medicine*, Philadelphia, 1984, Saunders.
13. Budassi-Sheehy S, Barber J: *Emergency nursing*, ed 2, St Louis, 1985, Mosby.
14. Bulkey BH: Pathology of coronary atherosclerotic heart disease. In Hurst JW, editor: *The heart*, ed 3, New York, 1986, McGraw-Hill.
15. Burney RE et al: Reperfusion arrhythmias during air transfer (abstract A-45), *Aeromed J* 3(5):41, 1988.
16. Coates AJ: ACE inhibitors after myocardial infarction: selection and treatment for all, *Brit Heart J* 73:395-396, 1995.
17. Cohn JN: Current therapy of the failing heart, *Circulation* 78(5):1099-1107, 1988.
18. Cooke JNC: Cardiac care. In Ernsting J, King P, editors: *Aviation medicine*, London, 1988, Butterworths.
19. Creswell LL et al: Revascularization after acute myocardial infarction. *Ann Thorac Surg* 60:19-26, 1995.
20. DeBakey ME et al: *Surgery* 92(6),1118-1132, 1982.
21. Dedrick D et al: Defibrillation safety in emergency helicopter transport, *Ann Emerg Med* 18(1):69-71, 1989.
22. Dehart RN: *Fundamentals of aerospace medicine*, Philadelphia, 1985, Lea & Febiger.
23. DeSanctis RW et al: Aortic dissection, *N Engl J Med* 317(17):1060-1066, 1987.
24. de Zwaan C et al: Effects of thrombolytic therapy in unstable agina: clinical and angiographic results, *J Am Coll Cardiol* 12(2):301-309, 1988.
25. Doyle J, Johantgen M, Vitello-Cicciu: Vascular disease. In Kinney MR, Packa DR, Dunbar SB, editors: *AACN's clinical reference for critical care nursing*, ed 2, New York, 1988, McGraw-Hill.
26. Dunn DL, Gregory JJ: Noninvasive temporary pacing: experience in a community hospital, *Heart Lung* 18(1): 23-28, 1989.
27. Eagle K et al: Aortic dissection. In Eagle K et al, editors: *The practice of cardiology*, ed 2, Boston, 1989, Little, Brown.
28. Ernsting J, King P, editors: *Aviation medicine*, London, 1988, Butterworths.
29. Ernsting J, Sharp GR: Air medical transport of the cardiac patient. In Ernsting J, King P, editors: *Aviation medicine*, London, 1988, Butterworths.
30. Feldman AJ: Thoracic and abdominal aortic aneurysms. In Tintinalli JE, Krome RL, Ruiz E, editors: *Emergency medicine: a comprehensive study*, New York, 1988, McGraw-Hill.
31. Ferguson JJ: Recent advances in the treatment of acute myocardial infarction, *Tex Heart Inst J* 22(1):5-9, 1995.

32. Ford PJ: Cardiovascular pathophysiology. In Price SA, Wilson LM, editors: *Pathophysiology: clinical concepts of disease processes,* ed 2, New York, 1982, McGraw-Hill.
33. Fowles RE: Myocardial infarction in the 90s, *Postgrad Med,* 97(6), 1995.
34. Goldschlager N: Acute pericarditis. In Luce JM, Pierson DJ, editors: *Critical care medicine,* Philadelphia, 1988, Saunders.
35. Goldschlager N: Aortic dissections. In Luce JM, Pierson DJ, editors: *Critical care medicine,* Philadelphia, 1988, Saunders.
36. Goldschlager N: Congestive heart failure. In Luce JM, Pierson DJ, editors: *Critical care medicine,* Philadelphia, 1988, Saunders.
37. Goldschlager N: Dysrhythmias. In Luce JM, Pierson DJ, editors: *Critical care medicine,* Philadelphia, 1988, Saunders.
38. Goldschlager N: Hemodynamic monitoring. In Luce JM, Pierson DJ, editors: *Critical care medicine,* Philadelphia, 1988, Saunders.
39. Goldschlager N: Hypertensive crisis. In Luce JM, Pierson DJ, editors: *Critical care medicine,* Philadelphia, 1988, Saunders.
40. Goldschlager N: Valvular disruption. In Luce JM, Pierson DJ, editors: *Critical care medicine,* Philadelphia, 1988, Saunders.
41. Gordon G, Silverstein S: Ischemic heart disease. In Rosen P et al, editors: *Emergency medicine: concepts and practice,* ed 2, St Louis, 1988, Mosby.
42. Guzy PM: Emergency cardiac pacing, *Emerg Med Clin North Am* 4(4):745-759, 1986.
43. Harwood-Nuss A, Luten RC: *Handbook of emergency medicine,* Philadelphia, 1995, Lippincott.
44. Jackson RE: Basic cardiopulmonary resuscitation. In Tintinalli J, Krome RL, Ruiz E, editors: *Emergency medicine: a comprehensive study guide (ACEP),* New York, 1988, McGraw-Hill.
45. Jackson RE: Hypertensive emergencies. In Tintinalli J, Krome RL, Ruiz E, editors: *Emergency medicine: a comprehensive study guide (ACEP),* New York, 1988, McGraw-Hill.
46. Jacobsen WK: Monitoring the critically ill surgery patient. In Ihde JK, Jacobsen WK, Briggs BA, editors: *Principles of critical care,* Philadelphia, 1987, Saunders.
47. Jones EL: Surgical revascularization during acute evolving myocardial infarction, *Circulation* 76(suppl 3):146-48, 1987.
48. Kaplan L, Walsh D, Burney RE: Emergency aeromedical transport of patients with acute myocardial infarction, *Ann Emerg Med* 16(1):55-57, 1987.
49. Keen J, Baird M, Allen J: *Critical care and emergency drug reference,* St Louis, 1994, Mosby.
50. Kinney M, Packa DR, Dunbar S: *AACN's clinical reference for critical care nursing,* ed 2, New York, 1988, McGraw-Hill.
51. Kochs M, Eggeling T, Homback V: Pharmacological therapy in coronary heart disease: prevention of life-threatening ventricular tachyarrhythmias and sudden cardiac death, *Eur Heart J* 14:107-119, 1993.
52. Kuhn LA: Acute and chronic cardiac tamponade, *Cardiovas Clin* 7:177-195, 1976.
53. Lamb J, Carlson V: *Handbook of cardiovascular nursing,* Philadelphia, 1986, Lippincott.
54. Lindsay HSJ, Zaman AG, Cowan JC: ACE inhibitors after myocardial infarction: patient selection or treatment for all? *Br Heart J* 73:397-400, 1995.
55. Lorell BH, Braunwald E: Pericardial disease. In Braunwald E, editor: *Heart disease,* ed 2, Philadelphia, 1984, Saunders.
56. Lough ME: Introduction to hemodynamic monitoring, *Nurs Clin North Am* 22(1):89-110, 1987.
57. Lynn-McHale DL: Interventions for acute myocardial infarction: PTCA and CABGS, *Crit Care Nurs Q* 12(2):38-48, 1989.
58. Manley N: Intra-aortic balloon pump, temperature and altitude effects during helicopter transport (abstract), *Aeromed J* 3(5):44, 1988.
59. Mathews J: Hypertension. In Rosen P et al, editors: *Emergency medicine: concepts and clinical practice,* ed 2, St Louis, 1988, Mosby.
60. Mayberry-Toth B, Landron S: Complications associated with acute myocardial infarction, *Crit Care Nurs Q* 12(2): 49-63, 1989.
61. Mertlich G, Quall SJ: Air transport of the patient requiring intra-aortic balloon pumping, *Crit Care Nurs Clin North Am* 1(3):443, 1989.
62. Miller C: Medications in angina, *Focus Crit Care* 15(4): 23-29, 1988.
63. Misinski M: Pathophysiology of acute myocadial infarction: a rationale for thrombolytic therapy, *Heart Lung* 17(6):743-750, 1988.
64. Mulford E: Nursing perspectives for the patient receiving postoperative ventricular assistance in the critical care unit, *Heart Lung* 16(3):246-255, 1987.
65. National Flight Nurses Association: *Practice standards for flight nursing,* St Louis, 1994, Mosby.
66. Niemann JT: The cardiomyopathies, myocarditis and pericardial disease. In Tintinalli JE, Krome RL, Ruiz E, editors: *Emergency medicine: a comprehensive study guide,* ed 2, New York, 1988, McGraw-Hill.

67. Niemyski P, Hellstedt L: Patient selection and management in thrombolytic therapy: nursing implications, *Crit Care Nurs Q* 12(2):8-24, 1989.
68. O'Donnell M et al: Autothrombotic therapy for acute MI, *J Am Coll Cardiol* 25:23S-9S, 1995.
69. Pandian N et al: Pericardial diseases. In Eagle K et al, editors: *The practice of cardiology,* Boston, 1989, Little, Brown.
70. Perchalski DL, Pepine CJ: Patient with coronary artery spasm and role of the critical care nurse, *Heart Lung* 16(4):392-402, 1987.
71. Pranicoff et al: Transport of unstable respiratory failure patients on extracorporeal life support. *Air Med J* 13(10): 431, 1994 (abstract).
72. Quaal S: Mechanical treatment of the failing heart. In Kern L, editor: *Cardiac critical care nursing,* Rockville, MD, 1988, Aspen.
73. Reimer KA, Jennings RB: The "wavefront phenomenon" of ischemic cell death in myocardial infarction size versus duration of coronary occlusion in dogs, *Circulation* 56: 768-794, 1977.
74. Ross R: The pathogenesis of atherosclerosis, *N Engl J Med* 314:488-500, 1986.
75. Ruzevich SA, Swartz MT, Pennington DG: Nursing care of the patient with a pneumatic ventricular assist device, *Heart Lung* 17(4):399-405, 1988.
76. Sheehy SB, Barber J: *Emergency nursing: principles and practice,* St Louis, 1985, Mosby.
77. Sheps DS, Heiss G: Sudden death and silent myocardial ischemia, *Am Heart J* 117(1):177-184, 1989.
78. Sherman CT et al: Coronary angioscopy in patients with unstable angina pectoris, *N Engl J Med* 315:913-919, 1986.
79. Slater EE, DeSanctis RW: Diseases of the aorta. In Braunwald E, editor: *Heart disease,* ed 2, Philadelphia, 1985, Saunders.
80. Sobel BE, Braunwald E: The management of acute myocardial infarction. In Braunwald E, editor: *Heart disease,* Philadelphia, 1984, Saunders.
81. Stine R, Chudnofsky C: *A practical approach to emergency medicine,* ed 2, Boston, 1994, Little, Brown.
82. Stults KR et al: Self-adhesive monitor/defibrillation success, *Ann Emerg Med* 16(8):872-877, 1987.
83. Thomas F, Clemmer TP: Hemodynamic assessment in aeromedical evacuation, Orem, Utah, 1984, H Collett.
84. Topol EJ: Thrombolytic intervention. In Topol EJ, editor: *Textbook of interventional cardiology,* Philadelphia, 1994, Saunders.
85. Topol E et al: Safety of helicopter transport and hospital intravenous fibrinolytic therapy in patients with evolving myocardial infarction, *Catheteriz Cardiovasc Diagnos* 12:151-155, 1986.
86. Vitello-Cecciu J: Anatomy and physiology of the cardiovascular system. In Kinney MR, Packa DR, Dunbar SB, editors: *AACN's clinical reference for critical care nursing,* ed 2, New York, 1988, McGraw-Hill.
87. Vitello-Cecciu J, Stewart SL, Griffin EL: Coronary artery disease. In Kinney MR, Packa DR, Dunbar SB, editors: *AACN's clinical reference for critical care nursing,* ed 2, New York, 1988, McGraw-Hill.
88. Wayne J, Braunwald E: The cardiomyopathies and myocarditides. In Braunwald E, editor: *Heart disease: a textbook of cardiovascular medicine,* Philadelphia, 1984, Saunders.
89. Wedige-Stecher T: In flight cardiac support-aeromedical transport of IABP and LVAD patients, *Hosp Aviation* 3(6): 16-19, 1988.

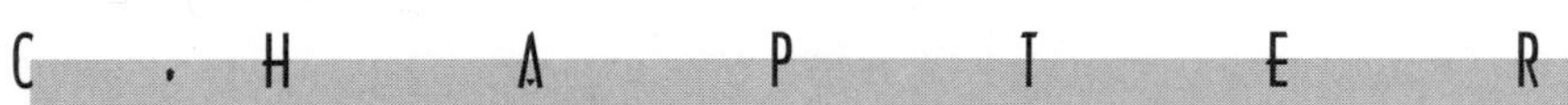

C H A P T E R 21

Pulmonary Emergencies

COMPETENCIES

1. Perform a thorough pretransport pulmonary physical examination.
2. Demonstrate the use of the following:
   - Oxygen therapy
   - Resuscitator bag
   - SpO_2 monitor
   - $ETCO_2$ monitor
   - $ETCO_2$ detector
3. Use targeted assessment skills and care/interventions before, during, and after transport for patients with the following conditions:
   - Acute respiratory failure
   - Adult respiratory distress syndrome
   - Chronic obstructive pulmonary disease
   - Spontaneous pneumothorax
   - Pulmonary emboli
   - Pneumonia
   - Carbon monoxide poisoning

The air transport of patients with medical disorders of the pulmonary system is of significant concern to flight nurses. Oxygenation in many patients with pulmonary system disease is already compromised, and altitude may have deleterious effects on patients with pulmonary conditions.[1] For the healthy person, alveolar oxygen tension (PaO_2) decreases to 65 mm Hg at 8000 feet with a decrease in arterial oxygen tension (PaO_2) to approximately 60 mm Hg.[2] Patients who have significant pulmonary disease may have signs of hypoxemia at altitudes well below 8000 feet. Severe tissue hypoxia can occur with minimal obvious clinical signs. Thorough physical assessment and the use of pulse oximetry may help the flight and transport nurse identify and intervene in impaired oxygenation.

Richards studied the effects of commercial air travel on people with cardiovascular disease and respiratory disease.[17] Of 71 passengers with chronic bronchitis and emphysema, 40.9% experienced dyspnea during flight. There were also three cases of heart failure after the flight, and four people experienced cyanotic episodes during flight. Of 42 patients with asthma, 11 experienced dyspnea in flight. A total of 23 people with postacute pulmonary infections were evaluated; 7 had adverse in-flight effects. None of the passengers was acutely ill, yet most experienced adverse effects from the flights.[3] Patients with acute illness or injury are commonly transported by flight nurses; the impact of pulmonary disease should be expected.

ANATOMY AND PHYSIOLOGY OVERVIEW

Anatomy

Airway

The upper airway consists of the nose, mouth, and pharynx. The pharynx extends from the nose to the larynx. The upper airway serves as a conducting system that warms, filters, and humidifies inspired air before it reaches the lungs. The pharynx branches into the larynx and the esophagus. The larynx contains the vocal apparatus, which includes the vocal cords, cartilage, and musculature. External landmarks of this area are the thyroid and cricoid cartilage, which can be palpated in the neck. The cricoid area is often the site for emergency surgical airway access. The epiglottis is a leaf-shaped, flexible cartilage that covers the larynx during swallowing. Its primary function is to prevent food and liquids from entering the trachea and lungs. The lower airway consists of the trachea, the right and left mainstem bronchi, bronchioles, terminal bronchioles, respiratory bronchioles, alveolar ducts, and alveolar sacs.[4]

The trachea originates at the distal margin of the cricoid cartilage at the level of the sixth cervical vertebra. It continues distally to the bifurcation, the carina, which is at the level of the fifth thoracic vertebra. In adults, the length of the trachea is approximately 11 cm with an internal diameter of 12 mm. The trachea accounts for approximately 20% of anatomic dead space (~30 ml).[4]

The mucosal surface of the trachea is made up of columnar epithelium and mucus-secreting cells. The carina branches into the left and right mainstem bronchi. The right mainstem bronchus is straighter and more in line with the trachea than the left mainstem. This may result in the catheter passing into the right mainstem rather than the left during intubation or suctioning.

The right and left mainstem bronchi branch into bronchioles. The bronchioles have some cartilage, but consist of less and less as the bronchioles progress distally. Further division gives rise to respiratory bronchioles that are the transitional zones between the bronchioles and the alveolar ducts. This is the transition between conducting airway and gas exchange areas. Alveolar sacs arise from the alveolar duct.[4]

The alveolar sac and pulmonary capillary are in close contact to facilitate gas exchange. The thin alveolar walls are made up of two types of epithelial cells, type I and type II. Type I cells are most abundant and are thin, flat squamous cells across which gas exchange occurs. Type II cells secrete surfactant, a lipoprotein that coats the alveoli. Surfactant facilitates gas exchange by lowering surface tension of the fluids lining the internal surface of the alveoli. This prevents alveolar collapse during expiration.[4]

Thoracic Cage

The boundaries of the thoracic cavity are the sternum, ribs, and costal cartilage anteriorly, and the ribs and thoracic vertebrae posteriorly. The superior and inferior boundaries are established by the clavicles and diaphragm. There are two layers of pleura lining the thorax. The visceral pleura covers the outer surface of each lung. The parietal pleura lines the inner surface of the thoracic cavity. Between the two layers of pleural tissue is the pleural space, a potential space containing a small amount of serous fluid. The fluid lubricates the two surfaces to facilitate ease of movement. It also creates a cohesive force that assists in maintaining the negative pressure that allows the lungs to remain inflated. Many organs are found within the thorax, including the heart, great vessels, trachea, esophagus, thymus gland, lymphatics, and nerves.

Muscles of Ventilation

Ventilation has two phases: inspiration and expiration. Inspiration is an active process. Contraction of the diaphragm and the external intercostal muscles increases the anterior posterior diameter of the thorax by raising the ribs and lowering the diaphragm. As chest cavity size increases, a negative pressure gradient is created and air is inspired. The muscles then relax and cause passive expiration.

The accessory muscles used in respiratory distress include the scalene and sternocleidomastoid muscles, which assist with inhalation. The abdominal wall muscles and the internal intercostal muscles are used during active exhalation.

Volumes and Capacities

To assess the events of pulmonary ventilation the air in the lungs has been divided into four different volumes and four different capacities.[4] Volumes are distinct measurements (Table 21-1). Total lung capacity (TLC) is the sum of the volumes. Capacities are combination of volumes (Table 21-2). Pulmonary volumes and capacities (Fig. 21-1) are approximately 20% to 25% less in women than in men.[4]

Physiology

Effective ventilation depends on an intact thoracic cage, patent airway, integrity of the alveolar-capillary membrane, normal compliance, normal airway resistance, and adequate nutrition.

Alveolar-Capillary Membrane

Gas exchange occurs in the alveolar-capillary membrane. Several structures are involved in this exchange (see box). Any change in these components alters gas movement across the respiratory capillary membrane.

TABLE 21-1

Lung volumes

Lung Volumes	Amount	Definition
Tidal volume	500 ml	Volume of air inspired or expired with a normal breath
Inspiratory reserve volume	3000 ml	Extra air that can be inspired in excess of normal tidal volume
Expiratory reserve volume	1100 ml	Amount of air that can be expired by forceful expiration after normal tidal volume
Residual volume	1200 ml in a 70 kg patient	Volume of air remaining at end of maximum expiration

STRUCTURES INVOLVED IN GAS EXCHANGE

Surfactant	Capillary membrane
Alveolar membrane	Plasma
Interstitial space	Red blood cells

The concepts integral to understanding gas exchange include diffusion, ventilation ($\dot{V}$), perfusion ($\dot{Q}$), ventilation-perfusion ($\dot{V}/\dot{Q}$) ratio, dead space, and shunts. Diffusion is the movement of gas from an area of higher pressure to an area of lower pressure, simply stated, from a greater concentration to a lesser concentration. Oxygen and carbon dioxide (CO_2) diffuse across the respiratory membrane.

Ventilation-Perfusion

Alveolar ventilation is the total volume of new air entering the alveoli each minute. In the normal adult man, alveolar ventilation is approximately 4 L/min.[4]

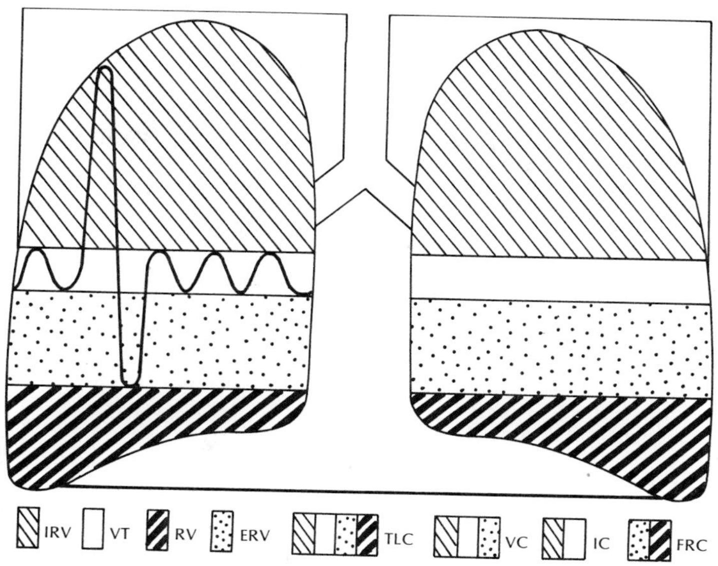

Fig. 21-1. Normal lung volumes and capacities. *IRV,* Inspiratory reserve volume; V_T, tidal volume; *RV,* residual volume; *ERV,* expiratory reserve volume; *TLC,* total lung capacity; *VC,* vital capacity; *IC,* inspiratory capacity; *FRC,* functional residual capacity. (From Des Jardins T and Burton CG: *Clinical manifestations and assessment of respiratory disease,* ed 3, St Louis, 1995, Mosby.)

TABLE 21-2

Capacities

Capacities	Amount	Definition
Inspiratory capacity	3500 ml (~50 ml/kg)	Tidal volume plus inspiratory reserve volume—the amount of air that can be breathed beginning at the normal expiratory level and distending lungs to maximum capacity
Functional residual capacity	2300 ml	Expiratory reserve volume plus residual volume—the amount of air remaining in the lungs at the end of normal exhalation
Vital capacity	4600 ml	Inspiratory reserve volume plus tidal volume—the maximum amount of air that can be expelled from the lungs after filling to the maximum and expiring maximally
Total lung capacity	5800 ml	Maximum volume lung expansion with greatest inspiratory effort

Perfusion is the amount of blood flow to the respiratory capillaries. Normally the amount of blood perfusing the alveoli is 5 L/min (i.e., cardiac output). In a perfect physiologic state, the ventilation of every alveolus is matched by an equivalent of perfusion, resulting in an equal $\dot{V}/\dot{Q}$ ratio.

Various physiologic conditions alter the ventilation and perfusion relationship. When ventilation is less than perfusion, as occurs in atelectasis, more unoxygenated blood enters the systemic circulation. Conditions that result in blood entering the system circulation without passing through a ventilated area of the lung are defined as shunt units.[6] Anatomic shunting is the effect of blood that has not been oxygenated by the lungs traveling from the right to the left side of the heart, as with bronchial circulation.[6] Anatomic shunting normally occurs to less than 5% of cardiac output. Inspiration of 100% oxygen does not correct the shunt unit because all blood does not come in contact with functional alveoli. Shunting is the single cause of hypoxemia that cannot be rectified by delivery of 100% oxygen.[6]

When ventilation is greater than perfusion, a ventilation-perfusion mismatch occurs. A disease state illustrating this situation is a pulmonary embolus. This physiologic occurrence is defined as a dead space unit.[6] Dead space is the inspired volume of air that does not come in contact with pulmonary capillary blood. Anatomic dead space is made up of the conducting airways and is normally 2 ml/kg of ideal body weight.[4]

In the setting of poorly ventilated arterioles, constriction occurs, thereby diverting the blood to better ventilated areas. Similarly, poorly perfused alveoli collapse, resulting in the diversion of airflow to more effectively perfused areas. This is termed a silent unit and helps to compensate for imbalanced $\dot{V}/\dot{Q}$ ratios (Fig. 21-2).

Transportation of Gases

Oxygen is transported in the blood as either bound to hemoglobin (97%) or dissolved in the plasma. The oxygen pressure (PO_2) reported on arterial blood gas analysis is a measure of dissolved oxygen only.

Oxygen-Hemoglobin Dissociation Curve

The oxygen-hemoglobin dissociation curve illustrates the relationship between hemoglobin saturation and PaO_2. This curve depicts the ability of hemoglobin to bind and to release oxygen into the tissues. The relationship between oxygen content and the pressure of oxygen in the blood is not linear (Fig. 21-3).

Various physiologic states change the relationship between hemoglobin saturation and PaO_2 (i.e., the oxygen-hemoglobin dissociation curve shifts in position.)[7]

A shift to the left indicates an increase in the affinity of oxygen and hemoglobin. Physiologically oxygen does not dissociate from the hemoglobin until tissue oxygen levels are very low because there must be a gradient. Situations that result in a left shift include alkalosis, hypocapnia, hypothermia, and decreased levels of 2,3-diphosphoglycerate (2,3-DPG). 2,3-DPG is an intermediate metabolite of glucose that assists in the dissociation of oxygen from hemoglobin at the tissue level. Levels of 2,3-DPG may be lower in patients who have received massive transfusions. This is related in part to the fact that stored blood is depleted of 2,3-DPG.[7]

The oxygen-hemoglobin curve shifts to the right in conditions that cause oxygen to dissociate more rapidly. In such cases, hemoglobin has a lessened affinity for oxygen, resulting in increased oxygen delivery at a cellular level. Physiologic conditions that result in a right shift include acidosis, hypercapnia, and hyperthermia (Fig. 21-3).

The understanding of this relationship is significant to the flight nurse to allow for the optimum intervention for patients. The amount of oxygen transported per minute is a product of oxygen content and cardiac output. This represents the quality of oxygen transported to the tissues per minute and is contingent on the interaction of the respiratory system, the circulatory system, and the erythropoietic system.[8] These relationships are defined in formula in the box on p. 423.

Oxygen Consumption

The arterial-mixed venous difference in oxygen content is the difference between the arterial oxygen content and the mixed venous oxygen content. This difference indicates the actual sum of oxygen removed from the blood during circulation through the tissue. Normal oxygen transport is 1000 to 1200 ml/min. In normal physiologic conditions, the tissues use 250 to 300 ml. Therefore normal oxygen consumption is 250 to 300 ml. Mixed venous oxygen content values are determined from blood samples from pulmonary artery catheters.[8]

Carbon Dioxide

Carbon dioxide is transported in the blood by three mechanisms. CO_2 is dissolved in the plasma.

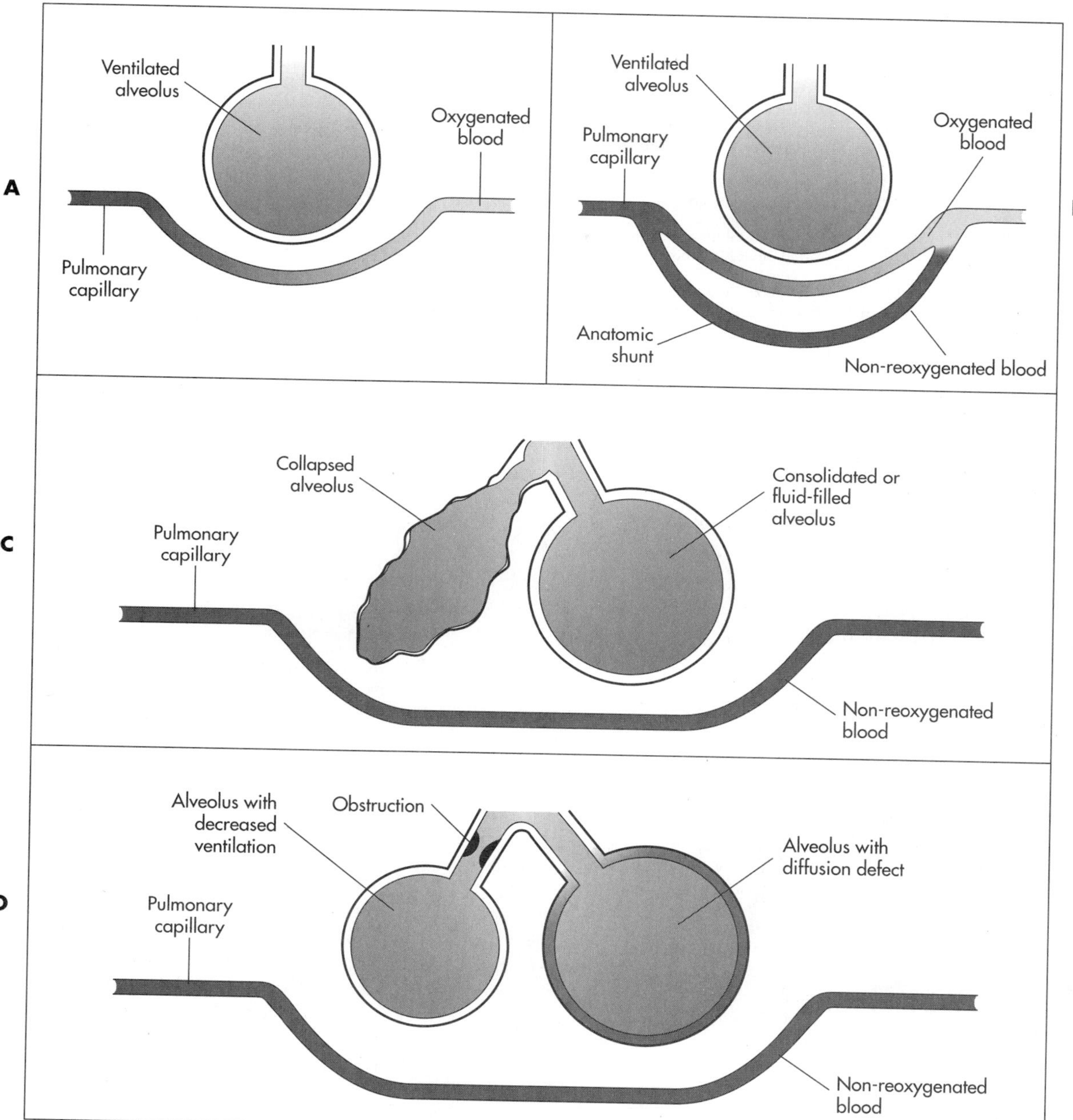

Fig. 21-2. Pulmonary shunting. **A,** Normal alveolar-capillary unit. **B,** Anatomic shunt. **C,** Types of capillary shunts. **D,** Types of shuntlike effects. (Modified From Des Jardins T: *Cardiopulmonary anatomy and physiology: essentials for respiratory care,* ed 2, Albany, NY, 1993, Delmar Publishers.)

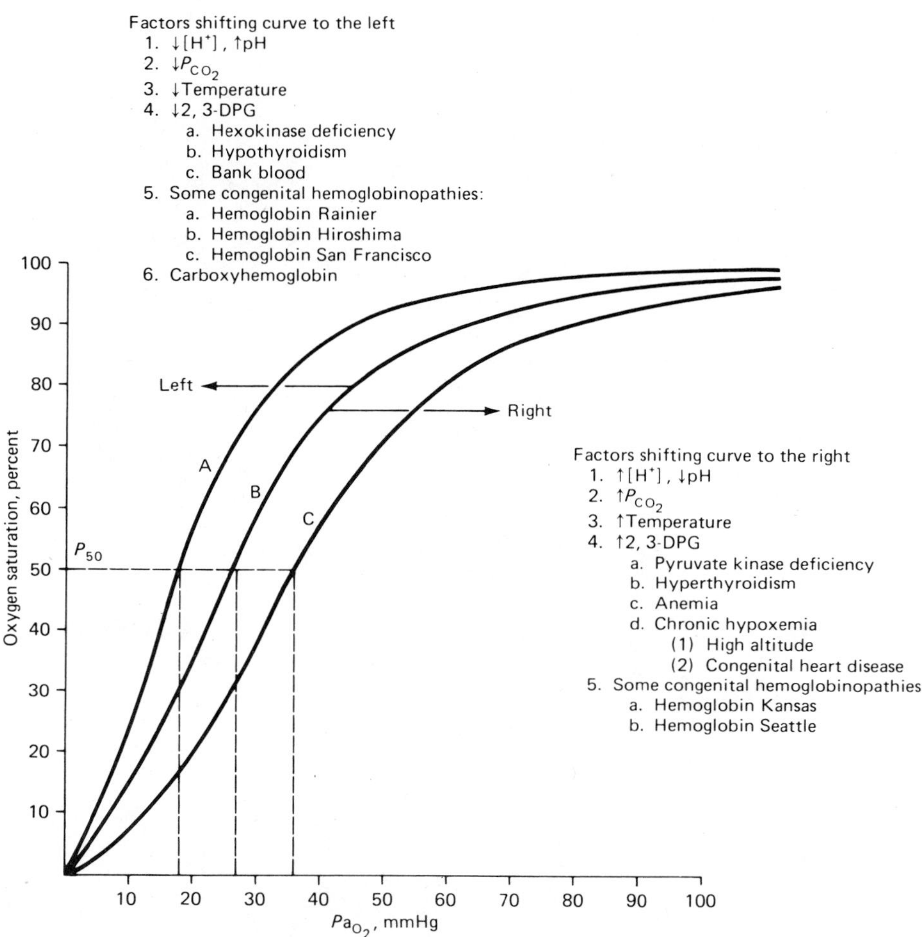

Fig. 21-3. Curve B is the standard oxyhemoglobin dissociation curve. Curve A shows the curve shifted to the left because of hemoglobin's increased affinity for oxygen. Curve C shows the curve shifted to the right because of hemoglobin's decreased affinity for oxygen. Factors responsible for shifting the curve are listed adjacent to curves A and C. (From Kinney MR et al: *AACN's clinical reference for critical care nursing,* St Louis, 1988, Mosby).

This represents 10% of the CO_2 transported in the blood. Carbon dioxide also is moved by a chemical association with hemoglobin, carbaminohemoglobin. This mechanism affects 30% of the CO_2 transported. It is a rapid system and can bind more CO_2 than oxyhemoglobin. The final and most significant mechanism is a conversion reaction as bicarbonate. This represents 70% of the CO_2 in the body. The bicarbonate reaction is slow in the plasma and rapid in the red blood cell.[8]

OXYGEN CONTENT COMPONENTS

Oxygen content = (Oxygen capacity × oxygen saturation) + (0.0031 × PaO_2)		
Oxygen capacity = Maximum amount O_2 blood can carry	Stated as milliliters of O_2 per 100 ml of blood (vol%)	Multiply hemoglobin by 1.34
Oxygen saturation = % of hemoglobin saturated with oxygen	Stated as percent	SpO_2 or SvO_2
Systemic oxygen transport (ml/min) = Arterial oxygen content (ml/100 ml) × cardiac output × 10 (conversion factor) = 1000 to 1200 ml/min		

RESPIRATORY SYSTEM SUPPORT

Oxygen Therapy

Many critically ill and injured patients require oxygen therapy to augment the delivery of adequate tissue oxygenation. The most frequently used initial therapy for hypoxia is oxygen therapy.

Oxygen delivery systems are classified in two categories: high-flow systems and low-flow systems. Low-flow systems include a nasal cannula and simple oxygen face masks. These low-flow systems allow the patient to draw a supplemental amount of oxygen from the apparatus while the majority of the inspired tidal volume comes from the room air within or around the apparatus. Therefore the amount of oxygen that is inspired varies depending on the patient. The flow of oxygen from a cannula or simple mask is constant. The concentration of inspired oxygen is variable and depends on the patient's minute ventilation[9] (Table 21-3). For example, a cardiac patient with a high minute ventilation inspires less oxygen than a patient with a lower minute ventilation because the patient with high minute ventilation uses a greater amount of room air per minute.[10]

High-flow oxygen systems include Venturi masks and non-rebreather masks. These devices result in the patient inspiring the total present fraction of inspired oxygen (FiO_2). Venturi masks operate by drawing oxygen through a narrow conduit that increases gas velocity and results in more room air being pulled into the mask. This high flow makes the concentration of inspired oxygen less dependent on the patient's ventilatory pattern. Venturi masks can render precise low concentrations of oxygen between 24% and 50%[9] (Fig. 21-4).

Non-rebreather masks have a reservoir bag that fills with 100% oxygen. These masks also use a one-way valve that allows inspiration from the reservoir and precludes inspiration of room air. The rebreather ensures that patients inhale basically 100% oxygen regardless of inspiratory effort[10] (Fig. 21-5).

TABLE 21-3

Low-flow oxygen systems

Apparatus	Oxygen flow rate	FIO_2
Nasal cannula	1-6 L/min	24%-45%
Simple face mask	4-6 L/min	35%-45%

Ventilatory Support

Many patients cared for by flight nurses require some type of ventilatory support. Patients usually have endotracheal tubes in place and require assistance with a manually powered, self-inflating positive-pressure resuscitator bag system. These bag-valve-mask systems afford the ability to deliver high FiO_2s and effective ventilation when used by experienced practitioners. The percentage of oxygen delivered by simple bags is limited to 40% to 60% because the bag inflation surpasses the oxygen flow rate, resulting

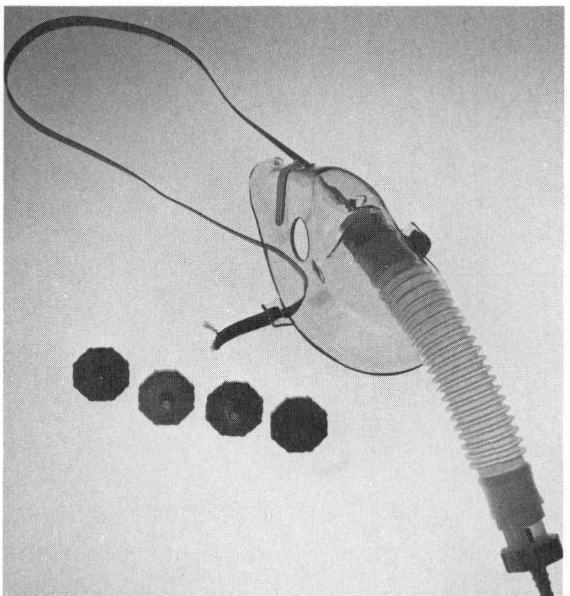

Fig. 21-4. Venturi mask and oxygen regulators. (Courtesy Richard Lazar, Stanford, Calif.)

in the entrainment of room air. Resuscitator bags with reservoirs are capable of delivering FiO_2s ≥90% provided that the oxygen flow rate exceeds minute ventilation.[11]

The effectiveness of ventilation with a manually powered, self-inflating resuscitator bag depends on the proficiency of the clinician. The flight nurse must constantly evaluate the compliance, resistance, chest rise, and other monitored parameters to appropriate tidal volume delivery. Spontaneous tidal volumes are approximately 500 ml; however, positive-pressure ventilation affects the distribution of gases in the bronchial tree. Therefore larger tidal volumes are necessary to maintain adequate alveolar ventilation. Typically 10 to 15 ml/kg is used adjusted according to peak inspiratory pressure,[4] with anatomic dead space of the conducting airways equaling 2 ml/kg of ideal body weight. For a 70 kg patient, these values calculate to 640 ml required to deliver one normal tidal volume. Most manually powered, self-inflating resuscitator bags inflate to 1000 ml; therefore 64% of the bag must be compressed to deliver an effective tidal volume.

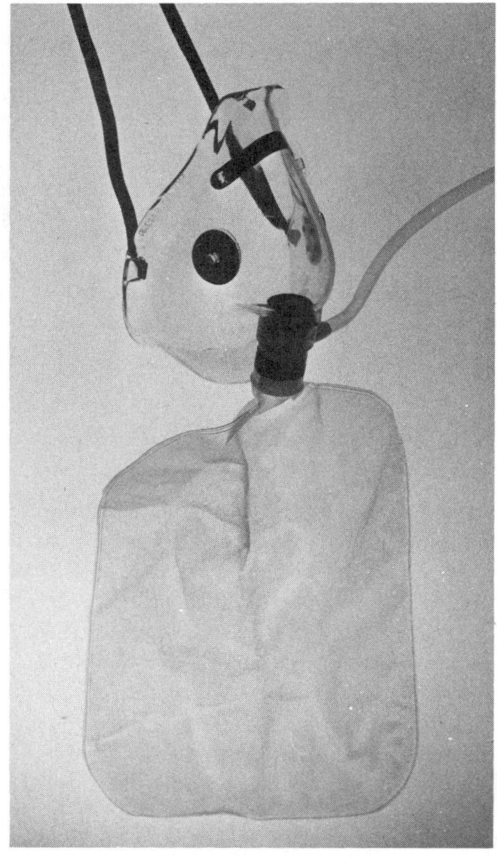

Fig. 21-5. Oxygen reservoir mask. (Courtesy Richard Lazar, Stanford, Calif.)

Numerous mechanical ventilators are available for in-flight use. The primary focus of the flight nurse must be clinical understanding of mechanical ventilation and operational knowledge of the particular ventilator used.

Respiratory Monitoring Methods

Measurement of respiratory function during transport assists the flight nurse in assessing acute changes in pulmonary function. Chapter 8 contains an in-depth discussion of current methods that can be used to monitor a patient's pulmonary status during transport.[15]

ACUTE RESPIRATORY FAILURE

Acute respiratory failure can occur when chronic pulmonary disease or other factors affect the patient's ability to maintain adequate ventilation. Acute respiratory failure is defined as PO_2 of less than 60 mm Hg and carbon dioxide pressure (PCO_2) greater than 45 to 50 mm Hg.[14] The flight nurse's initial concern is for adequate oxygenation and ventilation for the patient, followed by management of the underlying process that led to acute respiratory failure.

ADULT RESPIRATORY DISTRESS SYNDROME

Etiology

Adult respiratory distress syndrome (ARDS) is a lung injury that has many causes (Fig. 21-6). It may be a complication of other diseases or injuries. It is most commonly seen in patients with direct or indirect lung injury. Direct injuries may include gastric aspiration or inhalation injuries. Indirect injuries result in hypoperfusion of the lung. This may be the result of severe hemorrhage, major burns, sepsis, multiple transfusions, multiple trauma, head injury associated with a change in mental status, pulmonary contusion, multiple fractures, and acute pancreatitis. ARDS most commonly occurs in male subjects, and the mortality rate can be as high as 50%.[5]

Pathophysiology

ARDS results from a severe alteration in pulmonary vascular permeability, which leads to a change in lung structure and function. The outstanding characteristic is hypoxemia refractory to oxygen therapy. Fluids and proteins leak through the altered pulmonary capillary membrane, causing pulmonary edema and a decrease in lung compliance without concomitant congestive heart failure. Because ARDS is a complication of other illnesses or injuries, the flight nurse must also consider the pathophysiology of the underlying problem.

Assessment

Assessment of the patient with ARDS includes the history of the present illness to determine the predisposing factors leading up to the diagnosis. Patients with ARDS report sudden onset of dyspnea, cyanosis occurs, and intubation with mechanical ventilation often becomes necessary. The patient appears in obvious acute distress. If the flight nurse is using mechanical ventilatory support for the underlying illness or injury, pulmonary compliance may decrease.[8]

Chest radiographs reveal widespread pulmonary infiltrates. Hypoxemia is present and may be severe. As the process worsens, accumulation of fluid in the alveoli significantly reduces pulmonary compliance. The patient's condition may progress to hypercapnia respiratory failure as the ability to maintain an effective minute ventilation is lost.[9]

Intervention

Management of the patient with ARDS is a challenge. Positive end-expiratory pressure (PEEP) is added to mechanical ventilation in an attempt to improve arterial oxygenation. In addition, PEEP increases functional residual capacity (FRC). PEEP is measured in centimeters of water, and the lowest measurement possible should be used to restore FRC. As lung compliance decreases, higher levels of PEEP may be required to maintain oxygenation levels.[5,19]

Supplemental oxygen is required because hypoxemia is very significant. Use of 100% supplemental oxygen may be necessary during transport. The oxygen delivery system used depends on the patient's condition.

The use of the pulse oximeter can help the flight nurse to monitor the patient's oxygen status. Changes in oxygen saturation (SpO_2) will occur with ARDS, and subsequent changes may provide useful information for guiding other interventions. Ventilatory support with either with a mechanical ventilator or resuscitation bag is required for patients with endotracheal tubes in place. If a resuscitation bag is used, decreased lung compliance, decreased FRC, and impaired gas exchange may make adequate oxygenation difficult.

Fluids should be restricted unless shock is present. The impaired pulmonary capillary membrane allows fluids to leak into the alveoli. In the presence of shock, fluids must not be withheld. The main pulmonary system goal of air medical transport is to maintain adequate ventilation and oxygenation.

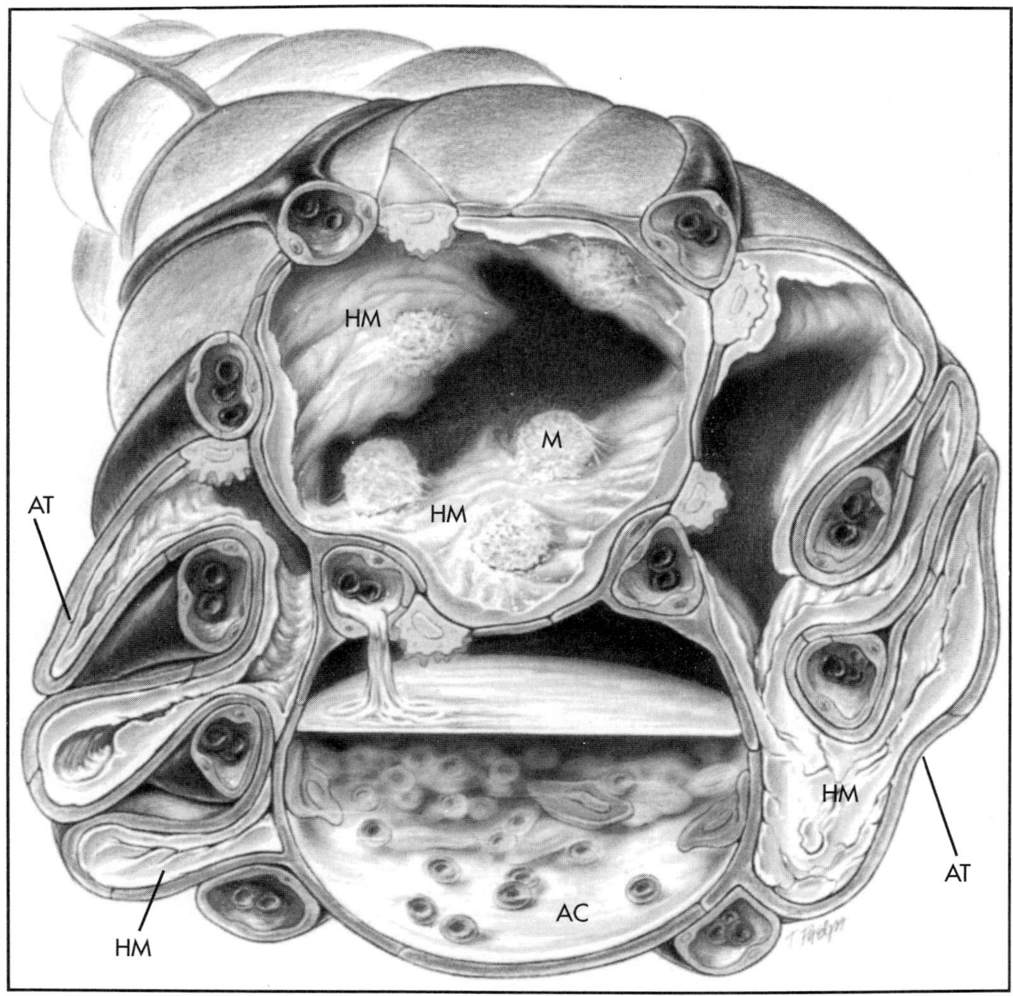

ADULT RESPIRATORY DISTRESS SYNDROME

Fig. 21-6. Cross-sectional view of alveoli in adult respiratory distress syndrome. *HM,* Hyaline membrane; *AT,* atelectasis; *AC,* alveolar consolidation; *M,* macrophage. (From Des Jardins T, Burton GG: *Clinical manifestations and assessment of respiratory disease,* ed 3, St Louis, 1995, Mosby.)

CHRONIC OBSTRUCTIVE PULMONARY DISEASE

Chronic obstructive pulmonary disease (COPD) can be considered a continuum with asthma on one end, chronic bronchitis in the middle, and emphysema on the opposite end.[14] It is not unusual for emphysema and chronic bronchitis to coexist in varying degrees. Although each entity is discussed separately, it is important to remember that different degrees of each can be present in the same patient.

One should not discount the effect of altitude on the patient with COPD. The ability of the patient with COPD to increase ventilation and cardiac output in response to stress is limited.[24]

Asthma

Etiology

Asthma is an obstructive pulmonary disorder that results from airway inflammation and airway smooth muscle contraction. Asthma may be either intrinsic or extrinsic. Intrinsic asthma is more difficult to treat and usually occurs in patients older than 35 years of age. It is nonatopic in nature and has an unpredictable pattern of occurrence. Skin test results are negative, and the IgE level is normal. Extrinsic asthma is usually of an allergic nature and occurs early in life. Serum IgE is elevated, skin test results are usually positive, and it has a typical seasonal occurrence. Extrinsic asthma is more responsive to therapy than is intrinsic asthma.[9]

Pathophysiology

Inhalation of pulmonary irritants and pulmonary infections stimulate bronchoconstriction, hypersecretion of mucosal cells, and edema of the airway mucosa (Fig. 21-7). The airflow path is narrowed, reversibly, and results in an increased airflow resistance; there is a resultant increased work of breathing leading to increased oxygen consumption and increased oxygen delivery requirements. Alveolar hypoventilation occurs, which leads to hypoxemia and eventually retention of CO_2. The hypoxemia stimulates hyperventilation with a resultant decrease in the P_{CO_2}. The obstruction of the lower airways by mucus plugs can lead to further alveolar hypoventilation.[23]

Assessment

The flight nurse should elicit a careful history to identify precipitating factors. For example, a viral illness may precede the acute exacerbation of asthma. The patient may report having a cough and dyspnea. A patient with a long history of asthma can usually rank the relative severity of the illness for the flight nurse. A thorough medication history with regard to timing and dosage is very helpful. For example, a patient who has been taking steroids will probably require additional steroids during an acute attack.[3]

The physical examination reveals different degrees of respiratory distress based on the severity of the current episode. Tachypnea, wheezing, and prolonged expiratory phase are not uncommon. If no wheezing is heard and the patient has difficulty talking, the flight nurse should consider the situation as emergent. Absence of wheezing may indicate that the patient is not able to ventilate sufficiently to produce breath sounds. Inspiratory retractions may be seen, as well as use of accessory muscles. The blood pressure is variable, and pulsus paradoxus may be present. Cyanosis and lethargy are late signs, and the presence of cyanosis or lethargy requires immediate attention.[3]

Diagnostic studies help determine the severity of the asthma. Resistance to airflow is measured by spirometry or a peak flow meter. Spirometric measurement of forced expiratory volume in 1 second (FEV_1) is done before and after treatment to ascertain treatment success. Peak expiratory flow rate (PEFR) can be accomplished with a handheld meter and has been used to determine whether arterial blood gas (ABG) measurement was necessary.[18,20]

In addition to measuring resistance to airflow, a chest radiograph may be done if other parameters are abnormal. Arterial blood gas measurement may be helpful in severe asthmatics. Table 21-4 illustrates the stages of asthma with corresponding ABG results.

Intervention

Ensuring an adequate airway and providing humidified supplemental oxygen are initial interventions. Pharmacologic therapy includes adrenergic agents, theophylline, a anticholinergics, and corticosteroids, which are discussed later in this chapter. Intubation and mechanical ventilation are used only in severe cases. The indications for intubation and mechanical ventilation are listed in the box. Mortality increases for asthma patients who require intubation.[21]

Evaluation

The flight nurse should evaluate the patient's condition at regular intervals to ensure success of therapy. A decrease in dyspnea or in degree of

TABLE 21-4

Stages of asthma

Stage	pH	P_{O_2}	P_{CO_2}	Interpretation
I	↑	Normal	↓	Hyperventilation: ED treatment
II	↑	↓	↓	Hyperventilation; ED treatment consists of correcting hypoxemia
III	Normal	↓	Normal	Obstruction prevents hyperventilation; patient may require hospitalization
IV	↓	↓↓	↑	Severe; ICU admission; may require mechanical support of respirations
V	↓	↓↓↓	↑↑	"Crossed" gases: $P_{CO_2} > P_{CO_2}$; hospitalization and mechanical support of respirations after intubation required

ED, Emergency department; *ICU,* Intensive care unit.
From Hammond BB, Lee G: *Quick reference to emergency nursing,* Philadelphia, 1984, Lippincott.

SEVEN INDICATIONS FOR INTUBATION AND MECHANICAL VENTILATION IN THE PATIENT WITH ASTHMA

1. Decreased level of consciousness
2. Progressive exhaustion
3. Absent breath sounds or severe wheezing despite therapy
4. pH 7.2
5. $P_{CO_2} > 55$ mm Hg
6. $P_{O_2} < 60$ mm Hg despite high-flow oxygen
7. Vital capacity decreases to level of tidal volume

tachycardia and absence of accessory muscle use are parameters to evaluate success of treatment. Obvious improvement in FEV_1 and PEFR measurements should occur. The patient should also be able to verbalize a subjective improvement in respiratory effort.

Chronic Bronchitis

Etiology

Chronic bronchitis is a chronic obstructive pulmonary disease that occurs most often as a result of cigarette smoking. Exposure to pollutants in the environment is also a contributor.

Pathophysiology

The bronchi are the site of illness in the patient with chronic bronchitis. The mucus-secreting cells of the bronchial walls hypersecrete copious amounts of sputum, which prevents airflow into the alveoli. The alveolar gas exchange is normal, but the alveoli are underventilated because of the obstruction of airflow. Hypoventilation results in hypercapnia and hypoxemia. Fig. 21-8 illustrates the pathophysiology of chronic bronchitis as well as emphysema.[14]

Emphysema

Etiology

Emphysema is a COPD that is defined anatomically as an irreversible increase in the size of air spaces distal to the terminal bronchioles. Most patients with emphysema are either current or past cigarette smokers. COPD develops in approximately 15% of smokers. There may also be a role of diantitrypsin in development of emphysema.[16]

Pathophysiology

Pathologic changes begin to occur years before the onset of obvious symptoms. The alveoli are destroyed, supporting structures fail to keep the alveoli open, and the air spaces beyond the terminal nonrespiratory

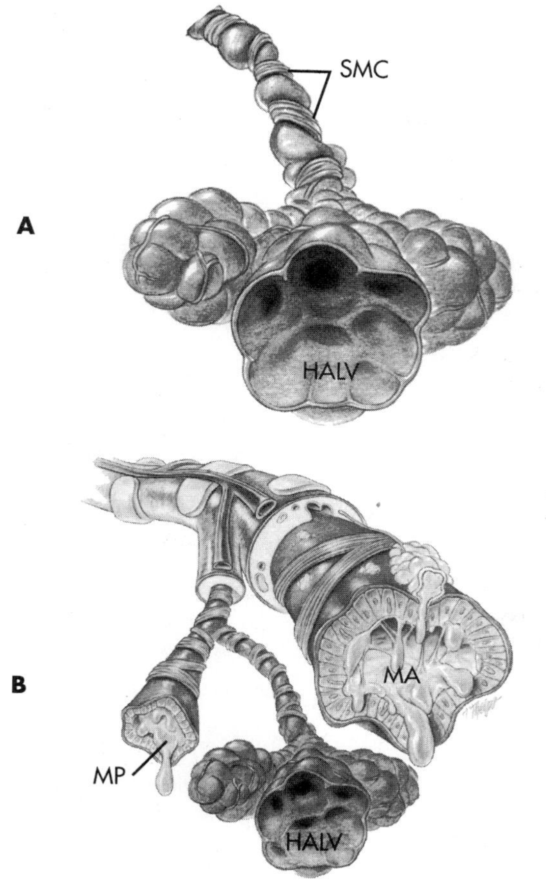

Fig. 21-7. Obstructive lung disorders. **A,** Bronchial smooth muscle constriction (*SMC*) accompanied by air trapping. **B,** Tracheobronchial inflammation accompanied by mucus accumulation (*MA*), partial airway obstruction, and air trapping. *MP,* Mucus plug. (From Des Jardins T, Burton GG: *Clinical manifestations and assessment of respiratory disease,* ed 3, St Louis, 1995, Mosby.)

bronchioles are increased in size. There is an increase in the ratio of air to lung tissue in the alveoli. The alveolar capillary interface area is decreased, resulting in a decrease in gas exchange. Air is trapped in the lungs, which increases residual volume. The expiratory phase increases as the increased resistance to airflow continues. The patient's vital capacity is close to normal until the disease has progressed to a severe stage. Retention of CO_2 is also a late finding. Fig. 21-8 illustrates the pathophysiology of emphysema.

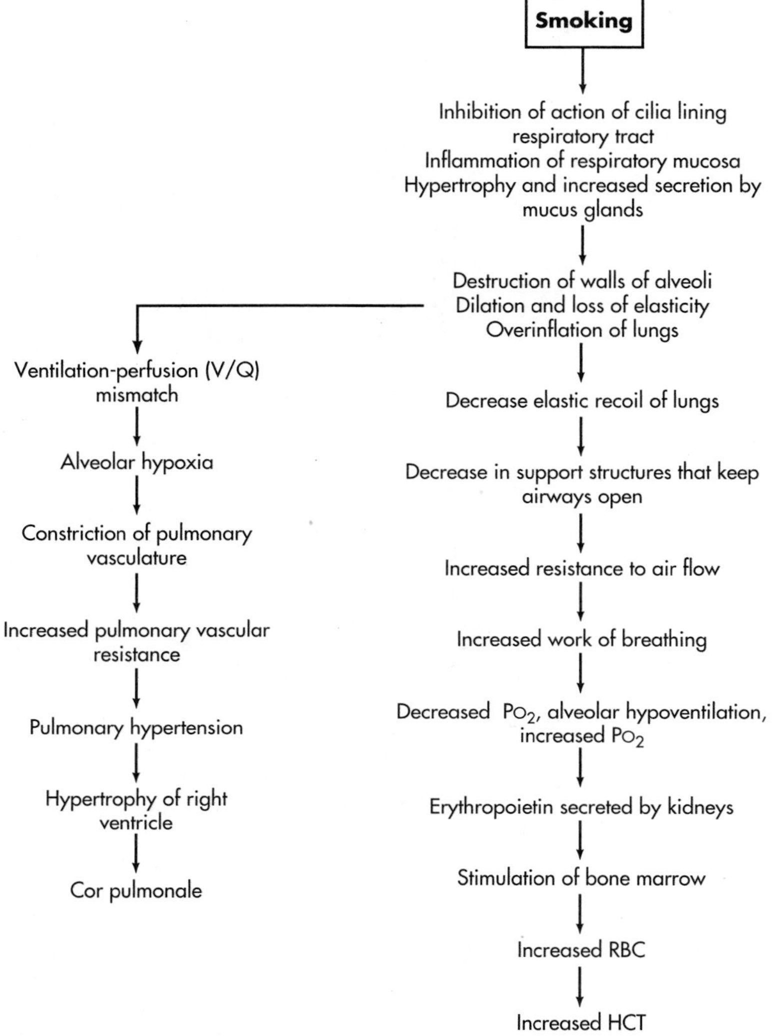

Fig. 21-8. Basic pathophysiology of chronic obstructive pulmonary disease.

Assessment of Chronic Bronchitis and Emphysema

The assessment of the patient with chronic bronchitis and emphysema is very similar, because the two entities often coexist in varying degrees. The history is important in determining the primary etiology of the disease. Exacerbations of stable states may occur with minor pulmonary infections, stress, change in weather, or continued exposure to environmental pollutants (including smoking). The patient's subjective assessment of his or her condition is important to determine the usual status of the disease. The patient may report increased dyspnea, increased or a change in sputum production, or an increase in the malaise that may accompany the disease.

Physical examination of the patient may reveal rhonchi and/or expiratory wheezes. Rales may be

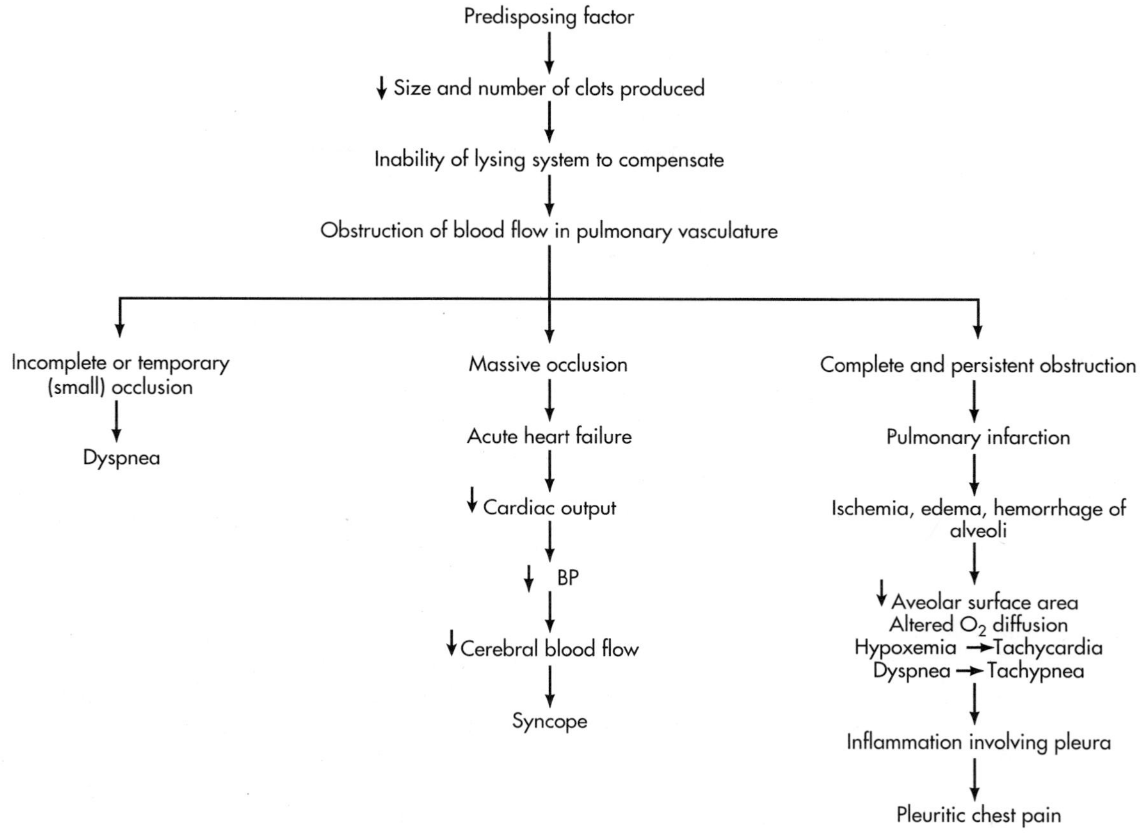

Fig. 21-9. Basic pathophysiology of pulmonary embolism.

present if the patient has an acute infection. The thorax is hyperresonant to percussion, and the anterior posterior diameter of the chest is increased. Observing the respiratory pattern of the patient reveals pursed lips and flaring nostrils. During acute exacerbations, every possible accessory muscle may be used because of the work of breathing. Patients with chronic bronchitis are frequently referred to as "blue bloaters" because they appear edematous and cyanotic. Conversely, emphysema patients are "pink puffers" because they are markedly dyspneic with a pink skin color. Tachycardia and the presence of dysrhythmias is also not uncommon. In the advanced stages of the disease, hemoptysis, fatigue, and weight loss may occur. Breath or heart sounds, or both, may be muffled because of the increased diameter of the patient's thoracic cavity. The patient frequently wants to sit and lean forward to better utilize accessory muscles.

The patient's mental status is an important component of the flight nurse's objective assessment of the patient. Retention of CO_2 occurs in the later stages of the disease process. Once the CO_2 level in the arterial circulation increases beyond the baseline level, one of the first signs is behavioral and emotional changes. The mental status changes may vary from confusion, irritability, and decrease in intellectual performance to obtundation.

Diagnostic studies include ABG measurement, chest radiograph, and ECG. The ABG results vary depending on the severity of the disease. It is normal for the patient with COPD to have a chronic respiratory acidosis compensated by metabolic alkalosis.[13] Chest x-ray reveals hyperinflation of the lungs, narrow and elongated heart shadow, increased anterior posterior diameter, and flattened hemidiaphragms in a lateral view.[16] The ECG findings are most often normal. However, some alterations that may exist include findings that may show low voltage (again, because of the barrel chest), large peaked P waves in the inferior leads, and right-axis deviation as a result of elongation of the heart, respiratory volume strain, and signs of cor pulmonale. It is not uncommon for atrial and ventricular arrhythmias to be noted on the ECG. Pulmonary studies are vital capacity and FEV_1. If either finding is less than 50% of normal for the patient, respiratory failure is present.

Intervention

Supplemental oxygen is given to attempt correction of the hypoxemia to the patient's baseline level. In the normal person, respirations are stimulated by CO_2 levels in the blood. In the patient with COPD, the retention of CO_2 has rendered this reflex ineffective, and the drive for respiration becomes hypoxemia. Thus administration of supplemental oxygen should be at low flow rates ($\leq$2 L/min) unless the patient is being assisted with respirations by means of a mechanical ventilator or resuscitation bag. Use of humidified oxygen is best to thin secretions.

The patient may require assistance with removal of tracheobronchial secretions. It may be necessary to administer IV fluids for rehydration. IV fluids should be administered cautiously because there is usually some degree of right heart failure. Cardiac monitoring is necessary to detect dysrhythmias. Often treatment with pharmacologic agents may cause dysrhythmia. Life-threatening dysrhythmias should be treated according to standard Advanced Cardiac Life Support (ACLS) protocols. Drug therapy is outlined in Table 21-5.[16]

Evaluation

Evaluation of the patient with COPD includes assessment of the patient's mental status for changes in baseline. Any alterations should be aggressively investigated. ABG results must be matched with the patient's clinical condition. Febrile illnesses are generally treated with antibiotics, and hospitalization may be necessary. If intubation and mechanical ventilation are necessary for respiratory failure in the patient with COPD, aggressive pulmonary toilet measures should be undertaken and evaluated for results.

SPONTANEOUS PNEUMOTHORAX

Etiology

A pneumothorax is defined as the accumulation of air or gas in the pleural space (Fig. 21-10). Spontaneous pneumothorax most frequently occurs in young adult men, but it is not uncommon in older patients who have an underlying obstructive pulmonary disease.[11]

Pathophysiology

Primary spontaneous pneumothorax most commonly occurs from the rupture of subpleural emphysematous blebs. The blebs are most often located in the apices of the lung.[12] The pathophysiology is similar to that of pneumothorax caused by thoracic trauma. The lung collapses in varying degrees, and hypoxemia may occur. If the pneumothorax is significant, a tension pneumothorax may occur when the air is trapped in the pleural space under pressure.

Assessment

Patients frequently have chest pain and dyspnea. The amount of pain may vary depending on the degree of lung collapse. In the patient with underlying COPD, the patient's condition deteriorates in spite of aggressive therapy. The breath sounds are decreased or absent on the affected side. In the patient with COPD, it may be difficult to determine any change in breath sounds because of the increased anterior posterior diameter. If the hypoxemia becomes severe, changes in mental status occur.

Intervention

In patients who are asymptomatic with a small collapse of the lung, usually admission to the hospital for observation is all that is necessary. Symp-

TABLE 21-5

Drugs used in chronic obstructive pulmonary disease

Beta Agonists
Bronchodilation, improve mucociliary clearance

Agent	Dose	Side effects
Epinephrine 1:1000	0.3 ml sc	Tremor, palpitations, headache, excitement, nausea
Terbutaline sulfate	0.25 mg sc	
Metaproterenol sulfate 5%	0.3 ml/inhaled, nebulizer	
Albuterol	0.5 ml/inhaled, nebulizer	
Isoetharine	0.5 ml/inhaled, nebulizer	

Methylxanthines
Bronchodilation, improve mucociliary clearance, improve diaphragmatic contractility, enhance myocardial contractility, decrease pulmonary vascular resistance and pulmonary artery pressure

Agent	Dose	Side effects
Aminophylline	5.6 mg/kg IV, loading dose 2.3 mg/kg IV, loading dose (on theophylline prep.) 0.2-0.9 mg/kg infusion	Nausea, vomiting, tachycardia, dysrhythmias, seizures, palpitations

Corticosteroids
Controversial in emphysema, chronic bronchitis; used in asthma; used in acute respiratory failure if pneumonia and sepsis ruled out

Agent	Dose	Side effects
Hydrocortisone	4-8 mg/kg, q6h	Cataracts, hypertension, diabetes, immunosuppression
Methylprednisolone	60-125 mg IV load 40-60 mg q6h	Adrenal insufficiency

Anticholinergics
Decrease in bronchomotor tone, smooth muscle relaxation

Agent	Dose	Side effects
Atropine	1.2-3.2 mg, nebulizer	Dry mouth, dizziness, blurred vision, urinary retention
Ipratropium bromide	40-80 μg q6h inhaler	Dry mouth

tomatic patients are usually treated with a tube thoracostomy. A chest tube is placed in the fourth intercostal space, with the anterior axillary line on the affected side.

The implications for flight nurses are significant. Gases expand at altitude. The flight nurse should not transport a patient with a pneumothorax, even in a helicopter at low altitudes, without inserting a chest tube. If a chest tube is not inserted before transport, the equipment should be readily available to perform

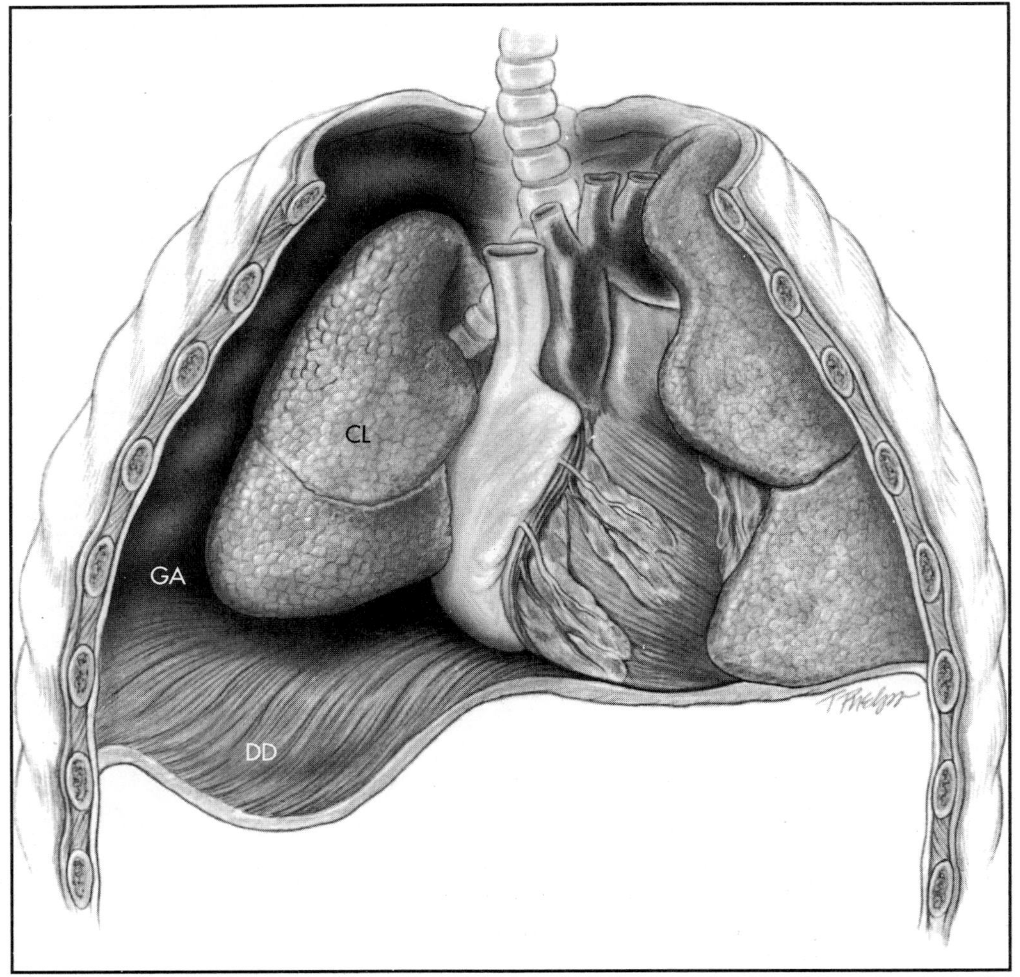

PNEUMOTHORAX

Fig. 21-10. Right-sided pneumothorax. *GA,* Gas accumulation; *DD,* depressed diaphragm; *CL,* collapsed lung. (From Des Jardins T, Burton GG: *Clinical manifestations and assessment of respiratory disease,* ed 3, St Louis, 1995, Mosby.)

a needle thoracostomy in flight should a tension pneumothorax occur.[1] In transporting a patient with COPD, baseline parameters should be closely assessed before transport. If the patient's condition deteriorates during flight, in spite of aggressive management, the possibility of a pneumothorax should be investigated.

Evaluation

The evaluation of a patient with a pneumothorax during transport includes reevaluation of mental status, observation of rise and fall of the thorax with respiratory movement, observation for changes in SpO_2, and ensuring patency of the chest tube (if present). Reports of chest pain and dyspnea should also be addressed and reevaluated. Sudden deterioration should lead to an evaluation of signs of tension pneumothorax (tracheal deviation, jugular venous distention, absent breath sounds, or chest movement on the affected side). Any interventions taken during flight should be constantly reassessed.

PULMONARY EMBOLISM

Etiology

Obstruction of pulmonary flow by emboli can result in alterations in lung tissue function, pulmonary circulation, and heart function. Pulmonary emboli contribute to the deaths of 50,000 to 100,000 patients annually and account for 5% to 10% of all the deaths in U.S. hospitals.[2] The risk factors include heart disease, cancer, immobility, estrogen therapy, disorders in clotting and fibrinolysis, multiple trauma, obesity, and childbirth.

Pathophysiology

Once the clot is produced, the lysing system is unable to compensate. The clot travels through the venous system to the right heart and on to the pulmonary vasculature. The obstruction of blood flow in the pulmonary vasculature may be small, massive, or complete. The results vary depending on the location and size of the clot. Fig. 21-9 illustrates the different types of emboli and the resulting symptoms and effects.

Assessment

Patients with pulmonary embolism report nonspecific and variable symptoms. Lower chest pain, dyspnea, cough, hemoptysis, anxiety, syncope, and diaphoresis are potential symptoms. The flight nurse should suspect pulmonary embolism in any patient when signs and symptoms of cardiorespiratory problems are not otherwise explained. A thorough history is necessary to determine risk factors.

Physical examination may reveal fever, pleural friction rub, tachypnea, tachycardia, and anxiety. Although the patient exhibits signs of hyperventilation, ABG values reveal hypoxemia. The usual diagnostic tests are generally inconclusive in the patient with pulmonary embolism. The ventilation-perfusion scan ($\dot{V}/\dot{Q}$ scan) is the test most often used to diagnose pulmonary embolism. To perform the scan, a small amount of radionuclide-labeled albumin is injected intravenously. After the injection, the labeled albumin particles attach to the pulmonary capillary bed. A pulmonary embolism reveals an area without radionuclide pickup, a perfusion deficit. The ventilation component of the scan assesses ventilatory function with the use of radioactive xenon. The perfusion and ventilation scans are compared. A perfusion deficit without a correlation on the ventilation scan in the same area is supportive of a pulmonary embolism. If there is low probability and a high index of clinical suspicion, or a high probability scan result, pulmonary angiography is done.

Intervention

Supplemental oxygen should be administered during the diagnostic phase. Cardiac monitoring should be continuous because these patients are at risk of cardiac dysrhythmias. Anticoagulation therapy is started once the diagnosis has been determined; the standard anticoagulant used in treatment is heparin. Some studies of pulmonary emboli reveal thrombolytic therapy is associated with more rapid clot lysis when compared with heparin. As shown in one study, a trend toward a decreased death rate appeared when pulmonary embolism was treated with urokinase followed by heparin compared with patients given heparin alone. However, many practitioners consider the benefits of thrombolytic therapy compared with heparin alone as yet unproved, therefore many patients are treated by anticoagulation therapy alone (current oxygen saturation [SpO_2]). Some physicians use thrombolytic therapy in patients with hypotension and low cardiac output in spite of treatments such as streptokinase, urokinase, and recombinant tissue plasminogen activator that have been used to treat pulmonary embolism. In patients whose conditions cannot be managed with heparin, thrombolytics, or a combination of these two therapies because of the massive size of pulmonary embolism, or contraindications to medications, surgical intervention may be required.[22] Intervention may include embolectomy or placement of an inferior vena caval umbrella filter.

TABLE 21-6

Pneumonias

***STREPTOCOCCUS* PNEUMONIA (PNEUMOCOCCAL)**

Organism

Streptococcus pneumoniae: Gram-positive, lancet-shaped *Diplococcus;* aerobe.

Risk factors

Young, elderly, immunosuppressed, alcoholic, COPD, cardiovascular disease, diabetes mellitus, hyposplenia; highest risk occurring in winter months

Pathophysiology

Bacteria is normal inhabitant of upper respiratory tract; aspiration, inhalation, or hematogenous seeding are routes of entry; damage occurs from overwhelming growth, which impairs gas exchange

Clinical manifestations

Malaise, sore throat, rhinorrhea, chills, fever, rust-colored sputum, pleuritic chest pain, nausea, vomiting, abdominal pain, tachycardia, tachypnea, dyspnea, decreased breath sounds, dullness, rales, pleural friction rub; in elderly patients change in mental status or congestive heart failure possible presentation

Diagnostic findings

Leukocytes up to 40,000 ml with left shift
Leukopenia
Liver function tests abnormal
CXR: Homogenous lobar or sublobular infiltrates

Treatment

Penicillin 6-12 million units/day, in presence of meningitis, another drug to be added

Continued.

Evaluation

Evaluation of the patient transported with pulmonary embolism includes a thorough history of illness and any treatment started. Samples for baseline coagulation studies should be obtained before the initiation of anticoagulant or thrombolytic therapy. The flight nurse should assess the patient's cardiopulmonary status constantly during the transport to allow immediate intervention should deterioration occurs.

PNEUMONIAS

Etiology

Pneumonia is an inflammation of the lung parenchyma, caused by either bacterium or viruses (Fig. 21-11). Table 21-6 lists the different types of pneumonia with the causative organism.

Pathophysiology

Lobar pneumonia is an inflammatory process in which the affected alveoli are diffusely involved. Bacteria, neutrophils, and protein pass from one alveolus to another, producing compact infiltrates. The dense alveolar consolidations prohibit volume loss and produce air bronchograms on chest radiography. *Streptococcus pneumoniae* and *Klebsiella pneumoniae* are the most common organisms that produce lobar pneumonia.

Bronchopneumonias occur with areas of normal lung parenchyma interspersed with affected lung parenchyma. It is multilobar and bilateral, with areas of atelectasis. *Staphylococcus aureus* is the most common organism. Interstitial pneumonia is the result of an inflammatory process that affects the support structures of the lung.

TABLE 21-6

Pneumonias—cont'd

STAPHYLOCOCCUS AUREUS

Organism

Staphylococcus aureus pneumonia: Gram-positive nonmotile spherical organism

Risk factors:

IV drug abuse, immunocompromised patients, and complication of influenza epidemic

Pathophysiology

Aspiration from upper respiratory tract leads to infections; growth occurs rapidly in the debilitated host; hematogenous seeding occurs in the dialysis patient or with IV drug use

CLINICAL MANIFESTATIONS:

Abrupt onset of fever, chills, cough, dyspnea, pleuritic chest pain; purulent sputum ranging from yellow to pink; frank hemoptysis common; toxic appearance; tachypnea, tachycardia, rales, rhonchi

Diagnostic findings

WBC > 150,000/ml

Positive blood cultures in 20% of cases

CXR: Bilateral lower lobe bronchopneumonia, early abscess formation or pleural effusion possible

Treatment

Hospitalization and treatment with penicillinase-resistant penicillin

Nafcillin, methicillin, or oxacillin, 1-2 g IV every 4 hr

Treatment period 2 wk unless bacteremia or emphysema occur, then 6 wk

KLEBSIELLA PNEUMONIAE

Organism

Klebsiella pneumoniae: Gram-negative, nonmotile, encapsulated rods

Risk factors

Men, over 50 years of age, alcoholic, heart disease, diabetes mellitus, COPD, aspiration

Pathophysiology

Results in necrosis of alveolar walls, multiple abscesses, loss of lung volume, friable blood vessels

Clinical manifestations

Fever, rigors, dyspnea, productive cough, hemoptysis, copious purulent sputum that is green or blood streaked

Diagnostic findings

Leukopenia or leukocytosis

CXR: Lobar consolidation, typically of right upper lobe; rapid appearance of lung abscesses; pleural effusion common; bronchopneumonia in lower lobes

Treatment

Aminoglycoside and third-generation cephalosporin (cefotaxime, ceftriaxone, cetizoxine)

Continued.

TABLE 21-6

Pneumonias—cont'd

PSEUDOMONAS AERUGINOSA

Organism:

Pseudomonas aeruginosa: Gram-negative motile rod, not encapsulated

Risk factor

Second most common nosocomial, decreased host defenses or antimicrobial therapy, alcoholism, diabetes mellitus

Pathophysiology

Aspiration, necrosis of alveolar walls, multiple abscesses, loss of lung volume, friable blood vessels

Clinical manifestations

Same as those for *Klebsiella* infection

Diagnostic findings

Leukocytosis with left shift
Arterial hypoxemia
Hypocapnia
Positive blood cultures in 33%-50% of cases
CXR: Patchy infiltrates in lower lobes; cavitation, empyema

Treatment

Antipseudomonas penicillin (azlocillin, piperacillin, ticarcillin) combined with aminolgycoside (tobramycin, amikacin)

HAEMOPHILUS INFLUENZAE

Organism

Haemophilus influenzae: Gram-negative, pleomorphic motile rod; encapsulated and nonencapsulated strains

Risk factors

50 years of age; >50% have alcoholism, COPD; URI 2-6 wk previously

Encapsulated strain: Alcoholism, diabetes mellitus, COPD, impaired immune system

Nonencapsulated strain: Exacerbation of bronchitis, nonbacteremic pneumonia

Nonbacteremic pneumonia

Pathophysiology

Bacterial infection that produces inflammation

Clinical manifestations

Minimal elevations in TPR, dyspnea, rales, rhonchi, pleuritic chest pain, nausea, vomiting

Diagnostic findings

Leukocytosis
CXR: Bronchopneumonia, lower lobe and multilobular pleural effusions

Treatment

Ampicillin; if organism ampicillin resistant, chloramphenicol

CXR, Chest x-ray; *TPR,* temperature, pulse, and respiration; *URI,* upper respiratory tract infection; *WBC,* white blood cell.
Modified from Carden DL, Smith JK: *Emerg Med Clin North Am* 7:255-278, 1989.

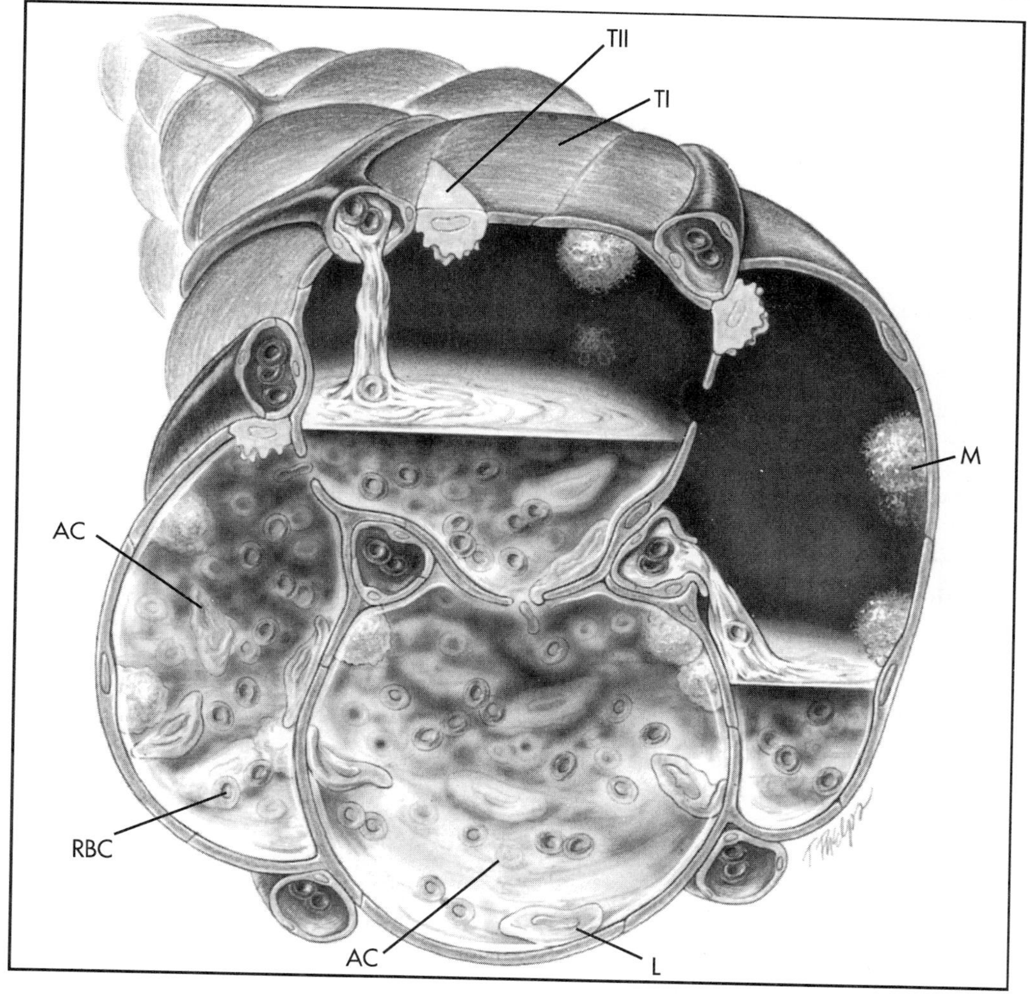

PNEUMONIA

Fig. 21-11. Cross-sectional view of alveolar consolidation in pneumonia. *TI,* Type I cell; *TII,* type II cell; *M,* macrophage; *AC,* alveolar consolidation; *L,* leukocyte; *RBC,* red blood cell. (From Des Jardins T, Burton GG: *Clinical manifestations and assessment of respiratory disease,* ed 3, St Louis, 1995, Mosby.)

Assessment

The history of the patient with suspected pneumonia includes fever and purulent sputum production. The specific signs and symptoms for different types of pneumonia are listed in Table 21-6. In addition to a careful history, physical examination should include not only a thorough pulmonary assessment but an assessment of the patient's overall health.

Intervention

The type-specific interventions are summarized in Table 21-6.

Evaluation

Pulmonary status should be constantly reevaluated during transport of the patient with pneumonia. Mental status, SpO_2 readings, cardiac monitoring, and adequate $\dot{V}/\dot{Q}$ parameters should be constantly assessed.

SUMMARY

The air medical transport of the patient with a pulmonary medical emergency requires knowledge of the common disease pathophysiologic changes. The effect of even low altitude on oxygenation in the patient with a chronic pulmonary problem cannot be overemphasized. The flight nurse combines the knowledge and skills to effect a safe, expeditious transport of a pulmonary patient to the appropriate facility.

PULMONARY SYSTEM CASE STUDY

HISTORY

Prehospital care providers were summoned to a small home of a retired woman. The weather in the area was unseasonably cold, and the woman's neighbors contacted the police when no one had been in contact with her for more than 24 hours. She was 65 years old with a history of coronary artery disease. The patient was found in bed and unresponsive with a heart rate of 68, blood pressure of 140/90, and a strong, radial pulse. She was breathing 16 breaths per minute. The cardiac monitor revealed a sinus rhythm with occasional premature ventricular contractions. A 100% nonrebreather oxygen mask and an intravenous line of lactated Ringer's was initiated. The patient was transported to the closest rural emergency department (ED). Upon arrive to the ED, the patient was placed on an oxygen saturation monitor which read 100%. Vital signs remained stable, and the EKG revealed no acute changes. The fire department then contacted the hospital and relayed that high levels of carbon monoxide were present in the house due to a malfunctioning furnace.

Carboxyhemoglobin levels were drawn and were 33%. The patient was intubated and a request was made for air medical transfer to a hyperbaric therapy center. The patient remained nonresponsive and vital signs were unchanged.

Carbon monoxide is a colorless, odorless, tasteless gas that results from incomplete combustion of carbonaceous material. The most common sources are car exhaust, defective heaters, and fires of all types. Carbon monoxide has an affinity to hemoglobin that is 240 times greater than that of oxygen. Because carbon monoxide binds to hemoglobin, oxygen delivery to the cells is altered and the patient suffers from tissue anoxia.[25] The symptoms vary depending on the amount and duration of exposure; symptoms include a slight headache, nausea, weakness, dizziness, dyspnea, cherry-red skin, confusion, respiratory depression, seizure, neurologic depression, cardiorespiratory failure, and death. Carbon monoxide poisoning is involved in approximately 50% of deaths due to burns.[4a] Normal carboxyhemoglobin levels for nonsmokers are 1% to 5%. Individuals who smoke may have levels of 5% to 10%. In patients who are injured by fires or are exposed to other carbon monoxide sources, symptoms may begin to present with levels of 10% or less.[17a] The appropriate initial intervention is to secure an airway. One hundred percent oxygen should be delivered by a non-rebreather face mask or endotracheal tube. Oxygen facilitates the breakdown of carboxyhemoglobin. Studies have shown that delivery of 100% oxygen reduces the half-life from approximately 5 hours in a room air setting to 30 to 150 minutes.[23a]

MEDICAL CREW ARRIVAL

On arrival, the medical crew assessed and resecured the airway. There were no difficulties ventilating and breath sounds were essentially clear. The patient's vital signs were stable and oxygen saturations continued to be 100%. All medical records were gathered and the air crew moved to the aircraft. The patient was secured for transport and the receiving center was notified of the estimated arrival time. The transport was uneventful. One hundred percent oxygen continued to be delivered via a resuscitator bag with a reservoir.

OUTCOME

The patient was delivered to the receiving center and a carboxyhemoglobin hemoglobin was drawn, resulting in a 23% reading. The decision was made to utilize hyperbaric oxygen therapy (HBO). The objective of this therapy is to reduce the half-life of the carboxyhemoglobin more rapidly. Many studies reveal a significant reduction in half-life. At 2.5 atm absolute, the half-life is reported to be 20 minutes.[23a]

Generally accepted criteria for HBO include syncope, neurologic impairment, seizure, persistent neurologic findings, signs of myocardial ischemia, and life-threatening cardiac dysrhythmia.[23a]

The patient underwent two HBO treatments. She became more responsive and was able to follow commands. Six months after the incident, the patient returned her preincident function level.

REFERENCES

1. American College of Surgeons: *Advanced trauma life support—skills procedure, chest trauma management, needle thoracentesis* (student manual), Chicago, 1993, American College of Surgeons.
2. Anderson FA, Wheeler HB: Venous thromboembolism risk factors and prophylaxis, *Clin Chest Med* 16(2):235-251, 1995.
3. Bates B: An approach to systems. In Bates B, editor, *A guide to physical examination and history taking,* ed 5, Philadelphia, 1991, Lippincott.
4. Bongard FS: Shock and resuscitation. In Bongard FS, Sue DY, editors: *Current critical care diagnosis and treatment,* Norwalk, Conn, 1994, Appleton & Lange.

4a. Bryant KK: Environmental emergencies. In Klein AR et al: *Emergency nursing core curriculum,* ed 4, Philadelphia, 1994, WB Saunders.

5. Chapman MJ: Adult respiratory distress syndrome—an update, *Anesth Inten Care* 22(3):255-266, 1994.
6. Cottrell JJ: Altitude exposures during aircraft flight, *Chest* 92:81-84, 1988.
7. Des Jardins T, Burton GG: *Clinical manifestations and assessment of respiratory disease,* ed 3, St Louis, 1995, Mosby.
8. Greene KE, Peters JI: Pathophysiology of acute respiratory failure, *Clin Chest Med* 15(1):1-11, 1994.
9. Grippi MA: Clinical presentations: pulmonary circulation and pulmonary edema. In Grippi MA, editor: *Lippincott's pathophysiology series pulmonary pathophysiology,* Philadelphia, 1992, Lippincott.
10. Guyton AC: *Textbook of medical physiology, pulmonary ventilation,* Philadelphia, 1986, Lippincott.
11. Jantz MA, Pierson DJ: Pneumothorax and barotrauma, *Clin Chest Med* 15(1):75-90, 1994.
12. Kirby TJ, Ginsberg RJ: Management of the pneumothorax and barotrauma, *Clin Chest Med* 13(1):97-112, 1992.
13. Mills FJ, Harding RM: Fitness to travel by air: physiological considerations, *Br Med J* 286:1269-1271, 1983.
14. Neagley SR: The pulmonary system. In Alspach JG, editor: *Core curriculum for critical care nursing,* Philadelphia, 1991, Saunders.
15. Oranato JP et al: Multicenter study of a portable hand-size colormetric end-tidal carbon detection device, *Ann Emerg Med* 21(5):518-523, 1992.
16. Panettieri RA: Chronic obstructive pulmonary disease. In Grippi MA, editor, *Lippincott's pathophysiology series pulmonary pathophysiology,* Philadelphia, 1992, Lippincott.
17. Richards PR: The effects of air travel on passengers with cardiovascular and respiratory disease, *Practitioner* 210: 232-241, 1973.

17a. Santa Clara Valley California Poison Control: *Patient management guidelines,* 1995, The Poison Control.

18. Scanlan CL, Spearman CB, Sheldon RL: *Egan's fundamentals of respiratory care,* St Louis, 1990, Mosby.
19. Schwartz AJ, Campbell FW: Cardiopulmonary resuscitation. In Barash PG, Cullen BF, Stoeling RK, editors: *Clinical anesthesia,* ed 2, Philadelphia, 1992, Lippincott.
20. Shapiro BA, Harrison RA, Walton JR: *Clinical application of blood gases,* St Louis, 1982, Mosby.
21. Sheehy SB: Pulmonary emergencies. In Sheehy SB, editor: *Emergency nursing: principles and practice,* ed 3, St Louis, 1992, Mosby.
22. Sue DY: Pulmonary disease. In Bongard FS, Sue DY, editors: *Current critical care diagnosis and treatment,* Norwalk, Conn, 1994, Appleton & Lange.
23. Sue DY: Respiratory failure. In Bongard FS, Sue DY, editors: *Current critical care diagnosis and treatment,* Norwalk, Conn, 1994, Appleton & Lange.

23a. Tomaszewski C: Carbon monoxide. In Goldfrank LR et al: *Goldfrank's toxicologic emergencies,* ed 5, Connecticut, 1994, Appleton and Lange.

24. Urden LD, Davie JK, Thelan LA: *Essentials of critical care nursing,* St Louis, 1992, Mosby.
25. Woolley S, Drueck C: Burn injuries. In Kitt S, Kaiser J: *Emergency nursing: a physiological and clinical perspective,* Philadelphia, 1990, WB Saunders.

CHAPTER 22

Gastrointestinal Medical Emergencies

COMPETENCIES

1. Perform a comprehensive abdominal assessment, including collection of subjective and objective data related to the patient's specific gastrointestinal emergency.
2. Initiate the appropriate nursing interventions on the basis of the patient's gastrointestinal medical emergency, including preparation of the patient for transport, insertion of gastric decompression devices, fluid volume resuscitation, and pain management.

The incidence of gastrointestinal (GI) disorders the flight nurse may encounter is relatively high. Regardless of whether the primary event arises from a GI disorder, most acutely ill patients sustain disruptive GI occurrences during the courses of their illnesses. Disorders encountered by air medical crews are esophageal obstruction and varices with rupture; stomach disorders such as gastric or duodenal hemorrhage, ulceration, or perforation, or pyloric obstruction; gallbladder and biliary tract disorders; liver disease; pancreatic disorders; and intestinal obstruction or rupture, ruptured diverticula, and acute appendicitis.

The aerodynamics and biophysics that govern air medical care are especially important in relation to the GI system, which encompasses 26 feet of liquid and gas-producing viscus. Careful patient history, assessment, and preflight planning are imperative for the patient transported by air.

ESOPHAGUS

The esophagus is a hollow tube of striated and smooth muscle that is approximately 10 inches long in an adult. Lying posteriorly to the trachea and closely aligning the left mainstem bronchus, the esophagus exits the thoracic cavity at the diaphragmatic hiatus, or approximately the T11 level. The esophagus provides the primary functions of peristaltic movement of food bolus, prevention of reflux by lower esophageal sphincter activity, and venting for gastric pressure changes.

Vascular supply to the esophagus is through branches of the descending thoracic aorta. Venous return from the esophagus is through the superior vena cava, azygos system, and portal vein system.

Neurologic intervention is initiated in the medulla and carried out by the vagus nerve. Because the esophagus lies in the thoracic cavity, under normal atmospheric conditions it maintains a subatmospheric pressure of −5 to −10 mm Hg, whereas the stomach, which is in the abdominal cavity, rests at an atmospheric pressure of +5 to +10 mm Hg. Acute esophageal occurrences are esophageal obstruction, esophageal varices, and esophageal rupture.

Esophageal Obstruction

Three areas in the esophagus are narrow and may be potential sites for obstruction and injury. These include the cricoid cartilage, the arch of aorta, and the point at which the esophagus passes through the diaphragm.[2]

Esophageal obstruction is fairly common. Strictures, webs, tumors, diverticula, foreign bodies, achalasia, and lower esophageal rings can all reduce or eliminate the venting property of the esophagus for the upper GI system. When air medical transport of obstructed patients is undertaken, intermittent exposure to variations in altitude is of great importance. Esophageal obstruction and an expanding gastrum can pose a serious threat if rapid decompression occurs at 35,000 feet. The venting property needs to be established before flight and depends on whether rotor-wing or fixed-wing transport is to be used.

Assessment

The flight nurse correlates careful physical assessment with interpretation of radiologic and laboratory data to plan air transportation and addresses the following topics that relate specifically to esophageal obstruction.

Subjective Data. The flight nurse must ascertain what brought the patient to seek medical care by either directly questioning the patient or asking the current care giver. Included in these subjective data should be the clinical course the patient has taken since the incident occurred.

Objective Data. The flight nurse performs a physical examination that includes assessment of the following:

- Patient's ability to speak
- Patient's ability to clear the airway of secretions
- Quality and location of pain
- Presence of a palpable mass or masses in the neck
- Signs or symptoms of fluid or electrolyte imbalance
- Time of patient's last meal
- Bowel sounds
- Patient's usual response to motion: airsickness, carsickness, or motion sickness of any kind

Diagnostic Tests

The flight nurse should know by what means the sending facility diagnosed the obstruction and what the estimated percentage of obstruction is. Which examination was performed to make the diagnosis should be noted on the flight record. A careful examination of the chest and kidney, ureter, and bladder (KUB) x-ray films is necessary for determination of adequate ventilation and dangerous air fluid levels before flight. Reviewing current electrolyte levels and complete blood counts will enable the flight nurse to determine and anticipate specific patient needs during the transport.

Plan and Implementation

The plan of care will depend on the anticipated transport altitude. The flight nurse establishes the ability of the patient to maintain his or her airway before flight. Even with aircraft pressurization, assurance of adequate gastric venting is extremely important if high altitude will be maintained. Preflight medications and antiemetic therapy are often helpful not only for the antiemetic effect but also for the associated drowsiness. A nasogastric (NG) tube should be placed and gastric contents emptied before and during flight, and the flight nurse must monitor these contents carefully to ensure blood consistency and patency throughout the flight. Continuous monitoring of respiratory status is also necessary.

Equipment. Adequate suctioning devices are essential to the air medical transport of patients. The flight nurse chooses an NG tube that has venting capabilities, such as a saline shunt; NG tubes that have only top and bottom ports can easily become obstructed. The flight nurse predetermines the amount of volume that would be necessary to volume resuscitate an active hemorrhage. In the occurrence of sudden hemorrhage, adequate volume resuscitation equipment *must be in the aircraft.* If a patient is actively vomiting and having difficulty with secretions, the airway must be protected.

Intervention

If the patient exhibits a trend of declining hematocrit levels, the flight nurse should ask that type-specific blood be prepared for transport. Caution must be exercised when a patient is placed on suction devices during transport; intermittent disconnection of suction from the NG tube allows the pressures to regurgitate and prevents extreme suction against the gastric wall.

Esophageal obstructions are a common occurrence, and most likely air medical transport is being requested because the patient has an acute condition. Flight nurses often encounter massive tumorous obstructions, hemorrhaging obstructions, or tracheal esophageal fistulas with multisystem failure.

Esophageal Varices

The most common cause of varices is hepatic congestion. Torturous, fragile dilated esophageal veins can bleed from spontaneous rupture caused by increased portal hypertension or physical or chemical trauma. Esophageal varices are usually associated with persons with cirrhosis. Varices occur frequently at the distal esophagus and hemorrhoidal plexus, and hemorrhagic shock from an esophageal bleed can occur rapidly.

Assessment

Sequential history of the patient with esophageal varices will help the flight nurse anticipate probable needs during transport.

Subjective Data. The flight nurse determines the cause of varices if possible and investigates previous documented bleeding episodes by asking whether the patient has ever had surgery for control of the varices or whether anything else has been done in the past to terminate hemorrhagic episodes. The flight nurse determines estimated blood loss and requests the appropriate fluids, blood, and blood products before transport.

Objective Data. Careful consideration of the patient's most recent preflight laboratory data (hematocrit and hemoglobin levels, PT/PTT, and electrolyte level) will help the flight nurse anticipate the patient's needs during transport. If the patient is transported directly from the scene, procurement of a blood bank specimen may be of use on admission.

If transport is between medical facilities, the flight nurse should review radiologic findings and ensure that adequate interventions have occurred. If a patient has undergone angiography, the flight nurse must secure the cannulization site before any patient movement and monitor the site frequently throughout the flight.

Plan and Implementation

The flight nurse's first priority is to ensure adequacy of the airway before transport. The flight nurse must estimate the volume needed in the event an acute hemorrhagic episode were to occur during flight. If saline lavage has been used, the flight nurse must estimate the volume of saline solution needed for the projected transport time. Continuous gastric suction can produce large volumes of secretions, and a system to adequately dispose of in-flight secretions needs to be ready, such as having available a supply of zip-lock bags or containers with tight seals.

As with all patient care, universal precautions should be observed; wearing protective goggles, masks, and gowns is imperative for the air medical crew. Adequate suction, IV fluids, blood, and irrigating fluid all need to be secured before flight. The flight nurse must maintain adequate care of esophageal tubes, such as the Sengstaken-Blakemore, Linton, or Minnesota tubes, if one is in place. Traction-dependent or specialized esophageal tubes can pose a problem for transport. Traction maintained with a football helmet can be used during air medical transport (Fig. 22-1). A plan of care must be predetermined in the event of airway loss. Airway loss from these particular types of tubes can be from either physiologic deterioration or tracheal obstruction. Saline solution, rather than air, can be used to inflate these cuffs to prevent further expansion during flight.

Intervention

If an acute hemorrhagic episode occurs, maintenance of airway and circulating volume is the first priority. Effective preflight planning to prevent vomiting and ensure adequate venous access and volume resuscitation is crucial.

Esophageal Rupture

Esophageal rupture commonly results from penetrating trauma but may also result from a blunt insult to the thorax. Rupture from invading lesions, tumors, or caustic exposure also occurs but to a lesser extent. If esophageal rupture has occurred, the venting properties and pathways have altered. During flight, and with possible altitude changes, the distribution and displacement of gases are no longer circumvented by the appropriate course. Complications of gastric pneumonitis, hemopneumothorax, and alteration in gas exchange may all occur.

Assessment

The flight nurse ascertains the history of incidents that led to the current episode. Drugs known to have corrosive effects on the esophagus are doxycycline, tetracycline, acetylsalicylic acid, clindamycin, potassium chloride, quinidine, and ferrous sulfate. Caustic substances can quickly lead to burning or complete erosion of the tissue. Estimation of the degree and size of burns is extremely difficult and can quickly compromise respiratory status. If the rupture is caused by an extravasating tumor, hemorrhage and airway control can become quite difficult.

Plan and Implementation

Priorities. The flight nurse's priorities are as follows:

1. Ascertain adequacy of airway and oxygenation
2. Maintain adequate venous access and volume support
3. Place NG tube with adequate suctioning
4. Assess patient's position to obtain highest level of hemodynamic stability

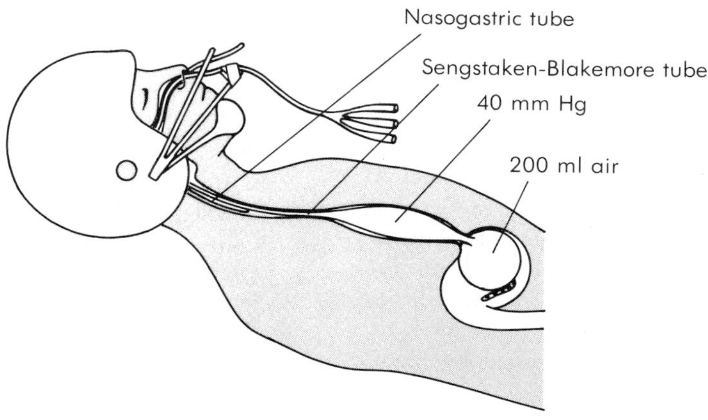

Fig. 22-1. Traction maintained with football helmet for Sengstaken-Blakemore tube.

STOMACH

The stomach lies beneath the diaphragm and is secured in the peritoneum by the lesser omentum. The stomach is subject to alterations in intraabdominal pressure, unlike the esophagus, which has negative atmospheric pressure. The cardiac sphincter separates the esophagus from the stomach. Vascular supply is from the celiac artery branches. Venous return is through the superior mesenteric, splenic, and portal veins.

The stomach functions as a receptacle of ingested substances and attempts to provide chemical and mechanical breakdown. As the stomach expands, peristaltic action increases. The average time of gastric emptying is 1 to 8 hours. Chyme is then propelled through the pyloric sphincter into the duodenum. Decreased gastric motility and alterations in altitude can lead to complications.

Acute Gastric Occurrences

Acute gastric occurrences can take the form of gastric duodenal hemorrhage, gastric perforation from both mechanical and chemical means, pyloric obstruction, and gastric and duodenal ulceration.

Bleeding from peptic or duodenal ulceration occurs more frequently than does esophageal variceal bleeding. Several methods may be used to manage the bleeding. Some of these methods include insertion of GI tubes, such as Linton or Minnesota tubes; injection sclerotherapy with a sclerosing agent such as Scleromate; thermal coagulation; and if bleeding is massive and cannot be controlled, surgery.[1]

Anticipatory planning and thorough preparation can ensure a safe patient transport.

Ulcerative lesions of the stomach or duodenum that lead to bleeding or perforation are in part caused by mucosal membrane erosion. The tissue beneath the mucosa is then subjected to general tissue corrosion. Ulcerations can lead to hemorrhage, perforation, or obstruction and may occur after an attempted repair. Gastric rupture caused by blunt trauma or penetrating trauma is discussed in Chapter 14.

Assessment

During assessment the flight nurse should do the following:

1. Ascertain significant medical history
2. Determine the occurrence that brought the patient to seek care
3. Elicit the number of days of hospitalization and progression or course of illness
4. Identify associated illness or trauma stress–related ulceration
5. Assess patient's psychologic stability

Diagnostic Tests

Two tests, which may not be readily available, are the gastric seriatim test and serum gastric level test. In addition, laboratory findings such as gastric pH, hematocrit level, trends, PT/PTT, and renal function test results will help determine the patient's physiologic condition. The flight nurse should also review radiographic studies.

Plan and Implementation

The flight nurse should develop the plan of care based on the assumption that bleeding could occur at any time during transport.

Priorities. The flight nurse's priorities for planning are in the following order:

1. Ensure adequate airway and circulatory access
2. Estimate volume (crystalloid/colloid) required for length of transport
3. Make available additional medications for supportive therapy, such as vasopressor, antiemetic, or whatever treatment has been initiated

Equipment. The flight nurse should make sure that the following equipment is readily available on the aircraft:

1. Airway equipment
2. NG tube to eliminate gastric contents (many varieties on the market) (NOTE: NG tubes without porting vent systems need to be monitored carefully and should be either at-

tached to suction or allowed to vent openly by gravity.)
3. Suction devices that offer high continuous or intermittent suction
4. Adequate volume resuscitation resources
5. Protective garments for implementation of universal precautions

Intervention

In the event of an acute hemorrhagic episode during flight, volume resuscitation and gastric saline lavage should be performed by the flight nurse, attempts to stop bleeding must be made, and individual flight programs should follow their set preestablished protocols. Complications may arise if the NG tube flow has been obstructed. Gastric dilation and excessive hydrochloric acid can cause nausea and vomiting, which may mechanically induce hemorrhage. Maintenance of adequate gastric venting is imperative throughout any altitude changes.

GALLBLADDER AND BILIARY TRACT

The primary function of the gallbladder and biliary tract is to receive approximately 2 L of bile a day from the liver. Bile, which is stimulated not only by food ingestion but also by stress and acute illness, flows into the duodenum through the common bile duct. Fluid and electrolyte reabsorption takes place in the gallbladder before the bile enters the duodenum; therefore, with generalized volume deficit, an even more concentrated efficacious bile enters the duodenum.

Bile, which is composed of fatty acids, bile salts, phospholipid, cholesterol, conjugated bilirubin, and water, mixes with the chyme to aid digestion.

The ampulla of Vater and Oddi's sphincter are common sites of disease or injury that dramatically affect the entire tract. The gallbladder and biliary tracts are stimulated sympathetically by the splanchnic nerve and parasympathetically by the vagus. Vascular supply is provided by the hepatic artery and cystic vein.

Gallbladder and biliary disorders that necessitate acute air medical transport are infrequent. However, necrotic gangrenous cholecystitis can progress to septicemia, acute pancreatitis, or gallbladder rupture, hepatic failure, or both, because of obstructional flow of bile production.

Plan and Implementation

Transport of patients with gallbladder and biliary tract disorders includes preflight evaluation and determination of adequate drainage of NG or T tubes or both. Careful observation during transport is imperative for prevention of flow obstruction. As with any major abdominal disease or trauma, effective pulmonary toilet must be maintained, and careful monitoring of oxygen tension and saturation should occur during flight.

Laboratory Data

Careful assessment of the laboratory data will give the flight nurse a clear picture of the acuity of the patient's condition and his or her probable needs during transport. Patients with severe obstructive necrotic processes that result in hepatic backup and failure will have serious complications related to electrolyte and volume balance, consumptive coagulopathies, and altered pharmacologic metabolism.

LIVER

The incidence of liver disease and its associated illnesses is relatively frequent. Often liver disease is induced by underlying disease processes, trauma, or chemical abuse.

An adult liver weighs approximately 3 pounds and is supplied by the hepatic artery and portal vein. The liver contains more than 50,000 lobules of hepatocyte.

Patients with liver disease who are most commonly encountered by air medical transport personnel are those who have cirrhosis, liver failure, or associated biliary atresia, or those who are candidates for liver transplantation.

Diagnostic Tests

The flight nurse should review results of liver function tests, hepatitis screening, coagulation studies, and radiography before transport.

Assessment

The flight nurse should find out whether hepatic failure is the primary or secondary event and assess respiratory component ascites leading to diaphragmatic elevation, which can worsen with altitude changes.

Plan and Implementation

In planning and treating the patient with liver disease, the flight nurse should apply, as with all patients, universal precautions. Specific actions should be taken to:

- Protect the patient from heat loss
- Obtain adequate venous access
- Monitor serial Glasgow Coma Scale scores
- Administer 100% FiO_2 during transport
- Replace colloid if recurrent associated hemorrhage episodes occur
- Use liver-metabolized antianxiety and pain medications cautiously

PANCREAS

The pancreas, a gland approximately 8 inches long in an adult, is located behind the spleen. The pancreatic body is positioned horizontally across the abdomen. Its vascular supply is through celiac and mesenteric arteries. The pancreas consists of endocrine, alpha, beta, and delta cells. Pancreatic disorders include pancreatitis and hemorrhagic pancreatitis, cancer, and damage caused by trauma. Devastation of this organ leads to difficult care management of fluid and electrolyte balance, hemodynamic stability, and pain control.

Diagnostic Tests

Amylase, creatinine clearance, electrolyte, and liver function test results require evaluation before transport, and radiographic studies, if available, should be reviewed.

Assessment

A sound history is helpful in determination of the cause of the pancreatic disease process. The flight nurse should also ensure proper airway and venous access before flight. Careful evaluation of electrolyte balance may help the flight nurse determine additional treatment. An NG tube must be in place before transport. If the patient has already undergone surgery and drains have been placed, the flight nurse must ensure proper venting for collection bulbs and surgical dressings. Pain management is an important flight-nursing intervention in the care of the patient with pancreatitis.

INTESTINES

The small intestine (duodenum, jejunum, and ileum) is approximately 23 inches long. The primary functions of the intestines are absorption and digestion. The large intestine is composed of the cecum, ascending colon, transverse colon, descending colon, and sigmoid colon. This extensive, enclosed, gas-producing system can pose many difficulties for the flight nurse transporting a patient who has either direct intestinal disease or general acute illness.

The intestinal problems most frequently encountered by flight nurses are obstructions, ruptures, ruptured diverticula, acute appendicitis, and mesenteric infarct.[5]

Assessment

A careful history is necessary for determination of whether the intestinal disease is a primary or secondary illness. A physical examination by the flight nurse should check specifically for abdominal distention, hyperactive high-pitched bowel sounds, and rectal blood, and the flight nurse should assess the patient for signs and symptoms of peritonitis or sepsis. The patient's temperature should be measured before transport.

Diagnostic Tests

Coagulation studies, electrolyte balance, and a complete blood count may demonstrate abnormal findings. The flight nurse should review radiographic studies of the abdomen to determine whether air fluid levels exist.

Plan and Implementation

The flight nurse should evaluate venous access and volume needs before the flight. The patient in shock may require fluid resuscitation and vasopressors to support his or her blood pressure.

During flight the flight nurse must ensure an adequate airway and provide oxygen, consider aircraft altitude or pressurization to reduce gas expansion, and ensure NG tube patency. Continuous NG tube suctioning is imperative throughout transport. Patients with stomas will need adequate collection-bag venting.

SUMMARY

Careful planning by the flight nurse before air medical transport helps provide effective, safe care. Flight nurses specialized in air medical transport should always be used; knowledge of aviation physiology is absolutely imperative for safe care.

Because patient problems are difficult to predict, flight nurses should plan for equipment and treatment modalities that can be applied easily to all patients before transport. Gases that expand with altitude are ever present in the GI system; proper venting mechanisms should be placed before flight, and backup devices should be available on the aircraft. Calculation of flight time, ground time, and unanticipated diversions will help the flight nurse estimate the amount of volume, battery time, capacities, and therapeutic support needed for the entire transport time.

Understanding the deviations that could occur at various altitudes helps the flight nurse to anticipate problems and be well prepared during flight.

GASTROINTESTINAL MEDICAL EMERGENCIES CASE STUDY

The helicopter was called to transport an 82-year-old man with an upper GI bleed from a community hospital to a tertiary-care center. Refractory massive hemorrhage had occurred during the previous 12 hours, and simple endoscopy by the local community hospital revealed what they believed to be a mass, greater than 13 cm, in the gastric pouch. Because of the size of the mass, clear visualization of the probable hemorrhagic sites was obstructed. This patient had a history of hospital admission 1 week before this occurrence for mild upper GI bleed brought on by food ingestion. A diagnosis of thrombocytopenia and hypertension was made at that time.

FLIGHT CREW EXAMINATION

The patient was a mildly obese man, who was pale and diaphoretic, in semi-Fowler's position on an emergency department stretcher. He was actively bleeding from an NG tube and periodically vomiting large amounts of bright red blood and clots. The patient was visibly anxious and expressed fear of dying.

Cardiovascular: Skin was pale, cool, and diaphoretic, with petechiae over chest, abdomen, and thighs anteriorly.

ECG: Global ischemia with occasional multifocal PVCs was noted. Two large-bore IVs were in upper extremities. PASG was in place with leg compartments inflated to 20 mm Hg.

Respiratory: Nasal cannula delivered 4 L/min. Breath sounds revealed faint rales at bilateral bases. Chest x-ray film revealed bilateral lower lobe infiltrates and a markedly distended gastrum elevating the left diaphragm. An approximate 13-cm mass with varying densities was seen.

GI-GU: Normoactive bowel sounds were auscultated, and a large mass was palpated in the left upper quadrant. A Foley catheter was in place and draining clear yellow urine. A no. 18 Salem sump was in place and lying posteriorly to the gastric mass draining bright red blood. Iced saline lavage was being performed by the emergency department staff.

Medications given before the flight crew's arrival were as follows:

Lasix 40 mg IVP
Valium 2 mg IVP
5 units of packed red blood cells
3200 ml of crystalloid

Laboratory data were as follows: Hct 27, PT 12.9, PTT 22.5; platelets 73,000; ABGs on 4 L/min nasal cannula O_2: pH 7.38, PO_2 68, PCO_2 32; vital signs: BP 110/68; AP 108; respiration 30; temperature 96° F, patient shivering.

INTERVENTIONS

The flight crew prepared the patient for transport and took iced saline solution in a cooler and 4 additional units of packed red blood cells. The stretcher was prepared with dry, warmed linen and a space blanket. The oxygen was changed to 100% nonrebreather mask, and the patient was given safety orientation before flight.

The flight time to the tertiary facility was 20 minutes. Vital signs remained stable, and the saline lavage was continued throughout the flight, with noted clearing on landing. Units no. 6 and no. 7 of red packed blood cells were infusing. Patency of the NG tube during air medical transport was crucial for this patient, and frequent manipulation of the tube was required to prevent occlusion.

Workup of this patient revealed that the gastric mass was a product of small bones, Styrofoam, hair, and paper products. The patient was taken to the operating room for removal of the foreign-body mass. It was noted at that time that the patient had no body hair.

DISCUSSION

Preflight planning for the needs of the patient for both the initial admission time and during the flight to the receiving facility is imperative. This patient continued to receive colloid replacement while being type- and cross-matched at the receiving facility.

The gastric bleeding was caused by mechanical lacerations from small bones. The patient has undergone surgical repair and psychiatric evaluation since admission. In this extremely complicated case, a diagnosis of bezoar was made, and further psychologic evaluations are to follow.

REFERENCES

1. Dinsdale-Novotny V, Andrews L: Gastrointestinal emergencies. In Kitt S et al, editors: *Emergency nursing,* Philadelphia, 1995, Saunders.
2. Finis NM: Abdominal trauma. In Kitt S et al, editors: *Emergency nursing,* Philadelphia, 1995, Saunders.
3. Mason PJ: Abdominal injuries. In Cardona V et al, editors: *Trauma nursing,* Philadelphia, 1988, Saunders.
4. McDonald M, Ralph D, Carithers R: Severe liver disease. In Ayres S, editor: *Textbook of critical care,* Philadelphia, 1995, Saunders.
5. White R: Diagnosis and therapy for emergent vascular disease. In Ayres S, editor: *Textbook of critical care,* Philadelphia, 1995, Saunders.

CHAPTER 23

Renal Medical Emergencies

COMPETENCIES

1. Perform a comprehensive assessment including the collection of subjective and objective data related to renal medical emergencies.
2. Identify the appropriate flight nursing interventions for the care of the patient with a renal medical emergency before and during transport.

Air transport of a patient for medical management of a long-standing renal condition only may be rare. However, several emergency situations are associated with sudden impairment in renal function that might require emergent air transport to a tertiary center for treatment. This chapter briefly reviews anatomy and physiology, disease states, and transplantation principles to aid flight nurses in caring for patients in acute and chronic renal failure.

INCIDENCE OF RENAL DISEASE

The incidence of chronic renal failure continues to increase yearly in the United States. In 1984, 78,483 patients with end-stage renal disease (ESRD) required dialysis. Between 1984 and 1994 this number increased to 186,822 patients.[1] Risk factors associated with chronic renal failure or ESRD include diabetes, hypertension, glomerulonephritis, polycystic kidney disease, interstitial nephritis, and obstructive nephropathy. According to 1991 statistics reported by the Health Care Financing Administration,[1] diabetes was listed as the primary diagnosis in 33% of patients with ESRD, hypertension in 27% of cases, and glomerulonephritis in 13%.[1] Recent investigations into slowing or improving the course of chronic renal failure in hypertensive patients has centered around the use of angiotensin-converting enzyme inhibitors and calcium antagonists.[4,7] Studies indicate that these drugs may exert a "renal protective" effect.

RENAL ANATOMY

The kidneys are situated in the posterior abdominal cavity in the retroperitoneal space. Because of the location of the liver, the right kidney sits slightly lower than the left. Each kidney weighs approximately 115 to 150 g and measures 11 to 13 cm long, 5 to 7 cm wide, and 2.5 cm thick. The kidneys receive 1.2 L of blood per minute or approximately 20% of the total cardiac output. The oxygen consumption rate per gram of kidney tissue is exceeded only by cardiac tissue. In the nondiseased kidney, blood flow remains relatively constant despite changes in arterial pressure, leading to the hypothesis that the kidney can "autoregulate" blood flow. The mechanism for autoregulation is not fully understood.

Blood supply to the kidneys is through a single renal artery that branches off the abdominal aorta and enters the kidney at the indentation called the *hilus.* At the hilus the renal artery divides into smaller arteries that travel throughout the kidney, where they eventually form multiple afferent arterioles and supply the glomerulus of the nephron. Nephrons are the structural and functional unit of the kidney, and each kidney contains about a million nephrons. Each nephron is composed of a glomerulus, a capillary filtering system composed of three different membrane types of various densities that allow for the passage of fluid and solutes from the blood into Bowman's space. The remaining structures of the nephron include the proximal convoluted tubule, loop of Henle, and distal convoluted tubule. The distal convoluted tubule enters a collection duct, which eventually merges with other collection ducts emptying into the renal calyx and eventually into the ureter.

After blood is delivered to the glomeruli by the afferent arterioles, the efferent arterioles drain the glomeruli. After flowing through a network of capillary vessels, which nourish the individual tubules of the nephron, the blood is returned to the inferior vena cava via the renal vein.

RENAL FUNCTION

The kidneys primarily function to eliminate nitrogenous wastes, toxins, and drugs from the body. Through this excretory function, they simultaneously maintain and regulate water and electrolyte balance and acid-base balance, which helps maintain body homeostasis. The kidneys also produce renin, an enzyme that helps regulate blood pressure and kidney function, and erythropoietin, a hormone that actively stimulates red blood cell production in the bone marrow. In addition, the kidneys metabolize vitamin D to its active form.

Urine formation begins with glomerular filtration. Glomerular filtration is a passive filtration process that allows approximately 120 ml of protein-free plasma to enter the nephrons each minute. This is known as the *glomerular filtration rate (GFR).* This high filtration rate is the result of the glomerular blood pressure, which is maintained at approximately 55 mm Hg (as opposed to the 15 to 20 mm Hg of other capillary beds), and the design of the filtration membrane of the glomerulus, which is thousands of times more permeable to water and solutes than other capillary membranes. In the proximal tubules most of the filtrate is reclaimed, together with the nutrients and some of the minerals. About one third of the original 120 ml of plasma that entered the proximal tubule passes on to the loop of Henle and the distal tubule for additional processing.

The GFR declines after age 40 to about half of normal by age 70. Although the cause for this reduced renal function is unknown, one possible result is that older patients may not recover as quickly from alterations in renal function.[2] The GFR normally depends on glomerular blood pressure, which is subject to intrinsic and extrinsic controls. One extrinsic condition occurs in hypovolemic shock. At the point in which systemic blood pressure equals normal glomerular filtration pressure (50 mm Hg), renal filtration stops and anuria results.

Measurement

Laboratory measurements of renal function reflects the GFR. Creatinine, a product of muscle metabolism, is released from muscle at a constant rate and excreted in the urine at the same rate; thus serum levels remain constant. The normal serum creatinine level is 0.6 to 1.4 mg/dl. However, because serum creatinine is the product of muscle metabolism, emaciated patients may have a "normal" creatinine of 0.3 mg/dl, and a serum value of 1 mg/dl may represent marked reduction in the GFR.[4] Another guide to GFR is the serum blood urea nitrogen (BUN) level. However, measurement of BUN value has limitations as an index of GFR. The level of urea in the blood is determined by factors other than renal function. A high protein diet, blood in the gastrointestinal tract, infection, the use of steroids, and certain medications may result in an increase in BUN value despite a normal GFR.

The most useful clinical guide to GFR is measurement of creatinine clearance. A 24-hour urine creatinine is collected and a serum measurement of creatinine is used to calculate the creatinine clearance value. The normal creatinine clearance value is 110 to 120 ml/min. Serum creatinine levels can then be used to monitor the patient's course, and the creatinine clearance can be repeated if the serum level changes appreciably.[2]

Urinalysis is also helpful in identifying pathologic processes of the kidney. Urine is normally pale to amber. Color changes (such as a change to red) may be caused by the presence of myoglobin and free hemoglobin. Red blood cells and heme pigments may cause urine color to range from pink to black. Malignant melanoma may also cause the urine to turn black. Patients with hepatic conditions may have yellow to brown or green urine. Certain medications and food dyes may cause urine to turn blue, orange, or bright yellow. Urine should also be clear. Cloudy urine may indicate the presence of epithelial cells or leukocytes and is associated with urinary tract infections.

The odor of urine may also furnish information about urine content. A sweet, fruity odor results from ketone formation, and certain conditions may cause urine to have a fishy or foul smell. Measurement of specific gravity indicates the density of dissolved substances in the urine, although a more accurate indicator of the kidney's ability to concentrate or dilute urine is osmolality. Specific gravity normally ranges from 1.003 to 1.030. A low specific gravity can be caused by overhydration, diuretic therapy, or alcohol or caffeine ingestion. Glucose or protein in large amounts may produce a high specific gravity.

The pH of urine normally ranges from 4.5 to 8.0 and largely depends on dietary intake. Undernutrition, diabetic ketosis, severe diarrhea, hyperkalemia, and respiratory alkalosis produce an acidic urine. Regulation of urine pH is beneficial in the treatment of chronic urinary tract infections and certain renal calculus. In addition, the alkalinization of urine is performed to enhance urinary excretion of salicylate in salicylate poisoning.

Normal urine should not contain protein; however, the urine of some patients may have a trace of protein. High levels of protein suggest renal or urinary tract disease. Conditions such as stress, aggressive exercise, febrile states, and exposure to extreme temperature changes may produce transient levels of proteinuria. A consistent elevated level of proteinuria is associated with the nephrotic syndrome, glomerulonephritis, lupus nephritis, and amyloidosis. Lower levels of proteinuria are associated with diabetic nephropathy, hypertension, polycystic kidney disease, and chronic pyelonephritis.

The urine microscopic examination can also be useful in identifying certain renal conditions. It identifies urinary sediment such as casts, cells, and crystals.

RENAL FAILURE

Acute Renal Failure

Acute renal failure is the acute cessation or impairment of renal function that leads to excessive accumulation of nitrogenous waste products in the serum. Depending on the amount of urine produced in 24 hours, acute renal failure is classified as *oliguric* if urine production is less than 500 ml and *nonoliguric* if urine production is greater than 500 ml.[5] Acute renal failure is the result of one of three conditions: prerenal, intrarenal, or postrenal.

Prerenal

Prerenal causes of acute renal failure are the result of conditions that impair or decrease blood flow to the kidneys. Hypovolemia from shock or dehydration, third spacing of fluids that occurs in burns or ascites, and circulatory conditions such as impaired cardiac function are examples of prerenal conditions leading to acute renal failure. Many cases of acute renal failure respond to fluids and are easily reversible. Treatment is aimed at restoring renal perfusion. When ischemia is severe or prolonged, the condition may lead to a more serious intrarenal condition: acute tubular necrosis.[2]

Intrarenal

Acute renal failure results from an intrarenal condition in which damage to the kidney, especially the nephron, occurs. Conditions such as acute glomerulonephritis resulting from infection or systemic lupus erythematosus, pyelonephritis, multiple myeloma, vascular diseases of the kidney, and acute tubular necrosis are examples of intrarenal causes of acute renal failure.

Approximately 75% of all acute renal failure is the result of acute tubular necrosis. The primary cause is drugs, especially the aminoglycosides. Other antibiotics also associated with acute tubular necrosis include the penicillins, cephalosporins, tetracyclines, amphotericin B, and the sulfonamides.[2] Additional causes are nonsteroidal antiinflammatory drugs, antineoplastic agents, radiographic contrast materials, organic solvents such as ethylene glycol (found in antifreeze), and heavy metals such as mercury, arsenic, lead, and uranium. Hemoglobinuria and myoglobinuria are also causes of acute tubular necrosis. The nonoliguric form of acute tubular necrosis has a better prognosis than the oliguric form.

The pathophysiologic processes that result in acute tubular necrosis are not fully understood. One popular theory is that the damaged tubular cells allow the normal filtrate to "leak back" into the efferent arterioles, thereby accounting for the decreased urine output or oliguria. The most recent theory is that the decreased urine state results from a profound reduction in glomerular filtration caused by afferent renal vasoconstriction.[2]

Early treatment of acute tubular necrosis includes inducing large volumes of urine through the administration of fluids and diuresis through the use of mannitol or furosemide. These measures are believed to improve interrenal circulation and perhaps "wash out" the nephrotoxins.

Postrenal

Postrenal conditions leading to acute renal failure are the result of obstructions to urine flow from the kidney to the urinary meatus. Total anuria is more suggestive of a mechanical obstruction than some other form of renal failure, although partial obstruction need not be accompanied by oliguria. Common causes of postrenal acute renal failure include bladder neck, urethral, and prostatic obstructions.

Chronic Renal Failure

Chronic renal failure is a slow, progressive loss of renal function in which the kidney is no longer able to maintain excretory and regulatory functions. The stages within the disease roughly reflect the total percentage of functional nephrons. The kidney can maintain function with a nephron loss as great as 80%.[6] The four stages of chronic renal failure are (1) diminished renal reserve, (2) renal insufficiency, (3) ESRD, and (4) the uremic syndrome.

In diminished renal reserve a 50% reduction in functional nephrons occurs and kidney function is only mildly or modestly reduced. Usually the patient has no symptoms. At 75% loss of nephron function, renal insufficiency results, producing only minimal abnormalities such as mild azotemia, a slightly impaired ability to concentrate urine, and anemia. The serum creatinine value may be as high as 5.0 mg/dl. If the patient becomes stressed by dehydration, infection, or heart failure, renal damage may be further exacerbated.

In ESRD the loss of functional nephrons is 90% and kidney function deteriorates to where dialysis or transplantation is necessary to maintain life. Serum creatinine values may be 10 mg/dl. Anemia secondary to decreased erythropoietin secretion is common, and typical hematocrit values can range from 20% to 30%. Blood transfusions may not be needed unless fatigue, activity intolerance, shortness of breath, or chest pain is experienced. With the availability of recombinant erythropoietin, the anemia can be successfully treated in most patients.[2] Administration of oxygen during transport is indicated, especially at high altitudes, because of correspondingly lowered hemoglobin levels that occur during flight.

The uremic syndrome is the final stage of chronic renal failure and is the systemic response of the body to the accumulation of uremic waste products. These symptoms involve the gastrointestinal tract, cardiovascular system, and nervous system. Characteristics of the uremic syndrome may include hypertension; peripheral, sacral, and periorbital edema; apathy and mental dullness; fatigue; anorexia; twitching and restlessness; muscle cramping; seizures; and pulmonary edema.

Anemia and metabolic and electrolyte disturbances are common to the patient with chronic renal failure. Patients on long-term dialysis are at a risk for developing cardiomyopathy, pleural effusions, pericarditis or pericardial effusions, and tamponades. Changes in personality, neuroses, and psychosis are also associated with the uremic syndrome, and extra precautions should be taken to maintain in-flight safety. Increasing the frequency of dialysis may help minimize the symptoms once they appear.[2,6]

Potassium Regulation

Hyperkalemia in chronic renal failure is much less common than in acute renal failure due to adaptive changes in the gut and the remaining nephrons that help eliminate potassium. In acute renal failure, hyperkalemia is much more common and can be exacerbated when it occurs in the presence of tissue injuries, which release quantities of intracellular potassium into the bloodstream. Signs and symptoms of hyperkalemia include serum potassium levels greater than 6 to 7 mEq/L, electrocardiogram (ECG) changes, and cardiac arrest. ECG findings are the single most important signs of hyperkalemia (Fig. 23-1). Emergency treatment of hyperkalemia includes the following:

1. Correction of metabolic acidosis with administration of IV sodium bicarbonate
2. Administration of IV calcium to antagonize cardiac effects of hyperkalemia
3. Hypertonic glucose and insulin to force potassium into cells
4. Administration of cation-exchange resin (Kayexalate)
5. Monitoring for hypokalemia caused by overtreatment
6. Preparation for dialysis as soon as possible

In chronic renal failure, glucose and sodium bicarbonate are of no value because the patient usually has normal stores of glycogen and is not acidotic. Emergency treatment of hyperkalemia in chronic renal failure consists of administration of IV calcium until dialysis can be instituted.[6]

DIALYSIS

Treatment of ESRD includes dialysis or kidney transplant. Some forms of acute renal failure are also treated with dialysis until the nephrons regain func-

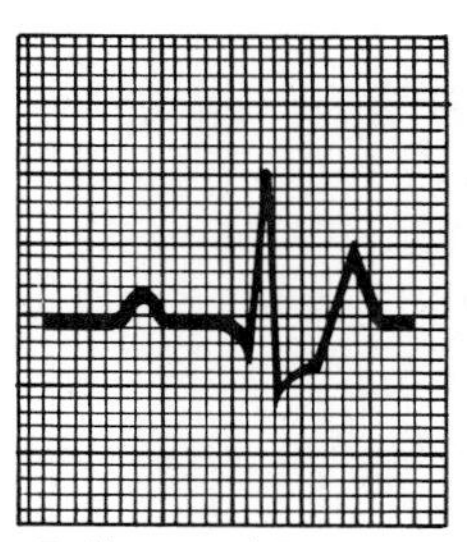

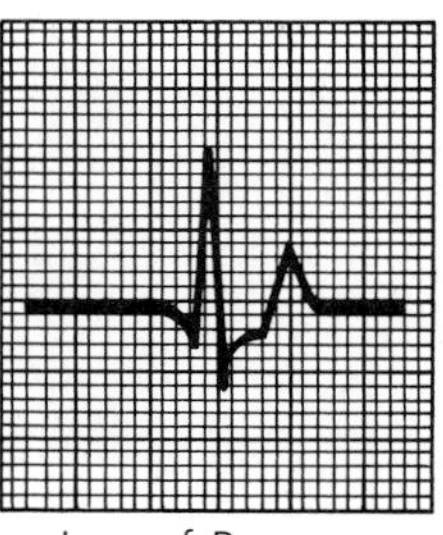

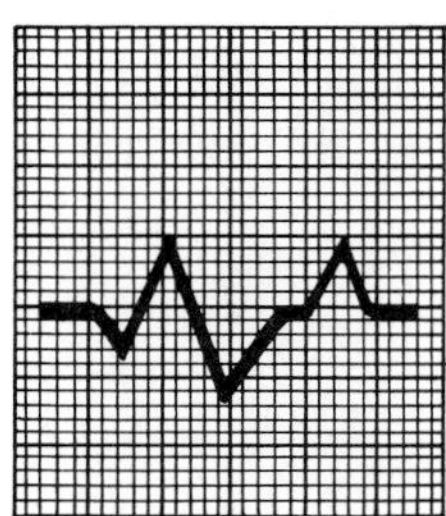

Fig. 23-1. ECG changes in hyperkalemia.

tion. In 1994 the number of dialysis patients in the United States was nearly 190,000. Nearly 80% of these patients were receiving hemodialysis; the remaining 20% were on some form of peritoneal dialysis.[1]

Hemodialysis

Patients who are receiving hemodialysis for acute renal failure or long-term dialysis for treatment of ESRD must have some form of vascular access. When emergency access is needed, the subclavian vein can be cannulated using a double-lumen catheter with flow controlled by a pump. In situations of acute or reversible renal failure and patients awaiting the maturation of an internal arteriovenous (AV) fistula, an external AV shunt may be inserted. Shunts are made by joining one 6-inch length of Silastic tubing to an artery and another one to a vein. A small amount of the tubing is tunneled subcutaneously and then brought to the external surface of the skin. The access site remains wrapped in a sterile dressing between treatments.

To assess the access site, the flight nurse should touch the loop of the site. The loop should feel slightly warm. A bruit, or "thrill" (buzzing sensation), may be felt over the blood vessel in the site. When auscultated with a stethoscope, the bruit is quite audible and distinctive.

More than likely a patient with chronic renal failure will have a surgical creation of an anastomosis between an artery and a vein. Thus the patient's own vessels provide the access for hemodialysis. The advantages of an internal AV fistula are that the fistula lasts longer than a shunt and has less of an infection rate, decreased clotting rates, and less likelihood of accidental dislodgment. The AV fistula is usually located in the inner aspect of the forearm but may be placed in the medial aspect of the tibial malleolus.

Another form of access is the AV fistula graft. The graft is placed in the same locations and for the same purposes as the AV fistula, but instead of the patient's own vessels being used, a synthetic material is grafted to the patient's artery and vein in a loop or straight line configuration. This synthetic area is the point at which the dialysis cannula is placed. On palpation, a graft feels much stiffer than a patient's own AV fistula.

Transport considerations for protection of the patient's hemodialysis access site include the following:

1. Protecting from cold—Exposure to weather or unusual cold (ice packs) may reduce blood flow and cause stasis and clotting in the site. If the extremity is injured, elevation without ice is the treatment of choice.
2. Protecting from pressure—Stasis factors such as positioning and placing of heavy equipment on the site may reduce flow and cause damage through clotting.
3. Limiting access—The site is the patient's "lifeline" and should not be used for routine IV access. In an absolute emergency situation, the fistula may be used. To gain IV access to the AV fistula or graft and to prevent damage, the flight nurse should use only metal needles.
4. Protecting the extremity harboring the site—Drawing blood or taking blood pressures should be performed on the extremities without the fistula, graft, or shunt.
5. Protecting shunt tubing from becoming disconnected—The patient could exsanguinate if the tubing disconnects. If it is disconnected, direct hand pressure over the bleeding site and a blood pressure cuff or tourniquet applied above the area will stop the bleeding.
6. Preventing erosion or infection of the skin at the access site—Long-term use increases the likelihood of erosion and infection at the access site. Breaks in skin integrity or infections should be reported to the accepting facility staff so that cultures and antibiotics may be started promptly.

When a graft is being accessed, the direction of the needle should always be the same as the direction of the blood flow through the graft. There are two types of grafts: straight and loop (Fig. 23-2). The direction of blood flow on a straight graft can be determined by remembering that the blood always flows from the distal end back toward the heart. On

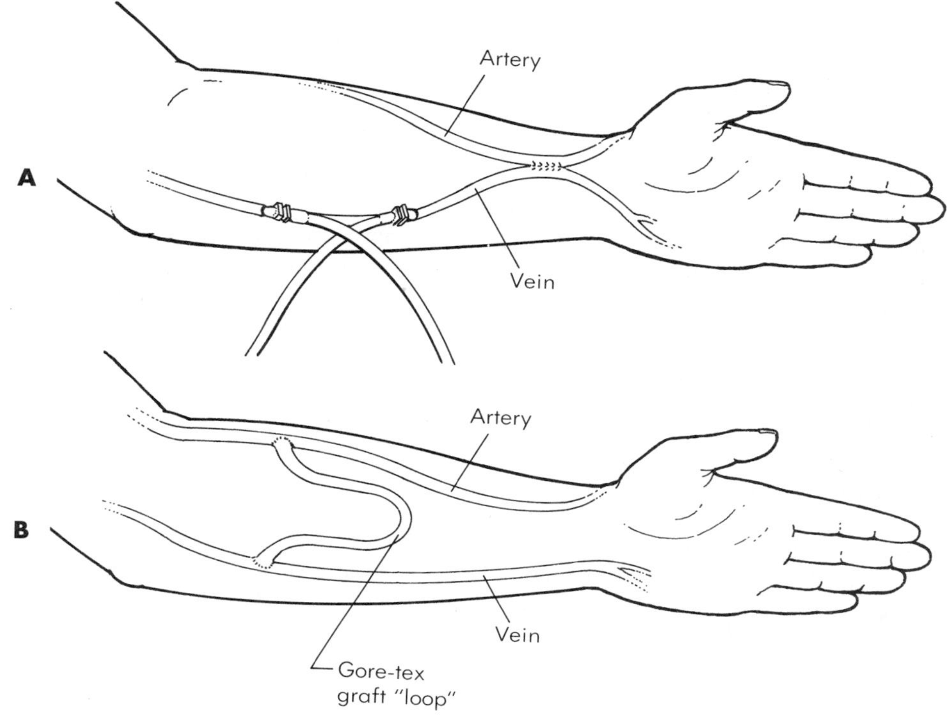

Fig. 23-2. Straight grafts (A) versus loop grafts (B).

a loop graft, blood flow direction can be determined by completely occluding one side of the loop of the graft at some point (any point) with a finger. Auscultation is then performed on either side of the finger. The softer sound is the blood flowing from the artery, and the louder sound is the blood flowing into the vein. This may sound "backward," so thinking of a finger occluding or plugging a hole in a dike and "softening" the flow through the hole is helpful. The loud-sounding venous side can be thought of as fluid gushing and breaking through the occlusion. The needle should be placed in the same direction as the blood flowing into the vein and back toward the heart.

Once the transport of the patient is complete, an alternative IV site, such as a central line, should be established. Care must be taken when the needle is removed from the fistula or graft. When the needle is being removed, the flight nurse should apply firm, direct pressure to the site and hold a fistula (the patient's own natural vessels) for 3 to 5 minutes and a graft (artificial material) for 8 to 15 minutes. Pressure should be maintained on both sides of the access site to ensure that bleeding has completely stopped. A pressure dressing should then be applied but not so tightly as to decrease the blood flow through the vessel.

Peritoneal Dialysis

In selected patients, peritoneal dialysis may be the preferred type of dialysis. The procedure involves the insertion of a catheter, which is tunneled through the subcutaneous tissue into the peritoneal cavity, and involves the principles of osmosis and diffusion. Dialysis is accomplished by cycling dialysis fluid through the peritoneal cavity, which allows movement of solutes across the peritoneal membrane from an area of higher concentration to an area of lower solute concentration. An exchange or a cycle is composed of the infusion, the dwell time, and the drainage. Typical adult infusion volumes are 2 L, and the fluid can be infused over 10 minutes. The dialysis fluid remains in the peritoneal cavity for 2 to 15 hours depending on the mode of dialysis. Modes of peritoneal dialysis include intermittent peritoneal dialysis, continuous cyclic peritoneal dialysis, and continuous ambulatory peritoneal dialysis. Modes differ by dwell times, cycles per exchange, and type of infusion.

Infection of the peritoneal membrane is the most frequent and critical complication in patients receiving chronic peritoneal dialysis. Renal patients on peritoneal dialysis who are initially seen with abdominal tenderness, particularly around the catheter site, decreased bowel sounds, and an elevated white blood cell count must be suspected of having peritonitis. In addition, a drained bag of dialysate should be used for analysis. Treatment may include the administration of antibiotics through the peritoneal catheter.

TRANSPLANT

Patients with ESRD may be transplanted with a kidney from a living donor or cadaver. In 1994, of the 11,368 kidney transplants, approximately 26% were from living donors. About 80% of the kidneys transplanted from cadavers are still functioning well 1 year after surgery. For kidneys transplanted from living related donors, the rate is 93% because of more closely matched organs.[3]

By federal mandate all states now have some form of "required request" legislation that mandates hospitals to set up a protocol for offering the next-of-kin of someone who has died the option of donating the organs and tissues of the deceased. By signing a uniform donor card (in most states on the back of the driver's license), individuals indicate their wish to be a donor. However, at the time of death, the person's next-of-kin is still asked to sign a consent form for donation. In most instances if the next-of-kin refuses, the organs are not harvested. This underscores the importance that persons who wish to be donors notify their families of their decision so that their wishes will be honored at the time of death. An estimated 35% of potential donors have organs that are never used because family members refuse to give consent.[3]

SUMMARY

Improved methods of treating chronic and acute renal failure have lead to a decrease in mortality, and an improvement in quality of life. As with many other conditions, the treatment and transport of renal failure patients require sound knowledge of the common pathophysiologic changes observed in this disease process.

RENAL MEDICAL EMERGENCIES CASE STUDY

An air medical team was dispatched to a town 40 miles northeast of the home base to transport a patient from the emergency department of a small rural hospital. The patient was one of three young men found in a van parked at a rest stop just off the interstate. The two other patients were reportedly pronounced dead at the scene from an apparent carbon monoxide poisoning. The youths were traveling cross country from Texas to Pennsylvania when it is believed they decided to pull over for some sleep. A kerosene heater with an empty fuel tank was found in the van. All three men were found lying on a mattress on the floor. A state trooper found the young men after noticing that the van, which he noted 4 hours earlier while driving through the rest stop, was parked in the same position and appeared abandoned. Basic EMTs transported the patient to the emergency department of the local hospital. The attending physician called for air medical transport immediately.

The flight team arrived 30 minutes after the patient arrived. They were directed to a young white man in his early twenties lying flat on a backboard with high-flow oxygen being delivered by nonrebreather mask. One large-bore IV was in place, and the patient was receiving normal saline at a brisk rate. The flight team's initial assessment revealed the following information:

Airway: Patient was unresponsive, breathing on his own. The upper airway was clear and free of obstruction, but dried blood and vomitus were noted on the face and in the hair.

Breathing: Respiratory rate 12/min, slow, and shallow. Bilateral chest expansion was noted with equal breath sounds. No subcutaneous air or crepitus noted. Oxygen was being administered by non-rebreather mask per high flow.

Circulation: Skin was natural, warm, and dry with 1+ peripheral pulses bilaterally. Cardiac monitor in place was showing sinus rhythm in 120s; no ectopy noted.

Deficit: No movement to pain stimuli seen. Pupils were fixed and sluggishly reactive. Glasgow Coma Scale value was 3.

Extremities: No obvious signs of injury seen. Large erythematous area was noted over right buttocks and posterior thigh area.

Treatment at the referring emergency department included high flow oxygen and one IV of normal saline and an ECG. The ECG showed a prolonged PR interval and tall, peaked T waves. Blood pressure at the scene was reported as 80/50, pulse 70, respirations 12-14. The present blood pressure was 96/60, pulse 100, respirations 12. Bloods were drawn, placed on ice, and given to the flight team. The flight team electively orally intubated the patient for airway protection, and while intubating the patient, the flight team established a second IV and inserted a Foley catheter. The patient was hyperventilated after successful intubation, and an IV bolus of 500 ml was administered. The urine obtained from the Foley catheter was noted to be cherry red, suggestive of myoglobinuria secondary to rhabdomyolysis. Two ampules of sodium bicarbonate were added to the IV bag, and IV mannitol 50 g was hung. In-flight hyperventilation was maintained with 100% oxygen. Brisk diuresis was noted with a gradual clearing of the red pigmented urine. The blood pressure on arrival at the receiving hospital was 130/80; pulse was 110. Neurologic exam findings were unchanged. Laboratory data from the bloods drawn at the referring institution revealed a carbon monoxide level of 55%. The serum potassium level initially was 5.6. The chest x-ray film showed early signs of aspiration pneumonia, and the head CT scan showed diffuse cerebral ischemia. The patient was treated aggressively with hyperbaric oxygen treatments immediately and over the next few days; however, clinical improvement was slow. Acute renal failure was averted by the prompt recognition and treatment of myoglobinuria. The patient was discharged to a long-term rehabilitation facility 45 days after treatment with significant memory loss and personality changes.

REFERENCES

1. Health Care Financing Administration, Bureau of Data Management and Strategy: Pub No 386 892/21246, Washington, DC, 1995, GPO.
2. Llach F: *Clinical nephrology,* ed 3, Boston, 1993, Little, Brown.
3. National Kidney Foundation: *Twenty five facts about organ donation and transplantation,* 1996, New York, The Foundation.
4. Neumayer HN, Gellert J, Luft FG: Calcium antagonists and renal protection, *Renal Failure* 15(3):353-358, 1993.
5. Rao KV: Emergency renal problems. In Tintinalli JE, Ruiz E, Krome RL, editors: *Emergency medicine: a comprehensive study guide,* New York, 1996, McGraw-Hill.
6. Weems J; *Quick reference to renal critical care nursing,* Gaithersburg, Md, 1991, Aspen.
7. Zucchelli P, Zuccala A: Blood pressure control effects on the progression of chronic renal failure, *Renal Failure* 15(3): 339-342, 1993.

CHAPTER 24

Metabolic and Acid-Base Emergencies

COMPETENCIES

1. Recognize alterations in the regulation of body fluids and electrolytes.
2. Perform analysis and interpretation of arterial blood gases.
3. Perform specific interventions to correct abnormalities in fluid and electrolyte imbalances.

In transporting critically ill patients, the flight nurse is likely to see many types of metabolic system and acid-base balance abnormalities. Those systems must be supported in the transport of every patient and, frequently, the flight nurse must provide critical intervention to change the outcome of events. For this reason, it is essential that the air medical personnel have a solid understanding of the body's normal fluid and electrolyte composition and hormonal regulation of homeostasis, and know how to interpret blood gas results. Transport personnel must be able to call on fine-tuned assessment skills in addition to clinical knowledge to correctly identify abnormalities and institute appropriate therapy.

OVERVIEW OF FLUID AND ELECTROLYTE BALANCE

The body's water compartments are generally differentiated into intracellular fluid (ICF) and extracellular fluid (ECF) spaces. The ECF then further divides into functional and nonfunctional components. Functional components are the interstitial fluid space (located between tissue cells) and the plasma (the fluid within the vascular space). There is also "nonfunctional" space, comprising the following transcellular fluids: pleural, peritoneal, joint, cerebrospinal, and the fluid in connective tissue, cartilage, and bone.

Total Body Water

Total body water (TBW) is variable and decreases progressively with increasing age. In newborns, TBW is very high, sometimes exceeding 70% to 80% of total body weight. The newborn needs more water because of the large body surface area (more water is lost) and because of immature kidneys that cannot concentrate urine. The TBW of an adult man is about 60%, of an adult woman 50% to 55%, and of older adults about 50% of total body weight. The greater the amount of fat related to muscle, the lower the percentage of TBW.

Intracellular Fluid

About 30% to 35% of a person's body weight actually consists of ICF (about 23 L of water). Because muscle comprises 40% of TBW, much of ICF is inside muscle cells. Muscle is 75% water, and fat is only 6% to 10% water; therefore the ICF compartment in men is usually larger. Women's ICF is generally 25% to 30% of total body weight.

Extracellular Fluid

The ECF averages 25% to 30% of TBW in both men and women. In a 70-kg person, ECF is approximately 19 L. This can be broken down into approximately 9 L of interstitial fluid (10% to 15% of body weight), 3 L of water in connective tissue (4% to 5% of body weight), 3 L of plasma (3% to 5% of body weight), and 1 L of transcellular fluid (1% to 2% of body weight).

The ECF can increase and decrease very rapidly in critically ill and injured patients. Because the intravascular volume is maintained at relatively constant levels, most of the changes occur in the interstitial fluid. These changes are important because a 10% loss of interstitial fluid is serious and 20% is usually fatal. The interstitial fluid, which surrounds tissue cells, represents three fourths—the largest part—of the ECF. Cell metabolism frequently suffers in the initial periods after trauma or blood loss. Diffusion into the interstitial space is impaired if inadequate quantities of fluid are provided to restore the interstitial fluid volume to normal.

Approximately 25% of the ECF is plasma. An average adult man's plasma volume is about 2800 ml, along with 2100 ml red blood cells, to equal about 5 L of total blood volume. The more muscular the individual, the greater the blood volume; the more obese, the lower the blood volume.

The transcellular component is neither interstitial nor intravascular and accounts for only a small portion of the body's total fluid volume, seldom exceeding 400 to 500 ml. The amount of fluid in the intestinal tract averages 500 ml but can be as high as 2 to 3 L after eating. In patients with a severe ileus or peritonitis, fluid in the intestinal lumen may be more than 8 to 10 L. This leaking of fluid occurs at the expense of interstitial and plasma volume if insufficient replacement is given (Table 24-1).

TABLE 24-1

Approximate electrolyte composition in the various fluid compartmens (mEq/L)

Ions	Plasma	Interstitial fluid	Intracellular fluid
Na^+	140	143	10
K^+	4.5	4	135
Ca^{++}	5	3	10
Mg^{++}	2.5	2	25
	152.0	152	180
Cl^-	101	113	5
HCO_3^-	24	27	10
HPO_4^-	2	2	100
SO_4^-	1	1	5
Organic acid	6	7	10
Protein	18	2	50
	152	152	180

Third Space

The concept of a third space is used to define fluid that is not intracellular and does not function as ECF. For example, the edema that occurs after trauma, fluid in the injured bowel, and ascitic fluid is not readily available to the circulation but can constitute a large portion of TBW. Third-space fluid often accumulates at the expense of the other two fluid spaces. If fluid is moved into the third space rapidly, severe hypovolemia can result. It is important that the third-space loss be considered when planning fluid therapy. Third spacing, although poorly understood, normally occurs in people after extended fixed-wing flights. Consideration for adequate fluids must therefore be given to the flight personnel and to the patient for extended flight in pressurized aircraft.

REGULATION OF BODY FLUIDS AND ELECTROLYTES

Electrolytes

Electrolyte concentrations play a major role in cellular function and the distribution of water in the various fluid spaces. An electrolyte, measured as a milliequivalent, is the measure of the chemical activity, or the chemical combining power, of an ion. In each fluid compartment the cations and anions must be balanced to achieve chemical neutrality. The amount and composition of fluids in each compartment remains relatively stable, but each compartment is constantly replacing and exchanging ions. These changes occur by diffusion, osmosis, active transport, and filtration.

Diffusion, Filtration, Active Transport, and Osmosis

Diffusion refers to the movement of substances from an area of higher concentration to an area of lower concentration. *Filtration* describes the movement of water and substances from an area of higher pressure to an area of lower pressure. *Active transport* requires energy expenditure to move ions from an area of lower concentration to an area of higher concentration. For example, sodium ions tend to diffuse from ECF into ICF (area of higher concentration to an area of lower concentration), and potassium ions tend to diffuse from ICF into ECF. The sodium-potassium pump actively transports the ions against a concentration gradient. *Osmosis* refers to the shift of water that occurs through a membrane that is impermeable to dissolved substances. The water moves from the area of lower solute concentration to the area of higher solute concentration. *Osmolality* is defined as the amount of dissolved solutes or particles in a unit of water (kg H_2O). The terms *osmolality* and *osmolarity* are used interchangeably in the literature. Osmolality is generally used to describe body fluids, whereas *osmolarity* is used to describe fluids outside the body such as normal saline. Osmolarity describes the numbers of particles in a unit of water (L H_2O).

Distribution of fluid between plasma and the interstitial fluid space is largely determined by the osmolarity (osmotic pressure) present in the spaces. An increased osmolality indicates decreased body water, and vice versa. The normal serum range is 280 to 294 μosm/kg/H_2O. Intracellular and extracellular osmolality are always equal, and the measurement indicates overall body hydration and the concentration of body fluids. Water diffuses from areas of low osmolality to high, and ICF rapidly reflects extracellular imbalance because of osmotic equilibrium.

In normal circumstances, the osmolality of body fluids is kept constant because of the free diffusion of water among vascular, interstitial, and cellular spaces. Because of the distribution of ions in various fluid compartments, sodium is the major determinant of osmolality of ECF, and potassium is the major determinant of osmolality of ICF. Glucose and urea also contribute to ECF osmolality, but in different ways. Urea slowly permeates most cell membranes; thus an elevated blood urea nitrogen (BUN) level will eventually raise both ECF and ICF osmolality without a net fluid shift. Glucose moves into cells much more slowly than urea. It increases serum osmolality and draws water out of the intracellular spaces.

When patients are transported by air from small hospitals with limited laboratory resources, the flight nurse can use the following formula to calculate serum osmolality by simple lab results:

Serum osmolality (μosm/L) =

$$2\text{ Na} = \frac{\text{Glucose (mg/100 ml)}}{18} + \frac{\text{BUN (mg/100 ml)}}{3}$$

An osmolality greater than 320 μosm/kg in critically ill patients is usually not well tolerated, and greater than 350 μosm/kg may result in coma.[4] The calculated osmolarity will usually be 5 to 8 μosm/kg less than the measured serum osmolality because of anions, such as lactate, in the blood.

Fluid Regulation

Serum osmolality is controlled by maintaining a balance between salt and water intake and output. The lungs and skin are important regulators, but the kidneys are the major controllers of fluid balance. The kidneys do this by regulating (1) concentration of certain electrolytes and osmolality of body fluids, (2) the volume of extracellular fluids, (3) blood volume, and (4) blood pH.

Kidney function is in turn controlled by the following:

1. Circulating blood volume
2. Antidiuretic hormone (ADH) secretion from the pituitary, which is initiated by the following:
   a. High plasma osmolality
   b. Low circulating blood volume
   c. Certain drugs and chemicals
   d. Intermittent positive pressure breathing
3. Adrenal cortex hormones

Normally the kidneys either rid the body of extra water and electrolytes or conserve them and return them to the circulation. However, nonosmotic stimuli, such as hypovolemia or pain, can override the osmotic stimuli. Another nonosmotic stimulus is stress, which causes the kidneys to retain sodium and excrete potassium. Therefore stress contributes to many of the electrolyte imbalances seen in ill patients. Even a patient who is hypotonic, indicated by a low osmolality, can retain even more water and become water toxic.

Normal Fluid Losses. The body normally loses some of its fluid each day through insensible (exhaled air and through skin), urine, and feces loss. The usual amounts are as follows:

Insensible loss: 600 ml/24 hr
Urine loss: 500 to 1000 ml/24 hr
Fecal loss: less than 100 ml/24 hr

This amount of fluid loss increases if the body temperature rises (50 ml/24 hr/degree of fever) and if the rate and depth of respiration is increased. Water is also lost through the skin in the form of sweat, which contains 5 to 50 mEq/L of sodium. The sodium concentration increases with sweating and adrenal insufficiency. Sweat is always hypotonic and leads to water deficits disproportionate to sodium losses.

To maintain a normal internal body environment, a minimum of 500 to 1000 ml urine output every 24 hours is necessary. The term *oliguria* indicates a urine volume of less than 600 ml/24 hr. Oliguria occurs when there is a functional deficit of at least 30% in the extracellular fluid. Urinary electrolyte losses can vary a great deal. In a patient who is severely stressed (e.g., burns, trauma, sepsis), urine contains almost no sodium because the body is conserving it to attempt to maintain hydration. In conditions of sodium loading, concentrations of up to 80 mEq/L might be seen. There is an obligatory loss of at least 30 mEq/L of potassium per day, but as much as 60 to 80 mEq/L/day can be lost.

Patients with vomiting or diarrhea, or those with some type of enterostomy, lose fluid essentially the same composition as that of ECF. These deficits should be replaced with IV fluid having similar electrolyte concentration (Table 24-2).

As altitude increases, relative humidity decreases. Longer flights in pressurized aircraft can increase dehydration through insensible loss because of cabin humidities of as low as 0.5% after 1 hour. All water reservoirs should be checked for evaporative losses, and maintenance fluid for the patient should be given either orally or IV as appropriate.

Antidiuretic Hormone. Increased plasma osmolality is the primary stimulus for ADH release.[4] Disorders of fluid regulation occur when antidiuretic hormone is not regulating normal homeostasis of fluid volume. Normally, ADH increases renal water reabsorption, and water loss is decreased, leading to an increase in the volume of ECF. This increase removes the stimulus that activates the volume or osmotic receptors, and ADH release is decreased. Produced by the hypothalamus, the absence of ADH synthesis or the absence of its release, produces cen-

TABLE 24-2

Composition of gastrointestinal drainage

Source of drainage	Na^+ (mEq/L)	K^+ (mEq/L)	Cl^- (mEq/L)	HCO_3^- (mEq/L)	pH	Average total daily secretion in adult (ml)
Saliva	25	20	30	15	7.0	1500
Acid-producing stomach	40-80	5-10	60-130	0	1-4	2500
Bile	120-140	5-15	90-100	15-30	7.4-7.6	500
Pancreatic fistula or upper jejunum	120-140	5-15	69-90	15-30	7.4-7.6	700-1500
Lower ileum ileostomy or rectal diarrhea	120-140	5-15	90-100	15-30	7.4-7.6	1000-1500

tral diabetes insipidus (DI). If a defect in the renal tubules exists, nephrogenic DI is diagnosed.

Any mechanism that alters ADH synthesis or its release prevents the patient from conserving water, and diuresis of large volumes (from 6 to 24 L/day) of unconcentrated urine occurs. Precipitating factors of central DI include (1) idiopathic, (2) familial, (3) brain tumor, (4) head trauma, (5) neurosurgery, (6) infection, and (7) medications. Approximately 50% of central DI cases are idiopathic, but head trauma and neurosurgical procedures in the area of the hypothalamus and pituitary are increasing causes of central DI and tend to be temporary.

Precipitating factors of nephrogenic DI include (1) idiopathic, (2) familial, (3) primary renal disease, (4) secondary renal disease, (5) electrolyte abnormalities, and (6) medications. Nephrogenic DI is associated with primary renal diseases such as pylonephritis, obstructive uropathy, tubular necrosis, and cysts, in which there is an alteration in the function or structure of the collecting tubules and ducts or a decrease in the glomerular filtration rate. Secondary lesions in the renal system from myeloma, sarcoidosis, and sickle cell disease can also cause nephrogenic DI. Electrolyte abnormalities such as hypercalcemia and hypokalemia have been associated with nephrogenic DI as a result of interference with the hypertonic medullary interstitium that results in impaired action of ADH. Starvation states can result because with reduced protein intake there is not enough urea provided to sufficiently maintain the hypertonic medullary interstitium necessary to concentrate urine.

FLUID AND ELECTROLYTE ABNORMALITIES

Syndrome of Inappropriate Antidiuretic Hormone

In the syndrome of inappropriate antidiuretic hormone (SIADH) the synthesis and release of ADH continue even though there is a reduced serum osmolality. Normally when the plasma osmolality falls there is decreased release of ADH, which results in diuresis. Therefore the term *SIADH* is used for the condition of elevated ADH in the presence of conditions that would normally decrease ADH release. This causes TBW increase. The increased volume inhibits the secretion of renin and aldosterone. This causes a retention of free water and no sodium. Therefore the patient has a high fluid volume and low serum sodium. This excess ECF lowers the osmotic pressure of the ECF. Fluid then moves into the intracellular space because of osmosis because the cells now have the greatest concentration. Therefore the result of SIADH is an intracellular accumulation of fluid. Pitting edema rarely occurs because water is retained in the ICF and not in the ECF. Death usually occurs from overhydration in ICF before ECF expansion is large enough to create edema.

Precipitating factors of SIADH include (1) central nervous system disorders, (2) pulmonary problems, (3) endocrine disorders, (4) tumors, (5) idiopathic, and

(6) medications. Central nervous system disorders of SIADH include brain tumors, head trauma, skull fractures, subarachnoid hemorrhage, subdural hematoma, infections (meningitis, encephalitis, abscesses), Guillain-Barré syndrome, Rocky Mountain spotted fever, and delirium tremens. Pulmonary conditions that can precipitate SIADH include pneumonia, cystic fibrosis, cavitation abscesses, empyema, pneumothorax, asthma, and positive-pressure breathing. Endocrine disorders such as chronic adrenal insufficiency, hypopituitarianism, and hypothyroidism may cause SIADH. The small cell cancer of the lung is well-known for secreting ectopic ADH.[3] It is independent of normal physiologic controls and may cause SIADH. Finally, many drugs can precipitate SIADH; morphine, meperidine, and tricyclic drugs are a few of them. SIADH may be permanent or transient.

The clinical manifestations of SIADH appear as the degree of water intoxication progresses and according to the rapidity with which the water intoxication has occurred. The signs and symptoms of SIADH are related to the hyponatremia, fluid overload, and low plasma osmolality.[3] The patient with SIADH is usually asymptomatic until the serum sodium has fallen below 120 mEq/L. When the patient has a serum sodium level of approximately 115 to 120 mEq/L, the symptoms are anorexia, nausea, headache, and weakness. As the serum sodium level decreases below 115 mEq/L, the patient experiences personality changes, irritability, lethargy, confusion, decreased reflexes, positive Babinski's sign, hypothermia, seizures, and coma. The cardiac monitor may reveal premature ventricular contractions as a sign of hypokalemia. Laboratory studies will reflect the hemodilution or water intoxication state with a low BUN, low creatinine, low serum sodium, and low serum osmolality.

Fluid Redistribution

Some disease processes cause fluid to be redistributed within the various body compartments. Because these fluids move out of the ECF, they cannot contribute to normal fluid balance, even though the electrolyte content of the redistributed fluid remains identical to the ECF. Often the amount of loss is much larger than that caused by intake and output imbalance. The redistribution of fluid does not appear as a change in the patient's weight or intake-and-output fluid record. As a result, detection is by physiologic changes in organ function.

Patients with mechanical obstruction or ileus can have many liters of ECF sequestered (third spacing). As an example, as little as 1 mm thickness of edema fluid is equivalent to several liters of ECF. The presence of an air-fluid level on an upright abdominal x-ray indicates that a minimum of 1500 ml is within the lumen of the intestine. Normally 8 to 10 L of gastrointestinal fluid are secreted each day. These secretions contain potassium, hydrogen ions, or bicarbonate in large amounts; thus depletion of the fluid from the appropriate fluid space can lead to potassium deficit and metabolic abnormalities along with significant volume depletion.

Critically ill patients often have impaired mechanisms for regulation of fluid balance. Examples would be injury to the hypothalamus so that body water regulation is impaired, injuries to the gastrointestinal (GI) tract that would lead to abnormal absorption of water, or kidney damage leading to problems with excretion of water and waste products. Many times all of these controls are damaged. Diagnosis is made more difficult because there are no laboratory tests that directly measure ECF volume or TBW. Tests that are available, such as electrolyte determinations, may be misleading and of little value. Consequently, unless there is a life-threatening abnormality that requires immediate correction, it is wise to watch for trends in laboratory results rather than basing all treatment on one set of laboratory tests.

Volume Depletion

Symptoms of volume depletion occur once the ECF loss has reached 25% to 30%. Symptoms such as postural hypotension, weak pulses, and tachycardia all indicate severe losses. Other indications of volume loss are apathy, weakness, anorexia, nausea, abdominal distention, ileus, decreased skin turgor, and ocular tension. A decreased urinary output (UO), high urine osmolality, and low urine sodium also indicate hypovolemia. Specific gravity may often be inaccurate because the results are altered if proteins and bacteria are present. With shifting of fluid from other compartments and the action of ADH, the patient becomes pale, and the skin becomes cool and diaphoretic. As acidosis progresses, the fluid pH cannot be compensated. There is more peripheral shutdown and more tissue selection for circulation, leading to deterioration in the patient's condition. In fact, the patient will certainly die if appropriate treatment is not instituted.

Volume Excess

Edema is generally considered to be a sign of volume excess, but in a critically ill patient it can be a misleading finding. Although volume excess can lead to the development of edema, other conditions can also cause it. Tissue damage from burns, contusions, and pancreatitis causes damage to capillary permeability, and protein leaks into the interstitial space (third-space loss). This can also occur with hyponatremia, hypotension, and hypoxia. Edema is obvious, although actual fluid volume in the vascular space is depleted. Rales and rhonchi in auscultating breath sounds may be a finding, with fluid excess in which edema does not appear obvious. In addition, the fluid volume necessary to promote adequate organ function may also be enough to produce edema. Generally, urine outputs of greater than 100 ml/hr indicate that the body is trying to rid itself of excess ECF. This should not be matched with an equally high IV replacement; in fact, the IV rate should be lowered, unless a diagnosis of DI has been rendered.

In summary, the optimal ECF is achieved when distribution of fluid between the vascular space and the interstitial space provides enough venous return to the heart so that a sufficient cardiac output can be maintained. Evidence of this is seen in adequate organ perfusion indicated by improved vital signs, mental function, UO, and signs of improved peripheral perfusion (decreased diaphoresis, increased warmth, lack of duskiness, improved capillary return, and stronger pulses).

Hyponatremia

A deficiency of the amount of sodium in relation to the amount of water in the extracellular compartment is called *hyponatremia.* A level of less than 135 mEq/L indicates a hyponatremic state. Hyponatremia may occur in association with low volume, normal volume, or high volume.[11] Causes of hyponatremia are dilutional, sodium loss, and factition. In dilutional cases, the TBW is increased, causing an expanded ECF. Some causes are as follows:

1. Excessive water intake orally or parenterally without enough salt intake
2. Congestive heart failure
3. Cirrhosis
4. SIADH
5. Acute renal failure with oliguria
6. Acute renal injury or sepsis

Sodium loss manifests as abnormal renal loss or extrarenal conditions that lead to dehydration and a resulting decreased ECF, caused by:

1. Severe diarrhea or vomiting, or sweating
2. Adrenal insufficiency (infrequent)
3. Salt wasting because of renal lesion (rare)

For example, factitious hyponatremia can be exemplified by hyperglycemia.

Some of the most frequent causes of actual sodium loss from the body are excessive diarrhea, sweating, or vomiting. In diabetes mellitus, serum sodium concentrations may be very low without excessive loss of sodium from the body and no increase of TBW, causing a "factitious hyponatremia." Each 100 mg/ml of glucose concentration above normal causes serum osmolality to increase by about 5.5 μosm/kg/H_2O, which reduces sodium concentration by about 2.2 mEq/L. The increased serum osmolality pulls water from the ICF into the extracellular space to dilute the sodium present. Once hyperglycemia is corrected, the ECF volume returns to normal, and serum sodium usually increases toward normal.

Signs and symptoms of hyponatremia are associated with increases in TBW. However, sudden decreases in serum sodium can cause neuromuscular irritability, restlessness, and convulsions, as described in the subsection on SIADH.

Hypernatremia

The cause of *hypernatremia,* a level of sodium greater than 145 mEq/L, is decreased body water resulting from poor fluid intake, excessive water losses, or sometimes following the use of osmotic diuretics. Occasionally increased ECF volume with sodium retention may also cause hypernatremia. Predisposing conditions are impaired thirst mechanism as a result of coma, response to the osmotic stimulus seen in diabetic ketoacidosis (DKA), nonketotic coma, mannitol usage, or administration of hypertonic tube feedings.

In patients in a dehydrated state, symptoms such as excessive thirst in responsive patients, mental irritability, fair to poor skin turgor, dry mucous membranes, fatigue, weakness, and negative fluid balance may be seen because of decreased ECF. In edematous states resulting from increased ECF, there may be weight gain, changes in mental status, and dyspnea.

Hypokalemia

A serum potassium level of less than 3.5 mEq/L is caused by increased potassium losses from the body, intracellular shifting of potassium secondary to alkalosis, and decreased intake. A rise of 0.1 in pH generally causes a 0.5 mEq/L fall in serum potassium. In alkalosis, as hydrogen moves out of the cell to bring the pH towards normal, potassium moves into the cell to maintain electroneutrality.[10] Therefore a low potassium state occurs in the ECF. Increased losses of potassium from the body can occur with excessive diuresis, vomiting, severe diarrhea, laxative abuse, severe trauma, excessive sweating, or excessive steroid use. Patients in DKA may have falsely high serum potassium levels because the potassium is driven out of the cells. During the osmotic diuresis in DKA, potassium is excreted. With insulin administration, glucose enters the cell and takes potassium back in with it. As the acidosis is corrected and the pH rises toward normal, serum potassium decreases and replacement is then generally necessary. These changes occur rapidly; careful continued assessment of the patient in ketoacidosis is essential. Decreased potassium intake may occur in alcoholics, older adults, or in hospitalized patients.

Symptoms usually occur because of disturbed muscle (GI, skeletal, and cardiac) function, and decreased deep tendon reflexes may be present. Hypokalemia should be suspected in patients who are weak, have a severe ileus, or have digitalis toxicity. The ECG typically shows low-voltage QRS complexes, flattened T waves (seen best in limb leads), depressed ST segments, U waves (seen best in precordial leads), and a prolonged QT interval. Associated dysrhythmias such as premature atrial contractions (PACs), premature ventricular contractions (PVCs), paroxysmal atrial tachycardia (PAT), sinus bradycardia, atrioventricular (AV) blocks, ventricular tachycardia, and fibrillation are the result of increased myocardial irritability that results from hypokalemia.

Hyperkalemia

A serum potassium concentration greater than 5.5 mEq/L is caused by the inability of the kidneys to excrete potassium ions because of tubule damage, salt depletion, increased potassium load, or decreased renal perfusion. The relation between plasma and cellular potassium is complex and is influenced by several factors, but acid-base balance is the most important. Hyperkalemia is most likely to occur because of oliguria, tissue breakdown, or excessive potassium intake. Each kilogram of lean muscle contains about 100 mEq of potassium. Consequently tissue breakdown after trauma or sepsis can release very large amounts of potassium into the blood. A similar problem may develop with hemolysis of blood from transfusion reactions. Hemolysis of blood as it is drawn from a patient may cause a factitious hyperkalemia. Under normal circumstances about 90% to 95% of potassium lost from the body is excreted from the urine; thus there is an inverse relationship between the serum potassium and UO. A low UO (oliguria) eventually leads to an elevated serum potassium, and a high UO usually leads to hypokalemia. Serum levels of potassium indicate hyperkalemia, but it should be suspected with oliguria, renal failure, and/or excessive tissue breakdown. Symptoms of hyperkalemia include flaccid paralysis of skeletal and smooth muscle, and ECG changes (PR lengthens, QRS widens, and P waves disappear).

Hypocalcemia

There are approximately 1 to 2 kg of calcium, 98% of which is skeletal, in the average adult body. The remaining calcium, located in the ECF, is critical for a variety of body functions, especially cardiac and neuromuscular function. The ECF is kept remarkably constant, the normal range being 8.8 to 10.4 mg/dl. Total serum calcium includes the three forms of calcium in the body (ionized, protein-bound, and complexed). The ionized calcium is the form primarily responsible for the signs and symptoms of hypocalcemia and hypercalcemia. Albumin levels alter the total calcium level. Therefore a corrected calcium concentration should be calculated to determine clinically significant calcium levels.[14] Corrected Ca^{++} = total Ca^{++} + 0.8 (4.0 − serum albumin).

Hypocalcemia occurs when the serum calcium level is below 8.5 mg/dl. The disorder may be seen with parathyroidism, osteomalacia, acute pancreatitis, chronic renal failure, vitamin D or magnesium deficiency, hyperphosphatemia, and increased thyrocalcitonin.

Decreased ionized calcium levels are seen most frequently in patients with hyperphosphatemia and alkalosis and in those who have massive, rapid transfusions, especially if shock is present. Banked blood contains citrate, which binds ionized calcium. Usually the body can mobilize ionized calcium easily and rapidly, but if the patient is in shock, the process is impeded, and ionized calcium levels fall below those needed for optimal cardiovascular function. One gram of calcium chloride IV is sometimes recommended to be given for every 3 to 4 units of blood given.

Decreased ionized calcium increases neuromuscular excitability and can cause tetany leading to peripheral and circumoral paresthesia, carpopedal spasm, intestinal cramps, and hyperactive deep tendon reflexes. Progressively more serious effects are seizures, bronchospasm, laryngospasm, Chvostek's and Trousseau's signs, and increasing QT intervals. Decreased ionized calcium also reduces the strength of muscle contraction, especially that of the myocardium. Levels less than 7.0 mg/dl are associated with a poor prognosis.

Hypercalcemia

The causes of hypercalcemia are increased mobilization of calcium from the bone by hyperparathyroidism, immobilization, thyrotoxicosis, excessive calcium intake, renal tubular acidosis, and chronic thiazide therapy. The most important concern for flight nurses is that patients taking digitalis preparations will have an enhanced calcium effect. ECG changes may include shortened ST segments, heart blocks, dysrhythmias, and cardiac arrest. Other less serious symptoms include anorexia, nausea, constipation, personality changes, lethargy, and coma. The major complications of hypercalcemia include neuropathies, renal calculi, and ventricular fibrillation.

ENDOCRINE FUNCTION

Overview

Regulation of the various organ systems of the body with their highly specialized functions is necessary to maintain homeostasis. The endocrine system is controlled by the metabolites in the ECF and also by the nervous system. Together the endocrine and nervous systems regulate the metabolic activities. The endocrine organs and their hormones of critical importance are listed in Table 24-3.

Hormones are chemical substances synthesized by groups of specialized cells. When needed they are secreted directly into the bloodstream and then transported by the circulatory system to target tissues. There they exert a physiologic effect that assists in the maintenance of homeostasis. When the physiologic effect has been accomplished, the endocrine organ diminishes the hormonal secretion. This control mechanism is called *negative feedback.* Once the physiologic effect has diminished, the endocrine gland is stimulated to once again secrete the hormone. Thus hormonal secretion is dependent on bodily requirements. Finally, the neural stimulation is diminished when the physiologic effect is noted by the nervous system. Homeostasis is maintained by this feedback system and allows adaptation to an excess or deficit of hormones. Life-threatening endocrine emergencies are infrequent, occurring only when the nervous system and negative feedback mechanism capabilities are exceeded. This usually occurs in the patient with known endocrine disease who is subjected to physiologic and psychologic stressors such as trauma, infection, or loss of a loved one.

Hormone abnormalities that cause crises such as adrenal crisis and thyroid storm are relatively rare in

TABLE 24-3

Nondiabetic endocrine system of significance, in summary

Endocrine gland and hormone	Principal actions	Hypersecretion	Hyposecretion
POSTERIOR PITUITARY			
Vasopressin Antidiuretic hormone	Elevates blood pressure through action on arterioles; promotes reabsorption of water by action on renal collecting ducts	Syndrome of inappropriate antidiuretic hormone	Diabetes insipidus
ADRENAL CORTEX			
Mineralocorticoid Aldosterone	Reabsorption of sodium; excretion of potassium	Conn's syndrome	Chronic adrenal insufficiency (Addison's disease); acute adrenal insufficiency (adrenal crisis)
Glucocorticoid Cortisol	Carbohydrate, protein, and fat metabolism; enhances stress response; antiinflammatory	Cushing's syndrome	Chronic adrenal insufficiency (Addison's disease); acute adrenal insufficiency (adrenal crisis)
ADRENAL MEDULLA			
Catecholamines Epinephrine	"Fight or flight" response to stress; actions on heart muscle, smooth muscle, and arterioles; increase serum glucose	Pheochromocytoma	Slight or no effect
Norepinephrine	Similar to epinephrine except not as intense on cardiac and metabolic functions; increase peripheral resistance	Pheochromocytoma	Slight or no effect
THYROID			
Thyroxine and triiodothyronine	Increase metabolic rate	Hyperthyroidism (hyperthyroid crisis, thyroid storm)	Hypothyroidism (myxedema coma, hypothyroid crisis)

patients who are transported. Patients with these diseases usually have chronic conditions. Once their disease is diagnosed, their conditions are usually well managed with medications. All of the hormone actions and fluid balance are interrelated.

Understanding the hormones is facilitated by dividing them into three functional categories: (1) releasing and inhibiting hormones, (2) tropic hormones, and (3) peripheral hormones (Table 24-4). Choreography of these hormones allows adaptation of the body to stress, as especially seen by the "fight or flight" set (catecholamines) (Fig. 24-1).

The releasing and inhibiting hormones are a group of hormones synthesized only by the hypothalamus and have only one target tissue, the anterior pituitary. When a physiologic effect is needed, the hypothalamus secretes the appropriate releasing or inhibiting hormone, which travels to the anterior pi-

TABLE 24-4

Hormonal functional categories

Hypothalamic releasing hormones	Pituitary tropic hormones	Peripheral hormones
Corticotropin-releasing hormone (CRH)	Adrenocorticotropin hormone (ACTH)	Cortisol, aldosterone
Thyrotropin-releasing hormone (TRH)	Thyroid-stimulating hormone (TSH)	Thyroxine, triiodothyronine

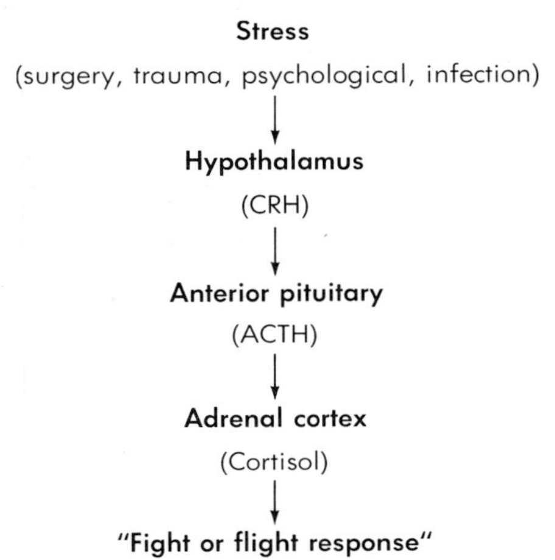

Fig. 24-1. Stimulation of cortisol secretion.

tuitary. The anterior pituitary in turn secretes the appropriate hormone (tropic hormone) to assist in exerting the needed physiologic effect and thus maintain homeostasis.

The tropic hormones are released into the bloodstream and carried to the appropriate target endocrine gland. The tropic hormones of importance are adrenocorticotropin (ACTH) and the thyrotropin-stimulating hormone (TSH).

Peripheral hormones act directly on the peripheral tissues to exert their physiologic effect. These hormones are secreted mostly by specific glands, but oxytocin and ADH are secreted by the posterior pituitary. The other hormones in this category are glucocorticoids (cortisol), mineralocorticoids (aldosterone), catecholamines (epinephrine, norepinephrine), thyroxine (T_4), triiodothyronine (T_3), ADH, glucagon, and insulin.

The glucocorticoids regulate fats, proteins, and carbohydrates. Cortisol is important in the stress response ("fight or flight") because of its physiologic effects on carbohydrate metabolism, the antiinflammatory response, and blood pressure maintenance. The catecholamines, released during the stress response, induce vasoconstriction. The blood pressure is elevated and cannot be maintained without the presence of cortisol. Mineralocorticoids were named for their influence on extracellular electrolytes, especially sodium and potassium. Aldosterone regulates the conservation of sodium, excretion of potassium, and maintenance of adequate ECF volume. The target tissues of aldosterone are the renal tubules, sweat glands, salivary glands, and intestine.

The physiologic effects of norepinephrine and epinephrine are related to the adrenergic receptors in the organs. Epinephrine excites alpha and beta receptors equally. Norepinephrine primarily excites alpha receptors but stimulates beta receptors slightly. Alpha-receptor site stimulation causes generalized vasoconstriction, pupil dilation, intestinal and bladder sphincter contraction, decreased gastrointestinal motility, pilomotor contraction, and decreased insulin secretion. $Beta_1$-receptor site stimulation causes increased heart rate, increased cardiac contractility, and lipolysis. $Beta_2$-receptor stimulation causes vasodilation in skeletal and cardiac muscles, bronchodilation, glycogenesis in liver and muscles, uterine relaxation, and decreased peristalsis in the GI tract.

The target sites of epinephrine include all body cells, especially the vascular beds and smooth muscles. Epinephrine provides for the "fight or flight" response to stress. It stimulates both alpha- and beta-adrenergic receptor sites. It has a greater effect on cardiac activity than norepinephrine, and therefore cardiac output is increased more with epinephrine than it is with norepinephrine. Norepinephrine has a greater vasoconstrictor activity in muscles, and therefore increases peripheral vascular resistance and arterial pressure more than epinephrine.

The thyroid hormones' target sites are all body cells. They increase metabolism except in the brain, spleen, lungs, retina, and testes. The pancreatic hormones from the islet cells of Langerhans produce glucagon and insulin, which raise and lower glucose levels. Abnormalities of these hormones are *frequently* seen by air medical transport teams. Normal activity of fluid, hormonal, and acid-base balance does not occur without this integrated balance of hormonal programming.

PANCREATIC HORMONE ABNORMALITIES

Hypoglycemic Coma

The brain receives glucose by dietary intake, glucogenesis, or glucogenolysis. Low blood glucose levels leave the brain vulnerable to irreversible damage because glucose is the primary energy source for the brain. Inadequate glucose stimulates the sympathetic nervous system to increase secretion of catecholamines and glucocorticoids, which increases blood glucose levels along with glucagon.

Hypoglycemia is characterized by a blood glucose level less than 50 mg%. It is the *most common cause of coma* in the diabetic patient and is the most common endocrine medical emergency.[12] It may be life threatening and requires prompt treatment. Rapid onset of hypoglycemia activates an adrenergic response, eliciting symptoms of hunger, tremulousness, palpitations, tachycardia, sweating, and pallor. In some persons symptoms may not develop even when the glucose level falls to as low as 30 to 35 mg/dl.[5] Slowly developing hypoglycemia is characterized by behavioral changes, irritability, and confusion. Many times the hypoglycemic symptoms resemble the behaviors of persons who have been drinking alcohol.[5] Of hypoglycemic patients, 12% have seizures.

Diabetic Ketoacidosis

Diabetic ketoacidosis is a life-threatening complication of insulin deficiency resulting in hyperglycemia, ketone formation, and metabolic acidosis. DKA has a 5% mortality rate.[7] The incidence of DKA requiring hospitalization has increased 21% in the past decade.[13] More than 160,000 hospital admissions can be attributed to DKA.[5] Prolonged or permanent brain damage is likely associated with the duration and severity of the low blood glucose.[12]

Precipitating factors of DKA are (1) endogenous insulin failure (previously unknown diabetic, pancreatitis, idiopathic, autoimmune); (2) hormonal insulin antagonist (Cushing's syndrome, hyperthyroidism, pheochromocytoma, acromegaly); (3) exogenous insulin failure (diet or exercise change, noncompliance, inadequate dosage or type of prescribed insulin, insulin antibodies); (4) increased insulin requirements (stress response, infection, pregnancy, myocardial infarction [MI], surgery, trauma, acute psychiatric illness); and (5) drug therapy (thiazide diuretics, glucocorticoids, phenytoin, sympathomimetics, diazoxide). The most frequent precipitating factors of DKA are noncompliance, infection, lack of or inadequate dose of insulin, and new-onset diabetes.[7]

Insulin deficiency affects carbohydrate, protein, and fat metabolism. Insulin deficiency causes decreased peripheral utilization of glucose because insulin is needed to transport the glucose into the cell. The liver increases gluconeogenesis in response to the starving cells. Fat metabolism is altered also, as evidenced by increased lipolysis and release of large amounts of fatty acids. These fatty acids are partially oxidized, which results in ketoacid formation. Protein metabolism alteration is characterized by increased catabolism. The altered metabolism results in hyperglycemia and ketoacidosis.

Hyperglycemia induces hyperosmolality, as evidenced by a 100-point rise in glucose, resulting in a 5-point rise in osmolality.[6] The hyperglycemia causes an osmotic diuresis resulting in a TBW deficit and electrolyte losses. With increased osmolality from hyperglycemia, sodium moves to the extracellular compartment and is lost in the diuresis. Therefore the patient in DKA will be hyponatremic.

Metabolic acidosis occurs as a result of the ketoacid formation. Acidosis shifts potassium from the intracellular to the extracellular space, resulting in a serum hyperkalemia. For each 0.1 decrease in pH, the potassium is artificially increased approximately 0.6. However, there is a total body deficit of potassium as a result of the osmotic diuresis. This is evident on rehydration of the patient as serum hypokalemia develops. The potassium deficit after DKA has been corrected may be in the range of 5 to 10 mEq/kg body weight.[7] In addition, the fluid deficit may be greater than 6 L or 10% of body weight for adults and 50 to 100 ml/kg in children.[6] Normal potassium is a grave finding and is usually only found when cardiac arrest is imminent.

In DKA, the patient has flushed dry skin, dry mucous membranes, decreased skin turgor, variable levels of consciousness (related to degree of acidity and hyperosmolarity), tachypnea, Kussmaul's respirations, acetone odor to the breath, vomiting, tachycardia (bradycardia if taking beta-blockers or an MI is in progress), and hypotension. If alert, the patient may complain of nausea and abdominal pain.

Laboratory findings when available reveal hyperglycemia (>250 mg/dl), glycosuria, metabolic acidosis, ketonuria, hyperkalemia, hyponatremia, and hyperosmolality. An elevated white blood cell (WBC) count reveals an infection.

Nonketotic Hypertonicity

Nonketotic hypertonicity (NKH) in diabetes is a life-threatening emergency that frequently occurs in older patients (mean age between 57 and 69 years) with type II diabetes or undiagnosed diabetes.[8] Although it shares many similarities with DKA, NKH does not present with ketosis[5]; however, some patients with NKH may develop a degree of ketosis. In the last 15 years the mortality rate associated with NKH has been reported as between 10% and 17%.[8]

Precipitating factors of NKH are (1) inadequate insulin secretion or action; (2) increased insulin requirements (stress response, infection, pancreatitis, uremia, burns, MI); (3) medications (thiazide diuretics, glucocorticoids, phenytoin, sympathomimetics, diazoxide, chlorpromazine, cimetidine, propranolol, immunosuppressives); and (4) supplemental parenteral and enteral feedings. Infection is the most common precipitating factor (32% to 60%) of NKH, with pneumonia (40% to 60%) being the most common precipitating infection.[8]

The relative insulin deficiency of NKH impairs glucose transport into the cells. However, it is theorized there is enough insulin present to prevent the development of ketones but not enough to prevent hyperglycemia.[6] The hyperglycemia produces a hyperosmolar state. An osmotic diuresis then occurs as a result of the hyperosmolarity. Dehydration and electrolyte losses then follow. The severe state of dehydration causes a decreased rate of glomerular filtration, which in turn decreases the amount of glucose excreted by the kidney. The level of blood glucose and serum osmolality increase further and a self-perpetuating cycle ensues.

The history of the patient with NKH includes the presence of a precipitating factor such as type II diabetes, old age, and preexisting cardiac or renal disease, or both. The patient reports weakness, thirst, frequent urination, and weight loss. The patient has signs and symptoms of extreme dehydration. The physical examination reveals flushed, dry skin, dry mucous membranes, decreased skin turgor, soft eyeballs, postural hypotension, altered level of consciousness, seizures, hemiparesis, tremors, nystagmus, tachycardia, hypotension, tachypnea, and shallow respirations. The patient may be obtunded when serum osmolality is greater than 350 μosm/L.[8]

Laboratory findings, when available, indicate glycosuria without ketonuria, hyperglycemia (greater than 600 mg%), hyperosmolality, hemoconcentration, elevated BUN, hypokalemia, and mild or no metabolic acidosis.

ACID-BASE REGULATION

The third component of maintaining neutral and optimal physiologic body function is acid-base balance. It is closely related to renal function and respiratory status, as well as the overall fluid and electrolyte status of the patient. A thorough understanding and confidence in interpreting arterial blood gas (ABG) results are imperative for flight nurses, because disastrous mistakes can result from carrying out incorrect treatment if blood gas analysis is incorrect.

Arterial blood gas values are obtained for two main reasons: (1) to determine the oxygenation of the blood, and (2) to show the status of acid-base regulation in the body. Results must be closely correlated with many factors, including interval since the test was done, any treatments instituted since the test results were obtained, the actual physical assessment of the patient, and any possibility of laboratory error.

Arterial blood is preferred because it gives the end result of pulmonary function as well as the composite acid-base status of all parts of the body. Venous blood may be used, but results from such samples provide information mostly about the extremity from which they were drawn.

Oxygenation

Table 24-5 illustrates that accepted arterial oxygen pressure (PaO_2) and oxygen saturation (SaO_2) levels vary depending on the altitude at which the patient is located. Patients with PaO_2 less than normal should receive supplemental oxygen therapy. What percentage of oxygen to use must be based on ABG results or pulse oximetry values, how much supplemental oxygen had been used previously, the patient's pathophysiologic processes, and physical presentation. Inspired oxygen content, ventilatory status, and the barometric pressure can vary the alveolar pressure of oxygen (PAO_2); thus it is important to take into account any altitude changes that will occur in transport. At increasing altitudes, more oxygen is indicated and must be correlated with oxygen deficits in relation to previous therapy. Since the advent of pulse oximeters (SpO_2), SaO_2 values are available in the prehospital setting. PaO_2 values may be estimated from the SpO_2 values of the pulse oximeter[2] (see box below). Delivery of oxygen is related to blood flow and hemoglobin levels.[1] SpO_2 values estimate only one component of the delivery of oxygen and thus sole reliance on the pulse oximeter can be misleading.[1] In addition, SpO_2 does not reflect acid-base status. Therefore the patient must be continually assessed for signs of adequate perfusion and oxygenation (mentation, skin color and condition, and pulse strength). It is essential that aggressive oxygen therapy be used for patients in any type of shock state to offset the pathophysiologic processes occurring. As people age, their blood gas values tend to move toward the lower normal range. This must also be kept in mind when planning oxygen therapy for any patient.[2]

TABLE 24-5

Normal blood gas results

	Arterial	Mixed venous
NORMAL BLOOD GAS VALUES (SEA LEVEL)		
pH	7.35-7.45	7.31-7.41
PaO_2	80-100	35-40
SaO_2	95% or greater	70%-75%
$PaCO_2$	35-45	41-51
HCO_3^-	22-26	22-26
Base excess	−2-+2	−2-+2
NORMAL BLOOD GAS VALUES (DENVER—5000 FEET ABOVE SEA LEVEL)		
pH	7.35-7.45	7.31-7.41
PaO_2	65-75	35-45
SaO_2	92%-94%	65%-75%
$PaCO_2$	34-38	40-44
HCO_3^-	22-26	22-26
Base excess	−2-+2	−2-+2

Definition of Terms

An *acid* is a substance that donates hydrogen (H^+) ions. A *base* is a substance that accepts hydrogen ions. When a base combines with an acid, a salt is formed.

ESTIMATION OF PO_2 VALUES FROM PULSE OXIMETRY

SO_2	PO_2
0.98	100
0.90	60
0.75	40
0.50	27

pH is the measurement of the negative logarithm of hydrogen ion concentration. Because it has a logarithmic derivation, it is important to understand that very small changes in pH represent marked changes in H^+ ion concentration. Measurement of the pH is the only laboratory method to determine if the body's acid-base regulation is being maintained in the necessary physiologic range.

The pH is determined by two factors: (1) processes that raise or lower the H^+ concentration, and (2) the body's buffer systems that respond to changes in the H^+ concentration to maintain the pH of body fluids at a normal value. There are several buffers, but the carbonic acid (H_2CO_3)–bicarbonate (HCO_3) buffer system is the most important for fine-tuning adjustments in the body pH. It requires adequate renal, pulmonary, and hemodynamic function to make the necessary adjustments.

Buffer systems usually consist of a weak acid or base in equilibrium with the salt of that acid or base:

Weak base + Strong acid = Neutral salt + Weak acid

If strong acids are released into the bloodstream, sodium bicarbonate (a weak base) will combine with the H^+ of the strong acid to form carbonic acid (a weaker acid) and a neutral salt. If the strong metabolic acid is lactic acid, this is the equation:

$$\leftrightharpoons \underset{\text{(Weak acid)}}{H_2CO_3} + \underset{\text{(Neutral salt)}}{\text{Nalactate}}$$

The hydrogen contributed to any strong acid can combine with HCO_3^- to form carbonic acid (H_2CO_3). This dissociates to release water (H_2O) and carbon dioxide (CO_2). For the carbonic acid system to function correctly, CO_2 must be delivered to the lungs. It must then cross the alveolar-capillary membrane into the alveolar space and be removed by ventilation. The two major factors that decrease the ability to efficiently remove the excess acid and change the body's pH are poor tissue or pulmonary circulation and inadequate ventilation.

The pH range for optimal body functioning is 7.35 to 7.45. *Acidemia* indicates an acid condition of the blood: the blood pH is less than 7.35. *Alkalemia* indicates an alkaline condition of the blood: the blood pH is greater than 7.45. *Acidosis* is the process that causes acidemia. *Alkalosis* is the process that causes alkalemia. *PaO_2* indicates the partial pressure of oxygen dissolved in the arterial blood. *$PaCO_2$* indicates the partial pressure of CO_2 dissolved in the arterial blood.

Respiratory Parameters

The $PaCO_2$ result is the respiratory parameter of the ABG results. CO_2 in the body comes from several sources. There are small amounts in the inspired air, and CO_2 is also a by-product of food metabolism. When the CO_2 in the body's cells exceeds the normal arterial value, it spills over into the plasma. In the plasma, some CO_2 combines with water to form carbonic acid (H_2CO_3), but the majority of CO_2 remains as a dissolved gas in the plasma. Excess CO_2 is then eliminated in one of two ways. Once formed, carbonic acid dissociates into hydrogen ions and bicarbonate. Much of the hydrogen is buffered by forming a loose association with the plasma proteins. It is also eliminated by the kidneys in the form of ammonia (NH_4^+). It is important to remember that this is a slow process that occurs over several days. The second, more efficient means of CO_2 elimination is via the respiratory system. Through ventilation, CO_2 is eliminated as a gas within minutes to hours (Fig. 24-2). It is helpful to think of CO_2 as an acid substance. As CO_2 continues to increase, the patient becomes acidotic, and pH therefore decreases.

The relationship between $PaCO_2$ and pH is shown in the box. However, if a more precise calculation is needed, the expected pH for any $PaCO_2$ value can be calculated as shown in the box. This calculation helps to determine if abnormal ABG results are caused totally or partially by respiratory abnormalities.

Respiratory Abnormalities

Respiratory Acidosis. The $PaCO_2$ is greater than 45 mm Hg at sea level, or greater than 38 mm Hg above 5000 feet with the pH less than 7.35. The cause of respiratory acidosis is hypoventilation, whether it has an acute or chronic etiology. Some examples of causes of respiratory acidosis are (1) obstructive lung diseases, such as emphysema,

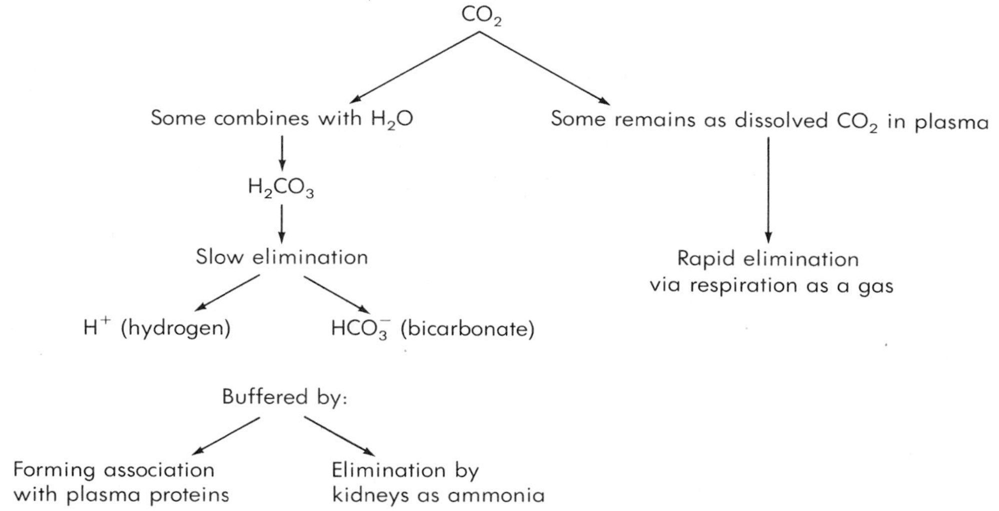

Fig. 24-2. Carbon dioxide elimination.

asthma, and chronic bronchitis; (2) conditions leading to respiratory center depression, such as head injury, oversedation, and drug overdose; (3) neuromuscular disease; and (4) inadequate mechanical ventilation. The treatment of respiratory acidosis is to improve ventilation by whatever means appropriate for the condition causing it (for example, increase bronchial hygiene, and improve oxygenation, suctioning, intubation, and hyperventilation).

Respiratory Alkalosis. The $Paco_2$ is less than 35 mm Hg at sea level or less than 34 mm Hg above 5000 feet, and the pH is greater than 7.45. The cause of respiratory alkalosis is hyperventilation. Some conditions leading to this are (1) hypoxia in the initial stages of lung disease, (2) high altitude, (3) nervousness and anxiety, (4) pulmonary embolus or fibrosis, (5) pregnancy, (6) central nervous system (CNS) injury, and (7) excessive mechanical ventilation. Treatment is to decrease the patient's minute volume by reassurance, sedation, and ventilatory control.

Metabolic Parameters

The bicarbonate value reported in blood gas results is the indicator of the body's metabolic processes. When these processes lead to the accumulation of acids or loss of bicarbonate in the body, bicar-

RELATIONSHIP BETWEEN $Paco_2$ AND pH[9]

CHANGE IN $Paco_2$	CHANGE IN pH
Decrease	*Increase*
1 mm Hg	0.01
10 mm Hg	0.10
Increase	*Decrease*
1 mm Hg	0.006
10 mm Hg	0.06

CALCULATING EXPECTED pH[9]

DECREASED $Paco_2$

Expected pH =

$$7.4 + (40 \text{ mm Hg} - Paco_2)\ 0.01$$

INCREASED $Paco_2$

Expected pH =

$$7.4 - (Paco_2 - 40 \text{ mm Hg})\ 0.006$$

bonate values drop below normal, and base deficit values are larger than normal. Conversely, if metabolic or iatrogenic processes cause loss of acid or accumulation of bicarbonate, the values rise above normal. The term *base excess* refers principally to bicarbonate but also comprises other bases in the blood such as plasma proteins and hemoglobin. Bicarbonate and bases are alkaline substances, and as they increase the pH does also. If bicarbonate or base increases, alkalosis occurs and causes pH to rise. If bicarbonate fails, acidosis occurs, and the pH falls. These changes have metabolic, not respiratory, causes.

For the body to function in a state of equilibrium, a certain metabolic ratio must be maintained. When electrolyte results are listed, often a CO_2 content is given. The substances constituting CO_2 content are mainly bicarbonate and, to a lesser extent, CO_2 gas.

	HCO_3^-	24.0 mEq/L
+	Dissolved CO_2 gas	1.2 mEq/L
	CO_2 content	25.2 mEq/L

The 1.2 mEq/L of dissolved CO_2 gas is the same as 40 mm Hg of dissolved CO_2 gas (the normal $PaCO_2$ value), merely expressed in different terminology. The ratio of bicarbonate (base) to CO_2 gas (acid) is as follows:

$$\frac{24\ \text{mEq/L}}{1.2\ \text{mEqL}} = \frac{20}{1}.$$

As long as the ratio remains 20 : 1, the pH remains in a normal range.

Metabolic Abnormalities

Metabolic Alkalosis. The bicarbonate is greater than 26 mEq/L, and the pH is greater than 7.45. The cause of metabolic alkalosis is accumulation of bases or loss of acids. Some conditions leading to metabolic alkalosis are (1) diuretic therapy, potassium deficiency, and administration of antacids; (2) Cushing's disease; (3) steroid treatment; (4) aldosteronism; and (5) loss of acid-containing fluid (chloride depletion) from the GI tract as a result of nasogastric (NG) suction, vomiting, or diarrhea. The cause of these problems is increased excretion of hydrogen, potassium, and chloride by the kidneys. By treating the patient with potassium chloride replenishment, the kidneys excrete potassium and chloride and stop excreting the body's own acid, leading to a correction of the metabolic alkalosis.

Metabolic Acidosis. The bicarbonate is less than 22 mEq/L, and the pH is less than 7.35. Acidemia may be caused by conditions that increase unmeasurable anions or by losses that will not change the anion gap. The term *anion gap* is simply the difference between the positively and negatively charged electrolytes measured by the lab. Determining the anion gap proves helpful when confronted with metabolic acidosis of unexplained etiology.

The total body base deficit can be calculated by multiplying the obtained base deficit per liter of ECF by the total number of liters of ECF. The total liters of ECF are equal to one-fourth the body weight in kilograms. The following formula will determine the total body bicarbonate deficit:

$$\text{Base Deficit} \times \frac{\text{Weight (kg)}}{4} = \text{mEq bicarbonate needed}$$

In a nonarrest state, sudden and total correction with boluses of bicarbonate are not indicated because of rapid ion shifts across the cell membranes that would be produced, increasing the risk of cardiac arrhythmias or convulsion, or both. It is safer to produce a 50% correction with boluses and infuse the remainder over longer periods of time. Repeat blood gas determinations are essential, and clinical application of data must be correlated with the patient's clinical status.

Blood Gas Analysis and Interpretation

Systematic Analysis

Blood gas analysis for determination of acid base status must be done in a systematic fashion so that all abnormalities are noted and treatment planned appropriately. The following sequence is helpful in recognizing and interpreting the major aspects of blood gas results.

1. First, note the pH result. If less than 7.35, an acidotic condition exists; if greater than 7.45, an alkalotic condition exists.
2. Next, determine the cause of an abnormal pH. The next result to note is the $PaCO_2$; if it is elevated, the cause is at least partially respiratory.

Compensation versus Correction

In both compensation and correction, an abnormal pH is returned toward normal in an attempt to maintain the 20:1 ratio necessary for optimal body functioning. In compensation, the body itself tries to correct the abnormal pH by altering the component not primarily affected. For example, if the $Paco_2$ is too high, bicarbonate is retained by the body to compensate for the acidosis caused by CO_2 buildup. The body usually does not overcompensate. It is important to remember that compensation is only an effort to return the pH toward normal, but the primary abnormality still exists. For instance, in the patient experiencing hypovolemic shock, it is common to see an attempt by the patient to compensate and bring his pH back to normal by increasing his respiratory rate to almost double the normal level. If he is unable to compensate, his condition will continue to deteriorate. Evidence of deterioration is seen in peripheral shutdown, oliguria, and deteriorating vital signs, along with restlessness and air hunger. There are decreased bicarbonate stores as a result of bicarbonate buffering the added hydrogen ions. Therefore the flight nurse may have to administer bicarbonate in transport to assist with that compensation for metabolic acidosis. It is common to see well-compensated blood gas results for patients with chronic obstructive pulmonary disease. An example is: pH 7.38, $Paco_2$ 55, base excess +7.

Correction, on the other hand, returns the pH to normal by altering the component primarily affected, and it is accomplished by medical therapies. As an example, an elevated $Paco_2$, indicating hypoventilation, would be corrected by an appropriate means of improved ventilation, such as by bronchial hygiene, intubation, and aggressive airway maintenance.

When analyzing blood gases, it is important to look at all aspects of the results. pH within the normal range does not necessarily indicate a normal underlying condition. There may be abnormalities for which the body is compensating. Using a pH of 7.40 as ideal, the flight nurse looks at the pH result to determine whether it is toward the alkalotic or the acidotic range. If above 7.40, the underlying process is alkalosis; if below 7.40, the underlying process is acidosis. For example:

pH 7.42 normal: toward alkalosis
$Paco_2$ 52: respiratory acidosis
Bicarbonate 33: metabolic alkalosis

There is combined respiratory acidosis and metabolic alkalosis. Because the pH tends toward alkalosis, the primary problem is metabolic alkalosis. To compensate, the body is hypoventilating, causing a respiratory acidosis to bring the pH toward normal. In this case, the compensation is complete because the pH is within the normal range.

Blood gas analysis need not be a complicated mystery. By remembering to use a systematic approach to interpretation of results, the flight nurse's assessment of the patient's acid-base status can be rapid, thorough, and accurate.

METABOLIC AND ACID-BASE EMERGENCIES CASE STUDY

The flight team was dispatched to a hospital to transport a victim of an explosion. The length of the flight was 1 hour. The patient's history obtained from the referring hospital included the following details: a 25-year-old white man had sustained burns, both second- and third-degree, over 60% total body surface area (TBSA). Both lower extremities had sustained open tibia/fibula fracture. Resuscitation was in progress and little information was available from the hospital during flight.

On arrival of the flight team, the flight team was told that the explosion had involved some sort of toxic chemical, but the barrels were not labeled. The emergency department personnel had followed their hazard material protocol and decontaminated the patient, washing him with soap and water.

When examining the patient, the flight team found him to be agitated, but alert and complaining of severe shortness of breath and pain. His face is swollen from second-degree burns of the midface area. His breath sounds are present and equal bilaterally. He has second- and third-degree burns of the chest, but in a scattered pattern. Chest expansion is equal, but shallow. His respiratory rate is 38 breaths/min. The patient has weak peripheral pulses and rapid central pulses. Both arms are burned on the front. His vital signs are blood pressure 80/52 mm Hg, pulse rate 160 beats/min and regular, respiratory rate of 38 breaths/min, and rectal temperature of 94° F.

Initial interventions by the referring institution included 100% oxygen by face mask and one large-bore intravenous line (staff members were concerned about starting another IV line because of the burn injury on his extremities); the patient has received 3 L of normal saline, and initial laboratory work has been obtained including arterial blood gases. They have administered 10 mg of morphine sulfate with little pain relief. Both lower extremities were wrapped with moist dressings, and the patient was placed in a pneumatic antishock garment with the legs inflated for immobilization.

A nasogastric tube and Foley catheter had been placed before the arrival of the flight team. The Foley catheter was draining dark brown urine and had tested positive for blood.

On secondary survey, the flight team had estimated 40% TBSA second-degree burns and 10% TBSA third-degree burns. Burned areas of the patient's body include his face, chest, both arms, abdomen, and upper and lower extremities.

The arterial blood gas values were pH 6.9, PO_2 90, PCO_2 22, and HCO_3 10. No other laboratory values were available. No care had been initiated to correct the patient's metabolic acidosis.

PLAN AND IMPLEMENTATION

Because of the length of the transport, the potential for inhalation injury and the patient's arterial oxygen concentration, the flight team performed a nasotracheal intubation. The patient was given 2 mg of midazolam and tolerated the procedure well. He was then given 5 mg of vecuronium, and hyperventilation was initiated by bag-valve-mask until the patient's ventilation could be mechanically supported by the aircraft ventilator.

Another large-bore IV line was inserted through burn tissue into the patient's left antecubital space and fluid resuscitation was continued. The burn surgeon was contacted and directed that the flight team continue fluid resuscitation, monitoring UO until the urine was clear.

Because the patient was in profound metabolic acidosis and a toxic exposure was suspected, the toxicologist directed the flight crew to initiate an IV therapy with normal saline and 1 ampule of sodium bicarbonate at an infusion rate of 100 ml/hr. They were also directed to administer 2 ampules before starting the infusion.

EVALUATION

The patient was monitored by the transport monitor so that cardiac rhythm and pulse oximetery could be monitored. The patient's SaO_2 remained at 90% despite hyperventilation with 100% oxygen during the transport. The patient was wrapped in a warm dry blanket. Morphine sulfate was administered during the flight for pain management. No acute changes occurred during transport. The patient's vital signs remained as follows: blood pressure 90/48 mm Hg, pulse 130 beats/min and regular, with mechanical hyperventilation.

On arrival at the referring facility, the patient was admitted to the burn unit. His condition continued to deteriorate despite aggressive resuscitation. During the course of his treatment he received 40 ampules of sodium bicarbonate and large amounts of fluid to correct the worsening metabolic acidosis. He died on the second day after his injury. Several chemicals in the barrel were suspect, although there was no labeling and no one seemed to know what could have been in them.

DISCUSSION

This case illustrates profound metabolic acidosis and some of the interventions that can be performed by the flight crew to correct the imbalance. There were several potential sources of this patient's acidosis, including shock and a toxic exposure. The coroner continues to investigate the case and the potential of sodium azide poisoning has been suggested.

REFERENCES

1. Ahrens T: Respiratory monitoring in critical care, *AACN Clin Issues Crit Care Nurs* 4(1):56-65, 1993.
2. Ahrens T: Changing perspectives in the assessment of oxygenation, *Crit Care Nurse* 13(4):78-83, 1993.
3. Batcheller J: Syndrome of inappropriate antidiuretic hormone secretion, *Crit Care Nurs Clin North Am* 6(4):687-692, 1994.
4. Bell TN: Diabetes insipidus, *Crit Care Nurs Clin North Am* 6(4):675-685, 1994.

5. Hudak CM, Gallo BM: Diabetic emergencies. In Hudak CM, Gallo BM, editors: *Critical care nursing,* Philadelphia, 1994, Lippincott.
6. Jones TL: From diabetic ketoacidosis to hyperglycemic hyperosmolar nonketotic syndrome: the spectrum of uncontrolled hyperglycemia in diabetes mellitus, *Crit Care Nurs Clin North Am* 6(4):703-720, 1994.
7. Kitabchi AE, Wall BM: Diabetic ketoacidosis, *Med Clin North Am* 79(1):9-37, 1995.
8. Lorber D: Nonketotic hypertonicity in diabetes mellitus, *Med Clin North Am* 79(1):39-52, 1995.
9. Malley WJ: *Clinical blood gases: application and noninvasive alternatives,* Philadelphia, 1990, Saunders.
10. Metheney NM: Potassium imbalances. In Metheney NM, editor: *Fluid and electrolyte balance—nursing considerations,* Philadelphia, 1987, Lippincott.
11. Mulloy AL, Caruana RJ: Hyponatremic emergencies, *Med Clin North Am* 79(1):155-168, 1995.
12. Service FJ: Hypoglycemia, *Med Clin North Am* 79(1):1-8, 1995.
13. Yealy DN, Wolfson AB: Hypoglycemia, *Emerg Med Clin North Am* 7(4):837-848, 1989.
14. Yuccha CB, Toto KH: Calcium and phosphorus derangements, *Crit Care Nurs Clin North Am* 6(4):747-766, 1994.

CHAPTER 25

Infectious Diseases

COMPETENCIES

1. Identify the modes of transmission of infection.
2. Describe the implications of the Occupational Safety and Health Administration (OSHA) guidelines to flight nursing practice.
3. Identify the appropriate equipment that should be used for patient care to prevent exposure during transport.

Encountering infectious diseases in transport presents a challenge. Infection is frequently not the primary disease and reason for transport but the complication that precipitated transport. The goal of transport is to access multidisciplinary resources not available to the referring hospital. The goals for transport personnel are to provide supportive care to the patient and to prevent the spread of the infectious process. Understanding the infectious process and some of the diseases that transport personnel encounter facilitates the accomplishment of these two goals.

THE CHAIN OF INFECTION

The causative agent (microbe) enters a reservoir, which provides an environment that encourages growth. Next, the agent must have a way to exit the reservoir and enter the next host. The means by which the agent exits one host and enters the next is called a *mode of transmission.* This chain of infection[34] is not only the sequential means that supports a disease but is also the easiest means of "curing" the disease process. Breaking the chain at any one of these intervals prevents the spread of infection (Fig. 25-1).

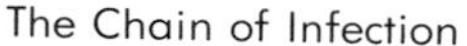

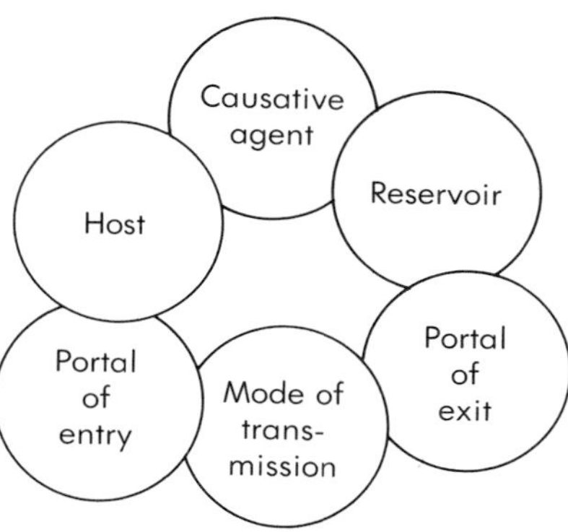

Fig. 25-1. The chain of infection. In the spread of infection, a causative agent passes from a reservoir (such as an infected person) to a susceptible host. The host may then become another reservoir from which the agent can spread.

MODES OF TRANSMISSION

Healthy skin and tissue are the biggest deterrents to infection. Normal bacteria reside on the skin and in other parts of the body (such as the nasopharynx and the gastrointestinal [GI] tract) as part of the "normal flora." As long as the balance of power is established, the patient does not have a problem with disease. For example, if the skin is healthy but is harboring staphylococci, no disease process is begun. Normal handwashing rids the skin of staphylococci, and the spread of disease is inhibited. If the skin is broken, the balance of power is upset. The microbes now have a mode of entry to a host, and disease processes are encouraged. Frequent handwashing becomes the "cure" for disease and the method to break the chain of infection. Common transmission modes for bacteria are direct contact, droplet infection exposure, organisms colonized on equipment, and percutaneous and mucocutaneous contact.

Nosocomial infections are those contracted in the hospital, and are estimated to occur about 2,000,000 times each year. Of these infections, 80% to 90% appear in one of four locations: the urinary tract, the respiratory system, the bloodstream (bacteremia), or a surgical wound. Most infections are acquired in the surgical suite.[2] Nosocomial infections are frequently established by direct contact. Sterilization easily prevents transmission of bacteria from equipment, but direct contact and droplet infection as modes of transmission are harder to contain. Staphylococci or other harmful microbes often are colonized in a host that exhibits no infectious process but can pass the disease to the next host. This carrier situation and poor aseptic technique are especially harmful in the hospital setting. There are personnel who are carriers of disease and who come in close contact with patients. Noncompliance with handwashing policies and droplet expulsion by coughing, sneezing, and talking can deliver germs to patients and enhance the spread of disease. An epidemic can be encountered from just one carrier of disease.

Whereas patients in the hospital may be susceptible to nosocomial infections, prehospital and hospital care providers are more susceptible to diseases transmitted by percutaneous and mucocutaneous methods. Hepatitis B virus (HBV), hepatitis C virus (HCV), human immunodeficiency virus (HIV), and human T-lymphotropic virus (HTLV-I-II) are contained in the blood of some of the patients health care providers encounter. When the patient harboring the organism sustains trauma, has extensive bleeding, or requires emergent procedures or resuscitation, the air medical crew member becomes susceptible to that microbial transmission. Minor areas of broken skin on the flight nurse can provide a mode of entry and be the reservoir for bacteria.

Any intervention that exposes the flight nurse to bloody secretions increases the risk of exposure to an infectious disease. The emergent nature and physical surroundings of the prehospital setting also increase that risk. The lack of light when giving care during the night prevents the nurse from determining if fluid contains blood. In most circumstances, the flight nurse should assume that all fluids are bloody, and the necessary precautions should be taken.

DISEASES AFFECTING TRANSPORT

Acquired Immunodeficiency Syndrome

Acquired immunodeficiency syndrome (AIDS) is caused by HIV. Because HIV attacks the white cells, it is characterized by profound immunologic abnormalities, multiple opportunistic infections, and unusual forms of certain malignant neoplasms.[33]

Clinical and laboratory investigators have isolated a human retrovirus as the causative agent in AIDS and have found that its mode of transmission in both blood and body fluids parallels that of HBV. Like HBV, HIV is transmitted percutaneously and mucocutaneously. It is transmitted through intravenous (IV) drug use, sexual intercourse with an infected person, from a mother to her unborn or newborn child, and through the major body fluids of blood plasma, semen, vaginal fluid, and possibly saliva. HIV has been isolated in cerebrospinal fluid, tears, breast milk, and saliva, although these have never been proved as sources of disease. The virus has been spread through blood transfusions in the past. New screening techniques were begun in 1985 that decrease the threat of infection through transfusion to only 1 in 50,000 units.[34]

The HIV is classified as a retrovirus, which descriptively carries its genetic material in ribonucleic acid (RNA) rather than deoxyribonucleic acid (DNA). The virus uses the host's reproductive apparatus to reproduce itself. It then kills the host cell and releases more of the virus into the body. The body will produce antibodies to the virus, but these are not protective; they only appear to be an indicator of active infection. Antibody to the virus has been consistently documented in patients with AIDS. It is almost always absent for individuals who are not in a risk category. Titers are usually lower in patients with advanced AIDS than in patients with AIDS-related complex (ARC).

One study found the seroprevalence of HIV 1 in emergency department (ED) patients who required resuscitation to be 4.1%.[20] Another study estimated that a prehospital care provider in their study would have 12.3 blood contacts, including a 0.2% percutaneous exposure per year.[22] A health care provider's risk of infection after percutaneous or mucocutaneous exposure to HIV 1–infected blood is between 0.3% and 0.5%.[20,26]

A report in *Morbidity and Mortality Weekly Report*[5] noted risk factors associated with infection after percutaneous exposure to HIV-infected blood. Three factors were statistically significant: (1) a larger quantity of blood indicated by visible blood on a device, (2) a procedure that involved a needle placed directly in a vein or artery, and (3) a deep injury. The risk was increased when the source patient had terminal illness. Postexposure use of zidovudine (formerly azidothymidine [AZT]) was associated with a lower risk for HIV transmission.

Occult HIV infection poses a risk to health care providers. The seroprevalence rate of ED patients in the study by Marcus et al.[22] was 4.1 to 8.3 per 100 patients. Prehospital care workers in that study did not know the HIV status of the patients they transferred 93.5% of the time. To adequately prevent the spread of infectious diseases, health care workers should assume that *every* patient is infectious and universal precautions should be used.

HTLV-I-II

Although the HIV retroviruses are more commonly known, there has been a growing concern over two other pathogenic retroviruses that cause malignant disease. These have been identified as HTLV-I and HTLV-II. Transmission of these viruses is through parenterally infected blood or body fluids, through sexual intercourse, or in utero. The $CD4^+$ and T lymphocytes (T4 cells) are infected by these viruses in the same manner as HIV infection. Retroviruses greatly increase the development of certain viruses by an indirect mechanism. The infected cell is not affected but can influence tumor development in an uninfected cell.[15]

HTLV-I infects the $CD4^+$ T cells, usually the lymphocytes, and is associated with a virulent adult T-cell leukemia/lymphoma and a demyelinating neurologic disease known as tropical spastic paresis (TSP) or HTLV-associated myelopathy (HAM). These latter diseases are progressive demyelinating diseases involving the upper motor neurons, characterized by lower extremity spasticity and sphincter dysfunction.[20]

Until recently HTLV-II was serologically indistinguishable from HTLV-I. When exposed to HTLV-II, the host is more capable of preventing pathogenic disease compared with exposure to HTLV-I. HTLV-II is not known to cause any specific disease, although it has been associated with hairy cell leukemia and some rare T-cell neoplasms. The transmission of HTLV-II is thought to be similar to that of HTLV-I.

The potential for exposure to HTLV-I-II has been documented, but there have been no occupational exposures.[17] Lewandowski et al.[20] found an HTLV-I-II seroprevalence of 1.9% in critically injured resuscitated ED patients. Coinfection of HIV I with HTLV-I-II may hasten the onset of AIDS.

Hepatitis

Viral hepatitis is a common infection of the liver caused by multiple viruses. Five distinct hepatitis viruses have been identified. HBV, HCV, and the hepatitis delta virus (HDV) are all three parenterally transmitted. The enterically transmitted hepatitis viruses are hepatitis A virus (HAV) and hepatitis E virus (HEV). The most accurate means to distinguish the various types of viral hepatitis involves specific serologic testing. Fewer than 5% of the patients initial signs and symptoms of acute viral hepatitis have not had serologic evidence of any of the five known hepatitis viruses. These patients have been classified as having non-ABCDE hepatitis. Serial transmission of such an agent in a primate model would be needed to prove that it is a new hepatitis virus capable of causing enterically transmitted disease.[1]

HAV is transmitted by the fecal-oral route. This transmission is enhanced by poor personal hygiene and intimate contact. In developed countries, exposure, infection, and subsequent immunity are almost universal in childhood. Childhood infections are frequently subclinical. Adults who contract the disease have symptoms that are more severe. The disease is usually self-limiting.

HBV is caused by a DNA virus that attacks the liver cells. Its incubation period is from 6 weeks to 6 months. Similar to the HIV, HBV is transmitted by percutaneous and mucocutaneous modes: IV needle use, sexual intercourse with an infected person, and from a mother to her unborn child through placental transmission, or her newborn through breast-milk contamination. The major body fluids of blood, plasma, semen, and vaginal fluid are the same primary contaminates as for AIDS. HBV is much more transmissible than HIV and is more environmentally stable. The risk of infection to a health care provider after percutaneous exposure of an infected source patient is approximately 30% if the exposure is to hepatitis B antigen–positive blood. As stated earlier, the risk of HIV after percutaneous exposure of an infected source patient is 0.3% to 0.5%.[26]

There are greater than 200 million carriers of hepatitis B surface antigen (HBsAg) in the world. Serum HBsAg is as infrequent as 0.1% to 0.5% in the normal population. HBV is found in 5% to 10% of the volunteer blood donor population. The existence of asymptomatic hepatitis B carriers with normal liver function suggests that the virus is not directly cytopathic. Patients with acute HBV report a percutaneous exposure only 50% of the time.[15] Chronic HBV is present in 5% of the world population. Despite the current focus on HIV risk, hepatitis infection risk is greater in health care providers because 200 die annually of complications of nosocomially acquired hepatitis B.[31] There has been a decline of HBV in heterosexuals and health care workers, but the overall incidence has remained constant.[36]

HCV is transmitted primarily through blood transfusions and other percutaneous routes. Other identified risk factors are heterosexual and homosexual contact, household exposure, hemodialysis, IV drug abuse, and occupational exposure. These risk factors parallel that of HBV and HIV. The period that a person can be an asymptomatic carrier without detectable levels of HCV is between 10 weeks and 1.5 years. Infection with HCV has been shown to have substantial morbidity, and 50% or more of these patients have chronic liver disease. One study demonstrated a prevalence of HCV as high as 7.7% in an adult trauma population.[16]

HDV is transmitted by nonpercutaneous means. It is endemic in those with HBV. There is a worldwide distribution of the HDV. The epidemiologic pattern is in the Mediterranean countries of Northern Africa, Southern Europe, and the Middle East. In the United States, the HDV is confined to those who are frequently exposed to blood and blood products, drug addicts, and patients with hemophilia.[15]

HEV is the enteric form of non-A, non-B hepatitis. It is rare for a person with HEV to spread the disease to close contacts. HEV occurs after contamination of water supplies. HEV is found primarily in India, Asia, Africa, and Central America. It is not known if HEV is found outside the endemic areas.[15]

The prophylaxis of hepatitis differs with each virus type. Knowledge of the transmission of each different type enlightens individuals to prevention of disease spread. Adherence to Occupational Safety and Health Administration (OSHA) standards decreases the possibility of contracting hepatitis when exposed. Immune globulins (IgG) have anti-HAV properties and are effective against HAV. Hepatitis B IgG is available for the prevention of HBV. OSHA standards require health care workers to receive hepatitis B vaccination. In 1992 Lamphear et al.[19] found that a program of hepatitis B immunization for health care providers was associated with a significant decline in clinical HBV infection despite continued exposure to patients positive for HBsAg.[19] IgGs are not recommended for HCV. An effective way to decrease the frequency of posttransfusion HCV is to eliminate commercially obtained donor blood. Vaccinating susceptible people with the hepatitis B vaccine does prevent HDV.

Tuberculosis

There has been a resurgence of tuberculosis (TB) in the world. The primary cause of this increase is linked to the AIDS epidemic. In 1953 the rate of TB cases was just 5% to 7% a year. In 1985 that rate started to rise and by 1991, the number of cases had increased to 23% to 25%.[15] In the United States the rate of increase of new TB cases averages 20% each year. In 1993 health care providers accounted for 3.2% of TB cases.[6]

The organism that causes TB is *Mycobacterium tuberculosis.* The mode of transmission is by droplet contamination through the respiratory tract. The organism is inhaled and then travels to the alveoli, which provide a good medium for growth of the organism. The risk for infection is proportional to the concentration and the length of the exposure. The *M. tuberculosis* organism is found in the lung about 85% of the time. The organism can also spread through the lymph system to other parts of the body. Tuberculosis has been found in the peritoneum, meninges, kidneys, and bones.[23]

Once the person is infected with TB, within 2 to 10 weeks cell-mediated immunity responds. The person will have a positive TB skin test result after this immune response is activated. If the immune system prevents further spread of the organism, the patient is said to have tuberculosis infection without the disease. Such patients are not infectious if they do not have the disease. They may be completely asymptomatic, or they may have mild coldlike symptoms. Even if the person is symptomatic, the chest x-ray film is often negative. Currently there are no sophisticated methods for diagnosing TB. Smears for acid-fast bacillus (AFB) cultures on patients with TB are estimated as being negative as frequently as 50% of the time.[28]

After exposure to the organism, TB can lie dormant for long periods. It is unclear why the disease becomes reactivated. Reactivation of the disease is more likely with people who have impaired cell-mediated immunity such as diabetes, renal failure, and HIV. There is a 5% chance of becoming infected within the first 2 years after exposure. The lifetime risk of acquiring active TB once infected is 5% to 10%.

There has been an increase of multidrug resistant TB (MDR-TB). MDR-TB is defined as any strain of *Mycobacterium tuberculosis* that is resistant to two or more of the five medications used for TB. Experts believe that MDR-TB is the reason that TB will become a bigger problem in the future. The resistant TB cases can be lethal if no medication is available to eradicate the organism. According to the Centers for Disease Control and Prevention (CDC), in 1991 at least 20 health care providers have nosocomially acquired MDR-TB and 9 of those have died.[8]

There is also an increase in TB in the AIDS population. It is estimated that 10% of all cases of HIV-infected persons in the world also have a coinfection with TB. This incidence is 500 times that of the general population.[23] The HIV destroys the hosts lymphocytes and monocytes early in the course of HIV. When this occurs, the person is unable to initiate a cell-mediated response to the *M. tuberculosis* organism when it is introduced into the body.

No health care provider is immune from exposure to tuberculosis. After TB outbreaks, Florida and Texas hospital employees had a skin test conversion rate of 20% to 50%.[8] This high rate of conversion indicates that the risk of exposure for health care workers is significant.

The CDC has issued guidelines to help prevent the spread of TB. First, health care workers should maintain a high degree of suspicion. Second, the infection should be identified early. Once identified, the infected person should be isolated and treated as early as possible. Most of the guidelines for preventing the spread of TB are directed toward health care providers who work in hospitals. Placing the person in the proper isolation room with proper airflow ventilation system is recommended. This type of isolation is not possible for infectious patients who require prehospital or interfacility transport.

The close proximity of the health care providers to the infectious patient in the transport vehicle puts these workers at an increased risk. The CDC[7] issued specific guidelines for prehospital personnel and others involved in transport. Because emergency medical services (EMS) and flight personnel work in close quarters, it is recommended that the windows of the vehicle or helicopter be opened whenever possible. If the heating or air conditioner is used, they should be set to nonrecirculating cycles.

If there is suspicion, or a patient has a confirmed case of TB, a mask should be placed over the patient's face. A conventional surgical mask does not filter 1- to 5-μm particles.[29] The size of the tuberculosis organism is small; therefore the only mask that filters small particles is the high-efficiency particulate respirator. Two disadvantages to using the particulate respirator are high costs ($5 to $7 per mask) and its tendency to be bulky. Even though it is bulky, it provides a better fit and protection than a surgical mask.

Different treatment options are available for health care providers who contract TB. The age of the person and the general health are taken into consideration. Isoniazid therapy is a treatment choice to prevent the reactivation of the disease. Careful monitoring for liver dysfunction is necessary for individuals receiving isoniazid therapy. Taking isoniazid is controversial after the age of 35 because the risk of hepatitis increases fourfold.[25]

An employee health physician is another good source of information on infectious diseases such as TB. These physicians have more experience with infectious diseases that are transmitted to the health care workers. They maintain current knowledge of the latest treatment modalities. The employee health physician can also be consulted when work practice controls to prevent the spread of infectious diseases are prepared.

Early identification of patients with TB and proper diagnosis prevent the spread of disease. Early drug therapy is essential for a person with TB. Initial steps toward the prevention of MDR-TB include patient education, stressing the importance of completing the drug therapy and appropriate follow-up. Education of health care workers on the transmission of TB assists them in taking the necessary precautions to avoid contracting or spreading the disease to others.

Bacterial Meningitis

Bacterial meningitis is a relatively common infection of adults and children. If left untreated, meningitis can be fatal in as few as 6 to 12 hours. The various organisms that cause meningitis, *Streptococcus pneumoniae* and *Neisseria meningitidis,* are the most common in infants of 1 month of age up to adults. Group B streptococci and aerobic gram-negative bacilli are common causes of bacterial meningitis in newborns. These organisms are causes of infection in that age group because individuals may be exposed to them when passing through the birth canal during vaginal deliveries. The incidence of *Haemophilus influenzae* has declined as a causative agent. This is thought to be related to the childhood immunization against *H. influenzae.*[12]

Exercising a high degree of caution when diagnosing or ruling out meningococcal meningitis is necessary. A missed diagnosis can have serious or even fatal repercussions. Classic signs of the disease are new seizure activity, headache, fever, and petechial rash. Absence of the rash does not exclude the diagnosis, because the rash may appear in only 50% of the patients. Nuchal rigidity, a positive Kernig's sign (back and leg pain on hip flexion/knee extension), or a positive Brudzinski's sign (back and leg pain on neck flexion) should heighten suspicion of the disease. These last three signs are unreliable in the infant population; therefore a lumbar puncture (LP) may be needed. A differential diagnosis of meningitis should always be considered in a person with an unexplained altered mental status change. This change could be as subtle as a flat affect.[18]

Fulminant meningococcal infection can lead to slight flattening of the gyri cerebri and to polymorphonuclear (PMN) leukocyte accumulation in the meninges and brain. Fibrin may build up in smaller vessels, creating an acute vasculitis resulting in petechial lesions of the meninges.[9] Inflammatory changes in the leptomeninges lead to PMN aggregates and resulting exudate invading the spinal fluid, limiting the entry of solutes, serum proteins, and some antibiotics. Glucose permeability is decreased. Symptoms suggesting this inflammatory process include lethargy and increased intracranial pressure (ICP). The results of fulminant infection can be development of shock, disseminated intravascular coagulopathy, respiratory failure, and electrolyte disturbances. Another nonspecific but important clue in the later stages of the disease is cold extremities caused by peripheral vasoconstriction. This is a compensatory mechanism to support normal central perfusion, and its presence may precede significant hypotension.

The bacterium that causes meningitis is very labile and may be cultured from the blood, spinal fluid, and other normally sterile media. Cultures from the nasopharynx are not helpful because healthy persons have a very high carrier rate. If a referring hospital has already administered antibiotic therapy, cultures should still be obtained from other normally sterile media, such as spinal fluid and blood. The culture results from these areas yield significant conclusive evidence that warrants obtaining them whenever possible. Gram stains help to direct the tertiary care personnel in the course of treatment.

Giving antibiotics to a person with suspected bacterial meningitis should be done as soon as possible. Parenteral antibiotics are recommended to be given 30 minutes after presentation. The transport team's medical control will discuss the case with the referring physician. This discussion can be instrumental in initiating the appropriate treatment of performing an LP, obtaining blood cultures, and administering antibiotics before the flight teams arrival. Although obtaining cultures should not delay the transport, antibiotic therapy should be initiated before departure from the referring facility. This is especially important when the disease has progressed to a shock state. It may be possible for the flight nurse, with assistance from the referring physician or nurse, to obtain specimens for blood cultures while the patient is being prepared for the transport.

Many physicians have concerns that the results of cultures can be altered if antibiotic therapy is initiated before obtaining specimens. Blazer et al.[4] found that cerebral spinal fluid (CSF) cell count and protein remained the same after 2 full days of parenteral antibiotics. This study demonstrated that antibiotics given before the LP does not affect the cell results but may decrease the culture yield. After 2 full days of antibiotic therapy, all of the study cultures were sterile.

The use of steroids in bacterial meningitis is controversial. It is theorized that central nervous system (CNS) damage after bacterial meningitis is related to an increased inflammatory response after the administration of the antibiotics. Researchers found that if steroids were given before antibiotics, there was a significant statistical difference in the neurologic sequelae, specifically the hearing loss.[11,27]

If bacterial meningitis is suspected, the flight team must properly protect themselves from transmission. This is particularly important because the patient care areas of helicopters and fixed-wing aircraft are small and have closed quarters. Masks and gloves should always be worn. Other personal protective equipment may be necessary, depending on the cause of the disease in each case.

Antibiotic therapy and supportive care must be instituted without delay. Morbidity and mortality are increased significantly with delays in treatment. Airway management is of great importance for patients with meningitis, especially in the presence of a decreasing level of consciousness. Mannitol may be given for signs of ICP. Fluid and electrolyte management are also of importance.

OSHA GUIDELINES

The OSHA of the Department of Labor has determined that health care providers face a significant health risk from the exposure to infectious bloodborne pathogens. OSHA officials believed that this risk could be significantly decreased or even eliminated by establishing work practice controls and guidelines. Therefore the *Occupational Exposure to Bloodborne Pathogens; Final Rule* was developed.[10] The effective date of the standard was March 6, 1992. Most institutions are governed by work practice laws enacted by OSHA. If OSHA officials find an institution in violation of any portion of the standard, the institution can be fined as little as $7000 up to as much as $70,000 for a single violation.[35] Flight programs may want to determine whether these laws affect their practice. In this chapter, this specific standard is referred to as the OSHA standard.

Every institution that falls under the jurisdiction of OSHA must have a formal infection control plan that covers all areas of the plan. If a flight program is hospital based, the program probably has a well-developed infection control plan that follows the OSHA standard. Flight programs can use the existing plan and modify it to encompass differences in flight nursing practice. Examples of how the OSHA standard is being adapted to flight nursing practice are throughout this chapter.

OSHA defines an *exposure* as a specific eye, mouth, other mucous membrane, nonintact skin, or parenteral contact with blood or other potentially infectious materials. Health care professionals need to be aware of what constitutes an exposure. Reporting an insignificant exposure such as splashes of blood on clothing is costly, time consuming, and nonproductive. Part of the required yearly training that OSHA mandates is dedicated to the epidemiology and the transmission of the bloodborne pathogens. With increased education, reporting of insignificant exposures should decline. The flight nurse can be a role model and disseminate information concerning a significant exposure to other medical employees and prehospital care providers. The flight nurse can assist them in determining the status of an exposure and reporting the significant exposures.

Exposure Documentation

Fig. 25-2 is an example of an exposure documentation form and a form to respond to the prehospital care provider's request for information from a Midwestern teaching hospital. With the information obtained from this form, the hospital can determine whether the exposure is significant enough to warrant further investigation. This facility does not begin testing of the source patient's blood unless the exposed health care provider completes the exposure documentation form and arranges for testing of his or her own blood. The reporting of insignificant exposures has decreased with this practice.

Formal documentation of this type is beneficial for the employer, employee, and the source patient. It is cost effective for the employer because it prevents the waste of time and money following up on insignificant exposures. Baseline data on infectivity status of health care providers help to prove or disprove that the infectious disease is work related. Patient confidentiality remains an important issue when testing the source patient for bloodborne infectious diseases. Random testing of source patients without justification is costly and may be psychologically difficult for the patient.

Formal documentation entails some responsibility by the employee to follow up on exposures. Health care providers frequently do not wish to have their own blood tested before they know the status of the source patient. This rationale does not consider the period required for seroconversion. Positive source patients motivate health care providers to have their own blood tested.

Universal Precautions

Use of universal precautions is one approach to infection control. According to OSHA definitions, *universal precautions* means that *all* human blood and certain human body fluids are treated as if known to be infectious for HIV, HBV, and other bloodborne pathogens. The emergent nature of care rendered to patients who are bloody makes use of universal precautions a prudent approach to infection control.

Text continued on p. 492.

UNIVERSITY OF CINCINNATI HOSPITAL

REQUEST NO. ________

REQUEST FOR INFORMATION BY EMERGENCY SERVICES WORKER

PLEASE PRINT - Use Blue or Black Ink - PRESS HARD

This form is for use by emergency care workers to request information on the presence of a contagious or infectious disease (if known) of a person, alive or dead, who has been treated, handled, or tranported to University Hospital by an emergency services worker.

Before you can be provided with this information, you must believe that you have suffered significant exposure through contact with the person about whom you are requesting the information. A significant exposure means:

> A percutaneous (break in skin or needle stick) or mucous membrane exposure (eyes, nose, mouth) to the blood, semen, vaginal secretions, or spinal, synovial (joint, bone, tendon), pleural (lung), peritoneal (abdomen), pericardial (heart), or amniotic fluid of another person.

Deposit top (white) copy in designated Emergency Department QA box. Submit yellow copy to your agency or employer. Retain pink copy.

1. Regarding the exposure, what was

   Name of patient: ____

   Date: ______________________ Time: ______________________

   Place: ____

   Manner of exposure:

   ________ Dirty needle stick ________ Broken skin exposure

   ________ Splash-eye, nose, mouth ________ Unprotected mouth to mouth

   ________ Other, describe: ________________________________

   ____

2. Your name: ____

3. Your address: ______________________________

City/State/Zip: ______________________________

4. Your telephone number: Home: ______________ Work: ______________

5. Have you completed more than two (2) injections in Hepatitis B series? Yes ______ No ______

6. Employer or volunteer agency for whom you were administering health care when exposure occurred:

Employer or agency: ______________________________

Address: ______________________________

City/State/Zip: ______________________ Phone: ______________

7. Name of your chief at above listed place of employment or volunteer agency: ______________

This is to attest that the above statements are true and correct to the best of my knowledge and belief.

Your signature: ______________________ Date: ______________

ACKNOWLEDGMENT

Name of person receiving request: ______________________________

Received: Date: ______________ Time: ______________

White-Emergency Department QA Box Yellow-Agency/Employer Pink-Requestor's Copy

Fig. 25-2. Example of an exposure documentation form.

Continued.

UNIVERSITY OF CINCINNATI HOSPITAL

REQUEST NO. ________

RESPONSE TO EMERGENCY SERVICES WORKER REQUEST FOR INFORMATION

PLEASE PRINT - Use Blue or Black Ink - PRESS HARD

THIS INFORMATION HAS BEEN DISCLOSED TO YOU FROM CONFIDENTIAL RECORDS PROTECTED FROM DISCLOSURE BY STATE LAW. YOU SHALL MAKE NO FURTHER DISCLOSURE OF THIS INFORMATION WITHOUT THE SPECIFIC, WRITTEN, AND INFORMED RELEASE OF THE INDIVIDUAL TO WHOM IT PERTAINS OR AS OTHERWISE PERMITTED BY STATE LAW. A GENERAL AUTHORIZATION FOR THE RELEASE OF MEDICAL OR OTHER INFORMATION IS NOT SUFFICIENT FOR THE PURPOSE OF THE RELEASE OF HIV TEST RESULTS OR DIAGNOSIS.

1. Date of oral report: ______________________ Name of ESW: ______________________

   Person giving report: ______________________

   Comments: ______________________

   ____

2. Date of written report: ______________________

   Report sent to worker ________ chief ________ chief's name ______________________

   Person sending report: ______________________

3. Your request for information has been received. It has been determined that:

   a. _____ There is no known presence of a contagious or infectious disease at this time based upon the following:

   _____ No tests were performed.

   _____ The following tests were performed with negative results:

   ______________________ ______________________
   ______________________ ______________________
   ______________________ ______________________

b. ____ There is the presence of a contagious or infectious disease. Testing on person in question was positive for:

____________________ ____________________
____________________ ____________________
____________________ ____________________

c. ____ The person in question has refused HIV testing.

d. ____ Patient discharged home.

e. ____ Patient discharged to health care facility/coroner's office/funeral home.
Address: ____________________

THIS RESPONSE PROVIDES ALL INFORMATION AVAILABLE AS OF THE DATE OF THIS WRITTEN RESPONSE.

4. Report included:

____	Name of disease	____	Suggested precautions for preventing transmission.
____	Signs and symptoms of disease	____	Recommended prophylaxis (if any)
____	Date of exposure	____	Suggested follow-up
____	Incubation period of disease	____	Appropriate counseling
____	Mode of transmission		

5. It is expected that the worker will consult a physician in cases of true disease exposure. It is understood by provider of report and recipients that decisions related to prophylaxis, treatment, and counseling will be at the discretion of that physician.

White-Requestor's Copy   Yellow-Agency/Employer   Pink-University Hospital Infection Control Committee/Prehospital Training

Fig. 25-2—cont'd. Example of a form responding to a prehospital care provider's request for information.

The standard specifies that employees wash hands and any other skin with soap and water or flush mucous membranes with water immediately or as soon as feasible after contact of such body areas with blood or other potentially infectious materials. Flight nurses do not have access to running water on aircraft; thus following this part of the standard becomes impossible. An alcohol-based foam soap product can be a replacement to water that can rapidly reduce transient bacteria and the risk of cross infection. The containers for these types of soap are small enough that they can be easily stored in a drawer of the aircraft. These products are antimicrobial and do not require water. After use, hands should be washed with soap and water as soon as possible. Alcare Plus is an example of an emollient ethyl alcohol that does not produce drying as with other alcohol products.

Frequent handwashing can compromise the epidermal barrier and leave the skin susceptible to irritation or allergic contact sensitization. A skin lotion from Healthpoint named Proshield Glove can be used to protect the hands. This cream is a water-in-oil emulsion that leaves a continuous film of protection on the skin after the water evaporates. The protection lasts through several handwashings. Studies from Healthpoint have demonstrated that the product does not support microbial growth even after a long shelf life. It actually has the potential to kill contaminating microorganisms.[13] The company has studied the effect of their product on chlorhexidine gluconate, which is an antimicrobial agent used in scrub cleansers such as Hibiclens. The study demonstrated that Proshield does not inhibit and may actually enhance chlorhexidine gluconate membrane penetration.[3]

Personal Protective Equipment

Personal protective equipment is meant to prevent blood or other potentially infectious materials from penetrating and reaching the employee's undergarments, skin, and mucous membrane. OSHA recommends masks with face shields and eye protection whenever splashes of blood or other potentially infectious materials may be anticipated. These devices should be worn *every time* an intubation or invasive procedure is performed. Even though it is fairly common to see prehospital care providers wearing gloves, these same workers rarely adhere to wearing masks and face shields.

Personal protective equipment (PPE) consists of specialized clothing or equipment employees wear to protect themselves against a hazard. The employer is required to supply PPE at no cost to the employee. If employees need special PPE, they are responsible for notifying the employer. The employer is required to purchase the necessary alternative equipment for all employees.

A flight nurse does not receive a detailed patient report before responding to the scene of a motor vehicle crash. The flight nurse has no way of knowing what care will be needed. With the emergent nature of flight nursing, it is fairly common to see flight nurses wearing gloves when they exit the aircraft to respond to a scene. Whatever PPE equipment the flight nurse brings out of the helicopter, and to the scene, is what is available for use. The vehicle's PPE can augment the flight nurse's equipment but not replace it. This differs from the hospital where PPE is readily available and can be obtained when the situation dictates. It is common practice for nurses and physicians practicing in EDs to don gowns, masks, face shields, and gloves when they know that a potentially bloody patient is being transported to their hospital.

There are several types of gloves that a person can choose to wear to prevent exposure. Disposable latex gloves are the most common choice. Sterile latex gloves do not offer any added protection over the disposable ones and only add to costs. A durable, nonstick glove that is changed frequently is best for the prehospital care provider. High-risk, infection control gloves that are thicker and longer are available for prehospital personnel. These gloves are commonly a blue or green color instead of the common flesh-colored disposable glove. Wearing a thicker glove may prevent cuts from glass at an accident crash site. A thick reusable glove is best for decontaminating equipment. These are the only types of glove that can be decontaminated for reuse.

The use of gloves is easy but not as efficient as one would think. In 1988 a test was completed on 600 gloves from five different manufacturers for visible defects. Visual inspection of the gloves, after the performance of normal tasks, resulted in dye penetration and bacteria penetration of a large percentage of gloves tested.

Latex allergies are becoming increasingly common among health care providers and patients since the institution and use of universal precautions. An increased demand for gloves may have changed the manufacturing procedure resulting in poor quality, highly allergenic gloves.[32] The protein in natural rubber is considered to be the responsible antigen.[30] The first documented case of a person with a reaction to latex gloves was in 1979. Approximately 1% of the general population is latex sensitive, and 7% to 10% of health care workers have a sensitivity. The incidence of sensitivity increases up to 12% for operating room personnel. A person with repeated exposure to latex has an increased risk of development of latex allergy. Genetic factors and allergies to certain foods predispose a person to latex allergies.

Reactions to latex range from contact and generalized urticaria to bronchospasm, anaphylaxis, and even death. Most (82%) of the reports are not serious and are classified as a type IV reaction, which presents clinically as contact dermatitis. Once a person has become sensitized to the allergen, repeated exposures are more severe. The more severe responses are cell mediated by IgE and are classified as type I reactions. Examples of type I reactions are asthma, anaphylaxis, and death.[32]

The treatment for allergies lies in the prevention of exposure. Nonlatex gloves can be worn. As with any allergic response, the person needs to remove the rubber gloves or, with severe reactions, leave the area of exposure. Latex proteins are easily absorbed by glove powders. Powder-free gloves are essential. Depending on the specific person's sensitization and reaction, other employees working with that individual also may have to wear powderless gloves. Cotton liners or barrier creams such as the Proshield help to decrease an allergic reaction. The employer is required to purchase special gloves for an allergic employee's use.

Gowns in the prehospital setting are the least effective method of protection; they are predictably soiled and soaked with blood or bodily fluids. A better option is to shower and change clothes as soon as possible after care is delivered.

Eye protection is recommended as protection against mucocutaneous contact with blood or body fluids through the conjunctiva. It is important to choose glasses that provide peripheral vision. This enhances safety in the air medical setting.

PPE should be removed as soon as possible when saturated with blood. It is difficult for the flight team to dispose of contaminated equipment in the helicopter. Bloody PPE can contaminate the helicopter. If bloody gloves are worn when entering the helicopter, the blood can contaminate the door handles, seatbelts, instrument controls, and headsets. A simple alternative is wearing two gloves to the scene. Before entering the helicopter, the outer bloody pair can be removed and the bottom layer remains in place for protection.

The OSHA standard stipulates that an employee has the right to temporarily decline the use of PPE if, in the employee's professional judgment, use of the PPE will hinder the delivery of health care. If a person makes this judgment, the employer must investigate the situation to determine what can be done to prevent this from occurring in the future.

Equipment

Recapping of needles increases the chance of a percutaneous stick. Experts believe that percutaneous needle sticks are underreported.[21] OSHA mandates that nurses shall *not* recap needles. Recapping needles is likely to be done and is often necessary in flight nursing practice. Because of the restrictions in space, only a limited amount of drugs can be stored in the aircraft. When needed, the medicine is drawn out of the ampule and into a syringe. If only a small amount of the drug is used, the nurse recaps the needle to keep the remaining drug sterile for future use.

If needles must be recapped, OSHA requires that it be accomplished through the use of a mechanical device or a one-handed technique. With a one-handed technique, the cap is placed on a surface and the syringe is placed inside the cap using one hand.

Needles must be placed in needle containers after use. A STIK-A-BRIK is a styrofoam, contaminated, single-use needle receptacle that is designed for transporting needles and syringes from a scene. This device is useful in a moving transport vehicle and is a suitable alternative to the traditional contaminated needle containers. It is quicker and easier to insert needles and syringes in the top of this device, than trying to find the opening of a plastic sharps container. The needles can then be transferred to an appropriate container after completion of the flight.

Leakproof sheets or body wraps can be used to contain blood during a flight. If a particular part of the patient's body is extremely bloody, that area can be wrapped with a plastic leakproof wrapping. With bloody gunshot wounds and amputations, the area can be surrounded with plastic and towels to absorb some of the blood and prevent it from spreading inside the aircraft.

Decontamination

Contaminated work surfaces must be cleaned as soon as possible after the incident. Flight nurses are frequently responsible for decontaminating their own equipment. Flight teams must work quickly after a flight to restock and clean the aircraft to return it to service. It may be necessary for the aircraft to be put on a short delay for the required decontamination. After flights involving the transport of extremely bloody patients, all of the equipment may have to be removed from the aircraft to adequately clean its interior surfaces. Fortunately HBV and HIV are known to live for only a short time on environmental surfaces. For decontamination to be successful, surfaces must be cleaned with the appropriate solution for decontamination. Running water from a hose may be necessary for cleanup of a large amount of blood.

Routine cleaning and disinfection of the air medical environment is also recommended on a regularly scheduled basis to prevent the transmission of disease. Buckets, mops, and brushes used for decontamination also need to be used on a rotating decontamination schedule. These items need to be clearly marked and used only for decontamination. A record of the cleaning schedules must be kept.

Flight programs frequently purchase specialized equipment that is exclusive for the needs of the flight team. Because of budget restraints, sometimes there are no backup pieces of the same equipment; therefore decontamination of the equipment must be done promptly to return it to service. If indicated, the central service department can be used for assistance in decontaminating equipment. If the equipment is specific to the flight program, the flight department's name should be clearly labeled on the equipment.

Solutions for disinfection vary in their use according to the equipment on which a particular solution is used. A knowledge of appropriate cleaning solutions and their use is necessary to ensure that adequate decontamination takes place. Bleach solution in 1:10 ml concentration is effective and safe on soft or hard plastic. The linoleum floors of the ambulance, helicopter, or airplane and the stretcher mattresses can be cleaned with this solution, providing the area is free from dirt and dried blood, although fabric will fade and discolor from use of the bleach solution.[2]

Glutaraldehyde 2% also can be used on plastics and vinyl without damage. Acid solutions should not be used around electronic equipment and on stainless steel because corrosion occurs on high-carbon metals with alkalinized solution. Glutaraldehyde should be mixed at the time of use because it is unstable in solution, even though it is very effective.[2] Alcohol is a very effective antiseptic. It is effective with very short contact on HIV, tubercle bacillus, fungi, and viruses. However, alcohol is flammable and very drying. Alcohol is not recommended for the hands. The surface being cleaned must be free of dirt and blood before use of alcohol can be effective.[14]

Iodoforms are safe, relatively fast, and effective against many organisms. Cleaning the patient's skin with iodoform and then with alcohol, and letting the area dry before an IV skin puncture, is often recommended to protect the skin from introduction of bacteria. IV tubings are becoming a source of infection more frequently because more medicines are being introduced into the catheters. Cleaning of the IV ports with alcohol or iodoforms or both definitely helps protect the patient from nosocomial infections.[14]

The pneumatic antishock garment, floor surfaces, and linens can be cleaned with detergent and water before disinfectant application. Cleaning of surfaces with one of the above proper chemical disinfectants removes the risk from the area.

Laryngoscope blades and handles are reusable and require decontamination after each use. These handles and blades can be properly decontaminated by soaking in an effective antimicrobial solution such as Metricide. This agent is a glutaraldehyde solution used for disinfecting and sterilizing inanimate objects. Surface particles must be cleaned before soaking. The amount of time that the object is soaked determines the effectiveness. HIV is completely inactivated after 10 minutes of soaking. The soaking time must be increased to 20 minutes to provide a 100% effective destruction of the mycobacterium. Because it is difficult to determine which organisms are on the objects, all items should be soaked for at least 20 minutes. Batteries must be removed from handles before soaking. In time, corrosion of various portions of the blade and handle can occur. Because the equipment must soak for 20 minutes, extra laryngoscope blades and handles will be needed for rotation back into the aircraft. Rotation of the blades and handles allows the aircraft to be restocked and promptly returned to service. When the blade and handle have been decontaminated, they must be rinsed thoroughly before they are returned to stock.

Disposable laryngoscope blades and handles are available. Disposing of these items after an intubation would definitely decrease the possibility of transmission of infectious organisms. The newer blades and handles are stronger than some of the older models. One disadvantage that may prevent some programs from using disposable laryngoscope blades and handles is their expensive cost.

Flight teams must be aware of other institutions' infection control policies. Contaminated equipment or laundry may need to be disposed of at other institutions. The flight nurse may have to ask questions at other institutions to be able to follow their specific policies. The development of the OSHA standard has given the industry some consistency and has made following other institutions' policies easier. When the flight team responds to a motor vehicle crash or other incidents where there is a large amount of blood, the site itself has to be decontaminated. Because the flight team is one of the first to leave the scene, the fire department must assume responsibility to overhaul and decontaminate the area to prevent transmission of infectious diseases to the public.

Compliance

Health care providers vary in their compliance of infection control practices. Education becomes paramount to increase their compliance. Compliance with infection control practices is directly proportional to the belief that there is a risk for exposure.

O'Boyle-Williams et al.[24] studied the variables influencing worker compliance with universal precautions. They found the health care workers were most likely to perform handwashing after contact with body fluids and to wear gloves if contact with blood was anticipated. Obstacles to compliance were listed as lack of time, interference with skills, and a perception that the patient was at low risk of having an infectious disease.

In one study, Kelen et al.[17] found that ED employees cited insufficient amount of time when they needed to give emergent care as a reason for their noncompliance with universal precautions. There was a decrease in use of universal precautions from 44% to 19% when the patient was profusely bleeding, and 65% during minor procedures to 16% during major invasive procedures. Wong et al.[36] showed that physicians used universal precautions less when they performed emergency procedures than when they performed nonemergency procedures. In both cases, the most critically injured patients, who were most likely to be bloody and were also most likely to be infectious, were the ones for whom health care workers were most likely to ignore use of universal precautions.

Training and Education

OSHA requires that training be provided at the time of the initial assignment. This training must be at no cost to the employee and be done on the employer's time. The extensive orientation that is required for a new flight nurse should encompass the infection control procedures that are different or in addition to the hospital's policies. An emphasis should be placed on how infection control practices differ in both the prehospital arena and the closed quarters of the aircraft.

All employees must have annual training. If the flight program is hospital based, the hospitalwide infection control program can be used to incorporate all of the teaching requirements of the OSHA standard. There must be a written exposure plan that is accessible to the flight nurse. This plan must be updated every year, or modified to reflect new tasks or procedures that affect occupational exposure. Additional training is required when there are changes or modifications of tasks. Flight nurses should take an active role in preparing and updating this plan so that it is appropriate for their use.

DISEASE PREVENTION

To break the sequence of events that cause disease and thereby protect the air medical crew and potential patients from infectious diseases, the flight personnel need to apply basic principles to control and reduce the number of infections. Following the OSHA guidelines is essential.

Handwashing is the single most important resource for preventing transmittal of disease; it systematically kills bacteria and is critical in the prevention of disease transmission. Handwashing is recommended before and after patient care in any category, including IV therapy, catheter insertion, and the administration of medication.

Hepatitis, measles, flu, and tetanus immunizations for the prehospital and hospital care provider are strongly recommended by the CDC for the prevention of disease, and yearly tuberculin testing also is recommended.

The HBV vaccination is required for health care providers in high-risk areas by the OSHA standard. The standard stipulates that the employer is required to notify the employee of the necessity of the vaccination. This vaccination shall be free of charge to the employee. If employees decline the HBV vaccine, they are required to sign a waiver stating their knowledge of the risks and their declination.

SUMMARY

Infectious diseases are a challenge for air medical personnel because of the multiple facets of involvement. Health care providers are inherently exposed to infectious diseases, and flight personnel have an increased risk because of the bloody injuries and the emergent resuscitative measures that their patients require. The close working quarters of helicopters and fixed-wing aircraft add to this risk.

Flight personnel can take up these challenges successfully by collaborative writing of infection control policies between the flight crew and the infection control department personnel. Following quality control procedures and enforcing OSHA standards will help to maintain surveillance, control, and prevention of infectious diseases in the air medical environment.

Knowledge of the epidemiology and the transmission of infectious diseases decreases the chance of exposure. Since the existence of the OSHA standard, infection control practices are well defined and universalized. Flight nurses must make adjustments from hospital to prehospital infection control practices. Use of universal precautions for *all* patient encounters is a prudent way to handle secretions and blood. Innovative infection control devices and competent performance of procedures help decrease the risk of exposure in the flight nursing environment. Careful assessment, planning, implementation, and evaluation of treatment is required for the successful outcome of transporting patients with infectious diseases.

INFECTIOUS DISEASES CASE STUDY #1

A request was received to transport a 3½-month-old female infant who had been admitted to the emergency department at the referring hospital with a history of poor feeding and lethargy the day of admission. The history was otherwise negative.

On admission, the patient's general appearance was that of a cyanotic, mottled infant. She was lethargic, her pupils were equal and sluggishly reactive, and the anterior fontanelle was soft and slightly depressed. She was tachycardic (pulse 210 beats/min), tachypneic (respirations 96 per minute), and hypotensive (30 mm Hg by palpation), and her rectal temperature was 100° F. Urine output was low the day of admission, and she had none after admission or during transport.

Initial treatment consisted of oxygen by mask at 10 L/min, an IV was started, laboratory results were obtained, including blood cultures, and a LP was performed. The infant was also given a fluid bolus for her hypotension.

The laboratory results were as follows:

CBC

WBC 3.9
Hgb 9.7
Hct 28.2
Poly 19.0
Band 6
Lymph 75

ELECTROLYTES

Na 131*
K^+ 5.5*
Cl 100
CO_2 14
Glucose 102
BUN 22

ABG

pH 7.15
Pco_2 17.7
Po_2 289.1
HCO_3^- 6.2
BE −20.7

SPINAL FLUID

WBC 14
  Mononuclear 9
  Polynuclear 5
RBC 6
Glucose 58 mg/dl
Protein 36 mg/dl

By the time the flight crew arrived, the patient's condition had obviously deteriorated. Their examination revealed the infant to be apneic with marked peripheral cyanosis, purpura, and mottling. Her pupils were 4 mm and fixed. She had marked rales and rhonchi bilaterally with a decrease in respiratory effort with a rate of 10 to 20 per minute. Other vital signs showed a regularly irregular heart rate of 105; her blood pressure had increased to 64 mm Hg after the second fluid bolus; and the rectal temperature had dropped to 97.2° F. The only other treatment before transport was intubation and oxygen delivery by bag-valve-mask at a rate of 28 with 100% oxygen.

During transport the infant had cardiac arrest and Advanced Cardiac Life Support protocols were instituted. On arrival at the receiving facility, all efforts to resuscitate the infant failed.

Her death was caused by an overwhelming sepsis caused by group A and group B-hemolytic *Streptococcus.*

*Repeat NA 125; repeat K^+ 5.0.

INFECTIOUS DISEASES CASE STUDY #2

The flight team responded to a small rural hospital to transport a 74-year-old woman with respiratory distress. Her medical history included frequent episodes of pneumonia.

On the helicopter's arrival, the woman was found to be in acute respiratory distress. She was coughing productively a thick purulent sputum. She had gasping breaths at a rate of 38 per minute. Her color was pale and her lips were cyanotic. She was diaphoretic and had a heart rate of 138 beats/min. Po_2 was 47 on 100% nonrebreather mask.

The flight team prepared the patient for intubation. The patient continued to cough productively and required oral tracheal suctioning. The flight team decided to intubate with rapid induction with succinylcholine. The intubation was uneventful and the team continued to prepare for the transport.

In flight the patient's color improved and her heart rate decreased. She continued to require endotracheal suctioning for copious amounts of yellow sputum. The remainder of the flight was uneventful, and the patient was admitted directly to the intensive care unit.

Follow-up of this patient indicated that her respiratory status had not markedly improved. Sputum culture results revealed *M. tuberculosis.* Antibiotic therapy was then changed to the appropriate drugs for TB.

Further discussion with the family revealed the patient's history of fatigue, weight loss, anorexia, and a persistent cough. The cough had progressed in severity for the last 2 weeks.

The flight nurse notified the flight physician of the TB diagnosis. Both members of the flight team were exposed to the sputum from the intubation and suctioning. Neither one of the staff used a mask during the intubation, and the physician did not wear gloves because of the emergent nature of the procedure. The team members did not have a high index of suspicion that the woman had an infectious disease such as TB, and therefore was not in any of the high-risk categories.

Both flight team members instituted personal follow-up on the exposure with employee health. The flight nurse called the referring hospital to inform them of the infectious disease so they could initiate their own follow-up.

REFERENCES

1. Arankalle VA et al: Non-ABCDE hepatitis: is there another enterically transmitted hepatitis virus? *Hepatology Elsewhere* 256-257.
2. Asepsis, *The Infection Control Forum* 2(2):2-10, 1989.
3. Baker JA: Effects of Proshield glove on chlorhexidine gluconate penetration, *Healthpoint Technical Bulletin,* no 2, Jan 1995.
4. Blazer S, Berant M, Alon U: Bacterial meningitis: effect of antibiotic treatment on cerebral spinal fluid, *Am J Clin Pathol* 80:386-387, 1983.
5. Case-control study of HIV seroconversion in health-care workers after percutaneous exposure to HIV-infected blood—France, United Kingdom, and United States, *MMWR Morbid Mortal Wkly Rep* 44(50), 1995.
6. Centers for Disease Control and Prevention: Expanded tuberculosis surveillance and tuberculosis morbidity—United States, *MMWR Morbid Mortal Wkly Rep* 43:361-366, 1994.
7. Centers for Disease Control and Prevention: Guidelines for preventing the transmission of *Mycobacterium tuberculosis* in health-care facilities [recommendation], *MMWR Morbid Mortal Wkly Rep* 43(RR-13):51, 1994.
8. Centers for Disease Control and Prevention: Nosocomial transmission of multidrug-resistant tuberculosis among HIV-infected persons—Florida and New York, 1988-1991, *MMWR Morbid Mortal Wkly Rep* 40:585-591, 1991.
9. Dagjartsson A, Ludvigsson P: Bacterial meningitis: diagnosis and initial antibiotic therapy, *Pediatr Clin North Am* 34(1):219, 1987.
10. Department of Labor: 29 CFR part 1910.1030: Occupational exposure to bloodborne pathogens [final rule], *Federal Register,* Dec 6, 1991.
11. Geiman BJ, Smith LS: Dexamethasone therapy for bacterial meningitis in children, *West J Med* 157:27-31, 1992.
12. Graham TP, Moran GJ: Meningitis update: pearls, pitfalls, guidelines, and controversies, *Emerg Med Rep* 16(22):213-223, 1995.
13. Hobson DW: Proshield glove: preservative efficacy, *Healthpoint Technical Bulletin,* no 1, Sept 21, 1994.
14. *Hospital Infection Control* 16(8):101-110, 1989.
15. Isselbacher KJ et al: *Harrison's principles of internal medicine,* New York, 1995, McGraw-Hill.
16. Kaplan AJ et al: The prevalence of hepatitis C in a regional level one trauma center population, *J Trauma* 33(1):126-129, 1992.
17. Kelen GD et al: Human T-lymphotropic virus (HTLV I-II): infection among patients in an inner-city emergency department, *Ann Intern Med* 113:368-372, 1990.
18. Klein NC, Cunha BA: Bacterial meningitis, *Emerg Med* 28-30, Feb 28, 1994.
19. Lamphear BP et al: Decline of clinical hepatitis B in workers at a general hospital: relation to increasing vaccine-induced immunity, *Clin Infect Dis* 16:10-14, 1993.
20. Lewandowski C et al: Health care worker exposure to HIV-1 and HTLV I-II in critically ill, resuscitated emergency department patients, *Ann Emerg Med* 21(11):1353-1359, 1992.
21. Mangione C, Gerberding J, Cummings S: Occupational exposure to HIV: frequency and rates of underreporting of percutaneous and mucocutaneous exposures by medical housestaff, *Am J Med* 90:85, 1991.
22. Marcus R et al: Occupational blood contact among prehospital providers, *Ann Emerg Med* 25:776-779, 1995.
23. Moran GJ: Recognizing and minimizing the risks, *Emerg Med* 37-42, Dec 1994.
24. O'Boyle-Williams C et al: Variables influencing worker compliance with universal precautions in the emergency department, *Am J Infect Control* 22:138-148, 1994.
25. *Physician's desk reference,* ed 49, Montvale, NJ, 1995, Medical Economics Data Production.
26. Robert LM, Bell DM: HIV transmission in the health-care setting risks to healthcare workers and patients, *Infect Dis Clin North Am* 8(2):319-329, 1994.
27. Schaad UB, Kaplan SL, McCracken GH: Steroid therapy for bacterial meningitis, *Clin Infect Dis* 20:685-690, 1995.
28. Schluger N, Rom W: Current approaches to the diagnosis of active pulmonary tuberculosis, *Am J Respir Crit Care Med* 149:264-267, 1994.

29. Sepkowitz KA: AIDS, tuberculosis, and the health care worker, *Clin Infect Dis* 20:232-242, 1995.
30. Simms J: Latex allergy alert, *Can Nurse* 91(2):27-30, 1995.
31. Sloan EP et al: Human immunodeficiency virus and hepatitis B virus seroprevalence in an urban trauma population, *J Trauma* 38(5):736-741, 1994.
32. Sussman GL, Beeshold DH: Allergy to latex rubber, *Ann Intern Med* 122(1):43-46, 1995.
33. CDC: Update: evaluation of human T-lymphotropic virus type III/lymphadenopathy-associated virus infection in health care personnel, *MMWR Morbid Mortal Wkly Rep* 31:507-514, 1985.
34. Update on infectious diseases, Baltimore, MD, Jan 1989, Maryland Institute of Emergency Medical Service Systems.
35. West K: The final word, *Emerg Med Serv* 40-46, 1992.
36. Wong JB et al: Cost-effectiveness of interferon-alpha 2b treatment for hepatitis B's antigen-positive chronic hepatitis B, *Ann Intern Med* 122(9):664-675, 1995.

CHAPTER 26

Pediatric Medical Emergencies

COMPETENCIES

1. Determine the flight nursing interventions for the pediatric patient with airway compromise.
2. List three major signs of respiratory distress in a child.
3. Describe the seven most important therapy modalities in the treatment of croup in the child.
4. Describe the flight nurse interventions for the two most frequent dysrhythmias in pediatrics.
5. List the single most important component in the resuscitation of a child.
6. Describe several special considerations necessary in the medical evacuation of a sick child.
7. Name three observations that can be made during assessment of the level of consciousness for an infant or preverbal toddler.
8. Estimate the fluid needs of a 9-kg infant (usual weight 10 kg) who is 10% dehydrated.
9. List the 10 clinical features used in the assessment of pediatric dehydration and how they are altered with mild (±5%), moderate (±10%), and severe (±15% to 20%) dehydration weight loss.

Faced with an age spectrum of infancy to mature adolescence, the flight nurse can encounter a wide variety of clinical entities in providing care for the pediatric population. Children are not miniature adults, and to approach them as such would be a disservice. A host of physiologic, psychologic, and anatomic differences must be recognized and respected for efficient, quality care to be provided.

ALTERATIONS IN RESPIRATORY STATUS

Disorders of the respiratory system are the most common pediatric complaint encountered by the flight team because these disorders account for approximately 50% of all clinical disease in children younger than 5 years and 30% in children between the ages of 5 and 12 years. Respiratory dysfunction is the most common cause of cardiac arrest in children. Therefore stabilization of the airway is the primary concern in the critically ill child.[8]

Although the pathophysiology of respiratory illness is for children and adults, the anatomic and developmental differences can have a significant effect on management. The airways, alveoli, and chest configuration change throughout the growth process of infancy and early childhood, requiring an approach to airway management that differs from that for adults.

Newborns and infants are obligated nose breathers for the first 4 months of life,[6] and respiratory distress can occur with the occlusion of the nares by secretions or with an anatomical malformation such as choanal atresia. The presence of a nasogastric tube also can intensify preexisting respiratory distress. The small upper airway in infants and young children also predisposes them to respiratory distress in the presence of mucosal swelling. A small reduction in the radius of the trachea or bronchus resulting from secretions or swelling greatly increases the resistance to air flow.

The infant larynx is cartilaginous and much softer than that of the adult or older child. As a result, airway compression can occur with hyperextension or flexion of the neck. A towel roll placed under the shoulders of an infant or young child creates a slight distention of the neck, maximizing airway size and reducing airway resistance. The cricoid ring is the narrowest portion of the child's larynx; this enables the use of an uncuffed endotracheal tube by providing for a natural seal. Cuffed endotracheal tubes are not considered for use in children under the age of 8, except in unusual circumstances.

Because the airway of the infant or child is shorter, with the right-mainstem bronchus at less of an angle then the left, it is more common to see right-mainstem intubations in children requiring endotracheal tubes. Tube placement should be carefully evaluated by means of auscultation and chest radiography before transport.

The chest wall of the infant or young child is thin, and auscultation of breath sounds can be misleading because of transference of sounds across the chest. In the evaluation of endotracheal tube placement, the examiner should listen at the midaxillary line and then check visually for equal chest expansion.

Infants and young children have cartilaginous ribs and sternum, with poorly developed accessory muscles for respiration, and are therefore more dependent on diaphragmatic excursion for adequate ventilation. Anything that disrupts or restricts diaphragmatic motion can intensify respiratory distress and should be eliminated when possible. An oral or nasogastric tube for gastric decompression should be used to treat or prevent abdominal distention. Position should also be carefully evaluated; a supine infant may undergo increased respiratory difficulties because of the increased pressure of the abdominal contents on the diaphragm.

The flight nurse should be able to recognize immediately the signs of respiratory distress in a child, which include the triad of nasal flaring, expiratory grunting, and retracting (especially in the intercostal, subcostal, and suprasternal regions). Tachypnea, tachycardia, and prolonged expiratory time are also associated with increased respiratory effort. Pallor may signal respiratory distress long before cyanosis appears. The cyanotic child is in grave respiratory distress.

Most often, ventilation (as opposed to perfusion, diffusion, and control of ventilation) is the component of respiration that suffers in the pediatric patient. Ventilation depends in part on adequate airway diameter and on the degree of resistance to ventilation. Airway resistance is related to airway radius. Specifically, a 1-mm reduction in the diameter of the adult trachea (caused by swelling or a foreign body) results in a 25% reduction in the cross-sectional area of the trachea. In the infant trachea, however, a 1-mm reduction in the trachea's diameter reduces the cross-sectional area of the trachea by a full 75%. This narrowing extends throughout the bronchi, bronchioles, and alveoli. Epiglottitis, croup, bronchiolitis, and asthma all have a component of airway edema. Because even minimal airway edema can significantly reduce the functional area of the airway, these diseases may cause serious respiratory distress.

Disorders of the Upper Airway

Croup (Laryngotracheobronchitis, or LTB)

Croup is an acute illness manifested by cough (frequently described as "barking") and inspiratory stridor. Croup occurs most commonly in children between the ages of 3 months and 3 years and most frequently during the late fall and early winter months. The organism responsible is usually the parainfluenza virus, although respiratory syncytial virus, rubeola, and adenovirus have also been implicated. The entire respiratory tract may be inflamed, but the symptoms of croup are caused by inflammation at the level of the larynx down to the cricoid cartilage. The disease is usually self-limiting and resolves within 3 to 7 days.

The child with croup presents with a history of upper respiratory infection for the past few days, with development of a barking cough with or without inspiratory stridor. Wheezing may be present if the lower airway is involved. Chest-wall retractions are often seen as well. A low-grade fever may be present.

The white blood cell (WBC) count is generally less than 10,000, without a left shift. Blood cultures are negative, and chest radiography findings are usually normal. The anteroposterior neck film will show significant subglottic narrowing. This is called the "steeple sign," referring to the steeplelike appearance of the airway as it narrows in the subglottic, inflamed soft tissues.

If the child with croup has significant airway obstruction, hypoxemia and hypercarbia may develop, and the child will eventually sustain complete airway obstruction. Cyanosis is a late sign of airway obstruction and should be considered with utmost gravity.

Treatment. The treatment for croup is as follows:

1. Minimize the child's anxiety and energy expenditure; consider bringing a parent along, if possible. Defer starting an IV line unless the child is in extremis.
2. Give oxygen by way of cool aerosol.
3. Give racemic epinephrine by nebulizer for the child who exhibits stridor at rest. Dilute 0.5 ml of racemic epinephrine of a 2.25% solution in 2.5 ml of sterile water or saline solution, and deliver the treatment by way of a handheld nebulizer over 4 to 5 minutes. Racemic epinephrine may bring about dramatic improvement in a severely distressed child, and it should be tried before intubation unless the child is in extremis. Rebound obstruction may occur within 30 to 60 minutes. A child who receives racemic epinephrine in flight or in the emergency department should be admitted for observation to the hospital because of the potential for rebound respiratory distress. If the transport is to exceed 20 minutes, be prepared to repeat the nebulized treatment in flight.
4. Administer steroids (dexamethasone 0.6 mg/kg IV or orally [if able]) if the transport is prolonged.[4] Regional practice will determine whether further doses should be ordered.[6]
5. Avoid sedating the unintubated patient. There is little value in turning an agitated, hypoxic child into an apneic, hypoxic child.
6. Remember that the child who remains in severe respiratory distress in spite of the preceding measures or who has diminished air entry, agitation, or lethargy, cyanosis or pallor, and significant stridor at rest will require intubation. Take the utmost caution to prevent airway injury, including nonreversible, fixed stenosis of the subglottic airway resulting from pressure from the endotracheal tube against the inflamed tracheal walls. The endotracheal tube should be a full size smaller than the one the child would normally require. It should be an uncuffed tube; if only cuffed tubes are available, the cuff should not be inflated. Generally, intubated patients with croup require only aerosol continuous positive airway pressure of 2 to 4 mm H_2O. However, be prepared to support ventilation

with a bag-valve device, especially if the patient is to be sedated. A nasogastric tube should be inserted in any intubated child for gastric decompression.

7. The intubated child with croup should be restrained to protect the endotracheal tube. The child may be sedated, if agitated, with diazepam (0.1 to 0.3 mg/kg) or lorazepam.
8. Reduce fever.

Epiglottitis

Epiglottitis is a rapidly progressing bacterial infection of the epiglottis and surrounding soft tissue. In addition to septic inflammation of the airway, bacteremia is usually present. Vaccination against *Haemophilus influenzae* has reduced the incidence of *H. influenzae* as a primary causative agent in epiglottitis. Group A β-hemolytic streptococcus organisms now predominate.[13] Epiglottitis occurs without respect for the season and usually affects children between the ages of 3 and 7.

The child with epiglottitis usually presents with an illness of sudden onset (within 6 to 8 hours of presentation), including symptoms of dysphagia, inspiratory stridor, hoarse or muffled voice, fever, and drooling (secretions may be necrotic or blood-tinged). A preference for sitting up and leaning forward may be noted.

The WBC count will be greater than 10,000, with a left shift. A lateral neck film will show the characteristic "thumbprint" sign because the usually slitlike epiglottis has enlarged to resemble a thumb encroaching on the upper airway.

A child with epiglottitis should be intubated by the most experienced health care provider available, preferably someone experienced in anesthesia or ear, nose, and throat work.

If the child is not in extremis and is to be transported before intubation, it is imperative to minimize agitation. The child should be allowed to choose the transport position, usually sitting up in the parent's lap and leaning slightly forward. Cool mist by way of mask may help minimize swelling. All patients should receive oxygen. Blow-by oxygen may be more readily tolerated. IV therapy should be deferred for the unintubated patient because starting an IV line could agitate or panic a child and result in complete upper-airway obstruction. If the child does sustain airway obstruction, positive pressure ventilation with 100% oxygen by way of a self-inflating bag can be performed until intubation is carried out.[1]

If the diagnosis of epiglottitis is strongly suspected at the referring hospital and the epiglottitis is to be visualized directly, it should be done by the personnel most skilled at managing the pediatric airway in the operating room. It is also advisable to be ready to perform tracheostomy should stimulation of the epiglottis cause laryngeal obstruction and resulting respiratory arrest. If the diagnosis is confirmed, the child should be intubated in the operating room by the most skilled person available, using an endotracheal tube a full size smaller than the one normally recommended for the child's weight and age. The tube should be very well secured, and the child should be physically restrained to prevent its being dislodged. If agitated, the child may be sedated with diazepam or lorazepam. The flight team should be prepared to support ventilation with a resuscitation bag if the child requires sedation. A nasogastric tube should be passed to allow gastric decompression.

IV access should be obtained only after the child has been intubated. Fluids and antibiotics should be started after samples for blood cultures are obtained. IV fluids should be 5% dextrose ¼ normal saline solution at a maintenance rate or 10 ml/kg lactated Ringer's solution or normal saline solution if child is hypovolemic or dehydrated. Repeat as needed. A third-generation cephalosporin is generally used for IV antibiotic coverage.

Fever is best managed with acetaminophen 15 mg/kg.

Foreign Body Aspiration

Children between the ages of 6 months and 4 years are at the highest risk for foreign body aspiration. The key to diagnosis is the discovery of a history of sudden onset of coughing or wheezing associated with an episode of choking. The child may also have a history of playing with a suspicious item (e.g., peanut, piece of popcorn, seed, or small toy) just before choking. The aspirated item need not be in the trachea to cause respiratory embarrassment;

large items lodged in the esophagus may compress the trachea forward, with resulting airway obstruction.

Signs and symptoms of foreign body aspiration are determined by the location of the aspirated item. If the foreign body is at the glottis, the child will be hoarse, with cough, aphonia, and generally decreased breath sounds. If the airway obstruction is significant, the child may be cyanotic. If the foreign body is below the vocal cords and lodged in the trachea, the child will cough persistently and have bilateral decreased breath sounds. There may be a palpable "thud" over the trachea because the foreign body operates as a ball valve, rising with inspiration and dropping back into place on expiration. If the aspirated item is in the bronchus (usually the right), the child coughs, wheezes, and has locally diminished breath sounds, asymmetric chest wall movement, and, possibly, fever and purulent sputum if the aspiration occurred hours or days before presentation.

If the foreign body is in the esophagus, the child may exhibit stridor and wheezing. In functioning as a ball valve, the aspirated item allows some air to pass distally on inspiration but prevents escape of air on exhalation. On radiography, this effect is manifested in distal hyperinflation resulting from air trapping. The most helpful radiographs in making the diagnosis of foreign body aspiration are forced expiratory films. The film will show a hyperexpanded lung on the involved side and a shift of the mediastinal structures toward the uninvolved side. If the aspirated item is a coin, its location may be determined on radiography. The coin's flat surface will appear on the lateral film if the coin is in the trachea, and the edge of the coin will be seen on the anteroposterior view. If the coin is in the esophagus, the reverse is true: the edge of the coin is seen on the lateral view and the flat surface on the anteroposterior view.

Appropriate treatment is determined by the degree of the child's respiratory distress. If the child is severely compromised and in respiratory failure, an airway must be established around the foreign body, displacing it distally if necessary. If the foreign body is below the glottis and completely obstructing the airway, the patient should be intubated, pushing the foreign body distally into the right mainstem bronchus. The endotracheal tube should then be pulled back into the trachea, where it provides for ventilation of the left lung, demonstrated by the presence of breath sounds on the left side.

The child in minimal to moderate distress can be safely transported, with the foreign body undisturbed, to a facility with pediatric bronchoscopy capabilities. Postural drainage and chest percussion should be avoided. If the foreign body is dislodged, it may travel to another segment of the airway. This would create two dysfunctional portions of the lung: the portion it had previously affected, which may be atelectatic and full of infiltrate, and the newly obstructed portion.

The patient should receive oxygen with cool mist, if available, during transport to help reduce inflammation of the airway. An intubated child may benefit from an IV insertion for venous access; for unintubated children, the IV access may be deferred if the transport time is short.

Disorders of the Intrathoracic Airway

Bronchiolitis

Bronchiolitis can be a severe infection in children younger than 2 years. It is characterized by widespread, generalized inflammation of the respiratory tract mucosa with exudate, mucosal edema, and airway narrowing. Bronchiolitis occurs during the winter months. It is a viral infection (respiratory syncytial virus, adenovirus, and parainfluenza or influenza viruses, or both). Bronchiolitis may also have an atopic component, especially if it is recurrent or if a strong family history of allergy exists.

The child with bronchiolitis presents with a history of rhinitis, gradual onset of cough, expiratory wheezing, and increasing respiratory distress manifested by retractions, tachypnea, nasal flaring, and cyanosis. In early infancy and especially in infants with history of premature birth, bronchiolitis may be associated with apnea, particularly when the infecting organism is respiratory syncytial virus.

The infant with bronchiolitis has a prolonged expiratory phase and exhibits air trapping and hyperinflation of the lungs. The hyperinflation may displace the diaphragm downward, forcing the liver edge below the right costal margin. The WBC count is rarely increased.

Oxygen therapy alone may ease the respiratory distress and resolve the apnea of young infants with bronchiolitis. Humidified oxygen is best. When allergy is a factor in the disease, a trial dose of subcutaneous epinephrine may be effective (0.01 ml/kg of 1:1000 epinephrine). Inhalation treatment with bronchodilators may be helpful for children older than 3 months, when bronchospasm is a factor in the disease.

Intubation and ventilation are indicated for children with significant apnea that fails to resolve with oxygen and stimulation. It is also indicated for patients who have demonstrated respiratory failure with respiratory acidosis that has not reversed with inhalation treatment and oxygen.

Respiratory Syncytial Virus

Respiratory syncytial virus (RSV) is the most frequent cause of viral respiratory illness in infants and children. It is the cause of 40% of all serious upper-respiratory infections and 70% of all cases of bronchiolitis.[9] RSV infection is an infection of early childhood, with most children acquiring antibodies to RSV by the age of 12 months. RSV is highly contagious, and care should be taken to prevent its spread.

Children with RSV infections present with a history of upper-respiratory symptoms including cough and fever. Premature and newborn infants highly susceptible to RSV infection exhibit a frequent complication of apnea. The child may have copious, thick nasal and pharyngeal secretions and conjunctivitis with yellow-green discharge. Respiratory distress may be exhibited in retractions, tachypnea, and grunting.

Overwhelming RSV infection has been implicated as a probable cause of death in some infants with sudden death. The mechanism of death may in fact be the RSV-related apnea of premature and young infants. Clues to the presence of RSV versus other viral infections are wheezing, cough, and fever. These three symptoms are particularly characteristic of RSV infections, although they are by no means diagnostic. Some evidence links RSV infections at a young age to the development of reactive airway disease later in life.

As for all children in respiratory distress, treatment focuses on preservation of the airway and on oxygenation. Humidified oxygen is recommended.

Asthma and Status Asthmaticus

Asthma is the most common medical reason for missed school days in children aged 6 to 16 years; it occurs in 3% of these children.[9] Up to 5% of the population is afflicted with asthma.[13] More than half of all asthma patients have onset of their disease before the age of 5 years. In children, twice as many boys as girls have asthma; by adolescence, the numbers have equilibrated.[9] Asthma is rarely found in infants younger than 6 months because of the young infant's relative lack of smooth muscle required for a bronchospastic response. The mortality rates in both adults and children with asthma are unfortunately increasing.

Asthma is defined as a disease characterized by increased responsiveness of the trachea and bronchi to various stimuli. This increased responsiveness is manifested in widespread airway narrowing, which changes in severity, either in response to treatment or spontaneously. Asthma is probably only partially reversible; many asthmatic patients have slightly abnormal pulmonary function even when well.[9]

The usual triggers for bronchospasm are dust, infection, cold air, exercise, and allergens such as food, dyes, dander, pollen, and feathers. Endocrine changes and stress are also implicated.

The pathophysiology of asthma includes three distinct processes: (1) bronchoconstriction/bronchospasm, (2) airway edema, and (3) increased mucus production. The most common autopsy finding in patients who have died of asthma is extensive mucus plugging of the small airways.[9]

Air trapping, which occurs in the distal airways because of mucus plugging, results in hyperexpansion of the lungs. In the infant or young child, the hyperexpanded lungs may displace the diaphragm downward, displacing the liver downward on the right side, below the costal margin. The respiratory distress seen in asthmatic patients involves difficulty in exhaling versus inhaling. Children display a prolonged expiratory phase early in the course of distress. They are rarely hypoxic in the early stages, and their PCO_2 is low as a result of hyperventilation.

As the disease progresses, the child's respiratory rate, initially increased to compensate for a decreased tidal volume, decreases as the child works harder to breathe. The PCO_2 begins to climb, and eventually the pH falls.

Grave signs in the pediatric asthmatic patient include the following:

1. The use of accessory muscles, especially sternocleidomastoid retractions, is evident.
2. Decreased depth of retractions, decreased wheezing, and minimal breath sounds are indicators that the lungs are maximally hyperinflated and that little air is moving. No wheezing in a previously compromised and wheezing child is an ominous sign.
3. Cyanosis is refractory to 100% oxygen.
4. Agitation or decreasing level of consciousness is present.
5. Pulsus paradoxicus (a decrease in the systolic blood pressure on inspiration of 10 mm Hg or more) is seen. This decrease reflects greatly increased intrathoracic pressure because of the hyperexpanded lungs. Effort to add even more volume by way of inspiration compresses the great vessels of the chest and produces diminished venous return to the heart, causing the blood pressure to decrease on inspiration. A paradoxic pulse can also be detected in a radial pulse that decreases in intensity on inspiration.

Status asthmaticus is asthma that does not respond to adrenergic drug therapy. It may be of sudden onset, resulting from spasm of the major airways; or it may be slower, precipitated by a viral respiratory infection.

Treatment of the asthmatic patient is determined by the severity of the disease. Oxygen is always indicated because of the patient's potential hypoxia. Epinephrine 1:1000, 0.01 mg/kg (0.01 ml/kg) should be given subcutaneously and may be repeated in 20 to 30 minutes. Children will generally tolerate the resulting tachycardia and transient hypertension better than adults.

Several adrenergic agents are available; if used early in the course of status asthmaticus they may obviate the need for a second dose of epinephrine. Albuterol should be first administered by nebulizer, in a dose of 0.5 ml (or if the child is >10 kg, give .25 ml) in 2 ml of normal saline solution. Asthma that fails to respond to initial albuterol treatments may respond to inhalational atropine 0.05 to 0.075 mg/kg in 2 ml normal saline solution or ipratropium bromide 500 μg unit dose inhalation (give 250 μg 710 kg 140).[7] Terbutaline may be used as an injection or for inhalation. The dose for subcutaneous injection is .01 mg/kg of 1:1000 solution. For inhalation, the dose is .1 mg/kg in 2 ml normal saline solution.

Aminophylline, now used less frequently than in the past, may be helpful for the child who is not currently receiving it, for the child who has been noncompliant in taking medications, or for the child who cannot take the medications because of illness. A loading dose of aminophylline, 5 mg/kg, should be infused over 20 to 30 minutes, in 50 to 100 ml of 5% dextrose in water. Following the loading dose, an aminophylline maintenance infusion should deliver 1 mg/kg/hr. Neither the loading dose nor the infusion should be started before the theophylline level is determined if the patient has taken theophylline in the recent past.

Isoproterenol as an IV infusion is indicated for status asthmaticus refractory to other medical management. If time and the patient's condition allow, it should be tried before the child is intubated. An isoproterenol infusion should begin at 0.1 μg/kg/min, with the rate titrated to the child's clinical response and with regard for the heart rate. Side effects include tachycardia, increased myocardial oxygen consumption, and peripheral vasodilatation. If isoproterenol is successful in relieving bronchospasm, the infusion rate should be decreased slowly (over 30 to 36 hours).

Starting an isoproterenol infusion is not recommended in the prehospital setting with an asthmatic patient in extremis. The drug's potent side effects preclude its administration. If the patient is moribund and in respiratory failure, intubation and ventilation should be undertaken with respect for the hyperexpanded lungs and tendency toward pneumothorax. A ventilatory rate that allows for a long expiratory time is the most efficient method of ventilation in the intubated asthmatic patient. Intubated asthmatic patients almost always require chemical paralysis and sedation for optimal ventilation.

Disorders of the Alveoli and Interstitium

Pneumonia

The characteristic adult pattern of lobar involvement with pneumonia is unusual in children. The pediatric disease is more diffuse and, with the airways more frequently involved, gives rise to the term *bronchial pneumonia.*

The child with pneumonia frequently presents with a history of upper-respiratory infection for 3 days or longer. There may be a sudden onset of fever and tachypnea. Bacterial pneumonia is one of the few causes of cough in the infant younger than 6 weeks. An infant younger than 6 weeks with cough should be presumed to have pneumonia until this diagnosis is proved otherwise on chest radiography.[9] A chest film will show loculated, focalized infiltrates with bacterial pneumonia. The pattern will be more diffuse with viral pneumonia.

The causes of pneumonia vary in different age groups. Newborns with pneumonia most typically have *Escherichia coli,* group B hemolytic streptococcus, gram-positive organisms, staphylococcus groups, and listena. *Chlamydia trachomatus* is a common offender in children up to 3 months of age. Immunosuppressed children are vulnerable to pneumonia, especially that caused by *Pneumocystis carinii.* For infants beyond the newborn period, the two organisms responsible for pediatric pneumonia are *Staphylococcus* and *Streptococcus pneumoniae.* Most pneumonia infections are viral. The incidence of *H. influenzae* as a causative agent has declined with the advent of *H. influenzae* vaccination.

Treatment in the air medical setting is supportive and should include improvement of oxygenation, fluid replacement for the dehydrated child, and fever control. The infant with severe pneumonia may require intubation and ventilation.

Pertussis

Pertussis is a highly communicable disease, prevalent in children younger than 2 years. Mortality is highest for children younger than 5 months. Before the development of the vaccine, pertussis was a major cause of death in infants, with seven times as many babies dying of pertussis as of meningitis.[9]

Adults and children over the age of 2 years usually have mild symptoms. These include low-grade fever and cough, which may be paroxysmal. In young infants, coughing paroxysms may be severe, not allowing for sufficient air movement. This gives rise to the inspiratory "whoop" as the child works to increase air intake. Coughing may be forceful enough to cause suffusion of the face, conjunctival hemorrhage, cyanosis, petechiae, and hypoxia-related seizures. Coughing may be accompanied by emesis, diaphoresis, and exhaustion. The acute phase of pertussis may last 1 to 2 weeks, followed by many weeks of resolving mild cough. The complete blood count of a child with pertussis is remarkable for lymphocytosis (70% to 80% lymphs) with a WBC count of 20,000 to 30,000/ml.

Complications of pertussis include secondary bacterial infections, especially pneumonia, apnea, and sudden death from severe paroxysms of cough.

Treatment of pertussis is symptomatic, focusing on preservation of the airway. Humidified oxygen should be administered. If the child is dehydrated, IV hydration may be indicated. Children who require intubation for pertussis will still have coughing episodes and may require chemical paralysis and sedation to achieve optimal ventilation.

Oral erythromycin 40 mg/kg/day for 96 hours is the antibiotic of choice.[11] Personnel who transport these children should be vaccinated themselves.

Apnea/Apparent Life-Threatening Event

Apnea in the infant is defined as the cessation of breathing for 20 seconds or longer, with or without slowing of the heart rate. Many preterm infants have apnea, which may persist up to several weeks past term.[15]

Apnea is further classified as *central apnea,* in which the infant does not make an effort to breathe; *obstructive apnea,* in which the chest moves but no air comes out of the mouth or nose; and *mixed apnea,* when obstructive apnea follows or is mixed with central apnea.[3]

Apnea accompanied by pallor, cyanosis, and bradycardia is always abnormal.

An apparent life-threatening event (ALTE), seen in children up to 6 months of age, consists of apnea, as described above; cyanosis, redness, or pallor; muscle tone alterations (usually limpness); and choking or gagging. It is frightening to the observer, who may think the infant has died. ALTEs are seen in 2% to 3% of the general population, with identifiable causes only about half of the time. These causes include infection, especially RSV; heart disease; infection; seizures; airway obstruction; choking; and breath-holding spells.[3] In the past ALTE was often labeled "aborted crib death" or "near-miss sudden infant death syndrome (SIDS)," terms that are now obsolete and misleading.[3]

Treatment in the transport setting is supportive, with cardiorespiratory monitoring, elevation of the head of the bed 20 to 30 degrees to minimize gastric reflux, intubation and ventilation as needed, and treatment of known underlying causes (e.g., control of seizures).

Sudden Infant Death Syndrome

SIDS is defined as the sudden, unexpected death of an infant in whom, on autopsy, no recognized lethal disorder is found.[1] It occurs most frequently in infants between the ages of 4 weeks and 1 year of age, with the incidence peaking at 2 to 3 months.[18] Of all cases, 88% to 91% occur in the first 6 months of life.[1] SIDS is the most frequent cause of death in children younger than 1 year, beyond the neonatal period.[9] The incidence of SIDS is 1.4 per 1000 live births.[10] Annually, 6000 to 7000 babies die of SIDS, with the highest incidence in the winter months. According to the Colorado SIDS Program (1988), boys die more frequently than girls by a ratio of 3:2.

Babies with associated contributing factors include those with history of premature birth, those who were of small size for gestational age, and those with subtle neurologic abnormalities.[11] Theories of cause are numerous and varied; they include immaturity of the central nervous system (CNS) resulting from an antenatal event, upper-airway obstruction, hyperactive upper-airway reflexes, cardiac conduction disorders, abnormal responses to hypoxia and hypercarbia, abnormal responses to hyperthermia, and alterations in fat metabolism.

On autopsy, 87% of babies found to have died of SIDS have intrathoracic petechiae, especially on the thymus, pleura, and pericardium.[9] Frequently, pulmonary edema is present, along with increased amounts of smooth muscle in the medial layer of the pulmonary arterioles.

Typically, the SIDS infant presents with a history of having been put to bed in good health, or possibly with a mild upper-respiratory infection. The infant is later found apneic and cyanotic. Generally these infants are in full arrest by the time they reach medical attention.

The relationship between apnea and SIDS is indistinct. Many babies are admitted for apnea workups, but very few go on to die of SIDS. Furthermore, the vast majority of infants who die of SIDS have no documented history of apnea.[9]

When the child's pupils are fixed and dilated, the cardiac rhythm is asystole, and rectal temperature is 35° C or lower, the prognosis is grim. Even if a rhythm is restored after prolonged arrest, CNS anoxic damage is significant.

Treatment of the infant who is potentially, or even questionably, viable should proceed in the same manner as for any infant in cardiac arrest. Studies have shown that the infant who does not respond to adequate ventilation and three rounds of drugs has a very poor prognosis, and resuscitation will probably not be successful.[9]

If the pulse returns with ventilation alone, the prognosis is much better.[12] This infant is one who is discovered in extremis, generally with cyanosis, bradycardia, pallor, and apnea. This is known as an *ALTE.* It is a risk factor for sudden death (including SIDS).[15] Depending on the duration of the respiratory arrest, the child may have pulmonary edema, aspiration pneumonia, and significant neurologic sequelae. SIDS itself, however, is irreversible respiratory and cardiac arrest. Even though the baby may regain a heartbeat and blood pressure in response to resuscitation, an ongoing process is at work and the child eventually will die.[1]

The medical community is rarely able to help the SIDS infant. Throughout the resuscitation, and afterward, the baby's family is as much a patient as the infant. The family may be helped tremendously by a few well-chosen words and the simple presence of a compassionate medical person. A direct, empathetic approach is usually best, and a relationship with the family should be initiated before resuscitation efforts are ceased.

The family should be provided a quiet, private place away from the hectic activity of rescue and emergency personnel, whether the resuscitative efforts take place in the home or in the emergency department.

If state law allows a nurse or emergency medical technician to pronounce a patient dead at the scene, the flight team should tell the family the truth about the child's death. If pronouncing a patient dead while at the scene is not legal, the baby must be transported. Involved explanations of SIDS are probably inappropriate and may be unwelcome. What is most appropriate is reassurance that the family could not have predicted or prevented the SIDS death. The family may not seem to listen to, or even hear, any words of comfort or explanation, but those words may bring relief weeks and months later.

Family members should be given the opportunity to see and hold the baby, after hearing a few preparatory words about how the infant will look and feel. Literature from the SIDS Foundation may be helpful. The flight team or the social worker at the receiving hospital should alert the local SIDS Foundation to the death so that it may offer support services.

ALTERATIONS IN CARDIAC FUNCTION

The two most important clues to the presence of heart disease in the child are also those two signs that are most apt to bring the child to the attention of emergency medical services: cyanosis and congestive heart failure.

Congenital heart defects and acquired heart disease are discussed in this section, as are the most common dysrhythmias of pediatrics, but an in-depth review of each of the defects is beyond the scope of this chapter. The discussion features the presentation of the child with a congenital defect, with defects organized according to the ages at which they most commonly become symptomatic.

By far, the most common causes of congestive heart failure in the child are congenital heart defects (producing volume overload, outflow obstruction, or impaired myocardial function), vascular defects (coarctation of the aorta), and acquired myocardial disease (myocarditis and rheumatic heart disease). Other causes of congestive failure include sepsis, acidosis, CNS disease, anemia, and hypoglycemia.

Elements of the child's history that should raise the flight nurse's suspicion of congestive heart failure include the following:

1. Poor feeding—The infant tires easily or feeds very slowly or becomes dusky while feeding.
2. Tachypnea—The infant has a respiratory rate above 60 breaths/min at rest.
3. Cyanosis—The infant's color may be grayer, or more ashen, than blue.
4. Hypoxemic spells, especially on awakening, after feeding, or after a bowel movement—The infant may become more tachypneic than usual and gray or blue. The infant may cry as if in pain.
5. Oliguria
6. Orthopnea and dyspnea
7. Growth retardation
8. Frequent pneumonias or upper-respiratory infections

Findings of the child's examination suggestive of congestive heart failure include the following:

1. Tachypnea, especially at rest
2. Rales, audible on auscultation of the chest
3. Edema, especially of the face, pretibial and presacral areas, and, later, the extremities
4. Hepatomegaly, possibly accompanied by splenomegaly; child's liver possibly palpable well below the right costal margin
5. Possible presence of clubbing, which implies the presence of long-standing tissue hypoxemia of pulmonary or cardiac origin
6. Cardiomegaly on chest radiography

The child with acquired heart disease may also present with congestive heart failure, cyanosis, or both. Children with myocarditis usually present with a history of upper-respiratory or gastrointestinal illness within 1 month of the gradual onset of cardiac symptoms, including dyspnea on exertion, and malaise. Radiography will demonstrate generalized cardiomegaly, and electrocardiography may show dysrhythmias and conduction delays. Viruses implicated in myocarditis are Coxsackie A and B, rubella, cytomegalovirus, mumps, herpes, and adenovirus.

Purulent pericarditis is the form of acquired heart disease most apt to be life threatening. It is virtually always the result of infection elsewhere in the body. Organisms responsible include *Pneumococcus, Streptococcus, Staphylococcus, Neisseria meningitidis,* and *H. influenzae.*

The child with purulent pericarditis will appear to have sepsis, with fever and, possibly, signs of cardiac tamponade. Prior treatment with antibiotics will sterilize the pericardial fluid but may not prevent a tamponade from developing. Pericardiocentesis in the child presenting with signs of tamponade and sepsis may be lifesaving.

Air medical treatment of the child with suspected or known congestive heart failure from either congenital or acquired heart disease is supportive. Medical therapy may include the following:

1. Furosemide, IV 1 mg/kg
2. Morphine, IV 0.1 mg/kg
3. Oxygen—Oxygen may not relieve the cyanosis of a child with a fixed right-to-left shunt, but should still be administered. Systemic PaO_2 may be increased by way of oxygen dissolved in the plasma, and pulmonary vasoconstriction may be partially relieved, decreasing the amount of right-to-left shunting.
4. Intubation and positive-pressure ventilation on 100% oxygen for the gravely ill child—PEEP, if initiated, should be performed very carefully, with consideration of the child's potentially decreased venous return resulting in compromised cardiac output.

The following congenital heart defects are grouped according to the ages at which they most frequently first present. They are listed in Table 26-1 in decreasing order of frequency.

Disorders of Cardiac Rate and Rhythm in the Child

Dysrhythmias in the pediatric population are more frequently caused by hypoxia, hypothermia, hypogly-

TABLE 26-1

Most frequently occurring heart defects grouped by age of most frequent onset

Birth-1 wk	1 wk-1 mo	1-6 mo	6-12 mo	5-15 yr
Hypoplastic left heart	Coarctation of the aorta	Endomyocardial disease	Ventricular septal defect	Rheumatic myocarditis
Aortic atresia	Transposition of the great vessels	Ventricular septal defect	Endomyocardial disease	Ventricular septal defect
Mitral atresia	Endomyocardial disease	Patent ductus arteriosus		Atrial septal defect
	Ventricular septal defect	Total anomalous pulmonary venous return		
	Patent ductus arteriosus	Coarctation of the aorta		
		Transposition of the great vessels		

cemia, electrolyte imbalance, or a malpositioned central venous pressure catheter than by primary myocardial or coronary artery disease. The two most frequent dysrhythmias are supraventricular tachycardias (SVTs) and asystole. Following is a discussion of these and other most frequently encountered dysrhythmias in the pediatric age group. A rule of thumb is that in the healthy child with a normal heart, a dysrhythmia is a sign of problems elsewhere in the body. The flight nurse should consider extracardiac causes of dysrhythmia.

Normal Sinus Rhythm

Normal sinus rhythm is characterized by a PR interval that is normal for age and heart rate (Table 26-2). The PR interval shortens with increased heart rates and increases with age. T-wave inversion is common in the limb leads and may be entirely normal.

Sinus Dysrhythmia

Sinus dysrhythmia is common in pediatrics, especially among adolescents. The heart rate varies with the phase of respiration, increasing during inspiration and decreasing during expiration. The underlying heart rate is within the normal limits for the child's age, and the PR interval is within normal limits.

Sinus Tachycardia

Tachycardia at rest or during feeding may be a clue to the presence of congestive heart failure. An increase in the heart rate of 20% above the baseline value is considered significant. Fever, anxiety, pain, hypovolemia, poisoning, and shock can cause sinus tachycardia. The highest sinus rate in children may be 210 to 220 per minute. Because of their normally healthy myocardiums, children usually tolerate tachycardias better than can most adults.

Treatment for sinus tachycardia is treatment of the underlying cause.

Sinus Bradycardia

Bradycardia in the child is frequently a serious, even ominous, warning sign of the need for prompt intervention. The child's history is an essential di-

TABLE 26-2

Maximum and minimum PR intervals

MAXIMUM PR INTERVALS (SEC)

Age	Heart rate (beats/min) 71-90	91-110	111-130	130-150	151+
Younger than 1 mo		0.11	0.11	0.11	0.11
1-9 mo		0.14	0.13	0.12	0.11
10-24 mo		0.15	0.14	0.14	0.10
3-5 yr	0.16	0.16	0.16		
6-13 yr	0.18	0.18	0.16	0.16	
Older than 16 yr	0.12		0.20		

MINIMUM PR INTERVALS ACCORDING TO AGE

Age	PR interval (sec)
Younger than 3 yr	0.08
3-16 yr	0.10
Older than 16 yr	0.12

agnostic tool in sorting out the causes. Most common are hypoxia, hypothermia, increased intracranial pressure (ICP), sick sinus syndrome, increased parasympathetic tone, and drug effects (digoxin, β-blockers).

The heart rate is less than normal for age. The PR interval is normal for age and heart rate, and P waves are present unless an escape rhythm (junctional or ventricular) takes over.

Treatment is removal of the underlying cause. If a prompt increase in heart rate is necessary to restore hemodynamic or neurologic stability, atropine, 0.01 to 0.03 IV mg/kg or by endotracheal tube; or isoproterenol, 0.1 to 1.0 μg/kg/min by IV infusion may be used to increase the heart rate while the cause of the bradycardia is being sorted out. If the patient is tolerating the bradycardia (has adequate peripheral pulses and stable blood pressure, and is alert), close observation is necessary with pharmacologic agents close at hand.

Premature Atrial Contractions

Premature atrial contractions (PACs) in the child may be an entirely normal finding, or they may be related to congestive heart failure or digoxin toxicity. PACs require no treatment unless they occur so frequently that the atrial contribution to ventricular filling is decreased and cardiac output falls. If treatment is required, digoxin is usually the drug of choice.

Supraventricular Tachycardias

SVTs originate at the bundle of His or above and result from an abnormal mechanism (versus a response to the body's need for a higher cardiac output). SVT is the most common symptomatic dysrhythmia in children.

At heart rates of 180 to 300 beats/min, it may be difficult to differentiate atrial from junctional and supraventricular from ventricular rhythms. These rhythms may be well tolerated, or they may cause hemodynamic compromise because of reduced atrial contribution to ventricular filling. The rapid ventricular rate may further decrease cardiac output by not allowing sufficient time for ventricular filling. Such children may present in congestive failure and simultaneous intravascular volume depletion.

Sinus tachycardia may be differentiated from supraventricular rhythms based on the following:

1. Sinus tachycardia rates rarely exceed 210 beats/min in children or 230 beats/min in infants.
2. Upright P waves in leads I, II, and AVF support a diagnosis of sinus tachycardia.
3. History may suggest one diagnosis versus the other (e.g., fever, dehydration, and sepsis suggest sinus tachycardia).
4. Response to medical treatment, such as a decrease in heart rate in response to volume or treatment of fever, favors sinus tachycardia.

Paroxysmal atrial tachycardia (PAT) is a supraventricular rhythm of sudden onset. About 10% to 20% of children with PAT have Wolff-Parkinson-White syndrome.

Treatment of SVT is determined by the child's status. Ocular pressure and carotid sinus massage are contraindicated in children. If treatment is required, it may be helpful to try an ice bag, placed firmly against the child's face and held in place for 10 to 15 seconds. This cooling of the face produces a transient Valsalva maneuver, central apnea, and shunting of blood to the vital organs. The shunting stimulates the baroreceptors, producing a decreased heart rate.

Adenosine given rapidly intravenously, followed by a saline bolus, can be effective in interrupting SVT. Cardioversion may be useful if the child is hemodynamically compromised. The dose is 0.5 to 1 J/kg, with lower dosages and much caution advised for digitalis-treated patients.

Digoxin may be more useful in narrow-complex tachycardias. In Wolff-Parkinson-White syndrome, digoxin may facilitate atrioventricular conduction and increase the ventricular rate. Verapamil has been noted to cause profound hypotension in children and should be used only in an intensive care setting.[12]

Atrial Fibrillation and Atrial Flutter

If the ventricular response to atrial fibrillation or flutter is regular, the irregularity may be a dysrhythmia of digoxin toxicity. If not, digoxin is the treatment of choice.

Both dysrhythmias are rare in the pediatric patient; they are usually associated with congenital heart lesions producing excessive atrial stretch, or are seen in patients who have undergone intraatrial manipulation.

Premature Ventricular Contractions and Ventricular Tachycardia

Differentiating ventricular tachycardia from supraventricular tachycardia with aberrancy may be difficult in children. Ventricular tachycardia may be an ominous dysrhythmia, progressing to fibrillation; or it may be well tolerated for 24 hours or longer. For this reason, perfusion deficits and changes in levels of consciousness are not always useful in deciding for or against ventricular tachycardia.

The most common causes of ventricular ectopy in children are hypoxia, hypokalemia, a malpositioned central venous pressure catheter, acidosis, and treatment with cardiotoxic chemotherapeutic drugs.

Treatment, if required, should begin with an IV bolus of lidocaine 1 mg/kg up to a total of 3 mg/kg, followed by continuous infusion at a rate of 20 to 50 μg/kg/min. Procainamide and phenytoin may also be useful. Cardioversion should be accompanied by administration of an antidysrhythmic drug. Ventricular tachycardia without a pulse should be defibrillated (versus cardioverted) at 1 to 4 J/kg.

Ventricular Fibrillation

Ventricular fibrillation is a rare dysrhythmia in pediatrics. It may occur after electrocution injuries or drownings, or as a result of severe metabolic imbalances (acidosis, hypoxia, and hypokalemia). It is often the preterminal dysrhythmia in severe acidosis.

Treatment, as for pulseless ventricular tachycardia, is immediate defibrillation with 1 to 4 J/kg.

Atrioventricular Conduction Blocks

Atrioventricular conduction blocks are rare in pediatrics. First-degree block may be entirely normal in pediatrics, or it may signify rheumatic heart disease, a congenital heart defect, or digoxin toxicity. No treatment is necessary unless the block signifies digoxin toxicity.

Second-degree blocks, both type 1 and type 2, have the same causes as first-degree block. Second-degree blocks may also be the result of increased parasympathetic tone.

Third-degree block may occur in the absence of any identifiable structural defects or with endocardial cushion defects, corrected transposition of the great vessels defect, and in babies whose history includes maternal lupus. Most infants tolerate third-degree heart block well, and few require pacemakers before the age of 2 years. The patient with symptoms of a low ventricular rate will benefit from a continuous IV infusion of isoproterenol.

Cardioversion and Defibrillation

Tachydysrhythmias requiring cardioversion and ventricular fibrillation are rare in pediatric patients. Synchronized cardioversion is used to convert SVT, atrial fibrillation, and flutter with hemodynamic compromise; and ventricular tachycardia with a pulse. The child, who may be awake, should be sedated with IV midazolam, diazepam, or lorazepam. One paddle should be placed to the right of the sternum at the level of the second rib and the other at the xiphoid level, in the midclavicular line on the left. For the infant, the paddles should have a diameter of about 4.5 cm; for older children, a diameter of 8.0 cm is adequate. The initial dose is 0.5 to 1.0 J/kg, with the defibrillator set in the "synch" mode.

For defibrillation, paddle placement is the same as for cardioversion. The dosage is 2 J/kg; if unsuccessful, double at 4 J/kg twice if necessary. If the patient remains in fibrillation or asystole, pH, oxygenation, temperature, and serum potassium should be reassessed.

Pediatric Cardiopulmonary Arrest

Effective pediatric resuscitation requires not only knowledge of appropriate drugs and CPR techniques but also an appreciation for the differences between the child and the adult and how those differences help determine the priorities for resuscitation.

The phenomenon of sudden cardiac death as defined by the American Heart Association is virtually unknown in the pediatric population. Airway obstruction, anoxia, or both are the precipitating event in fully 90% of all pediatric arrests.[9] The remaining 10% are associated mainly with congenital heart disease and the resulting dysrhythmias. The child's airway is at risk not only from accidental injuries (motor vehicle, drowning, and mechanical suffocation), but also from the two nearly exclusive pediatric disease entities, croup and epiglottitis. The most crucial step in pediatric resuscitation is the establishment of a patent airway and adequate ventilation. Frequently ventilation and reoxygenation alone will restore a normal heart rate and blood pressure.

Ventilation

The single most important component in the resuscitation of a child is the reestablishment of adequate ventilation and oxygenation. Anoxia or airway obstruction is nearly always the precipitating event in pediatric arrest. The following sequence of events for cardiac arrest resulting from respiratory failure has been suggested[5]:

1. Increased respiratory effort produces
2. Increased oxygen consumption, and
3. Increased fatigue, with early metabolic acidosis, which, coupled with
4. Increased respiratory acidosis and hypoxia, creates
5. Enzyme system dysfunction, which in turn leads to
6. Decreased myocardial contractility and decreased cardiac output, with resulting
7. Cerebral ischemia and respiratory center depression, followed by
8. Respiratory arrest and then cardiac arrest

Not all children will require intubation and ventilation; often, repositioning to open the airway is sufficient. The trachea in infants and children has not yet developed the firm cartilaginous support of the adult trachea, and for this reason, hyperextension of the head and neck may collapse the trachea. The child should be placed in a "sniffing" position, with the occiput elevated slightly on a small towel or blanket. Pulling the mandible forward usually relieves upper-airway obstruction by the tongue. If the child does not resume breathing at this point, bag-mask ventilation should begin promptly, using 100% O_2. Sufficient tidal volume is that volume required to make the chest rise; a guideline for calculating this volume for ventilator placement is 10 ml/kg. Nearly any pediatric patient, aside from those with airway obstruction by a foreign body, can be well ventilated with a bag mask, including the epiglottitis patient. Just as in the adult patient, intubation may cause dysrhythmias in the hypoxic, acidotic child. It should not be the first line of airway management used.

If endotracheal intubation is required, it should be done by the most experienced person at the scene, and only after the child has been oxygenated and ventilated with the bag mask. The most frequent short-term complications of intubation are vagally induced bradycardia and asystole. Both usually resolve with ventilation and oxygenation. Atropine also given before intubation may be helpful in avoiding vagally induced bradycardia and diminishing secretions.

Ideally, any child younger than 8 years should be intubated with an uncuffed tube. If only cuffed tubes are available, the cuff should be left uninflated. When there is doubt about the child's size, it is best to intubate with an uncuffed tube.

Any pediatric patient being ventilated with a bag mask or bag endotracheal tube should have a pressure manometer in line if available. Inspiratory pressures should not exceed 30 mm Hg in the child with normal pulmonary function.

Oxygen delivery should always be at 100% during resuscitation. Retrolental fibroplasia is virtually unknown beyond 42 weeks of gestation. Hypoxia-based respiratory drive is very rare in children, as is pulmonary fibrosis resulting from oxygen toxicity. The child undergoing optimal cardiopulmonary resuscitation (CPR) has a cardiac output only 25% to 30% of normal. Mixed venous blood is markedly desaturated, and, as a result of intrapulmonary shunting, arterial oxygen saturation also falls off. The benefits of 100% oxygen in an arrest situation clearly outweigh the risks. Either a nasogastric or an orogastric tube should be placed as soon as possible. This will help decrease the risk of vomiting and aspiration, particularly during transport.

Frequently, establishing an airway and ventilating the child will reestablish circulation. If the child remains pulseless, however, or if the heart rate is less than 50% of the normal rate for the appropriate age group, CPR should be initiated to restore cardiac output. A child's pulse is best checked at the brachial and femoral arteries.

Precordial thumps are not used in pediatric resuscitation because of the substantial risk of injury to the relatively larger liver. Ventricular fibrillation is a rare dysrhythmia in children and is as likely to be converted by CPR as by a precordial thump.

In the infant, CPR is performed with two or three fingers over the lower third of the sternum or by encircling the infant's chest with both hands and compressing the lower third of the sternum with both thumbs, at a rate of 100 to 120 compressions/min.

In the older child, the heel of one hand is used to compress the lower third of the sternum 80 to 100 times/min. In adolescents, the technique is the same as that for adults.

Intravenous Access

Establishing an IV line may well be the most difficult step in a pediatric resuscitation. The most accessible vein that does not require interruption of CPR is ideal. In the infant and young child, the femoral vein may be the best candidate, although it should be reserved for emergency situations only because cannulation of this vein is associated with many complications, including septic arthritis of the hip.

Other sites include the scalp veins in infants, the veins of the dorsum of the hand, the antecubital veins, the external jugular veins, and the saphenous vein and veins of the foot. The optimal vein to be cannulated will vary with the child and the diagnosis.

Another option for the critically ill child is an intraosseous line. This line uses a steel needle (a bone-marrow needle, spinal needle with a stylet, or an intraosseous needle designed specifically for this procedure) that is inserted through the bony cortex into the bone marrow of the tibia, femur, or anterior iliac crest for the purpose of infusing drugs, fluids, or blood (Fig. 26-1). Circulation times for drugs infused via intraosseous lines are comparable to those for IV lines. Unlike peripheral veins, intramedullary vessels do not collapse in the patient in shock because they are protected by hard, noncollapsible bony walls.

The best sites for intraosseous line placement are those where the bone marrow is most plentiful and most accessible. The most commonly used sites are (1) the proximal tibia 1 to 2 cm below the tubercle, on the anteromedial surface; (2) the distal femur 2 to 3 cm above the external condyle, in the anterior midline of the femur; and (3) the anterior surface of the iliac crest.

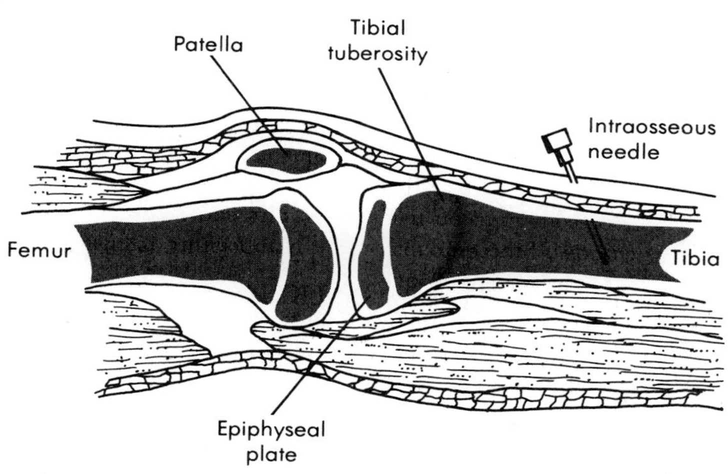

Fig. 26-1. Intraosseous insertion of needle. (From Barkin RM, Rosen P: *Emergency pediatrics,* ed 4, St Louis, 1994, Mosby.)

The needle should be inserted at a 90-degree angle to the skin and, on resistance, should be advanced with a boring or screwing motion; when decreased resistance or "give" is encountered, the needle has penetrated the bone marrow. The stylet is removed. Marrow should be aspirated through the needle to verify intramedullary placement, and then the line should be flushed with normal saline solution to clear it of bone, clot, or debris. IV tubing is attached and the infusion started. Because of the force required to insert this line and the pain that the patient suffers, intraosseus lines are not recommended for use in conscious patients.

Complications of intraosseous lines include subperiosteal and subcutaneous infusions, osteomyelitis (in only 0.6% of all cases reported in which an intraosseous line was in use), and decreased cellularity of the bone marrow of young infants after infusions of strongly alkaline solutions or very hypertonic substances (e.g., 8.4% sodium bicarbonate or dextrose 50%). Dilution of these two drugs on a ratio of 1:1 with sterile water is recommended for infants.

Pharmacologic Therapy

Sodium Bicarbonate. The role of sodium bicarbonate in resuscitation merits critical review. Effective ventilation with the goal of creating a mild-to-moderate respiratory alkalosis may counteract substantial metabolic acidosis. On the other hand, the indiscriminate use of sodium bicarbonate may produce metabolic alkalosis (a potent myocardial depressant, especially at a pH greater than 7.60), as well as hypernatremia, and a hyperosmolar state. Both of the latter conditions have been implicated in intraventricular hemorrhage in infants. Severely hyperosmolar states may themselves be lethal. The aggressive use of sodium bicarbonate may contribute significantly to morbidity of the child.

In addition, pediatric patients may in fact be less sensitive to the effects of metabolic acidosis than adults. Data have shown that the average adult patient demonstrates disturbances in cardiovascular function at a pH of 7.20 or less. Children may not exhibit the same disturbances unless the pH is 6.9 or lower.[17]

Sodium bicarbonate dosages are ideally determined on the basis of arterial blood gas (ABG) values and the patient's kilogram weight. If ABG values are not available and the patient has had an unwitnessed arrest, the initial dose is 1 mEq/kg, repeated every 10 minutes with half of the initial dose.

If the patient's arrest is of short duration, or witnessed, and adequate ventilation is reestablished quickly, sodium bicarbonate should not be given until ABG results are known.

When ABG results are available, doses are based on the following formula:

$$\text{Base deficit} \times 0.3 \times \text{Patient's weight (kg)} = \text{Amount of bicarbonate to be administered}$$

Half of this amount should be replaced at once, with the other half given over the following hour, to avoid rapid changes in pH and serum osmolarity.[5]

In the newborn infant up to the age of 30 days, only half-strength sodium bicarbonate (i.e., 4.2%) should be given. If the commercially prepared form is not available, 8.4% should be diluted in an equal volume of sterile water.

Atropine. Atropine is one of the most useful and benign drugs in the resuscitation of children. The child generally tolerates the atropine-generated tachycardia and increased myocardial oxygen demands better than the adult with some degree of coronary artery disease. The child's physiologic response to severe hypoxia, hypercarbia, or both is usually bradycardia. Atropine is useful in the treatment of bradycardia (sinus and second-degree and proximal third-degree heart block) and asystole. It is also useful in the pretreatment of patients who require intubation to prevent the reflex bradycardia that occurs in response to instrumentation of the airway. The dose of atropine is 0.02 mg/kg. A complete vagolytic dose in young children is 1.0 mg; in older children and adolescents, it is 2.0 mg. In insufficient doses (less than completely vagolytic doses), atropine may cause a paradoxical bradycardia. The American Heart Association recommends giving at least 0.15 mg as a minimum dosage.[14]

Epinephrine. Epinephrine's most important contribution in cardiac arrest is its peripheral vasoconstrictive properties. In addition, it increases the perfusion pressure generated during cardiac massage, improves myocardial contractility, and stimulates spontaneous cardiac activity.

The dose of epinephrine is 0.1 ml/kg (0.01 mg/kg) of 1 : 10,000-diluted epinephrine. The dilution strength of 1 : 1000 should not be used in resuscitation; if it is the only strength available, it should be diluted in 9 ml of sterile saline solution to yield a 1 : 10,000 dilution.

Epinephrine may be administered by the endotracheal tube or intravenously. Absorption of epinephrine from the trachea is rapid, and new studies have demonstrated a more sustained, long-lasting release of epinephrine from the lungs as opposed to that from an IV bolus.[19] Epinephrine by either route has a short duration of action and should be repeated every 5 minutes.

Dextrose. The child who sustains an arrest may well have depleted energy stores and may benefit from supplemental dextrose. In addition to supplying the brain and myocardial cells with substrate, glucose is a myocardial stimulant that may act synergistically with epinephrine to increase myocardial contractility.

The dose of dextrose is 500 mg/kg, and it should be diluted from 50% dextrose to 25% dextrose in 0.9 normal saline solution to reduce its viscosity.

Lidocaine. Children rarely have ventricular dysrhythmias; therefore lidocaine is rarely a first-line drug in pediatric arrest. Most ventricular dysrhythmias in pediatrics are a result of hypoxia, hypokalemia, or a misplaced central venous catheter that is irritating the myocardium.

Lidocaine is used to increase the ventricular fibrillation threshold and to control ventricular ectopy. Ectopy significant enough to merit the use of lidocaine may be demonstrated in the following:

1. Bigeminal rhythms
2. Trigeminal rhythms
3. Multifocal premature ventricular contractions (PVCs) occurring at a rate of more than 10/min
4. Runs of more than three PVCs
5. Any significant level of ectopy accompanied by hypotension

Once the treatable causes of ventricular dysrhythmias have been ruled out and lidocaine is indicated, a loading dose of 1 mg/kg is given. This dose may be repeated every 10 to 15 minutes until ectopy diminishes or until a total of 3.0 mg/kg has been given. Because the half-life of lidocaine is about 20 minutes, the bolus should be followed with an infusion at 20 to 50 μg/kg/min.

Lidocaine is metabolized by the liver, and serum levels reflect not only the dose administered but also hepatic metabolism. If the child has liver disease or congestive heart failure, with its resulting liver dysfunction, any lidocaine administered after the initial loading dose should be given cautiously.

Calcium. Calcium plays a controversial role in resuscitation today. It may be that calcium has a negative effect on cell survival and neurologic function after resuscitation. In the digitalis-treated patient, calcium may potentiate digitalis-induced dysrhythmias and induce asystole refractory to all resuscitation. Calcium is probably most useful in cases of documented hypocalcemia and hyperkalemia.

In an arrest situation, calcium chloride is preferred to calcium gluconate because it is ionized and immediately available to the body for use. (The less sclerosing calcium gluconate must first be metabolized by the liver, which, in an arrest situation, is not well perfused.)

The dose of calcium chloride is 20 to 30 mg/kg for emergencies other than an arrest; the dose of calcium gluconate is 100 mg/kg. Both drugs should be administered slowly, with continuous ECG monitoring, and only with absolutely certain IV line placement.

Dopamine. Dopamine is useful for both its α-adrenergic and β-adrenergic effects, after a spontaneous heart rate is reestablished. The usual starting dose for dopamine is 10 to 15 μg/kg/min; dosages in this range cause increased heart rate, increased cardiac output, and increased blood pressure. At higher doses (20 μg/kg/min or more), dopamine is frequently paired with a peripheral vasodilator such as isoproterenol or sodium nitroprusside.

Isoproterenol. Isoproterenol is a potent, exclusively β-stimulant that increases the contractile force and rate of the heart and acts as a peripheral vasodilator. The child with inadequate preload may become hypotensive in response to isoproterenol. The dose range is 0.1 to 1.0 μg/kg/min.

Cerebral Resuscitation

Any discussion of pediatric resuscitation is incomplete without the inclusion of cerebral resuscitation. The child who has sustained cardiac arrest can be presumed to have at least minimal anoxic brain injury. Some simple, effective things can be done to preserve cerebral function. The first is to avoid giving the child free water in IV fluids. Cerebral volume has been shown to increase, specifically by an increase in cerebrospinal fluid (CSF) production, when free water instead of lactated Ringer's solution is infused. Although D_5W is the usual fluid given to adults with medical problems or cardiac arrest (as opposed to trauma), it has virtually no place in pediatrics. Far better choices are D_5.25NS, D_5.9NS, lactated Ringer's solution, and 0.9 normal saline solution.

Second, the patient's temperature should be maintained in the normal range. Studies of pharmacologically paralyzed patients have demonstrated a direct linear relationship between body temperature and cerebral metabolic rate. For every degree centigrade of fever above 37°C, there is a concomitant 5% increase in cerebral metabolic rate.[12] Aggressive control of fever with acetaminophen and sponging should be instituted whenever possible in the child with increased ICP.

Third, the head should be kept in the midline and elevated 30 degrees. There are no valves in the venous system from the right atrium to the cerebral veins; as a result, increases in intrathoracic pressure are directly transmitted to the brain, resulting in increased ICP. Elevating the head guards against this phenomenon; keeping the head in the midline promotes optimal venous return from the head by allowing unimpeded flow through the jugular veins.

ALTERATIONS IN NEUROLOGIC FUNCTION

Assessment of the child with an alteration of neurologic function can present a special challenge to the flight team. Although diagnosis in older children can be based on assessment skills similar to those used for the adult population, the presentation of the infant and toddler with incomplete verbal skills requires different assessment criteria.

Of primary importance in the physical examination in an infant younger than 18 months is the assessment of the fontanelles. The skull of the infant is not the enclosed structure of the adult; rather it comprises separate cranial bones that are not normally fused until 18 months of age. The resulting "soft spot," or fontanelle, can provide important information on both the hydration of the infant and possible alterations in cerebral pressure.

Palpation of the fontanelle should reveal a soft firm surface that is even with the adjoining cranial bones. A normal variation of this finding will be the bulging that is noticeable with any increase of superior vena cava pressure, such as that which occurs with vigorous crying or a supine position.[8] Abnormal findings are the sunken fontanelle, which is indicative of dehydration, and the tense, bulging fontanelle, which is the hallmark of the infant with increased ICP.

An additional assessment parameter in the examination of the infant with a suspected increase in ICP is the accurate measurement of head circumference. However, because this measurement is most meaningful when gathered over several days, it may not be helpful as a diagnostic tool during the initial physical examination.

Accurate assessment of level of consciousness for the infant or nonverbal toddler is based on evaluation of alertness, level of activity, and response to environment and to significant others.[8] Normal infants will focus on objects, and visually track them from side to side. They are interested in their surroundings without exhibiting undue irritability or lethargy when stimulated. Parents can elicit a social smile in their infants, whereas toddlers frequently exhibit shyness when confronted by strangers. In addition, the cry of the child with a neurologic disorder frequently has a high-pitched, irritating quality that is difficult to overlook.

Following is a list of signs and symptoms of increased ICP, most of which are the same for infants, children, and adults.[8]

1. Deterioration of level of consciousness
2. Changes in pupil size, decreased response to light, or both
3. Increased systolic pressure, with a widened pulse pressure, followed by the late change of a decrease in systolic pressure
4. Tachycardia, followed by bradycardia as the pressure increases
5. Irregular respiratory rate
6. Hyperthermia (hypothermia may also be a finding in infants)
7. Loss of motor or sensory function, or both
8. Headache
9. Vomiting in infants and children
10. Papilledema, if increased pressure is of longer duration

Seizures

The incidence of seizures in children ranges from 1 in 15 during the first 7 years of life[16] to 1 in 10 by the age of 15 years.[9] Seizures are defined as an abnormal electrical discharge from the brain, usually resulting in altered mental status, and manifesting as abnormal muscle movements, psychic alterations, or both. True status epilepticus consists of prolonged seizure activity (duration of greater than 30 minutes) or a series of closely spaced seizures from which consciousness is not regained.[14] Status epilepticus is considered a medical emergency, with a mortality rate of 10% to 15%.[16]

Causes of nonfebrile seizures beyond the neonatal period include systemic and CNS infections such as meningitis, as well as head trauma, congenital malformations, metabolic and electrolyte disturbances, and idiopathic origins. An additional precipitating event is a change or withdrawal of medication in children with a known seizure disorder. Other rare causes are mass lesions, poisonings, toxic ingestions, and breath-holding episodes.

Seizures precipitated by a febrile episode are the main type of seizures seen during the first 5 to 6 years of life, with 40% of all first-time seizures falling into this classification.[9] Of those children who have had febrile seizures in childhood, most do not exhibit seizure disorders as adults.[9]

Febrile seizures are commonly seen in the age range of 3 months to 6 years, with a peak incidence of 8 to 20 months.[1] Even though the rectal temperature of these children normally reaches 39°C, the intensity of the seizure is not associated with the severity of the fever. The usual finding during history and physical examination is the presence of an underlying infection, most frequently of the upper-respiratory tract. Although underlying metabolic and neurologic disorders are unusual with this presentation, they must be ruled out. A differential diagnosis to rule out meningitis must also be made, even though the incidence is small.[1]

Management of the child in active seizures requires initial attention to basic life support measures. The child should be positioned in a semiprone or lateral position to protect the airway from vomitus and secretions. FiO_2 100% should be administered when the child is in seizure, with assistance to ventilatory effort by a bag-valve–mask device if necessary.

Intubation may be required, and flight personnel should be ready with the appropriate equipment and tube sizes.

Although IV access should be established as quickly as possible, action should be directed mainly toward halting the seizure. Many of the diazepams can be given rectally with excellent, rapid absorption. This route should be used if prior IV access has not been established. The dosages for this route are .5 mg/kg (maximum, 20 mg). Some centers also use intranasal versed (.2 to .23 mg/kg) if IV access is difficult in the first minutes.[2]

Glucose levels should be checked with a rapid determination method for any child who presents with any alteration in level of consciousness. If the level is below 40 mg/dl, administration of 2 to 4 ml/kg of 10% dextrose (D_{10}) in the infant and 1 to 2 ml/kg of 25% glucose in the older child is indicated. Maintenance IV fluids with glucose should be hung of any solution containing sodium. Rapid infusion of D_5W or $D_{10}W$ can have a dilutional effect on the serum sodium and can further contribute to seizures.

Correction of the underlying cause of the seizure is the most important weapon in the anticonvulsant arsenal. Prolonged seizures, especially grand mal, must be halted to prevent untoward neurologic sequelae. Determining the cause, however, is often difficult in the transport setting, and the use of anticonvulsants is indicated for the child in seizure. IV diazepam 0.1 to 0.3 mg/kg can be administered slowly and can be repeated at 15-minute intervals. Lorazepam .5 mg/kg can also be administered. Both of these drugs can be given rectally or by IV. Phenobarbital 10 to 20 mg/kg IV may be used if seizures do not respond to the diazepams alone; however, the combination of these two agents may cause either respiratory depression or respiratory arrest, and the flight team should be prepared to intubate the child. Phenobarbital may also cause hypotension and may necessitate administration of a fluid bolus of 10 to 20 ml/kg of normal saline or lactated Ringer's solution.

Pyridoxine 100 mg IV may be useful in the hospital setting for persistent seizure activity.[2] For seizures associated with head injuries, IV phenytoin 10 to 20 mg/kg is the drug of choice because this medication does not affect level of consciousness as drastically as phenobarbital or the diazepams.

Meningitis

Meningitis continues to be one of the most serious and frequent infections of infancy and childhood. Neurologic, audiologic, and learning deficits are often unfortunate sequelae of this disease. Occasionally, despite antibiotic therapy, meningitis is rapidly fatal.

Meningitis can be attributed to viral (aseptic), bacterial (septic), or, rarely, fungal origins. Most commonly seen in the transport setting is purulent, bacterial meningitis. The type of bacteria encountered, and the corresponding chemotherapy, tend to be related to the child's age. The predominant organisms in children older than 2 months of age are *N. meningitidis* (meningococcal) and *S. pneumoniae* (pneumococcal). An *H. influenzae* vaccine is available for immunization of the child older than 2 months and has been effective in reducing the incidence of *H. influenzae*–caused disease. It is not as prevalent as in recent years but may still be found as a causative agent. Enteroviruses and, occasionally, echoviruses are frequent causes of viral (aseptic) meningitis.[9]

Medical personnel should have a high index of suspicion for meningitis when a young infant presents with poor feeding, with or without vomiting; lethargy; and irritability. In the young infant, specific signs of meningal irritation are often absent. Kernig's and Brudzinski's signs may be elicited in the older child but may be delayed for several hours as the disease progresses.[9] Other signs and symptoms include headache, fever, drowsiness, lethargy, bulging fontanelle, seizures, and alterations in level of consciousness. Respiratory distress, cyanosis, and petechiae, especially, should be assessed. Petechiae and purpura are associated with fulminant meningococcemia, which is a true medical emergency.

Lumbar puncture and identification of the responsible organism in the CSF by Gram staining provides the definitive diagnosis. Other CSF biochemical values can provide prognostic indicators. Although it is unnecessary to delay an emergency transport or resuscitative measures to perform lumbar puncture in a clinically symptomatic child, it is imperative that antibiotics be administered expediently. Obtaining a blood culture to rule out sepsis can often easily be accomplished while the IV line is started before antibiotics are given.

Treatment or emergency transport should never be delayed for lumbar puncture or blood cultures. Initial resuscitation is of prime concern. Counterimmunoelectrophoresis can be used after stabilization to detect the capsular antigens of the responsible organism, and lumbar puncture can still be performed after antibiotics are administered.

Shock and hypovolemia must be attended to urgently. Gram-negative sepsis, especially that associated with meningococcemia, may accompany meningitis. Low blood pressure, a classic sign of shock in the adult, is frequently the last vital sign change to appear in the critically ill child. As the child mounts a sympathetic response in the face of vascular disaster, shock will manifest in poor perfusion, mottling, diminished urine output, and tachycardia.

IV access must be established immediately after appropriate airway and breathing support is initiated. Depleted intravascular volume may be replaced with a rapid infusion of 10 to 20 ml/kg of 0.9% normal saline solution or 5% albumin. The fluid bolus may need to be repeated until perfusion is improved and mottling and tachycardia have diminished. The child must not be overloaded with fluid, and frequent checks of glucose levels are important because glucose stores may be depleted.

Dopamine 5 to 10 μg/kg/min may be necessary to improve perfusion and blood pressure after fluid resuscitation. Fever must be reduced and seizures stopped.

As a result of hypothalamic irritation from meningeal inflammation, *water intoxication,* or *syndrome of inappropriate secretion of antidiuretic hormone* (SIADH), may occur with meningitis. In these cases, and without presentation of dehydration or shock, fluids must be restricted to about two thirds to 80% of maintenance requirements.

FLUID AND ELECTROLYTE THERAPY

Fluid and electrolyte management in infants and children must be meticulously managed to restore and maintain precise equilibrium. The main basis for fluid calculation and administration in the pediatric patient is the weight of the child. If the exact weight is not known, estimation of average weight in kilograms, based on the age of the average child, can easily be established (box).

The distribution of total body weight varies drastically from infancy to adulthood. Newborn infants consist of as much as 77% to 80% total body weight, which gradually tapers to 58% by adulthood.[9] This has important implications for the types of IV solutions used. The younger the child, the more rapidly sodium abnormalities will develop. Therefore plain D_5W is rarely appropriate as the primary IV solution for children. Overzealous use can lead to such undesired sequelae as rapid serum sodium shifts precipitating seizures or pulmonary edema. D_5 in 0.2% normal saline solution is usually more appropriate as the minimum sodium concentration.

The amount of fluid a child needs in a 24-hour period, or maintenance fluid (and then divided by 24 hours for hourly requirements) can be quickly determined (box). In addition to maintenance fluid requirements, replacement of deficit and ongoing losses must be considered. Deficit losses are replaced over a 24- to 48-hour period, with half of the deficit administered over the first 8 hours. Ongoing losses are usually replaced over a 4-hour period to avoid fluid overloading. Obviously, shock must be attended to immediately with 10 to 20 ml/kg lactated Ringer's or normal saline solution, repeated once or twice until signs and symptoms of shock have abated. Improvements in capillary refill, perfusion, pulses, urine output, and diminished tachycardia will be noted.

The reasons for fluid and electrolyte imbalances are many, including diarrhea and vomiting, decreased oral intake, fever, burns, diabetes, and shock resulting from hemorrhagic losses, sepsis, or both. Diarrhea and vomiting losses can result in hypertonic (serum sodium greater than 150 mEq/L), hypotonic (serum sodium less than 130 mEq/L), or isotonic (serum sodium 130 to 150 mEq/L) dehydration states.[16]

In the hospital setting, sodium replacement must be carefully calculated and administered. For the transport setting, it is important to remember that even children with hypertonic dehydration will need sodium in their IV solutions to prevent rapid fluid shifts leading to cerebral edema and seizures. Losses are corrected over 48 to 72 hours.[11]

In certain conditions such as congestive heart failure, increased ICP, and kidney failure, maintenance fluid rates may need to be less than maintenance levels once an euvolemic state is achieved.

Estimation of percentage of dehydration can be determined by knowing the child's predehydration

ESTIMATION OF WEIGHT BASED ON AGE OF AVERAGE CHILD

Newborn:	3 kg (6 lb, 10 oz)
6 months:	7 kg (15 lb, 6 oz)
1 year:	10 kg (22 lb)
3 years	15 kg (33 lb)
5 years:	20 kg (44 lb)
8 years:	25 kg (55 lb)
10 years:	30 kg (66 lb)
12 years:	40 kg (88 lb)
14 years:	50 kg (110 lb)

Modified from Wellington et al: *Guidelines for pediatric emergency drugs and equipment,* St Louis, 1994, Cracom.

CALCULATING MAINTENANCE FLUID RATES

$<$10 kg weight = 100 ml/kg/24 hr

$$11 \text{ to } 20 \text{ kg} = 1000 \text{ ml} + \frac{50 \text{ ml/kg/24 hr for each kg over 10 kg}}{24 \text{ hr}}$$

$>$20 kg = 1500 ml + (20 ml/kg/24 hr for each kg over 20 kg)

For fever: Increase by 7 ml/kg/24 hr for each degree over 99°F

ESTIMATING FLUID/H_2O DEFICIT

1. Using known recent weight:
   Previous Weight (kg) − Current Weight (kg) = H_2O (L)
2. Estimate percentage of dehydration from clinical features and lab values.
3. $$\text{Rehydrated Weight (kg)} = \frac{\text{Current Weight (kg)}}{1 - \text{Percentage of Dehydration}}$$
   Example: 9-kg infant with estimated 10% dehydration
   $$x = \frac{9}{1 - 0.10} = \frac{9}{0.9} = 10 \text{ kg}$$
   10 kg − 9 kg = 1 L or 1000-ml deficit

weight and current dehydrated weight and calculating the percent difference (box). Various signs and symptoms are related to percentages of dehydration. Components to assess include heart rate, pulse condition, blood pressure, skin turgor/elasticity, color and perfusion, neurologic status, mucous membranes, fontanelle (if open), urine output, condition of eyes, and presence of tears (Table 26-3).

Questions to ask include the child's recent fluid intake, recent urine output with time of most recent void, and other fluid losses (e.g., hemorrhage, vomiting, diarrhea).

Restoration of airway, breathing, and circulation is the first priority. Next, establishment of a secure, patent IV line is essential; this may be extremely difficult in the shocky child. A cutdown procedure may be indicated. In extremis, intraosseous infusion may be considered. Lactated Ringer's or normal saline solution is the initial solution of choice. D_5 with lactated Ringer's or normal saline solution may be indicated in the younger child. It is always prudent to check the glucose with a fingerstick by means of the rapid-determination method. Dosage of 20 ml/kg over 45 to 60 minutes must be administered to improve perfusion and level of consciousness and restore urine flow. This may be repeated with 10 ml/kg as necessary.[1] Potassium should not be added to the IV until urine flow has been established.

After circulation is restored, the remaining deficit is gradually replaced over the next 48 hours. Fluid amounts will include maintenance fluid plus deficit replacements plus ongoing losses.

SPECIAL CONSIDERATIONS IN TRANSPORTING CHILDREN

Temperature regulation is of utmost concern in the care and transport of the critically ill infant or child. All resuscitative efforts will be of diminished value if the child is hypothermic or hyperthermic. In the frenzy of resuscitation, normothermia can be dif-

TABLE 26-3

Correlation of clinical features with percent dehydration

Clinical feature	Percent dehydration (isotonic) Mild (±5%) weight loss	Moderate (±10%) weight loss	Severe (±15%-20%) weight loss
Heart rate/pulse	Normal or fast	Tachycardic	Tachycardic, weak pulses
Blood pressure	Normal	Possibly normal	Low, possibly in shock
Skin turgor	Diminished	More diminished, doughy	Doughy, tenting
Skin color and perfusion	Pale	Gray	Mottled
Eyes/tears	Normal eyes/dry	Sunken eyes/no tears	Very sunken eyes/no tears
Mucous membranes	Dry	Very dry	Parched
Urine output	Diminished specific gravity ±1.020	Oliguric, less than 1 ml/kg/hr, specific gravity >1.030	Marked oliguria and azotemia, specific gravity >1.035
Fontanelle (last to change)	Probably normal	Flat	Sunken
Neurologic status	Apathetic, hypotonic	Lethargic, possible high-pitched cry	Comatose, seizures

ficult to achieve, maintain, and control. However, because infants and children suffer more rapidly from the effects of heat loss and are more likely to exhibit high fevers special attention must be paid to the maintenance of normothermia.

The child's ratio of surface area to body mass contributes to the rapid loss of heat. Shivering is absent or insufficient in infants younger than 6 months.[8] Brown fat, present for several months after birth and found around the kidney and under the scapula and thorax, should not be relied on as a source of internal heat production. In addition, the use of brown fat as a source of heat increases the infant's oxygen consumption by increasing the metabolic load. Although normal infants can tolerate this increased consumption, the already stressed infant may not be able to effectively increase oxygen available for normal cellular metabolism. As a result, cold stress can produce lactic acidosis and hypoxemia.[8]

Caloric needs of children are higher than those of adults, and glucose is of prime importance in brain metabolism. Children become hypoglycemic and ketonuric much faster than adults because their stores of protein and fat are considerably smaller. As a result, those conditions that raise metabolic activity will diminish those stores and place the child at risk for a hypoglycemic event. All children transported with an altered level of consciousness should undergo glucose measurement by the fastest means available. Glucose determination should also be performed and rechecked frequently for all infants younger than 1 year. Especially at risk for hypoglycemia are children with seizures, meningitis, congenital heart disease, Reye's syndrome, sepsis, toxic ingestions, adrenal insufficiency, apnea, insulin reactions, and liver failure.

Hypoglycemia should be considered in infants or children with pallor, tachycardia, sweating, seizures, hunger, coma, and neurologic alterations. A serum glucose of less than 40 mg/dl must be treated promptly with an IV bolus of 25% dextrose at 1 to 2 ml/kg. A maintenance IV solution of a least D_5 with 0.2% normal saline solution should be started to maintain blood sugar.

SUMMARY

The flight nurse plays a crucial role in the transport of pediatric patients with acute medical emergencies. Special skills and knowledge are used to ensure a safe, expeditious transport. Children are not small adults, and attention must be given to their unique physiologic, psychologic, and anatomic differences.

PEDIATRIC EMERGENCY CASE STUDY #1

The pediatric transport team received a call from a nearby community hospital to transport a 9-month-old, 10-kg, male infant with dehydration, shock, and a possible bowel obstruction. The patient had been brought to the emergency department (ED) with a 4-day history of vomiting and diarrhea. After home remedies had been unsuccessful, the parents were persuaded by a relative to take the baby to the ED. In the ED he was noted to be in shock with respiratory failure. He was immediately intubated with a 4.5 oral endotracheal tube, given 100% oxygen at a rate of 60 breaths/min, pressures 24 cm H_2O, and a PEEP of 3. On his initial ABG analysis, pH was 6.88, P_{CO_2} 11, BE −31, and P_{O_2} 322. A repeat ABG showed a pH of 6.79, P_{CO_2} of 11, and a BE −34. IV access was accomplished with difficulty, and two intraosseous lines failed. The infant was given 35 ml/kg of normal saline solution with 80 mEq/L sodium bicarbonate. A nasogastric tube drained 48 ml of green bile. The patient was catheterized with a small feeding tube, but no urine was obtained. The serum glucose level was 187 mg/dl. An abdominal radiograph was interpreted as significant for an ileus. IV ampicillin (50 mg/kg), gentamicin (2.5 mg/kg), and clindamicin (5 mg/kg) were administered.

The pediatric transport team arrived to find a cold, mottled, tachypneic, and poorly perfused infant. The baby's pupils were equal and reactive to light, and he responded to stimulation with brief eye-opening and withdrawal of extremities. He had spontaneous respirations in addition to assisted ventilations, with an oxygen saturation of 99% on pulse oximetry. During the flight the baby remained on assisted ventilation. His color continued to be pink, with 100% saturation. However, he remained tachycardic with a heart rate of 160, blood pressure 84/56 mm Hg with poor perfusion. The blood pressure increased after the bolus to 93/63 mm Hg; heart rate was 166. A portawarm mattress was placed under the infant to correct his hypothermia. At arrival to the pediatric intensive care unit, his temperature was normal. He had voided a loose diarrheal stool.

The patient's hospital course was uneventful. He did receive an additional 28 ml/kg of IV fluid in the pediatric intensive care unit. This represented a total of 80 ml/kg resuscitation fluid given. After 24 hours the patient was extubated. On discharge, his diagnosis was hypovolemic shock resulting from dehydration from viral gastroenteritis.

Prompt attention to the basics in pediatric resuscitation resulted in a positive outcome for this severely ill patient. The flight team optimized his resuscitation by assisting ventilation, continuing to meet his massive fluid needs, and resolving thermoregulation problems. Although care needs to be taken to avoid fluid overload in children, it is imperative that assessment and interventions be precise and quantified to each patient's particular requirements.

PEDIATRIC EMERGENCY CASE STUDY #2

A 5-month-old, 7-kg female Hispanic infant presented to a local emergency department with a 2-day history of increasing irritability, lethargy, diminished oral intake, decreased urine output, and a rash. In the ED she was noted to have a bulging, tense fontanelle, petechiae, and obtundation. The patient was afebrile and tachycardic (heart rate, 176 beats/min) and appeared dehydrated. Peripheral pulses were strong and good perfusion was noted.

On the arrival of the pediatric transport team, the infant was being given 1 L of O_2 per nasal cannula with oxygen saturations 98% to 99% (altitude, 5,280 ft). A normal saline bolus of 8.5 ml/kg was given. IV ceftriaxone 50 mg/kg and IV dexamethasone 0.15 mg/kg/dose were given. Blood cultures were drawn after the antibiotic had been administered. The child's condition was stable, and no further stabilization was necessary.

During transport, rapid determination of glucose was within normal limits, and an IV of normal saline solution was infused at 1.5 times the maintenance rate for the mild dehydration and decreased urine output. After the arrival to the pediatric intensive care unit, a lumbar puncture was performed, revealing moderate gram-negative diplococci. A diagnosis was made of meningococcemia/meningitis caused by *N. meningitidis.* Further inquiry revealed that the patient had visited Mexico recently and had been exposed to an ill male child who had died after exhibiting a similar, but more severe rash.

After admission to the pediatric intensive care unit, the patient was placed on low dose (renal) dopamine with subsequent improvement of urine output. Mild disseminated intravascular coagulation was created with a heparin drip. Before discharge, CT showed bilateral subdural effusions with mild prominence of ventricular size. Renal scanning revealed an anomalous right kidney. The patient was discharged home in good condition after receiving a 10-day course of penicillin and rifampin. Close contacts, including the transport team, also received a course of prophylactic rifampin.

This disease process can be frightening, fulminating, and overwhelming. This child was fortunate and did not succumb to a potentially fatal illness. Attention to the basics in pediatric care can truly be lifesaving. Prompt administration of IV antibiotics and an approximate 10 ml/kg fluid bolus (keeping in mind the need to be cautious with the potential for increased intracranial pressure in a child with a bulging fontanelle) was instrumental in her resuscitation. Diagnostic interventions must wait until the life-threatening concerns are addressed.

REFERENCES

1. Barkin RM, Rosen P: *Emergency pediatrics: a guide to ambulatory care,* St Louis, 1994, Mosby.
2. Battan KF: Personal communication, 1995.
3. Brooks JC: *Fact sheet: facts about apnea and other apparent life-threatening events,* McLean, Va, 1987, National Sudden Infant Death Syndrome Clearinghouse.
4. Carpenter T: Personal communication, May 8, 1995.
5. Dobrin RS: Personal communication, 1980.
6. Fleisher GR et al: *Textbook of emergency medicine,* ed 3, Baltimore, 1993, Williams & Wilkins.
7. Griebel J: *Respiratory medication recommendations,* Denver, 1994, Children's Hospital.
8. Hazinski MF: *Nursing care of the critically ill child,* ed 2, St Louis, 1992, Mosby.
9. Kempe C et al: *Current pediatric diagnosis and treatment,* ed 9, Los Altos, Calif, 1987, Lange Medical.
10. Klonoff-Cohen HS, Edelstan SL: A case-control study of routine and death scene sleep position and sudden infant death syndrome in California, *JAMA* 273(10), 1995.
11. Levin DL, Morriss FC: *Essentials of pediatric intensive care,* St Louis, 1990, Quality Medical.
12. Loftness S: Personal communication, 1986.
13. McCloskey KAL, Orr RA: *Pediatric transport medicine,* St Louis, 1995, Mosby.
14. McIntyre KM, Lewis AJ: *Textbook of advanced cardiac life support,* Dallas, 1983, American Heart Association.
15. National Institutes of Health: *Infantile apnea and home monitoring,* National Institutes of Health Consensus Development Conference Statement, vol 6, no 6, Oct 1986.
16. Oppenheimer EY, Rosman NP: Seizures. In Reece RM: *Manual of emergency pediatrics,* ed 3, Philadelphia, 1984, Saunders.
17. Orlowski JP: Pediatric cardiopulmonary resuscitation, *Emerg Med Clin North Am* 1(1), 1983.
18. Reece RH: *Manual of emergency pediatrics,* ed 4, Philadelphia, 1992, Saunders/Harcourt Brace Jovanovich.
19. Standards and guidelines for cardiopulmonary resuscitation and emergency cardiac care, *JAMA* 255(21), 1986.
20. Wellington et al: *Guidelines for pediatric emergency drugs and equipment,* St Louis, 1994, Cracom.

CHAPTER 27

Cold-Related Emergencies

COMPETENCIES

1. Define mild, moderate, and severe hypothermia.
2. Describe thermoregulation and mechanisms of heat loss.
3. Identify methods to prevent heat loss in the injured patient.

Hannibal started over the Pyrenean Alps in 218 BC with an army of 46,000, but within 15 days lost more than 20,000 men to the cold.[3] Statistics have not significantly improved since Hannibal's time. United States' soldiers sustained 90,000 cold-related injuries in World War II, and Germany more, with 100,000. During two winter months in 1942, the Germans performed 15,000 cold-related amputations.[44] During the Korean War, the United States had a 10% cold-related casualty rate.[27,30]

Flight personnel must be aware of the risk of hypothermia regardless of the climate or terrain. A summer-day hiker in the Rocky Mountains, an older person in an unheated home in the Sun Belt, and a sailor stranded off the warm Florida coast are all at equal risk of hypothermia. Studies have shown that cold contributes to 16% of all recreational boating fatalities and 20% of all scuba-diving fatalities.[21,38]

HYPOTHERMIA DEFINED

Hypothermia, defined as a core body temperature of less than 35° C, occurs because the body can no longer generate sufficient heat to maintain body functions.[3] Accidental hypothermia, in contrast to iatrogenic hypothermia, is the unintentional decrease in core temperature associated with trauma or exposure to the environment.[3] Core body temperature can be measured at the rectum, the esophagus, the tympanic membrane, or the bloodstream. Rectal thermometers provide the least reliable measurement of core body temperature. The esophageal and tympanic thermometers are more reliable. However, these devices may not be practical for field use. The use of thermometers that measure the temperature in the external auditory canal is now being explored.[3] Should these thermometers be found reliable, they would be of great use in the field. Table 27-1 lists thermometric equivalents for Fahrenheit and Celsius temperatures.[9]

Classification

Hypothermia is classified into three categories. *Mild hypothermia* is defined as a core body temperature greater than 32° C and less than 35° C and is associated with low morbidity and mortality. *Moderate hypothermia* occurs when the core body temperature is greater than 28° C but less than 32° C. Finally, severe hypothermia is defined as a core body temperature of 28° C or less and is associated with a higher morbidity and mortality.[14] The classification distinction at 32° C is not arbitrary but is based on profound metabolic and physiologic changes. Heat can still be conserved by vasoconstriction and produced by shivering at core temperatures of 35° C to 32° C. At a core temperature below 32° C, the body no longer tries to conserve or produce heat. At 28° C the body can no longer generate heat by itself and is essentially poikilothermic.[14] These changes are summarized in Table 27-2. The lower limit of survival according to Caroline[1] is 23° C, although she reported one isolated patient who survived a core temperature of 10° C after being in cardiac arrest for 1 hour.[13,25]

Hypothermia can also be classified as acute or chronic, according to length of exposure. Acute hypothermia occurs when body heat is lost over a period of less than 6 hours. Immersion in water colder than 21° C is a common cause of acute hypothermia because water accelerates conductive heat loss. Chronic hypothermia occurs when the patient is exposed to cold for more than 24 hours, and it occurs more frequently on land. Urban hypothermia is a form of chronic hypothermia that is associated with factors such as age, debilitation, drug and alcohol use, predisposing disease, and decreased level of consciousness.[22]

TABLE 27-1

Thermometric equivalents (Celsius and Fahrenheit)

Celsius	Fahrenheit
15.0	59.0
16.0	60.8
17.0	62.6
18.0	64.4
19.0	66.2
20.0	68.0
21.0	69.8
22.0	71.6
23.0	73.4
24.0	75.2
25.0	77.0
26.0	78.8
27.0	80.6
28.0	82.4
29.0	84.2
30.0	86.0
31.0	87.8
32.0	89.6
33.0	91.4
34.0	93.2
35.0	95.0
36.0	96.8
37.0	98.6
38.0	100.4
39.0	102.2
40.0	104.0

Mortality

The mortality rate for severe hypothermia cited in the literature varies from 0% to 50%.[3] Many factors influence the mortality rate, including degree and

TABLE 27-2

Physiologic changes related to temperature

Celsius	Fahrenheit	Symptoms
38.0	99.6	Normal rectal temperature
37.0	98.6	Normal oral temperature
MILD		
36.0	96.8	Increased basal metabolic rate in an attempt to balance heat loss, tachycardia, increased cardiac output
35.0	95.0	Shivering at the maximum, usually still responsive, but level of consciousness beginning to decrease, regulatory systems beginning to falter
34.0	93.2	Dysarthria, amnesia, blood pressure still normal, oxyhemoglobin curve begins to shift to the left
32.0	91.4	Heart rate decreases to 50-60 beats/min, ataxia, poor coordination, apathy, lethargy
MODERATE		
32.0	89.6	Vasoconstriction level of consciousness progressively falls
31.0	87.8	Shivering stops, respirations and blood pressure may be difficult to obtain
30.0	86.0	Mental confusion, delirium, increased muscle rigidity; heart rate and cardiac output begin to decrease, arrhythmias begin to develop (atrial fibrillation)
29.0	84.2	Acidosis, hyperglycemia, metabolic rate decreased by 50%, decreased respirations, bradycardia, decreased stroke volume, decreased cardiac output, pupils dilated
SEVERE		
28.0	82.4	Hypotension, loss of vasoconstrictive capabilities, ventricular fibrillation if patient handled roughly, increased myocardial irritability
27.0	80.6	Prolonged PR, QRS, and QT intervals; muscle flaccidity; no voluntary movement (appears dead); no pupillary reactions
26.0	78.8	Seldom conscious, areflexic
25.0	77.0	Stuporous, hypoventilation, ventricular fibrillation may appear spontaneously, cerebral blood flow one third of normal, cardiac output 45% of normal
24.0	75.2	Coma, pulmonary edema, respiratory arrest
23.0	73.4	No spontaneous movement, rigor mortis appearance, no corneal reflexes
22.0	71.6	Maximum risk of ventricular fibrillation, 75% decrease in oxygen consumption
21.0	69.8	Apnea
20.0	68.0	Ventricular fibrillation, cardiac standstill/asystole
17.0	62.6	Isoelectric electroencephalogram

duration of hypothermia, age, poverty, predisposing disease, and complications. Most victims die of cardiac dysrhythmias. The presence of a severe underlying disease is almost always associated with increased mortality. Rankin and Rae[32] noted no correlation between the severity of hypothermia or the rate of rewarming and the clinical outcome but, rather, that mortality was correlated with the presence or absence of severe underlying disease.

NORMAL TEMPERATURE REGULATION

Human beings become uncomfortable with even a small deviation in core body temperature from

37.6° C. In *De Re Medicina,* Aurelius Cornelius Celsus described in AD 25 the universal discomfort of cold temperatures as "hurtful to an old or slender man, to a wound, to the precordia, intestines, bladder, ears, hips, shoulders, private parts, teeth, bones, nerves, womb and brain. It also renders the surface of the skin pale, dry, hard and black. From this proceed shudderings and tremors."[2] Normal body temperature is maintained in a narrow range by a delicate balance of heat loss and heat production regulated by a "thermostat" in the preoptic anterior hypothalamus. The hypothalamus is sensitive to temperature changes as small as 0.5° C.[4] Stimuli sent from the hypothalamus to the sympathetic nervous system increase heart rate and dilate muscle blood vessels to increase heat production. In addition, shivering generates heat by increasing muscle activity. At the same time, cutaneous vasoconstriction reduces heat loss by shunting blood from the periphery to the core.[45]

The ability to shiver is affected by hypoglycemia, hypoxia, fatigue, alcohol, and drugs. Shivering is the body's main mechanism of heat production and its strongest defense against hypothermia. However, shivering requires increased blood flow to peripheral muscles and consequently results in a 25% heat loss. Preshivering increases heat production by 50% to 100%. Visible shivering increases heat production by 500%. An average 70-kg person produces about 100 kcal of heat/hr under basal conditions and up to 500 kcal/hr when shivering.[3] This degree of heat production, however, cannot be sustained for long because the patient becomes fatigued once glycogen stores are depleted. Maximum shivering occurs at 35° C and stops below 32° C. Cessation of shivering is a sign that the patient has made the transition from mild to severe hypothermia.

Hypothermia results when the thermoregulation system becomes overwhelmed or damaged centrally at the hypothalamic level or systemically by a decrease in heat production or an increase in heat loss. Thermoregulation is disrupted at the hypothalamic level by head trauma, cerebral neoplasms, cerebrovascular accidents, acute poisoning, acid-base imbalance, Parkinson's disease, and Wernicke's encephalopathy. Acute spinal transection can eliminate vasoconstrictive control by the hypothalamus. Heat production is decreased by malnutrition, hypothyroidism, hypopituitarism, and rheumatoid arthritis. Normally, 90% of the heat produced by the body is lost to the environment by way of conduction, convection, radiation, and evaporation.

Methods of Heat Loss

Conduction, together with convection, accounts for 15% of heat loss.[13] Conduction occurs when the body comes into direct contact with a heat conductor. Examples of good conductors are water, snow, metal, and damp ground. Normally, conduction plays a minor role in heat loss but is an important factor when the patient has been immersed in cold water, lying in a snowbank, or wandering without shoes for an extended period. Heat loss in water is approximately 25 times greater than heat loss in air of the same temperature.[3] Immersion in water in temperatures less than 10° C causes hypothermia in only a few minutes,[3] in contrast to more than an hour in air.

Heat loss by convection occurs when either air or water moves over the patient or the patient moves through air or water. Heat loss is accelerated by increasing air movement (forced convection). The wind, the rotating blades of the helicopter, and the movement required to transport the patient to the aircraft all contribute to forced convective heat loss. Fig. 27-1 lists temperature differences related to wind-chill factors.

Body heat lost by radiation is 45%.[3] Radiant heat transfer occurs when a difference exists between body temperature and ambient temperature. The body absorbs heat when the ambient temperature is higher and emits heat when the ambient temperature is lower. Radiant heat loss, as convection, is directly related to dermal blood flow and percentage of skin surface exposed. Radiant heat loss is accelerated at night or when the sky is overcast.

Evaporation occurs when water on the body surface is converted from a liquid state to a gaseous state.[3] The body is cooled as the vapor moves off the body into the air. The evaporative process accounts for about 25% of heat loss[3] and occurs normally through the skin, lungs, and upper airway. Burns and various skin lesions expose more open, moist surface area and thereby increase evaporative

Wind in m.p.h.	Local Temperature in Degrees Fahrenheit									
	32	23	14	5	−4	−13	−22	−31	−40	−49	−58
	Equivalent Temperature (Wind Plus Local Temperature)										
Calm	32	23	14	5	−4	−13	−22	−31	−40	−49	−58
5	29	20	10	1	−9	−18	−28	−37	−47	−56	−65
10	18	7	−4	−15	−26	−37	−48	−59	−70	−81	−92
15	13	−1	−13	−25	−37	−49	−61	−73	−88	−97	−109
20	7	−6	−19	−32	−44	−57	−70	−83	−98	−109	−121
25	3	−10	−24	−37	−50	−64	−77	−90	−104	−117	−130
30	1	−13	−27	−41	−54	−68	−82	−97	−109	−123	−137
35	−1	−15	−29	−43	−57	−71	−85	−99	−113	−127	−142
40	−3	−17	−31	−45	−59	−74	−87	−102	−116	−131	−145
45	−3	−18	−32	−46	−61	−75	−89	−104	−118	−132	−147
50	−4	−18	−33	−47	−62	−76	−91	−105	−120	−134	−148
	little danger for those properly clothed →		**considerable danger** →			**extreme danger** →					

Fig. 27-1. Chill factor: temperature plus wind. (From Vaughn PB: *Milit Med* 5:307, 1980.)

losses. In addition, evaporation increases when the patient is wearing damp clothing or is covered with blood.

Heat loss is inversely proportional to body size and body fat. Fat insulates because it has less blood flow and consequently has less of an ability to vasodilate and lose heat. Consequently, large people conserve heat better than small people, obese people better than thin people, and adults better than children.

PHYSIOLOGIC RESPONSE TO HYPOTHERMIA

Metabolic Derangements

Complications of hypothermia result mainly from the sequelae of metabolic derangements. Initially metabolism increases to generate heat. Optimal metabolism begins to decrease at 35° C. Symptoms of mild hypothermia consequently include shivering, hypoglycemia, and increased respiratory rate, heart rate, and cardiac output. A dramatic decrease in metabolic rate occurs between 30° C and 33° C as the patient makes the transition from moderate to severe hypothermia. Every 10° C decrease in temperature decreases metabolism by half.[3] At 28° C all thermoregulation ceases. The metabolic functions of the liver also begin to falter at temperatures below 33° C. The liver no longer efficiently metabolizes fats, proteins, and carbohydrates; or drugs, alcohol, and lactic acid. Symptoms of severe hypothermia include absence of shivering, hyperglycemia, and decreased respiratory rate, heart rate, and cardiac output. Bowel sounds are decreased, if not absent, as a result of decreased gastric motility and gastric dilation.[16]

Hypoglycemia is associated with chronic mild hypothermia, whereas hyperglycemia is associated with acute severe hypothermia. Glucose and glucose stored in the form of glycogen are depleted by long-term shivering. Shivering can stop at temperatures greater than 33° C if glucose or glycogen stores are depleted or if insulin is no longer available. Shivering begins again when the core body temperature increases to 32° C if depleted glucose is replaced. Hyperglycemia occurs at temperatures below 30° C because insulin no longer promotes glucose transport into cells once metabolism significantly decreases.[3,14] Hyperglycemia will not occur if glucose and glycogen stores have been previously depleted but not replaced.

Oxygenation and Acid-Base Disorders

Respiratory rate initially increases after sudden exposure to cold but then decreases as body temperature and metabolism decrease.[3,14] At temperatures above 32° C, ventilation is usually adequate. At 30° C, respirations are shallow and difficult to observe. Apnea and respiratory arrest commonly occur at temperatures between 21° C and 24° C. Although carbon dioxide production also decreases to about half the basal level with each 8° C drop in temperature,[14] the decreased respiratory rate is inadequate to effectively excrete CO_2 at a temperature below 33° C. Consequently, a respiratory acidosis develops in the hypothermia victim.

Cellular respiration is impaired by the decrease in metabolism, drop in cardiac output, and left shift on the oxyhemoglobin dissociation curve. Hypothermia decreases cardiac output by decreasing heart rate and circulating blood volume, as well as by increasing blood viscosity and peripheral vascular resistance. Blood shifting to the core results in a perceived "overhydration," and the body responds by removing the "extra" volume through diuresis. Prolonged hypothermia also causes plasma to leak from the capillaries, thereby increasing blood viscosity by 2% for every 1° C decline.[3,14,40]

Hypothermia begins to shift the oxyhemoglobin dissociation curve to the left at 34° C. Oxygen then binds tenaciously with hemoglobin, resulting in reduced tissue oxygen delivery. In addition, Biddle has noted that oxygen consumption was half of normal at 27° C and at 17° C had fallen to one quarter the normal value.[3,14] Anaerobic metabolism and lactic acid production increases from the combination of decreased cardiac output, oxygen delivery, and oxygen consumption. The increase in lactic acid leads to cardiac dysrhythmias and death.

The cardiovascular system is more sensitive to the effects of acid-base disturbances than any other body system. Acidosis is commonly associated with asystole, and alkalosis is associated with ventricular fibrillation.[3,14,15] Hypoventilation and lactic acid production lead to respiratory and metabolic acidosis. Acidosis usually corrects itself once the patient is rewarmed. Hyperkalemia is associated with metabolic acidosis, as well as with muscle damage and kidney failure, which may all be present in the rewarmed hypothermic patient. Iatrogenic respiratory and metabolic alkalosis is difficult to treat and should be avoided.

Central Nervous System

The central nervous system (CNS) displays some of the most impressive sequelae in the hypothermic patient. Complete recovery is possible even after prolonged cardiac arrest. Hypothermia protects CNS integrity and allows the brain to withstand long periods of anoxia.[19] Cerebral blood flow decreases 6% to 7% for every 1° C decline until 25° C is reached.[3,7,14] Cerebral oxygen requirements decrease to 50% of normal at 28° C, to 25% of normal at 22° C,[7,33] and to 12.5% of normal at 16° C.[49] Caroline[1] noted that the brain can survive without perfusion for about 10 minutes at 30° C, whereas it can survive for up to 25 to 30 minutes at 20° C.[10] Remarkably, Steinman noted that at 16° C the brain can survive without oxygen for up to 32 to 48 minutes.[39]

Mildly hypothermic patients are clumsy, apathetic, withdrawn, and irritable. Reflexes are hyperactive at temperatures above 32° C. Level of consciousness begins to decrease markedly at 32° C, and the patient becomes lethargic or disoriented and begins to hallucinate. Hypothermia victims will even remove jackets, gloves, shoes, and other protective clothing; "paradoxical undressing" is often one of the first signs that the patient is becoming severely hypothermic. The cough reflex is absent at decreased temperatures, and aspiration of stomach contents can occur. Coma develops between 28° C and 30° C. At temperatures below 30° C, the pupils dilate and become nonreactive. In addition, corneal and deep-tendon reflexes may be absent. The hypothermic patient must be carefully examined to rule out rigor mortis or death. At temperatures below 20° C, the electroencephalogram, if it were available, would be flat.[28]

Cardiac Dysrhythmias

The effects of hypothermia on heart rhythm were noted as early as 1912 to produce bradycardia progressing to asystole.[3,14] In 1923, subjects reportedly showed T-wave changes on their ECGs after drinking 600 ml of icewater.[47] It is believed that up to 90% of all hypothermic patients have some electrocardiographic abnormality.[26,42]

The heart initially responds to mild hypothermia with an increase in heart rate as a result of sympathetic stimulation; this response is short lived. Heart rate then decreases to 50 to 60 beats/min at 33° C and at lower temperatures decreases to 20 beats/min.[3,14] Atrial fibrillation with a slow ventricular rate is common at temperatures below 29° C. Okada[24] recently noted that atrial fibrillation was unusual in mild hypothermia (temperature greater than 32° C) and that it was often observed in moderate (32° C to 26° C) and moderately deep (less than 26° C) hypothermia. About half of the cases studied in moderately deep hypothermia remained in sinus, atrial, or junctional rhythm. Okada also noted that atrial fibrillation usually converted to sinus rhythm spontaneously after return to normothermia.[24]

Changes in the conduction system begin at 27° C and may be observed as a widened QRS interval and prolonged PR and QT intervals. The Osborne or J wave is seen clearly at 25° C. The J wave is described as an extra deflection at the junction of the QRS and ST segments (Fig. 27-2). The origin of the J wave is unknown. According to Okada, Nishimura, and Yoshiro, the prolongation of the Q-T interval and the presence of J waves are directly related to the severity of the hypothermia.[25] Large J waves are

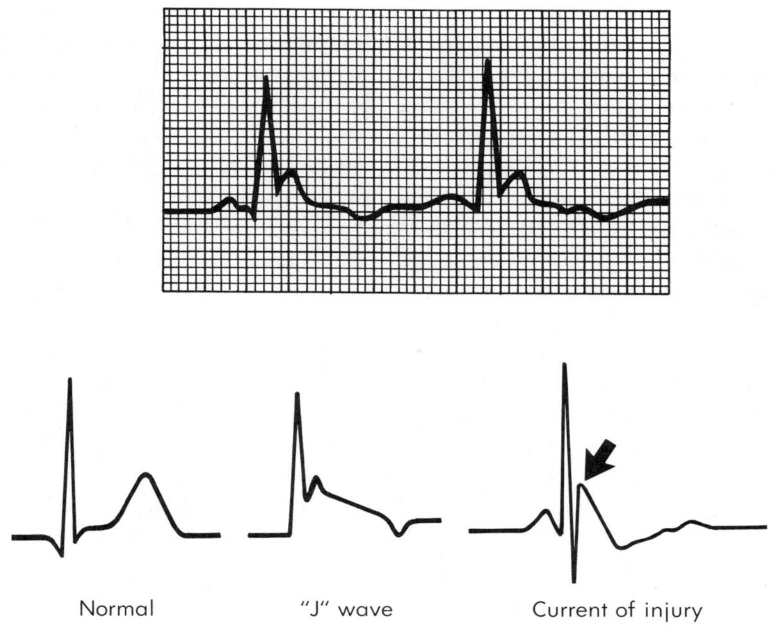

Fig. 27-2. An ECG tracing showing the characteristic J or Osborne wave of hypothermia.

seen at temperatures of less than 30° C, whereas small J waves are seen at higher temperatures.

Several theories have been offered for the presence of J waves in hypothermia. The J wave may represent hypothermia-induced ion fluxes that cause delayed depolarization or early repolarization of the left ventricle. The J wave may also be a hypothalamic or neurogenic factor. It is important to note that J waves may also be seen in patients with central nervous system lesions or cardiac ischemia or who are septic, or even in young healthy people.[14]

Ventricular irritability, occurring at temperatures less than 30° C, is commonly associated with alkalosis and is the most lethal cardiovascular response to hypothermia. At 28° C the heart can be irritated by rough handling, careless intubation, or cardiac compressions. Ventricular fibrillation can occur spontaneously at 25° C. Unfortunately, dysrhythmias at temperatures below 30° C become increasingly refractory to drugs and defibrillation.

Asystole occurs at 20° C but has a surprisingly good prognosis if the patient is rewarmed quickly. Asystole is associated with acidosis and appears to be the primary arrhythmia in accidental hypothermia. Rankin and Rae[32] found that asystole was the terminal rhythm in all 22 patients they studied.

Frostnip and Frostbite

Frostnip, a superficial form of frostbite usually found on the face, nose, and ears, is manifested by numbness and pallor of the exposed skin. Management consists of warming the area with a warm hand or wrapping or covering the area for protection.

Frostbite most often involves the distal extremities. Destruction of the skin produces a more severe injury than frostnip. Although frostbite is commonly associated with below-freezing temperatures, it can be produced at above-freezing temperatures by wind, altitude, humidity, and prolonged exposure and exacerbated by impaired vascular integrity and decreased cardiac output.[29,46]

The injury caused by frostbite has been divided into four phases. These are the prefreeze phase: the freeze-thaw phase, the vascular stasis phase, and the late ischemic phases. This pathophysiology results in both intracellular and extracellular formation, cell dehydration and shrinkage, abnormal intracellular electrolyte imbalances, thermal shock, and denaturation of the lipid-protein complexes.[20]

Blood cells "sludge" within the vessels, and eventually circulation to the tissue ceases.[54]

Frostbite is classified as first, second, or third degree. First-degree injury, superficial freezing without blistering or peeling, is characterized by hyperemia and edema. The tissue becomes mottled, cyanotic, and painful after rewarming. Second-degree frostbite produces blistering or peeling of the skin and is characterized by hyperemia and vesicle/bleb formation. When rewarmed, the skin is deep red, hot, and dry to touch. Third-degree frostbite is characterized by death of the dermis and even deeper tissue such as muscle and bone.[43]

Frostbite management has three stages.[3] The first stage is the most crucial and includes protection of the affected area from trauma or partial thawing. The second stage, rapid rewarming in a whirlpool bath, must occur in a controlled setting with constant observation. The third stage involves provisions for long-term care and follow-up.[41]

Air medical care focuses on protecting the affected area from trauma and partial thawing. The affected area should be kept frozen if there is any possibility that it will be refrozen. It must never be massaged. The patient should not be allowed to walk if the legs are involved. Narcotics should be used for pain management.

EPIDEMIOLOGY

Any individual will become hypothermic given the proper circumstances, but specific groups are particularly vulnerable: infants, older individuals, alcoholic subjects, trauma victims, outdoor people, and those with CNS dysfunction.[8,11,12,15,19] The flight nurse must always consider hypothermia when assessing patients in these high-risk groups.

Infants

Infants and neonates are particularly vulnerable to hypothermia. Mortality rates for neonatal cold injury range from 26% to 45%.[14] Hypothermia must be considered a threat in all out-of-hospital deliveries. The high mortality rate of infants is attributed to several causes:

1. The infant has less tissue insulation than the adult.
2. The large head in proportion to body size allows for greater heat loss.
3. Shivering occurs only at extreme degrees of hypothermia and may go undetected.
4. Limited energy stores are quickly exhausted.
5. Poor motor development may prevent infants from curling into a fetal position for protection.

In addition, the signs and symptoms of hypothermia in the infant are different from the adult and include lethargy, decreased appetite, facial and limb edema, and erythemic rather than blanching skin.

Older Subjects

Accidental hypothermia is common and often fatal in older subjects. Urban hypothermia is commonly seen in older subjects who do not have enough money for heat or warm clothing. People 75 years and older are estimated to have a five times greater chance of death from hypothermia than those younger than 75.[14,31] The reasons for the increased susceptibility of the elderly are many:

1. Older subjects normally have a lower basal metabolic rate and body temperature.
2. Older subjects have a decreased ability to adapt to temperature changes by vasoconstriction and shivering.
3. Older subjects have a diminished perception of heat and cold.
4. Older subjects are predisposed to other diseases such as diabetes or pneumonia that make them more susceptible to hypothermia.
5. Older subjects are more susceptible to chronic dehydration.

All confused and lethargic older patients should be assessed for hypothermia in addition to other problems such as cerebrovascular accident or hypoglycemia.

Alcohol and Other Toxic States

Alcohol ingestion has been found to cause serious problems with thermoregulation. Many people consume alcohol with the mistaken belief that it will "warm" them. Many homeless people who become hypothermic are also intoxicated. Alcohol causes vasodilation, which contributes to additional heat loss. Alcohol ingestion also causes the patient to feel warm, perhaps by altering perception. Hypoglycemia is caused by alcohol ingestion and decreases the patient's ability to shiver and conserve heat. The effects of alcohol on thermoregulation are moderated by the temperature, the amount of alcohol ingested, the patient's nutritional status and body composition, and the patient's ability to tolerate the amount of alcohol ingested.[20]

It is important that alcohol intoxication be recognized as a dangerous cofactor for the hypothermic patient. It is not uncommon for trauma patients to be intoxicated.[8,15]

Other medications also cause hypothermia by impairing centrally mediated vasoconstriction. Barbiturates induce hypothermia in greater than therapeutic doses, whereas phenothiazines induce hypothermia even at therapeutic doses. Other drugs that can contribute to hypothermia include general anesthetics and tricyclic antidepressants. The toxic effects of any drug may not be significant while the person is hypothermic but will become evident when liver, kidney, and metabolic function increase with rewarming. Interestingly, a combination of alcohol, barbiturates, and hypothermia prolongs brain survival even further than hypothermia alone.[48]

Trauma Victims

Trauma victims are especially susceptible to hypothermia. Long delays in response time, extrications, stabilization at the scene, and transportation to the hospital contribute to the development of hypothermia. In addition, cold oxygen and IV fluids, removal of clothing, and continuous evaluations by numerous medical personnel add to the problem. The ability of trauma patients to thermoregulate may be disrupted by hypovolemia or head injuries. Burn patients are at high risk because skin integrity has been interrupted. All trauma victims should have temperature closely monitored.[11,12,15,19]

Outdoor People

Boaters, campers, sailors, hikers, anglers, mountaineers, and other outdoor people are at risk for hypothermia. Generally such people are healthy but become victims of the environment, physical exhaustion, or their own carelessness. Outdoor hypothermia is categorized in two groups: immersion and nonimmersion. Examples of nonimmersion hypothermia include exposure to wind, rain, snow, and freezing temperatures. Immersion hypothermia occurs more rapidly than nonimmersion hypothermia; heat loss is 35% higher if the patient swims or treads water rather than stays still.[6] A person with immersion hypothermia may drown sooner because the level of consciousness decreases at 30° C.

Central Nervous System Dysfunction

Not only does CNS dysfunction increase susceptibility to hypothermia, hypothermia mimics the symptoms of CNS dysfunction. Cerebrovascular accidents are the most common CNS dysfunction to cause hypothermia. It is important for the flight nurse to determine if the suspected cerebrovascular accident patient is hypothermic. Schizophrenia and senile dementia are occasionally accompanied by hypothermia. It is unclear whether hypothermia in these states is a consequence of hypothalamic dysfunction[14] or of psychosocial factors such as homelessness and inattention to potential environmental danger.

REWARMING TECHNIQUES

Both Edwards[14] and Bangs and McCauley[20] note that careful review of the literature reveals no evidence supporting one rewarming technique over another. The consensus is that the patient should be rewarmed as quickly as possible because the myocardium is refractory to therapy below 30° C. There are three techniques for rewarming: passive external, active external, and active internal. Only passive external, active external, and limited forms of active internal rewarming can be initiated in the air medical setting. Consequently, rapid transportation to a facility that can provide more extensive rewarming techniques is imperative. Flight personnel must be aware of the existence of these facilities in their service areas.

Passive External Rewarming

Passive external rewarming is simple, inexpensive, and easily instituted. It is used only in mild hypothermia and when the patient can generate heat by shivering and vasoconstriction. The patient is placed in a warm environment, covered with blankets, and allowed to rewarm naturally. Passive external rewarming is available in any aircraft with the use of a blanket and a heater. Long-term alcoholic patients have a lower mortality rate when passive external rewarming is used. Passive external rewarming increases core body temperature by 1° C per hour.

Active External Rewarming

Active external rewarming involves placing heat on the external surface of the body. Heated baths, thermal blankets, and packs to the groin, neck, and axilla are examples of active rewarming.

Afterdrop is a dangerous phenomenon that can occur in the initial stages of passive and active external rewarming. Afterdrop is defined as a decline of 1° C to 2° C in the core body temperature when cool blood from the extremities moves to the core.[48] Any action that moves blood rapidly from the extremities to the heart, including moving the patient or injudiciously applying heat to the periphery, can cause afterdrop and precipitate ventricular fibrillation. Savard et al.[34] suggested another possible explanation for the afterdrop phenomenon: the myocardial irritability of afterdrop is caused by a blood chemical shift and not necessarily from a blood temperature shift.

Active Internal Rewarming

Active internal rewarming delivers heat directly to the body core, thereby avoiding the dangers of afterdrop. The heart, lungs, and brain are warmed first and in turn rewarm of the rest of the body. Heated oxygen, IV fluids, hemodialysis and peritoneal dialysis, gastric lavage, mediastinal lavage (after thoracotomy), and cardiopulmonary bypass are all examples of active internal rewarming. The least invasive method of active internal rewarming is used when the patient has severe hypothermia but is cardiovascularly stable. On the other hand, the most rapid active internal rewarming methods, such as cardiopulmonary bypass, are recommended if the patient has severe hypothermia and is unstable with cardiovascular collapse unresponsive to drugs and defibrillation.

AIR MEDICAL MANAGEMENT

Management of hypothermia has been controversial since Napoleon's chief surgeon, Baron Larrey, noted that hypothermic soldiers closest to the fire were the ones who died.[3,14] Hypothermia experiments in human subjects can be safely performed only to 35° C, and those in animals are not equivalent because the physiologic response of animals to hypothermia is different from that of human beings. Consequently, current air medical management of the hypothermic patient is based mainly on anecdotal reports in the literature.

All hypothermic patients must be transported, regardless of cardiopulmonary status. The old adage "A patient is not dead until warm and dead"[10,37] holds true. "Warm" is defined as 32° C. Severe hypothermia takes priority over any other problem except obstructed airway or major trauma with rapid exsanguination.

Management of the mildly hypothermic patient is relatively uncomplicated; further heat loss is prevented by covering the patient with blankets and allowing the patient to warm naturally. Management of the severely hypothermic patient is more complicated and will test the expertise and knowledge of flight personnel.

Gentle Handling

The patient must be handled gently during transport, and stimulation should be minimized. Any movement, including lifting, has been shown to precipitate ventricular fibrillation. Rubbing or massaging the patient is contraindicated. Air medical personnel should always cut clothing rather than pull it off. A mildly hypothermic patient must be kept quiet and not allowed to walk or stand. Aircraft vibration can also, theoretically, add to stimulation, but its effects have not been investigated.

Preventing Further Heat Loss

Prevention of further heat loss is paramount in the management of the hypothermic patient. Limited exposure during assessment will prevent heat loss during examination. The patient's wet clothing should be removed immediately to prevent conductive heat loss. The patient should be removed or protected from any wind source—including helicopter turbulence, which can produce wind up to 100 mph. Insulated and windproofed blankets should be placed under and over the patient, leaving the face exposed, while the patient's head is protected with a wool hat. An electric blanket is contraindicated because this form of active external rewarming can precipitate afterdrop. The cold railings of the stretcher conduct heat and should not be allowed to touch the patient during transport. Warm oral fluids should be considered for the conscious patient only after assessment for an active gag reflex. Aspiration can be a problem, especially if the size of aircraft does not permit the patient to sit upright or at least at a 45-degree angle. Beverages containing alcohol are contraindicated.

Active Internal Rewarming

The respiratory tract is a major area of heat exchange and evaporative loss. Administration of warm humidified oxygen effectively rewarms the heart, lungs, and brain by way of the bronchial circulation. In addition, the cilia will become more active while being rewarmed and humidified and can assist in decreasing and mobilizing secretions. Warm, humidified oxygen is easy to administer, safe, effective, noninvasive, and readily available in the air medical setting. One hundred percent warm humidified oxygen should be administered by mask or bag-valve apparatus at 42° C to 46° C. The rate of rewarming varies from 0.5° C to 2.0° C/hr[17] to 3.5° C in 20 minutes.[18] A high flow rate is essential for this method to be effective. Core temperature increases an additional 0.3° C/hr by increasing ventilatory rate by 10 liters per minute.[23] McCauley,[20] Danzl,[3] and Slovis and Bachvarov[36] have described various commercial products available.

Rehydration of the hypothermic patient with warm IV fluids increases blood flow to the heart and decreases blood viscosity, vasoconstriction, potential of afterdrop, and the likelihood of cardiac arrhythmias.[3] Hypothermic patients appear to have a better chance of survival when a bolus of warm IV normal saline solution is given before the patient is moved or externally rewarmed.[3] The flight nurse should establish an IV line in the largest vein available. If needed, a small amount of heat may be applied to the area to facilitate venous access. Five percent dextrose in normal saline solution (D_5NS) is the fluid of choice because lactated Ringer's solution is not fully metabolized by the liver in severe hypothermia.[3] D_5NS can be made by adding 2 amps of D50 to 900 ml of normal saline solution. An adult patient may be infused with at least 200 ml/hr and the pediatric patient with at least 4 ml/kg/hr, with adjustment if the patient requires additional fluid resuscitation. Pulmonary edema, jugular vein distention, and other problems associated with fluid overload are monitored. IV fluids are administered at a temperature of 40° C. Fluids can be warmed en route by wrapping them in a shirt, jacket, towel, or an electric blanket or other commercial warming devices. Some aircraft now come with environmental drawers that keep fluids warm during transport.

Monitoring Vital Signs

The patient's rectal temperature, heart rate, and respirations should be monitored carefully and on a regular basis. A special thermometer capable of registering to 20° C is required for the hypothermic patient. An esophageal or tympanic thermometer is preferable, but they are impractical in the air medical setting. Danzl[3] noted that rectal temperature lags behind actual core temperature and is influenced by leg temperature and placement of the rectal probe. Volunteers were placed in freezing-cold water for 15 minutes and noted all the classic signs of hypothermia; however, he discovered the body was able to compensate and core body temperature remained unchanged for at least 15 to 20 minutes.[20]

Inaccurate assessment of the patient's respirations can lead to improper management and can precipitate life-threatening arrhythmias. The patient must be observed carefully for at least 1 full minute for the presence of respirations to be determined. A spontaneous respiratory rate of 4 to 6 breaths/min is adequate in hypothermia. An effective cardiac rhythm may be assumed if the patient is breathing spontaneously. Cardiac monitoring may be difficult because of muscle tremors. In fact, baseline oscillations on the ECG may be the only sign that the patient is shivering. Blood pressure may not be obtainable or may be inaccurate because of vasoconstriction. An ultrasound stethoscope may be of use in assessing the presence of a pulse or heartbeat.

Airway

The airway is opened without the use of adjuncts when possible and intubation only if airway reflexes are absent. Blind nasal intubation may be necessary if trismus is present.[3] The risk of cardiac arrhythmia may be decreased during intubation with preoxygenation and careful technique. Hyperventilation must be avoided because respiratory alkalosis can precipitate ventricular fibrillation. Fewer than 10 breaths/min will successfully oxygenate the hypothermic patient without causing respiratory alkalosis.[3]

Cardiac Resuscitation

Cardiac resuscitation in the hypothermia patient is a controversial topic. The main concern is that chest compressions could be initiated on a patient with a slow but viable rhythm. External cardiac massage on a hypothermic bradycardic heart can precipitate ventricular fibrillation. Established ventricular fibrillation or asystole on the heart monitor is the only indication for prehospital cardiopulmonary resuscitation (CPR) of the severely hypothermic patient.[1,5]

Some investigators believe that chest compressions should be withheld in any patient with a core temperature of less than 28° C.[14] Others believe that chest compressions should be reduced to half the recommended rate because metabolic demands are decreased in the hypothermic brain.[1,5] Strong evidence supporting these deviations from Advanced Cardiac Life Support (ACLS) guidelines for CPR is lacking. Although hypothermia does protect the brain from anoxic damage, this "safe period" has not been established, and brain damage will occur after cardiac arrest unless CPR is started.[39] Therefore cardiac compressions should be started according to ACLS guidelines once ventricular fibrillation or asystole is established. If spontaneous respirations are present at any rate, a viable rhythm may be assumed and CPR may be deferred. Danzl and Pozos[4] proposed that CPR be initiated in all cases except the following: (1) a do-not-resuscitate order is confirmed, (2) obviously lethal injuries are noted, (3) chest-wall compression is impossible, (4) rescuers are jeopardized during evacuation, or (5) signs of life are present. Again, a careful assessment of respirations and pulse for at least 1 full minute is imperative to avoid unnecessary and dangerous CPR.

Defibrillation is usually not effective until core temperature is greater than 28° C. However, it is recommended that defibrillation at 200 W seconds be attempted twice, then deferred until the patient is rewarmed.

Pharmacologic Therapy

Little clinical evidence to confirm or rule out the effectiveness or complications of pharmacologic therapy has been noted.[3] Medications should be used with extreme caution. Decreased circulation pools medications in the extremities; a toxic reaction can occur when the patient is rewarmed and medication flows to the core. In light of this possibility, several authors have suggested withholding all medications from the hypothermic patient.[1,3] The flight nurse should give sodium bicarbonate judiciously (0.5 to 1 mEq/kg) and only in documented severe metabolic acidosis uncorrected by rewarming.[3] Overzealous correction can precipitate ventricular fibrillation.

A glucometer may be consulted, if available, and treatment initiated according to the results. Otherwise adults can be given 1 amp of D50 and pediatric patients 2 ml/kg of D25 (dilute D50 to half strength) if the blood sugar level is unknown.

Pharmacologic manipulation of pulse, blood pressure, and respiratory rate should be avoided.[3] The value of naloxone, lidocaine, and propranolol is under investigation. Bretylium has shown a protective effect against ventricular fibrillation experimentally in animals by decreasing the temperature threshold at which ventricular fibrillation occurs.[3] Routine administration of steroids and antibiotics is not recommended.[3] Empiric treatment of hypothermia with thyroxine is appropriate in myxedema coma.[3] Medications should not be given orally or intramuscularly because of decreased absorption rates. Other medications should be deferred until the core temperature is 30° C.

Special Considerations

The following principles should be considered by air medical personnel in the management of cold-related emergencies:

1. Treat major trauma as the first priority and hypothermia as the second.
2. Notify the receiving facility while en route to the scene, clinic, or hospital to give the receiving facility time to activate appropriate resources.
3. Insert a Foley catheter and nasogastric tube for long transports.
4. Avoid vasopressors. Consider them only if rewarming shock is unresponsive to fluids.
5. Continue CPR until the patient is rewarmed to 32° C.

DOCUMENTATION

The history of the incident should be documented, including the time and type of exposure, whether the patient was in cardiopulmonary arrest on arrival of the first responder, what management was initiated before the arrival of flight personnel, and the heart rhythm, drug therapy, and rewarming techniques. Past medical history is important if it is readily available.

Written assessment of the hypothermic patient consists of an initial head-to-toe evaluation including all pertinent findings. The vital signs should be monitored and charted on a regular basis, preferably every 10 to 15 minutes, and should include rectal temperature and heart rhythm with strip readout. The patient and the rewarming techniques should be assessed continually during flight.

SUMMARY

Almost any treatment mode will suffice in managing the mildly hypothermic patient. Expertise of flight personnel will be tested when presented with a severely hypothermic patient. Management requires gentle handling, accurate assessment of cardiopulmonary status, passive external rewarming to prevent further heat loss, and active internal rewarming with heated humidified oxygen and IV fluids.

COLD-RELATED EMERGENCIES CASE STUDY

A 7-year-old male passenger in an automobile was thrown from the car, landing in a river. Paramedics were at the scene when the patient was extricated 1 hour later, and primary assessment revealed no breathing and no carotid or femoral pulse. The patient was gently moved to the ambulance, where CPR and ACLS procedures were initiated immediately. The patient was orally intubated using careful technique, and ventilations were assisted with a bag-valve mask. Two IV lines were started: one in the right jugular vein and one in the right antecubital space. The following medications were given: sodium bicarbonate 50 mEq, atropine 1 mg, epinephrine 2 mg, and dextrose 50% 15 ml. Warm packs were placed in the groin and armpits to initiate active external rewarming. A nasogastric tube was placed and a small amount of pale yellow liquid evacuated. Air medical transport of the patient was ordered immediately by personnel at the scene.

On the arrival of the flight team, reassessment revealed a young male patient (30 kg) lying supine on a backboard in the back of the ambulance; CPR was in progress, the skin was pale and cold to touch, and no capillary refill noted. The patient was orally intubated, with ventilations assisted every third compression. Ventilation with a bag-valve mask at 100% oxygen with fair lung compliance was performed. Cardiac monitor displayed pulseless electrical activity rhythm with a rate of 60 to 70 beats/min with no associated femoral or carotid pulses. Rectal temperature was 24° C.

Physical examination revealed the following findings.

Neurologic: Pupils were fixed and dilated at 8 cm. There was no spontaneous movement of extremities, the child was areflexic, and GCS was 3.

Head: Skull and facial bones were grossly intact. The patient had no visible sign of trauma, the nose and ears were clear, and the cervical spine had no palpable deformities. A small amount of pink frothy sputum from the endotracheal tube was seen, and the IV line to the right jugular vein was patent and secure.

Chest: Breath sounds were equal, with scattered rales. The chest wall was intact with no visible trauma.

Abdomen: The abdomen was distended and tense. Nasogastric tube placement was confirmed and secured.

Extremities: The long bones were grossly intact, IV to right antecubital patent and secure.

The patient was gently loaded into the helicopter during continuing CPR and assisted ventilations. The pilot radioed to alert the emergency department of the patient's condition and requested the hypothermia team to remain on standby. In flight the patient was managed in the following manner:

1. Continuous reassessment of condition
2. Continued CPR and assisted ventilations
3. Warm, humidified oxygen administered by bag-valve mask
4. Warm IV fluid provided at a keep-vein-open rate
5. Blankets added to prevent further heat loss
6. Nasogastric tube to suction
7. D50 additional 15 ml given to bring patient to 1 ml/kg dose
8. Cervical spine immobilization

During the flight, the patient remained clinically unchanged. Agonal respirations were noted toward the end of the flight, and ventilations were assisted. Rectal temperature rose to 28° C.

On arrival at the emergency department, the patient had a blood pressure of 98/60 mm Hg, with agonal respirations. Rectal temperature was 30° C. An increase in pink frothy sputum from the endotracheal tube was noted, and 3 cm of positive end expiratory pressure (PEEP) was added to the ventilator. A dopamine drip was started by pump at 16.6 μg/kg/min to maintain a systolic blood pressure between 90 and 100 mm Hg. All fluids were placed on IV warmers. The heart monitor displayed sinus tachycardia with palpable femoral and brachial pulses. Peritoneal lavage was started with warmed normal saline solution as a check for abdominal bleeding and to initiate active internal rewarming.

Initially, arterial blood gas (ABG) values (adjusted for rectal temperature) were pH 7.13, P_{CO_2}

32, Po_2 50, actual HCO_3 11, base deficit 20, O_2 calculated 91, O_2 actual 89, K 2.9.

Sodium 10 mEq was given along with potassium chloride 10 mEq IV. Peritoneal lavage was negative for blood. Chest radiography revealed right pneumothorax, which was treated with a chest tube. Computed tomography of the head and neck was negative. The patient was transported to the intensive care unit in fairly stable condition.

In the intensive care unit the patient was maintained on the ventilator with warm humidified oxygen. The dopamine drip was continued to maintain a stable blood pressure between 90 and 100 mm Hg systolic. The patient was placed between hypothermia blankets. The pupils remained fixed and dilated at 8 cm; no corneal reflex was present. There was slight spontaneous flailing of all extremities. ABGs were stabilized throughout the evening with small doses of sodium bicarbonate. The patient's blood pressure was stabilized with 18 μg/kg/min dopamine. Rectal temperature increased slowly, finally stabilizing at 37° C. Four hours after admission to the intensive care unit, the patient suddenly deoxygenated, with the heart monitor displaying bradycardia. The patient's rhythm quickly deteriorated to ventricular fibrillation, and a cardiac arrest situation was called. Unfortunately, efforts failed, and the patient was pronounced dead after 1 hour of aggressive resuscitation.

REFERENCES

1. Caroline NL: *Emergency care in the streets,* ed 2, Boston, 1983, Little, Brown.
2. Collins KJ: *Hypothermia: the facts,* New York, 1983, Oxford University Press.
3. Danzl DF, Pozos RS: Multicenter hypothermia survey, *Ann Emerg Med* 16(9):1042, 1987.
4. Danzl D, Pozos R, Hamlet M: Accidental hypothermia. In Auerbach P, editor: *Wilderness medicine,* St Louis, 1995, Mosby.
5. Davies DM, Miller EJ, Miller IA: Accidental hypothermia treated by extracorporeal blood-warming, *Lancet* May 13, 1967, p 1036.
6. Department of Transportation/United States Coast Guard: *Hypothermia and cold water survival,* Washington, DC, 1980, GPO.
7. Ehrmantraut WR, Ticktin HE, Fazekras JF: Cerebral hemodynamics and metabolism in accidental hypothermia, *Arch Intern Med* 99:57, 1957.
8. Freund B, O'Brien C, Young A: Alcohol ingestion and temperature regulation during cold exposure, *J Wilderness Med* 5:88-98, 1994.
9. Gordon AS: Cerebral blood flow and temperature during deep hypothermia for cardiovascular surgery, *J Cardiovasc Surg* 3:299, 1962.
10. Gregory RT, Patton JF: Treatment after exposure to cold, *Lancet* 1:377, 1972.
11. Gregory J, Flanbaum I, Townsend M: Incidence and timing of hypothermia in trauma patients, *J Trauma* 31:795-800, 1991.
12. Hauty M, Esrig B, Long W: Prognostic factors in severe accidental hypothermia: experience from the Mt. Hood tragedy, *J Trauma* 27:1107-1112, 1987.
13. International Commission of Alpine Rescue, Subcommission of Medicine: *Field and base treatment of cold injuries.* Presented at the Fifth International Symposium on Mountain Medicine, Innsbruck, Austria, Nov 13, 1976.
14. Jolly T, Ghezzi K: Accidental hypothermia, *Emerg Med Clin North Am* 10(2):311-328, 1992.
15. Jurkovich G, Gaser W, Luterman A: Hypothermia in trauma victims: an ominous sign, *J Trauma* 27:1019-1024, 1987.
16. Knowlton FP, Starling EH: The influence of variations in temperatures and blood pressure on the performance of the isolated mammalian heart, *J Physiol* 44:206, 1912.
17. Lloyd EL: Accidental hypothermia treated by central rewarming through the airway, *Br J Anaesth* 45:41, 1973.
18. Lloyd EL, Frankland JC: Accidental hypothermia: central rewarming in the field (correspondence), *Br Med J* 4:717, 1974.
19. Luna G, Maier R, Pavlin E: Incidence and effect of hypothermia in seriously injured patients, *J Trauma* 27:1014-1018, 1987.
20. McCauley RL et al: Frostbite and other cold-induced injuries. In Auerbach P, editor: *Wilderness medicine,* St Louis, 1995, Mosby.
21. McAniff JJ: The incidence of hypothermia in scuba-diving fatalities, First International Hypothermia Conference, Kingston, Jamaica, Jan 23-27, 1980.
22. Miller JW, Danzl DF, Thomas DM: Urban accidental hypothermia: 135 cases, *Ann Emerg Med* 9:456, 1980.
23. Morrison JB, Conn ML, Hayward JS: Thermal increment provided by inhalation rewarming from hypothermia, *J Appl Physiol* 46:1061, 1979.
24. Okada M: The cardiac rhythm in accidental hypothermia, *J Electrocardiol* 17:123, 1984.

25. Okada M, Nishimura F, Yoshiro H: The J-wave in accidental hypothermia, *J Electrocardiol* 16:23, 1983.
26. O'Keefe KM: Accidental hypothermia: a review of 62 cases, *JACEP* 6:491, 1977.
27. Orr KD, Fainer DC: *Cold injuries in Korea during winter of 1950-1951,* Fort Knox, Ky, 1951, US Army Medical Research Laboratory.
28. Proehl J: Environmental emergencies. In Kitt S et al, editors: *Emergency nursing,* Philadelphia, 1995, Saunders.
29. Purdue GF, Hunt JL: Cold injury: a collective review, *J Burn Care Rehabil* 7(4):331, 1986.
30. Rango N: Exposure-related hypothermia mortality in the United States, 1970-1979, *Am J Public Health* 74:1159, 1984.
31. Rango N: Old and cold: hypothermia in the elderly, *Geriatrics* 35(11):93, 1980.
32. Rankin AC, Rae AP: Cardiac arrhythmias during rewarming of patients with accidental hypothermia, *Br Med J* 289:874, 1984.
33. Reuler JB: Hypothermia: pathophysiology, clinical settings and management, *Ann Intern Med* 89:519, 1978.
34. Savard GK et al: Peripheral blood flow during rewarming from mild hypothermia in humans, *J Appl Physiol* 58:4, 1985.
35. Semonin-Holleran R: *Prehospital nursing,* St Louis, 1994, Mosby.
36. Slovis CM, Bachvarov HL: Heated inhalation treatment of hypothermia, *Am J Emerg Med* 2:533, 1984.
37. Smith DS: Accidental hypothermia: giving "dead" victims the benefit of the doubt, *Postgrad Med* 81(3):38, 1987.
38. Smith DS: The cold water connection, First International Hypothermia Conference, Kingston, Jamaica, Jan 23-27, 1980.
39. Steinman AM: The hypothermic code: CPR controversy revisited, *JEMS* 8(10):32, 1983.
40. Steinmann S, Shackford S, Davis J: Implications of admission hypothermia in trauma patients, *J Trauma* 30: 200-202, 1990.
41. Tek D, Mackey S: Non-freezing cold injury in a marine infantry battalion, *J Wilderness Med* 4:353-357, 1993.
42. Tolman KG, Cohen A: Accidental hypothermia, *Can Med Asso J* 103:1357, 1970.
43. United States Coast Guard Station, UCN 0075, New York, Apr 5, 1982.
44. Vaughn PB: Local cold injury—menace to military operations: a review, *Milit Med* 145:305, 1980.
45. Weast RC, editor: *Handbook of chemistry and physics,* ed 55, Cleveland, Ohio, 1974, CRC Press.
46. Wilkerson JA, Bangs CC, Hayward JS: *Hypothermia, frostbite and other cold injuries,* Seattle, 1986, Mountaineers.
47. Wilson FN, Finch R: The effect of drinking iced water upon the form of the T deflection of the electrocardiogram, *Heart* 10:275, 1923.
48. White JD: Hypothermia: the Bellevue experience, *Ann Emerg Med* 11:417, 1982.

CHAPTER 28

Heat-Related Emergencies

COMPETENCIES

1. Identify risk factors that contribute to heat-related illnesses.
2. Distinguish between the different types of heat-related illnesses, including heat exhaustion and heat stroke.
3. Initiate rapid cooling measures to decrease the body temperature of patients experiencing heat stroke.

Deaths attributed to heat-related illnesses have been reported for centuries. The Bible refers to persons who had heat stroke after working in hot fields 2000 years ago. In 24 BC, a Roman army was annihilated in the heat of the Arabian desert. The warriors of the Crusades were ultimately beaten in the Holy Land by heat and fever.[12] Incarceration in the infamous "Black Hole of Calcutta" resulted in high numbers of heat-related deaths.[8] During the summers of 1980, 1983, and 1988, severe heat waves in the United States resulted in 1700, 556, and 454 deaths, respectively, from heat stroke.[1] Recent data related to heat illness have been obtained from pilgrims in Mecca, Saudia Arabia, in 1984 and 1985,[9,20] and military experience has provided extensive data on heat illness and the effect of heat on human physiology.[16]

Heat stroke is a true medical emergency that requires rapid diagnosis and treatment. The longer the body remains hyperthermic, the greater the damage and consequent increase in morbidity and mortality. The flight nurse, by quickly recognizing and immediately treating the heat illness, can do much to combat permanent organ damage and the sequelae of untreated or undertreated hyperthermia.

INCIDENCE AND CAUSATIVE FACTORS

The very young and the elderly are at greatest risk of being afflicted with heat-related illness. Moderate forms of heat-related illness can cause discomfort but are of relatively short duration, with rare sequelae. Heat exhaustion and heat stroke are the two serious, pathologic states of heat illness.

Even in relatively mild weather, heat illness can affect persons with predisposing risk factors; it can also affect persons who are unacclimatized or unconditioned and who are then pushed rapidly beyond their tolerance or physical capability, as can happen in military "boot camp" and with novice joggers. Even well-conditioned athletes are subject to heat illness if they are not properly acclimatized. Heat illness is second only to head injuries as a cause of death of U.S. athletes.[11,16]

The mortality and morbidity statistics for heat illness do not reflect the true impact of this illness on the civilian population. Civilian statistics can be inferred from military experience. Records show that heat exhaustion affects 280 of 100,000 military recruits undergoing basic training in South Carolina.[11,16]

Many times, death from heat stroke goes unrecorded during heat waves. The patient often has an underlying cardiovascular, pulmonary, renal, or neurologic pathology. During heat waves, deaths from myocardial infarction, pneumonia, kidney failure, and stroke climb sharply; these are recorded as the cause of death. Thus the estimate of heat illness is a "dramatic underrepresentation" of the true magnitude of this problem.[8]

Infants have a relatively small surface area with which to dissipate heat. Parents often prevent heat loss by wrapping infants in blankets and in clothing that is too heavy for a hot environment. The thermoregulatory ability of children lags behind other body systems in maturity and functional ability. Therefore children are more predisposed to heat illness, and recognition and diagnosis of heat pathology are often made more difficult.

Heat illness can develop in elderly persons under conditions that would not generally affect younger persons. As a person's age increases, physiologic ability to regulate temperature decreases. Older persons often do not notice temperature changes less than 2.3° C, probably because of sensory afferent deterioration.[2] The elderly population generally has a higher rate of cardiovascular and pulmonary disease, diabetes, and neurologic pathology, and often use multiple drugs. All of these conditions contribute to the increased likelihood of heat illness in persons in this age group.

A person who is obese also has a higher risk of experiencing heat illness. Heat loss is inversely proportional to body size and body weight. Adipose tissue has less ability to lose heat compared with nonadipose tissue because of decreased vascularity. Fat serves as an insulator, which is not conducive to heat loss.

Dehydration occurs because of a decrease in body water. As heat illness progresses, the circulatory blood volume decreases. When heat illness is superimposed on preexisting dehydration, the body has a severely limited volume reserve. The more severe the dehydration, the faster the physiologic compensation will be exhausted. Fluid intake is crucial for the prevention of heat illness.

An increased endogenous heat load will limit the body's ability to maintain normothermia in a hot environment. A classic endogenous heat source is fever. Fever is generally caused by pyrogens released from bacteria or viruses or by breakdown of cells caused by the infectious organism.

It is important to note that two different mechanisms are involved in fever and heat illness. With fever, the thermal set point is elevated because of the induction of prostaglandin synthesis in the thermoregulatory center. Salicylates work well to inhibit the reactions that lead to elevation of the thermal set point and thus relieve hyperthermia caused by fever. With heat illness, the thermal set point remains normal. Hyperthermia occurs because of the body's inability to dissipate heat; normal defense mechanisms designed to protect the set point are overwhelmed. Salicylates do not work well in this setting and should not be used.[8]

Hyperactive states demand more energy. The increasing energy demand is met by an increase in metabolic activity. Endogenous heat increases as a by-product of the increased metabolic rate. Strenuous physical exercise and seizures are examples of hyperactive states. Drugs can also lead to a hyperactive state and increase endogenous heat production.

Muscular exertion increases endogenous heat because of increased metabolic demand. Skeletal muscle is one of the major sources of heat production in the body. Muscular exertion often occurs outdoors under conditions in which the ambient temperature exceeds body temperature and high humidity is present. Hyperthermia can occur in this setting. "Weekend warriors," novice hard laborers, military inductees in physical training, football players who practice in the heat, and persons who use hot tubs unwisely can all predispose their bodies to heat illness.

Use of many prescription drugs and alcohol can also predispose a person to heat illness. Anticholinergic drugs reduce sweat gland secretions because of the blocking action of anticholinergics on transmission of sympathetic postganglionic nerve impulses to sweat glands. This cessation of sweating removes the body's chief agent of heat dissipation. Use of tricyclic antidepressants, phenothiazines, butyrophenones, thiothixenes, diuretics, and β-blockers predispose the patient to heat illness.[8,11]

Other drugs associated with hyperthermia are glutethimide, those that induce hypersensitivity or idiosyncratic reactions (antibiotics, anticonvulsants, and hypertensives), and those that induce direct pyrogenic stimulation (bleomycin).[4,8,10]

Psychiatric patients often take anticholinergic drugs. Lithium and haloperidol have been reported to cause fatal hyperthermia. Haloperidol may reduce awareness or recognition of thirst.[9] Thioridazine (Mellaril) overdose is documented to cause hyperthermia.[1] The interaction of monamine oxidase inhibitors with amphetamines, tricyclic antidepressants, or phenothiazines is a well-documented cause of hyperthermia. Psychiatric patients may lack the awareness or desire to care for themselves properly in hot environments.

Alcohol use is known to predispose most persons to heat illness.[8] The exact mechanisms of this phenomenon are complex. Alcohol is a vasodilator and may enhance external heat absorption. Use of alcohol interferes with the judgment and mental acuity necessary to care for oneself. Use of cocaine and LSD has also been documented to cause fatal hyperthermia.[8]

One of the major organs that must be functional if heat is to be dissipated is the skin. Any pathologic process that disrupts skin integrity, interrupts normal physiologic functions, or both conditions will sharply limit heat dissipation. Sunburn and heat rash are relatively minor conditions that can have a drastic impact on physiologic compensation for heat stress. Major burns cause partial to total loss of skin function. Lack of ability to regulate body temperature is a complication of burn injury. Obviously the burn victim may be a candidate for heat illness.[14]

Patients with cystic fibrosis have a striking elevation of sweat electrolytes; the sodium and chloride content of their sweat is two to five times greater than that of healthy control subjects, and this occurs in 98% to 99% of affected children. These children are subject to massive sodium depletion in hot weather. Today, because of improved early diagnostic measures and treatment, many more patients with cystic fibrosis are living into early adulthood.

Lack of acclimatization predisposes a person to heat illness. On entering a warmer climate, exercise and general activity levels must be gradually increased. Persons vacationing in warm climates often overexert. Even well-conditioned athletes can be affected by heat-related illness if their training programs do not allow sufficient acclimatization before vigorous physical activity in hot, humid weather.

Persons can become acclimated to a hot climate within 10 days with daily exposure to moderate work and heat.[8] With a less zealous routine acclimatization will occur within a period of several weeks. The recognition of the principle of acclimatization has led to a reduction of the incidence of heat illness for those who are exposed to hot or high-risk environments. Acclimatization can occur at any age; however, its effectiveness can be limited by any of the aforementioned predisposing factors.

The most important physiologic adaptations during the acclimatization period include retention of salt and water, expansion of extracellular fluid volumes, and slight hemodilution.[8] Through these processes, sweating mechanisms improve. This is characterized by early onset of sweating, an increase in the volume of sweat, and a lowering of electrolyte concentration in the sweat.[8]

The increase in the volume of sweat accompanied by a lowering of the threshold for the onset of sweating results in better heat dissipation. An increase in aldosterone production lowers the sodium content of sweat. Combined with a 7% increase in total body water, the increase in aldosterone lowers sodium content of sweat from 100 mEq/L to 70 mEq/L.[2] The chloride concentration in sweat falls from 40 or 45 mEq/L to as low as 15 or 20 mEq/L, and sweat volume rises from 1 to 3 L/hr.[8]

After acclimatization, cardiovascular and metabolic proficiency is improved. Vasodilation occurs earlier and in greater magnitude. The heart rate is lower with a higher stroke volume, thus increasing cardiac output. Biochemical efficiency at the cellular level improves to the point that heat production for a given amount of work is less than in an unacclimatized person. Storage and utilization of glycogen are improved, thus delaying the onset of anaerobic metabolism with resultant lactic acidosis.

PATHOPHYSIOLOGY

Normal Thermogenesis

Human core temperature is closely regulated by a number of mechanisms to maintain a body core temperature of between 36° and 38° C. Processes that alter temperature homeostasis result in pathologic changes at the cellular level. Rising body temperature, if unregulated, can exceed the "critical thermal maximum" and cause irreversible organ damage; death quickly ensues. It is well documented that the human thermal maximum is 43° C.

Body core temperature is a species-specific, genetically determined set point that is regulated by the hypothalamus. Temperature regulation is quite precise, with response to temperature changes as small as 0.2° C (1.6° F).[8] A "thermostat" in the preoptic anterior portion of the hypothalamus receives information from various body thermoregulators. Peripheral and core temperature sensors in the skin, viscera, and nervous system tissues produce both thermal and endocrine signals. These signals are transmitted to the hypothalamus via neuronal and circulatory pathways. The "thermostat" then responds through a variety of negative feedback mechanisms to activate processes by which heat is lost or gained. These responses are mediated by means of the sympathetic nervous system.

Body heat production occurs because of two separate processes: endogenous metabolic processes and exogenous environmental exposure. Close regulation of body temperature is critical because the human body is dependent on relatively low temperature biochemical reactions at the microcellular level to sustain life.

Every body process produces exothermic heat. Normal basal cellular metabolism generates 50 to 60 kcal/hr and would cause a rise of 1° C/hr if not dissipated by compensatory mechanisms.[8] Digestion of food is the source of body heat. Major heat-producing organs are the liver and skeletal muscle. Body temperature is raised by increasing body work. Maximum sustained exercise produces 600 to 900 kcal/hr, raising body core temperature 5° C/hr without functional compensatory mechanisms.[16]

Exogenous (external) heat comes from the environment. Exposure to direct sunlight raises body core temperature 150 kcal/hr. The amount of humidity present in the air directly affects the body's ability to disperse heat. Humidity limits cooling by evaporation, which is caused by a lack of an evaporation gradient from skin surface to air.

Methods of Heat Loss

Thermoregulation by the hypothalamus maintains normothermia by balancing heat production and heat loss. When thermoregulation breaks down because of excess heat generation (endogenous), inability to dissipate heat (pathophysiologic), overwhelming environmental conditions (high ambient temperature with high humidity), or a combination of these factors, hyperthermia results. Under normal conditions, 90% of the heat produced by the body is lost to the environment via the skin surface by conduction, radiation, convection, and evaporation.

Environmental temperature obviously has a direct effect on the patient. The higher the temperature, the more external heat is present. When the environmental temperature is equals or greater than the body's temperature, passive heat loss through the means of conduction and radiation is decreased. Radiant heat loss occurs when the ambient temperature is lower than the body's temperature; conversely, the body readily absorbs radiant heat from the environment.

When air or water moves across the body surface, heat is lost by convection. Increasing the amount of air moving over the skin (forced convection) increases the amount of heat loss. The drier the air, the better the skin surface to air gradient, and the more heat that is lost.

The primary mechanism for heat dissipation is the evaporation of sweat. Through vaporization from the body surface, loss of 1 ml of sweat reduces body heat load by 1.7 kcal.[8,14,16,18] Under conditions of high ambient temperature and high ambient humidity, the skin is unable to provide effective cooling as the evaporation gradient is lost. At 75% humidity, evaporation decreases; at 90% to 95% humidity, evaporation ceases.[8]

The average person can produce up to 1.5 L of sweat per hour. Through conditioning and acclimatization, sweat production increases. The well-trained athlete can produce up to 3 L/hr.[8,11,16]

Insensible heat loss also occurs; heat is lost with passage of urine and feces, and the respiratory tract can dissipate heat by convection and evaporation.

Physiologic Compensation

Physiologic compensation begins in the hypothalamus. The exact chemical nature of thermoregulation is not yet fully understood. As endocrine and thermal sensors arrive from the heated periphery and core, the hypothalamic "thermostat" reduces bio-amine concentrations. Final common pathway effectors probably include prostaglandins, central nervous system amines, and a host of other hypothesized candidates.[8]

Upon reception of effector "messages" from the hypothalamus and peripheral thermoreceptors, the cardiovascular system responds with peripheral vasodilation. Vasodilation maximizes the cooling surface and greatly decreases peripheral vascular resistance. In this manner, the cardiovasculature conducts heat to the surface of the body, where it can be released to the environment. When skin vessels dilate, blood flow shunted through the area can exceed 4 L/min.[8] With this increased flow, 97% of cooling occurs at the skin surface.[12]

Heat Pathophysiology

On exposure to heat, the body initiates compensation by decreasing peripheral vascular resistance, thus shunting blood to the periphery. This action causes an increase in stroke volume and cardiac output, thus increasing demand on the heart. The healthy cardiovascular system can sustain this hyperdynamic state for a limited time; however, it will eventually tax the myocardium.

The purpose of this response is to cool the body. Heat is lost from the skin surface by evaporation of sweat. In severe heat stress, the body loses as much as 1.5 L/hr and even 3 L/hr in extreme cases.[8] Over a period of time, the circulating blood volume is reduced.

The cardiac output continues to drop as a result of the ensuing hypovolemia. Homeostasis becomes compromised. An altered hemodynamic state may develop that mimics high-output failure, such as that seen in sepsis. This results in hyperdynamic failure. In persons who undergo heat stroke, structural damage to the heart is common, although not extensive. Rarely, acute transmural myocardial infarction or widespread myocardial damage may occur.[8]

Cardiac dysrhythmias and myocardial damage may occur because of subendocardial hemorrhage, rupture of muscle fibers, necrosis, and infarction. This pathology is second to increased cardiac workload, thereby increasing myocardial oxygen demand. Not enough oxygen is available because of disruption of oxidative phosphorylation and a resulting shock state. Hypotension is usually a sign of severe or premorbid heat illness.[8]

The respiratory system initially responds with an increase in respiratory rate and depth to meet increased oxygen demand. This hyperventilation results in an initial heat loss from an increased volume of air moved over and through the respiratory tract. This evaporative loss decreases with increased respiratory fatigue. A high ambient humidity also limits this evaporative loss. An initial respiratory alkalosis develops as a result of the hyperventilation, with concurrent hypocarbia and the traditional muscle tetany. This tetany is the pathophysiologic basis for the ill-defined syndrome of heat tetany.

Ataxia, dysmetria, and dysarthria may be seen early in the onset of heat stroke because the Purkinje cells of the cerebellum are particularly sensitive to the toxic effects of high temperature. Because these changes are seen in other neurologic events, such as stroke, heat stroke may not be recognized initially.

Cerebral edema with associated diffuse petechial hemorrhages are often found in fatal cases.

When the hyperthermic insult is associated with status epilepticus and profound hypotension, the energy requirements of the brain increase. This in turn contributes to the spiraling core temperature, increasing up to four times the metabolic rate of the brain. The cerebral vessels dilate maximally, and thus the blood flow is dependent on mean arterial pressure. The added effects of dehydration (hypovolemic source) produce a pathophysiologic state conducive to brain death and damage.

Kidney function is altered from the loss of sodium and water in sweat. The kidneys retain sodium, and thus they retain water and excrete potassium. Renal dysfunction occurs because of hypovolemia and hypoperfusion. Urinary output drops, and acute renal tubular necrosis may ensue. If sodium losses are of sufficient severity, signs of hyponatremia may appear. There is a risk that hypokalemia may develop because of the excretion of potassium in the urine.

The liver, which is particularly sensitive to temperature damage, is affected in nearly every case.[7,8] Liver function decreases by 20%. This decrease in function theoretically should aid in heat reduction, because the liver is one of the major heat-producing organs. Prothrombin times become prolonged.[3] Reduced hepatic perfusion caused by shunting of blood to the periphery leads to hypoglycemia in 20% of patients with exertional heat stroke.[9] Interestingly, the pancreas is the only organ not damaged by the toxic effects of heat stress.[4]

During heat stress, the gastrointestinal tract undergoes direct thermotoxicity and relative hypoperfusion because of the shunt of blood to the periphery. Ischemic intestinal ulceration can occur, which may lead to frank gastrointestinal bleeding.[4]

Muscle damage is evidenced by rhabdomyolysis. Muscle degeneration and necrosis occur as a direct result of extremely elevated temperature. Elevated creatine phosphokinase (CPK) values are a diagnostic hallmark of heat stroke because of this rhabdomyolytic process. The release of destructive lysosomal enzymes occurs as a result of extensive skeletal muscle damage. The release of lysosomal enzymes into the circulation may cause widespread capillary injury, leading to disseminated intravascular coagulation, acute respiratory distress syndrome, and acute renal tubular necrosis.[9] Muscle enzymes are greatly elevated.

ASSESSMENT PARAMETERS

The most common forms of heat illness, from least to most severe, are heat cramps, heat exhaustion, and heat stroke.

Heat Cramps

Heat cramps of heavily exercised muscle occur during and after exercise in a hot environment and are an extreme inconvenience to the patient. These cramps usually occur in trained athletes and in physically fit, acclimatized persons. These persons sweat profusely and characteristically replace sweat losses with water and inadequate amounts of salt. Hyponatremia ensues, which hinders muscle relaxation mechanisms. Usually the muscles will show the fasciculations of fatigue. A slight or moderate rise in CPK enzymes in serum is often observed. This rhabdomyolysis has not been shown to constitute an important clinical problem.[9] No permanent effects have been demonstrated from heat cramps.

Heat cramps involve exquisitely painful sustained muscular contractions, most commonly involving the muscles of the lower extremity; however, any muscle group in the body can be affected. The patient usually reports heavy exercise in a hot environment, with onset of cramping after rest.

Heat Exhaustion

Heat exhaustion is an ill-defined syndrome that can affects anyone. Hubbard et al.[8] define it as "a derangement of body function encountered when the body temperature is elevated, usually in the 39° to

41° C [102.2° to 105.8° F] range." The typical victim of heat exhaustion is usually unacclimatized to the environment and has worked in the heat for several days. Both infants and elderly bedridden patients are at higher risk of experiencing heat exhaustion because of their impaired ability to dissipate heat and communicate thirst.

Heat exhaustion, if allowed to proceed, will result in heat stroke. An essential distinction between the two entities is that cerebral function is unimpaired in persons with heat exhaustion, aside from minor irritability and poor judgment. Body temperatures are lower and the symptoms are less severe in persons experiencing heat exhaustion.

This syndrome results from loss of water, loss of salt, or both. Pure forms of single loss of either water or sodium are rare. Water-depletion heat exhaustion, which results from inadequate fluid replacement, is more serious and develops within a few hours. Salt-depletion heat exhaustion develops over the course of several days.

Heat exhaustion is largely a manifestation of the strain placed on the cardiovascular system when it is attempting to maintain normothermia. With sodium and water loss the patient becomes dehydrated, tachycardic, and syncopal, with orthostatic hypotension. The patient's temperature is usually less than 38° to 39° C (100.4° to 102.2° F) and is often normal. The patient retains the ability to sweat, which gives rise to cool, clammy skin. Headache and euphoria commonly occur because of dehydration and hypoperfusion. Mental status remains intact, although minor aberrations may be manifested. Flu-like symptoms of nausea, vomiting, and diarrhea with muscle cramps may be present. Subjective complaints include intense thirst, vague malaise, myalgias, and dizziness.

Laboratory values show classic signs of dehydration (elevated hematocrit, blood urea nitrogen [BUN], serum protein, and concentrated urine levels) with hyponatremia and hypokalemia. Moderate elevations (to several thousands) of muscle enzymes CPK, serum glutamate oxaloacetate transaminase (SGOT), serum glutamate pyruvate transaminase (SGPT), and lactate dehydrogenase (LDH) occur as a result of muscle cell damage.

Heat Stroke

Heat stroke is a life-threatening medical emergency in which the body's physiologic heat dissipating mechanisms fail and body temperature rises rapidly and uncontrollably. The central core temperature exceeds 42° C. At 42° C and above, cellular oxygen demands surpass the oxygen supply and oxidative phosphorylation is disrupted, causing cell and organ damage throughout the body. The duration of the hyperthermic episode and the temperature reached may be the single most important factors in patient survival and prognosis.

The resultant damage of such severe hyperthermia has many causes. Central nervous system disruption with altered mental status is a key diagnostic criterion in heat stroke. Early in the course of heat stroke, some persons appear confused and demonstrate irrational behavior, or even frank psychosis; others become comatose or have seizures.

The patient may have hot, flushed skin, with or without sweating, vomiting, and diarrhea. Hyperventilation at rates up to 60 is universally seen. Respiratory alkalosis is often present with tetany and hypokalemia. Pulmonary edema is not uncommon.

The cardiovascular system responds by reaching maximum stroke volume. Because of the shunt through the dilated periphery, tachycardia (up to 180) is the only way to increase cardiac output. Heat stroke results in high output failure, with cardiac output of 20 L or more. Central venous pressure readings are elevated despite hypotension caused by decreased ventricular contractility over 40° C. The hyperdynamic state persists even after cooling. The ECG generally shows nonspecific ST-T changes with various atrial and ventricular dysrhythmias.[8]

Blood studies should include arterial blood gas, complete blood cell count, platelets, prothrombin time/partial thromboplastin time (PT/PTT), electrolytes, BUN, creatinine, glucose, CPK, SGOT, SGPT, LDH, and a urinalysis. White blood counts of 30,000 to 50,000 are not uncommon. The platelet count and PT/PTT are monitored for onset of hypocoagulability. Hypofibrinogenemia and fibrinolysis may occur and progress to frank DIC.

The muscle enzymes (CPK, SGOT, SGPT, and LDH) in heat stroke are elevated in the tens of thousands—a diagnostic hallmark of heat stroke. Muscle breakdown occurs from direct thermal injury, clonic muscle activity, or tissue ischemia. In exertional heat stroke, CPK levels up to 1,500,000 IU/L have been reported. CPK levels greater than 20,000 are ominous and are indicative of later DIC, acute kidney failure, and potentially dangerous hyperkalemia.[6,8]

Reduced renal blood flow from shock and dehydration leads to ischemic kidneys. Concentration of the urine may lead to accumulation of uric acid and myoglobin, which have the capacity to crystallize in renal tubules. Crystallization may lead to obstructive uropathy and the development of acute tubular necrosis. BUN levels are frequently elevated. Low serum osmolarity, moderate proteinuria, and machine oil appearance of the urine occurs in patients with exertional heat stroke.[6,8,16]

The liver is frequently damaged, and frank jaundice is noted. The development of early jaundice, less than 24 hours after onset, has a worse prognosis than delayed jaundice. The engorged vessels of the gastrointestinal tract may become ulcerated and hemorrhage massively.

PATTERNS OF HEAT STROKE PRESENTATION

Heat stroke is manifested in three distinct patterns: classic, exertional, and drug induced. The three essential elements in the diagnosis of heat stroke are exposure to heat stress, internal or external; central nervous system dysfunction; and increased body temperature greater than 40° C.

Classic heat stroke, which tends to occur in the elderly, the ill, and infants, develops over a period of several days. It often occurs during heat waves and affects persons who do not have access to a cooler environment and fluids. Often the patient is discovered in bed and is unresponsive. In these cases the patient has hot, red, or flushed skin, has usually ceased sweating, and is significantly dehydrated.

Initial symptoms of classic heat stroke are similar to those of heat exhaustion: dizziness, headache, and malaise, progressing to frank confusion and coma. Fever, tachycardia, and hypotension are additional presenting signs. These patients also hyperventilate, which gives rise to respiratory alkalosis.

Exertional heat stroke usually occurs in young, fit, but unacclimatized persons who are often male athletes. Many such patients perform in hot and humid weather conditions that prevent adequate dissipation of generated heat. Of these patients, 50% still sweat profusely from the rapid onset; severe dehydration has not yet had time to occur.

Exertional heat stroke has a prodrome of chills, nausea, throbbing pressure in the head, and piloerection on the chest and upper arms. Concentration wanes, a subjective sense of physical deterioration is noticed, and the person feels increasingly hot, with decreased sweat production. Parasthesia is noted in the hands and feet.

Onset of irrational behavior then occurs. The face turns ashen gray and the skin may feel relatively cool if sweat is still being produced. This is followed by seizures and collapse. Patients who have exertional heat stroke often have severe respiratory acidosis from lactate caused by muscle exertion and volume depletion. They also have significant rhabdomyolysis.[8,16]

Drugs that predispose a person to heat stroke have been previously identified. Anticholinergic drugs such as phenothiazines, tricyclic antidepressants, antihistamines, antiparkinsonian agents, antispasmodics, and glutethimide inhibit sweating, thus interfering with heat dissipation. The side effects of some anticholinergic drugs include hyperkinesis and agitation, resulting in an increase in body temperature. Drugs with cardiovascular actions (β-blockers, diuretics, and antihypertensives) can inhibit or depress cardiovascular performance during increased demand resulting from heat stress. Diuretics, especially if abused, can lead to dehydration. Amphetamines, neuroleptics, and possibly tricyclic antidepressants induce heat stroke because they increase the endogenous heat load.[16] Hyperthermia resulting from interaction of monoamine oxidase inhibitors with tricyclic antidepressants and amphetamines has been noted.

Patients with drug-induced heat stroke have classic signs of heat stroke; the main difficulty is identifying the causative agent. Management should *never* be delayed by attempts to elucidate a comprehensive drug history.

INTERVENTION AND TREATMENT

Priorities

The most critical goal and life-saving measure in heat illness is cooling the victim to *rapidly decrease body temperature.* Immediate treatment often leads to prompt recovery. The more rapid the cooling, the lower the risk of mortality. Morbidity and mortality are directly related to the duration and intensity (temperature maximum) of hyperthermia.

While the patient is being cooled as rapidly as possible, maintenance of the "ABCs" of emergency care must not be forgotten. Because the patient may not have the ability to protect his or her airway, the flight nurse must effectively ventilate the lungs, oxygenate the blood, and maintain an adequate circulatory volume with an intact pump while carrying out continuous astute assessment through the duration of required therapy.

Equipment

No special equipment is required to effectively treat patients with heat illness. Standard equipment required for the provision of advanced life-support measures must be available.

Methods for cooling a patient range from use of simple ice packs to elaborate cooling tables. At this time, no method has proved to be superior to any other method. Recognition of the illness and prompt initiation of treatment are the most important tools in the management of heat illness.

Interventions—Mild to Invasive

Cooling can be accomplished in the prehospital setting first by removing the patient from the hot environment and especially moving him or her away from hot surfaces, such as concrete and pavement, even if no shaded area is nearby. The flight nurse should remove the patient's clothing and wet down the patient.

Covering the patient with cool fluid and increasing the movement of air over the patient enhance heat loss by increasing the evaporative gradient. The flight nurse should open the windows of the ambulance or make use of the air circulation of helicopter rotors during transport to further increase air movement over the patient. In one study of three cases of heat stroke, the patients were sprayed with lukewarm water while they were exposed to the downwash of a helicopter's rotors.[13,15]

Heat cramps constitute a mild form of heat illness. Treatment consists of salt replacement. Oral replacement of salt with a 0.1% salt solution (¼ teaspoon in 1 qt of water) and rest in a cool environment quickly resolves the cramping. If oral intake is contraindicated, 1000 ml of normal saline solution is administered intravenously over a 1- to 3-hour period. Mild forms of heat exhaustion are treated in a similar manner. If the patient's body temperature is elevated, the flight nurse should cool the skin with fans and cool compresses.[6,18]

More severe cases of heat exhaustion require rehydration. Laboratory values (renal electrolytes, BUN, and hematocrit) are best used to guide replacement of salt and water. Fluid is titrated to cardiovascular status. Normal saline solution, half-normal saline solution, and dextrose–half-normal saline solution have all been used; no evidence exists of a clear superiority of any one of these fluids.[6,18] Within 12 hours patients generally should feel well with normal vital signs and can be discharged without sequelae.

Heat exhaustion must be regarded on a continuum from the mild case, treated by simple cooling measures, to the severe case, which progresses to full-blown heat stroke. The most important treatment for heat illness is recognizing the hyperthermic insult and rapidly initiating cooling.

Controversy surrounds the question of which method is ideal for cooling the patient with heatstroke. Several methods are considered to be of therapeutic benefit. Packing the patient in ice and immersing the body in cold water are historic methods of cooling.[8] More recent therapy involves the use of warm water evaporated from the victim's skin surface by circulating air from a fan. The field treatment measure of ice packs placed in areas of maximum heat transfer (neck, axillae, and inguinal area) may also be continued.

Recent studies have revealed that dropping the skin surface temperature below 22° to 28° C may actually inhibit cooling because of peripheral vasoconstriction with a marked decrease in cutaneous blood flow. At or below these skin temperatures there is a sevenfold reduction in heat transfer from the body to the environment.[12] Counterproductive shivering may also occur at these skin temperatures. Recent research has demonstrated that if a patient's temperature has not been decreased within 30 minutes, cold water immersion should be seriously considered.[8,17]

Use of the warm water evaporation method of cooling is easier to accomplish and allows easier access to the patient should more invasive support methods be required. Warm water is used because it improves the vapor pressure gradient from air to skin. The ideal method seems to be to use room temperature water mist sprayed on the skin surface while a fan is used to promote evaporation. The optimal temperature for the moving column of air from the fan appears to be 45° C.[12] This temperature enhances evaporation and helps reduce patient discomfort and shivering.

Shivering, frank shaking, seizures, vomiting, and defecation can be expected during the cooling process. Shivering is counterproductive because it increases endogenous heat production. Chlorpromazine (Thorazine) in doses of 10 to 50 mg administered intravenously is the drug of choice to terminate shivering. This drug decreases metabolic oxygen consumption and dilates skin vessels, which further promotes cooling.[7-9]

Cooling measures are ceased when body core temperature reaches 39° C (102° F). The core temperature will then continue to fall to the normal range. If normal thermoregulatory mechanisms have been damaged by the thermic insult, a hypothermic overshot could result from further active cooling measures.[7]

Refractory hyperthermia will require more aggressive invasive methods. Ice-water gastric lavage has been reported to be effective both in a controlled canine model[12] and in actual victim treatment.[8] Gastric lavage has the advantages of rapid cooling and effective use of readily available equipment. Iced peritoneal lavage, hemodialysis, and cardiopulmonary bypass have been used as end attempts in severely refractory cases.[8] These increasingly invasive, operative methods obviously require a great commitment of resources and have higher degrees of risk and complication rates.

DEFINITIVE CARE (TRANSPORT CARE)

Heat stroke presents a complex patient management picture. If, when the flight nurse arrives, cooling measures have not been implemented or require augmentation, institution of the previously discussed interventions must be of the highest priority. As in any life-threatening case, a secured airway, institution of oxygenation, ventilation, and stabilization of cardiovascular status are mandated.

Endotracheal intubation is indicated for any patient who has a depressed sensorium because of the risk of emesis, aspiration, and seizure activity.

Patients with heat stroke are often hypotensive because of dehydration and the physiologic compensation of extreme vasodilation. In the vast number of cases, the hypotension will respond to cooling. Large amounts of fluids and inotropic agents are required only when cooling results in no response.

The choice of intravenous fluid is open to debate. In normotensive patients or those in whom hypotension is readily resolved with cooling, Ringer's lactate or normal saline solution is most often recommended.[8] Isoproterenol is frequently recommended because vasoconstriction does not occur when it is used. Metaraminol and dopamine have been used with desired effect. Because of complications of impaired cardiac function, pulmonary edema, congestive heart failure, adult respiratory distress syndrome, and acute kidney failure, fluid replacement is best guided by placement of a Swan-Ganz or CVP line. Field guidelines for fluid replacement recommend infusion of normal saline solution until a systolic blood pressure of 90 is obtained.[8]

In the light of the axiom that "the best defense is a good offense," monitoring the patient for multiple organ failure and prompt intervention upon clinical manifestation of such failure are of utmost importance. Placement of a nasogastric tube accomplishes gastric decompression and monitors for the onset of gastrointestinal bleeding. Antacids or intravenous cimetidine may be administered to keep the gastric pH above 4.[12]

An in-dwelling Foley catheter should be inserted to monitor hourly urinary output. Because of the possibility of kidney impairment, the flight nurse must closely monitor and support kidney function. Furosemide is commonly used to maintain urinary output. In the face of kidney failure, short- or long-term dialysis is often required.

Liver failure is a frequent complication of heat stroke. When liver failure is combined with kidney failure, the choice of drugs used in treatment becomes difficult. DIC occurs in severe cases; most patients who die from heat stroke have evidence of DIC.[8] Standard treatment measures are instituted.[7]

Electrolyte and acid-base imbalances may be manifested. Patients with low serum glucose levels are treated with D50 administration. Hyper- and hypokalemia are common. Hypokalemia with respiratory alkalosis is transient and requires no treatment; hypokalemia with acidosis requires replacement therapy.[8] Hyperkalemia reflects cellular damage and acidosis.[12]

The recurrence of seizure activity during and after cooling is treated with intravenously administered diazepam or lorazepam. Use of prophylactic treatment has been considered because seizures may increase heat production, metabolic acidosis, and hypoxia.

MALIGNANT HYPERTHERMIA

Malignant hyperthermia is chemically induced either by anesthetic agents or by catecholamine release in stress.[5,8,19] This disease is a genetic myopathy transmitted by an autosomal dominant gene. Malignant hyperthermia occurs in anesthetized patients at a ratio of approximately 1:15,000 in children and 1:50,000 in adults.[2,5] It is most common in male patients between age 15 and 30 years. Malignant hyperthermia has been reported in all races but with less frequency in blacks; a muscle-mass sex influence increases the incidence in men. It is uncommon in patients over the age of 50 years and under the age of 2 years.[2,5] The triggering agents are anesthetics: potent inhalant agents (often Halothane) and skeletal muscle relaxants (succinylcholine chloride and amide local agents).

The primary disorder is a defect in the sarcoplasmic reticulum in skeletal muscle metabolism. The sarcoplasmic reticulum is a reservoir for calcium storage in the muscle cell. Under normal conditions, the sarcoplasmic reticulum releases calcium ions into the myoplasm, causing skeletal muscle contractions. Contraction is sustained as long as a high concentration of calcium ions exists in the myoplasm. Relaxation occurs when a constantly functional calcium pump in the wall of the sarcoplasmic reticulum pumps calcium ions back into the reticulum.

In malignant hyperthermia, either the sarcoplasmic reticulum is unable to reaccumulate calcium or an accelerated release of calcium occurs. The increase in intracellular calcium results in sustained muscle contractions, and hypermetabolic state ensues. Increased oxygen consumption leads to decreased tissue oxygen saturation, causing metabolic and respiratory acidosis. Increased heat production leads to hyperthermia.

The loss of muscle cell membrane integrity occurs, which complicates the existing problem. The cell ions and molecules follow their concentration gradients. Calcium continues to move into the myoplasm, sustaining and worsening the muscle contractions. Hyperkalemia, myoglobinemia, and elevated CPK levels occur in the serum.

Malignant hyperthermia is characterized by hyperthermia, sustained tetanic muscle rigidity and contractions, hypermetabolism, and muscle cell destruction. Signs and symptoms are dependent on the use or nonuse of succinylcholine chloride.

With the administration of succinylcholine chloride at induction, rigidity of the masseter muscle may make intubation impossible. Additional doses will only worsen the rigidity. Muscle fasciculations normally observed with use of the drug may not occur. Unmovable joints with hard unindentible bellies may be noted.

Tachycardia is the most consistent first sign of malignant hyperthermia with the use of potent inhalation agents. Tachypnea, which results from hyperventilation caused by increasing acidosis, is the second sign. If the patient is not completely paralyzed, he or she may exhibit ventilatory efforts. Instability of systolic blood pressure is another consistent sign. Cardiac dysrhythmias and ensuing profound hypotension may occur. Cyanotic mottling of the skin, dark blood in the surgical field, and fever are late signs and indicate that the patient is already in crisis.

Immediate reversal of anesthesia and termination of surgery are mandated. Dantrolene sodium (Dantrium) is administered to maximize the survival of the patient. Dantrium, a skeletal muscle relaxant that acts by preventing the release of calcium ions from the sarcoplasmic reticulum, is the drug of choice. Dosage is 1 to 3 mg/kg initially to a maximum dose of 10 mg/kg.

Procainamide is the drug of choice for ventricular dysrhythmias because it does not affect myoplasmic calcium. Lidocaine and cardiac glycosides are contraindicated because they increase myoplasmic calcium. Hyperthermia is treated with previously described cooling methods. The standard therapy for hyperkalemia is indicated. Late complications can include pulmonary edema, DIC, kidney failure, and recurrence of malignant hyperthermia that was initially responsive to treatment measures.

SUMMARY

Heat illness presents as a continuum from mild to severe. Heat exhaustion, if untreated, may proceed to frank heat stroke, which is a life-threatening medical emergency. Causes of heat illness encompass endogenous, environmental, and drug-related pathologies. Malignant hyperthermia rarely occurs but has deadly consequences.

Prompt recognition of the problem and rapid cooling limit the severe sequelae associated with heat toxicity. Various cooling methods are used to limit the duration of exposure to hyperthermia. Research shows the length of exposure and maximum temperature reached are two critical criteria in the survival and recovery of patients with heat stroke.

Complications of heat stroke affect every organ system and can lead to multiple organ system failure. Liver and kidney failure are common. Neurologic complications are usually rare with prompt cooling to achieve euthermia. Cerebellar effects are the residual pathologies most often seen.

The onset of DIC, coma lasting more than 8 hours, cardiac dysfunction, hypotension, and high lactate and CPK levels are ominous signs and are usually predictive of mortality. Prevention of heat illness with adequate hydration, recognition of environmental, exertional, and physiologic risk factors, and proper acclimatization are important educational tools for the flight nurse and potential patients.

HEAT-RELATED EMERGENCIES CASE STUDY

The helicopter flight crew was dispatched immediately to a rural hospital a distance of 60 miles from their base hospital. The dispatch information stated that a female patient in her middle 60s had collapsed and was unresponsive. The basic life-support unit reported seizure activity with no change in her level of consciousness after tonic-clonic motor activity. Because the facility has no CT scan or neurosurgical capabilities, the rural physician was requesting that she be transferred. The patient had not yet arrived at the rural hospital.

The past week had been hot, with temperatures hovering between 90° and 110° F and humidity registering 80% to 85%.

On arrival at the hospital, the patient's husband reported that they had arrived early that morning at an outlying lake for a fishing trip. He stated that their boat trailer became stuck on the ramp; as a result, he and the patient had to walk about 1¼ miles to get assistance to launch the boat. The patient tired and sat in the truck while the boat was launched.

After 2 hours of fishing, the patient complained of a headache and nausea, which lasted for an hour. Her husband then noted "really strange behavior—she was talking funny and didn't remember she was in the boat." By the time he reached the shore, the patient was unresponsive. She subsequently had a seizure when the ground ambulance arrived. Because of the location of the boat dock, the weight of the patient, and the ground response time, the patient had been unresponsive for an hour before arrival at the rural hospital.

Physical Findings

Obese female, weight 100 kg, age 64 years, supine on ED cart with red, flushed skin surfaces. No response noted to any stimuli.

Vital signs: BP 106/62; pulse 152/minute regular in rate and rhythm, sinus tachycardia; respirations 40/minute; temperature 105.5° F rectally.

HEENT: PERRLA, neck supple, mucous membranes dry, tongue leathery in appearance, upper airway patent.

Thorax: Symmetric expansion on inspiration, breath sounds clear and equal bilaterally, heart sounds normal S_1 and S_2, no murmur or rub noted, no trauma noted.

Abdomen: Obese, soft, no apparent guarding or tenderness, bowel sounds present but decreased, no organomegaly.

Extremities: No obvious trauma, no edema.

Neurologic: Glasgow Coma Score 4 (1-2-1), flaccid tone, no focal deficits noted, Babinski negative bilaterally.

Skin: Hot, dry, red in color, no rashes or other abnormalities noted.

Current interventions: Oxygen 8 L by plain face mask; in-dwelling Foley inserted; patient covered with damp bath blanket.

The patient's husband stated she has no medical allergies; she occasionally takes Lasix for "fluid build-up"; her only past medical history is mild heart failure.

Laboratory and X-Ray Data

CBC: WBC 22,100; RBC 4.2; Hgb/Hct 14.6/42; differential normal.

ABG: pH 7.54; Pco_2 26; Po_2 97; HCO_3 26; O_2 sat 94: B.E. + 2; Na 142; K 3.2; Cl 100; CO_2 17; BUN 32; glucose 62; creatinine 1.2; CPK 25,000; LDH 730; amylase 142.

Urinalysis: Color dark greenish-brown; specific gravity 1.042; pH 7; ketones 3+; protein 2+.

PT/PTT and platelets: Within normal limits.

Chest x-ray: Within normal limits with heart size upper side of normal.

ECG (12 lead): Sinus tachycardia without ectopy; nonspecific ST-T changes.

Flight Nurse Interventions

Before take-off, the patient was endotracheally intubated because of neurologic depression and to prevent aspiration; she was placed on a T-piece for supplemental oxygenation. Concurrently with cooling measures, an NG tube was placed for stomach decompression and ECG monitoring was instituted.

Immediate cooling measures consisted of stripping the patient and covering her with a wet sheet. Ice-packs placed in the axilla, neck, and inguinal areas were promptly replaced when they became warm.

Two large-bore lines were started for IV access because fluid replacement is best guided by central monitoring; central venous access may be desirable at this time, especially if the flight team has monitoring equipment available for in-flight use.

An in-dwelling Foley catheter was placed by the referral facility. UO over the last hour was 20 ml. Because of decreased UO and abnormal urine character as a result of muscle rhabdomyolysis, renal diuresis was indicated; mannitol (1 mg/kg) was given to maintain adequate urine flow.

Further initial treatment was based on a review of the laboratory values. Respiratory alkalosis with hypokalemia was present; hypokalemia should clear with cooling. If signs of hypercarbia became evident the patient would require ventilatory intervention. Hypoglycemia was corrected with the administration of dextrose (D50). CPK values over 20,000 alerted the flight nurse to the probability of the development of DIC and ARDS. Amylase was slightly elevated, perhaps indicative of pending liver failure.

In-Flight Assessment

Continuous assessment of this patient for further signs of multiple organ failure was mandatory. Reassessment of the efficacy of cooling measures, airway patency, and neurologic status was especially important in the care of this patient. If seizure activity reoccurred, prompt termination with diazepam would be indicated. Chlorpromazine, 10 to 50 mg, was prepared to be given as a prophylactic measure.

While in flight the patient was kept moist with water and evaporation that was enhanced by directing air vents onto the body and flying with the windows open (permitted by the rotorcraft's design). The wet sheet was removed once the patient was loaded because it was warm and prevented evaporation. Ice-packs were replaced as needed. When the patient's temperature reached 39° C (102° F), cooling measures were stopped.

Airway patency was ensured by frequent suctioning of the endotracheal tube and continuous assessment of respiratory status. If respiratory fatigue had become evident, ventilatory assistance would have been required. Oxygenation was assessed and titrated by pulse oximetry. Observation for increased pulmonary secretions, indicating pulmonary edema, was done in flight.

ECG monitoring was required; ACLS protocol was followed in the event of dysrhythmia occurrence. Nasogastric output was observed for the presence of blood because GI bleeding is a frequent complication. Urine character and output were monitored to assess renal function.

Close attention and continuous, ongoing assessment of the patient's condition for presenting signs of possible complications allowed the flight nurse to promptly initiate corrective and supportive care measures.

REFERENCES

1. Heat-related illnesses and deaths—United States, 1994-1995, *MMWR* 44(25):465, 1995.
2. Ayers SM, Keenan RL: The hyperthermic syndromes. In Ayers SM et al, editors: *Textbook of critical care,* Philadelphia, 1995, Saunders.
3. Baker PS et al: Hyperthermia, hypertension, hypertonia, and coma in massive thyriodazine overdose, *Am J Emerg Med* 4:346, 1988.
4. Drake DK, Nettina SM: Recognition and management of heat-related illness, *Nurse Pract* 19(8):43, 1994.
5. Greany D, Brown MM: Malignant hyperthermia: a concern for critical care patients, *Focus Crit Care* 15:49, 1988.
6. Harker J, Gibson P: Heat-stroke: a review of rapid cooling techniques, *Intensive Crit Care Nurs* 11(4):198, 1995.
7. Hart LH, Dennis SL: Two hypothermias prevalent in the intensive care unit: fever and heatstroke, *Focus Crit Care* 15(49):235-237, 1988.
8. Hubbard RW, Gaffin SL, Squire DL: Heat-related illnesses. In Auerbach P, editor: *Wilderness medicine,* St Louis, 1995, Mosby.
9. Karrimi FA et al: Adult respiratory distress syndrome and disseminated intravascular coagulation complicating heat stroke, *Chest* 9(4):571, 1986.
10. Lee-Chiong TL, Stitt JT: Heatstroke and other heat-related illnesses: the maladies of summer, *Postgrad Med* 98(1):26, 1995.
11. Lim MK: Occupational heat stress, *Ann Acad Med* (Singapore) 23(5):719, 1994.
12. O'Brien DJ: Heat illness, *J Aeromed Healthcare* 2:6, 1985.
13. Pouton TJ, Walker RA: Helicopter cooling of heat stroke victims, *Aviation, Space Environ Med* 58:358, 1987.
14. Proehl J: Environmental emergencies. In Kitt S et al, editors: *Emergency nursing,* Philadelphia, 1995, Saunders.
15. Semonin-Holleran R: *Prehospital nursing: a collaborative approach,* St Louis, 1994, Mosby.
16. Sidman RD, Gallagher EJ: Exertional heat stroke in a young woman: gender differences in response to thermal stress, *Acad Emerg Med* 2(4):315, 1995.
17. Syverud SA et al: Iced gastric lavage for treatment of heat stroke: efficacy in a canine model, *Ann Emerg Med* 14:424, 1985.
18. Tek D, Olshaker JS: Heat illness, *Emerg Med Clin North Am* 10(2):299, 1992.
19. Tomarken JL, Britt BA: Malignant hyperthermia, *Ann Emerg Med* 16:1253, 1987.
20. Yaqua BA et al: Heat stroke and the Mekkah pilgrimage: clinical characteristics and course of 30 patients, *Q J Med* 59:523, 1986.

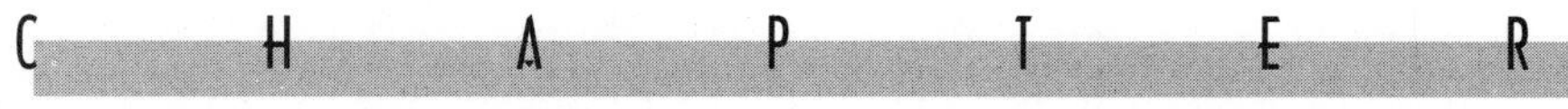

CHAPTER 29

Drowning and Near Drowning

COMPETENCIES

1. Perform a complete assessment of the patient who has experienced a near drowning.
2. Obtain a history related to the near-drowning incident.
3. Identify complications related to near drowning in the pulmonary, cardiovascular, renal, and neurologic systems.

Drowning, which is a leading cause of accidental death in the United States, claims between 5500 and 7000 lives each year.[3,7] More than half of the victims of drowning and near drowning (also known as *submersion emergencies*) are under the age of 30 years.[7]

Drowning is the second most common cause of accidental death in children, second only to motor vehicle accidents. More than 25% of those who drown are under the age of 5 years, and boys are three times more likely to drown than girls.[7]

A person can be submerged in numerous substances, such as water, grains, or chemicals; however, two thirds of all submersion emergencies occur in fresh water. Backyard pools, bathtubs, open bodies of water, and buckets of water are common sites of drowning or near drowning.[9] Many children who drown do so with an adult nearby.

RISK FACTORS

Multiple risk factors are involved in submersion emergencies, including age (generally toddlers or teenagers), location (home, swimming pools), gender (male), race (African-American children being at greater risk than children of other races), and ability to swim.[7] Two specific risk factors that should always be considered by the flight nurse are the presence of drugs, particularly alcohol, and the possibility of child maltreatment. Approximately 6% of drownings involve child maltreatment, and this possibility must be eliminated, especially when toddlers "accidentally" drown at home. Alcohol and other drugs are often associated with drownings as well.[7]

Finally, the flight nurse must consider the possibility of injuries or diseases associated with the near drowning. For example, a swimmer who has experienced drowning or near drowning may have a cervical spine injury. An elderly person found drowned may have had a cerebral vascular accident or cardiac dysrhythmia.

PATHOPHYSIOLOGY

A number of classic definitions of submersion incidents involving suffocation have evolved in the literature. Modell[6] proposed the clearest and most consistent definitions in 1981:

1. Drowning: death from suffocation after submersion in a fluid medium
2. Near drowning: survival at least 24 hours after suffocation by submersion in a fluid medium
3. Secondary drowning: death that occurs more than 24 hours after a submersion injury as a result of progressive pulmonary dysfunction despite successful initial resuscitation

Robinson and Seward,[11] on the other hand, believe that secondary drowning is simply a general category for pulmonary complications of near drowning and could more correctly be identified as pulmonary edema or adult respiratory distress syndrome.

Drowning typically begins with an attempt by the person involved to hold his or her breath. As carbon monoxide builds, hypoxia progresses, followed by a profound hunger for air. The person panics and struggles violently to emerge from the fluid medium and obtain air. Gasping inspiration causes either aspiration of fluid (seen in 85% of all victims) or intractable laryngospasm (seen in 15% of all victims).[7,11]

Dry Versus Wet Drowning

To appreciate the course of the pathophysiologic events that unfold in the person who experiences near drowning, a distinction should be made between persons who have no evidence of aspiration at autopsy ("dry" drowning victims) and those in whom aspiration has accompanied drowning ("wet" drowning victims). After the initial period when the person holds his or her breath, large quantities of fluids are swallowed, and the stomach distends until regurgitation occurs. Laryngospasm follows the first aspiration of fluid as the victim gasps. Unconsciousness ensues, and airway reflexes are abolished. Fluid then passively enters the airway, resulting in cardiorespiratory arrest. If aspiration occurs, the prognosis is complicated by the amount and type of material taken into the respiratory tract. Pulmonary edema will follow prolonged hypoxia, regardless of the matter aspirated; this results in persistent hypoxemia and metabolic acidosis that continue well after ventilation has been restored.

Salt Versus Fresh Water

Until recently, a great deal of emphasis was placed on the pathophysiology of drowning in salt water versus drowning in fresh water. These distinctions referred to blood volume shifts, electrolyte disturbances, and cardiac dysfunction. However, the most important problem experienced by persons who have nearly drowned is hypoxia; the other disturbances are of less significance in determining prognosis. Hypoxemia is the most life-threatening consequence of near drowning. The flight nurse should never waste time attempting to determine the extent of fluid or electrolyte derangements, because they are not the cause of death. The objective of therapy is to maintain oxygenation and preserve cerebral perfusion. Respiratory failure, which commonly follows submersion incidents, is a consequence of fluid-filled and poorly ventilated alveoli that continue to be perfused by pulmonary arterial blood. The pathophysiologic mechanisms triggering respiratory failure differ slightly in fresh water versus salt water immersion. Fresh water washes pulmonary surfactant from the alveoli. The decreased level of surfactant changes the surface tension actions of the alveoli, which leads to alveolar collapse. These atelectatic areas are not ventilated but continue to be bathed by pulmonary arterial blood, resulting in intrapulmonary shunting and hypoxemia.

Furthermore, the aspirate within the alveoli produces ventilation-perfusion abnormalities, which in turn further exacerbate intrapulmonic shunting. Salt water aspiration causes diffuse alveolar flooding, which leads to physiologic shunting. Whether because of physiologic shunting or surfactant inactivation and diffuse atelectasis, the end result is hypoxemia; however, either physiologic disturbance may be reversed with the use of positive-pressure breathing in the form of positive end expiratory pressure (PEEP) or continuous positive airway pressure.[4,7]

Clinical Manifestations

General

Clinical signs and symptoms in persons who experience near drowning are variable and depend on many factors, such as the amount and type of fluid aspirated and the time lag before resuscitation is initiated. The most frequent signs of near drowning are pulmonary and neurologic abnormalities. Other types of lung injury causing hypoxemia depend on the osmolarity and chemical characteristics of the fluid. The presence of chlorine in water will not affect the outcome of the person who experiences near drowning.[9]

Pulmonary

Hypoxia and the direct effect of aspirated water produce noncardiogenic pulmonary edema in approximately 5% of all near-drowning cases, which also includes persons who initially have few or no symptoms.[9] Pneumonia may result from aspiration of contaminated material. Both fresh and salt water cause injury to the lung by causing a movement of protein-rich fluid into the alveoli, by decreasing the level of available surfactant, or both. This leads to reflex airway resistance, which results in intrapulmonary shunting and hypoxia. Aspiration of as little as 2 ml/kg is sufficient to produce injury; however, significant changes in intravascular volume do not occur until more than 10 ml/kg is aspirated.[11] Vomiting, which frequently occurs during and after resuscitation, is usually caused by gastric distention that occurs when large quantities of fluid and air are swallowed during the submersion incident.

Cardiovascular

Profound cardiovascular dysfunction often follows near drowning. In the past, severe electrolyte abnormalities were blamed for ventricular fibrillation and asystole; however, in fact they rarely occur in the clinical setting. Cardiac dysrhythmias are usually caused by hypoxemia. Cardiogenic shock may result from hypoxic damage to the myocardium, with acidosis further impairing the function of myocardial tissue. Atrial fibrillation and premature ventricular contractions are the most frequently seen dysrhythmias, but they are usually abolished when hypoxemia and acidosis are corrected. Pump failure resulting from myocardial ischemia and acutely expanded blood volume is unusual. More frequently, pulmonary edema and restricted cardiac output result from the pulmonary injury caused by water aspiration.[7]

Neurologic

The neurologic status of a person who has nearly drowned can vary widely, ranging from slightly altered mental status to grand mal seizures and coma. The neurologic status of a person who has nearly drowned usually does not deteriorate after he or she has been admitted to a hospital unless there has been a preceding deterioration in pulmonary function. Patients who have a deteriorating mental status must therefore be scrupulously evaluated for trauma associated with the drowning incident. Approximately 80% of patients who arrive at the emergency facility with a score of 5 or less on the Glasgow Coma Scale generally have a poor prognosis.[6,11] Many patients with a score of 8 or greater on the Glasgow Coma Scale are likely to make a full recovery. When assessing and treating all drowning victims, a cervical spine injury should always be assumed until proven otherwise by a complete c-spine x-ray series encompassing all seven cervical vertebrae. In general, good prognosticators are spontaneous movements and respirations at the time of recovery and quick physiologic response to medical interventions.

Renal

Kidney failure is not common in persons who have experienced near drowning, but when it occurs it is generally the result of hypoxic insult. Kidney failure may be precipitated by hemoglobinuria or myoglobinuria. Free hemoglobin (the by-product of damaged red blood cells) or myoglobin (from damaged muscle tissue), hypoperfusion, acidosis, and hypoxia all have profound damaging effects on the kidneys.

Metabolic

Metabolic acidosis occurs rapidly and may have profound consequences. Hypernatremia has been reported as a result of drownings in salt water. Acidosis is common and may be either respiratory, metabolic, or both. The partial pressure of carbon dioxide (PCO_2) can rise precipitately during apnea or hypoventilation. After resuscitation the PCO_2 will often be normal to low, whereas the pH will remain low because the metabolic component is of longer duration.[7]

Temperature Derangements

Mild hypothermia has a protective effect; it decreases consumption of oxygen and glucose and results in an improved prognosis. The protective effect of hypothermia on the cerebrum is considered to be a factor that contributes to survival. Persons submerged in cold water for as long as 20 minutes may have a survival rate equal to that of persons submerged in warm water for 10 minutes. Hypothermia, defined as a core temperature of 27° to 35° C, usually follows immersion in cold water.[10] Loss of body heat in water is about 30 times greater than loss of body heat in air. A person may survive immersion in 60° F water for 6 hours, but exposure to water at a temperature of 40° F can precipitate asystole in 10 minutes. A core temperature of 28° C causes ventricular fibrillation or heart block, and thus death may occur from immersion hypothermia rather than from drowning *per se.* Children are very susceptible to hypothermia because they have less body fat and a high ratio of body surface in relation to water mass.

The Diving Reflex

Some human beings have a protective mechanism against submersion hypoxia that is referred to as the "diving reflex"; this resembles the diving reflex observed in seals and other mammals that breathe air.[2,4] This oxygen-conserving response, which is commonly seen in diving mammals, allows them to remain submerged for up to 30 minutes with no untoward effect. Immersion in cold water induces a reflex mechanism of apnea, bradycardia, and significant peripheral vasoconstriction with shunting of circulation to the heart, brain, and lungs, while tissues resistant to hypoxia (gut, skin, and muscle) temporarily receive a markedly reduced blood supply. A similar but less intensive reflex response has been seen in humans, and survival has been attributed to this response. The diving reflex is usually seen in young children and is rarely present in adolescents and adults. Hypothermia increases the viscosity of the blood, and thus the movement of blood in the coronary vessels and other vascular beds is decreased. Cardiac output is profoundly reduced as a result. Bradycardia follows, resulting in reduced cardiac output with no excessive rise in blood pressure in response to the hypoxia. The flight nurse performing cardiopulmonary resuscitation (CPR) should be aware of this reflex because the victim may exhibit profound bradycardia with nonpalpable pulses caused by vasoconstriction and, in fact, may appear to be dead. Pupils will dilate when the core temperature reaches 32° C. The patient may appear areflexic. For this reason, the patient should be warmed to at least 32° C before a decision is made whether to continue resuscitation efforts.

Outcome Scores

Two scoring systems have been developed that help evaluate the outcome of patients who have experienced a submersion incident: the Orlowski Score[10] (summarized in the first box) and the Submersion Outcome Score (summarized in the second box). Both of these scores offer guidelines for predicting the possible outcome of patients who have had a submersion incident.

History

The flight nurse may be unable to obtain a complete history at the scene because of patient acuity. Ideally, caregivers should attempt to obtain information that will affect management and prognosis, such as the following: (1) estimated time and length of submersion, (2) type and estimated temperature of water, (3) type of resuscitative measures used,

ORLOWSKI SCORE: PROGNOSTIC FACTORS IN PEDIATRIC CASES OF DROWNING AND NEAR DROWNING

1. Age < 3 years
2. Estimated maximum submersion < 5 minutes
3. No attempt at resuscitation for at least 10 minutes after rescue
4. Patient in a coma on admission to the emergency department
5. Arterial blood gas pH ≤ 7.10

One point is awarded for each unfavorable prognostic factor

A score of ≤ 2 = a 90% chance of recovery

A score of ≥ 3 = a 5% chance of recovery

From Orlowski J: Prognostic factors in pediatric cases of drowning and near-drowning, *J Am Coll Emerg Med* 8:176, 1979.

SUBMERSION OUTCOME SCORE

1. Arterial pH ≤ 7.10
2. PaO_2 ≤ 0.35
3. Anion gap ≥ 15

One point awarded for each variable present

A score of ≥ 2 predicts poor outcome, that is, death or permanent neurologic sequelae

From Anderson K, Roy T, Danzl D: Submersion incidents: a review of 39 cases and development of the submersion outcome score, *J Wilderness Med* 2:27, 1991.

PaO_2, Partial pressure of oxygen, arterial.

(4) how soon after rescue the victim gasped for air, and (5) previous history of medical conditions such as epilepsy, cardiac conditions, and diabetes, or consumption of alcohol or drugs.

PATIENT CARE

At the Scene

Performing immediate, appropriate emergency resuscitation measures can have significant bearing on the outcome of the patient. The major objectives of care are oxygenation, ventilation, perfusion, stabilization of associated injuries, and prevention of further trauma.

The standards for CPR as set forth by the American Heart Association are the standard of medical care for the patient. Mouth-to-mouth-resuscitation should begin in the water if at all possible and if this poses no danger to the rescuers. Otherwise, resuscitation measures should be initiated as soon as the victim reaches land. Intubation and ventilation with 100% oxygen via Ambu should be initiated as soon as possible, with cervical spine immobilization if c-spine injury is suspected.

In the Emergency Department

The first priority in treating a patient is to maintain an airway and breathing. The airway must be patent and secure, with equal breath sounds auscultated. A cervical spine injury must be assumed in all drowning cases until proven otherwise, and thus cervical immobilization devices should be used and well secured. In addition, the patient should be immobilized on a firm surface, such as a backboard. The backboard serves a dual purpose, because it both protects the vertebral column from further injury and provides a firm surface should it become necessary to perform CPR. Ventilation should be accomplished with use of 100% oxygen. A nasogastric tube should be inserted and any gastric contents evacuated. The tube should be left open to the atmosphere or connected to suction during flight. Circulation should be assessed and pulses should be checked for quality, rate, and rhythm. A heart monitor should be used, and the heart rate and rhythm should be monitored and recorded. Intravenous fluid boluses should be administered as indicated. PALS guidelines should be followed for pediatric resuscitation.

The peripheral pulses will be the best indicator of circulating blood volume. Vasopressors are indicated if the patient is unresponsive to fluid challenge. Advanced cardiac life support (ACLS) protocols should be used, and defibrillation or cardioversion should be performed if indicated. Resuscitation medications should be administered as indicated. Arterial blood gas results should be carefully monitored, with oxygenation and ventilation used as the chief means of combating acidosis. Once CPR is initiated, it must be continued until the patient is warmed to at least 94° F. If resuscitation attempts are unsuccessful after rewarming, the patient may be pronounced dead according to protocol. Otherwise, treatment is continued, the patient is constantly monitored, and trends are recorded. Treatment should be continued as follows:

Oxygenate and ventilate with 100% oxygen.

Give PEEP as needed, starting with 5 cm H_2O for children. PEEP and continuous positive airway pressure may reduce ventilation/perfusion mismatching in near-drowning patients by preventing premature airway closure and alveolar collapse and by increasing absorption of alveolar fluid. The usual indication for PEEP is inability to maintain an arterial oxygen pressure of greater than 60 torr. PEEP should be used when extensive interstitial or frank pulmonary edema occurs.

Insert a nasogastric/orogastric tube to decrease gastric distention and increase ventilation capacity.

Administer other cardiotonic drugs using ACLS guidelines. Mannitol, 0.5 to 1.0 gm/kg, or furosemide, 1 mg/kg, may be administered to decrease free water and treat cerebral edema as indicated by neurologic protocols.[8]

Dopamine, 5 to 20 μg/kg per minute administered by intravenous drip, may be used to treat continued hypotension that has not been corrected by fluid administration.

Assess the patient for any other injuries and provide appropriate treatment. Neurologic assessment should include use of the Glasgow Coma Scale.

Record the approximate temperature of the water.

Obtain a water sample if possible. Patients submerged in salt water or water in a swimming pool are less likely to aspirate water contaminated with bacteria, but those pulled from lakes, ponds, and stagnant water often are infected with such pathogens as *Pseudomonas* and coliform bacteria.

Before the Flight

The care that the patient receives at a hospital before the arrival of the flight team will vary according to that institution's capabilities and staffing. The flight crew should be considered a part of the team providing continuing care for the patient and should attempt to complement that care in every way possible. The flight nurse should provide thoughtful explanations about patient care that is provided so that the needs of the patient are met and the hospital's efforts are respected.

Before air medical transport from a hospital to another institution, the patient should be prepared for flight so that the likelihood of untoward events such as inadvertent extubation or unpredicted rapid deterioration is minimized. Many things can go wrong if a rapid but thorough assessment is not performed before lift-off. Airway/breathing with c-spine control remains a priority. The airway must be patent and secure. The flight nurse should auscultate breath sounds and note findings. If available, a chest x-ray film should be checked for proper endotracheal placement. The flight nurse should carefully note the placement markings on the endotracheal tube so that periodic visual inspections can be made to ensure that the tube has not slipped. If the patient is being ventilated, the flight nurse should note the current ventilation parameters. The initial and latest arterial blood gases should be noted. If acidosis is present, the flight nurse should note the treatment in progress, that is, whether the gases are moving back toward normal range. If the P_{CO_2} is elevated, he or she notes whether ventilation was increased and by how much. If hypoxemia is present, the flight nurse should record the fraction of inspired oxygen that is present and indicate whether PEEP has been used. A nasogastric tube for gastric decompression should be inserted if this has not already been done. Patients believed to have hypoxic cerebral injury should be hyperventilated, and their P_{CO_2} should be maintained between 25 and 30 torr. Peripheral and cerebral pulses should be assessed for rate and quality, and the patient should be connected to a heart monitor. Dysrhythmias should be treated according to ACLS protocols. Before transport, at least one large-bore intravenous line should be inserted. Vital sign trends should be noted and recorded at least every 15 minutes. If a fluid challenge was given, the flight nurse should note the amount and results. If vasopressors are needed, he or she should note what was administered and the result. The initial neurologic examination should note spontaneous movements and spontaneous respirations. A baseline neurologic assessment including the Glasgow Coma Scale should be performed, and the flight nurse should record whether the pupils are fixed, dilated, midposition, reactive, or nonreactive and note any change.

The flight nurse should examine the c-spine x-ray film for clear visualization of all seven cervical vertebrae and maintain cervical spine immobilization if there is any doubt regarding the condition of the cervical spine. If any active rewarming was performed, the flight nurse should note the type of rewarming that was used, when it was started, and the results. Rewarming efforts should be continued or other measures instituted as appropriate. If no rewarming was done, the flight nurse should institute rewarming procedures. Rewarming should proceed no faster than 1° C per hour, and the patient should be strictly monitored to avoid dysrhythmias and hypotension caused by peripheral vasodilation. Hyperthermic patients should continue to be cooled with use of appropriate measures described earlier. If the patient is hyperkalemic, the flight nurse should correct the acidosis and discontinue K+ in intravenous lines as directed. If the patient was given mannitol or furosemide, the flight nurse should note amounts given and results. He or she should also note any change in neurologic status, record urinary output, and record vasopressors given and the result.

In-Flight Treatment

The flight nurse should perform the following procedures during the flight:

1. Maintain a patent and secure airway.
2. Administer 100% oxygen, warmed and humidified if possible. Hyperventilation should be performed if indicated, using PEEP cautiously, starting at 5 cm H_2O pressure for all ages.
3. Monitor cardiac status during flight.
4. Maintain intravenous line patency.
5. Treat hypotension if symptomatic (poor perfusion, reduced urinary output). If indicated, the flight nurse should give a fluid challenge of lactated Ringer's solution or normal saline solution. If there is no response to fluid challenge, the flight nurse should consider use of vasopressors, remembering that vasopressors do not work well in an acid environment. Fluid challenge should be given before vasopressors are administered.
6. Monitor and record vital signs at least every 15 minutes.
7. Keep ACLS resuscitation medications readily available to treat cardiac dysrhythmias.
8. Continue efforts at restoring normal body temperature.
9. Maintain serial neurologic and pupil checks with vital signs. If the patient deteriorates in flight, the flight nurse should consider administration of mannitol, 1 g/kg per protocol, and hyperventilate at 24 to 28 per minute. Response should be noted and recorded.
10. Treat agitation and combativeness in the intubated patient after double-checking for patency and security of the endotracheal tube. The flight nurse should administer medication for sedation or consider neuromuscular blockade with sedation.

Postflight Follow-Up

After reaching their destination, the designated flight crew member should give a complete, concise report to the receiving medical/nursing team. The flight crew should remain at the receiving facility for an appropriate period of time and assist the receiving medical team as appropriate. Finally, the flight crew should give family members a brief report regarding the patient's status in flight and the current plan for continued treatment as appropriate.

NEAR DROWNING CASE STUDY

At approximately 11:00 AM, on January 13, 1995, a pick-up truck estimated to be traveling at 45 mph was witnessed swerving back and forth down a straight road. The truck, which carried only the driver, traveled off the road and down a slight incline and came to rest in a lake. The truck sank quickly. The witness to the accident stopped immediately, and the passenger in the car jumped in the lake to recover the driver. Passengers in other cars stopped to assist. One passerby used his car phone to call 911 for assistance. Approximately 4 to 5 minutes from the time of the accident, a man who was approximately 18 to 20 years old was pulled from the lake by the rescuer. Mouth-to-mouth resuscitation was immediately initiated because of the absence of spontaneous respirations. A radial pulse was thought to be palpated.

Because of the nature of the 911 call, a flight team was placed on standby by the rescue squad. The rescue squad arrived within 6 minutes of the initial 911 call. A quick assessment was performed and the flight team was activated.

When the rescue squad arrived, ventilations were taken over with a bag-valve mask using 100% oxygen. Peripheral access was obtained with use of a 16-gauge Angiocath. At this point the patient was noted to be having occasional spontaneous respirations. The Glasgow Coma Scale score was E = 1 + 1 + 3 = 5. At the time of venous access, a Philadelphia collar was applied for cervical spine immobilization. The patient was then carefully logrolled onto a backboard.

The flight team arrived 6 minutes later and rapidly assessed the victim. Because of the unsecured airway, intubation was accomplished with a No. 8.0 endotracheal tube at 23 cm lip line with use of inline traction. Breath sounds were auscultated bilaterally to confirm placement. The victim was hyperventilated en route to the helicopter.

There was an 8-minute estimated time of arrival to the hospital. Vital signs in flight were as follows: blood pressure, 90/60; pulse, 128; respirations, 22 (assisted). Two minutes into the flight, spontaneous respirations increased and the patient had spontaneous eye opening. Pupils were 4 mm, midpoint, and reactive bilaterally. A normal saline solution bolus of 500 ml was initiated with warm fluids.

On arrival at the emergency department, the Glasgow Coma Scale was E = 2 V = 1 M = 5 = 8. The patient was breathing spontaneously and moving purposefully. His core temperature was 93° F on arrival. Active rewarming was instituted. Repeat vital signs were as follows: blood pressure, 110/60; pulse, 104; respirations, 18 (spontaneous).

When the patient's family arrived, a more detailed past medical history was obtained, which included epilepsy. The family disclosed that the patient had not been compliant with anticonvulsant medications for the past month.

Further work up in the emergency department included complete spine films, which were negative. Peritoneal lavage was negative. The patient was admitted to the hospital for a total of 4 days. He was sent home with specific instructions, which included compliance with taking anticonvulsant medication.

REFERENCES

1. Anderson K, Roy T, Danzl D: Submersion incidents: a review of 39 cases and development of the submersion outcome score, *J Wilderness Med* 2:27, 1991.
2. Astrup J: Energy-requiring cell functions in the ischemic brain: their critical supply and possible inhibition in protective therapy, *J Neurosurg* 56:482, 1982.
3. Bolte RG et al: The use of extracorporeal rewarming in a child submerged for 66 minutes, *JAMA* 260:377, 1988.
4. Gonzalez BA: Drowning and the diving reflex in man, *Med J Aust* 2:583, 1972.
6. Modell JH: Drowning versus near drowning: a discussion of definitions, *Crit Care Med* 4:351, 1981.
7. Newman A: Submersion incidents. In Auerbach P, editor: *Wilderness medicine,* St Louis, 1995, Mosby.
8. Nussbaum E, Galent SP: Intracranial pressure monitoring as a guide to prognosis in the nearly drowned, severely comatose child, *J Pediatr* 102:215, 1983.
9. Olshaker J: Near drowning, *Emerg Med Clin North Am* 10: 339, 1992.
10. Orlowski J: Prognostic factors in pediatric cases of drowning and near drowning, *J Am Coll Emerg Med* 8:176, 1979.
11. Robinson MD, Seward P: Submersion injury in children, *Pediat Emerg Care* 3:1, 1987.

CHAPTER 30

Diving Emergencies

COMPETENCIES

1. Perform a comprehensive assessment of the patient, including the collection of subjective and objective data on the patient who has sustained a diving emergency.
2. Anticipate and plan for the effects of air medical transport on the patient with decompression illness.

Scuba (from "self-contained underwater breathing apparatus") diving is an increasingly popular pastime. It is estimated that there are now more than 4 million recreational scuba divers in the United States, with about 400,000 joining their ranks every year.[12] Diving activities are no longer restricted to coastal resorts, but can be found in just about any body of water large enough to hold a diver and equipment, such as lakes, streams, quarries, and swimming pools. Not surprisingly, this increase in popularity has brought about a concomitant increase in scuba diving injuries.[18] In 1994, more than 1100 serious diving medical emergencies were reported to the National Divers Alert Network (DAN).[8]

Manifestations of diving injuries may not be noticed by the diver for 24 to 48 hours after a dive and may, in fact, be seriously potentiated by air travel. Thus patients may present with diving-related problems many hours and many thousands of miles from the original dive site.

Air medical personnel encounter many types of scuba-related diving injuries such as marine envenomation, near-drowning, decompression illness, arterial gas embolism (AGE), middle-ear squeeze, and other forms of barotrauma. Of these diving injuries, decompression illness and AGE are medical emergencies requiring immediate recompression treatment. Air medical transport of the patient to a hyperbaric chamber is often necessary to avoid the significant morbidity and mortality resulting from delays in treatment of these disorders. Air medical personnel must therefore be able to diagnose and manage these diving emergencies in a timely manner.

This chapter provides a brief discussion of diving principles and the pathophysiology, clinical manifestations, and management of diving emergencies likely to be encountered by air medical flight crews.

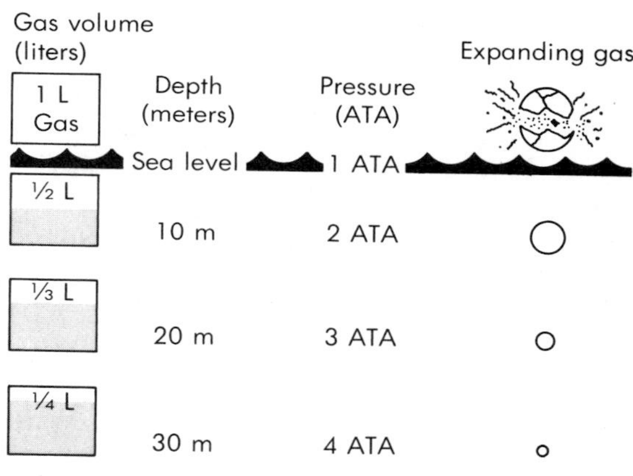

Fig. 30-1. Boyle's Law.

DIVING PRINCIPLES

To gain a thorough understanding of the pathophysiology underlying decompression illness and air embolism, it is necessary to include a brief discussion of a few physical properties inherent to scuba diving.

At sea level, a 1-sq-inch column of air extending upward from the earth's surface to the edge of the atmosphere would weigh 14.7 lb. Thus the pressure exerted by this column of air at sea level is 14.7 lb per sq inch (psi) or 760 mm Hg, which is defined as 1 atmosphere of pressure (ATM). As altitude increases, the column of air becomes shorter and the air pressure decreases. For example, at an altitude of 18,000 feet, the atmospheric pressure is half that at sea level: 380 mm Hg, or 0.5 ATM. On the other hand, water is much denser than air, and a similar 1-sq-in column in seawater would only have to be 33 feet (10 m) to exert the same amount of pressure as a 1-sq-inch column of air. Because the density of water is uniform throughout, the proportional relationship of pressure and depth remains constant: pressure increases 1 ATM for every 33-foot (10-m) column of seawater (Fig. 30-1). For the scuba diver, the combined weights of the air and water columns must be taken into consideration. At a given depth underwater, the total pressure will be the sum of the barometric pressure exerted by the column of air above plus the hydrostatic pressure exerted by the column of water. This is the concept of absolute pressure or atmospheres absolute (ATA). Therefore a scuba diver at a depth of 33 feet will experience an ambient pressure of 2 ATM absolute pressure, or 2 ATA. Similarly, a scuba diver at 66 feet will experience an ambient pressure of 3 ATA.

As the diver descends from the water's surface the effects of increasing ambient pressure on the scuba diver involve an understanding of the behavior of gases under conditions of varying pressure and volume. The following is a brief discussion of the primary gas laws of diving.

Boyle's Law

The first gas law is Boyle's Law, which states that at a constant temperature and mass the volume of a gas is inversely proportional to the total pressure. Simply stated, volume decreases as pressure increases; conversely, the volume increases as pressure decreases. Fig. 30-1 depicts the increase of gas volume as the pressure and depth decrease.

Henry's Law

The second gas principle is Henry's Law, which states that solubility is proportional to the partial pressure of a gas. As the pressure increases or decreases, the gas goes into or comes out of solution accordingly. This is the "soda bottle" phenomenon. When you release the pressure from the bottle by removing the cap, the dissolved gas comes out of solution (Fig. 30-2).

Dalton's Law

The last gas principle is Dalton's Law of partial pressures, which states that the total pressure of a mixture of gases equals the sum of partial pressures exerted by the constituent gases. The partial pressure is the pressure exerted by a single gas in a mixture as if it were the only gas in the mixture. Air comprises approximately 78% nitrogen, 21% oxygen, and 1% other gases. As illustrated in Fig. 30-3, by increasing the total pressure of the mixture, the pressure of each constituent gas is increased proportionately. At a depth of 99 feet (30 m), a scuba diver is under an ambient pressure of 4 ATA and is breathing compressed air with partial pressures of nitrogen and oxygen four times their value at the surface.

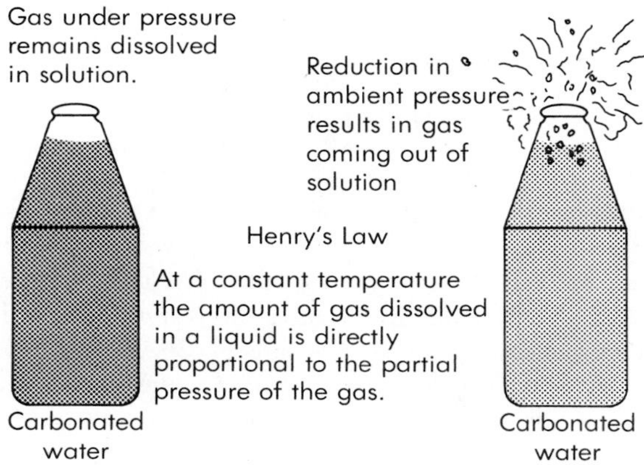

Fig. 30-2. Henry's Law.

PATHOPHYSIOLOGY

Nitrogen is a relatively inert gas that is driven into solution as the diver descends according to Henry's Law. The saturation of tissues with nitrogen depends on intrinsic properties, including tissue perfusion and solubility coefficients of the various tissues.[21] The quantity of dissolved nitrogen in the tissues increases with the duration and depth of the dive. If ascent of the scuba diver is too fast or the tissues are oversaturated with gas, the nitrogen is separated from solution rather than being safely transported to the lungs for elimination. Tissue desaturation of nitrogen results in the formation of inert gas bubbles in venous blood and tissues on reduction in ambient pressure.[6]

Decompression Illness

The lesion resulting from decompression illness has been a subject of debate for many years, although

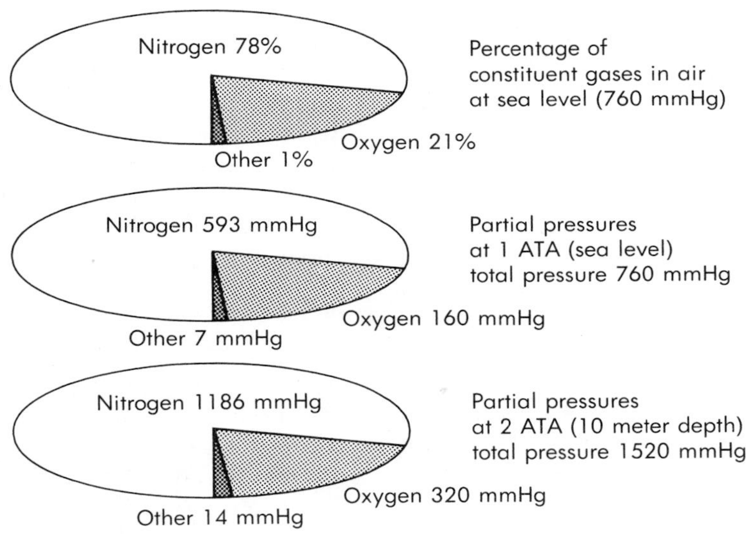

Fig. 30-3. Dalton's Law.

it is generally accepted that tissue ischemia is the final common pathway.[12] Hallenbeck demonstrated venous congestion by gas bubbles in the epidural venous plexus system of the spinal cord, most frequently in the lumbosacral region. The location of the intravascular lesion was consistent with the corresponding neurologic symptoms.[10] The formation of bubbles in tissues and venous blood has multiple mechanical and physiologic consequences. Mechanical effects of bubble formation include intravascular or intralymphatic obstruction, cellular distention and rupture, and stretching of ligaments and tendons. These effects result in ischemia or infarction, edema formation, cell death, and pain. The physiologic consequences include activation of the intrinsic clotting pathway, kinins, and the complement system, all resulting in platelet aggregation, increased vascular permeability and microvascular sludging. The end results of all of these events are decreased tissue perfusion and ischemia.[12]

Arterial Gas Embolization

By far the most serious manifestation of pressure related injuries or barotrauma is the arterial gas embolism (AGE). AGE is a leading cause of death among scuba divers.[4]

In accordance with Boyle's Law, gases in the lungs of a scuba diver expand as ambient pressure decreases during ascent. The greatest changes in pressure and volume occur at shallower depths. Pulmonary overpressurization syndrome and alveolar rupture can occur during an ascent from a depth as shallow as 4 feet if compressed air is held in the lungs.[1] Breath-holding during an ascent, as with a panicked diver, or air-trapping in a diseased lung results in lung overexpansion and rupture of alveoli. Air bubbles from the ruptured alveoli are free to enter the pulmonary venous return to the left side of the heart for subsequent dissemination through the systemic circulation. Air bubbles can track in the lung parenchyma and tissue planes. The result may be interstitial and mediastinal emphysema or pneumothorax.[1]

Gas bubbles may enter the coronary arteries and produce myocardial ischemia or infarction. However, bubbles most often enter the carotid circulation, producing multiple areas of circulatory occlusion in the brain with resulting ischemia and infarction.

Because multiple cerebrovascular watersheds may be affected, a confusing clinical picture with multiple neurologic deficits may result.

CLINICAL MANIFESTATIONS

Diagnosis of a diving injury is usually made on the basis of the patient's history and clinical presentation.[16] Unfortunately, many of the signs and symptoms of decompression sickness (DCS) and AGE are nonspecific and may mimic other disease processes such as low back pain, arthritis, tendinitis, bronchospasm, stroke, and myocardial infarction. Because of the high morbidity and mortality that can result when treatment of DCS and AGE is delayed, diving accidents and injuries must be treated aggressively. The most common management error of these diving emergencies is failure to treat borderline cases.[16]

Decompression Sickness

The signs and symptoms of DCS depend on the size and location of the ischemic insult. The most common presentation of decompression sickness may comprise headache, fatigue, limb or joint pain, skin rash and pruritus, and localized swelling. This collection of localized symptomatology is referred to as "pain-only" or type I DCS. The joints commonly affected in type I DCS are the shoulders, elbows, hips, knees, and ankles. The box shows a classification scheme based on the systems or tissues involved.[15]

Type II DCS comprises the more serious manifestations. Symptoms may involve any, or combinations of, the following symptoms: sensory and visual disturbances; dyspnea and nonproductive cough; paresthesia; paresis; fatigue and weakness; headache and nausea; chest, abdominal, or back pain; bowel and bladder dysfunction; shock; and loss of consciousness.

Pulmonary Decompression Illness

Otherwise known as the "chokes" or type IV DCS, pulmonary decompression illness is the result of large volumes of emboli occluding end arteries in the pulmonary circulation. If the lesion is large enough, pulmonary artery pressure increases, result-

CLASSIFICATION OF DECOMPRESSION SICKNESS

Type I

Local effects only: limb bends (joint or limb pain), skin bends (skin rash or itch), lymphatic obstruction effects

Type II

Cerebral manifestations: fatigue, malaise, visual disturbances, headache, impaired coordination, motor and sensory disturbances ranging from minor neurologic impairment to major deficits (e.g., paraplegia, quadriplegia, hemiplegia, altered states of consciousness ranging from drowsiness to coma, convulsions, and death)

Type III

Spinal manifestations: any degree of any motor and sensory modality impairment, but commonly weakness and numbness of lower limbs and bladder and sphincter impairment

Type IV

Pulmonary chokes: pulmonary dyspnea, pain, cough, altered gas exchange

Type V

Staggers: mild to severe impairment of balance and coordination, often debilitating

Type VI

Dysbaric osteonecrosis: lytic bone lesions resulting from long-term exposure to diving

From Otton J: *Aust Fam Phys* 18(6):674-685, 1989.

ing in symptoms of dyspnea, chest pain, and nonproductive cough.[13] Pulmonary DCS is a rare but life-threatening manifestation of DCS that progresses rapidly to shock unless immediate hyperbaric treatment is administered.[6]

Arterial Gas Embolism

Manifestations of AGE usually begin during or within minutes of ascent. As described earlier, AGE is a result of pulmonary overpressurization. Therefore symptoms occur at or shortly after the time of the insult. The manifestations of AGE are consistent with strokelike phenomena, and almost any sign of cerebral damage may be observed, ranging from mild dizziness, motor and sensory deficits to severe impairment, coma, and death.[16] In a series of 42 cases analyzed by Kizer[11], the most common symptom was asymmetric multiplegia or paralysis involving the lower extremities. Other signs of AGE include altered mental status and personality changes, syncope, vertigo, dizziness, cardiac dysrhythmia or cardiac arrest, chest pain, apnea, cough, hemoptysis, and epistaxis.[4,11,17] Air medical personnel should always suspect AGE whenever a scuba diver presents with an altered level of consciousness, respiratory distress, or signs of cerebral decompression illness.

MANAGEMENT

Air embolism and decompression illness are medical emergencies and are managed similarly.[11] Recompression in a hyperbaric chamber is the only effective treatment for these diving emergencies. The DAN, located at Duke University in Durham, North Carolina, can be reached by telephone at (919) 684-8111. DAN provides assistance in diagnosis and treatment, as well as in locating the nearest treatment facility. DAN may assist in making ground and air transport arrangements.[3]

The immediate treatment for a patient who is experiencing a diving emergency takes the following sequence:

1. Establish basic life support measures.
2. Place the patient in a supine position. The head-down (Trendelenburg) position and the head-down left lateral decubitus position (Durante position) have been recommended to minimize further passage of air emboli to the brain. The head-down position is no longer recommended for two reasons. First, a patient placed in a head-down position will sustain an increase in intracranial pressure, which may exacerbate cerebral edema and ischemia. Second, the passage of air emboli throughout the circu-

latory system is probably more dependent on flow dynamics than on gravity.

3. Administer 100% oxygen at high flow rates (10 to 15 L/min) through a face mask to create a gradient for increased elimination of excess nitrogen.
4. Administer fluid with 5% dextrose in normal saline solution or lactated Ringer's solution to correct underlying fluid deficits and maintain an adequate intravascular.
5. Protect the patient against hypothermia or hyperthermia.
6. Monitor pulmonary, cardiovascular, and neurologic status. Treat developing complications (e.g., pneumothorax, shock, seizures).
7. Avoid rough or excessive handling.
8. Give analgesics as needed.
9. The use of corticosteroids for cerebral edema and endothelial stabilization remains controversial. The recommendation is a combination of dexamethasone and a rapid-acting steroid such as methylprednisolone or hydrocortisone.
10. Transport patient to the nearest hyperbaric treatment facility.
11. Provide the hyperbaric medical personnel with a detailed history of the dive (e.g., depth and duration of dive), timing and onset of symptoms or complications, and treatment rendered. This information will aid the hyperbaric medical personnel in determining proper management such as time and pressure profiles.
12. Always consider the possibility of DCS or AGE in the patient's diving partners as well.

AIR MEDICAL TRANSPORT

Air medical transport of the patient to a hyperbaric chamber is often necessary to avoid significant morbidity and mortality resulting from delays in treatment. However, transportation by air ambulance or even ground ambulance over elevated terrain may exacerbate the patient's condition.[2] Patients should be transported in aircraft with cabins pressurized to 1 ATA—such as the Lear jet, Hercules C-130, Cessna Citation, or many commercial aircraft—but this may require flight at a lower altitude, at considerable fuel expense. If the aircraft cannot be pressurized to 1 ATA (e.g., a helicopter), it should be flown at the lowest and safest altitude possible, preferably below 1,000 feet above sea level.[2] In some locations, a portable recompression chamber can be used to transport the patient from the field to the hyperbaric treatment center in a nonpressurized aircraft. The portable unit (with the patient inside) is mated to the larger static hyperbaric chamber while the patient is maintained under pressure.[15]

SUMMARY

The number of scuba-related injuries grows with the increasing number of scuba divers. Of these injuries, DCS and AGE are true medical emergencies that require immediate treatment in the nearest hyperbaric chamber. Delays in the treatment of these diving injuries may result in significant morbidity and mortality. Air medical flight crews may be called on to rapidly assess, manage, and transport patients with these life-threatening injuries. Knowledge of diving principles, pathophysiology, and manifestations of AGE and DCS will aid air medical personnel in developing proper management strategies.

DIVING EMERGENCIES CASE STUDY

An air ambulance was dispatched to the scene, where a 19-year-old woman was reported to be unconscious. On arrival the patient was found in a left lateral Trendelenburg position. Bystanders reported that the patient was an inexperienced diver with a history of asthma. She had been scuba diving in a 12-foot swimming pool.

The patient was lethargic and incoherent. Her airway was patent with an intact gag reflex. Her color was pale with no cyanosis. She was dyspneic, with a respiratory rate of 40 breaths/min, heart rate of 120 beats/min, and blood pressure of 150/90 mm Hg. She also had symptoms of a left cerebral infarction including impaired speech, right-sided paresthesia, and decreased motor strength in the right arm. Breath sounds were diminished over the right apex, with occasional expiratory wheezes.

Immediate management included 100% oxygen by mask, IV lactated Ringer's solution at 125 mL/hr, and continuous cardiac, neurologic, and pulmonary monitoring. The patient was placed in a supine position. Cerebral AGE was the most likely diagnosis, but flight personnel observed the patient for a possible closed-head injury as well. The patient was 10 minutes from the nearest recompression chamber, and the decision was made to immediately transport her by helicopter at a low altitude. Initial diagnosis by flight personnel was based solely on history and clinical findings.

On the patient's arrival at the emergency department, assessment remained unchanged. The patient had a blood pressure of 140/86 mm Hg, heart rate of 116 beats/min, and respiratory rate of 42 breaths/min, with an intact airway. Neurologic examination findings were unchanged. Cervical spine radiographs and computed tomography of the head were negative. The emergency physician confirmed a cerebral AGE. Endotracheal intubation was deferred because the airway was adequate, and the patient was taken immediately to the hyperbaric chamber.

Initial recompression therapy was performed to a depth of 6 ATA. The patient became increasingly coherent, with return of feeling to her right side. Vital signs remained stable during recompression therapy, and a patent airway was maintained. The patient required two additional recompression treatments to a depth of 3 ATA and made a full recovery.

Recreational divers are found in every part of the country. In particular, knowledge of AGE embolism and decompression illness, the two most dangerous diving emergencies, is essential. Before embarking on any flight involving a diving emergency, flight personnel must know the location of the recompression chamber nearest the patient, along with transportation alternatives. This information can be obtained 24 hours a day by calling DAN at (919) 684-8111.

REFERENCES

1. Arthur DC, Margulies RA: A short course in diving medicine, *Ann Emerg Med* 16:689-701, 1987.
2. Bennett PB et al: Flying after diving: 1987 accidents, *Alert Diver* 5(1):1, 1989.
3. Bennett PB et al: DAN position statement: injury risk in sport diving, *Sources* 1(2), 1989.
4. Boettger ML: Scuba diving emergencies: pulmonary overpressure accidents and decompression sickness, *Ann Emerg Med* 12:563-567, 1983.
5. Bove AA, Davis JC: *Diving medicine,* ed 2, Philadelphia, 1995, Saunders.
6. Davis JC: Decompression sickness in sport scuba diving, *Phys Sportsmed* 16(2):108-122, 1988.
7. Dick AP, Massey EW: Neurologic presentation of decompression sickness and air embolism in sport divers, *Neurology* 35:667-671, 1985.
8. Dovenbarger J: Report on diving accidents and fatalities, DAN: the annual review of recreational scuba diving injuries and deaths, 1996 ed, 1996.
9. Francis TJ, Dutka AJ, Flynn ET: Experimental determination of latency, severity, and outcome in CNS decompression sickness, *Undersea Biomed Res* 15(6):419-427, 1989.
10. Hallenbeck JM, Bove AA, Elliott DH: Mechanisms underlying spinal cord damage in decompression sickness, *Neurology* 25:308-316, 1975.
11. Kizer KW: Disorders of the deep, *Emerg Med* 18-58, 1984.
12. Kizer KW: Scuba diving and dysbarism. In Auerback P, editor: *Wilderness medicine,* ed 3, St Louis, 1995, Mosby.
13. Leveritt SO, Bitter HL, McIver L: *Studies in decompression sickness: circulatory and respiratory changes associated with decompression sickness in anesthetized dogs,* TDR 63-67, Brooks AFB, 1963, TX USAF School of Aerospace Medicine.
14. Mebane GY, Dick AP: *Underwater diving accident manual,* ed 2, Durham, NC, 1982, National Divers Alert Network.
15. Orton J: Medical problems of recreational diving, *Aust Fam Phys* 18:674-685, 1989.
16. Repogle WH et al: Scuba diving injuries, *Am Fam Pract* 37:135-142, 1988.
17. Spencer MP: Decompression limits for compressed air determined by ultrasonically detected blood bubbles, *J Appl Physiol* 40:229-235, 1976.
18. Strauss RH: Diving medicine, *Am Rev Respir Dis* 119: 1001-1023, 1979.
19. Ward CA, McCullough D, Fraser WD: Relation between complement activation and susceptibility to decompression sickness, *J Appl Physiol* 62:1160-1166, 1987.
20. Warren JP Jr et al: Neuroimaging of scuba diving injuries to the CNS, *AJR Am J Roentgenol* 151:1003-1008, 1988.
21. Workman RD: Calculation of decompression schedules for nitrogen-oxygen and helium-oxygen dives, Washington, DC, 1965, US Navy Experimental Diving Unit, Washington Navy Yard.

CHAPTER 31

Toxicology

COMPETENCIES

1. Identify three common sources of poison.
2. Provide care for the initial management of the poisoned patient.
3. Name three antidotes for specific poisons.
4. Identify a nonvenomous snake.
5. Provide care for specific poisonings such as carbon monoxide, envenomation, and cocaine overdose.

In 1994, 1,926,438 human poison exposures were reported to the American Association of Poison Control Centers (AAPCC). The AAPCC compiles the Toxic Exposure Surveillance System (TESS), the largest database of information about toxic exposures in the United States. More than 90% of these exposures occurred in the victim's home. Others occurred in locations such as the workplace (2.9%), health care facilities (0.4%), schools (1.2%), and public areas (1.3%).[23]

The human environment contains natural and manufactured toxins including plants, animals, chemicals, drugs, and chemotherapeutic agents. Even though there are multiple substances and various sources of toxins and poisons, only a limited number of antidotes are available. Table 31-1 lists most of the available antidotes that may be useful in the management of the poisoned patient.

The most important concept in the care of the patient who has been poisoned is supportive care. In addition to maintenance of the patient's airway, breathing, and circulation, the poisoned patient must be discovered quickly to prevent further harm to the patient and those providing care to the patient.

TABLE 31-1

Antidotes for selected poisonings

Toxin	Antidote
Opiates	Naloxone
Carbon monoxide	Oxygen
Cyanide	Amyl nitrate Sodium nitrate Sodium thiosulfate
Anticholinesterase Organophosphates Carbamates	Atropine
Methemoglobinemic agents Nitrates Chlorates Nitrobenzene	Methylene blue
Ethylene glycol	Ethanol
Acetaminophen	*N*-Acetylcysteine
Heavy metals	BAL Disodium edetate Penicillamine
Iron	Deferoxamine
Anticholinergics Diphenhydramine Benzotropine	Physostigmine
Anticoagulants Coumadin Heparin	 Vitamin K
Cardiac medications β-Adrenergic blockers	Protamine
Calcium-channel blockers	Glucagon
Digoxin	Calcium
Tricyclic antidepressants	Digoxin Fab antibodies Sodium bicarbonate

From Wright RO et al: Poison antidotes: guidelines for rational use in the emergency department, *Emerg Med Rep* 16(21):201-211, 1995.

The general purpose of this chapter is to discuss the general management of the poisoned patient, identify the pathophysiology of selected drugs, and describe the flight nursing care involved in the management of the poisoned patient.

GENERAL CONSIDERATIONS

Intentional and Unintentional Poisoning

Ingestion of or exposure to a toxic substance is intentional or unintentional. It is important to determine why the patient has become poisoned because it could make a difference in the care of the patient. In 1994 the AAPCC reported that 86.4% of the human exposures reported were unintentional, 11.1% intentional. Sources of unintentional exposure included therapeutic error (taking too much of a medication), bites and stings, environmental exposures, and food poisoning. Intentional poison exposures resulted from suicide attempts, abuse, and intentional misuse of medications.[23]

The word *poisoning* denotes a toxic exposure that can be intentional, unintentional, or unknown to the patient. A patient or family member may have misread a label, taken too much of a drug, and accidentally become poisoned. A child may climb up and get into a medicine cabinet, ingest a bottle of aspirin, and be unintentionally poisoned. Poisonous substances are not often used by criminals as a method of injuring or killing.[11,13]

An intentional overmedication or ingestion of a toxic substance is considered an *overdose.*[14] Poisoning generally occurs in the pediatric population. Patients who have overdosed or intentionally poisoned themselves are usually 12 years or older, although some cases suggest that children 5 years and older should be evaluated for intentional ingestion.[13]

It is important to make the distinction between accidental and intentional toxic exposure. If the patient is suicidal, the flight nurse should take additional precautions to ensure a safe environment for the flight crew and the patient during transport.

GENERAL MANAGEMENT OF THE POISONED PATIENT

The initial management of any poisoned patient includes securing of the airway, ventilation, and maintenance of adequate circulation. Further evaluation consists of obtaining a detailed history about the event that led to the poisoning, a thorough physical examination, administration of antidotes as indicated, and transport to an appropriate health care facility for definitive care. The patient's family should be a part of the initial care because they may be able to offer important information about the incident. The emotional support of the patient, particularly a patient who has attempted suicide, should be included in the planning of care.

Initial Management

As with any other critically ill or injured patient, the ABCs (airway-breathing-circulation) take initial precedence. One exception in the case of the poisoned patient is the need to remove the victim from a toxic environment or toxic source before the ABCs can be attended to. If the patient has been sprayed with a toxic substance, or the snake that caused envenomation is still in the immediate vicinity, the environment must be controlled and made safe before patient management so that the air medical crew will not be injured or poisoned.

Many toxins and poisons alter mental status and therefore may compromise the airway. A protected airway is particularly important if the toxin is going to be removed by gastric lavage. Mouth-to-mouth resuscitation should always be avoided because of the possibility of contamination of the rescuer with the toxic substance. Endotracheal or nasotracheal intubation is the preferred method of protecting the airway and preventing the possibility of aspiration. Protection of the airway is particularly important before and during patient transport.

If the patient is found unconscious and the history of what has happened is not clear, initial management should include administration of 50% dextrose in normal saline solution, naloxone (if narcotic overdose is suspected), and oxygen in the appropriate dosages based on the patient's age and weight. If possible, blood samples should be drawn before these drugs are given.[26]

Alterations in the patient's circulatory status may be profound and life threatening. A largebore IV catheter and appropriate IV fluids should be initiated before transport. In the extremely hypotensive patient, fluid delivery is the mainstay of therapy. Once the vascular compartment is filled, pressor agents should be used to chemically reverse hypotension. Hypertensive crisis should be managed with afterload reducers or negative inotropic agents.

Depending on the type of poison or toxic exposure, decontamination may need to be carried out before the patient can be transported. Generally, decontamination of the patient can be accomplished by using soap and water. However, there are some toxins that require specific decontaminates. It is important for the flight team to know and follow appropriate procedures to protect both themselves and the patient.[36]

Assessment

History

The history of the toxic exposure provides a significant way to identify the type of substance responsible for the patient's symptoms. Poisoning or an overdose should be suspected in the following types of patients: a psychiatric patient, a trauma victim, a comatose patient with an unknown cause of coma, a young person with a life-threatening dysrhythmia of undetermined origin, a patient rescued from a fire, a child with unexplained lethargy, and any person exhibiting suspicious or unusual behavior.[13] The history should include the type of substance or suspected substance that was taken, the exposure route (e.g., IV, oral, nasal, rectal, dermal, or bite), the time of the exposure, and size or dosage of the exposure.

If a thorough history cannot be obtained, the environment in which the patient was found should be explored for clues to what may have caused the poisoning. The air medical crew should look for bottles, containers, drug paraphernalia, animals, or items that may provide additional information about a suspected or unknown toxic substance. These items should be transported with the patient. Identification of witnesses to the event can add more information concerning what may have happened to cause the poisoning or toxic exposure.[13]

Past medical history such as allergic reactions, previous surgeries, and past hospitalizations should be noted. When possible, it is important to assess whether the patient has attempted suicide in the past.

In the care of the pediatric or elderly patient, the possibility of abuse or neglect must be kept in mind. A referral may be necessary to outside agencies—perhaps even the police—so that the patient's environment may be evaluated to see if it is appropriate and safe.[14]

Symptoms of Poisoning and Toxic Exposures

Certain symptoms without a clear cause may suggest poisoning or overdose. Severe poisoning symptoms include coma, cardiac dysrhythmia, metabolic acidosis, seizures, and GI disturbances.[13,36] Many disease states may mimic overdose and should be considered in the differential diagnoses. It is important to keep in mind that head injuries, encephalitis, metabolic disturbances, and psychiatric diseases are easily mistaken for poisoning.

Physical Examination

The physical examination of a poisoned patient should include assessment of general appearance and pulmonary, cardiovascular, abdominal, and neurologic systems. The information obtained from physical examination will not only help determine the source of the toxic substance but also provide baseline data to follow the effects of the toxic substance and the particular interventions that have been initiated.

Baseline assessment data are particularly important in the determination of any changes in the patient's condition during transport. During flight the toxic effects of the substance should be considered, as well as the success or failure of initial treatments on the patient's condition.

The physical appearance of the patient may give a clue to the type of poison or overdose the patient has taken. The presence of needle tracks, burns, bruises, lacerations, cutaneous bullae, erythema, petechiae, cyanosis, flushed skin, or bite marks may provide information to help diagnose the poison or toxic exposure.[5,14] Breath odors may suggest possible poisoning or help rule it out to another cause. For example, a sweet fruity odor may indicate Placidyl poisoning. Table 31-2 lists odors associated with certain poisonings.[13,20,33]

Respiratory rate and pattern are important assessment parameters. Auscultation of breath sounds is also included in this assessment. Many toxins can cause respiratory arrest, as well as hamper the airway, yielding the potential for aspiration.

The mental status assessment of the poisoned or overdose patient is secondary only to the patient's respiratory assessment and may reveal a spectrum of altered sensorium. Hyperactivity, psychosis, somnolence, or coma may be manifested. Generalized seizures have been reported in many different cases of poisoning or overdose. Level of consciousness, pupillary response, motor and sensory function, and vital signs should be included in the assessment.

An assessment of the patient's level of consciousness should go beyond orientation to person, place, and time. The patient's interaction with the environment can yield useful information about the patient's level of consciousness. Many drugs and toxic substances cause visual, auditory, or other sensory hallucinations, as well as alter the patient's personality.

Pupil size, shape, and reaction are parts of the neurologic assessment. Constricted or dilated pupils may indicate drug or treatment effects. Motor and sensory function are usually assessed together and may vary from normal activity to no movement at all. Seizure activity is not an uncommon complication from toxins and should be appropriately documented and treated.

The presence or possibility of these mental status changes occurring requires appropriate safety measures for air medical transport. Restraints and, in some cases, chemical restraint may be warranted to ensure safe transport by air.

Cardiac monitoring should be performed and blood pressure and pulse quality frequently checked during transport. Hypotension, premature ventricular contractions, prolonged QT intervals, and a widened QRS complex are examples of some of the cardiac

TABLE 31-2

Odors associated with poisonings

Odor	Possible poison
Sweet	Placidyl
	Acetone
	Chloroform
Bitter almond	Cyanide
Pear	Chloral hydrate
Garlic	Arsenic
Wintergreen	Methylsalicylate

dysrhythmias that may occur because of cardiac toxicity related to poisoning or overdose.

Certain toxic substances cause GI disturbances such as nausea, vomiting, and severe abdominal pain. Iron, lithium, mercury, phosphorus, arsenic, mushrooms, organophosphates, and fluoride are examples of toxic substances that can cause GI disturbances. Phosphorus poisoning can cause luminescent vomit and flatus.[13] A nasogastric tube should be inserted before flight to prevent aspiration.

Laboratory Studies

Many substances responsible for adverse reactions, intoxications, and poisoning are difficult to identify. Serum levels are not reflective of tissue concentration or receptor interactions. Therefore levels of specific toxins may be incongruous with clinical manifestations.[14]

Laboratory evaluations such as complete blood count, electrolytes and glucose determinations, and coagulation studies are frequently helpful. Many toxins are associated with leukocytosis or electrolyte alterations. An example is the hypokalemia associated with theophylline toxicity. Arterial blood gas are beneficial in determining acidosis or alkalosis. Acidosis can be appreciated in late methanol or ethylene glycol poisoning, whereas alkalosis occurs in early salicylate intoxication.[13]

The treatment of poisoning with some drugs such as acetaminophen and aspirin necessitates determination of baseline serum levels and a repeat of these levels 3 to 6 hours after ingestion. Levels of some drugs may have to be monitored for several days after ingestion to ensure that they have been eliminated. Any blood, gastric contents, and urine that have been obtained for toxic analysis should accompany the patient for transport.

Removal, Elimination, or Disruption of the Toxin

Ingestion, parenteral injection, ocular contamination, dermal exposure, inhalation, and envenomation are the major routes of intoxication.[13,23] The method of exposure must be established so that a method of removal or interruption can be chosen. Methods for reversal of the clinical effects of poisons include the use of antidotes, antivenin, supportive therapy, forced diuresis, charcoal, cathartics, sorbent hemoperfusion, and dialysis.[13,20,30] The most common methods of removal are gastric lavage followed by administration of charcoal and cathartics.

Two types of forced diuresis may be used to enhance the elimination of specific poisons: diuresis with ion-trapping and diuresis without ion-trapping. In diuresis without ion-trapping, the patient is given IV fluid to maintain urine output of 5 ml/min or 300 ml/hr. This method can be dangerous to the patient with any renal or cardiovascular disease.[36]

Ion-trapping diuresis is accomplished by alkalinization and acidification of the poisoned patient's urine. To achieve alkalinization of urine, sodium bicarbonate is added to IV solution, and fluids are administered to yield a urine pH of 7.5. In the assessment for complications, invasive monitoring devices such as a Swan-Ganz catheter may be useful.[36]

If the toxin has been inhaled, the individual should be removed from the source of the exposure. Administration of oxygen may be of use, particularly for the patient who has sustained carbon monoxide (CO) poisoning.

Contact poisons or toxins may enter the body through the skin, eyes, or mucous membranes. Removing the patient from the toxic environment, taking off the patient's clothes, and cleansing the affected area are the most important steps in the initial removal of the poison or toxic substance. It is important to use the correct irrigation fluid or fluids to prevent further injury to the patient. Attention also must be given to the proper disposal of the contaminated fluid and materials to prevent poisoning of air medical personnel and the surrounding environment—particularly in the helicopter or airplane.

Antivenin administration, hemoperfusion, and dialysis should all be performed under the direction of a trained toxicologist or other health care professional acquainted with each procedure.

Supportive and Emotional Care of the Poisoned Patient

As noted earlier, specific antidotes are limited compared with the numbers of the poisons and toxic substances disseminated in the environment. Frequently, supportive care directed at preventing complications from the poison or toxic substance is the most that can be done for the patient.[20] A part of this supportive care may be the air transport of the patient to a specific center with additional methods of caring for the patient. Supportive care is based on the previous discussion of initial management, physical examination, and removal, elimination, or interruption of the toxic sequence.

The emotional care of the poisoned patient can be difficult. If the poisoning is intentional, the motive must be quickly discovered so that proper psychiatric and social care can be rendered. All procedures should be explained to the patient and a nonjudgmental attitude imparted when care is provided. If possible, the patient's family should be given some time with the patient before transport.

Protection of the patient from complications and respect for the patient as a human being are important components of the flight nursing care of the poisoned patient. E.J. Daniels noted how insensitive nursing care can affect the poisoned patient[7]:

> The curtains hadn't been completely closed, and anyone and everyone walking by peered in, adding to my humiliation. I tried staring at everything but Brenda and the gaggy network of tubes in an attempt to keep my mind off the nauseating trauma. Alright. I have to put some medications down you. Try not to gag on it, because you really need it, keep this down. I'd never heard of any medicine that was pitch black! I felt like she had been flushing me out for hours. She hooked up a huge syringe to the end of the tube down inside of me. The thought of the tar going down my throat into my stomach was more repulsive than the gurgling sensation of lavage.

Safety Issues in the Transport of the Poisoned Patient

Safety is one of the most important issues to be addressed in the flight care of a poisoned patient. Many intoxicants can cause hallucinations or violent behavior. Physical or chemical restraint to ensure safety of the flight team must be initiated during preparation of the patient for transfer.

Both physical and chemical (i.e., medications) restraints provide means of safely controlling the patient for transport. Decreasing excessive stimulation during flight with ear protectors may also reduce the possibility of dangerous or threatening patient behavior during flight.

Summary

The flight nursing care of the poisoned patient begins with management of the patient's airway and ventilation and maintenance of the cardiovascular system. Physical examination, including the patient's general appearance; assessment of the neurologic, respiratory, cardiovascular, and gastrointestinal systems; removal, elimination, or interruption of the toxic sequence; and supportive and emotional care are other important components of care of the poisoned patient.

Preparation for the transport of the poisoned patient includes decontamination; sampling of the toxic substance; transfer of laboratory work such as blood, urine, or vomitus; and informing the family of the transport destination.

The following box summarizes flight nursing care for the poisoned patient. It is critical to approach the care of the poisoned patient in an organized

CARE OF THE POISONED PATIENT BY THE FLIGHT NURSE

1. Provide basic and advanced life support.
2. Remove the patient from the toxic environment.
3. When indicated, remove the toxin from the patient by removing clothing and washing off toxin.
4. Administer appropriate antidote when indicated.
5. Assess respiratory, neurologic, and cardiovascular system frequently.
6. Document or obtain baseline data.
7. Ensure the patient and flight team's safety in transport with the use of soft restraints or sedating or neuromuscular blocking agents.
8. Explain to the patient and family what is happening.
9. Transfer appropriate records and specimens.
10. Inform the patient's family of the patient's destination.

manner to provide supportive care and prevent complications.

PHARMACOLOGIC PROPERTIES OF DRUGS

Therapeutic dose responses are affected by multiple variables including the rate of absorption, distribution, binding, or localization in tissues and inactivation and excretion. The rate of absorption is defined as the time needed for the chemotherapeutic agent to cross the enterovascular barriers and circulate in the cardiovascular system. Agents dissolved in solution are absorbed more rapidly than those in solid forms. Timed-release, enteric-coated products are engineered to greatly decrease the absorption rate. Medications given in higher concentration are absorbed more rapidly.

Gastric pH may deactivate or precipitate a drug. Areas of increased vascularity such as the vagina or rectum tend to absorb agents more rapidly. Topical exposure or inhalation of poisons reaches toxic levels quickly because of the large surface areas exposed to the intoxicants.

The vast majority of drugs are administered orally. Sites of absorption include the oral mucous membranes, stomach, duodenum, and small intestine. Sublingual administration usually promotes quick dissolution and rapid absorption. Absorption in the stomach is a passive process mediated by dissolution and diffusion. The nonionized form of a dissolved medication passes the mucosal barriers and enters the vascular compartment. Most drugs are either weak bases or weak acids. Gastric pH affects both dissolution and diffusion. Weak acids such as salicylates and barbiturates are predominantly nonionized in a strongly acidic environment. Therefore they are readily absorbed. Weak bases are in an ionized form in the stomach and are poorly absorbed. The intestinal pH is less acidic than the stomach (pH = 5.3). Weak bases are readily absorbed, but weak acids cross the mucosal barrier less readily. In addition, the gastric mucosa is a lipoid membrane, which absorbs lipid soluble substances, such as alcohol, rapidly. Factors that change gastric emptying time also alter the rate of absorption of a drug. IV injection is the most immediate and consistent blood concentration for any drug. After injection, a redistribution phase may significantly decrease the blood level of the drug. Absorption of medication given subcutaneously or intramuscularly depends on the site of injection, solubility of the drug, and vascularity of the injection area.

Once the drug is absorbed into the cardiovascular compartment, a redistribution occurs throughout the body. Agents enter or pass through the various body-fluid compartments (plasma, interstitial, transcellular, vitreous, and cellular fluids). Medications are restricted in distribution by their ability to pass through cellular membranes.

Drugs may accumulate in storage depots because of protein binding, fat accumulation, and active transport. Medications are stored in equilibrium and released as plasma concentrations are reduced. Storage depots permit maintenance of plasma levels for long periods, prolonging pharmacologic effects. Anatomic components that act as storage depots include plasma proteins, connective tissues, tissue constituents (such as proteins, phospholipids, or nucleoproteins), adipose tissue, and transcellular fluids.

The mechanism responsible for drug transport across cell membranes may be an active or passive process. Passive transfer is diffusion driven by concentration gradients. Active transport is mediated by a carrier and requires expenditure of energy. The ultimate fate of a drug is metabolism and excretion. Biotransformation involves chemical reactions, classified as nonsynthetic and synthetic. The nonsynthetic class involves oxidation, reduction, and hydrolysis. The parent drug is changed to a more active, a less active, or an inactive metabolite. Most nonsynthetic reactions are mediated by hepatocytic enzymes. Exceptions include nonenzymatic hydrolysis in the plasma, plasma cholinesterase and pseudocholinesterase, and synaptic metabolism of neurotransmitter analogs.

Synthetic reactions or conjugation occur in the liver or kidney. The process couples parent drug or its metabolites to endogenous substrates (usually carbohydrates, amino acids, or inorganic sulfates). Conjugated drugs form inactive, highly ionized, water-soluble substances that are excreted in the urine. Conjugation is an active process requiring adenine triphosphate expenditure.

Active parent drugs and metabolites are excreted in the urine as a primary route of disposal. Drugs are also eliminated through excretion of feces. Metabolites are dissolved in bile, secreted into the alimentary tract, and passed through the GI tract. In addition, the unabsorbed parent is removed with fecal passage.

This discussion has focused on the incidence of poisoning; general considerations in the care of the poisoned patient; general management of the poisoned patient; signs and symptoms of toxicity; physical examination of the poisoned patient; useful laboratory studies; removal, elimination, or disruption of the poison; supportive and emotional care of the poisoned patient; flight nursing care of the poisoned patient; and the pharmacologic properties of drugs. The next part of this chapter focuses on the toxicity and treatment of toxicity of specific drugs. Information about each of these drugs is presented for quick reference.

TOXICITY AND TREATMENT OF POISONING BY SPECIFIC DRUGS

Acetylsalicylic Acid (Aspirin)

Aspirin is one of the oldest nonprescription pharmaceutical agents. Its therapeutic popularity is mainly a result of its antipyretic and analgesic effects. Aspirin can be taken orally, topically, or rectally. The most common route of toxicity is by ingestion. It is very important to keep in mind that many over-the-counter medications contain aspirin and that multiple sources of poisoning may be involved. Table 31-3 describes a method of assessing the severity of salicylate intoxication.

Salicylate toxicity initially manifests in an increased respiratory rate and hyperventilation. Blood gas analysis usually reflects respiratory alkalosis. Clinical manifestations of mild intoxication include headache, vertigo, tinnitus, mental confusion, sweating, thirst, hyperventilation, nausea, vomiting, and drowsiness. Severe intoxication produces similar symptoms combined with base/electrolyte imbalances. Patients are agitated, restless, and uncommunicative and may have seizures or become comatose. Pulmonary edema is observed in severe poisoning, whereas bleeding diatheses are less common.[31]

TABLE 31-3

Assessment of the severity of salicylate intoxication based on the estimated dose ingested

Ingested dose (mg/kg)*	Estimated severity
<150	No toxic reaction expected
150-300	Mild to moderate toxic reaction
300-500	Serious toxic reaction
>500	Potentially lethal toxic reaction

From Haddad L, Winchester J: *Clinical management of poisoning and drug overdose*, Philadelphia, 1990, Saunders.
*Number of tablets ingested times the milligrams of aspirin per tablet divided by patient weight in kilograms equals the acute ingested dose. If a patient has received aspirin therapeutically in the preceding 24 hours, the potential toxicity of the acutely ingested dose will be increased.

Treatment of salicylate poisoning involves gastric emptying, administration of oral-activated charcoal, and alkaline diuresis. Charcoal administration without gastric emptying has been found effective in the management of salicylate toxicity.[1,36]

Alkaline diuresis is performed to increase the pH of the patient's urine to improve free salicylate excretion. Supportive care and maintenance of vital functions are mainstays of treatment in this type of poisoning.[20]

Acetaminophen (Tylenol)

Acetaminophen, similar to aspirin, has antipyretic and analgesic properties. It is not chemically related to the salicylates. Acetaminophen has become a useful alternative to aspirin because it does not cause the GI and bleeding complications that can occur with aspirin use. Like aspirin, acetaminophen is contained in many over-the-counter drugs and may be administered orally or rectally. The main site of absorption is the small intestine, and the drug is uniformly distributed throughout most body fluids.[19]

The classic clinical course of toxic acute acetaminophen poisoning occurs in four stages. The initial stage of toxicity occurs 30 minutes to 24 hours after ingestion and produces anorexia, nausea, vomiting, malaise, pallor, and diaphoresis.

The second stage begins 24 to 48 hours after ingestion. Right upper quadrant pain and tenderness may result from liver enlargement. The levels of liver enzymes, serum bilirubin, and prothrombin time begin to increase 36 hours after ingestion. Oliguria may result from acute tubular necrosis.

The third stage begins 72 to 96 hours after ingestion and is the time of peak liver-function abnormalities. Anorexia, nausea, vomiting, and malaise return; jaundice becomes apparent. Fatalities from acetaminophen poisoning usually occur during this stage and result from fulminant hepatic necrosis.

The fourth stage or "resolution period" occurs 4 days to 2 weeks after poisoning. Patients are asymptomatic, and liver function parameters return to baseline values.[32,36]

Ingestions of more than 7.5 g or 150 mg/kg are considered potentially toxic. The serum level of acetaminophen should be measured 4 hours after ingestion in any person who has ingested a potentially toxic dose of acetaminophen. If the acetaminophen level is still toxic at 4 hours after ingestion or the level cannot be assayed before 10 hours have passed since ingestion and the history suggests a toxic ingestion, *N*-acetylcysteine (NAC) should be administered. NAC is administered orally at an initial dose of 140 mg/kg. A maintenance dose of 70 mg/kg every 4 hours for 17 doses is then given.[32,36] Research is being conducted in the administration of NAC by the IV route. This is already done in Great Britain and Australia.[34] It is important to ensure that the patient retain this medication. Antiemetics may be necessary before flight.

Antidepressants (Tricyclics)

Tricyclic antidepressants (TCAs) are widely prescribed in the United States. Their primary use is in the treatment of endogenous depression in adults; however, recent study has increased their use for school phobia, pain control, obsessive-compulsive behavior, and sleep disorders in children.[17] Overdose statistics show cyclic antidepressants as one of the most deadly types of poisoning, with a high degree of morbidity and mortality in significant overdoses. Many tricyclic antidepressants are available throughout the United States.[23]

TCAs are well absorbed in the GI tract. The parent compound and active metabolites are quickly bound to plasma proteins. TCAs exert their effects by inhibiting the amine pump mechanism responsible for the reuptake of norepinephrine and serotonin in adrenergic and serotonergic neurons. Cyclic antidepressants also block cholinergic receptors in the parasympathetic nervous system and exert antihistaminic properties.[4,9,13]

The clinical manifestations of TCA poisoning include mydriasis, tachycardia, dry mucous membranes, urine retention, and decreased peristalsis. Central nervous system (CNS) signs include confusion, agitation, hallucinations, seizures, and coma. Twitching, jerking, and myoclonic movements have also been reported. Grand mal seizures are reported in 1% to 20% of TCA poisoning cases. Respiratory depression is common. The enhanced adrenergic stimulation of the myocardium and direct toxic effects of these agents result in many cardiovascular effects. Sinus tachycardia and mild hypertension occur early in poisoning. TCAs exert a quinidine-like cardiac action that depresses conduction velocity. QRS-interval widening, right bundle-branch block, and first-degree heart block are common findings. Acidosis occurs because of cardiac and respiratory depression.[4,9,13]

In TCA poisoning, support of vital functions is essential. Hypotension is initially managed with an IV infusion of saline solution. Pressor agents are used if hypotension is refractory to fluid challenges. α-Adrenergic agents are preferred. Physostigmine is not an antidote to cyclic antidepressant poisoning and should not be used for these patients.

Benzodiazepines

Benzodiazepines became available in the United States in 1963 to control anxiety. These drugs are now used to decrease anxiety, as sedative-hypnotics, muscle-relaxants, and anticonvulsants. Generally, a toxic level of benzodiazepines must be quite high; however, benzodiazepines are often taken in combination with other poisons, such as alcohol, that can cause death.[19]

The syndrome of benzodiazepine toxicity is nonspecific. The clinical picture is usually mild compared with those of other sedative-hypnotic poisonings. Most oral poisonings result in drowsiness and coma.

In contrast, IV diazepam use has been associated with a 1.7% incidence of life-threatening reactions, including hypotension and cardiorespiratory arrest. Diazepam toxicity is markedly increased by the concomitant use of other drugs, particularly alcohol.

The treatment of benzodiazepine poisoning begins with management of the patient's ABCs. Flumazenil can be administered to reverse the sedative, ataxic, anxiolytic, and muscle-relaxant effects of a toxic benzodiazepine ingestion. However, this drug must be administered with caution because many patients who take overdoses take combinations of drugs, some of which may cause seizures at toxic levels, such as TCAs. Flumazenil reverses the anticonvulsant effects of benzodiazepines, which leaves patients with polyoverdoses at risk for lack of seizure management.[36]

Digitalis

The term *cardiac glycoside* is used to describe a large group of drugs prescribed to treat heart failure. These drugs have been used throughout history, with early mention of the compound found in ancient writings in the year 1500 BC. Digitalis has become the most familiar of the group. It is derived from the dried leaf of the foxglove plant *Digitalis purpurea.*[13]

Several factors contribute to digitalis poisoning. These include the patient's age, severe heart disease, electrolyte imbalances, and drug therapy such as the use of diuretics.[13]

Clinical manifestations of digitalis toxicity are divided into cardiac and noncardiac. Cardiac manifestations are the result of depression through the sinoatrial and atrioventricular nodes and alteration of impulse formation. Noncardiac signs and symptoms include fatigue, vascular weakness, anorexia, nausea, vomiting, diarrhea, confusion, restlessness, insomnia, drowsiness, hallucinations, frank psychosis, blurred vision, photophobia, and yellow-halo visual effects.[13]

Treatment of digitalis toxicity includes support of vital functions and possible correction of the underlying cause (e.g., correction of an electrolyte imbalance). Advances in immunotherapy have yielded digoxin-specific antibody fragments (Fab), which neutralize digoxin toxicity. Fab fragments are indicated if conventional supportive care to life-threatening dysrhythmias and hyperkalemia fails. Fab fragments bind to digoxin, and the fab-digoxin complex is excreted in the urine.[35,36]

Street Drugs

Cocaine

Cocaine use has reached epidemic proportions in the United States. It has been estimated that more than 30 million Americans have tried cocaine and that about 5 million use it regularly. It was one of the most popular drugs in the 1980s. Thirty percent of men and 20% of women between the ages of 24 and 34 have used cocaine at least once.[17] The cocaine problem varies with geographic location; however, probably few places in the United States have escaped difficulties related to illegal drug use.

Cocaine is a naturally occurring alkaloid, the only source of which is the leaves of the evergreen shrub *Erythroxylon coca.* The leaves contain 0.5% to 2.5% cocaine. The plant is native to Peru, Bolivia, and Colombia but is now a major cultivated cash crop in many Central and South American countries. The crystallized cocaine is extracted from the coca leaf in the hydrochloride salt form. Cocaine hydrochloride is usually transported in a 90% to 95% pure form until it reaches its intended destination, where the drug is diluted and adulterated for street sale. Street cocaine generally varies in potency from 2% to 30% purity. Common adulterants are mannitol, lactose, and local anesthetics such as lidocaine, procaine, and tetracaine. Many times street samples contain no cocaine at all, but are combinations of caffeine, amphetamines, codeine, phencyclidine (PCP), and other local anesthetics.[3,12,26]

There are several routes of cocaine abuse. The easiest and most popular method of misuse is nasal inhalation or "snorting." The blood concentration increases rapidly after snorting for approximately 20 minutes, peaks at 1 hour, and then slowly subsides for several hours.

Cocaine may also be injected intravenously. Because blood levels peak after 3 to 5 minutes, this method can be very toxic and lethal. In addition, cocaine is mixed in a mixture that may contain a flammable solvent that is ignited. Smoking cocaine not only may lead to toxicity but also to severe burn injuries.[13]

Crack is the "cooked and dried" version of free-base cocaine. When cocaine is mixed with baking soda and water and then heated in an ordinary pot, the impurities used to cut the drug are removed. The resulting mixture dries into a hard substance that is broken into small chunks or "rocks," which are white or yellowish-white in color. The user then smokes the rocks.[26]

Ingestion of cocaine is not a popular method of abuse. However, oral exposure and poisoning have been observed in the "body-packer" or smuggler. In an effort to hide the illegal substance from authorities, the runner ingests a large supply of cocaine that has been packaged in rubber, latex, or similar material. Each individual package may contain 2 to 10 g of pure cocaine; up to 175 bags have been swallowed. If the bag leaks or ruptures, absorption of the cocaine is rapid and often lethal.[5,10,13]

Another popular method of cocaine use is for the male to apply the drug topically to his penis before sexual intercourse. Because cocaine is a local anesthetic, the desired effect of this practice is prolonged erection. Cocaine is absorbed in the female's vagina, and intoxication can occur.[3]

The drug is metabolized by the liver and excreted by the kidney.[13,17] Cocaine stimulates both the peripheral and central adrenergic nervous systems. Cocaine produces an euphoria and a mild-to-moderate CNS stimulation manifested by decreased fatigue, excitement, and a general feeling of well-being. The user generally tends to be talkative, physically active, and sociable and may experience a slight tachycardia, mydriasis, slight diaphoresis, and tremor.

Death from cocaine results from cardiovascular and respiratory collapse. Metabolic acidosis, hyperthermia, status epilepticus, or ventricular dysrhythmias are seen in the severely poisoned patient. Fatalities may occur from any method of abuse. Unexplained sudden death may occur after IV injection, but most fatal cases follow a progressive downhill course over 30 to 60 minutes. Death can also occur as a result of the effects of agents used to mitigate cocaine effects (especially heroin) or from the untoward effects of adulterants or substituted drugs.[21]

The main objectives in treating acute cocaine poisoning are to support the respiratory system, control hypertension, suppress malignant cardiac dysrhythmias, correct metabolic acidosis, reduce hyperthermia, and minimize seizure activity.[3]

Hallucinogens

Two types of drug poisoning that cause hallucinations are PCP and lysergic acid diethylamide (LSD). PCP was initially developed as a general anesthetic in 1958. Because of the postanesthetic reactions that occurred with its use, it has not been used legally since 1965. PCP now is manufactured in "kitchen" laboratories.

The drug may be smoked, snorted, or ingested. The drug is distributed to all tissue compartments, metabolized by the liver, and excreted through the kidneys. Its effects can last up to 48 hours.[14] PCP can produce bizarre and dangerous behavior. In larger doses it can cause psychosis, hostility, and coma. A common neurologic sign of PCP intoxication is nystagmus.[5,36]

Treatment consists of supportive care. Air transportation of patients who have taken PCP demands close observation. Patients may become hostile, belligerent, and destructive. Sedative or neuromuscular blocking agents with airway control may be necessary to safely transport these patients.

LSD is the most potent hallucinogen known. The drug was initially used by psychiatrists in the 1950s as an aid in clinical psychotherapy. Abuse became popular during the 1960s, with illicit use reaching epidemic proportions in 1965.[5,36]

LSD can be taken both orally and nasally. The dose required to produce hallucinations is between 0.5 and 1.0 $\mu g/kg$, and the intensity of its effect is dose dependent.[11] Absorption of the drug is rapid, and LSD is distributed to all tissues, including the brain. Initial effects occur within 30 to 40 minutes, and peak effects occur within 1 to 2 hours. LSD is metabolized in the liver, and small amounts of it are excreted unchanged in urine.[13]

Psychologic effects follow ingestion of LSD within 30 to 90 minutes. These effects are generally pleasurable, and the person is usually able to function and is aware that he or she is experiencing a drug-induced illusion. Occasionally a person may have an intense panic reaction ("bad trip"), which includes frightening hallucinations and loss of the knowledge that the symptoms are caused by a transient drug effect. Such a person may become confused, aggressive, suicidal, or violent. Particularly frightening and uncontrollable experiences are linked to the contamination of LSD with other drugs such as amphetamines.[13]

As with the patient who has taken PCP, extreme caution should be taken during the air transport of these patients. Use of ear protectors and sedation, as well as prophylactic restraints, may be necessary before transport.

Alcohol

Alcohol (ethanol) is the most widely used and abused drug in America. It is often involved in poison emergencies because it is frequently used with other drugs.

Ethanol alcohol is rapidly absorbed from the stomach, small intestine, and colon. Food reduces the rate of absorption by 2 to 6 hours. Once ethanol is ingested, equilibration is rapid, and distribution uniformly occurs throughout all bodily tissues and fluids. Passage across the placenta has been documented.[36]

Ethanol metabolism occurs mainly in the liver. Ethanol is oxidized by alcohol. Alcohol is a CNS depressant. Acute intoxication produces psychomotor retardation, reflex slowing, lethargy, sleep, and, ultimately, coma and death. Initially, respirations are stimulated as a result of the production of carbon dioxide. However, with increasing concentrations of alcohol, respirations are dangerously depressed. Ethanol enhances cutaneous blood flow, which causes heat loss through vasodilation. Excessive amounts depress the central thermoregulatory mechanism, adding to the hypothermia effects. Ethanol stimulates gastric secretions, which causes an irritation of the gastric mucosa. In addition, ethanol causes diuresis mediated through inhibition of antidiuretic hormone, which decreases renal tubular reabsorption of water.[13,36]

Patients respond differently to alcohol poisoning. Table 31-4 correlates signs and symptoms of alcohol intoxication with blood alcohol levels.[13] The lethal dose of alcohol in children is considered 3 gm/kg and in adults 5 to 8 gm/kg.

Care of the alcohol-poisoned patient consists of supportive care. Such patients may become combative, and precaution should be taken for appropriate restraint before flight.

Ethylene Glycol

Ethylene glycol is an odorless, water-soluble solvent most commonly used in permanent-type antifreezes and coolants. Ingestion usually occurs in the inquisitive toddler or the subject desperate to commit suicide. Ethylene glycol is rapidly absorbed and reaches peak blood levels in 1 to 4 hours after ingestion. Large doses result in an inebriated patient without the odor of alcohol. Ethylene glycol approximates ethanol in CNS toxicity; however, its metabolites produce profound systemic effects.[13,36]

Ethylene glycol is hepatically metabolized. It eventually breaks down into four main by-products that include formic and oxalic acid. Most believe that these by-products are responsible for the pathology seen in ethylene glycol toxicity.[13,36]

Signs and symptoms of ethylene glycol ingestion include nausea, vomiting, ataxia, stupor, coma, convulsions, nystagmus, depressed deep-tendon reflexes, myoclonic jerks, hypothermia, and low-grade fever. A profound anion-gap metabolic acidosis is a hallmark of this poisoning, but it occurs after metabolism has begun. Severe hypocalcemia resulting from chelation of calcium may produce tetany, as well as cardiac compromise. Other complications of ethylene glycol poisoning include kidney failure and pulmonary edema.[21,36]

Treatment for ethylene glycol ingestion is guided by serum/blood levels. If history suggests a significant ingestion, an IV ethanol drip should be initiated before the ethylene glycol level is determined. Ethanol blocks the conversion of ethylene glycol to its toxic form. Dialysis is used to remove the ethylene glycol because metabolism is retarded and renal excretion of the parent compound is poor. Thiamine and pyridoxine have also been used to treat ethylene glycol toxicity. Thiamine is administered at 100 μm and pyroxidine is administered at 50 mgm either intravenously or intramuscularly. There are also case reports of the use of

TABLE 31-4

Signs and symptoms of alcohol intoxication by blood alcohol level

Blood alcohol level	Signs and symptoms
Mild (0.5%-0.15%) 0.5-1.5 mg/ml	Decreased inhibitions Slight visual impairments Slight muscular incoordination Slowing of reaction time
Moderate (0.15%-0.3%) 1.5-3 mg/ml	Definite visual impairment Sensory loss Muscular incoordination Slowing of reaction time Slurred speech
Severe (0.3%-0.5%) 3-5 mg/ml	Marked muscular incoordination Blurred or double vision Approaching stupor Sometimes hypoglycemia with hypothermia Conjugate deviation of the eyes Extensor rigidity of the extremities Unilateral or bilateral Babinski's sign Convulsions and trismus Fatalities begin to occur
Coma (>0.5%) > 5 mg/ml	Unconsciousness Depressed respirations Decreased reflexes and complete loss of sensation Deaths are frequent

From Dreisbach RH, Robertson WO: *Handbook of poisoning: prevention, diagnosis and treatment,* Norwalk, Conn, 1987, Appleton & Lange.

4-methylpyrazole, a potent inhibitor of alcohol dehydrogenase that prevents the metabolism of methanol and ethylene glycol.[34]

Carbon Monoxide

CO is a colorless, odorless, tasteless gas yielded by the incomplete combustion of carbonaceous material. Sources include car exhaust, space heaters, defective fireplace flues, flame-type water heaters, improperly vented gas ranges and furnaces, coal and oil furnaces, poorly ventilated charcoal and gas grills, and fires of all types.[36]

CO combines with the hemoglobin molecule in the red blood cell. The affinity of hemoglobin for CO is approximately 200 times that for oxygen. Not only does CO compete with oxygen for hemoglobin, but the presence of carboxyhemoglobin also greatly impedes the dissociation of oxygen from hemoglobin. This leads to a decreased partial pressure of oxygen in the blood and diminished gradient for oxygen diffusion from the red blood cell to the tissues, resulting in tissue anoxia. Arterial hypoxia results from any of the following reasons: pulmonary venous admixture from an uneven ventilation/perfusion relationship; marked inhibition of the circulatory system; direct effect of CO on the pulmonary tissue, which results in increased capillary permeability and decreased production of surfactant; and a change in the oxyhemoglobin dissociation curve with a shift to the left.[36]

Some authorities believe that the concentration of CO in the blood relates poorly to the clinical

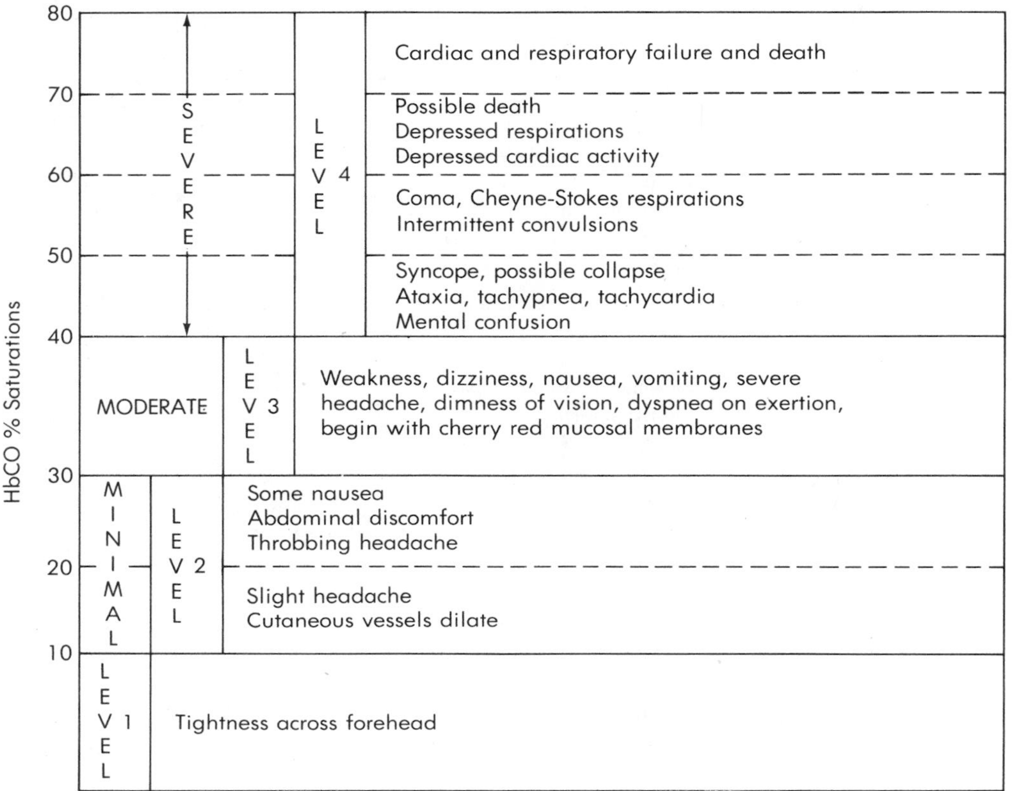

Fig. 31-1. Signs and symptoms of various blood levels of HbCO. (Modified from Elo T: *Carbon monoxide: quick reference to clinical toxicology,* Philadelphia, 1980, Lippincott.)

features observed in the person who has been exposed. Fig. 31-1 describes the symptomatology of CO poisoning related to CO saturation in the blood.[36]

The treatment of acute CO exposure is oxygen delivery. Carboxyhemoglobin will dissociate and convert to oxyhemoglobin if high concentrations of oxygen are provided. Hyperbaric therapy has also been found to be extremely successful for patients with levels of 40% at the exposure site and emergency unit levels of 25%.[36]

The treatment of the patient in flight with CO poisoning includes stabilization of the patient's airway so that high-flow O_2 can be delivered. In addition, the patient must be observed and treated for such hypoxic side effects as seizures.

SNAKEBITES

Responding to the needs of a victim of a snakebite may not be one of the most common flights encountered by the flight nurse; however, knowledge of how to care for the patient can decrease complications and save lives. Approximately 40,000 to 50,000 snakebites occur in the United States each year. About 7,000 to 8,000 are inflicted by venomous snakes; 12 to 15 deaths result yearly.[2,6,18,28]

Venom is a special category of poison that must be injected by one organism into another to produce a harmful effect.[14] It is secreted by special epithelial cells in certain organisms and is stored in the lumina or exocrine glands. It comprises multiple substances, some of them toxic. The toxins may affect particular body systems such as the neurologic, hematologic, and cardiovascular systems.[2,22,28]

The most prevalent venomous snakes in the United States are the pit vipers, which include the true rattlesnakes, the copperheads, and water moccasins. These snakes are found throughout the country with the exception of Maine, Alaska, and Hawaii.[2,28]

The coral snake is another kind of venomous snake found in the United States. The eastern coral snake is found in North and South Carolina, Florida, Louisiana, Mississippi, Georgia, and Texas.

In addition to the venomous snakes native to the United States, poisonous snakes have been collected from all over the world. A bite from any one of these snakes may be fraught with complications or may even be instantly fatal.

The following subsections describe the venomous snakes, the initial treatment of snakebites, flight nursing care of snake-bitten patients, and the role of flight transport in the care of these victims.

Recognition of Venomous Bites

Fig. 31-2 compares venomous and nonvenomous snakes. The most prevalent type of venomous snake in the United States is the pit viper. Only trained people should handle live snakes; even a dead snake can envenomate a careless person.[22,28]

Pit vipers, who belong to the Crotalidae family (as shown in Fig. 31-2), have a pit midway between the eye and nostril on each side of the head. This pit is a heat-sensing organ that helps the snake locate its prey. This particular characteristic, unlike others in Fig. 31-2, is a 100% consistent characteristic in the identification of pit vipers.[22,28]

Envenomation by a pit viper usually results in symptoms of localized pain, swelling, and edema in the bitten area. Other symptoms include diaphoresis and chills, paresthesia, nausea, hypotension, faintness, weakness, muscle fasciculations, local ecchymosis, and coagulopathies.[22,28]

The second largest family of snakes in the world are the Elapidae, which contain some deadly species. These include cobras, mambas, and the eastern coral snakes. One of the distinguishing characteristics of these snakes is their color.

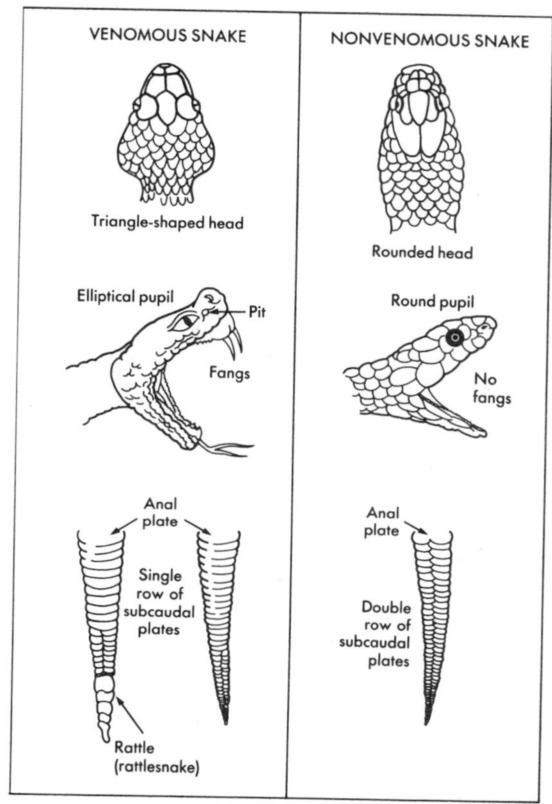

Fig. 31-2. Venomous and nonvenomous snakes. (From Otten M: Venomous animal injuries. In Rosen P et al, editors: *Emergency medicine,* vol 1, ed 2, St Louis, 1988, Mosby.)

Envenomation by a coral snake may result in a neurotoxic course. Systemic manifestations include drowsiness, euphoria, weakness, nausea, vomiting, fasciculations, dysphagia, salivation, extraocular muscle paresis, hypotension, and cardiopulmonary failure.[22,28]

Initial Management of Snakebites

Just because a person has been bitten by a snake, it does not always mean that envemonation has occurred. It has been estimated that 20% to 30% of crotalid bites and 50% of elapid bites do not result in penetration; such bites are called "dry bites."[22] There is lengthy and controversial discussion in the literature over the appropriate management of a snakebite. As noted by Kunkel,[22] many an emotional discussion has occurred over the appropriate management of a snakebite. In the following discussion of the general management of snakebite patients, it is important to emphasize that experts should be consulted when questions arise about the care of snake-bitten patients. Many of the authors cited in this chapter are available for consultation, as is the local poison control center.

If the snake has not been secured, the patient should be moved to a safe environment. It is important to keep the patient calm and to immobilize the affected part. These two interventions decrease the circulation of venom throughout the patient's system. Specific prehospital care of the snakebite patient is based on the type of envenomation that has occurred. For elapid envenomation the wound should be cleansed, a compressive bandage applied, the extremity immobilized, and the patient transported. The care of viper envenomation should include cleansing of the wound, immobilization of the affected part, no use of compression techniques, and transport of the patient.[2,22,28]

The airway, ventilatory, and circulatory status of the patient should be constantly evaluated. Two large-bore IV lines should be started, preferably in an area away from the bite. The patient must be observed closely for progression of symptoms from a localized reaction at the wound site to a systemic reaction.

When possible, blood samples for baseline laboratory work should be drawn before transport. These may include a complete blood count, coagulation studies, electrolytes, blood urea nitrogen, creatinine, and urinalysis. Included in the coagulation studies should be fibrin split products and fibrinogen levels.[2,22,28]

If the patient exhibits signs of severe envenomation—such as edema that has progressed 30 cm within 1 hour of the bite, shock, kidney failure, pulmonary edema, bleeding, or paralysis—administration of antivenin should be started.[2,22,28] The size of the patient needs to be considered in relation to the amount of venom that the person may be able to tolerate. A child or small adult may be more severely affected.

Snake antivenin is prepared from the serum of horses hyperimmunized against a specific venom or venoms. Unlike other drugs, the dosage of antivenin should be based on clinical findings rather than on the age and weight of the patient. Skin testing for hypersensitivity with epinephrine at the patient's bedside should be performed before antivenin is administered.[2,28]

When antivenin is given, the package instructions should be followed and resuscitation equipment kept in close range. Patients should be monitored continuously for anaphylactic reactions.

Serum sickness may develop after antivenin administration. The incidence of serum sickness varies from 10% to 80% of all patients given antivenin therapy.[16] The symptoms of serum sickness have occurred up to 3 weeks after antivenin administration. They include fever, rash, nausea, vomiting, and neurologic symptoms. Treatment of serum sickness includes antihistamines and steroids.[2,28]

Flight Nurse Care of Snakebite

The flight nurse may become involved in the care of the patient with a snakebite by directly responding to the scene of the injury or by transporting the patient to a center for care. Experts in the care of

FLIGHT NURSE CARE OF THE SNAKEBITTEN PATIENT

1. Provide a safe environment for the patient.
2. Provide basic life support.
3. If possible, obtain information about the type of snake.
4. Immobilize the affected part.
5. Keep the patient calm.
6. Initiate advanced life support as indicated.
7. Establish a large-bore IV line.
8. Watch local and systemic effects from the snakebite.
9. Administer analgesia for pain.
10. Consult an expert if questions arise.
11. Bring the dead snake in a secure container for identification if possible.
12. When indicated and if available, administer antivenin.

snakebites note that rapid transport of these patients to a hospital or to a person who can manage their injury is imperative in saving lives and preventing complications. The box summarizes nursing care to be provided by the flight nurse for the patient bitten by a snake.[2,28]

TOXICOLOGY CASE STUDY #1

Hallucinogenic Toxicity

A 16-year-old boy ingested a plant known as monkshood after being told by his friends that he would have a "good trip." The plant that he ingested was a potent alkaloid. He immediately began hallucinating and then went into status epilepticus. The flight team was dispatched to assist in patient care and transport the patient.

On the arrival of the flight team, the patient's seizures had subsided after administration of 5 mg diazepam. However, the patient was screaming and had be physically restrained. An IV line was started and the patient was intubated with the use of rapid sequence induction. Ten milligrams of vecuronium and 2 mg lorazepam were given for safety and sedation.

Blood pressure was 80 mm Hg systolic by palpation, pulse was 130 beats/min and irregular (the monitor showed atrial fibrillation), and respirations were being assisted because of the vecuronium. A fluid bolus of 200 ml of normal saline solution was infused. The patient's blood pressure increased to 100/50 mm Hg. The patient was prepared for transport. Restraints were applied and a headset placed on the patient to decrease outside stimulation.

During transport, the patient sustained cardiac arrest, going into coarse ventricular fibrillation. He was successfully electroconverted with 360 W/sec. Atrial fibrillation continued after resuscitation. A lidocaine bolus was administered and a lidocaine drip initiated per Advanced Cardiac Life Support protocol.

The patient experienced no additional problems during transport and was admitted to the medical intensive care unit of the receiving facility. The toxicologist continued supportive care, including correction of the metabolic acidosis and maintenance of sedation. The patient regained consciousness 48 hours later and was discharged home within 5 days of the incident.

TOXICOLOGY CASE STUDY #2

Victim of a Snakebite

The flight team was asked to transport by helicopter a 4-year-old boy who had sustained a snakebite. The child stated he had been playing in a field when a "brown snake with sharp teeth bit him." This incident was not witnessed by an adult.

The child was alert and oriented. His vital signs were stable. The referring physician reported that the child had two puncture wounds at the side of his right foot. Localized swelling was also noted.

The care of this patient included assessment of whether the bite was venomous. Because copperheads are native to the area and fang marks were visible, the flight nurse had to assume that the child had been bitten by a pit viper. The wound had been cleansed and immobilized. The flight nurse placed an IV line and started a cardiac monitor. A tetanus shot was administered because the child had never been immunized.

During flight, the flight nurse monitored the child for signs and symptoms of localized and systemic poisoning including increasing edema in the bitten extremity, nausea and vomiting, hypotension, and excessive bleeding.

An important role for the flight team in the care of snakebite envenomation is the timely delivery and initiation of antivenin in areas where it is not readily available. However, this child, as in about 50% of snake bites, only sustained a dry bite. He was admitted for observation and discharged later without complications.

REFERENCES

1. Albertson TE et al: Superiority of activated charcoal alone compared with ipecac and activated charcoal in the treatment of acute toxic ingestions, *Ann Emerg Med* 18(1): 56-59, 1989.
2. Auerbach P: *Wilderness medicine,* St Louis, 1995, Mosby.

3. Brabowski J: *Cocaine pharmacology: effects and treatment of abuses,* National Institute on Drug Abuse Research Monograph series, Washington, DC, NIDA Research Monograph 50, 1984.
4. Braden NJ, Jackson JE, Walson PD: Tricyclic antidepressant overdose, *Pediatr Clin North Am* 33:691-701, 1986.
5. Brent J: Drugs of abuse: an update, *Emerg Med* 7:56-70, 1995.
6. Curry S et al: The legitimacy of rattlesnake bites in central Arizona, *Ann Emerg Med* 18:658-663, 1989.
7. Daniels EJ: *Any other song,* Bowie, Md, 1980, Brady.
8. Elo T: Carbon monoxide. In Hanenson IB, editor: *Quick reference to clinical toxicology,* Philadelphia, 1980, Lippincott.
9. Foulke GE: Identifying toxicity risk early after antidepressant overdose, *Am J Emerg Med* 13(2):123-126, 1995.
10. Gay G: Clinical management of acute and chronic cocaine poisoning, *Ann Emerg Med* 11:562, 1982.
11. Geiderman J: Adverse drug reactions: an emergency department view, *Topics Emerg Med* 1-11, 1986.
12. Goodman L, Gilman A, editors: *The pharmacological basis of therapeutics,* ed 2, New York, 1991, Macmillan.
13. Haddad L, Winchester J: *Clinical management of poisonings and drug overdose,* Philadelphia, 1990, Saunders.
14. Haley K, Baker P: *Emergency nursing pediatric course,* Park Ridge, Ill, 1993, Emergency Nurses Association.
15. Higgins R: Cocaine abuse: what every nurse should know, *J Emerg Nurs* 15:318-323, 1989.
16. Hoffman RS, Goldfrank LR: The poisoned patient with altered consciousness: controversies in the use of a "coma cocktail," *JAMA* 274(7):562-569, 1995.
17. Hollander J: The management of cocaine associated myocardial ischemia, *JAMA* 333(19):1267-1272, 1995.
18. Jurkovich G et al: Complications of Crotalidae antivenin therapy, *J Trauma* 28:1032-1037, 1988.
19. Karb V, Queener S, Freeman J: *Handbook of drugs for nursing practice,* ed 2, St Louis, 1996, Mosby.
20. Kitt S et al: *Emergency nursing: a physiologic and clinical perspective,* Philadelphia, 1995, Saunders.
21. Kulberg A: Substance abuse: clinical identification and management, *Pediatr Clin North Am* 33:325-355, 1986.
22. Kunkel D et al: Reptile envenomation, *J Toxicol Clin Toxicol* 21:503-526, 1984.
23. Litovitz T et al: Annual report of the American Association of Poison Control Centers toxic exposure surveillance system, *Am J Emerg Med* 13(5):551-558, 1995.
24. Matyunas NJ: *Tricyclic antidepressant poisoning,* clinical paper, Lexington, Ky, 1986, Kentucky Regional Poison Center.
25. Mendenhall CL, Weesner RE: Alcohols and glycols. In Haneson IB, editor: *Quick reference to clinical toxicology,* Philadelphia, 1980, Lippincott.
26. Merigian KS, Roberts JR: *Cocaine,* clinical paper, Cincinnati, 1987, University of Cincinnati Medical Center Department of Emergency Medicine.
27. Merigian KS, Roberts JR: *LSD,* clinical paper, Cincinnati, 1986, University of Cincinnati Medical Center Department of Emergency Medicine.
28. Norris RL, Ling LJ, Wang R: Snake venom poisoning in the United States: assessment and management, *Emerg Med Rep* 16(10):87-94, 1995.
29. Olson KR et al: Seizures associated with poisoning and drug overdose. *Am J Emerg Med* 11(6):565-568, 1993.
30. Perrone J, Hoffman RS, Goldfrank LR: Special considerations in gastrointestinal decontamination, *Emerg Med Clin North Am* 12(2):285-299, 1994.
31. Riggs B: Acetaminophen. In Noji E, Kelen G, editors: *Handbook of toxicologic emergencies,* Chicago, 1989, Year Book.
32. Riggs B: Salicylates. In Nofi E, Kelen G, editors: *Manual of toxicologic emergencies,* Chicago, 1989, Year Book.
33. Sheehy S, Barber J: *Emergency nursing principles and practice,* ed 3, St Louis, 1992, Mosby.
34. Stolpe M et al: Preliminary observations on the effects of hyperbaric oxygen therapy on western diamondback rattlesnake *(Crotalus atrox)* venom poisoning in the rabbit model, *Ann Emerg Med* 18:871-874, 1989.
35. Sullivan J: Immunotherapy in the poisoned patient: overview of present applications and future trends, *Med Toxicol* 24:47-60, 1986.
36. Wright RO et al: Poison antidotes: guidelines for rational use in the emergency department, *Emerg Med Rep* 16(21): 201-211, 1995.

CHAPTER 32

Gynecologic Emergencies

COMPETENCIES

1. Perform a focused assessment for the patient with a gynecologic emergency, including the collection of subjective and objective data related to each specific emergency.
2. Identify life-threatening gynecologic emergencies such as ectopic pregnancy.
3. Initiate the appropriate interventions for the patient with a gynecologic emergency before and during transport.

A woman who presents to a medical facility with the complaint of abdominal pain, pelvic pain, or both must be evaluated carefully and efficiently. Any delay may compromise the care of the presenting problem, may jeopardize the future reproductive capabilities of the patient, and may result in death in extreme cases. This chapter addresses the emergency and potential emergent gynecologic emergencies that the flight nurse may encounter.

GENERAL EVALUATION

Evaluation of acute abdominal pain and gynecologic problems requiring rapid intervention should always be approached in the same manner. Maintaining a high level of suspicion and using a systematic method of evaluation and assessment will help ensure that a potentially life-threatening condition or a condition that threatens a patient's future reproductive capabilities is not overlooked.

On initial contact with the patient, a primary survey should be conducted and the resuscitation phase initiated. At the time of the secondary survey, the abdomen can be evaluated more thoroughly—the specific diagnosis is not as important as recognizing that an abdominal catastrophe has occurred and requires definitive intervention. Once the initial physical evaluation and history have been completed, a more in-depth abdominal evaluation is indicated. The findings of a pelvic and breast examination, if these surveys are performed before the arrival of the flight nurse, will aid in the differential diagnosis and must be included in the report given to the receiving facility.

A brief, accurate gynecologic and menstrual history must be obtained for the correct diagnosis to be made. To determine normal menses, the timing of not only the last menstrual period (LMP) must be determined but also the two previous menstrual periods. The length of the LMP and the volume of flow, determined by the number of pads or tampons used, is also useful information. A soaked pad suggests 20 to 30 ml of blood loss.

Information about complications encountered in previous pregnancies may suggest the possibility of a specific pregnancy complication because it is common for recurrent episodes to be clinically similar to a previous episode. Spontaneous abortions and ectopic pregnancies have minimum recurrence risks of 15% and 12%, respectively.[5]

It has been proved many times over that although contraception minimizes the risk of pregnancy, it does not completely eliminate it. The failure rate for contraception varies from less than 0.5% for tubal ligation to as much as 30% to 40% for such methods as withdrawal, douching, and rhythm.[8] It is important to determine whether sexual intercourse occurred in conjunction with the use of effective and reliable contraception methods.

Understanding the pathophysiology of the following conditions will aid in the interpretation of the data obtained in the evaluation of a patient experiencing a gynecologic emergency. The often-subtle differences that may be encountered could very easily be overlooked or misinterpreted, possibly delaying appropriate intervention. The flight nurse must know all of the diagnostic procedures that may be used in making a differential diagnosis, although many of these procedures may not have been performed prior to transport.

ECTOPIC PREGNANCY

In every patient with a clinical scenario including lower abdominal or pelvic pain and vaginal bleeding, the possibility of ectopic pregnancy should be considered in the differential diagnosis. Ectopic pregnancy, or a pregnancy in which the fertilized ovum implants itself in a site other than the usual endometrium, accounts for nearly 13% of all maternal deaths and is the leading cause of maternal deaths in the first trimester.[8] The ectopic pregnancy rate is 16.8 per 1000 pregnancies.[2] Of ectopic pregnancies, 98% occur in the fallopian tubes, with the rest occurring in the abdomen, on the ovary, or on the cervix.[3]

Predisposing factors of ectopic pregnancy include previous infections, previous ectopic pregnancy, previous abdominal or tubal surgeries, intrauterine device (IUD) use, and history of tubal ligation. At one time, infections tended to completely occlude the fallopian tubes with scarring. It is now believed that with the widespread use of antibiotics, the ciliated epithelium is not normally regenerated, leaving the tube functionally impaired, even though total scarring is avoided. With the current methods of tubal ligation, the incidence of pregnancy is less than 1%, but should pregnancy occur the risk of ectopic pregnancy approaches 50%.[8] Ectopic pregnancy reoccurs in 10% of women. The incidence of ectopic pregnancies has tripled over the past decade; it is now believed that ectopic pregnancy accounts for 1% to 2% of all pregnancies.[5]

Most ectopic pregnancies occur between the fifth and eighth weeks after the last menstrual period. A positive pregnancy test confirms the diagnosis of pregnancy, whether intrauterine or ectopic. Human chorionic gonadotropin (HCG), produced by the placenta, can be detected in the serum in a normal pregnancy; HCG blood levels double every 2 days for the first 6 to 8 weeks. In early pregnancy, a quantitative HCG level that does not increase by 66% in 48 hours is a strong indicator of ectopic pregnancy.

Hall and Todd[5] discovered that 200 (or 40%) of 500 patients with the confirmed diagnosis of ectopic pregnancy were seen by medical personnel and initially given another diagnosis. Many times the complaints associated with an ectopic pregnancy bring to mind pelvic inflammatory disease (PID) or menstrual cramping. It is very important to determine the location of the pain experienced by the patient at the onset of symptoms. The pain associated with ectopic pregnancy is initially localized and unilateral, usually described as intermittent and crampy. As the pregnancy progresses, the tube ruptures or abortion occurs from the fimbriated end, causing diffuse pain across the entire lower abdomen and pelvis. If rupture and hemoperitoneum have occurred, palpation elicits severe pain with rebound tenderness throughout the lower abdomen. The complaint of shoulder pain during examination, especially while the patient is in the supine position, strongly suggests the presence of a significant hemoperitoneum.

The uterus is of normal size or, if enlarged, smaller than gestational dates would indicate. The increase in size of the uterus during an ectopic pregnancy is caused by increased vascularity rather than by hypertrophy. The cervix undergoes minimal changes and almost never attains the soft texture typical of an intrauterine pregnancy. There may be pain on cervical motion (Chandelier's sign), especially if intraperitoneal hemorrhage has occurred. Cul-de-sac fullness or bulging sometimes can be palpated, but an adnexal mass is only found in 40% to 50% of patients.

Speculum examination may be normal or may reveal a reddish-brown discharge caused by the sloughing of the decidua. Abnormal vaginal bleeding associated with ectopic pregnancy most likely follows the event that disrupted the tubal implantation site. The endometrial mucosa responds to the hormonal stimulus of pregnancy by forming decidua that will continue to grow until the embryo dies. Once the embryo dies, the decidual cast is shed and passed vaginally, often mistaken for an aborted fetus. It may be detected only on the pathology report that a decidual cast rather than an aborted fetus was passed.

Any patient with a small uterus and irregular vaginal bleeding should undergo sonography if any suspicion of ectopic pregnancy exists, even in the face of a negative pregnancy test result. Although a positive pregnancy test result confirms the diagnosis of pregnancy, further localization of the pregnancy can be attempted by sonogram. At or about the fifth week, a gestational sac with a fetal pole can usually be visualized. An embryonic mass with cardiac motion is usually apparent by the seventh week.

A negative culdocentesis may rule out hemoperitoneum but not the possibility of an ectopic pregnancy. Aspiration of blood—clotting or nonclotting—along with the clinical picture of an ectopic pregnancy, mandates further evaluation by laparoscopy, sonography, or exploratory laparotomy.

PELVIC INFLAMMATORY DISEASE

PID is a polymicrobial infection that involves the cervix and endometrium, resulting in infection of the fallopian tubes and ovaries. It is the most common serious infection found among reproductive-age women.[1] The most frequently found causative pathogens include *Neisseria gonorrhoeae, Chlamydia, Peptostreptococcus,* and *E. coli.*[4]

Chlamydial infection is now one of the most common sexually transmitted diseases that can cause PID. Chlamydia was isolated from the fallopian tubes or cervix in 20% to 40% of the women with salpingitis confirmed by laparoscopy in a study done in the United States and Sweden.[10] It has been suggested that chlamydia may cause salpingitis that is clinically subacute but severe enough to cause tubal damage. Risk factors include:

1. History of previous PID
2. History of sexual activity with multiple partners
3. Use of IUD for birth control
4. Any recent instrumentation of the uterine cavity or cervix, such as endometrial biopsy or curettage
5. Chlamydia and other sexually transmitted diseases, such as syphilis and gonorrhea

Few physical examination findings are specific for salpingitis. A patient may present with a variety of clinical symptoms. Symptoms are usually noticed during the menstrual cycle from ovarian activity. Onset of pain frequently occurs after a menstrual flow. Uterine bleeding abnormalities are unusual. GI symptoms such as nausea and anorexia are common and may suggest appendicitis or viral gastroenteritis, which will always enter into the differential diagnosis of abdominal pain. Symptoms include lower abdominal pain with possible rebound tenderness, cervical motion tenderness, and adnexal tenderness. The patient will appear to have discomfort during ambulation, causing a slow gait often referred to as the "PID shuffle."

Discharge of pus from the fallopian tubes onto the adjacent peritoneal tissues or around the liver may cause a more localized pain of pelvic peritonitis with rebound tenderness or perihepatitis (Fitz-Hugh–Curtis syndrome). A micropurulent discharge from the cervix is commonly found; it may be foul-smelling, depending on the causative agent. Fever may be present, and the white blood cell (WBC) count increased, but it is not uncommon for the patient to be afebrile or have a normal WBC count.

Findings of a unilateral or bilateral adnexal or cul-de-sac mass strongly suggest the presence of a tubo-ovarian abscess or pelvic abscess. Tuboovarian or pelvic abscess is a frequent complication among patients with acute salpingitis, especially when treatment has been delayed. PID is usually a bilateral process, but the development of an abscess is primarily unilateral. Abscess formation usually occurs in patients in the 30- to 40-year-old range but may be seen at any time during the reproductive years.[4] The challenge is to determine if the abscess has ruptured. In the absence of rupture or leakage, nonsurgical management with the appropriate antibiotic therapy is successful in 33% to 74% of cases.[7] Leakage or rupture of a tuboovarian abscess is a surgical emergency.

The clinical picture of a ruptured pelvic abscess is highly variable. Fever is usually present, but may be only of low grade. Among 57 patients with the confirmed diagnosis of ruptured abscess, 35% were afebrile and 23% had a normal WBC.[4] In the absence of rupture, careful examination usually demonstrates that any signs of peritonitis become more intense as palpation approaches the pelvic brim and significantly increases in intensity deep in the pelvis. When the intensity of the peritonitis increases as palpation progresses away from the pelvic brim, especially on the right side, it is circumstantial evidence that the inflammatory process is coming from an intraabdominal source, rather than a pelvic source. In some instances, the patient will demonstrate a full picture of shock. During the operative and postoperative phases, large fluid shifts into the peritoneal space are common. A postoperative ileus is expected and usually requires nasogastric drainage.

OVARIAN CYSTS

Two types of ovarian cysts normally occur with each menstrual cycle. In the first 2 weeks, follicular cysts occur; in the second 2 weeks, the corpus luteum is present. The corpus luteum of pregnancy persists through the first month, secreting progesterone. Ovarian cysts are almost asymptomatic until complications such as torsion, rupture, or hemorrhage ensue.

In most cases, the symptoms will begin at or after ovulation, with pain as the main presenting symptom. Rupture of an ovarian cyst is frequently associated with exercise or intercourse, causing a sudden, sharp, well-defined unilateral pelvic pain. Timing in the menstrual cycle can give a clue to the type of cyst that ruptures. A follicular cyst rupture occurs mid-cycle with the extrusion of the ovum from the ovary and may be accompanied by slight bleeding from the surface of the ovary. This is referred to as *mittelschmerz* and is experienced by as many as 25% of all ovulating women.[7] A rupture of the corpus luteum cyst exhibits the same clinical picture, except that it occurs just before the onset of menses.

Ovarian cysts can also be endometriotic in nature, meaning that there are endometrial implants within the ovary itself. Ectopic endometrial tissue responds to hormonal stimulation just like normal endometrial tissue. During the latter half of the menstrual cycle, the endometrial tissue proliferates and may cause a steadily progressing ache.

Duration and severity of the pain experienced when an ovarian cyst ruptures are directly related to the contents of the cyst. The rupture of an endometrial cyst will cause the spread of "chocolate fluid," which results in severe, prolonged pelvic pain caused by the chemical peritonitis that will occur. The pain caused by the rupture of a functional serous cyst usually resolves spontaneously and requires only observation and reassurance. The rupture of an endometrial cyst often requires exploratory laparotomy and peritoneal cleansing.

Ovarian hemorrhage is intraovarian or extraovarian in nature. Intraovarian hemorrhage distends the ovarian capsule, causing sharp, unilateral pain. Extraovarian hemorrhage, caused by rupture, results in bilateral pelvic pain caused by the resultant hemoperitoneum.

The presence of hemorrhagic shock depends on the size of the torn vessel. On occasion, the hemorrhage is severe enough to produce abdominal distention and hypovolemic shock. If the patient is hemodynamically unstable, laparotomy is necessary to ligate the bleeding vessel. Pain resulting from the rupture of a blood-filled corpus luteum is often indistinguishable from signs and symptoms associated with a ruptured ectopic pregnancy or a ruptured ovarian cyst.

OVARIAN TORSION

Torsion of a normal fallopian tube or ovary around the vascular pedicle is possible, but it more often involves a pathologically large simple cyst. The onset of pain is often sudden and may be intermittent. There may be a dull ache with sharp exacerbations. Associated nausea and vomiting occur simultaneously with the onset of pain, whereas nausea and vomiting precede the pain in the case of appendicitis. It is important to keep in mind that the patient may not appear acutely ill early in the course of the event.

Findings on physical assessment vary from slight unilateral lower abdominal tenderness to signs of frank peritonitis. The pain described may be out of proportion to the physical findings. Most patients exhibit cervical motion tenderness. A mass may not be discernible at first but may become easily palpable when occlusion of venous drainage occurs, resulting in edema.

Diagnostic laparoscopy is usually required to make the diagnosis of ovarian torsion, but once the diagnosis is made, laparotomy is required. The consequences of a missed diagnosis, or a tardy one, will vary from scarred fallopian tube to necrosis of the ovary with peritonitis and shock.

TOXIC SHOCK SYNDROME

Although toxic shock syndrome (TSS) is not usually considered a true gynecologic event, it is discussed in this chapter because of the high incidence of TSS associated with the use of tampons.

TSS was first described by Todd in 1978 as a clinical syndrome involving the development of a high fever, myalgias, rash, and hypotension.[9] This syndrome is thought to be caused by toxins produced by *Staphylococcus aureus*. After the initial report was published, the Centers for Disease Control reported 55 cases of TSS in 13 states over the next 2 months.[10] Most of the cases involved menstruating women, with a fatality rate of 13%.[11] The outbreak was associated with the use of super-absorbent tampons, but since the removal of Rely brand tampons from the market in 1980, the number of cases has decreased.

The incidence of TSS is still highest in menstruating women, but TSS has been known to occur in a wide variety of clinical conditions, including surgical infections, nasal packing, postpartum infections, diaphragm use, burns, and many other conditions. *S. aureus* has been isolated in virtually all cases of menstrual and nonmenstrual TSS.

The patient presents with a 1- to 4-day history of fever, chills, myalgias, vomiting, diarrhea, headache, and hypotension. Nonpitting edema of the face, eyelids, and the extremities is also frequently observed. A diffuse rash described as similar to a sunburn is usually present with the initial presentation but usually fades in about 3 days.

Hypotension or orthostatic changes are seen in all patients with TSS by definition. This is thought to be caused by gastrointestinal losses, vasodilatation, and third-space effect. Pelvic examination may reveal a malodorous discharge along with the menstrual flow. Bilateral adnexal tenderness may also be present.

There is no definitive test for TSS, and the diagnosis is based on clinical criteria. Management includes hemodynamic support and removal of the source of the infection. Fluid resuscitation should be accomplished with crystalloids. Dopamine, dobutamine, or epinephrine may be needed to support the blood pressure if there is no response to fluid resuscitation.

Definitive patient management may require invasive hemodynamic monitoring along with ventilatory support. Antistaphylococcal antibiotics are indicated to decrease the incidence of recurrence, but treatment of TSS is directed mainly at fluid resuscitation and supportive care.

TRANSPORT CONSIDERATIONS

Expedient evaluation and preparation are always indicated to ensure that the patient receives definitive care in a timely manner. The priorities when transporting a patient experiencing a gynecologic emergency are to first ensure a patent airway and then maintain adequate oxygenation and circulation. Preparation for transport should include the following:

1. Oxygen administration
2. Pulse oximetry
3. At least two large-bore IV lines
4. PASG suit in place, inflated if indicated
5. Cross-matched blood, if available, for infusion en route, if necessary

Although the patient may be hemodynamically stable at the time of the initial evaluation, frequent reassessment is imperative. In transit, frequent evaluation of vital signs and level of consciousness will alert the flight nurse to any changes in the hemodynamic status of the patient and permit immediate intervention. One of the most common complications during transport is hypovolemic shock. Being prepared with large-bore IV lines and the PASG will allow for immediate intervention in the event of shock.

Most patients requiring transport because of a gynecologic emergency experience varying degrees of abdominal pain. It is important that the symptoms not be masked by the injudicious use of analgesics. The patient will benefit from frequent reassurance and the use of comfort measures. If narcotic analgesia is indicated, small doses of IV narcotics should be administered.

Transport in Fowler's position will minimize the spread of peritoneal irritation and infection, especially in the instance of PID or ruptured ovarian abscess. If the patient has experienced any nausea or vomiting, placement of a nasogastric tube will minimize the incidence of vomiting and help protect the airway.

If pregnancy enters into the diagnosis and the patient is known to be Rh negative, RhoGam administration should be considered. Antibiotic therapy, once instituted, must be maintained and the patient observed closely for allergic reaction.

The results of all diagnostic studies and assessments made before transport, along with records of any interventions, should be copied and transported with the patient. Complete records of the patient's status before transport and in transport will aid in maintaining continuity and quality of care.

SUMMARY

Immediate intervention and expedient transport to a facility able to provide definitive care can mean the difference between continued reproductive capabilities and impaired fertility or possible death.

GYNECOLOGIC EMERGENCIES CASE STUDY

A 34-year-old woman went to a small clinic for the evaluation of bilateral low abdominal pain that had been increasing in severity for approximately 24 hours. On further questioning, it was established that the pain had initially been located mainly on the right side but was thought to be cramping that the patient often experienced at the onset of her menstrual period.

The patient had been experiencing irregular menstrual periods for the last several years and was unsure of the exact date of her last menstrual period. She was sexually active and used a diaphragm and spermicidal jelly for birth control. Her past gynecologic history was negative for ectopic pregnancies or PID, but she had used an IUD for 2 years in her early twenties. Her only pregnancy, 6 years previously, resulted in a normal vaginal delivery without complications.

The patient's initial physical evaluation revealed a well-nourished woman in moderate distress with diffuse pain across the lower abdomen. The speculum examination was negative for cervical discharge or bleeding. The examiner was unable to palpate an adnexal mass, but the patient experienced a significant increase in pain when the cervix was moved.

When the patient stood, her blood pressure was 112/86 mm Hg; and her pulse, 102 beats/min. She did experience slight dizziness and nausea. Laboratory studies revealed HCG, with hemoglobin and hematocrit within normal limits. Sonography was not available at this facility, and it was decided to transport the patient by helicopter to a hospital for further evaluation and possible laparotomy for a suspected ectopic pregnancy.

On arrival of the flight crew, the patient was given one IV infusing and initial fluid challenge of 300 ml of lactated Ringer's solution. The evaluation by the flight nurse revealed that the patient was still experiencing diffuse lower abdominal pain and was also complaining of an aching in her shoulders. Her systolic blood pressure remained between 110 and 118 mm Hg, and her pulse was 100 to 110 beats/min while she was supine. Physical examination revealed neurologic status was normal, and the skin was warm and dry. Capillary refill time was less than 2 seconds, and peripheral pulses were easily palpated in all extremities.

A second large-bore IV line was started, and the patient was given another fluid challenge of 500 ml. The PASG was placed on the patient but not inflated. Because the patient was experiencing an increasing amount of nausea, especially on movement, a nasogastric tube was inserted. The patient was then loaded into the helicopter. Oxygen was started by nasal cannula at 4 L/min. The patient's blood pressure and pulse were checked every 5 minutes. The nasogastric tube was attached to low suction and kept patent.

The flight was 20 minutes long. Eight minutes before landing, the patient's blood pressure dropped to 70 mm Hg systolic. Both IV lines were immediately opened, and the patient was given another fluid challenge of 500 ml and given high-flow oxygen by nonrebreather mask. Her blood pressure responded to the fluid administration and remained over 100 mm Hg systolic for the duration of the flight.

On arrival at the receiving facility, the patient was briefly evaluated and then taken to the operating room. Laparotomy revealed a ruptured ectopic pregnancy with a significant hemoperitoneum. The patient had a stable recovery and was discharged from the hospital several days later.

REFERENCES

1. Brown MA: Diseases causing abdominal pain. In Parker JG, editor: *Emergency nursing: guide to comprehensive care,* New York, 1984, John Wiley & Sons.
2. Buckley K, Kulb NW: *High risk maternity nursing manual,* Baltimore, 1993, Williams & Wilkins.
3. Budassi D, Barber J: *Mosby's manual of emergency care, practices and procedures,* St Louis, 1984, Mosby.
4. Burnett LS: Gynecological causes of acute abdomen, *Surg Clin North Am* 68:2, 1984.
5. Honigmen B: Pelvic pain. In Rosen P, editor: *Emergency medicine concepts and clinical practice,* St Louis, 1988, Mosby.
6. Landers DV, Sweet RL: Tubo-ovarian abscess: contemporary approach to management, *Rev Infect Dis* 5:876, 1983.
7. Musick JR: Gynecologic emergencies. In Tintinalli J et al, editors: *Emergency medicine: a comprehensive study guide,* New York, 1988, McGraw-Hill.
8. Thomas D, Worthington DS: Toxic shock syndrome: a review of the literature, *Ann Emerg Med* 17:3, 1988.
9. Walters CL et al: Antibodies to *Chlamydia trachomatis* and risk for tubal pregnancy, *Am J Obstet Gynecol* 159:4, 1988.
10. Wright SW, Trott A: Toxic shock syndrome: a review, *Ann Emerg Med* 17:3, 1988.
11. Young G: Pelvic pain. In Rosen P, editor: *Emergency medicine: concepts and clinical practice,* St Louis, 1988, Mosby.

CHAPTER 33

Obstetric Emergencies

COMPETENCIES

1. Perform a focused assessment of the pregnant patient, which includes collecting subjective and objective data related to the patient's pregnancy.
2. Perform a focused assessment of the fetus before and during transport.
3. Initiate appropriate interventions for the patient in preterm labor.

Complications that arise during pregnancy and place the obstetric patient at risk have many causes. Some complications may be related to the pregnancy itself, others are related to preexisting medical conditions that may be aggravated by the pregnancy, and yet others may be related directly to the fetus.

Flight nurses who provide care for the obstetric patient at risk must be prepared to assess obstetric factors so that stabilizing care can be provided in preparation for transport. The well-being of the fetus as well as the mother must be considered. Identification of risk factors, early detection of possible complications, and interventions by the flight nurse during the transport can ensure a more favorable outcome for both the mother and the fetus. The flight nurse must be prepared to perform a general obstetric assessment, determine strategies for transport, perform fetal monitoring, and intervene as the situation requires. Complications discovered can include amniotic fluid embolism, delivery complications, diabetes in pregnancy, hemorrhagic complications, multiple gestation, pregnancy-induced hypertension (PIH) and related disorders, preterm labor (PTL) and related issues, and trauma in pregnancy.[4] The information gained by the general obstetric assessment (box) will aid the flight nurse in setting priorities for nursing care during the transport.[2,3,7,11]

GENERAL OBSTETRIC ASSESSMENT

1. Age of patient: Age (for teenagers and women over age 35 years) predisposes the obstetric patient to many complications.
2. Gravida/para: How many times has the patient been pregnant? How many deliveries has she had at or beyond 20 weeks gestation? (Parity is not greater if twins are delivered or less if the fetus is stillborn.)
3. Estimated date of confinement (EDC): The EDC can be estimated from the first day of the last menstrual period (LMP) by using Nägele's rule: Count back 3 months from the LMP and then add 7 days. The due date is accurate within 2 weeks.
4. Ultrasound: Has the patient had an ultrasound? How many? In the event of an uncertain or unknown LMP or irregular menses, an early ultrasound performed between 12 and 30 weeks is reliable for dating the pregnancy within 2 weeks. An ultrasound can confirm the EDC estimated by the LMP. An ultrasound is invaluable if there is any question about placental location, amount of amniotic fluid present, fetal presentation, expected fetal growth, or anomalies.
5. In addition to inquiry into medical history and allergies, obstetric history is of particular significance. The following information may be of some predictive value for the outcome of the current pregnancy:
   a. Did the patient deliver vaginally or by cesarean section? Has she had a vaginal birth after a cesarean section? Observe for the location and extent of any abdominal scars.
   b. Did she herself or the baby experience any delivery complications?
   c. Did she experience any complications associated with any past pregnancies?
   d. Has she had any preterm deliveries? At what gestation did she deliver, and what was the outcome?
   e. Has she had either spontaneous or elective abortions? Was a dilation and curettage required?
   f. How many living children does she have? What were the birth weight and sex of each child?
   g. Has there been less than 1 year between the last delivery and commencement of the current pregnancy?
   h. What was the length of her last labor?
6. Pertaining to the current pregnancy:
   a. Is the patient having contractions? If so, when did the contractions begin? Has there been a change in the intensity or frequency of contractions? Is there accompanying backache, pelvic, or rectal pressure?
   b. Is any vaginal bleeding or "bloody show" present? Is there active bleeding? Attempt to help the patient quantify the bleeding by the number of towels, pads, or amount of clothing soaked before arrival and observe for evidence of dried blood on the perineum, legs, and soles of the feet. Was the bleeding painless or associated with contractions or abdominal pain? Was the blood bright red or dark? Was mucus combined with the blood (bloody show)? When did the bleeding begin? Was there any previous activity that may have precipitated the bleeding?
   c. Does the patient believe her "bag of waters" has ruptured? Was there a gush or an intermittent trickle? A small leakage of clear fluid may be confused with urinary incontinence. leakage of amniotic fluid is uncontrollable. What time did it happen? What color was the fluid—meconium-stained, dark (presence of blood in the fluid), or clear? Was an odor present? Is the chux under the patient wet or pooling with fluid?
   d. Does the patient smoke? If so, how much? Is there any evidence of alcohol or substance abuse? Attempt to ascertain from the patient the frequency and time of last usage.
   e. Has the patient had an adequate weight gain? Does she appear malnourished or obese?

Continued.

GENERAL OBSTETRIC ASSESSMENT—cont'd

f. Has the patient had consistent prenatal care, no prenatal care, or limited prenatal care (three or fewer visits)?
g. Has there been any change in fetal activity in the past several days?
h. Is the patient currently taking any medications? If so, what is she taking and when was the last dosage?
i. Is the patient having any current medical problems or problems with this pregnancy?
j. Have any diagnostic tests been done?

7. Assess initial vital signs, including temperature; the blood pressure (BP), pulse, and respirations should be assessed every 15 minutes or as indicated. The obstetric patient should be positioned in the left lateral recumbent position before the BP is taken. When the patient is in the supine position, the gravid uterus may cause obstruction of the inferior vena cava, diminishing venous return to the heart, and this may lead to supine hypotension. Consequently, uteroplacental blood flow is decreased, placing the fetus at risk for compromise.
8. Fetal heart tones (FHT): If the patient is currently being monitored with electronic fetal monitoring (EFM), evaluate the fetal heart rate (FHR) baseline and variability, observing for accelerations and decelerations. FHR should be assessed by Doppler if EFM is unavailable. FHR auscultations should be assessed every 15 minutes or less if any irregularities are noted. For strip interpretation, refer to the discussion in this chapter on fetal monitoring.
9. Fundal height (FH): FH should be measured in centimeters from the symphysis to the fundus. The fundal height roughly correlates to the gestation of the pregnancy in weeks. In the presence of hydramnios, multiple gestation, a large-for-gestation fetus, or a fetus with intrauterine growth retardation, the fundal height may not correlate with the gestation, signaling the possibility of complications.
10. Lightly palpate the fundus for strength, frequency, and duration of contractions. The fingertips can indent the fundus freely with mild contractions and slightly with moderate contractions; firm tension will be noted with strong contractions. Between contractions, palpate the abdomen for localized or generalized tenderness and observe the patient's coping response to the contractions. Gestures, posture, and facial expressions in response to contractions as well as verbal description should be noted. If the patient is in labor, observe for indications of advancing labor such as apprehension, restlessness, increasing difficulty coping with the contractions, screaming, nausea and vomiting, bearing-down effort, increase in bloody show, or a bulging perineum.
11. Roughly determine the fetal position by abdominal palpation: With the fingertips and palms, lightly palpate the fundus for the head or buttocks, moving down the sides to identify the fetal spine and small parts, and palpate the lower uterine segment for the presenting part. If the fetal position remains unclear, the fetus may be in a transverse lie. The FHT will be heard most clearly over the fetal spine.
12. Assess cervical status as indicated by the presence of contractions. If the amniotic membranes are intact, cervical status just before departure should be documented. If the membranes are ruptured, a sterile vaginal examination (SVE) should never be attempted unless delivery is deemed imminent. In the presence of hemorrhage, an SVE should never be attempted unless a placenta previa has been ruled out by ultrasound. During transport, an SVE is not indicated unless signs of advancing labor are noted.
13. Observe for the presence of other risk factors that predispose the obstetric patient to complications.

GENERAL STRATEGIES FOR TRANSPORT

The primary survey and obstetric physical assessment can be completed in a very short time. Pertinent information obtained from the patient may be gathered as the situation permits during the course of the transport. In a life-threatening situation for either the mother, the fetus, or both, life-saving measures must take precedence. During transport, the flight nurse should perform the following assessments and interventions[9]:

1. Place the patient in a left lateral recumbent position or displace the uterus with a wedge if the patient cannot be turned. By displacing the uterus from the inferior vena cava, venous return to the heart is improved.
2. Note the patient's temperature. If possible, assess vital signs every 15 minutes.
3. Note fetal heart tones (FHTs). Initiate continuous electronic fetal monitoring (EFM) if available, or use a Doppler for fetal heart rate (FHR) assessment at least every 15 minutes. Note fetal movement and any contractions.
4. Start an intravenous line with a large-bore 18- or 16-gauge catheter and blood tubing. Use lactated Ringer's solution with an infusion rate of up to 125 ml/hr depending on hydration and renal, cardiac, and pulmonary status.
5. Provide supplemental oxygen with use of a face mask as indicated by FHR pattern or maternal condition.
6. Monitor oxygen status by pulse oximetry, maintaining a level of 98% to 100%.
7. Assess uterine contractions and cervical status.
8. Note and quantify any bleeding or leaking of fluid.

Emotional and psychological support provided to the obstetric patient at risk and her family is as vital an aspect of flight nursing as the emergency care provided. The flight nurse should encourage the patient to express and verbalize her anxiety, fear for the fetus, and concern regarding the complications she is experiencing. The flight nurse should assess the patient's knowledge of the situation, encourage questions, and use the opportunity for patient education. The vocabulary used should be based on the education and employment background of the patient. Because most patients have never been transported by air ambulance, the flight nurse should explain all medications, procedures, and equipment to allay apprehension about the unfamiliar circumstances. The flight nurse should also reassure family members about the current condition of the patient and answer any questions they may have regarding the diagnosis, treatment, or destination.

FETAL MONITORING

Fetal monitoring may be accomplished by intermittent Doppler auscultation, which is used most frequently for short transports, and by EFM, used for longer transports (approximately 30 minutes or longer in duration). An external ultrasonographic device records FHTs, and a tocodynamometer detects uterine activity.[8]

Assessment of fetal well-being is best accomplished through the use of EFM. FHTs are recorded simultaneously with uterine activity. Subtle changes in the FHT are often the earliest indication of hypoxia caused by uteroplacental insufficiency or umbilical cord compression.

Recognition of normal FHR tracing permits abnormalities to be realized quickly; appropriate intervention should be aimed at correcting or alleviating the source of insult. Baseline FHR (the average FHR) during a 10-minute period should be between 120 and 160.

Fetal Heart Rate Abnormalities

Variability

Fluctuations in the FHR reflect an interplay between the sympathetic and parasympathetic branches of the autonomic nervous system. Normal variability is indicative of an adequately oxygenated autonomic nervous system. Variability is the single most important factor in predicting fetal well-being. Short-term variability is the beat-to-beat irregularity of the FHR and is dominated by the parasympathetic branch; it is described as present or absent. The parasympathetic branch is more susceptible to hypoxia. Absent short-term variability may be the first indicator of possible fetal hypoxia. The presence of short-term variability has been associated with normal acid-base balance at delivery. Long-term variability is the waviness of the FHR tracing and is dominated by the sympathetic branch; it normally varies from 6 to 25 beats above and below the baseline.[10]

Decreased variability (Fig. 33-1), as demonstrated by absent short-term variability or less than 5 beats during a long-term period, may be precipitated by fetal hypoxia, administration of drugs to the mother, smoking, extreme prematurity, and fetal sleep. The fetus will have frequent sleep periods ranging from 20 to 40 minutes. Increased or marked long-term variability of more than 25 beats may be one of the earliest signs of hypoxia.

When an ultrasound transducer is used, a greater degree of variability may be recorded than is actually present. If there is any question regarding the presence of long-term or short-term variability, use of a fetal scalp electrode is recommended. If the patient has intact membranes, is preterm, or has any other condition that contraindicates internal monitoring at the referring facility, the questionable variability should be presumed to be decreased, with interventions made accordingly. When EFM is used during the transport of an obstetric patient, it is external monitoring that will most frequently be used. The flight nurse should keep in mind that a greater degree of variability may be recorded than is actually present when an ultrasound transducer is used. Because short-term variability cannot be accurately documented, it is not evaluated. Special notice of long-term variability and other reassuring signs must be made. The long-term variability can be assessed as present or absent and is reflected in the baseline range.

Periodic Changes

Periodic changes in the FHR occur in response to stimulation, such as fetal movement and uterine contractions. The FHR may accelerate, decelerate, or not respond.

Acceleration (Fig. 33-2). Accelerations above the baseline are usually associated with fetal movement

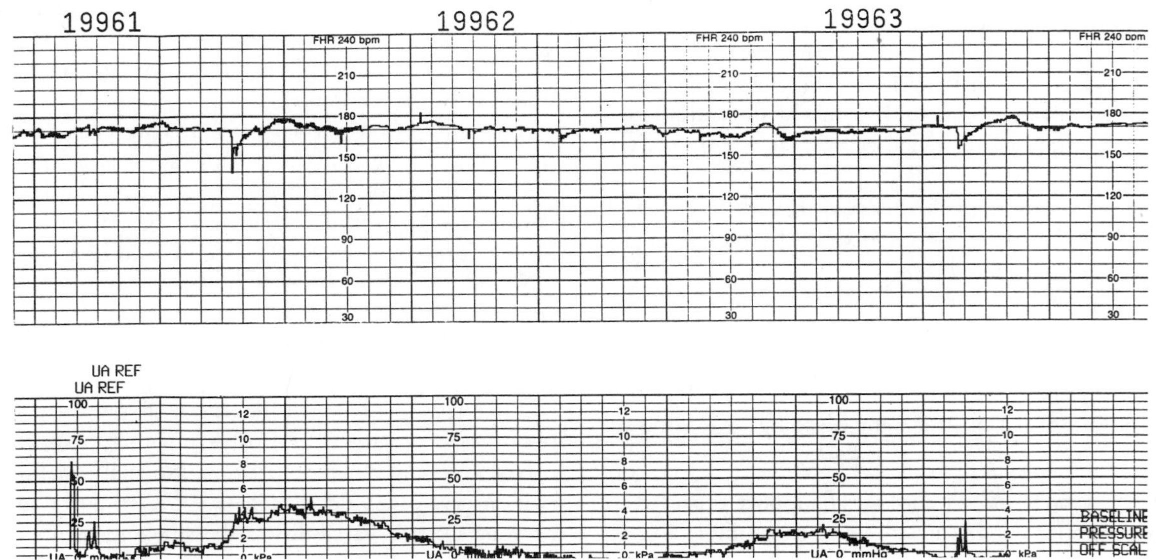

Fig. 33-1. Reduced variability and tachycardia. Note the almost absent beat-to-beat variability and reduced long-term variability as recorded by a fetal scalp electrode; also note the tachycardic baseline.

but may occur during contractions. A hypoxic fetus experiencing metabolic acidosis is unable to accelerate its heart rate. The flight nurse should take note of fetal movements, whether the mother has noticed a decrease, increase, or no change in fetal movement. Decreased fetal movement is indicative of hypoxia.

Variable Deceleration (Fig. 33-3). Variable decelerations can occur at any time during a contraction. The shape may also vary and is frequently V-shaped or W-shaped. Cord compression is responsible for these decelerations, which have a very characteristic appearance; frequently a short acceleration is observed, followed by a rapid deceleration for some seconds, then a rapid rise and a short acceleration, before there is a return to the FHR baseline. Cord compression may occur in a variety of circumstances. After the membranes rupture, there is less fluid to cushion the cord. Variables usually occur in response to uterine contractions but also may occur in response to fetal movement in the absence of contractions when membranes are ruptured. If a nuchal cord, short cord, or cord entanglement is present, variables usually result.

These decelerations have commonly been described as mild, moderate, or severe, depending on the drop in FHR. However, it is more conclusive to describe the deceleration. A better indicator of the fetal response is reflected in the FHR baseline, variability, and changes in the variable decelerations. Signs that the fetus is losing its ability to tolerate the stress of repeated cord compression or that the cord compression is becoming more severe include a deeper deceleration that lasts longer, a slow return to baseline, an "overshoot" increase in FHR baseline immediately after the deceleration, loss of shoulders, and decreased variability, especially short-term variability. In interpreting the tracing, careful observations of any changes in FHT will reveal more than what has just occurred during the last contraction. The flight nurse should look for answers to these questions: Do the variables occur with every contraction? Were they intermittent for some time? Is the variability decreased? Are the decelerations smoother in appearance? Are shoulders now absent? Does it look as if the FHR attempted to accelerate following the variable and that the baseline is grad-

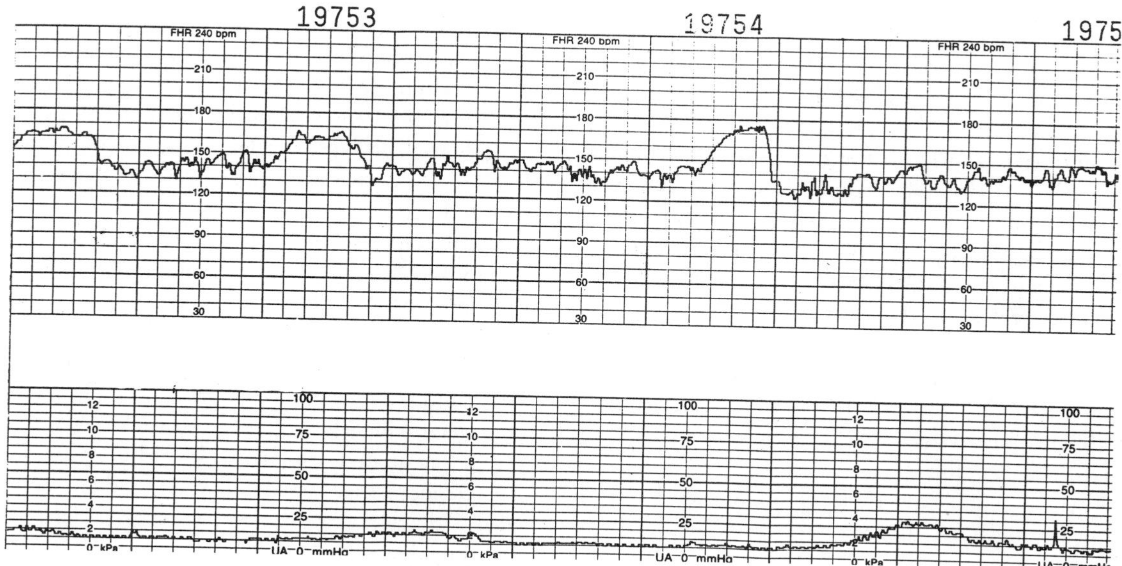

Fig. 33-2. Accelerations. With use of an ultrasound transducer, accelerations of approximately 20 beats above the baseline may be noted. Long-term variability is present, and the FHR baseline range is approximately 135 to 145.

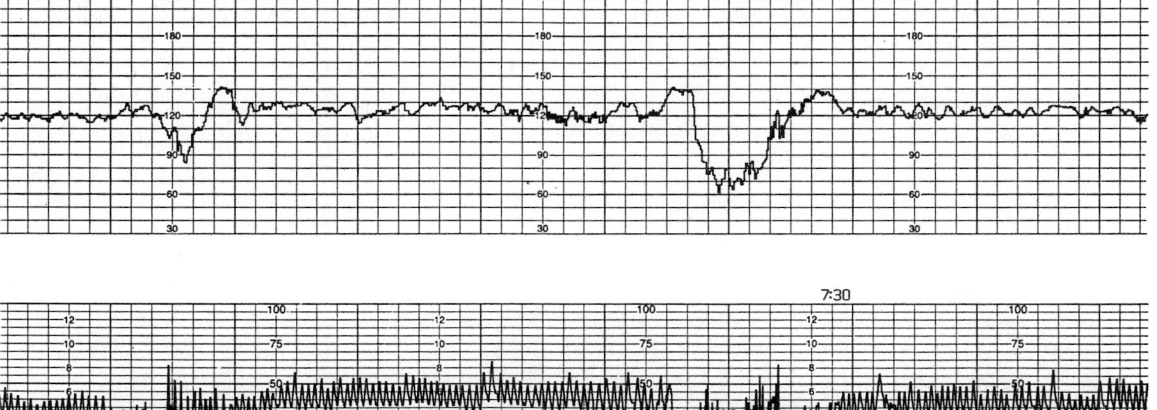

Fig. 33-3. Variable decelerations. Note the variable decelerations in the presence of average variability. The accelerations before and after the deceleration (also called shoulders) are a reflection of adequate variability.

ually rising? Is the FHR drop during the deceleration lasting longer? Is it a deeper drop?

Late Decelerations (Fig. 33-4). In reference to the onset of the deceleration in relation to the contraction, a late deceleration is one that begins close to the apex of the contraction, gradually decelerates, and gradually returns to the FHR baseline after the contraction is over. Late decelerations always mean uteroplacental insufficiency; there is inadequate oxygen exchange within the placenta during a contraction. When a contraction is stronger, the insufficiency is greater and the deceleration is proportional.

With severe hypoxia, the myocardial depression may be such that the heart is unable to decelerate in response to the stress of the contraction, and very subtle late decelerations will be seen accompanied by a flat FHR baseline.

Uteroplacental insufficiency may result from pregnancy-induced hypertension (PIH), diabetes mellitus (DM), cardiovascular or kidney disease, chorioamnionitis, smoking, and a fetus that is past maturity. Uteroplacental insufficiency may also result from decreased placental perfusion in placental abruption or previa, uterine hypertonus as a result of oxytocin stimulation, and hypotension. As with variable decelerations, evaluation of late decelerations with respect to FHR baseline, variability, and changes noted over time is necessary in evaluating the well-being of the fetus. Signs of fetal decompensation include back-to-back decelerations, loss of variability, lack of spontaneous accelerations, tachycardia, and subtle decelerations.

Early Decelerations. Early decelerations are innocuous decelerations that begin very close to the beginning of the contraction, appear almost as a mirror image of the contraction, and end close to the end of the contraction. Head compression with vagus stimulation causes the deceleration. These decelerations frequently occur in active labor when the cervix has dilated 4 to 7 cm. In FHR interpretation, it is essential that late decelerations not be confused with early decelerations. Accurate placement of the tocotransducer over the fundus ensures that contractions are recorded correctly.

Sinusoidal. A uniform sine wave pattern indicates fetal hypovolemia or anemia and may occur in cases

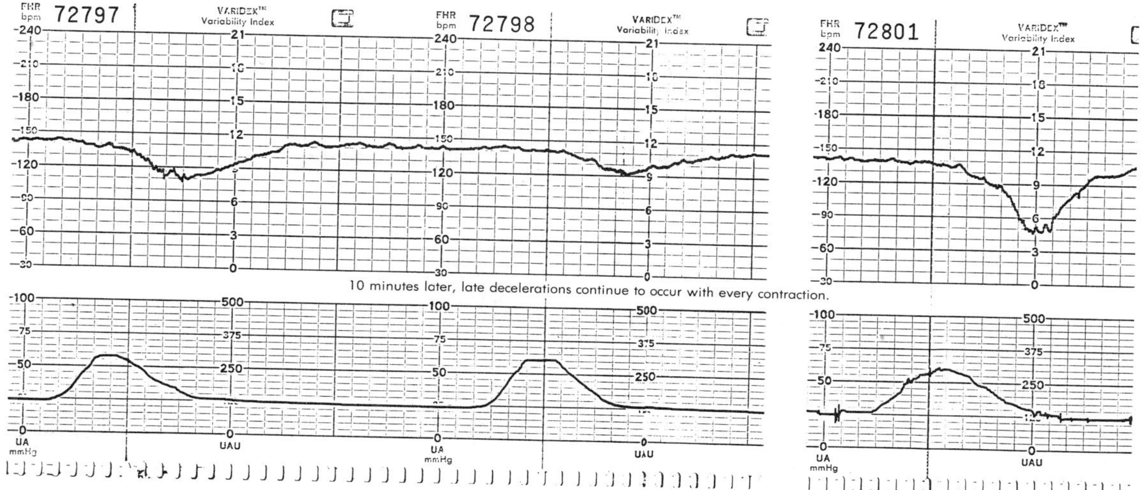

Fig. 33-4. Late decelerations. Note the onset of deceleration at the apex of the contraction. Also note the minimal variability, slow recovery, and the proportional deceleration observed.

of erythroblastosis fetalis, accidental tap of the umbilical cord during amniocentesis, fetomaternal transfusion, placental abruption, or another type of accident. Variability will be absent or minimal, and accelerations are not seen. When this pattern is recognized, rapid delivery is usually recommended. However, a pseudosinusoidal or undulating pattern (Fig. 33-5) may be identified and linked to maternal drug administration.

Bradycardia. An FHR of less than 120 for a period of 5 to 10 minutes or longer is defined as bradycardia. However, many term fetuses and those past maturity may have a stable baseline between 100 and 120, reflecting a more mature fetal neurologic system. In the absence of hypoxia, adequate variability and accelerations will also be noted.

Bradycardia is a response of increased parasympathetic tone and is reflected by a decrease in fetal cardiac output in the presence of hypoxia. The fetus can tolerate sustained bradycardia for only a short length of time before becoming acidotic. Bradycardia can be a result of severe cord compression and can occur minutes before delivery, when the cord is drawn into the pelvis in the second stage, or with a cord prolapse. Bradycardia can also occur with hypertonic or tetanic contractions and maternal hypotension. When it is a result of chronic hypoxia, bradycardia is usually a late occurrence.

Occasionally, a sterile vaginal examination or application of a fetal electrode will induce a prolonged deceleration, caused by vagal stimulation. The deceleration rarely lasts longer than 90 to 120 seconds. Pushing during the second stage of labor may precipitate end-stage bradycardia, which is characterized by a rapid drop in the FHR baseline. Delivery usually follows within a few minutes. Evaluation of variability will determine how the fetus is tolerating the stress.

Tachycardia. An FHR of more than 160 for a period of 10 minutes or longer is considered tachycardia. Tachycardia is a response of increased sympathetic tone and is reflected by a compensatory mechanism to increase cardiac output in the presence of transient hypoxia. A decrease in variability is generally associated with tachycardia. Factors that contribute to tachycardia include smoking, maternal fever, use of β-sympathomimetic agents, fetal anemia, fetal hypovolemia, chorioamnionitis, and maternal hyperthyroidism. Fetal distress is a loose term implying that there are grounds for believing that the fetus is in danger of hypoxia and metabolic acidosis. Late and variable decelerations are sources of stress

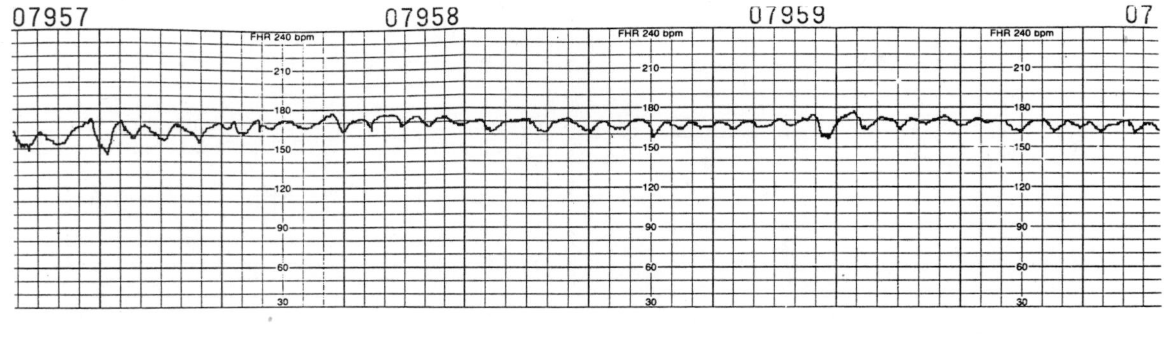

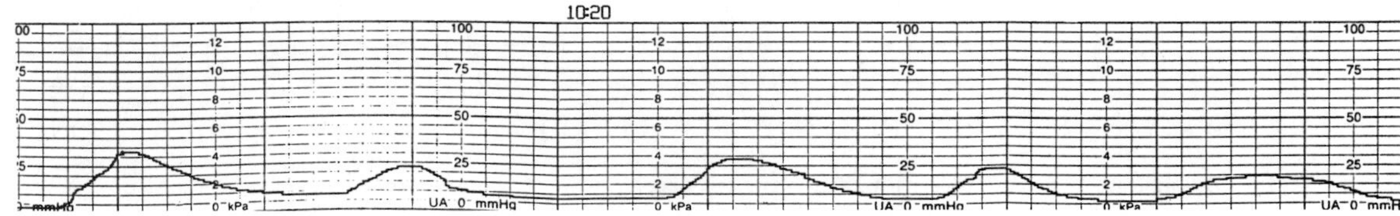

Fig. 33-5. Sinusoidal pattern. Note the jagged, nonuniform pattern observed after intravenous administration of Stadol, 1 mg, which resolved spontaneously after 20 minutes.

to the fetus, whereas variability is an indicator of how the fetus is tolerating the stress. Thus, in ruling out fetal distress, the flight nurse can ask these questions to evaluate the tracing for the following reassuring signs of fetal well-being:

1. Is the baseline FHR within normal range? If so, the fetus is maintaining an adequate cardiac output.
2. Is adequate variability present? If so, the fetus is receiving an adequate oxygen supply.
3. Are any accelerations present? If so, metabolic acidosis can be ruled out.
4. In the presence of tachycardia or bradycardia, is adequate variability present? Are accelerations present? In the presence of late or variable decelerations, assessment of the reassuring signs of fetal well-being can indicate how the fetus is tolerating the stress of the decelerations. If after applying these criteria the flight nurse is not confident of the well-being of the fetus, before considering the transport of the obstetrical patient, scalp stimulation may be attempted (Fig. 33-6).

   Pressure to the fetal scalp with the fingertips may produce a brisk acceleration of the FHR. Accelerations in response to scalp stimulation have been demonstrated only when a normal acid-base balance is present. Fetal response may also be elicited with acoustic or abdominal stimulation.

Nonreassuring signs of fetal well-being include a significant increase or decrease in the FHR baseline during a period of several hours, a wandering baseline, a spontaneous decrease in variability or a decrease in variability as labor progresses, bradycardia or tachycardia with reduced variability, subtle late decelerations, or any combination of these signs.

Abnormal FHR tracings will be observed in situations of congenital anomalies. Frequently, variability will be reduced or absent, and tachycardia or bradycardia may be noted. Table 33-1 summarizes comparative signs of acute and chronic distress. Whatever the mechanism of insult to the fetus, the plan of action when presented with possible fetal distress is intrauterine resuscitation.

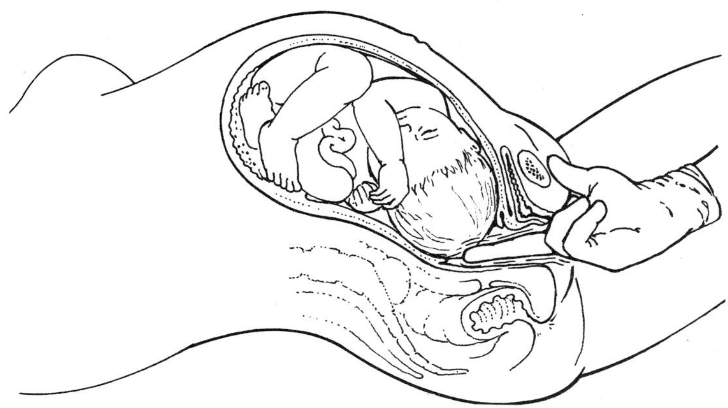

Fig. 33-6. Technique for scalp stimulation.

TABLE 33-1

Comparison of signs of chronic and acute distress

Chronic distress (occurs over time)	Acute distress (occurs suddenly)
MECHANISM OF INSULT	
Uteroplacental insufficiency	Umbilical cord compression or uteroplacental insufficiency
Signs of IUGR, decreased fetal movements	Initially no indication of fetal compromise
CONTRIBUTING FACTORS	
PIH (Preeclampsia)	Cord prolapse
Cardiac or kidney disease	Placental abruption
Severe anemia	Hypotension (vena cava compression, epidural anesthesia, hemorrhage)
DM (Class B-R)	Hypertonic contractions
Post date pregnancy	Placenta previa with hemorrhage
Rh isoimmunization	
Chorioamnionitis	
Smoking	
FETAL RESPONSE (PROGRESSION DIFFERS DEPENDING ON CIRCUMSTANCES)	
Tachycardia	Variable decelerations
Increased variability	Prolonged decelerations
Decreased variability	Tachycardia
Late decelerations	Increased variability
Bradycardia	Decreased variability
	Late decelerations
	Bradycardia

IUGR, Intrauterine growth retardation.

The "Key" formula (LOCK) is as follows:

"L" Place the patient in the left lateral recumbent position;
"O" Provide supplemental oxygen, 100%, with use of a tight face mask, at 8 to 10 L per minute;
"C" Correct or improve contributing factors; and
"K" Keep reassessing the FHR and intervene when indicated.

Contributing Factors to Fetal Distress

Interventions that must be performed by the flight nurse when signs and symptoms of fetal distress are present are as follows:

1. Hypotension: Initiate a 500 ml intravenous fluid bolus, depending on the condition of the patient, or correct for supine hypotension with a change to the left lateral position or uterine displacement, if this has not already been done.
2. Hypertonic or tetanic contractions: Discontinue the oxytocin infusion. Oxytocin has a short half-life of approximately 3 minutes, and circulating levels diminish rapidly. Consider use of terbutaline, 0.25 mg administered subcutaneously or by intravenous push. Check to ensure that the patient's heart rate is under 120 before administering the medication.
3. Rule out cord prolapse. A sterile vaginal examination will confirm the presence of a cord. Lift the presenting part off the cord to relieve the cord compression and reposition the patient, following recommendations provided in this chapter.
4. Assess for placental abruption or other complications that may affect the FHR.
5. Change the position of the mother. If the left lateral position does not relieve the cord compression as indicated by continued variable decelerations, reposition the mother to the right side, to the hands and knees, or, last, to the knee-chest position.

If the patient is located in an outlying area where the transport time is expected to be lengthy, evaluation of the FHT for reassuring signs of fetal well-being will aid in the decision to transport the mother or to deliver the fetus at the referring facility to increase the chance of fetal survival. Likewise, if the transport is expected to be short and the time required by the referring facility to prepare for a cesarean section is longer than the estimated transport time, maternal transport is recommended. The intent of the transport is to attain the most expedient delivery of the fetus in a facility most capable of dealing with the fetus at risk.

The flight nurse may consider use of Doppler auscultations for all rotor-wing transports and EFM for all fixed-wing transports. However, EFM should be considered for rotor-wing transports longer than 30 minutes; it can be beneficial, even when factoring in the presence of turbulence in strip interpretation, for a more significant assessment of fetal well-being.

COMPLICATIONS OF PREGNANCY AND DELIVERY

In the following discussions regarding complications of pregnancy and delivery, it is assumed that a general obstetric assessment and implementation of general guidelines for transport have already been performed, including assessment of fetal well-being.

Amniotic Fluid Embolism

Amniotic fluid embolism occurs when amniotic fluid gains access to the maternal circulation during labor or delivery or immediately after delivery, resulting in obstruction of the pulmonary vasculature. In addition to amniotic fluid, particulate matter in the fluid such as meconium, lanugo hairs, fetal squamous cells, bile, fat, and mucin may also embolize. In the United States, amniotic fluid embolism occurs in 1 in 20,000 to 30,000 deliveries.[1] It is a very rare complication and is frequently fatal, with a maternal mortality rate nearing 90%. Amniotic fluid embolism is probably often misdiagnosed, as indicated by the vague clinical picture of surviving patients and missed autopsy findings in fatal cases.

Etiology and Pathophysiology

The route by which amniotic fluid enters the circulatory system of the mother is not clear. The most frequently suggested sites of entry are lacerations in the endocervical veins during cervical dilation and lacerations in the lower uterine segment, the placental site, and uterine veins at sites of uterine trauma. Under the pressure of uterine contractions, amniotic fluid gains access to the circulatory system of the mother and travels quickly to the pulmonary vasculature, where embolization quickly ensues.

Factors that have been associated with amniotic fluid embolism include uterine rupture, cesarean section, and the use of uterine stimulants to induce labor, which produces hypertonic contractions. Other factors that place the obstetric patient at risk are a large fetus, placenta previa, placental abruption, intrauterine fetal death, meconium in the amniotic fluid, multiparity, precipitous delivery, knee-chest position, and maternal age over 30 years.

Disseminated intravascular coagulation (DIC) is a complication that can be expected, although the pathway is unclear. Uterine atony and postpartum hemorrhage are also frequent complications. Acute cor pulmonale, right heart failure, and pulmonary edema follow.

Assessment

Of the predisposing factors that the patient may have, sudden acute dyspnea is the most characteristic symptom, which is followed by profound cyanosis and sudden shock. Other symptoms may include chest pain, restlessness, anxiety, coughing, vomiting, pulmonary edema with pink, frothy sputum, seizures that are frequently confused with eclamptic seizures, and coma. If the patient has delivered, the flight nurse should watch for symptoms of postpartum hemorrhage caused by uterine atony.

Because of the extremely rare occurrence of amniotic fluid embolism and the rapidity of onset of symptoms with deterioration, the flight nurse may be unsure of the clinical picture. If dyspnea appears in a patient who is in a tumultuous labor with ruptured membranes, it is recommended that amniotic fluid embolism be suspected. Tachycardia, hypotension, and tachypnea indicate the severity of the embolic process. Urine output may be decreased (less than 30 ml/hr), indicating inadequate renal perfusion. Blood is shunted away from the uterus to the vital organs, and FHR changes indicative of placental insufficiency will be observed. Severe fetal distress may be present. DIC can be suspected if petechiae, hematuria, bruising, or bleeding from intravenous sites is observed. Coagulation studies confirm DIC. Chest x-ray films may show infiltrates.

Strategies for Transport

In the event that an obstetric patient with amniotic fluid embolism is transported, supportive care should be provided. Although the clinical picture may not be clear, treatment focuses on the alleviation of presenting symptoms. The flight nurse should provide supplemental oxygen with use of a tight nonrebreather face mask at 10 L and be prepared to intubate if necessary. Positive end-expiratory pressure may be required. The flight nurse can provide circulatory support with additional intravenous fluids and should consider starting a second intravenous line. The flight nurse may initiate blood replacement in an attempt to correct hypovolemia and blood loss. FHTs should be monitored for signs of severe distress.

If the fetus has been delivered, oxytocin, 20 to 40 units, may be added to 1000 ml intravenous solution for uterine atony. Frequent fundal massage should be performed by supporting the lower uterine segment with one hand while massaging the fundus with the other. Morphine, 2 to 5 mg administered intravenously over a 1 to 2 minute period, may be considered for apprehension and dyspnea. The flight nurse should expedite the transport in any way possible; he or she can initiate a patch informing the medical director and receiving hospital of the situation and requesting that immediate physician support be available on arrival.

Delivery Complications

Delivery complications can be predicted in some situations and may be quite unforeseen in others. A neonatal flight nurse should always be included on flights when delivery is a possibility. In this case, a nurse with high-risk obstetrics knowledge or skills would be useful.

The information about assessment and suggested transport care that follows makes specific reference to the complication only. It is assumed that general obstetric assessment and guidelines for transport care will be considered by the flight nurse as well.

Breech Presentation

Presentation refers to the portion of the body of the fetus that is within the bony pelvis or is in closest proximity to it and can be felt through the cervix on vaginal examination. With a breech presentation, the buttocks may descend first, with the legs flexed on the fetal abdomen and the feet alongside the buttocks (complete breech); the legs may also be extended upward (frank breech), or one or both feet or knees may be present (footling or incomplete breech). At or near term, the incidence of breech is 3% to 4%. However, before 34 weeks gestation, the incidence is considerably higher.

Etiology and Pathophysiology. Breech presentation is more likely to occur in situations in which there are uterine abnormalities, such as a septum extending part or all of the way from the fundus to the cervix (septate uterus), or when the uterus is Y-shaped (bicornuate uterus). It is believed that as the pregnancy progresses the uterine cavity provides the most room for the fetus's bulkier and more movable parts, with the extremities in the fundus of the uterus and the cephalic presenting. Before 34 weeks gestation, the head of the fetus is disproportionately larger than the body, favoring the breech presentation. For the same reason, the hydrocephalic fetus has a high incidence of breech presentation.

Other factors that appear to predispose to the breech presentation are grand multiparity, a previous breech delivery, multiple gestation, hydramnios, oligohydramnios, placenta previa, uterine tumors, congenital anomalies, and implantation of the placenta in either fundal region that is close to the fallopian tube.

Complications associated with breech presentation are inherent because of the position of the fetus. With the buttocks and lower extremities presenting, cord prolapse, cord entanglement around the extremities, and cord compression are more likely to occur. When delivery is managed too forcefully, birth trauma may result. Trauma to the fetal cervical spine, and brachial plexus and fractures of the humerus, clavicle, skull, and neck may occur.

The fetus in breech presentation is at higher risk for birth asphyxia (hypoxia, hypercapnia, and metabolic acidosis) compared with the fetus that has a vertex presentation. Head entrapment is a complication that occurs when the buttocks and lower extremities of the premature fetus pass through a cervix that is not completely dilated and is inadequate for the head to be delivered without trauma, asphyxiation, or both for the infant.

Assessment. While the possibility of breech presentation may be determined either through vaginal

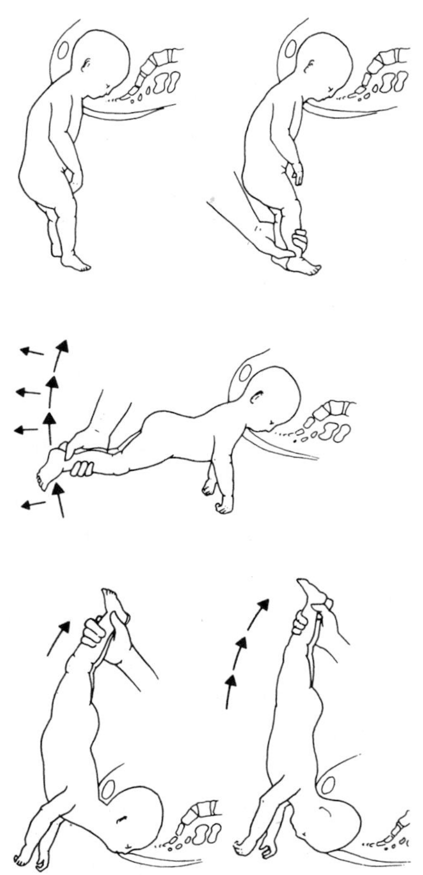

Fig. 33-7. Breech extraction: upward traction to effect delivery of the posterior shoulder, followed by freeing the posterior arm. (From Hickman M: *Midwifery,* ed 2, Oxford, England, 1985, Blackwell Scientific Publications.)

examination or ultrasound, this does not have any bearing on the transport of the obstetric patient unless the patient is in active labor or the membranes are ruptured. Labor is frequently slower with a breech presentation, and thus rapid transport should be considered. In the event that vaginal delivery is inevitable, the flight nurse must be prepared to assist in the delivery. Vaginal delivery is imminent when the buttocks are bulging the perineum and one or both legs are visible.

Strategies for Delivery. Essentially, the fetus in a breech presentation should not be touched until the umbilicus has spontaneously delivered. At that time the lower end of the scapula will be visible. The flight nurse should disengage the legs if one or both have not delivered spontaneously. The cord can be palpated at the umbilicus for the FHR. At this point the arms can usually be delivered by hooking the index finger over each of the baby's shoulders in turn (Fig. 33-7). After the shoulders have been delivered, the baby's trunk is rotated so that the back is anterior, and gentle steady downward traction is applied until the hairline is visible. The body can now rest on the palm of one hand and forearm with the index and middle fingers supporting the baby's mouth and chin to maintain flexion of the head. With the other hand supporting the back and shoulders, the body can then gently be brought upward while another member of the air medical crew applies suprapubic pressure to facilitate the delivery of the head with a minimum amount of neck traction (Fig. 33-8). Care must be taken to achieve slow and controlled delivery of the head, allowing the chin, face, and brow to sweep over the perineum. As soon as the baby's mouth has been delivered, the flight nurse should clear the airway with a bulb syringe and then gently and slowly deliver the rest of the head.

Because breech delivery is a rare occurrence for the flight nurse, there may be a tendency to act in haste when this situation arises. The flight nurse should guard against haste because it increases the risk for birth trauma.

Hemorrhagic Delivery Complications

Once excessive bleeding occurs, it is necessary to move quickly to minimize further blood loss. Postpartum hemorrhage, uterine inversion, and uterine rupture are delivery complications that predispose the patient to hypovolemic shock. In addition to proceeding according to the following specific recommendations, the flight nurse should treat the patient for hypovolemic shock and observe for symptoms of DIC as a complication of hemorrhage.

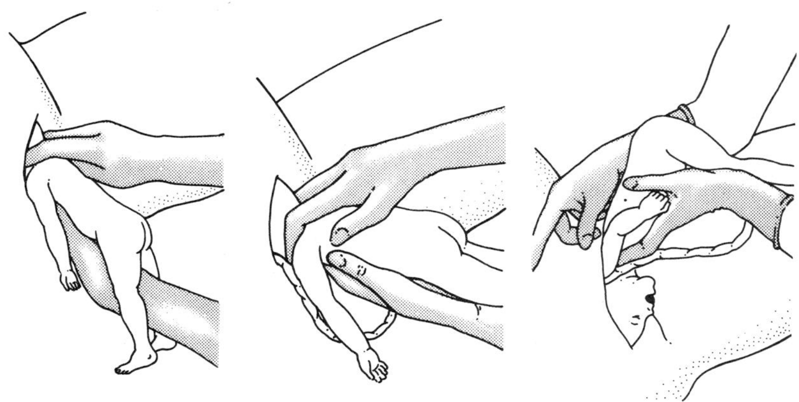

Fig. 33-8. Delivery of aftercoming head with use of Mauriceau's maneuver. Note that as the fetal head is being delivered, flexion of the head is maintained by suprapubic pressure provided by an assistant and simultaneously by pressure on the maxilla *(insert)* by the operator as traction is applied. (From Hickman M: *Midwifery,* ed 2, Oxford, England, 1985, Blackwell Scientific Publications.)

Postpartum Hemorrhage

Blood loss in excess of 500 ml after delivery is defined as postpartum hemorrhage (PPH). The blood loss frequently occurs within the first few hours after delivery but can occur more than 24 hours later. The incidence of PPH occurs in approximately 5% of all deliveries.

Etiology/Pathophysiology. A blood loss of 500 ml or more frequently results from vaginal delivery and is not necessarily an abnormal event. Estimates of blood loss must be accurate. Some studies have shown that estimated blood loss was approximately half the amount actually lost.

Uterine atony is the major cause of postpartum hemorrhage. Normally, bleeding from the placental site is controlled when the interlacing muscle fibers of the uterus contract and retract in conjunction with platelet aggregation and clot formation in the vessels of the decidua. Factors that predispose to uterine atony and prevent compression of the vessels at the implantation site predispose to postpartum hemorrhage. Uterine atony can occur after a prolonged or tumultuous labor or after general anesthetic is used. The uterus that is overdistended as a result of multiple gestation, uterine tumors, hydramnios, or a large fetus is more likely to be hypotonic after delivery. Multiparity, chorioamnionitis, previous PPH, placenta previa, and use of labor stimulants place the obstetric patient at increased risk for uterine atony and PPH.

As the uterus fills with clots, it is increasingly unable to contract and retract normally, compounding the problem of hemorrhage. In addition, when the placenta and membranes are retained the same circumstances are created. An abnormally adherent placenta (placenta accreta) or incomplete separation may be the cause.

Another common cause of PPH is lacerations that result from delivery. Undetected lacerations of the cervix, vagina, perineum, or lower uterine segment are all sources for hemorrhage. Hemorrhage as a result of lacerations is usually limited and is rarely severe. However, constant seepage over a few hours can amount to an appreciable loss. Application of forceps may be the reason for the hemorrhage. When a patient has had a previous cesarean section followed by a vaginal delivery, dehiscence of an old uterine scar with hemorrhage may result. Lacerations should be suspected when hemorrhaging occurs in the presence of a firmly contracted uterus. Coagulopathy associated with DIC, placental abruption, and PIH are other causes of PPH. Idiopathic thrombocytopenia or von Willebrand's disease as preexisting coagulopathies predispose to PPH.

Hemorrhage may also result from a combination of sources. Hemorrhage from uterine atony may be coupled with hemorrhage from a cervical laceration.

Assessment. The flight nurse should determine the source of the hemorrhage. Abdominal palpation may reveal a boggy, enlarged, and soft uterus. Persistent vaginal bleeding from slight to profuse will be noted with uterine atony. The flight nurse should also examine the patient for the presence of lacerations in the perineal, cervical, vaginal, and lower uterine segment.

Strategies for Transport. The flight nurse should palpate and vigorously massage the fundus. One hand should cup the fundus and the other provide support to the lower uterine segment just above the symphysis pubis. Frequently clots will be expressed, and frequent massage alone may be all the stimulation that is required for the uterus to adequately contract and retract. Fundal massage should be performed at least every 5 to 15 minutes, and the location of fundus in relation to the level of the umbilicus, the degree of firmness, and the vaginal flow should be noted.

Rapid infusion of 20 to 40 units of oxytocin in 1000 ml lactated Ringer's solution and/or methylergonovine, 0.2 mg administered intramuscularly or intravenously, is recommended. The flight nurse should use methylergonovine cautiously in patients with PIH because of the pressor effects that may result in further elevated blood pressure.

The integrity of the cervix, vagina, perineum, and lower uterine segment should be documented at the referring facility. Inspection of the placenta after delivery will reveal missing fragments, membranes, or both that may be retained. The flight nurse should assess blood loss and inspect the perineum; little external bleeding will be observed in the presence of a pelvic hematoma. Blood from lacerations tends to be brighter red.

If atony persists, bimanual uterine compression is recommended. To perform this compression, the uterus is compressed between one hand on the abdomen with the other hand clenched as a fist in the vagina; the pressure is maintained for approximately 2 to 5 minutes (Fig. 33-9).

Uterine Inversion

Complete inversion of the uterus occurs when the entire uterus turns inside out, extending out through the cervix and into the vagina, and is visible. The uterus can partially invert with the fundus turned inside out. Partial inversion is not as obvious and may initially be more difficult to determine. The rate of inversion occurs in approximately 1 in 20,000 to 1 in 60,000 deliveries.

Etiology and Pathophysiology

Inversion may occur spontaneously after a contraction or with increased abdominal pressure caused by coughing or sneezing, and it often occurs as the result of overly aggressive management of the third stage of delivery. Predisposing factors include excessive cord traction, fundal pressure, excessive cord traction with a placenta accreta, fundal implantation of the placenta, and uterine atony.

Assessment

Vaginal bleeding, which may be profuse after delivery and accompanied by sudden and severe lower abdominal pain, may be caused by uterine inversion. Abdominal palpation may reveal a defect in the fundus, or it may not be palpable at all, being nonglobular in shape. Signs of hypovolemic shock may develop quickly.

Strategies for Transport

If uterine inversion is recognized immediately before the uterus has had a chance to contract down and the cervix to constrict, manual replacement can generally be accomplished easily. Without attempting to remove the placenta, the flight nurse should apply pressure with the fingertips and palm of the hand to push the fundus upward and through the cervical canal (Fig. 33-10). This procedure can be extremely painful for the patient. The flight nurse should consider administering analgesics and should explain the procedure and the necessity for it to the patient while the attempt at manual replacement is being made.

If the uterus has contracted, a tocolytic agent such as 10 to 20 mg magnesium sulfate administered in-

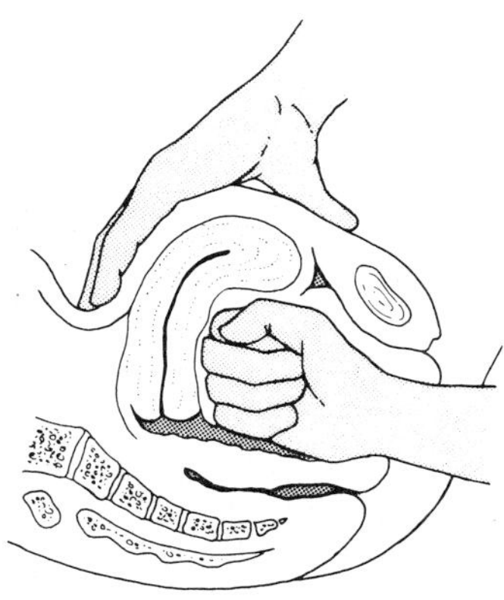

Fig. 33-9. This technique is very invasive; hence, the flight nurse may avoid use of this procedure. It is a last line of action but is usually effective in controlling PPH as a result of uterine atony. Note the placement of the fist in the anterior fornix. (From Hickman M: *Midwifery,* ed 2, Oxford, England, 1985, Blackwell Scientific Publications.)

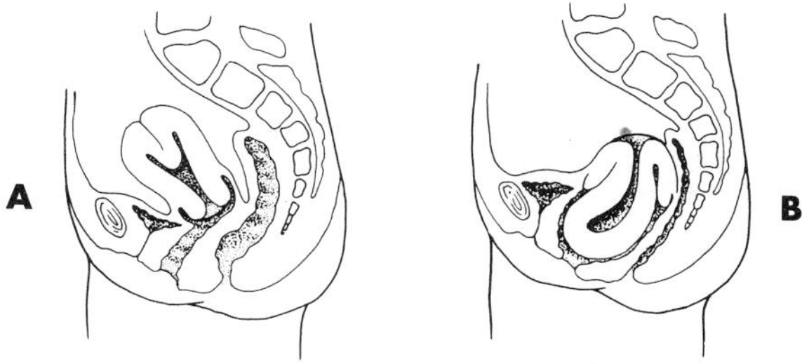

Fig. 33-10. A, First degree; **B,** second degree. Note the abdominal depression where the fundus would normally be and vaginal palpation of the fundus at the cervical opening. Continued pressure with the fingertips will encourage reversion of the fundus. Note the stages of inversion in the inset. (From Hickman M: *Midwifery,* ed 2, Oxford, England, 1985, Blackwell Scientific Publications.)

travenously over a 5-minute period will relax the uterus to allow replacement. If the diagnosis is delayed or if the uterus is difficult to replace, anesthesia and surgical management will be required. Rapid transport is recommended.

Removing the placenta before attempting to replace the uterus may increase the hemorrhaging. The placenta will deliver unless there is some degree of placenta accreta, and oxytocin should be administered immediately. The best preventive measure is allowing spontaneous delivery of the placenta.

Uterine Rupture

A spontaneous or traumatic disruption of the uterine wall, known as uterine rupture, can occur. If the laceration is extensive and comes in direct contact with the peritoneal cavity, it is a complete rupture. The rupture most frequently occurs in a weak area of the myometrium, usually at the site of a previous incision. Uterine rupture occurs in approximately 1 in 100 to 1 in 11,000 deliveries.

Etiology and Pathophysiology

Before further discussion of uterine rupture, it is necessary to differentiate between "rupture" and "dehiscence" of a scar. Rupture refers to the separation of an old incision and possibly an extension into previously uninvolved myometrium, with rupture of membranes. Fetal parts may extend through the rupture into the peritoneal cavity. Hemorrhage is usually present from the edges of the separation and may be massive. A dehiscence does not involve the fetal membranes and may not even involve all of the previous scar. Bleeding may be minimal or bloodless. Dehiscence occurs gradually, whereas rupture occurs as a sudden event. A dehiscence may become a rupture with labor or trauma.

Factors that predispose to uterine rupture include previous surgery involving the myometrium, previous cesarean section with a higher incidence of a "classic" vertical scar being involved, use of labor stimulants, trauma, previous rupture, overdistention of the uterus as a result of multiple gestation or hydramnios, for example, and grand multiparity. Uterine rupture usually occurs during labor but can occur before the onset of labor, with unstimulated labor, with an unscarred uterus, after blunt trauma, or after other internal trauma such as perforation with an instrument or difficult forceps delivery, external pressure such as from an external version of the breech fetus, or overvigorous fundal pressure during delivery attempts.

In situations in which the patient has had a previous cesarean section, the probability of rupture is much greater when the scar traverses the body of the uterus vertically than when the scar involves the lower uterine section transversely. Dehiscence occurs more frequently without subsequent complications when the scar is low and transverse.

The degree of hemorrhage and extent of possible complications depend on the location and extent of the rupture. If the rupture does not involve the large arteries, the hemorrhage will be less severe. If the rupture is complete, the mortality rate for the fetus is high. Postpartum infection, injury to the bladder, sterility as a result of hysterectomy if the rupture is unable to be adequately repaired, hypovolemic shock, kidney failure, DIC, and death may result.

Assessment

Signs and symptoms of uterine rupture include severe, sudden, continual abdominal pain and signs of hypovolemic shock. Contractions may cease or may increase in intensity and frequency. Shoulder or chest pain as a result of the collection of blood under the diaphragm, generalized tenderness with rebound, an abdominal mass with fetal parts easily felt, or vaginal bleeding is likely when the rupture occurs in the lower uterine segment. Most bleeding is intraabdominal, and the abdomen may be distended.

Strategies for Transport

Rapid recognition of the signs and symptoms of uterine rupture will often mean the difference between life and death for the obstetric patient. Surgical intervention is required, and nursing care is supportive. Oxytocin, 20 to 40 units in a 1000 ml solution administered intravenously, may incite uterine contraction with vessel constriction and reduce the bleeding. Serial abdominal measurements can be made to further assess intraabdominal bleeding.

Acute fetal distress with increasingly severe, variable decelerations or absent FHT will be observed.

A history of previous cesarean sections and observation of abdominal scar is of primary importance. Although the scar noted may be low and transverse, documentation is required to determine the location of the scar on the uterus. For the patient in labor who has had a previous cesarean section, the sign of placental abruption may actually be rupture.

Meconium Staining

Meconium staining refers to the presence of meconium in the amniotic fluid. With light meconium staining the fluid is yellow or light green in appearance. With heavy meconium staining the fluid is dark green and may be thick in the presence of oligohydramnios. The incidence of meconium-stained amniotic fluid during labor has been documented in 8% to 22% of all deliveries. Meconium aspiration syndrome develops in approximately 2% of the infants born through meconium-stained fluid.

Etiology and Pathophysiology

Passage of meconium by the fetus has been most frequently associated with a hypoxic event. The fetus responds with hyperperistalsis of the intestine and relaxation of the anal sphincter. Once the meconium has been passed, fetal gasping may lead to meconium aspiration either in utero or at delivery. The FHT may reflect uteroplacental insufficiency with late decelerations, cord compression with variable decelerations caused by oligohydramnios, or both. Bradycardia may be present. Decreased variability indicates a continuing hypoxic insult to the fetus.

Conditions that predispose to meconium staining include postterm pregnancy, preeclampsia, PIH, anemia, cardiovascular or kidney disease, and other complications associated with uteroplacental insufficiency. Situations that cause severe cord compression may also predispose to meconium staining.

Assessment

Once meconium has been observed in the amniotic fluid, intervention is aimed at preventing aspiration or minimizing the insult. Early passage of meconium can be noted when rupture of the amniotic membranes occurs, signifying a hypoxic event, with passage either before the onset of labor or during labor.

Late meconium passage can be noted during the second stage of labor, when the fluid was previously clear; this signifies a later hypoxic event, frequently severe cord compression.

Strategies for Delivery

The incidence of meconium aspiration can be high if the infant's trachea is not immediately suctioned at birth. After delivery the flight nurse must avoid stimulating the infant, because crying may result in aspiration. A DeLee suction device should be available for suctioning of the nares and mouth immediately after delivery of the head so the neonatal flight nurse can visualize the vocal cords and suction the trachea.

Precipitate Delivery

Precipitate delivery occurs when the labor is abnormally rapid with strong contractions and rapid cervical dilation and descent of the presenting part. Delivery usually occurs within 2 hours from the start of contractions. The flight nurse's goal is to prevent an expulsive delivery and minimize trauma to both the mother and the fetus. Possible complications include uterine rupture, amniotic fluid embolism, PPH, and lacerations.

Retained Placenta

Normally, the placenta separates spontaneously within 5 to 20 minutes after delivery of the fetus. Signs of separation include lengthening of the exposed cord and a gush of blood; the uterus appears to "ball up." Slow, gentle, downward traction is usually all that is required to assist the delivery of the placenta. When no signs of separation occur and hemorrhage is not evident, transport can be accomplished with the placenta retained. When the placenta is partially retained, postpartum hemorrhage will result.

Shoulder Dystocia

After delivery of the head, the anterior shoulder pushes against the symphysis, creating a situation commonly referred to as *shoulder dystocia.* The condition becomes apparent when the head is pulled down against the perineum and the shoulders do not follow with gentle traction. The incidence of shoulder dystocia increases significantly with birth weight. The rate of shoulder dystocia is approximately 1 in 333 births for infants weighing between 2500 and 4000 g, 1 in 21 births for infants weighing more than 4000 g, and 1 in 11 births for infants weighing more than 4500 g.

Etiology and Pathophysiology

Several predisposing factors have been linked to shoulder dystocia. However, shoulder dystocia can occur quite unexpectedly without obvious associated factors. The complication occurs more frequently with the presence of a large fetus, a macrosomia fetus of a patient with gestational diabetes, a contracted pelvis, maternal obesity, after a prolonged second stage of labor, or after instrumental delivery following a prolonged second stage of labor.

Possible complications of shoulder dystocia include brachial plexus damage and a fractured fetal clavicle. Fetal hypoxia can occur when the cord is drawn into the pelvis and compressed.

Assessment

In any situation of imminent delivery, unless the fetus is expected to weigh 2500 g or less, shoulder dystocia is a possibility. After the head has been delivered and inspection for a nuchal cord has been performed, the delivery of the anterior shoulder should be accomplished before the nares and mouth are suctioned. Otherwise, precious time may be wasted suctioning before realizing that the shoulder is affected, and because of cord compression, time is of the essence.

Unnecessary haste and overly aggressive force should be avoided because of the increased possibility of birth trauma to the fetus. Excessive lateral flexion of the neck and overly vigorous traction of the head and neck increase the risk of damage to the brachial plexus.

Strategies for Delivery

Once the flight nurse is aware of the situation, he or she may observe the head retract against the perineum. Fundal pressure aggravates the shoulder impaction and should be avoided. If an episiotomy has not been made, a generous mediolateral episiotomy is recommended. A combination of suprapubic pressure applied by another member of the air medical crew (the shoulder can be palpated suprapubicly) and gentle downward traction of the head should be tried first. The flight nurse should not persist if the shoulder does not slip under the symphysis.

The McRoberts maneuver, a simple maneuver that increases the diameter of the pelvis by stretching the pelvic joints, should be tried next. With the patient's legs flexed at the knees, the flight nurse should help the patient draw her knees up and toward the chest (dorsal knee-chest position) and continue, with gentle downward traction of the head. Once the anterior shoulder clears the symphysis, the posterior shoulder usually delivers without resistance.

Delivery of the posterior shoulder can also be attempted by rotation of the posterior shoulder downward and into the left posterior quadrant. With release of the posterior arm and shoulder, the anterior shoulder will follow. As a last resort, the infant's clavicle may be deliberately broken; however, when this is done the chance of damage to the brachial plexus is increased.

Umbilical Cord Prolapse

Overt cord prolapse occurs when the cord slips down into the vagina or appears externally after the amniotic membranes have ruptured. When the cord slips down into or near the pelvis, lying adjacent to the presenting part, it is not palpable on vaginal examination (occult prolapse). The cord may also have slipped down to where it is palpable through the cervix, but within intact membranes (forelying prolapse). Varying degrees of prolapse may occur. Cord prolapse occurs in approximately 1 in 200 deliveries.

Etiology

Circumstances that cause maladaptation of the presenting part to the lower uterine segment or prevent descent of the presenting part into the pelvis predispose the obstetric patient to cord prolapse. These factors include breech presentation, transverse lie, premature rupture of membrane (PROM), a contracted pelvis, unengaged large fetus multiparity, hydramnios, multiple gestation, a long cord, and preterm labor. Complications include severe fetal distress and fetal death.

Assessment

Cord prolapse occurs suddenly and requires quick identification of the problem and quick action. Identifying the obstetric patient who is vulnerable to cord prolapse is of primary importance. Clinical signs of prolapse include sudden fetal bradycardia and/or severe recurrent variable decelerations that do not respond to change in maternal position, administration of oxygen, and hydration. Compression of the cord between the presenting part and the pelvic tissues causes the FHT patterns that are observed.

Strategies for Transport

Actions to take in the event of cord prolapse include elevating the presenting part off the cord with a hand in the vagina to prevent further cord compression and positioning the patient in a Trendelenburg's or knee-chest position to further reduce pressure on the cord. The cord may spontaneously retract, depending on the degree of prolapse, but should never be manually replaced because severe compression may occur. Intervention to elevate the presenting part off the cord must be maintained during the transport.

The flight nurse should provide supplemental oxygen by nonrebreather mask at 8 to 10 L/min. A tocolytic agent, such as terbutaline, 0.25 mg administered subcutaneously or by intravenous push, should be given to slow the contractions and reduce the pressure on the cord during contractions. When the cord compression is relieved the fetus will be able to recover from the hypoxic event in utero as long as the compression does not recur.

If cord prolapse occurs when the patient is en route, the receiving facility should be alerted to prepare for an emergency cesarean section. On occasion the FHR pattern will be normal or show minimal abnormalities, and the only symptom evident is the prolapsed cord; however, the interventions are the same.

Diabetes in Pregnancy

Basically, DM is a disease in which the body is unable to produce or sufficiently use insulin to metabolize glucose. The disease is complicated by faulty metabolism of fats and proteins for energy. The course and outcome of a pregnancy complicated by diabetes depend on the severity of the disease process. Diabetes occurs in approximately 1% to 2% of the pregnant population.[6]

Etiology and Pathophysiology

This discussion of diabetes in pregnancy is limited primarily to how diabetes, whether gestational or as a preexisting condition, is affected by the pregnancy and how the pregnancy affects the patient with diabetes. Pregnancy is considered a diabetogenic state in which the patient has an increased need for glucose and protein and fat are metabolized to aid in the demand for higher glucose levels. During pregnancy, the metabolism of the mother adapts to provide fuel for the growing fetus and for the pregnant woman. Early in pregnancy, during the period of rapid growth of the embryo, the mother's blood glucose level decreases. The obstetric patient who has diabetes may exhibit hypoglycemia.

At approximately 24 weeks gestation, the diabetogenic effects of pregnancy begin. Increased hormonal activity exerts an antiinsulin effect that results in a decreased responsiveness to insulin and a rise in the level of blood glucose. Increased production of insulin by the pancreas counteracts the antiinsulin effects of the hormones, and normal blood glucose levels are maintained. If, as a result of an acquired or inherited defect in beta cell function, maternal insulin secretion fails to keep pace with the demand, a further increase in blood glucose levels will occur. At this point in the pregnancy, gestational diabetes is frequently recognized and diagnosed. For the woman who is already diabetic, an increase in insulin requirement occurs and remains increased until after delivery.

The obstetric patient with a pregnancy complicated by DM is at an increased risk compared with the remainder of the pregnant population for developing PIH and related disorders, hydramnios, infections such as vaginitis, urinary tract infections, and pyelonephritis. Delivery by cesarean section and preterm delivery also occur with increased frequency because of macrosomia or fetal distress.

The fetus is at increased risk as well when the mother has diabetes. Complications associated with the fetus include congenital anomalies, intrauterine growth retardation (IUGR), macrosomia, delivery trauma, fetal distress, hypoglycemia, hypocalcemia, hyperbilirubinemia, respiratory distress, and intrauterine death. Macrosomia refers to a fetus that is large for gestational age with increased fat deposition and an enlarged spleen and liver. Macrosomia is seen more commonly when the mother has gestational DM or DM without vasculopathy. Congenital anomalies are seen more frequently when pregnant diabetic women are in poor control of their diabetes.

Assessment

Assessment of the patient with diabetes includes screening for the presence of risk factors linked to DM. All pregnant women with diabetes need to be assessed so their disease can be classified. Assessment by the flight nurse should include the following:

1. Obstetric history: Assess for the possibility that a previous pregnancy was complicated by undiagnosed diabetes. Has the patient had gestational DM with a previous pregnancy, or is there a family history of DM? Has she delivered an infant weighing more than 4000 g? Has she had unexplained perinatal losses, stillbirth, or traumatic delivery? Has more than one pregnancy been complicated by PIH? PIH as a multipara? Does she have a history of hydramnios or preterm delivery? Is she older than 35 years?
2. Current pregnancy: Does the patient have signs and symptoms of DM? Is glycosuria present? Are results of a glucose challenge test abnormal? Is the patient obese? Has the patient had recurrent urinary tract infections or vaginitis? Does the patient have chronic hypertension? What are the results of ultrasounds or other diagnostic tests? Is the diabetes controlled by diet or insulin? What is the patient's current insulin regimen?
3. History of preexisting condition: What class is the DM, as determined by the age of onset, duration of the disease, and evidence of vasculopathy? Does the patient have cardiovascular or kidney disease? Has there been good control of the diabetes during the pregnancy? What is the patient's current insulin regimen?

Strategies for Transport

In addition to following the general guidelines for transport care, careful assessment is required of the obstetric patient with gestational DM or the diabetic obstetric patient because of changing metabolic demands. The flight nurse should obtain a diabetic history from the patient and assess for complications associated with DM in pregnancy. It is also important to record the time of her last meal and last insulin injection.

If the patient is in labor, simultaneous continuous insulin and glucose infusions will stabilize maternal levels and may reduce neonatal hyperglycemia. The insulin may be adjusted after delivery on the basis of blood sugar levels, and the insulin demand will decrease after delivery. Five units of regular insulin is added to 500 ml of dextrose 5% and delivered by infusion pump. An initial rate of 1 unit of insulin and 5 g of glucose per hour is initiated. The patient is given nothing by mouth. Blood glucose levels are evaluated every 1 to 2 hours and maintained at a level of 80 to 120 mg/dl.

The mainline intravenous solution used should be lactated Ringer's or normal saline solution, a solution without glucose, to prevent accidental infusion of a large amount of intravenous fluid containing glucose. The flight nurse should obtain a blood glucose reading just prior to transport. Because labor increases metabolic needs, the flight nurse should be aware of the signs and symptoms of hypoglycemia and hyperglycemia and should never administer terbutaline to an insulin-dependent diabetic because of the transient hyperglycemic response seen with terbutaline.

Hemorrhagic Complications

Placental Abruption

Placental abruption can be defined as the premature detachment of a normally implanted placenta from the uterine wall. The separation may occur over a small area with little evidence or can separate totally with devastating results. The incidence of abruption varies widely, depending on the source. Placental abruption in 1 in 55 deliveries to 1 in 250 or even more deliveries has been documented, with differing criteria used for diagnosis. Of considerable significance is the incidence of recurrence with subsequent pregnancies, which is about 1 in 18 deliveries.

Etiology. The primary cause of placental abruption is largely unknown. Hypertension, whether chronic or PIH, and previous abruption are two factors that are known to greatly increase the risk of placental abruption. Other factors that place the obstetric patient at risk include abdominal trauma, an unusually short umbilical cord, amniocentesis, multiparity, age over 35 years, uterine anomalies or tumors, sudden uterine decompression when a twin is delivered and the remaining twin is placed at risk or immediately before delivery of single fetus, cigarette smoking, and substance abuse, especially abuse of cocaine.

Pathophysiology. Hemorrhage occurs from the arterioles that supply the decidua (lining of uterus), causing a retroplacental hematoma. Placental separation takes place at that site and may continue as the hemorrhage continues. As the hemorrhage continues, more vessels are disrupted, leading to increased hemorrhage and further separation. Placental separation can be an avalanche that continues to total separation or suddenly stops for reasons unknown. Sometimes a clot blocks the hemorrhage. The decidua is rich in thromboplastin, and clotting occurs rapidly. When vaginal bleeding is observed, the blood is usually dark because of the rapid clotting. If separation occurs at the margin of the placenta (Fig. 33-11) or if the amniotic membranes are dissected from the decidua as a result of the hemorrhage, vaginal bleeding will be observed. No vaginal bleeding will be observed if the hemorrhage is completely concealed behind the placenta.

As the hemorrhage continues and a retroplacental clot forms, enough pressure may be exerted to force blood through the membranes, giving the amniotic

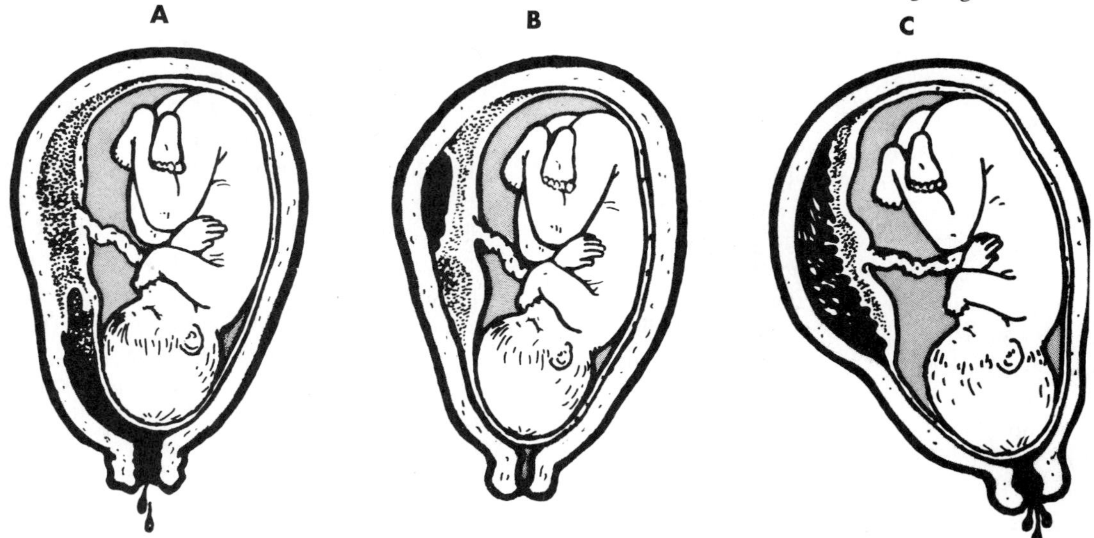

Fig. 33-11. Examples of placental abruption. **A,** Placental separation occurs at the margin of the placenta; **B** and **C,** separation originates from a central area behind the placenta. (Illustrated by Vincenza Genovese, Phoenix, Arizona. From Gilbert ES, Harmon JS: *High-risk pregnancy and delivery,* St Louis, 1986, Mosby.)

fluid a port wine color, or into the myometrium, causing a condition called Couvelaire uterus. The uterine tone is increased, and irritability will be noted. Contractions will frequently be present.

A common complication of placental abruption is DIC. Other complications include postpartum hemorrhage, anemia, postpartum infection, hypovolemic shock, kidney failure, and fetal distress or death. The factors that predispose to placental abruption may occur preterm, predisposing to preterm delivery.

Placenta Previa

Placenta previa occurs when the placenta becomes implanted in the lower uterine segment and as a result covers or partially covers the internal cervical os. A marginal or low-lying previa extends to or close to but does not cover any part of the internal os. Placenta previa occurs approximately once in every 200 to 400 deliveries. The incidence of placenta previa is higher preterm. As the pregnancy progresses, however, the fundus hypertrophies, the lower uterine segment elongates, and the placenta grows, allowing for placental migration away from the internal os toward the fundus.

Etiology. Although the exact cause is unknown, there is a higher incidence of placenta previa where uterine scarring is evident. A previous cesarean section or dilatation and curettage, increased parity, multiparity with short intervals, and a previous occurrence of placenta previa can scar the uterus. Other factors that place the obstetric patient at risk for placenta previa include previous chorioamnionitis, multiple gestation for which there is a larger surface area covered by the placenta, fetal erythroblastosis, maternal age over age 35 years, substance abuse, and uterine tumors.

Pathophysiology. Normal placental implantation usually occurs in the fundus or body segment of the uterus. It has been suggested that defective perfusion of the decidua may favor implantation of the placenta in the lower uterine segment. Because there is less vascularization in the lower uterine segment, the placenta compensates and tends to grow thinner and larger, thus covering a larger area and thereby increasing perfusion.

Before the onset of labor, the cervix begins to soften, efface, and dilate. These cervical changes disrupt the placental attachment, tearing the vessels, and hemorrhage results. Bright red vaginal bleeding will be observed; it is usually painless and is not initially associated with contractions. The initial episode is usually slight (less than 250 ml of blood is shed) and tends to cease spontaneously as clot formation occurs. Recurrence is unpredictable. Generally, the greater the extent to which the internal os is covered, the sooner the initial episode occurs.

Potential complications of placenta previa include complications similar to those of placental abruption, such as DIC, hypovolemic shock, kidney damage, anemia, postpartum infection, postpartum hemorrhage, and fetal distress or death. Because hemorrhage may occur at any time without warning or precipitating events, the risk is increased with premature delivery. Furthermore, placenta accreta is a rare complication of placenta previa.

Assessment of Placental Abruption and Placenta Previa

Generally, the clinical findings of placental abruption vary in degree with the extent of the placental separation and clot formation behind the placenta. Onset of symptoms may be gradual in mild cases to sudden and without warning in severe situations. In cases of vaginal bleeding after 20 weeks gestation, placenta previa should be considered.

Uterine Assessment (Placental Abruption). Symptoms of placental abruption may range from slight abdominal tenderness and lower back discomfort with a mild abruption to severe unceasing abdominal pain in a severe situation. Sudden severe pain may be indicative of retroplacental hemorrhage into the myometrium. The intensity, frequency, and duration of contractions may vary, from contractions with a slight increase in uterine tone to hypertonic (Fig. 33-12) or tetanic contractions (lasting longer than 90 seconds) with a boardlike uterus that fails to relax. With severe abruption, labor tends to progress rapidly. Abdominal palpation for intensity, length, and frequency of contractions, as well as observation of any sustained tone between contractions, will aid in the assessment. If it is difficult to determine when a contraction begins or ends and the ab-

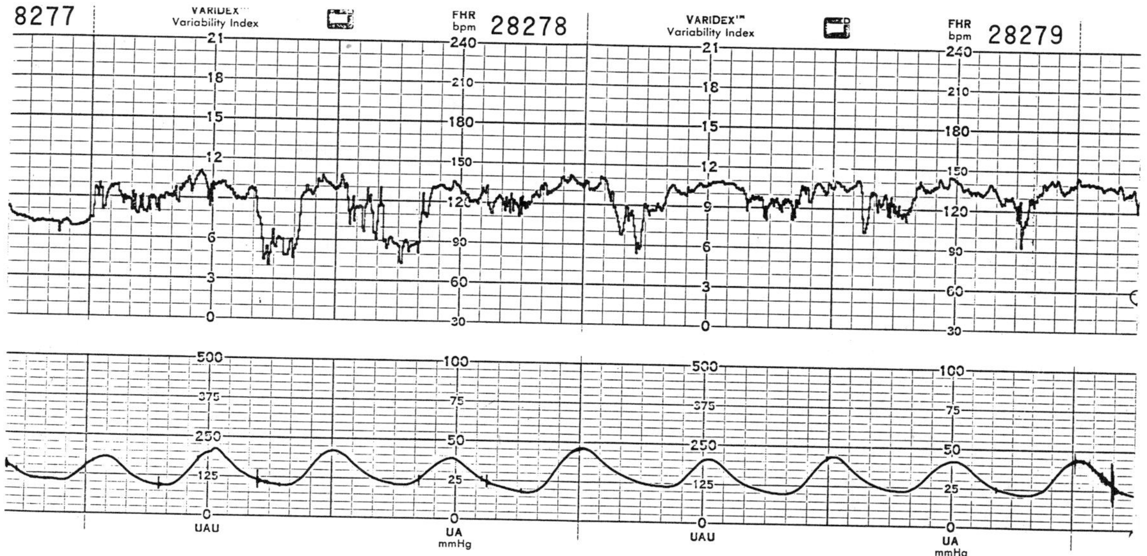

Fig. 33-12. Abruption pattern. Note the increased uterine tone documented with the use of an internal uterine pressure catheter (IUPC). Hypertonic contractions are occurring approximately every minute with virtually no period of relaxation between contractions. Note the distressed fetal response. An emergency cesarean section was performed with Apgar scores of 2 and 7 at 1 and 5 minutes, respectively.

domen is rigid, a severe placental separation should be suspected. Unless an internal uterine pressure catheter has been placed, increased tone or intensity of contractions cannot accurately be assessed with EFM.

Uterine Assessment (Placenta Previa). Contractions may or may not be present with placenta previa. The onset usually occurs during or after the hemorrhage because of increased uterine irritability.

Assessment of Blood Loss (Placental Abruption). When placental abruption occurs, vaginal bleeding may be absent or minimal to profuse. It is essential to realize that the amount of vaginal bleeding is not an indicator of the degree of separation or of total blood loss but of the location of the separation. Assessment of a concealed hemorrhage includes noting any change in fundal height as an indication of continued hemorrhage. The fundus can be marked, providing a quick visual indicator of increasing uterine size. The bleeding usually continues until delivery of the placenta, when the uterus can contract sufficiently to close off the open vessels.

Assessment of Blood Loss (Placenta Previa). Blood loss can be more accurately estimated with placenta previa, for which only external hemorrhage will be observed. Placenta previa is characterized by repetitive and frequently more extensive bleeding episodes.

Ultrasound. An ultrasound can confirm the location of the placenta. If ultrasound is not available, a previa cannot be ruled out. A sterile vaginal examination may stimulate profuse bleeding by dislodging a clot and *should never be done.* With cervical changes that accompany active labor, an increase in bloody show will be noted and may appear excessive, leading the flight nurse to believe that a placenta previa is present. A very gentle examination may be attempted only if delivery appears imminent. An ultrasound can also rule out the presence of an abruption.

Assessment of Vital Signs. Signs of hypovolemic shock may not be present until a blood loss of approximately 30% has occurred. However, before any change in vital signs, shunting away from the placenta occurs, and FHT indicative of placental insufficiency will occur.

Assessment of FHT. Fetal distress as a result of placental separation or placenta previa occurs primarily from placental insufficiency (hypertonic uterus, maternal hemorrhage, or decreased placental perfusion) or fetal hemorrhage as a consequence of placental separation. The flight nurse must observe for late decelerations and bradycardia.

Assessment of Urinary Output. Urinary output of 60 to 100 ml per hour suggests adequate renal perfusion and, indirectly, adequate circulating blood volume. Urinary output of less than 30 ml per hour suggests decreased circulatory volume, in which case insertion of a Foley catheter is recommended.

Assessment of Coagulopathy. The flight nurse should observe for petechiae, hematuria, bruising, or bleeding from intravenous sites.

Assessment for Impending Shock. Because of the normal physiologic changes of pregnancy, early symptoms of hypovolemia may be masked. Careful assessment of serial vital signs will aid in differentiating expected blood pressure, pulse, and respirations from symptoms of impending shock. Symptoms include tachypnea, decreased blood pressure, increased pulse rate (rapid and thready), oliguria, cyanosis, pallor, and clamminess.

Strategies for Transport (Abruption and Previa)

The flight nurse should implement the following strategies for transport of patients with abruption or previa:

1. Implement general guidelines for transport care after the primary survey and obstetric assessment are completed. Assess for contractions, the extent of hemorrhage, and estimated blood loss specific to abruption or previa. Determine fundal height or mark the fundus, reassessing frequently. Recognition of concealed bleeding will be confirmed by noting an increase in the fundal height.
2. Administer tocolytics as recommended. Refer to the discussion in this chapter regarding preterm labor for specifics about labor suppressants. Terbutaline and ritodrine administered intravenously are contraindicated in the presence of hemorrhage because of the fetal stimulation with resulting tachycardia.
3. Assess vital signs every 15 minutes or more frequently as needed. Note any subtle changes that may indicate hypovolemia. Check capillary refill as needed to assess for peripheral perfusion. Initiate EFM, if available, to monitor FHT for changes indicative of impending fetal distress. Frequent Doppler evaluations of the FHR during shorter rotor-wing flights are acceptable. Provide supplemental oxygen, 100%, with use of a face mask at 10 L/min.
4. Observe for signs of DIC. In the event of a longer transport, a clot-retraction test can indicate the presence of coagulopathy. In a red-top tube, draw at least 5 ml of blood and tape it upright to the wall of the aircraft. If no clot develops within 6 to 12 minutes, abnormalities may be present. Consider starting a second intravenous line if hypovolemia is suspected. Provide fluid replacement with lactated Ringer's solution to maintain blood pressure, uteroplacental perfusion, and urinary output greater than 30 ml/hr. Consider blood replacement, if available, and plasma expanders, such as 50 ml of albumin 25%. Place a Foley catheter for accurate determination of hourly urinary output if necessary. In the event of suspected hypovolemic shock, elevate the patient's feet and apply a pneumatic antishock garment, avoiding inflation of the abdominal flap. Vasopressors will further compromise uterine perfusion. Ephedrine, an alpha and beta stimulant that vasoconstricts but has some β_2 receptors that spare the uterus, may be considered at 25 mg, administered slowly by an intravenous route.
5. Expedite transport if the patient's condition deteriorates. If the transport service has a fixed wing aircraft, consider a rotor-wing transport from the airport to the receiving facility. Notify the medical director and re-

ceiving hospital to prepare for a possible emergency cesarean section delivery.

Disseminated Intravascular Coagulation

DIC is a serious and deleterious complication of pregnancy. When accelerated coagulation and activation of the fibrinolytic system occur simultaneously in pregnancy, DIC occurs as a secondary event activated by hemorrhagic complications such as placental abruption and placenta previa, or by delivery complications such as a ruptured uterus, uterine inversion, postpartum hemorrhage, traumatic labor and delivery, amniotic fluid embolism, and sepsis. DIC is also a complication of trauma in pregnancy, retained dead fetus syndrome (over 3 weeks since intrauterine death), and hydatidiform mole.

After the delivery of the fetus and after the patient's primary complication has been eliminated or improved, further intervention may not be needed unless the hemorrhage has been severe. For a more detailed discussion, please refer to Chapter 9.

Multiple Gestation

A pregnancy with more than one fetus is a multiple gestation. Twins occur in 1 in 80 to 90 births, and triplets occur in 1 in 8000 births.

Etiology

Embryologically, twins may result from multiple ovulation, in which two distinct ova are fertilized (dizygotic, or fraternal), or from one separate ovum that subsequently divides into two (monozygotic, or identical). Either or both processes can also result in triplets, quadruplets, and so on. The incidence of dizygotic twins is influenced by heredity, maternal age, race, and treatment for infertility, whereas the frequency of monozygotic twins is relatively constant.

Previous delivery of twins or a maternal family history of delivering fraternal twins increases the chance of delivering twins.

Pathophysiology

Pathophysiology is related to the complications associated with multiple gestation. The large area of the uterine surface covered by the placentas is suspected in several complications. Portions are more likely to implant in the lower uterine segment where there is less vascularity, increasing the chances of IUGR, or at or near the cervical os, increasing the chances of placenta previa. The superabundance of chorionic villi appears to predispose the obstetric patient to PIH, especially if it is her first pregnancy.

Other complications may be caused by uterine overdistention and hemodynamic and endocrinologic changes associated with multiple gestation. The mother is placed at risk for anemia, glucose intolerance, hydramnios, dysfunctional labor associated with uterine overdistention, and dystocia. In addition, multiple gestation predisposes to PROM, preterm labor and delivery, placental abruption, cesarean section, uterine atony and resulting postpartum hemorrhage, and malpresentations. The fetuses are at risk for congenital anomalies, cord prolapse or entanglement, vasa previa, twin-twin transfusion, discordant fetal growth, and intrauterine death.

The greatest threat to multiple gestation is premature labor and delivery. The average gestational age for onset of labor is about 36 weeks.[5] Rarer but serious complications include conjoined twins, monoamniotic twins (with a mortality rate of approximately 50% because of knotting and tangling of the cord), and twins locked or compacted, preventing descent or engagement of either twin.

Assessment

Multiple gestation is usually suspected when a discrepancy develops between the gestational age determined by the obstetric patient's last monthly period and the uterine size determined by regular fundal measurements. When the expected size of approximately 1 cm per week of gestation is exceeded, investigation may be warranted. If twinning is suspected, an ultrasound will confirm or disprove the presence of more than one fetus.

Strategies for Transport

The flight nurse must be aware that any multiple gestation is a pregnancy at risk and must assess for additional risk factors associated with a multiple gestation.

The primary survey, including general obstetric assessment, is completed initially, followed by the general guidelines for transport care. The fundal height should be noted. EFM should include continuous monitoring, alternating fetuses, unless the transport is of short duration. The FHR of the fetus not currently being monitored can be determined with Doppler auscultation.

The drug of choice in the treatment of preterm labor is $MgSO_4$, because it has been observed that an increased incidence of pulmonary edema is associated with use of β-sympathomimetic agents in women with multiple gestations.

PIH AND RELATED DISORDERS

PIH refers to a group of hypertensive disorders that have their onset during pregnancy and resolve after pregnancy. Gestational hypertension develops after 20 weeks gestation without evidence of hypertension. Preeclampsia is characterized by hypertension, proteinuria, and edema. PIH may develop before 20 weeks gestation in cases of trophoblastic disease. Eclampsia refers to the development of clonic and tonic seizures in a preeclamptic patient. Persistent hypertension not associated with pregnancy that develops before 20 weeks gestation is considered to be chronic. Chronic hypertension as a preexisting condition may be complicated during pregnancy by superimposed preeclampsia. HELLP syndrome (*h*emolysis, *el*evated *l*iver enzymes, and *l*ow *p*latelets) is considered a complication of severe preeclampsia. The incidence of PIH in the United States is 4% to 7%. The progression to eclampsia occurs in 1 in every 1000 to 1500 deliveries.

Etiology

The absolute cause of PIH is unknown. Current theories point to nutritional deficiencies, immunologic deficiencies, genetic predisposition, response to chorionic villi exposure, chronic intravascular coagulation, and other factors. Certain factors are known to predispose the obstetrical patient to development of PIH. Primarily, PIH is a disease of the primigravida, the teenaged primigravida, or the primigravida over 35 years of age. The patient with DM, preexisting cardiovascular or kidney disease, hydramnios, family history of PIH, or no prenatal care is also at risk. Other predisposing factors include the pregnancy exposed to a superabundance of chorionic villi, such as with multiple gestation, hydatidiform mole or fetal hydrops, or a poor nutritional status, large fetus, or Rh incompatibility.

Pathophysiology

To understand the pathophysiology of PIH, it is necessary to have a basic understanding of the magnitude of physiologic changes that normally occur in pregnancy, specifically those pertaining to the pathophysiology of PIH. Briefly, blood volume increases almost 50%, hemodilution occurs, the pulse rate increases, cardiac output increases, and the glomerular filtration rate increases. Increased vasodilation is seen, peripheral resistance drops, and blood pressure decreases in the second trimester and returns to normal near term. A fluid shift from the intravascular space to the extracellular space in dependent limbs occurs, and the potential for coagulation increases. Resistance to the pressor effects of angiotensin II also occurs.

In patients with PIH, the disease process actually begins many weeks before the onset of any symptoms. A chain reaction of events is initiated as, for unknown reasons, an increased sensitivity to angiotensin II develops. As a result, vasospasm occurs, particularly arteriolar vasospasm, which initiates vasoconstriction, which leads to increased peripheral resistance and eventually hypertension. Blood perfusion to all body organs is decreased, and the function of the placenta, kidneys, liver, and brain is significantly impaired. While not forgetting the essential problem of vasospasm, the following pathophysiology is characteristic of PIH.

Uteroplacental Changes

Compromised uterine and placental blood flow can lead to degeneration of the placenta and necrosis. With chronic decreased blood perfusion, IUGR can result. During labor, fetal distress caused by uteroplacental insufficiency (late decelerations) will frequently be seen. As a consequence of decreased uterine blood flow, uterine activity is increased and uterine irritability and preterm labor may be seen.

Renal Changes

Decreased renal blood flow decreases glomerular filtration rate and decreases urinary output. Cellular changes are observed in the glomerular capillary endothelial cells. The cells swell, producing narrowing of the capillary lumens, and lesions develop, causing the proteinuria (primarily albumin) seen in preeclampsia. Plasma uric acid is typically elevated as a result of the decreased uric acid clearance by the kidneys. In addition, creatinine clearance and blood urea nitrogen aid in the evaluation of kidney function. With decreased kidney function, sodium and water are retained. In conjunction with a decreased circulating albumin and a decrease in colloid osmotic pressure, fluid is shifted from the intravascular space to the extracellular space, giving rise to edema, which may be slight to severe.

Hematologic Changes

Because of fluid shifts, hemoconcentration is seen, with a rise in hematocrit levels. An increase in the hematocrit level is noted after an initial assessment may signal a deteriorating condition. The normal hypervolemia of pregnancy is decreased or nearly absent when preeclampsia is present. Also observed is intravascular platelet and fibrin deposition that occurs in response to vessel wall damage as the disease progresses. In addition, there is some evidence of hemolysis and coagulopathy in patients with severe preeclampsia that is more frequently associated with HELLP syndrome and the development of DIC as severe complications of preeclampsia.

Hepatic Changes

Reduction in blood flow to the liver impairs liver function. Swelling of the capsule (the fibrous sheath that completely covers the liver) and subcapsular hemorrhage may occur. Necrosis and damage to liver tissue are demonstrated by elevated liver enzymes. In rare cases, subcapsular hemorrhage can be so extensive that the liver capsule can rupture with massive hemorrhage into the peritoneal cavity. Epigastric pain (right upper quadrant pain) is associated with hepatic swelling and subcapsular hemorrhage.

Cerebral Changes

Although cerebral perfusion is not impaired, vasospasm gives rise to cerebral edema, hemorrhage, and central nervous system irritability, which is evidenced by hyperreflexia, headaches, ankle clonus, nausea and vomiting, and clonic and tonic seizures.

Retinal Changes

Retinal arteriolar spasms, ischemia, and edema as a result of decreased perfusion are the sources of the visual disturbances seen in preeclampsia. Blurring and scotoma (blind or twinkling spots in the vision) and diplopia (double vision) may occur. Retinal detachment is a rare occurrence.

Pulmonary Changes

Changes in pulmonary capillary permeability can occur, predisposing to pulmonary edema in severe cases of PIH.

Complications

Complications of PIH, some of which have already been discussed, include eclampsia, placental abruption, pulmonary edema, DIC, HELLP syndrome, hemolytic anemia, thrombocytopenia, preterm delivery and prematurity, and IUGR. Seldom observed and grave complications include retinal detachment, kidney failure, cerebral hemorrhage, liver rupture, heart failure, intrauterine death, and, rarely, maternal death.

As a general rule, the predisposition for the development of complications increases as the disease state deteriorates. Though prompt treatment should stabilize the patient with PIH, complications and progression to eclampsia can occur.

Eclampsia

Eclampsia can occur before labor, during labor, or early into the postpartum period. Headache, visual disturbances, epigastric pain, apprehension, anxiety, and hyperreflexia with clonus in a patient with severe preeclampsia are signs of impending eclampsia.

Seizures are characterized by clonic and tonic activity and usually begin around the mouth in the form of facial twitchings. The seizure may be so

TABLE 33-2

General guidelines for determining the severity of the disease process*

	Mild	Severe	Impending eclampsia
Blood pressure	≥140/90 Diastolic increases ≥ 15 mm Hg	Diastolic > 100 mm Hg	Diastolic > 100 mm Hg
Proteinuria (dipstick)	2+/3+	3+/4+	3+/4+
Urinary output	> 30 ml/hr	<20-30 ml/hr	<20-30 ml/hr
Edema	+1/+2	+3/+4	+3/+4
Pulmonary edema	Not present	May be present	Present
Headache	Not present	May be present	Present
Visual disturbances	Not present	May be present	Present
Epigastric pain	Not present	May be present	Present
Hyperreflexia and clonus	Not present	May be present	Present

Modified from Gilbert E, Harmon J: *High-risk pregnancy and delivery,* St Louis, 1986, Mosby.
*Some crossover of clinical findings can occur, and not all findings are absolute for each category.

forceful that the patient may fall from the bed. Respirations cease during the seizure but spontaneously resume as the seizure activity quiets. Coma frequently ensues, and the patient remembers little of the events immediately before and after the seizure. The length of the coma varies, with the patient gradually becoming responsive. Frequently, labor spontaneously begins and progresses rapidly. Pulmonary edema may develop. Massive cerebral hemorrhage and death can occur as a result of eclampsia, but the incidence is very rare (Table 33-2).

HELLP Syndrome

The HELLP syndrome was first identified and described as a serious complication of preeclampsia by Weinstein in 1982. *H* stands for *h*emolysis, which is confirmed by the evidence of red cell fragments and irregularly shaped red cells on peripheral blood smears. It is believed that as red cells pass through the constricted vessels that have sustained wall damage with platelet and fibrin deposition, red cell integrity is altered and many cells are lysed. As a result, hyperbilirubinemia is frequently seen. *EL* stands for *e*levated *l*iver enzymes. Elevated serum glutamic-oxaloacetic transaminase and serum glutamic-pyruvic transaminase are observed. *LP* stands for *l*ow *p*latelet count. Consumptive thrombocytopenia (a platelet count lower than 100,000/mm^3) unaccompanied by any other coagulation factor abnormalities is characteristic of the HELLP syndrome.

Assessment

The "Big Three" in assessing PIH includes hypertension, edema, and proteinuria.

Hypertension

Hypertension is a rise in systolic pressure of 30 mm Hg or a rise in diastolic pressure of 15 mm Hg on the basis of previously known pressures, or a blood pressure of 140/90 or higher. The diastolic pressure is a more reliable predictor of the disease process. The blood pressure should be taken with the patient in the left lateral recumbent position. Hypertension associated with PIH is labile and may change in the time it takes to retake the blood pressure.

Edema

A sudden excessive weight gain of more than 2 lb in a week or 6 lb in a month is primarily attributable to fluid retention. Nondependent edema of the eyelids, face, and hands is characteristic of PIH. Pitting edema of the lower extremities is common. For evaluation of edema, see Table 33-3.

TABLE 33-3

Assessment of edema and hyperreflexia

Evaluation of edema	Score
Minimal edema of lower extremities	+1
Marked edema of lower extremities	+2
Edema of lower extremities, face, and hands	+3
Generalized massive edema including the abdomen and sacrum	+4

Assessment of edema should include description and scoring with regard to location, onset, and duration, any sudden increase in swelling noticed, and any pitting edema.

Evaluation of hyperreflexia	Grade
None elicited	0
Sluggish or dull	+1
Active, normal	+2
Brisk	+3
Brisk with transient clonus	+4
Brisk with sustained clonus	+5

Assessment of hyperreflexia is usually accomplished by eliciting patellar deep-tendon reflexes. Clonus can be assessed at the same time by swift dorsiflexion of the foot. Clonus indicates neuromuscular irritability, and each beat should be counted.

Modified from Gilbert E, Harmon J: *High-risk pregnancy and delivery,* St Louis, 1986, Mosby.

Proteinuria

Proteinuria usually develops after hypertension, and edema is evident when proteinuria is present. The flight nurse should observe the patient for evidence of the following: (1) central nervous system irritability (headache, hyperreflexia evaluated by deep tendon reflexes and ankle clonus [see Table 33-3], nausea, vomiting, apprehension, and anxiety); (2) impaired renal function (oliguria and proteinuria); and (3) hepatic involvement (epigastric pain [unmistakable from uterine contractions], malaise, nausea, vomiting, and jaundice).

The flight nurse should also assess fetal status by EFM evaluations of FHR baseline, variability, acceleration, and deceleration patterns; observe for fetal activity; observe for evidence of pulmonary involvement (moist rales on auscultation, dyspnea, tachypnea, tachycardia, wheezing or cough, and anxiety), and identify evidence of evolving or impending eclampsia, placental abruption, HELLP syndrome, and DIC.

Strategies for Transport

Protecting the obstetric patient from the effects of vasospasm and hypertension and preventing seizures and other complications are critical. Maintaining or improving uteroplacental blood flow minimizes the risk of insult to the fetus.

The primary survey, including obstetric assessment, is done initially. The flight nurse should follow general guidelines for transport care and assess for PIH and risk factors and complications associated with PIH. Obtaining a history of the onset of any symptoms provides insight in the consideration of the clinical picture.

The fetus is at increased risk for uteroplacental insufficiency. The flight nurse should observe for late decelerations and reduced variability while monitoring and take note of fetal movement.

The flight nurse should place a Foley catheter to monitor urinary output and proteinuria when symptoms indicate severe preeclampsia. When assessing for proteinuria, the flight nurse should avoid contamination with vaginal discharge (blood, amniotic fluid, and bacteria) to avoid inaccurate results.

Sensory stimulation should be decreased during transport by keeping lights and voices low and sirens turned off, or by turning the cardiac monitor audible signal to low or off. The flight nurse must be prepared to intervene in the event of an eclamptic seizure. $MgSO_4$, diazepam, airway aids, available suction equipment and oxygen, syringes and needles, calcium gluconate, and a padded tongue blade must be close at hand during the transport.

A coagulopathy is suspected if petechiae, hematuria, bruising, or bleeding from intravenous sites is noted. Symptoms of shock may rapidly ensue. A gross evaluation of clotting time by a clot retraction test can be done in the aircraft. In a red-top tube, the flight nurse can draw at least 5 ml of blood and tape it upright to the wall of the aircraft. If no clot develops within 6 to 12 minutes, then abnormalities may exist in the clotting mechanism.

The flight nurse should evaluate pulmonary status for signs of pulmonary edema. If acute pulmonary edema with respiratory distress occurs, morphine (2 to 5 mg administered intravenously over 1 to 2 minutes) and furosemide (20 to 40 mg administered intravenously over 2 to 3 minutes) can be given. The medical plan to control the disease includes a thorough knowledge of the action, dosage, administration, and adverse reactions of the following medications used most frequently in the transport of obstetric patients with PIH: $MgSO_4$, calcium gluconate, hydralazine, and diazepam.

Magnesium Sulfate

$MgSO_4$ acts at the neuromuscular junction to slow transmission of impulses. By displacing calcium it interferes with the release of acetylcholine, blocking nerve transmission to the muscle, and thereby preventing the seizure. Fifty grams of $MgSO_4$ can be added to 500 ml lactated Ringer's solution (or 40 g added to 1000 ml) with a bolus of 4 to 6 g given slowly over 15 to 30 minutes, followed by 2 g per hour, preferably by infusion pump. Therapeutic serum magnesium levels to prevent seizures range from approximately 4 to 8 mEq/L (1.5 to 2.5 mEq/L is normal). When therapeutic levels are achieved, deep tendon reflexes will be depressed but not absent. Loss of deep tendon reflexes indicates a toxic level. Respiratory arrest and cardiac arrest are seen with highly toxic levels (greater than 15 mEq/L). While a patient is receiving intravenous $MgSO_4$, frequent assessment of deep tendon reflexes is essential. Respirations should also be closely monitored and the infusion stopped if less than 12 per minute is observed. Pulse oximetry should be used during transport.

The antidote for magnesium toxicity is calcium gluconate. Calcium stimulates the release of acetylcholine, stimulating nerve transmission to the muscle. The recommended dosage of calcium gluconate is 1 g of a 10% solution administered intravenously over at least 3 minutes. If administered too rapidly, bradycardia and arrhythmias may occur.

$MgSO_4$ is not an antihypertensive agent. However, a transient drop in blood pressure after initiation of treatment is frequently seen and can be attributed to smooth muscle relaxation. Adverse reactions include flushing, sweating, nausea and vomiting, and drowsiness. A decrease in FHR variability may be observed. Because $MgSO_4$ is primarily excreted in the urine, toxicity may develop rather rapidly in the patient with significantly impaired kidney function. The urinary output should exceed 30 ml per hour while the patient is receiving $MgSO_4$. The infusion should be decreased or stopped if urinary output drops below 30 ml per hour. In cases of kidney or heart disease, $MgSO_4$ should be used cautiously.

Labetalol

Labetalol is a selective β-blocking agent that decreases systemic vascular resistance without changing cardiac output. The standard dosage, 20 mg administered by intravenous push over 2 minutes, may be repeated every 10 minutes with 40 to 80 mg until the maximum dosage of 300 mg has been given.

Hydralazine

Hydralazine acts by relaxing arterioles and decreasing vasospasm, and as a result, it reduces blood pressure and stimulates cardiac output. Blood perfusion to the brain, kidneys, liver, and uterus is thus improved. To prevent a cerebrovascular accident, hydralazine is recommended when the diastolic pressure is 110 mm Hg or greater. Two milligrams administered intravenously every 5 minutes until the diastolic pressure is within the 90 to 100 mm Hg range is the standard dosage. During administration, the blood pressure should be taken every couple of minutes, because the onset of action is 5 to 10 minutes. If the diastolic pressure falls below 90 mm Hg, uterine blood flow may be further reduced, placing the fetus at risk. Adverse reactions include reflex tachycardia, headache, palpitations, dizziness, nausea, and vomiting. Hydralazine is contraindicated in cases of lupus erythematosus and tachycardia.

Diazepam

Diazepam is classified as an antianxiety drug, but it is known to prevent or arrest seizure activity, although the exact mode of action is not known. It also produces mild sedation and muscular relaxation. The standard dose is 5 to 10 mg administered intravenously, not to exceed 5 mg over 1 minute. It should be injected through the intravenous tubing as close to the vein insertion as possible. Adverse reactions include transient bradycardia and hypotension.

The box outlines the quick actions required on the part of the flight nurse in the event of an eclamptic seizure.

PRIORITIES IN THE EVENT OF AN ECLAMPTIC SEIZURE

1. The first priority in the event of an eclamptic seizure is to maintain a patent airway. Lower and turn the patient's head to the side to reduce the threat of aspiration. Suction oral passages as needed.
2. Insert a padded tongue blade between the teeth to prevent injury to the tongue.
3. Diazepam, 5 to 10 mg administered by slow intravenous push, or $MgSO_4$, 4 to 6 g administered intravenously over 5 to 10 minutes, will in most cases arrest seizure activity. If a seizure begins while the patient is receiving $MgSO_4$ therapy, administer another bolus with 2 to 4 g. Use of amobarbital sodium, a barbiturate, is not recommended during transport because of the high incidence of respiratory arrest that follows administration of this drug.
4. After the seizure stops, insert an airway. The tongue blade may facilitate the insertion; the tongue blade should then be removed. Administer supplemental oxygen to improve oxygenation after the apnea observed during the seizure.
5. Initiate $MgSO_4$ therapy at 2 to 3 g/hr.
6. Assess and record fetal response to the seizure with EFM. Bradycardia can occur but usually resolves. The patient should remain in the left recumbent position.
7. Record the time, duration, and description of seizure activity and significant events before the seizure, if any.
8. Assess the patient's level of consciousness and watch for signs of increasing responsiveness.
9. In the event of a recurrent seizure, repeat the previous instructions. Be prepared to intubate and provide ventilator support if necessary.
10. Continue to provide nursing care of the patient with PIH as outlined.

PRETERM LABOR AND RELATED ISSUES

Regular and rhythmic contractions that produce progressive cervical changes after the 20th week of gestation and before the 37th week are considered to be preterm labor. Preterm delivery occurs in 6% to 9% of all deliveries. Preterm labor does not always result in preterm delivery; however, the rate of preterm delivery has changed little in recent years. With improved prenatal care, elimination or improvement of risk factors, patient education, and earlier diagnosis and treatment of preterm labor, the next decade may realize a decrease in the rate of preterm delivery.

Etiology

Although many factors predispose the obstetric patient to preterm labor, a few single identifiable causes exist. Infection has been recognized as a primary cause of preterm labor. Although the pathways frequently differ, sources of infection may include urinary tract infection, pyelonephritis, vaginitis (particularly bacterial), chorioamnionitis, and viral infection. Another identifiable cause is PROM (spontaneous rupture before the onset of contractions and before the 37th week). Other factors include previous preterm delivery (the single most frequent contributing factor), uterine anomalies, poor nutritional status, poor perineal hygiene, poor weight gain, no prenatal care, less than 1 year between the last delivery and commencement of the current pregnancy, substance abuse, PIH, cigarette smoking, diabetes, chronic cardiovascular or kidney disease, previous induced or spontaneous abortion, abdominal trauma, a long commute to work, a high stress level at work or home, physical stress, overdistention of the uterus as a result of multiple gestation, hydramnios, uterine tumors, age (teenage or over 40 years), placenta previa or placental abruption, cervical incompetence, women exposed to diethystilbestrol in utero, a retained intrauterine device, a history of pelvic inflammatory disease, and fetal anomalies, distress, or death.

Only a few or many factors may be implicated in each instance of preterm labor. When multiple factors are present, the obstetric patient is at greater risk.

Pathophysiology

In any situation in which uterine blood flow is reduced or impaired, an increase in uterine irritability can be noted and may result in the onset of labor. Viral infections with symptoms of fever, nausea, vomiting, or diarrhea may predispose to preterm labor primarily because of dehydration, which reduces uterine blood flow. Other similar conditions in which uteroplacental perfusion is compromised include PIH, diabetes, cardiovascular or kidney disease, overdistention of the uterus, heavy smoking, placental abruption, or placenta previa.

Hormonal influence contributes to increased uterine activity and the onset of labor. Prostaglandin release is associated with PROM, bacterial infections, abdominal trauma, and overdistention of the uterus. In at least half of the patients who have PROM, labor begins within 48 hours. Meconium-stained amniotic fluid (indicating possible fetal distress) contains high levels of oxytocin, which can initiate labor.

When a patient has cervical incompetence, the cervix is unable to support and maintain the growing pregnancy to term and often dilates without perceptible contractions. Cervical incompetence is characterized by premature, painless, bloodless cervical dilation in which the membranes bulge and rupture and delivery rapidly follows. Congenital defects and traumatic injury to the cervix may result in cervical incompetence. Probable causes of cervical injury include trauma during a previous childbirth, cervical dilation after elective or spontaneous abortions, or gynecologic procedures. Other physiologic abnormalities where preterm labor (PTL) is known to occur, especially if it does not allow for uterine growth and expansion during the course of the pregnancy, include exposure to diethystilbesterol and uterine anomalies.

For many identified risk factors, no single physiologic factor or other pathology can be identified. It appears that numerous issues are involved. Consequently, for many patients, the cause of preterm labor cannot be identified.

The complications associated with preterm labor and delivery predominantly affect the fetus. Birth trauma and the complications associated with the transition to extrauterine life for the premature infant are primary. Neonatal sepsis can result from PROM. The severity of the complications seen depend in a great measure on the gestational age of the neonate.

Maternal complications include adverse reactions to labor-suppressing agents, complications associated with cesarean section (increased incidence with preterm labor), endometritis, septicemia and septic shock related to prolonged PROM and chorioamnionitis, or other complications associated with preexisting conditions or the current pregnancy.

Assessment

Preterm labor should be suspected if the patient has a history of contractions 10 minutes apart or less for a period of 1 hour or longer. The flight nurse should assess for factors associated with preterm labor, remembering that the incidence of preterm labor increases with the number of predisposing factors.

Spontaneous Rupture of Membranes

To assess the status of the amniotic membranes, the flight nurse should ask the following question: Did contractions begin before or after rupture? If there is any history of possible spontaneous rupture, a sterile speculum examination (SSE) will verify the presence of amniotic fluid leaking from the cervix and collecting in the posterior fornix of the vagina (the area underneath the cervix posteriorly). If an SSE has already been performed, the flight nurse should note documented results. Three factors, positive pooling, positive nitrazine, and positive ferning, will definitely confirm spontaneous rupture of the membranes (SROM). Pooling of fluid will be seen in the vaginal vault. If none is seen, the flight nurse may encourage the patient to cough; the increased pressure will usually result in the release of amniotic fluid. A sample from a site as close to the posterior fornix as possible will turn nitrazine paper dark blue (alkaline) in the presence of amniotic fluid. Vaginal secretions are acidic in nature and will not affect the paper. The flight nurse should use caution because blood, cervical mucus, and betadine are alkaline in nature and can give a false-positive reading. Finally, a small amount of the fluid can be spread on a slide and allowed to dry completely. A frond crystallization pattern of dried amniotic fluid (with a high concentration of sodium chloride) will be seen under microscopic examination; it looks very similar to a Boston fern in appearance. Because a microscope may not be available in small outlying areas and there may not be time to perform this procedure, the flight nurse must depend on the presence of pooling and positive results of a test for nitrazine. If rupture is confirmed, avoid performing a sterile vaginal examination (SVE) unless delivery appears imminent; this will prevent introducing microbes from the vagina into the cervical canal, which can place the patient at an increased risk for infection. If a gross rupture has occurred, if the patient has a history of a large volume loss, or if continual leaking is observed, a sterile speculum examination is not necessary if it does not alter the plan for nursing care. The flight nurse should keep in mind that with a decreased amount of amniotic fluid the umbilical cord is at risk for compression and variable decelerations may be seen, with or without contractions.

If a rupture has not occurred, an SVE will confirm if any cervical changes have taken place. The cervix does not have to dilate before changes can be noted. Normally, the cervix is firm, long, and closed. Any softening or effacing, which frequently occurs before dilation, indicates cervical changes.

If this is not the initial episode of preterm labor, the flight nurse should assess for the history of onset, current medications, other treatment such as home monitoring or bed rest, and patient compliance. Frequently the present episode can be linked to increased activity, failure to take medication altogether, or inconsistency in following the medication regimen.

The flight nurse should observe the patient for any indications of the presence of infection. Symptoms of a urinary tract infection, pyelonephritis, or both include dysuria, frequency of urination, fever, and flank tenderness, pain, or both. Evidence of poor perineal hygiene may be a factor not only in the development of a urinary tract infection but in vaginal infections and chorioamnionitis as well. The flight nurse should obtain a catheterized urine specimen for urinalysis, culture, and sensitivity, observing for cloudiness and color as an indication of concentration.

The flight nurse may assess the patient for possible chorioamnionitis; symptoms include fever, tachycardia, fetal tachycardia, uterine tenderness not associated with contractions, purulent vaginal discharge, and an elevated white blood cell count. If results of laboratory tests done by a referring facility are available, the labs indicated are a complete blood count with differential and cervical cultures for β-strep (hemolytic streptococcus) and *Neisseria gonorrhoeae.* However, most are asymptomatic. The most common route for infection is the ascending route from the vagina to the cervix. Evidence indicates that the presence of bacteria in the vagina may locally dissolve the membrane; the bacteria then gain access to the fluid and cause a chorioamnionitis that dissolves the membrane, and SROM results. With no evidence of prior infection, the incidence of infection after SROM greatly increases if the membranes have been ruptured longer than 24 hours.

A history of flulike symptoms and persistent nausea with vomiting, fever, or diarrhea may precipitate PTL, in which case fluid and electrolyte replacement is needed.

The flight nurse should assess the patient for cervical incompetence. A history of previous pregnancy losses, especially associated with "painless labors," is suspect. Vaginal mucus may be the first sign of cervical dilation. The mucus plug that fills the cervical canal can be dislodged by cervical changes. Other symptoms include lower abdominal discomfort or a sensation of fullness in the vagina. Vague symptoms should not be taken lightly. The flight nurse may ask the patient if a cervical cerclage is present; the sutures are designed to reinforce the weak cervix in hopes of retaining the pregnancy to term. After the procedure, the patient is at increased risk for PROM and infection. A cerclage will fail in the presence of perceptible contractions unless tocolytic agents are successful in arresting labor. If labor continues, there is a threat of cervical lacerations as dilation occurs.

Strategies for Transport

Protection of the obstetric patient and the fetus from the threat of preterm delivery is accomplished primarily by supporting the medical plan to suppress labor, maintaining or improving uterine perfusion, and investigating for causes.

The primary survey, including general obstetric assessment, should be done first. The flight nurse should then follow these general guidelines for transport care:

1. Determine the contraction pattern: Determine the phase of labor and assess whether transport can safely be attempted or whether delivery should be accomplished at the referring facility. In the event of an imminent delivery, call for the neonate team, notify the medical director, and help the referring facility prepare for delivery.
2. Determine the status of the amniotic membranes: If there is questionable history of fluid leakage and contractions have slowed or stopped altogether, absolute determination of rupture is not required before transport if it does not alter the plan for nursing care.
3. Determine cervical status: Determine the number of SSEs done at the referring facility, especially if an SSE was done in the presence of ruptured membranes. Assess the amount of cervical change accomplished since admission to the referring facility. Remember that once labor is established, the multiparous woman will frequently progress at a faster rate than a primipara and may require rapid transport.
4. Maintain the patient in the left lateral position: Not only does the left lateral position improve uterine perfusion, thus decreasing uterine irritability, but it decreases pressure on the cervix from the presenting part and may protect against further cervical changes. Having the patient stand, sit, or bend can place pressure against the cervix and should be avoided during transport.
5. Assess for infection: Observe for symptoms of urinary tract infection, pyelonephritis, vaginitis, chorioamnionitis, or signs of a viral infection.
6. Assess for cervical incompetence: An incompetent cervix can be suspected if the patient has vague symptoms accompanied by disproportionate cervical changes. Obstetric history in these cases is of particular importance. Placing these patients in the left lateral position in a slight Trendelenburg's position, or with hips slightly elevated, may further reduce any pressure on the cervix.
7. Administer tocolytic agents: Suppression of labor is always attempted to "buy time" for the transport. Optimal neonatal outcome can be anticipated when the delivery occurs in a hospital that is prepared for the intensive care of premature infants. If hydration and positioning to the left lateral have not slowed or arrested labor, tocolytic agents can be administered. The medications used most frequently in suppressing labor are $MgSO_4$ or terbutaline sulfate, procardia, and ritodrine.
   a. Magnesium sulfate
   $MgSO_4$, discussed in detail in reference to PIH, is now being used successfully in the treatment of preterm labor with less adverse reactions than the β-sympathomimetic agents. $MgSO_4$, as opposed to intravenously administered terbutaline or ritodrine, is recommended during transport. In addition to relaxing smooth muscle, it improves uterine perfusion, decreases uterine irritability, and further suppresses labor. Dosage, administration, and therapeutic levels are the same as in the treatment of PIH.
   b. Terbutaline H sulfate and ritodrine
   Both terbutaline sulfate and ritodrine are β-sympathomimetic agents and can be discussed simultaneously. Both stimulate β_1 receptors (producing cardiac stimulation with tachycardia and increased

myocardial contractility), and β_2 receptors (producing primarily uterine and bronchial relaxation, peripheral vasodilation, and decreased intestinal motility). With stimulation to the β_2 receptors more predominate, uterine relaxation can be achieved if the patient tolerates the dose without the development of adverse reactions.

Terbutaline may be administered intravenously. The dose is increased every 10 to 15 minutes until the contractions stop, intolerable reactions develop, or the maximum safe dose is reached. With the initiation of β-sympathomimetic therapy before or during transport, cardiac monitoring per continuous ECG is highly recommended.

Terbutaline may be administered subcutaneously, 0.25 mg, or intravenously and may be repeated in 15 minutes to 1 hour until a pulse rate of 120 is achieved or contractions decrease. Subcutaneously administered terbutaline is the drug of choice when the contractions are occurring every 10 minutes or less. With terbutaline on board, $MgSO_4$ or another tocolytic agent can be prepared for intravenous infusion.

Once the patient is stabilized with the intravenous infusion, terbutaline, 2.5 to 5 mg administered orally every 4 hours, or ritodrine, 10 mg administered every 4 hours, may maintain tocolysis.

Side effects include tachycardia, palpitations, and widening of the pulse pressure. It is not uncommon to see a blood pressure of 110/50 or 100/40 caused by a drop in the diastolic pressure. Nausea and vomiting, tremors, and feelings of restlessness are common. Fetal tachycardia is seen. Decreased serum potassium levels may be seen as a result of a shift to the intracellular; however, supplemental potassium is usually not necessary, because the potassium levels normalize soon after discontinuing the intravenous therapy.

Intravenous infusion should be discontinued if the heart rate reaches 140 or higher, FHR reaches 180 or higher, or the blood pressure drops below 90/60. Symptoms of pulmonary edema can occur, usually as a result of fluid overload. Chest pain or cardiac arrhythmias such as premature ventricular contractions, supraventricular tachycardia, or atrial fibrillation are also indications for discontinuing the infusion.

In addition to stopping the infusion, supplemental oxygen should be provided. Propranolol hydrochloride (a β-blocker), 0.5 to 1.0 mg, administered slowly and intravenously, or verapamil hydrochloride (a slow channel blocker), 5 to 10 mg, administered slowly and intravenously, counteracts the effects of terbutaline and ritodrine, with improvement seen within a short length of time.

Terbutaline or ritodrine is contraindicated in patients with suspected chorioamnionitis or multiple gestation because of an increased incidence of pulmonary edema among these patients when β-sympathomimetic agents are used. In patients who are insulin-dependent diabetics, it is contraindicated because of transient hyperglycemia seen with treatment. Any patient with chronic hypertension or cardiac disease should not be treated with β-sympathomimetics if at all possible. If hemorrhage is present, it is advisable not to administer terbutaline or ritodrine, because the cardiac stimulation may increase the hemorrhage.

If contractions have not appreciably slowed, even with use of labor suppressants, and the patient is in active labor, the dosage and administration of the tocolytic agent may have been inadequate; administering another bolus or increasing the dosage of the current drug may be effective.

c. Procardia

Procardia is a calcium channel-blocking agent. The loading dose is 60 mg sublingually and 20 mg every 6 hours. Side effects of procardia include maternal hypotension and possible fetal compromise. Vital signs along with fetal heart rate and oxygen saturation should be checked every 5 to 20 minutes.

TRAUMA IN PREGNANCY

Minor accidental injuries are common during pregnancy. The gravid uterus, loosened joints, altered center of gravity, shortness of breath, dizziness, increased fatigue, and edema all contribute to minor accidents.

Serious accidental injuries during pregnancy place not only the obstetric patient but the fetus at risk. The fetus is well protected within the confines of the uterus as it is surrounded by amniotic fluid, which serves as an excellent shock absorber. It is extremely rare for a fetus to experience physical trauma except as a result of direct penetrating wounds or extensive blunt trauma. The fetus is at greatest risk for fetal distress and intrauterine death as a result of maternal trauma and death. The obstetric patient is more vulnerable to hemorrhage because of the increased vascularity surrounding the gravid uterus. Early signs and symptoms of hypovolemia may be masked by the normal physiologic changes of pregnancy. As a result, blood is shunted away from nonvital organs, including the uterus, threatening the well-being of the fetus. In dealing with a trauma patient who is pregnant, the best interest of the fetus is served by prompt assessment and interventions on behalf of the mother. When the situation is life-threatening, the pregnancy should be ignored. Chapter 14 features a detailed discussion on trauma in pregnancy.

OBSTETRIC EMERGENCIES CASE STUDY

The air medical crew received a call at 1926 hours to pick up a 19-year-old woman, G4/P2, approximately 31 to 32 weeks gestation, twins, PROM, not in active labor, and currently receiving $MgSO_4$ per IV infusion. A follow-up call to the physician at the referring facility confirmed the report. He reported doing an SSE with rupture of membranes confirmed by positive nitrazine and positive pooling. The cervix was not visualized. No SVE had been done. He reported that the patient had gestational diabetes, controlled by diet. Because of the distance from the airport to the clinic (about 30 minutes), the physician decided to transport the patient by ambulance to the airport to meet the flight crew there.

The patient had come to a clinic in a small outlying area at approximately 1800 hours with the chief complaint of ruptured membranes, which occurred at approximately 1730 hours, with clear fluid noted. Soon thereafter the patient reported that contractions began. Terbutaline, 0.25 mg, was administered subcutaneously at 1940 hours. An IV was started in the left hand with an 18-gauge catheter and a 6 g $MgSO_4$ bolus was administered, followed by an infusion, 2 g per hour.

Less than 30 minutes after the call was received by the flight crew, the plane lifted off at 1947 hours, and landed at the referring airport after approximately 50 minutes.

FLIGHT CREW ARRIVAL AND EVALUATION

Clinical findings: The ambulance arrived at the airport with the patient, who was accompanied by an LPN. A brief history provided by the nurse included EDC by US with LMP unknown and no significant medical history. Obstetrical history included spontaneous vaginal deliveries in 1986 and 1988 without complications, and a spontaneous abortion in 1986. The current pregnancy was complicated by preterm labor 1 month ago, and the patient was currently being treated with terbutaline, 5 mg every 4 hours, with last dose 2 days ago. The patient states, "I ran out of medicine." The patient was found in the left recumbent position, and appeared to be uncomfortable during contractions. Contractions were palpated firm, lasting approximately 60 seconds, with a frequency of every 2 minutes. It was noted that the mainline IV of lactated Ringer's solution contained 700 ml with an attached burette containing 2 g of $MgSO_4$ in 50 ml that was not infusing. The patient began to complain of pelvic and rectal pressure with lower back discomfort. A slight amount of bloody show was observed on the perineum. The LPN reported that contractions at the clinic were irregular, occurring every 5 to 15 minutes. An SVE by the flight nurse revealed complete dilation with the breech presenting at a +2 to +3 station.

Laboratory and x-ray findings: No laboratory

tests or x-rays were done with the exception of a cervical culture done for *Neisseria gonorrhoeae* and *Chlamydia,* with a culture and sensitivity pending.

Provisional diagnosis: Twin gestation, active PTL, delivery imminent, breech presentation, PROM, gestational diabetes controlled by diet.

TRANSPORT CARE AND INTERVENTIONS BY FLIGHT NURSE

1. Terbutaline, 0.25 mg, was administered SQ at 2050 hours.
2. Radio contact was made with the referring facility via ambulance radio regarding the possibility of returning to the facility for possible delivery. The physician recommended against returning because of the 30-minute time factor if there was another facility closer by air that was better equipped to deal with premature twins.
3. The decision was made to air transport the patient, diverting from the original destination to a level II facility approximately 30 minutes away.
4. Airborne at 2055 hours, radio contact was made with the communications department informing them of a change of destination and need for an ambulance to be waiting at the airport upon arrival. The receiving facility was notified of the condition of the patient, and preparations were made.
5. Aggressive coaching took precedence over all other nursing actions. The situation was explained to the patient, with the patient expressing desire to cooperate in any way possible to prevent delivery while en route. The patient was encouraged to pant and breathe during contractions and not to bear down.
6. While en route, preparations were made for an emergency delivery and infant resuscitation.
7. Between contractions, the IV was switched over to blood tubing with 1000 ml lactated Ringer's solution at a rate of 125 ml per hour. Supplemental oxygen was administered per nonrebreather face mask at 12 L/min. The patient was maintained in the left lateral position.
8. During contractions, the flight nurse was breathing with the patient for encouragement, providing support as needed. Contractions of strong intensity continued every 2 to 3 minutes.
9. Vital signs and FHT were evaluated every 15 minutes as tolerated by the patient. FHT remained stable with no irregularities identified by Doppler auscultation. An SVE was done at 2105 hours with no further descent of the breech noted. Frequent visual evaluations of the perineum were done to note any indication of imminent delivery such as increased bloody show, bulging of the perineum, or crowning of the breech.
10. Upon arrival at the receiving airport at 2128 hours, an ambulance with a paramedic crew was waiting. The patient was transported to the hospital with lights and sirens, and arrived at 2145 hours.

PATIENT OUTCOME

The flight nurse was greeted at the labor and delivery unit by an obstetrician and pediatrician. At that time the patient was having an increasingly strong urge to bear down, and just following transfer to the delivery table by a sheet pull, twin A spontaneously delivered over an intact perineum assisted by the flight nurse at 2150 hours. The cord was clamped and cut, and the infant was immediately attended to by the pediatrician and nursery personnel in the resuscitation area of the delivery room. The FHT of twin B remained stable at 154 per Doppler auscultation after delivery of twin A. EFM of the remaining twin was initiated at that time. Apgars were 6 and 7, at 1 minute and 5 minutes, respectively. Twin A, a boy, weighed 1700 g (3 lb, 12 oz).

Twin B presented as a footling breech, and the decision was made to deliver by cesarean section. At this point the medical director was called, and after conferring with the obstetrician and pediatrician, a neonate team was dispatched for the transport of both twins to a level I facility. Twin B, also a boy, was born at 2230 hours with Apgars of 7 and 7, weighing 1673 g (3 lb, 11 oz).

DISCUSSION

This case had the potential for a disastrous outcome. The possibility of the breech delivery of a preterm infant and possibly twins in an ambulance at least 30 minutes away from the closest facility is not an appealing situation. One of the most alarming facts of this case was the misinformation provided by the referring physician that the patient was not in labor. Under the presumption that the patient was stable, receiving tocolytics, and that labor had been successfully arrested, there was no need for the flight nurse to be accompanied by other flight personnel. However, on a call where there is any possibility of a delivery, especially on a longer transport, a neonate flight nurse is a crucial member of the flight crew.

The flight nurse accurately assessed the danger of the situation and opted for immediate air transport to the nearest facility, which was a level II facility. Even when faced with imminent delivery, tocolytics were considered. Tocolytics may or may not slow the progression of labor at that late phase; if it does, it allows precious time to get a patient to a receiving facility undelivered. This transport revealed how important it can be to coach the obstetric patient. Provision of support may have aided the patient as much as the terbutaline. Had the flight nurse been at the referring facility when the situation presented as it did, the transport would not have proceeded as planned. It would have been safer for both mother and fetuses to deliver at the referring facility, however inadequate, and immediately call for a neonate team, than to risk delivery en route. A flight crew consisting of a flight nurse and another crew member should have been considered. The flight nurse on this transport expressed concern that had twin A delivered, she only had two hands with which to work, considering the obstetrical care the patient required, the possible resuscitation of twin A, and concern for the well-being of twin B.

Communications during this flight among the pilot, flight nurse, and the communications department were pivotal in expediting completion of the flight. When the patch was made, the receiving hospital was given adequate time to prepare for the delivery of preterm twins, the ambulance that was notified arrived ahead of time to be prepared in the event of a delivery en route, and the medical director was made aware of the situation and the change in destination. The medical director was consulted after the flight nurse arrived at the receiving hospital, was given an update of the outcome of the transport, and was asked for further recommendations. The medical director should be consulted when the flight team is presented with an unexpected event or when the patient is not stable for transport.

In this situation, intervention by the flight nurse ensured a favorable outcome for both the mother and the fetuses. It also demonstrated how, in a very short period of time, the obstetrical and fetal assessment was made and a successful plan of nursing action was developed.

REFERENCES

1. Arnone B: Amniotic fluid embolism: a case report, *J Nurse Midwifery* 34:92, 1989.
2. Benorub GI: *Obstetric and gynecologic emergencies,* Philadelphia, 1993, Lippincott.
3. Buckley K, Klub N: *High risk pregnancy manual,* Baltimore, 1993, Williams & Wilkins.
4. Clark SL, Cotton DB: *Handbook of critical care obstetrics,* Boston, 1994, Blackwell.
5. Cunningham GF et al: *Williams obstetrics,* ed 19, East Norwalk, Conn, 1993, Appleton-Century-Crofts.
6. Gilbert E, Harmon J: *High-risk pregnancy and delivery: nursing perspectives,* St Louis, 1986, Mosby.
7. Harvey CJ: *Critical care obstetrical nursing,* Gaithersburg, Md, 1991, Aspen.
8. Mandeville LK, Troiano NH: *High risk intrapartum nursing,* Philadelphia, 1992, Lippincott.
9. Mattson S, Smith JE: *Core curriculum for maternal newborn nursing,* Philadelphia, 1993, Saunders.
10. Pritchard JA, MacDonald PC, Gant NF: *Williams obstetrics,* ed 17, East Norwalk, Conn, 1985, Appleton-Century-Crofts.
11. Smith J: The dangers of prenatal cocaine use, *Matern Child Nurs J* 13:174, 1988.

CHAPTER 34

Care and Transport of the Neonate

COMPETENCIES

1. Execute a complete initial assessment of the neonate.
2. Perform the necessary interventions to maintain the neonate's airway, breathing, and circulation after delivery.
3. Prepare the neonate for transport using the appropriate equipment for size and need.

The neonate has a unique anatomy, physiology, and pathophysiology. The depth of knowledge required by transport personnel is directly related to the mission of the team as it pertains to the care of neonates. In the case of the infant requiring care in a nonmedical environment, including a home, car, and so on, the needs of the infant are for basic resuscitation and stabilization and expedient transport to the nearest appropriate medical facility. In the case of interfacility transport of newborns, the emphasis should be on providing a level of care during stabilization and transport equivalent to the level of care the infant will obtain at the receiving hospital. This implies that the combined expertise of the referring staff and the transport team can provide that level of assessment and care. The final step in ensuring quality care should include review of all neonatal protocols, procedures, and cases by a designated individual with recognized expertise in that field.

FETAL CIRCULATION AND TRANSITION

The scope of this chapter allows only a brief overview of the fetal circulation and transition to extrauterine life. The umbilical vein carries blood with the highest oxygen saturation back to the right atrium via the ductus venosus and the inferior vena cava. A large percentage of this blood is directed across the foramen ovale to the left atrium, left ventricle, and ascending aorta, thus perfusing the coronary arteries and the brain with the most highly oxygenated blood in the fetal circulation. Some of the blood coming from the umbilical vein along with blood returning from the superior vena cava flows through the tricuspid valve to the right ventricle and out through the pulmonary valve. Because of the high resistance in the peripheral pulmonary vasculature, most of the blood flow from the right ventricle

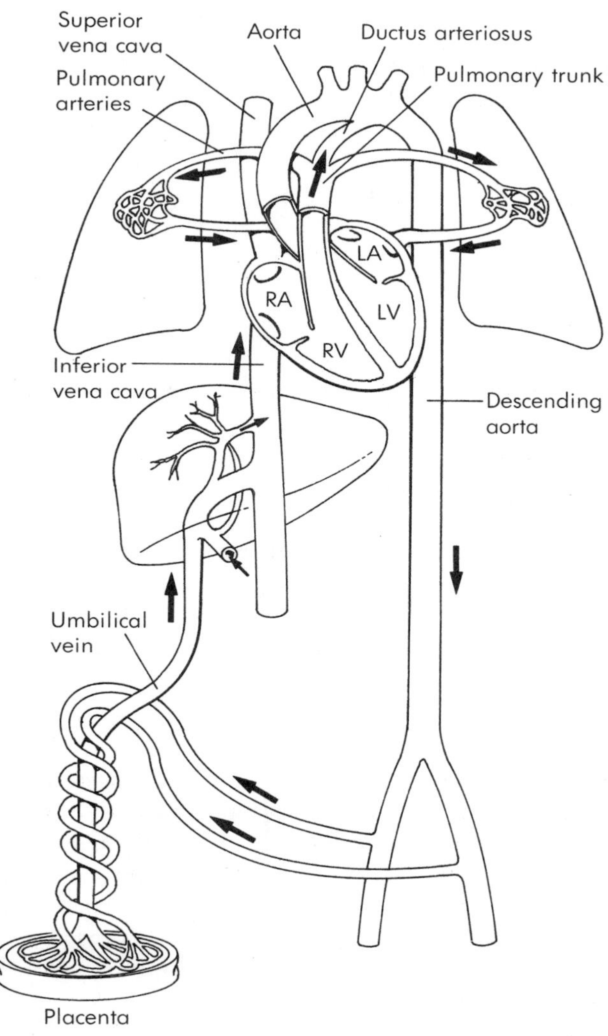

Fig. 34-1. The normal fetal circulation and major fetal flow patterns. (From Heymann MA: Biophysical evaluation of fetal status: fetal cardiovascular physiology. In Creasy RK, Resnik R, editors: *Maternal fetal medicine,* Philadelphia, 1984, Saunders.)

passes from the pulmonary artery through the ductus arteriosus and into the descending aorta, mixing with the remainder of the blood coming from the left side of the heart. In utero, the right and left ventricles both pump at systemic pressures into the aorta (Fig. 34-1).[21]

With the expansion of the lungs and improved oxygenation at birth, the pulmonary vascular resistance falls, allowing a rapid increase in pulmonary blood flow and a consequent decrease in flow across the ductus arteriosus. Simultaneously, the umbilical cord is clamped, removing the low-resistance placental circuit and increasing systemic resistance. This increase in afterload, as well as increased return to the left atrium from the pulmonary circuit, closes the flaplike foramen ovale. Neonatal hypoxia, hypoglycemia, hypothermia, sepsis, and acidosis can all interfere with the normal progression of this transition period.[15,31,33] Therefore careful ongoing assessment and early intervention are critical during this time period. Common findings at this time include intermittent grunting, mild retracting, and tachypnea.[39] The infant should be observed closely until all these symptoms have resolved.

DELIVERY ROOM MANAGEMENT

Assessment

Traditional delivery room assessment includes the assignments of the Apgar score developed in 1953 by Dr. Virginia Apgar (Table 34-1).[1] The Apgar score is a basic rapid evaluation of the infant's immediate adaptation to extrauterine life. The Apgar score evaluates color, respiratory effort, heart rate, body tone, and responsiveness to stimuli. It is routinely measured at 1 and 5 minutes after birth. If, however, the infant continues to be depressed after 5 minutes of age, it can be useful to continue assigning Apgar scores until accurate and comprehensive nursing notes are begun. Early studies correlated low 5-minute Apgar scores with poor neurologic outcome.[13] However, later studies have shown that the Apgar score is not an accurate indicator of neonatal asphyxia as defined by metabolic acidosis.[30,40] In the case of a depressed infant, cord gases should be evaluated whenever possible for the presence of metabolic acidosis. The Apgar score remains, however, an excellent tool for assessing perinatal depression, which may be the result of to a number of etiologies. In addition to perinatal asphyxia, the Apgar score can be affected by maternal medications, prematurity, neuromuscular disorders, previous intrauterine cerebral insults, and central nervous system (CNS) abnormalities, among others. The use of the Apgar score is most helpful in directing the level of intervention required by the infant.

CLEAR THE AIRWAY

Immediately on delivery of the head, the airway should be cleared with either bulb, DeLee, or mechanical suction. The oropharynx should normally be cleared before suctioning of the nose because stimulation of the nares may cause the infant to gasp and

TABLE 34-1

The Apgar score

Score	Sign		
	0	1	2
*A*ppearance, color	Blue, pale	Centrally pink	Completely pink
*P*ulse, heart rate	None	Less than 100 beats/min	Greater than 100 beats/min
*G*rimace, reflex	No response	Grimace	Cough, gag, cry
*A*ctivity/attitude	Flaccid/limp muscle tone	Some flexion	Well-flexed/active motion
*R*espiratory, effort	None, irritability	Weak/irregular	Good, crying

aspirate secretions present in the oropharynx. Stimulation of the vagus nerve resulting in severe bradycardia can result from suctioning too vigorously and too deeply. Therefore suctioning after the initial clearing of the airway should be done strictly on an as-needed basis.

It is essential that thorough suctioning of the oropharynx and nasopharynx be completed before the delivery of the thorax and the infant's first breath. The aspiration by the infant of meconium-stained fluid into distal airways contributes significantly to morbidity and mortality. The more heavily stained the fluid, the higher the risk of significant pulmonary disease. The incidence of this complication can be greatly reduced by effective clearing of the airway.[11,43] After delivery, if the infant is depressed or has respiratory distress or heavily stained amniotic fluid, the trachea should be intubated and suctioned before positive-pressure ventilation is used.

Maintain Body Temperature

As soon as possible after delivery the infant should be dried and a heat source provided. The use of a stocking cap can greatly decrease heat losses. The only circumstance in which drying of the infant should be delayed is in the presence of meconium-stained fluid. In this situation, the baby should not be stimulated until the airway has been cleared, possibly including direct suctioning of the trachea.

Initiate Breathing

The baby's head should be maintained in the sniffing position and blow-by oxygen may be supplied until the infant is centrally pink. If the infant does not begin spontaneous respirations or the heart rate remains below 100 beats/min after clearing of the airway and stimulating the infant, ventilation should be initiated at a rate of 40 to 60 breaths/min. During the resuscitation stage, 100% oxygen should always be used. Face-mask and anesthesia-bag ventilation should be tried initially. Adequate ventilation should be evaluated by auscultating breath sounds and observing chest excursion. The infant will respond to adequate ventilation with an improvement in color, heart rate, and tone. Ventilating pressures should always be monitored with a manometer. Although pressures up to 30 to 40 cm H_2O may be required in the initial breaths to open the lungs, the lowest pressures possible to maintain good ventilation should be used. Newborn infants are at high risk for pulmonary air leak during mechanical ventilation. Once the infant has established spontaneous respirations, a heart rate >100 beats/min, and is centrally pink, the flight nurse reevaluates for the amount of support required. Support may include blow-by oxygen, face-mask continuous positive airway pressure (CPAP), continued ventilation, or no additional oxygen.

If there is no response in heart rate and color after 30 seconds to 1 minute of bag and mask ventilation, then the flight nurse should place an endotracheal tube (Table 34-2). Because there is little room for error in the placement of the endotracheal tube, careful and immediate evaluation for right-mainstem or esophageal intubation should be done, and adequacy of ventilation should be as-

TABLE 34-2

Endotracheal tube size selection

Weight (kg)	Endotracheal tube (size)	Depth of insertion (cm from upper lip)	Suction cath size
1	2.5	7	5 Fr
2	3.0	8	6 Fr
3	3.5	9	8 Fr
4	4.0	10	8–10 Fr

sessed again. Ventilation should be continued until effective spontaneous respirations have been established.

Chest Compressions

If the heart rate remains below 60 beats/min or between 60 and 80 beats/min and does not increase after 15 to 30 seconds of ventilation, the flight nurse should initiate chest compressions. The lower third of the sternum should be depressed ½ to ¾ inch at a rate of 90 compressions per minute interposing 30 breaths per minute for a 3 : 1 ratio.[3] Recheck the heart rate after 30 seconds and again at 1 minute. The infant should be evaluated at least once per minute for heart rate, perfusion, pulses, color, and respiratory effort. Once the heart rate has returned to greater than 80 beats/min cardiac massage may be discontinued.

DRUG SUPPORT

Drugs are rarely needed in the delivery room resuscitation of the newborn if adequate ventilation has been established (Table 34-3). If the heart rate continues below 80 beats/min despite adequate ventilation and compressions for a minimum of 30 seconds, or if there is no heart rate, the flight nurse should instill 0.1 to 0.3 ml per kg of 1 : 10,000 solution of epinephrine down the endotracheal tube. To ensure that the epinephrine reaches the lungs, it may be diluted in or flushed with 1 to 2 ml of normal saline. IV access should be attained as soon as possible. During delivery room resuscitation the umbilical vein is the most accessible parenteral route (box). If the heart rate remains below 80 beats/min, a second dose of epinephrine may be given through the endotracheal tube or through the established IV line. Hypovolemia should be suspected when there is a history of bleeding or if the infant demonstrates poor response to resuscitation, pallor, or poor pulse volume despite adequate ventilation. If hypovolemia is thought to be a problem, volume expanders should be given. Once adequate ventilation and tissue perfusion have been established, the flight nurse may administer sodium bicarbonate 4.2% solution in a dose of 2 mEq/kg slowly over 2 to 3 minutes for documented metabolic acidosis. Under transport conditions, documenting blood gas status may be impossible. A decision to administer sodium bicarbonate in the presence of prolonged asphyxia/resuscitation may be made after the earlier steps have been adequately completed. As soon as possible a blood sample should be evaluated for partial pressure of oxygen (PaO_2), partial pressure of carbon dioxide ($PaCO_2$), and pH. If an arterial sample is not available, a venous sample is still valuable, particularly for

TABLE 34-3

Neonatal emergency drug dosages

Drug	Indication	Dose	Route*
Naloxone (neonatal Narcan)	Narcotic depression	0.1 mg/kg	IV/UVC/IM/ETT
Epinephrine (1 : 10,000)	Bradycardia, cardiac arrest	0.1-0.3 ml/kg	ETT/UVC/IV
Sodium bicarbonate, 4.2% (0.5 mEq/ml)	Metabolic acidosis	2 mEq/kg over 2-3 minutes	UVC/IV (always clear line before and after administration)
5% Albumin	Hypotension volume restoration	10 ml/kg over 5-10 minutes	UVC/IV
Lactated Ringer's	Hypotension volume restoration	10 ml/kg over 5-10 minutes	UVC/IV
Dextrose 10%	Hypoglycemia	2-4 ml/kg	UVC/IV

**IV,* Intravenous; *IM,* intramuscular; *UVC,* umbilical venous catheter.

UMBILICAL VEIN CATHETERIZATION

The flight nurse should place the umbilical vein catheter under aseptic technique. The umbilical stump and surrounding skin should first be cleansed with three applications of povidone-iodine (Betadine), which is allowed to dry and then removed with either alcohol or sterile water. Drapes are then placed to provide a sterile field. A no. 5 Fr. catheter is usually adequate and can normally be placed in all sizes of infants; it is prepared by either attaching the catheter directly to a three-way stopcock or trimming the flared end of the catheter and inserting a blunt needle adapter. The blunt needle adapter would then be connected to the three-way stopcock and flushed with solution.

Umbilical tape is tied snugly around the base of the cord to provide control of bleeding during the procedure. The umbilical stump can then be cut approximately 1 cm above the skin line. The flight nurse can then identify the two thick-walled constricted arteries and the thinner-walled larger vein. A pair of curved iris forceps may be helpful in identifying and opening the lumen of the vein.

The flight nurse then inserts the catheter tip in the lumen and gently advances it. It may be helpful to stabilize the cord by gently holding the cord at the base or applying traction with a clamp on the Wharton's jelly. The umbilical vein normally runs in a cephalad direction. Directing the catheter in that line may assist in ease of entry. The venous catheter should be inserted only as far as necessary to obtain blood return, which is normally 2 to 3 cm. Advancing the catheter further may result in a placement in the liver and consequent hepatic damage from medication injections.

The umbilical catheter can then be secured with a tape bridge. A purse-string suture around the Wharton's jelly and then tied to the catheter will control bleeding, as well as assist in securing the catheter.

Complications of this procedure include infection, hemorrhage, air emboli, and thrombus formation. Therefore the procedure should only be undertaken after appropriate training under supervision and then performed with extreme care.

$PaCO_2$ and pH. If the heart rate has not responded to the above therapy, epinephrine may be repeated every 5 minutes and sodium bicarbonate as indicated by blood gas determination. For narcotic depression, naloxone 0.1 mg/kg can be given IV, IM, SQ, or via the endotracheal tube. These infants, however, should respond to ventilation with improved heart rate and color despite their respiratory depression. Naloxone may precipitate severe withdrawal in the infant of a mother with narcotic addiction and should be used with extreme caution if the flight nurse suspects this situation.

Evaluation

If the infant has not responded to the measures just discussed, the flight nurse must reevaluate the clinical assessment and management of the infant. Common reasons for an inadequate response to resuscitation include:

1. Mechanical problems
   a. Inadequate oxygen supply
   b. Inadequate ventilatory pressures
2. Tube malposition
   a. Tube in esophagus
   b. Tube in right mainstem
   c. Blocked tube
3. Unrecognized clinical problem
   a. Pneumothorax
   b. Diaphragmatic hernia
   c. Hypoplastic lungs

STABILIZATION BASICS

The goal of stabilization is an infant who has normal vital signs, normal blood pressure (BP), normal perfusion, normal blood gases, and normal glucose and electrolyte levels. This goal is not always attainable, but every attempt should be made to achieve it before transport.

Thermoregulation

Because of the large surface area compared to body mass and poor thermal insulation, the infant is at high risk for hypothermia. Hypothermia in the neonate can be lethal. It is usually an iatrogenic condition and is almost always preventable. Compared with the adult, the newborn has limited ability to produce heat by shivering. Similarly, the hyperthermic infant has an increased oxygen consumption and a limited ability to dissipate heat through sweating. It is therefore essential to understand the mechanisms of heat production and loss and interventions for maintaining a neutral thermal environment. The neutral thermal environment is that range of environmental temperature at which the baby can maintain a normal body temperature with minimal metabolic activity and oxygen consumption.[8,12,38]

The optimal temperature ranges for the newborn are:

Skin temperature 36.0° to 36.5° C
Axillary 36.5° to 37.0° C
Rectal 36.5° to 37.0° C

It is essential that skin temperature be monitored in the newborn in addition to either axillary or rectal temperature. An infant can have a normal central temperature using axillary or rectal measurements and still be cold stressed with a cool skin temperature. Cold stress increases mortality and morbidity. Side effects of cold stress and hypothermia include increased oxygen consumption, hypoxemia, acidosis, and pulmonary vasoconstriction. In addition, the infant increases his or her glucose consumption, which may result in hypoglycemia. Release of free fatty acids into the blood may contribute to the development of kernicterus at low levels of indirect hyperbilirubinemia.

The neonate maintains his or her body temperature through basal metabolism, muscular activity, and chemical thermogenesis. The infant's primary mechanism of heat production in response to cold stress is chemical thermogenesis using his or her brown fat stores. This process requires increased oxygen consumption.[23] In the presence of decreased brown fat stores (i.e., prematurity) or hypoxia, his or her ability to generate heat production is severely limited.[37]

Heat losses occur through convection, conduction, evaporation, and radiation, as follows:

Radiation: Heat transfer between the body and surrounding objects (for example, isolette walls)
Convection: Heat transfer dependent on air flow over the body (for example, a cold delivery room)
Evaporation: Heat transfer to water in the state change from liquid to gas (for example, a wet infant)
Conduction: Heat transfer between the body and objects in contact (for example, a scale)

The latter is the least important mechanism of heat loss in newborns. The management of the infant's thermal environment requires a careful balancing of heat losses and heat sources. Interventions for blocking heat loss include keeping the infant dry; swaddling in blankets, foil, or plastic; using heat shields and stocking caps; and preventing drafts. Heat sources may be most effective when used in combination. Available sources include radiant heat, warmed air, and warming pads. During transport the flight nurse must anticipate the effects of weather conditions. The newborn can lose significant amounts of heat through radiation to cold isolette walls. Therefore continuous temperature monitoring during transport is preferable. Lacking this capability, the temperature should be assessed at 15-minute intervals as a minimum standard.

Fluids, Calories, and Electrolytes

Maintaining fluid, electrolyte, and glucose balance in the newborn requires an initial educated guess as to the individual infant's requirements followed by close observation and evaluation. The main components of fluid loss in the newborn are through insensible water loss and urinary output (UO). In the sick newborn, UO should be measured as accurately as possible, by means of urine bags, diaper weights, catheterization, and so on. Insensible water loss increases significantly as the level of prematurity increases. Radiant warmers, elevated environmental temperatures, and respiratory distress increase insensible water loss. On the other hand, use of heat shields and warm humidified inspired air on the ventilator can significantly decrease these losses. Fluid balance in newborns on IV therapy should be monitored with daily body weights, UO, specific gravities, and serum electrolytes. The need for electrolyte evaluation before transport must be determined based on the age of the newborn, the length of the transport, and the presence of risk factors for electrolyte imbalance.

The newborn infant normally has a fluid requirement of approximately 60 to 80 ml/kg/day on the first day of life. This requirement increases approximately 10 ml/kg/day on subsequent days of life. In the premature infant, particularly <1500 g, special consideration should be given to potential increased fluid needs. The use of the radiant warmer or phototherapy in these infants can increase fluid requirements by as much as 50% for each.[5] As mentioned, use of heat shields or clear plastic covers over the infants may help to control these losses. With appropriate fluid intake, UO should be 1 to 2 ml/kg/hr with specific gravities of approximately 1.008 to 1.012. During the first week of life it should be anticipated that the infant will lose 5% to 15% of birth weight.[5] Subsequent changes in the baby's fluid intake are based on evaluation of these criteria.

The addition of electrolytes to IV fluids is usually not necessary in the first 12 to 24 hours. Serum electrolyte levels should be checked before additions. Potassium should not be added until after the infant has voided. Normal electrolyte supplementation is approximately 3 to 4 mEq/kg/day of sodium and 2 to 3 mEq/kg/day of potassium. Because of the immaturity of the renal system, the premature infant may have comparatively larger sodium losses requiring a corresponding increase in sodium supplementation. In the term infant, normal sodium level is 135 to 145 mEq/L with a normal serum potassium of 3.5 to 6.0 mEq/L. The preterm infant frequently has a serum sodium as low as 130 mEq/L. The flight nurse must precisely calculate the infant's fluid requirement, including any abnormal losses, because either too much or too little fluid can be detrimental to the progress of the infant. High fluid intake in these infants contributes to an increased incidence of patent ductus arteriosus.[5] The extremely low birth weight infant of less than 1000 g may require recalculation of fluid and electrolyte requirements two to three times per day.

Glucose Requirements

Newborns are susceptible to hypoglycemia because of immature glucose control mechanisms, decreased glucose substrate stores, or both. The definition of hypoglycemia in the newborn may be variable depending on the reference. In actual practice most clinicians consider a serum glucose of less than 40 mg/dl to represent hypoglycemia.[32,35] The healthy term infant normally reaches the nadir of his or her serum glucose level at approximately 2 hours after birth. It is therefore recommended that glucose screening be conducted in all healthy term infants at 1 to 2 hours of age. However, in the transport setting, the population is generally at higher risk for developing hypoglycemia (box). These high-risk infants should have screening glucose levels as soon as possible after delivery and at appropriate intervals thereafter. Most newborns can be maintained on IV fluids of 10% dextrose in water at the fluid levels recommended in the previous section. Glucose levels should be checked every 30 minutes to 1 hour until

RISK FACTORS FOR HYPOGLYCEMIA

Small for gestational age (SGA)
Hypothermia or cold stress
Respiratory distress
Congenital heart disease
Large for gestational age (LGA)
Infant of a diabetic mother
Rh incompatibility
Beckwith-Wiedemann syndrome
Nesidioblastosis
Islet-cell adenomas
Sepsis
Asphyxia

it has been demonstrated that the amount of glucose provided is adequate to maintain normal serum levels. The infant weighing less than 1000 g should receive 5% dextrose in water because of his or her intolerance of the higher glucose loads, resulting in hyperglycemia.

Any bedside glucose screening strip indicating an abnormal glucose reading should be double-checked and then confirmed with a blood or plasma glucose determination if possible. Hypoglycemia may be treated in several ways depending on the severity of the deficiency. A bolus of 200 to 400 mg/kg (2 to 4 ml/kg) of 10% dextrose in water may be given to return the serum glucose to the normal range. It can then be maintained with maintenance IV fluids. If the hypoglycemia is not profound, the flight nurse may elect to respond by increasing the maintenance fluids to increase glucose delivery without the use of a bolus. A decision as to whether to increase fluid rate or dextrose concentration must be made on the basis of the fluid tolerance of the individual baby. A peripheral vein may be used for glucose concentrations of up to 12.5% dextrose. At concentrations of 12.5% dextrose and higher, a central venous line should be considered. Treatment of extremely resistant hypoglycemia may include the use of corticosteroids, glucagon, epinephrine, and diazoxide. Administration of these drugs, however, is beyond the scope of this chapter.

Hyperglycemia, blood glucose levels greater than 125 mg/dl, is most commonly seen in the infant weighing less than 1000 g or in infants whose hypoglycemia has been overcorrected. Management of hyperglycemia in infants $<$1000 g can usually be handled with the use of 5% dextrose as a maintenance fluid. Hyperglycemia in the infant who is being treated for hypoglycemia can be avoided by administering the appropriate amount of glucose. In general, hyperglycemia is not a problem that requires further management during transport.

Respiratory Management: General Considerations

Because most ill neonates requiring transport have some degree of respiratory compromise, it is essential that the flight nurse perform careful and continuous assessment of their respiratory status. Assessment must include both physical assessment and blood gas and radiographic studies. The presence of retractions, grunting, and flaring indicates a decrease in lung compliance. Both central and peripheral color should be evaluated for the presence of cyanosis. The presence of adequate central oxygenation indicates adequate pulmonary blood flow and gas exchange. The peripheral color may reflect problems with either oxygenation or perfusion. If the infant is centrally oxygenated but peripherally cyanotic, then he or she should be evaluated to determine the cause of the poor perfusion. This may include poor cardiac output or vasoconstriction. Auscultation reveals adequacy of air entry and the presence or absence of fluid in the bronchial tree.

The primary component of respiratory management is ensuring correct positioning and clearing of the airway. As a basic principle, sufficient oxygen should be supplied to ensure central oxygenation. Adequacy of central oxygenation should be checked by evaluating mucous membranes of the mouth and the tongue. Oxygen should be considered a drug, with risks and side effects associated with its use. These risks need to be weighed against the complications of hypoxemia in determining what percentage of oxygen to supply. The term or near-term infant is at increased risk for persistent pulmonary hypertension in the presence of hypoxemia while having a very low risk for the development of retrolental fibroplasia from hyperoxia. It is prudent to err on the side of hyperoxia in the infant of 35 weeks and greater gestation. The infant of 34 weeks or less gestational age has a decreased incidence of persistent pulmonary hypertension. However, there is an increased concern of irreversible side effects if these newborns are maintained in a hyperoxic state. It is therefore important to ensure adequate oxygenation in these infants without sustaining long periods of hyperoxia. Current technology including use of transcutaneous monitor and pulse oximetry greatly enhances the ability to supply oxygen for the newborn within an appropriate range.

Oxygen can be supplied by a number of methods. Blow-by or free-flow oxygen near the baby's face can be used on a short-term basis but has severe drawbacks. First, it is impossible to accurately measure the exact percentage of oxygen that the baby is receiving on a continuous basis. Second, the flow of cold oxygen onto the cold-sensitive face may result in increased inappropriate heat-generating maneuvers on the part of the baby. Hood oxygen allows for the accurate measurement and stabilization of oxygen supply to the newborn. Its drawback is the lack of accessibility to the newborn's head without disturbing the oxygen concentration. Continuous positive airway pressure can be delivered via alternate modes including nasal prongs, nasopharyngeal tube, and endotracheal tube. An endotracheal tube obviously provides the most effective delivery of CPAP but requires the invasive procedure of intubation. Positive-pressure ventilation requires the placement of an endotracheal tube, with its inherent potential complications, but it can be done safely in the hands of a skilled practitioner. In selecting the mode of oxygen delivery, the flight nurse must weigh both the benefits to be gained and the risks incurred by the selected approach. These are addressed in this chapter under the various disease entities.

Once respiratory support has begun, continuous observation and reevaluation must be accomplished to maintain the correct level of support. Adjustments must be made to accommodate changes in the infant's pulmonary compliance. Diminishing compliance without an appropriate adjustment in oxygen support may result in hypoxia with hypercarbia. Improvement in compliance could result in hyperoxia, hypocarbia, and potentially tamponade with a resultant decrease in cardiac output. Any infant treated with positive pressure is at an automatic increased risk for air leaks including pneumothorax, pneumomediastinum, and pulmonary interstitial emphysema. Uncommonly, pneumoperitoneum and pneumopericardium could also occur. Any sudden deterioration in an infant receiving positive-pressure ventilation should prompt immediate evaluation for pulmonary air leaks. Evaluation should include assessment of breath sounds, shifting of the point of maximal intensity (PMI), transillumination of the chest, and chest x-ray.[39] Mechanical problems with the oxygen delivery system should also be immediately ruled out. It is always important after bag-mask ventilation to ensure that excess air is removed from the stomach, because a distended stomach could interfere with adequate ventilation.

Blood Pressure and Perfusion

Hypotension, poor perfusion, or both are also common problems in the neonate. Assessment of this problem should begin with an evaluation of the obstetric history, which would suggest a cause for either hypovolemia or myocardial dysfunction. Historical facts suggestive of hypovolemia as a basis for poor perfusion would include compression of the cord, preferentially obstructing flow to the baby through the umbilical veins while allowing flow from the baby to the placenta through the firm-walled umbilical arteries, and a history of blood loss during the pregnancy, labor, or delivery.

Infants with a history of asphyxia may well have both hypovolemia and myocardial dysfunction. Assessment would include aortic pressures, central venous pressures, extremity versus core temperatures, a capillary refill greater than 3 seconds in the presence of a normal temperature, and evaluation of pulse volume. The presence of a progressive metabolic acidosis in a well-ventilated and oxygenated infant and evidence of cardiomegaly on x-ray films may be indicative of an asphyxial cardiomyopathy.

Treatment is aimed at the return to adequate perfusion of the tissues to prevent continued metabolic acidosis. If the flight nurse suspects hypovolemia, the treatment would include careful transfusion with whole blood, fresh-frozen plasma, 5% salt-poor albumin, lactated Ringer's, or normal saline. Rapid increase in systemic blood pressure carries the risk of sudden rise in pressure in vascular beds. This could cause capillary rupture and hemorrhage and result in intracranial bleeding. If myocardial dysfunction is suspected, the flight nurse may consider administering inotropic agents. Whichever treatment is instituted, careful monitoring of arterial pressures is essential both to monitor results and to prevent complications.

ASSESSMENT OF THE NEWBORN

Assessment of the newborn includes historical information, clinical examination, and laboratory data. Obstetric information obtained should include the estimated day of confinement (EDC) based on the mother's dates and clinical data, maternal age, gravity, parity, abortions, fetal demises, neonatal deaths, number of living children, length of rupture of membranes, and complications of the pregnancy, labor, or delivery. Neonatal history would include Apgar scores, resuscitation required, initial physical examination, and subsequent course. Laboratory data and radiographic studies must also be reviewed.

Gestational Age Examination

Both Dubowitz[14] and Cappurro[10] have developed assessment tools for gestational aging of the newborn. Cappurro's scale is reproduced here (Fig. 34-2). In 1977 Hittner published an assessment of gestational age using the examination of the anterior vascular capsule of the lens.[2] This examination is especially helpful for assessing infants between 27 and 34 weeks gestation. For the infant less than 34 weeks of age, Jacinto Hernandez at The Children's Hospital in Denver, Colorado, has developed a system correlating foot length with gestational age. Using this measurement, the foot is measured from the heel to the tip of the longest toe. A 4.5 cm measurement would equal 25 weeks. For each additional 0.5 cm of length, 2 weeks is added to the gestational age. These measurements have been well correlated in preterm infants less than or equal to 34 weeks gestation using the Dubowitz examination. However, it is not reliable in the small-for-gestational-age infant. Once the gestational age has been determined according to both historical and clinical data, the weight, length, and head circumference of the infant should be plotted on standardized growth charts.[2,34] The infant with a weight less than the 10th percentile for gestational age is classified as small for gestational age. The infant with a weight greater than 90th percentile for gestational age is classified as large for gestational age. All infants between the 10th and the 90th percentile are classified as appropriate for gestational age.[4,6,28,29]

Physical Examination

A considerable amount of information can be obtained strictly through observation of the infant. The observation should include:

1. Signs and symptoms of distress
2. Nutritional state
3. Morphology
4. Color
5. Respiratory effort
6. Posture and tone
7. Cry
8. Activity level/behavioral state

Before disturbing the baby by handling, the flight nurse should evaluate those things for which a quiet infant is required, including:

1. Heart: Rate, rhythm, heart sounds, murmurs, extra sounds
2. Chest: Symmetry and adequacy of air entry, rales, rhonchi, wheezes
3. Abdomen: Bowel sounds, organomegaly, masses
4. Femoral pulses: Volume

It is then important to complete the rest of the examination in an organized, systematic approach. For example, the flight nurse might examine the infant beginning from the head and working downward. The rest of the examination is outlined as follows:

1. Head: Symmetry, shape, caput succedaneum, cephalhematoma
2. Fontanelles/sutures: Fontanelle number, fullness, depression, and size; suture mobility
3. Symmetry of face: Development, shape, movement
4. Eyes: Shape, position, size, pupils, hemorrhages
5. Mouth: Clefts, teeth, movement of tongue
6. Neck: Webbing, length
7. Nose: Symmetry, septum, patency
8. Clavicles: Masses, intactness
9. Chest: Size, symmetry, shape
10. Umbilical cord: Number of vessels
11. Genitals: development, testes, urethral and vaginal openings
12. Anus: Patency
13. Spine: masses, symmetry, dimples
14. Extremities: symmetry, development, movement, pulses

	A.	VARIABLES					
B. SOMATIC AND NEUROLOGICAL K=200 days	SOMATIC K=204 days	Nipple formation	Nipple barely visible; no areola 0	Well-defined nipple; areola <0.75 cm 5	Areola stippled not raised >0.75 cm 10	Areola raised >0.75 cm 15	
		Skin texture	Thin, gelatinous 0	Thin and smooth 5	Smooth, medium thickness, superficial peeling 10	Slight thickening, superficial cracking & peeling of hands & feet 15	Thick and parchment like 20
		Ear form	Pinna flat & shapeless 0	Incurving of part of edge 8	Partial incurving of whole of upper pinna 16	Well-defined incurving of pinna 24	
		Breast size	No breast tissue 6	Diameter <0.5 cm 5	Diameter 0.5–1 cm 10	Diameter >1 cm 15	
		Plantar creases	No creases 0	Faint red marks over anterior ½ 5	Definite red marks over anterior ½, indentations over anterior ⅓ 10	Indentations over anterior ½ 15	Deep indentations over more than anterior ½ 20
		Scarf sign	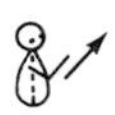 0	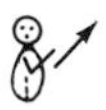 6	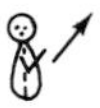 12	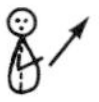 18	
		Head lag	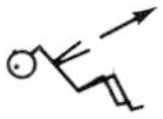 0	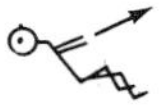 4	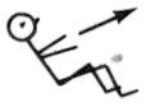 8	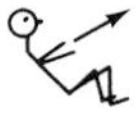 12	

Variables and assigned scores in the modified Dubowitz method for assessment of gestational age. A. Gestational age in days = 204 + total somatic score (for neurologically depressed infants). *B.* Gestational = 200 + total combined somatic and neurologic score (for healthy infants).

Fig. 34-2. Cappurro's method for assessing gestational age. (From Cappurro H et al: A simplified method for diagnosis of gestational age in the newborn infant, *J Pediatr* 93:121, 1978.)

15. Hips: Range of motion
16. Reflexes: Root, suck, Moro's, grasp
17. Tone: Head control when pulled to sit, jitteriness, flexion

In the transport setting, the potential value of each part of the examination must be weighed against any stress it may cause to an already compromised infant.

PATHOLOGIC CONDITIONS OF THE NEONATE

One of the major roles of the transport team is to assist in the development of the differential diagnosis and management plan for the newborn requiring transport. In the development of this plan, steps outlined in the section "Assessment of the Newborn" serve as the basics for the differential diagnosis. The history obtained must include the development and timing of symptomatology and the progress of the condition. Integration of historical data with the physical examination and evaluation of laboratory and x-ray data is essential.

Respiratory Disorders

Diaphragmatic Hernia

Diaphragmatic hernia is caused early in gestation when the pleuroperitoneal cavity fails to close. Abdominal contents migrate into the thoracic cavity, compressing developing lungs and causing pulmonary hypoplasia.

Early detection of this defect is essential to the initiation of appropriate therapy. Classic presentation by these infants includes early onset of respiratory distress with deterioration between the 1- and 5-minute Apgar scores in the delivery room. Clinical signs include dyspnea, unequal breath sounds, a shift in the PMI, and potentially scaphoid abdomen. Although scaphoid abdomen is listed as a classic sign, it is frequently not evident in the delivery room. Because any distention of the bowel further compromises respiratory function, the flight nurse should insert a gastric tube and initiate suction. Positive-pressure ventilation with a face mask should be avoided. When ventilation is required, the flight nurse should perform immediate endotracheal intubation.

Diaphragmatic hernia used to be considered a "surgical emergency." Recent studies have supported delaying surgery to allow for a period of physiologic stabilization.[27] The efforts of preoperative stabilization are aimed at optimizing oxygenation, maintaining an adequate systemic blood pressure, and reducing the associated pulmonary hypertension.

These infants are at high risk of severe hypercarbia and pneumothoraces. Therefore ventilatory management is aimed at maximizing ventilation while minimizing barotrauma, if possible. Persistent pulmonary hypertension and shock frequently complicate the management of these infants. In the transport setting, an additional member should be added to the team if it would decrease the stabilization time.

Aspiration Pneumonias

Although aspiration of meconium is the most severe form of aspiration pneumonia, the infant may also aspirate amniotic fluid or blood at the time of delivery. The presence of meconium in the amniotic fluid should alert the medical team to the possibility of acute or chronic in utero asphyxia. The airway should be cleared as discussed previously in this chapter. Meconium can be aspirated in utero and therefore may be impossible to prevent in the presence of severe asphyxia. The flight nurse should attempt to clear the meconium from the airway. The presence of meconium in the bronchial tree causes obstruction to airflow and pneumonitis. These infants are usually term or postterm. Common complications in meconium aspiration syndrome include pulmonary air leak and persistent pulmonary hypertension. Therefore the goals of respiratory management are the maintenance of oxygenation, avoiding acidosis, and minimizing high airway pressures. Antibiotic therapy is frequently started in these infants to prevent a secondary bacterial pneumonia. Common symptoms in these newborns include the appearance of a hyperinflated chest and tachypnea. X-ray findings can contribute significantly by revealing patchy densities bilaterally.

Surfactant Deficiency

The most common cause of respiratory distress in the preterm infant is hyaline membrane disease (HMD). This condition is primarily caused by a deficiency of surfactant. A deficiency of surfactant may also occur in the presence of extreme stress such as severe hypoxia. Surfactant decreases surface tension in the alveolus during expiration, allowing the alveolus to maintain a functional residual capacity. The absence of surfactant results in poor lung compliance and atelectasis. Infants with surfactant deficiency demonstrate progressive increase in symptoms as a result of poor lung compliance. This progression is evidenced by increasing effort at breathing with intercostal retractions, flaring, and grunting. Oxygen requirements continue to increase to maintain an adequate arterial oxygen level. The increased respiratory effort required results in increasing lethargy. Characteristic x-ray findings include reticular granular pattern in the lungs and hypoexpansion. The severity of the illness varies from requiring minimal respiratory support by hood oxygen to maximal support with the ventilator.

The cornerstone of treatment for HMD is supplemental oxygen to maintain a PaO_2 of 60 to 70 mm Hg and an arterial saturation of 92% to 95%.[42] Intubation and ventilation should be undertaken for signs of worsening respiratory distress including partial pressure of oxygen (PaO_2) <60 mm Hg in 70% to 80% fraction of inspired oxygen (FiO_2) or a partial pressure of carbon dioxide ($PaCO_2$) >50 mm Hg. Continuous positive airway pressure, administered either nasally or by endotracheal tube, can be tried if the infant is older than 30 weeks of gestation. Ventilation should be instituted if the infant becomes fatigued, as indicated by worsening arterial blood gases.[7]

Exogenous surfactant was approved for use by the Food and Drug Administration (FDA) in 1990. Ten years of extensive clinical studies before then showed that exogenous surfactant treatment substantially reduces mortality and the incidence of air leak, although it does not appear to reduce other complications such as bronchopulmonary dysplasia and intraventricular hemorrhage. There are both natural surfactant extracts and synthetic preparations. The primary function of lung surfactant is to lower surface tension at the air-water interface of the alveoli, thereby preventing atelectasis and improving compliance. Administration of exogenous surfactant may result in rapid changes in lung compliance, subsequent overventilation, and air leaks unless close monitoring and adjusting of ventilator settings occur.

Pulmonary interstitial emphysema is common in those infants requiring high levels of ventilatory support. Added complications of the disease include development of chronic lung disease as a result of ventilatory support and a patent ductus arteriosus. These complications may be decreased by using the lowest possible ventilatory settings and avoiding excessive fluid administration during transport.[6,18,20]

Pneumonia

Pneumonia is often associated with a history of prolonged rupture of membranes of at least 12 hours before delivery. However, respiratory infection can occur in the fetus even in the presence of intact membranes. Symptoms of amnionitis and fetal infection including maternal fever or elevated white count, purulent or foul-smelling fluid, fetal tachycardia, loss of beat-to-beat variability, or premature labor are also very suggestive. Signs of infection in infants may be present immediately at birth or be delayed for 1 to 2 days. In addition to respiratory symptoms of tachypnea, apnea, grunting, flaring, or retracting systemic symptoms may also be present. These may include hypotonia, hypotension, poor perfusion, lethargy, and seizures. An elevated or extremely low white blood cell count may or may not be present. Radiographic examination may resemble either HMD with a uniform granularity or aspiration with patchy lung fields. Management includes maintaining adequate oxygenation and ventilation, antibiotic therapy, and cardiovascular support.

Pulmonary Air Leaks

Air leaks including pulmonary interstitial emphysema (PIE), pneumothorax, and pneumomediastinum are most commonly related to excessive positive-pressure ventilation used during resuscitation or the use of positive airway pressure treatments.[36] The infant with an air leak may appear nearly asymptomatic, with only muffled heart tones, or the infant's condition may deteriorate rapidly, requiring immediate intervention. Assessment includes evaluation of breath sounds, location of PMI, transillumination of the chest, and x-ray. In the infant requiring immediate resuscitation, there may be no opportunity to delay for x-ray diagnosis, and a diagnostic thoracentesis must be performed. In the milder form with minimal symptoms, no treatment may be necessary, or a one-time needle thoracentesis and hood oxygen may be adequate. In the clinically significant tension pneumothorax, the placement of a chest tube is usually required. In the transport setting, air medical personnel must anticipate increasing symptoms from an untapped pneumothorax if the transport requires moving the child at altitude. Before departing the referring hospital, the flight nurse must also evaluate the effectiveness of the use of either a one-way valve or suction on the chest tube.

Neonatal Heart Disease

The diagnosis and management of the infant with congenital heart disease can be a major challenge in the transport setting. Frequently, the referring staff and transport team do not have the benefit of echocardiography and must rely on history, clinical examination, laboratory, and x-ray results. The initial symptoms of serious congenital heart disease in the newborn, in order of frequency, are cyanosis, cyanosis with heart failure, heart failure without cyanosis, cardiogenic shock, and arrhythmias. Because the early signs of congestive heart failure are tachypnea and tachycardia, it is easy to understand the potential difficulty in distinguishing pulmonary from cardiac disease in the cyanotic, tachypneic newborn.

In the transport setting, the critical issues include the differentiation of pulmonary from cardiac disease and the determination of those heart lesions that are dependent on ductal flow. Once the determination has been made that cyanosis in the newborn is caused by a fixed right-to-left shunt, the flight nurse must still differentiate between shunting caused by persistent pulmonary hypertension and anatomic heart disease. A history containing high-risk factors for persistent pulmonary hypertension and a clinical course demonstrating previous adequate oxygenation in room air is helpful.

It is essential to obtain a detailed history of the onset of symptoms from the referring staff (Table 34-4). The referring nursing staff can frequently provide the most detailed chronologic report. Immediate onset of respiratory symptoms at birth is likely to indicate the presence of pulmonary disease because few babies are born in active heart failure. An obstetric history that would indicate an infant at risk for pulmonary disease is also important to elicit. High-risk factors for pulmonary disease would include prematurity, postmaturity, meconium-stained fluid, prolonged rupture of membranes, maternal diabetes, neonatal asphyxia, or cesarean section.

Clinical examination includes a complete examination of the cardiorespiratory system and a search for evidence of other anomalies. Findings suggestive of cardiac disease include cardiac murmur, hepatomegaly, decreased or unequal pulses, hyperactive pericardium, arrhythmias, and poor perfusion. Tachypnea without other signs of respiratory distress such as grunting and retracting may also be an indication of early heart failure. Clinical signs suggestive of respiratory disease include retractions, grunting, poor air exchange, and unequal air entry.

TABLE 34-4

The top five diagnoses presenting at different ages

AGE ON ADMISSION: 0-6 DAYS (N = 537)	
Diagnosis	**%**
D-Transposition of great arteries	19
Hypoplastic left ventricle	14
Tetralogy of Fallot	8
Coarctation of aorta	7
Ventricular septal defect	3
Others	49
Total	100
AGE ON ADMISSION: 7-13 DAYS (N = 195)	
Diagnosis	**%**
Coarction of aorta	16
Ventricular septal defect	14
Hypoplastic left ventricle	8
D-Transposition of great arteries	7
Tetralogy of Fallot	7
Others	48
Total	100
AGE ON ADMISSION: 14-28 DAYS (N = 177)	
Diagnosis	**%**
Ventricular septal defect	16
Tetralogy of Fallot	7
Coarctation of aorta	12
D-Transposition of great arteries	7
Patent ductus arteriosus	5
Others	53
Total	100

From Fyler D, Lang P: Neonatal heart disease. In Avery GB, editor: *Neonatology,* Philadelphia, 1987, Lippincott.

Laboratory data that may be helpful include a comparison of oxygenation in room air and 100% oxygen. The infant who is hypoxic in room air but demonstrates a partial pressure of oxygen (Po_2), greater than 150 in 100% oxygen is more likely to have pulmonary disease than heart disease with a fixed right-to-left shunt. Comparison of simultaneous arterial blood gases demonstrating a Pao_2 at least 10 mm higher from a preductal site versus a postductal site indicates right-to-left shunting of desaturated blood at the ductal level.[24]

Those heart defects that may be dependent on ductal patency for pulmonary blood flow would include transposition without ventricular septal defect (VSD), pulmonary or tricuspid atresia, and critical pulmonary stenosis including tetralogy of Fallot. Coarctation of the aorta and hypoplastic left heart syndrome may also require the use of prostaglandin E_1 for stabilization for transport.[17] In these situations the prostaglandins are required to maintain adequate systemic blood flow. Prostaglandins are normally used during transport when the patient's condition is deteriorating, as indicated by the presence of metabolic acidosis, or when deterioration is anticipated before completion of the transport. The most common side effect complicating transport with the use of prostaglandin E_1 is apnea or hypoventilation. The length of the transport and the difficulty of placing an endotracheal tube during transport must be considered in the decision as to whether to place an endotracheal tube before transport when prostaglandins are begun. Other side effects with the use of prostaglandin E_1 include fever, vasodilation with flushing, and diarrhea. Uncommonly, the vasodilation may result in systemic hypotension requiring intervention.

Management of the infant with congenital heart disease during transport involves treatment of the symptomatic failing heart. The presence of clinical and laboratory evidence of heart failure dictates the interventions to stabilize the patient's condition during transport. Clinical symptoms would include hepatomegaly, decreased pulses, capillary refill greater than 3 seconds, mottled color, peripheral cyanosis, tachycardia, and cool extremities. Laboratory indications would include cardiomegaly on x-ray findings and metabolic acidosis. The primary intervention available for the failing myocardium is inotropic drug support.

Persistent Pulmonary Hypertension in the Newborn (PPHN)

PPHN is a syndrome characterized by persistent elevated pulmonary vascular resistance resulting in right-to-left shunt at the ductus arteriosus or the foramen ovale leading to hypoxemia in the presence of a structurally normal heart.[16] This disease process is most commonly seen in near-term infants with severe asphyxia, meconium-aspiration syndrome, congenital diaphragmatic hernia sepsis, or other respiratory distress resulting in hypoxia. It can be very difficult in the transport setting to make the clinical differentiation between cyanotic heart disease and PPHN. Demonstration of right-to-left shunting at the ductus using preductal and postductal simultaneous arterial blood gas levels is helpful in the diagnosis of this problem. Treatment is aimed at maintaining adequate oxygenation until the pulmonary vasculature resistance begins to drop. This normally occurs within the first several days. The more severely affected infants may require extremely high inspiratory pressures and rates to maintain adequate oxygenation. Current treatment therapies include maintaining the infant in an alkalemic state through hyperventilation and the use of blood buffers, sedation or paralysis, and cardiotonic drugs. Alkalemia is believed to enhance the decrease in pulmonary vasculature resistance. Maintenance of the systemic BP discourages right-to-left shunting. Intravenous vasodilators including tolazoline and nitroprusside have had limited success primarily because of the complication of systemic hypotension resulting increased right-to-left shunting.[34] New studies of the pulmonary vasodilatory effects of inhaled nitric oxide have been promising; however, nitric oxide remains an investigational drug at this time.[25]

Complications of the ventilatory therapy include pulmonary air leaks and chronic lung disease.

Gastrointestinal Disorders

The transport team deals primarily with gastrointestinal disorders related to obstruction, either functional or anatomic, infection, or externalized abdominal contents. Obstructions of the gastrointestinal (GI) tract can occur anywhere from the esophagus through the anus. The management of all of these disorders primarily centers around decompression of the bowel, fluid management, antibiotic therapy, and respiratory support.

Esophageal Atresia

Findings related to identification of esophageal atresia include inability to pass an oral gastric tube to the stomach, excessive oral secretions, and feeding intolerance. An obstetric history of polyhydramnios should increase suspicion of upper GI obstruction. Of patients with esophageal atresia, 92% have an associated tracheoesophageal fistula. Approximately 85% of fistulas occur between the lower esophageal pouch and the trachea. This fistula allows air to pass from the respiratory tree into the stomach and gastric acids to reflux into the bronchial tree. These infants are at high risk for aspiration either from the oropharynx refluxing from the upper esophageal pouch or aspiration of gastric contents from the lower tracheoesophageal fistula. A flight nurse who suspects that an infant has esophageal atresia should immediately elevate the head of the bed and place a double-lumen suction tube in the upper esophageal pouch. This tube should be placed to continuous suction. Diagnosis can be confirmed with x-rays taken while having a radiopaque catheter curled in the upper esophageal pouch. The presence of air in the stomach or intestines would confirm the presence of a lower esophageal fistula. Management of these infants during transport should feature the following:

1. Intermittent suction of the upper esophageal pouch
2. Elevation of the head of the bed to prevent gastric reflux
3. Intravenous fluid therapy for fluids and glucose

Positive-pressure ventilation distends the stomach via the fistula and may interfere with ventilation or result in gastric perforation.

Approximately 8% of infants with esophageal atresia have no tracheoesophageal fistula. Esophageal atresia with a fistula to the tracheal tree from both the upper and the lower pouch occurs approximately 1% of the time. An H-type fistula that connects an intact esophagus and tracheal tree occurs approximately 4% of the time. These conditions may be more difficult to diagnose, with more subtle initial symptoms of choking or coughing during feedings. They also require more detailed x-ray studies using a contrast-medium dye; this should not be attempted in the transport setting. The infant with esophageal atresia and without air in the abdomen may be considered for transport either prone or even with the head slightly lowered to encourage effective evacuation of the upper esophageal pouch. Careful evaluation of the rest of the GI tract, the cardiovascular system, and the genitourinary system should be completed because of frequent associated anomalies.[19]

Intestinal Obstructions

Common initial symptoms for intestinal obstruction include bilious vomiting, abdominal distention, feeding intolerance, large quantities of gastric contents at delivery, absence of an anal opening, and lack of stooling in the first 24 hours. Obstetric history with a high obstruction may reveal polyhydramnios. Although the presence of bilious vomiting may be related to other causes, intestinal obstruction should be presumed until ruled out. Abdominal distention may be present depending on the level of the obstruction. Presence of tenderness, metabolic acidosis, or decreasing platelets may indicate a bowel necrosis or peritonitis and should be treated as an urgent problem.

Diagnosis can usually be made through x-ray evaluation. Contrast studies are rarely, if ever, indicated on transport. X-ray studies should be carefully evaluated for perforation of the bowel. Urgent cases include malrotations with volvulus and those with associated peritonitis, perforation, or suspected bowel necrosis.

Management includes decompression of the bowel with intermittent large-bore gastric suction, IV fluids, antibiotic therapy as indicated, and respiratory support. These infants may have large fluid requirements because of large interstitial fluid losses. Severe abdominal distention may compromise respiratory status. Evaluation of these children should include assessment of their oxygen needs and ventilatory capacity with appropriate measures taken to correct deficits. In severe cases of peritonitis, sepsis and shock may also be present and should be treated appropriately.

Necrotizing Enterocolitis

Although the cause of necrotizing enterocolitis (NEC) remains controversial, ischemia of the bowel predisposes the infant to this disease process. Infants at particular risk include those with asphyxia, especially the small, ill, preterm infant.[9] Early recognition of risk factors and symptoms allows for early treatment, minimizing the incidence of necrosis of the bowel. Early symptoms include feeding intolerance with increased gastric aspirates, bile-stained gastric aspirates, abdominal distention, and hematest-positive stools. Progression of the disease results in increasing abdominal distention to the point of tautness, grossly bloody stools, abdominal wall erythema, and abdominal tenderness. X-ray findings include intestinal distention, thickening of the bowel wall, and the classic sign of air in the bowel wall (pneumatosis intestinalis). The absence of this finding, however, does not rule out the diagnosis of necrotizing enterocolitis. These infants are at risk for peritonitis, bowel perforation, and disseminated intravascular coagulation.

The infant at risk for NEC as a result of severe birth asphyxia should be maintained on NPO status on IV fluids to allow the bowel to recover. Symptomatic infants should also be placed on NPO status on IV fluids and antibiotics. Any abdominal distention should be treated with intermittent gastric suction to keep the bowel decompressed. The presence of thrombocytopenia may indicate an underlying disseminated intravascular coagulation and may require treatment with platelet infusions.

Omphalocele/Gastroschisis

Although omphalocele and gastroschisis are two separate entities, their treatment during transport is essentially the same. An omphalocele is an arrest of development of the abdominal wall, with the abdominal contents remaining externalized. The defect remains covered by a membrane in utero although the sac may be broken during delivery. The size of the defect may vary from a small hernia to inclusion of a large percentage of the abdominal contents. Gastroschisis, on the other hand, is a defect in the abdominal wall that has otherwise completed its development. The defect allows for protrusion of abdominal contents. Because the defect is normally very close to the umbilicus, it is frequently mistaken for an omphalocele. This defect, however, is not covered by a membrane. If the defect occurred early in gestation and the intestines have been floating in the amniotic fluid for some time, they may appear very edematous with adhesions.

Both groups of infants are at risk for infection, large fluid losses, impaired bowel perfusion, and hypothermia. Treatment includes immediate wrapping of the defect with moist saline gauze and plastic wrap or, alternatively, placing the defect in a bowel bag to prevent fluid losses. The infant must obviously remain on NPO status, and gastric suction should be applied to maintain decompression of the bowel. If the abdominal opening is extremely small, the patient may be at a high risk for bowel ischemia as a result of the constriction of blood flow. Caring for the child on his or her side may help to reduce tension on the bowel and improve circulation. Careful monitoring and maintenance of temperature within normal range are essential in the management of these children. This increased need for thermogenesis also places them at risk for hypoglycemia and requires closer observation of blood glucose. They may also require increased fluid intake, particularly in the case of the gastroschisis or omphalocele with ruptured membranes.

Neonatal Infections

The most common neonatal infections requiring treatment on transport include pneumonia, both viral and bacterial, sepsis, and, infrequently, meningitis. Pneumonia has been addressed in the subsections featuring respiratory illnesses. The infant with sepsis may have very mild and subtle onset of symptoms or a fulminating course resulting in rapid progression to shock. Symptoms include temperature instability, either hypothermia or hyperthermia, lethargy, poor feeding, tachypnea, hypoglycemia, or cyanosis. An infant with any of these symptoms must be evaluated for potential sepsis. If the infant has meningitis, seizures must be added to the list of common presenting signs.

Evaluation of these infants includes a complete blood cell count with differential. A low absolute neutrophil count and elevated ratio of immature to total neutrophils, although not diagnostic, increases the level of suspicion for bacterial sepsis. Samples for blood cultures should be obtained using strict aseptic technique. Although the definitive diagnosis of septicemia requires positive blood culture results, infants with highly suspicious signs should be started on an appropriate antibiotic regimen. In addition to antibiotic therapy, supportive therapy should be provided as needed. Infants with overwhelming sepsis may be in shock, requiring support of blood volume and myocardial function. In the case of meningitis with seizures, examination of the cerebrospinal fluid is indicated but usually can be delayed until after the transport. However, antibiotic therapy and treatment for the seizures should be begun as soon as possible on transport.

Neurologic Disorders

The primary neurologic disorders requiring therapy during transport include cranial enlargement, neural tube defects, and seizures.

Cranial Enlargement

Cranial enlargement may either be benign or caused by a number of pathologic conditions that include hydrocephalus, intracranial hemorrhage, intracranial cysts and tumors, or other encephalopathy. Differentiation of etiology requires careful evaluation of history, skull films, computed tomographic (CT) scan, and transillumination. If the history indicates a difficult delivery and intracranial bleeding is suspected, the infant should be evaluated for anemia. From a transport perspective, management of these disorders is primarily supportive, responding to secondary dysfunctions in the respiratory or cardiovascular systems.

Neural Tube Defects/Encephaloceles

Failure of development of the neural tube early in gestation may result in a number of defects including anencephaly, meningomyelocele, meningocele, and encephalocele. These defects may include nervous tissue. The primary concern during transport is to prevent infection in the case of the open lesion. A moist, sterile dressing should be applied. Otherwise, transport management includes normal supportive therapy. Antibiotics may or may not be ordered.

Seizures

Seizures occur frequently in ill newborns, either as a primary or secondary disorder. Because of the immature nervous system of the newborn, they rarely exhibit the generalized tonic-clonic seizures seen in adults and older children. Seizures in the newborn can be divided into four categories[22]:

1. *Subtle.* This type of seizure is frequently overlooked by caretakers. It may consist of repetitive mouth or tongue movement, bicycling movements, eye deviation, repetitive blinking, staring, or apnea.
2. *Clonic* (multifocal or focal). Clonic seizures are characterized by repetitive jerky movements of the limb(s), which may move from limb-to-limb in a disorganized fashion.
3. *Tonic* (generalized or focal). Tonic seizures may resemble posturing seen in older infants and children and be accompanied by disturbed respiratory patterns, and may include tonic extension of limb or limbs or tonic flexion of upper limbs and extension of lower limbs.
4. *Myoclonic.* Myoclonic seizures are characterized by multiple jerking motions of the upper (common) or lower (rare) extremities.

Seizure activity is frequently confused with jitteriness in the newborn. Jitteriness may be distinguished from seizures in the following ways:

1. Jitteriness is sensitive to stimulus, whereas seizures are not.
2. Jitteriness is characterized by tremors rather than the slow and fast phases of seizure activity.

3. Jitteriness can normally be stopped by flexing the limb, as opposed to seizures that will not respond to this maneuver.

To treat neonatal seizures, it is important to attempt to identify the cause (box). Careful examination of the obstetric and neonatal history may reveal risk factors for seizure disorders. Physical examination should be performed, along with laboratory studies including glucose, calcium, phosphorus, magnesium, sodium, and potassium. The glucose level should be checked immediately with the bedside test strip. If hypoglycemia is present, it should be corrected immediately with an infusion of glucose. If a correctable metabolic cause is not identified, seizures should be treated according to established protocols or after consultation with the appropriate physician. A number of medications including phenobarbital, phenytoin (Dilantin), and diazepam (Valium) may be used. Serious side effects from these drugs may include respiratory or cardiovascular depression.

CAUSES OF NEONATAL SEIZURES

Birth trauma/intracranial hemorrhage
Hypoxic/ischemic encephalopathy
Hypoglycemia
Hypocalcemia
Hypomagnesemia
Hypophosphatemia
Hyponatremia/hypernatremia
Pyridoxine deficiency
Amino acid disturbances
Neonatal injection of caine derivatives
Bacterial meningitis
CNS abnormalities
Drug withdrawal

EQUIPMENT

The transport of the neonate requires a skilled team and proper equipment. The box contains a list of neonatal equipment designed for critical care interfacility neonatal transport. The equipment selected for a scene-response team could be much abbreviated.

NEONATAL EQUIPMENT INVENTORY

Respiratory Equipment

Laryngoscope handle with blades, sizes Miller 0 and Miller 1
Spare laryngoscope bulbs and batteries
Endotracheal tube stylet
Anesthesia bag (500 ml) with manometer
Face masks, sizes 0 and 1
Endotracheal tube sizes 2.5, 3.0, and 3.5
Suction catheter and glove sets sizes nos. 5/6 Fr, 8 Fr, and 10 Fr
Thoracentesis setups:
- 60 ml syringe
- 3-way stopcock
- 23-gauge butterfly
- Alcohol and povidone-iodine (Betadine) prep

Heimlich valve setups
Argyle trocar cannulae, nos. 10 Fr and 12 Fr

Intravenous Therapy Equipment

250 ml bags of D_5W and $D_{10}W$
IV pump tubing
IV filters
Platelet and blood infusion sets
Umbilical artery catheters, sizes 3½ and 5 Fr
IV extension tubing
T-connectors
Steri drape
3-tail connector
Syringes, sizes from 1 ml through 60 ml
Needles, assorted sizes 18-gauge through 25-gauge
3-way stopcock and stopcock plugs

NEONATAL EQUIPMENT INVENTORY—cont'd

Betadine and alcohol wipes
Scalp vein needles, sizes 23- and 25-gauge
Quick catheters, sizes 22- and 24-gauge
Medication additive labels
Disposable razors
Paper tape measure
Tongue blades
Armboards, sizes premature and infant
Assorted tape
Umbilical tape
Betadine and alcohol, one bottle each
4.0 silk suture with curved needle
Umbilical artery catheterization/thoracotomy set including: 2 sterile drapes, iris forceps, needle holders, scissors, curved forceps, tongue tissue forceps, sterile 2 × 2s, umbilical tape, scalpel, and blade
Blunt end adapters, sizes 17-, 18-, and 20-gauge

Thermoregulation and Monitoring Equipment

Stocking hat
Plastic wrap
Portawarm
Silver swaddler
Thermometers
Limb leads
Chest electrodes
Heart monitor lead wires
Capillary tubes
Chemstrips
Lancets
Arterial transducer tubing

Miscellaneous

Blood culture bottles
Scissors and hemostat
Flashlight
2 × 2s
Limb restraints
Safety pins
Rubber bands
Pacifier
Cotton balls
Benzoin
Christmas tree adapters
No. 8 Fr feeding tubes
Germicidal cleaning cloth
Salem sump tubes, No. 10 Fr and No. 12 Fr
Replogle tube 10 Fr
Sterile glove packs
Sphygmomanometer with cuffs, sizes premature, newborn, and infant
Neonatal stethoscope
Trash bag

Medications

Epinephrine 1:10,000
$NaHCO_3$ 4.2%
Narcan
$NaHCO_3$ 8.4%
Dopamine
Dobutamine
Isuprel
Priscoline
Phenobarbital
Dilantin
Valium
Fentanyl
Pavulon
Concentrated sodium chloride and potassium acetate
Xylocaine 1%
Chloral hydrate
Morphine sulfate
Heparin 1000/ml
0.9% normal saline dilutent
Sterile water dilutent
Flush solution
Antibiotics
5% albumin
$D_{50}W$
Wydase
Atropine
Calcium gluconate 10%
Prostaglandin E_1
Exogenous surfactant
Glass filter needles

NEONATAL CASE STUDIES

CASE 1

Baby B was a 38-week, 3200 gram, appropriate-for-gestational age female born to a 24-year-old gravida 1, para 1 (now 2), living child 1 (now 2), A+ married woman. Previous medical history unremarkable. Normal prenatal course during this pregnancy. At 38 weeks by date, an elective repeat cesarean section was performed. Membranes were ruptured at delivery with clear fluid. Apgar scores were 7 at 1 minute and 9 at 5 minutes, requiring suctioning, O_2 blow-by, and stimulation in the delivery room. Baby's early course was reported to be unremarkable in level I. She was breastfeeding in room air. Transport was called at 18 hours of age for sudden deterioration with respiratory rate of 78, pale, cyanotic, poorly perfused infant with diminished pulses. Lower extremity pulses appeared to be weaker than upper extremity pulses. Arterial blood gas in 40% oxygen by hood, PO_2 of 52, PCO_2 of 38, pH 7.28, with a base deficit of 11. Complete blood cell count with differential was within normal limits. Provisional diagnosis was coarctation of the aorta with a closing ductus.

Predeparture differential diagnosis by the transport nurse included:

1. Rule out sepsis
2. Respiratory distress/rule out pneumonia vs. PPHN vs. aspiration
3. Rule out congenital heart disease

Transport considerations included the distance of the trip, which was 1600 miles round trip, with an approximate trip time of 8 hours. Prostaglandin E_1 would be taken in the event the child had a ductal-dependent congenital heart defect. The transport team anticipated the need for full support; a neonatal nurse practitioner and a respiratory therapist were dispatched.

Upon arrival at the referring hospital, the infant was observed to be pale pink in a 78% hood in a crib. Further history from the nursing staff included an early nursery course remarkable for intermittent mild tachypnea with respiratory rates in the 60s and slight duskiness with agitation. The chest x-ray findings at 18 hours of age revealed increased perihilar streaking, fluid in the right fissure, and a normal cardiothoracic ratio. The x-ray film was otherwise unremarkable. Both history and x-ray findings were consistent with mild retained fetal lung fluid and borderline oxygenation.

The infant was placed on a radiant warmer with automatic temperature control. Transcutaneous PO_2 and PCO_2 monitors were placed. Physical examination was remarkable for a lethargic term infant who was pale pink in 78% oxygen by hood. Pulses were decreased in all extremities but equal with upper extremity blood pressures of 52 mm Hg by palpation and lower blood pressure extremities of 58 mm Hg by palpation. Capillary refill was 4 seconds with slight mottling. Heart tones were normal with no murmur or extra sounds noted. Respiratory rate was 82, breath sounds were equal and clear with shallow air exchange. Peripheral IV was infusing with $D_{10}W$ at 80 ml/kg/day. Blood glucose level was 60. O_2 was increased to 85%, secondary to transcutaneous PO_2 of 50 with an increase to PO_2 of 54 and PCO_2 of 36. After consultation with the attending physician at the receiving hospital, 10 ml/kg of 5% albumin was begun by slow push through the peripheral IV. An umbilical artery catheter was placed and blood culture obtained. Continuous blood pressure monitoring was begun via umbilical catheter. Blood pressure after volume was 64/42 mm Hg, capillary refill 3+ seconds. Simultaneous preductal and postductal pulse oximeters were placed with results of 93% preductal and 85% postductal, indicating a shunting of blood at the ductal level.

Oxygen was increased to 100% by hood with no increase in transcutaneous PO_2. Baby was given 2 mEq/kg of sodium bicarbonate. Blood pressure remained at 60/36 mm Hg. A second 10 ml/kg of 5% albumin was administered with increase in blood pressure to 72/45 mm Hg and decrease in capillary refill time to 3 seconds.

An endotracheal tube was inserted and hand ventilation was used to test for response to hyperventilation with decrease of $PaCO_2$ to 26. TCM began to increase, rising to transcutaneous PaO_2 of 78, with a transcutaneous $PaCO_2$ of 26. The patient was placed on 24 over 4, a rate of 60, and a 100% attempting to match hand ventilation. Arterial blood gas results revealed a PO_2 of 80, PCO_2 of 25, pH 7.43, and a base deficit of 6.

Transport diagnoses included:

1. Health care maintenance for a 38-week appropriate-for-gestational female. *Plan:* Fluids of $D_{10}W$ were continued at 80 ml/kg, and blood

glucose levels were checked every 1 to 2 hours and remained stable throughout.

2. Respiratory distress; rule out PPHN. *Plan:* Blood pressure was monitored continuously throughout transport with a plan to support blood pressure with dopamine and volume as needed to prevent right-to-left shunting. Continued to hyperventilate, maintaining P_{CO_2} in the mid 20s and P_{O_2} > 60.
3. Rule out sepsis. *Plan:* Antibiotics begun before transport.

Care during transport included cardiorespiratory monitor, continuous skin temperature monitoring, continuous blood pressure monitoring, continuous transcutaneous P_{O_2} and P_{O_2} monitoring, vital signs with axillary temperature every half hour throughout trip. Oral gastric tube was placed before transport to empty the stomach of any air or contents. The neonatal nurse practitioner and the referring physician spoke with the family, updating the patient's condition, current treatment, potential complications, and risks of transport. Transport consent was signed. The parents were also provided with information regarding intensive care nurseries and the specific information on the receiving nursery, including phone numbers, the attending physician, the policies regarding phone information, and visiting. A Polaroid photograph of the baby was left with the parents. After the baby was put in the transport isolette, she was taken to the parents' room where the parents were encouraged to see her and touch her before departure. The parents were offered the option of having one parent accompany the baby to the receiving hospital, but this was declined. The baby was in stable condition tolerating the transport well.

CASE 2

Baby H. was a 28-week, 1430 g, appropriate-for-gestational age male born to a gravida 5, para 3, who had no prenatal care. Previous history includes maternal IV drug abuse, but denied use during pregnancy. The mother smokes a half pack of cigarettes per day. Prenatal laboratory data were unavailable.

The mother came to the emergency department in labor, where she was completely dilated with bulging membranes. Terbutaline was given 1 hour before delivery but did not stop labor. Phenobarbital was also given before delivery. The membranes were ruptured 30 minutes before delivery and an attempt was made at a vaginal delivery, but the baby's presentation had changed to a transverse lie. A cesarean section was performed with the mother receiving epidural anesthesia.

Infant cried spontaneously and appeared to be about 28 weeks of gestational age by examination. Apgar scores were 6 at 1 minute and 8 at 5 minutes. A 2.5 endotracheal tube (ETT) was inserted. Initial ventilator settings were 20/4, rate 50, 100% F_{IO_2}; arterial blood gases were pH 7.18, P_{CO_2} 59, P_{O_2} 43. Umbilical artery and umbilical vein catheters were placed. Initial chest x-ray films revealed ETT down the left mainstem and air leak around ETT; reintubation with 3.0 ETT. Second chest x-ray film revealed bilateral reticular granular pattern with ETT down the right mainstem; ETT pulled back. The umbilical venous catheter was in the liver and was discontinued. Blood samples for culture and complete blood cell count were sent to the laboratory with these findings: complete blood cell count: white blood cell count 10.1 with 26% neutrophils, 61% leukocytes, 12M 1B, hematocrit 51, hemoglobin 17.1%, platelets 278,000. Initial blood glucose level 80. Ampicillin and Claforan given at 3:30 AM.

Attending physician called for transport because of inability to care for a premature infant on a ventilator. Transport team arrived 1 hour and 19 minutes after transport initiated. Predeparture differential diagnosis by transport nurse included:

1. Premature appropriate-for-gestational age male infant
2. Respiratory distress, probable HMD vs. group B streptococcal pneumonia
3. Rule out sepsis
4. Rule out maternal drug use

Transport considerations included ventilatory management and thermoregulation because of the infant's extreme prematurity.

On arrival at the referring hospital, the patient was on a radiant warmer with temperature 37°C axillary, heart rate 163 beats/min, RR with ventilator, blood pressure 46/18 mm Hg. Ventilator settings were 24/4, rate 60, 60% F_{IO_2} with arterial blood gases of pH 7.37, P_{CO_2} 34, P_{O_2} 288. Pulse oximeter reading was 99. The team received report and x-ray films were viewed.

Because the umbilical venous catheter was discontinued, the neonatal nurse practitioner began a peripheral IV for maintenance fluids. After discussion with the attending physician, it was decided to give exogenous surfactant. In-house time is lengthened because the patient's condition should be monitored in-house for at least a half hour after surfactant is given. Patient's ventilator settings were weaned using physical parameters (i.e., chest excursion, auscultation, and by monitoring transcutaneous readings and pulse oximetry). A second sample was sent for determination of arterial blood gas values 20 minutes after the surfactant. The values were as follows: ph 7.40, Pco_2 29, Po_2 142 on 22/4, rate 50, 40% Fio_2.

Transport diagnosis included:

1. Health care maintenance for a 28-week appropriate-for-gestational age male. *Plan:* Fluids of $D_{10}W$ in the PIV and normal saline solution in the umbilical artery catheter continued at 80 ml/kg/day. Blood glucose levels were checked every 1 to 2 hours and remained stable throughout.
2. Respiratory distress, presumed HMD. *Plan:* Continue to wean ventilator as indicated by above physical and monitor observations.
3. Rule out sepsis. *Plan:* Antibiotics were begun during transport.
4. Rule out maternal drug use. *Plan:* A urine toxicology screen would be sent when patient voided.

Care during transport included all measures mentioned in Case 1. The patient's condition was stable, but he became agitated and began breathing against the ventilator. Fentanyl was given for sedation and the patient did not "fight the vent." On arrival at the hospital, report was given to the attending physician and bedside nurse. Care was transferred to the staff.

REFERENCES

1. Apgar V: A proposal for new method of evaluation of the newborn infant, *Anesth/Analg* 32:260-267, 1953.
2. American Academy of Pediatrics: Emergency drug doses for infants and children and Naloxone use in newborns: clarification, *Pediatrics* 83(5):803, 1989.
3. American Academy of Pediatrics and American Heart Association: *Textbook of neonatal resuscitation*, Dallas, 1994, The Associations.
4. Babson SG, Behrman RE, Lessel R: Live-born birth weights for gestational age of white middle class infants, *Pediatrics* 45:937-944, 1970.
5. Bell EF, Oh W: Fluid and electrolyte management. In Avery GB, Fletcher MA, MacDonald M, editors: *Neonatology*, ed 4, Philadelphia, 1994, Lippincott.
6. Bell EF et al: Effect of fluid administration on the development of symptomatic patent ductus arteriosus and congestive heart failure in premature infants, *N Engl J Med* 302:598-604, 1980.
7. Berg TJ et al: Bronchopulmonary dysplasia and lung rupture in hyaline membrane disease: influence of continuous distending pressure, *Pediatrics* 55:51-53, 1975.
8. Buetow KC, Klein SW: Effect of maintenance of normal skin temperature on survival of infants of low birthweight, *Pediatrics* 34:163-170, 1964.
9. Caplan MS, MacKendrick W: Necrotizing enterocolitis: a review of pathogenetic mechanisms and implications for prevention, *Pediatr Pathol* 13:357-369, 1993.
10. Cappurro H et al: A simplified method for diagnosis of gestational age in the newborn infant, *J Pediatr* 93:120-122, 1978.
11. Carson BS et al: Combined obstetric and pediatric approach to prevent meconium aspiration syndrome, *Am J Obstet Gynecol* 126:712-715, 1976.
12. Day RL et al: Body temperature and survival of premature infants, *Pediatrics* 34:171-181, 1964.
13. Drage JS et al: The Apgar score as an index of infant morbidity: a report from the Collaborative Study of Cerebral Palsy, *Dev Med Child Neurol* 8:141-148, 1966.
14. Dubowitz LMS, Dubowitz V, Goldberg C: Clinical assessment of gestational age in the newborn infant, *J Pediatr* 77:1-10, 1970.
15. Flanagan MF, Fyler DC: Cardiac disease. In Avery G, Fletcher MA, MacDonald M, editors: *Neonatology*, ed 4, Philadelphia, 1994, Lippincott.
16. Fox WW, Duara S: Persistent pulmonary hypertension in the neonate: diagnosis and management, *J Pediatr* 98: 505-514, 1983.
17. Freed MD et al: Prostaglandin E1 in infants with ductus arteriosus-dependent congenital heart disease, *Circulation* 64:899-905, 1981.
18. Greenough A, Dixon AK, Roberton NRC: Pulmonary interstitial emphysema, *Arch Dis Child* 59:1046-1051, 1984.
19. Guzzetta PC et al: Surgery of the neonate. In Avery GB, editor: *Neonatology*, ed 3, Philadelphia, 1987, Lippincott.
20. Hart SM et al: Pulmonary interstitial emphysema in very low birthweight infants, *Arch Dis Child* 58:612-615, 1983.

21. Heyman MA: Biophysical evaluation of fetal status: fetal cardiovascular physiology. In Creasy RK, Resnik R editors: *Maternal fetal medicine,* Philadelphia, 1984, Saunders.
22. Hill A, Volpe JJ: Neurologic disorders. In Avery G, Fletcher MA, MacDonald M, editors: *Neonatology,* ed 4, Philadelphia, 1994, Lippincott.
23. Hill JR, Rahimtulla KA: Heat balance and the metabolic rate of newborn babies in relation to environmental temperature, and the effect of age and weight on basal metabolic rate, *J Physiol* 180:239-265, 1965.
24. Jacob J et al: The contribution of PDA in the neonate with severe RDS, *J Pediatr* 96:79-87, 1980.
25. Kinsella JP, Abman SH: Recent development in the pathophysiology and treatment of persistent pulmonary hypertension of the newborn, *J Pediatr* 126:853-864, 1995.
26. Koops BL, Morgan LJ, Battaglia FC: Neonatal mortality risk in relation to birth weight and gestational age: update, *J Pediatr* 101:969-977, 1982.
27. Langer J et al: Timing of surgery for congenital diaphragmatic hernia: is emergency operation necessary? *J Pediatr Surg* 23:731-734, 1988.
28. Lubchenco LO, Hansman C, Boyd E: Intrauterine growth in length and head circumference as estimated from live births at gestational ages from 26 to 42 weeks, *Pediatrics* 37:403-408, 1966.
29. Lubchenco LO, Searls DT, Brazie JV: Neonatal mortality rate: relationship to birth weight and gestational age, *J Pediatr* 81:814-822, 1972.
30. Martin M, Paes BA: Birth asphyxia: does the Apgar score have diagnostic value? *Obstet Gynecol* 72:120, 1989.
31. Nelson N: Physiology of transition. In Avery G, Fletcher MA, MacDonald M, editors: *Neonatology,* ed 4, Philadelphia, 1994, Lippincott.
32. Pagliari AS et al: Hypoglycemia in infancy and childhood, *J Pediatr* 82:365-379, 1973.
33. Phibbs RH: Delivery room management. In Avery G, Fletcher MA, MacDonald M, editors: *Neonatology,* ed 4, Philadelphia, 1994, Lippincott.
34. Philips JB, editor: Neonatal pulmonary hypertension, *Clin Perinatol* 11:515-776, 1984.
35. Pildes R et al: The incidence of neonatal hypoglycemia—a completed survey, *J Pediatr* 70:76-80, 1967.
36. Primhak RA: Factors associated with pulmonary air leak in premature infants receiving mechanical ventilation, *J Pediatr* 102:764-768, 1983.
37. Scopes JW, Ahmed I: Range of critical temperatures in sick and premature newborn babies, *Arch Dis Child* 41: 417-419, 1966.
38. Silverman WA, Fertig JW, Berger AP: The influence of the thermal environment upon the survival of newly born premature infants, *Pediatrics* 22:876-886, 1958.
39. Streeter NS: *High-risk neonatal care,* Rockville, MD, 1986, Aspen.
40. Sykes GS et al: Do Apgar scores indicate asphyxia? *Lancet* 1:494-496, 1982.
41. Whitfield JM: Neonatal transport. In McCloskey KAL, Orr RA, editors: *Pediatric transport medicine,* St Louis, 1995, Mosby.
42. Whitsett J et al: Acute respiratory disorders. In Avery G, Fletcher MA, MacDonald M, editors: *Neonatology,* ed 4, Philadelphia, 1994, Lippincott.
43. Wiswell TE, Tuggle JM, Turner BS: Meconium aspiration syndrome: have we made a difference? *Pediatrics* 85: 5, 1990.

CHAPTER 35

Risk Management in Air Medical Practice

COMPETENCIES

1. Identify the elements of malpractice.
2. Describe the impact of COBRA on patient transport.
3. Identify the components of professional flight nursing practice.

Risk management and continuous quality improvement (CQI) go hand in hand in reducing the risks of legal actions against an air medical program. Risk management focuses on the individual patient and his or her family, evaluating events related to an individual patient's perception, and intervening to prevent a lawsuit.[4] CQI looks at the process of transport including personnel and systems, and assesses patterns and trends. The two efforts, when combined, identify, analyze, and treat potential hazards to prevent deleterious effects.[4]

Knowledge of legal principles is necessary to a viable risk management program. Flight nurses practice in a unique setting. There are myriad legal principles with which one must become familiar. In addition to nursing practice issues, Federal Aviation Administration (FAA) and Federal Communications Commission (FCC) regulations may be applicable in certain circumstances. The education and training of flight nurses must include information on the various laws and regulations pertinent to a flight nurse's practice. Specific laws such as the Consolidated Omnibus Reconcilation Act (COBRA) provide guidelines and regulations that the flight nurse must be aware of to provide safe and competent patient care.

AN OVERVIEW OF THE LAW

Law comprises all of the rules and regulations by which a society is governed. Statutes are laws made by governmental bodies, and they vary from state to state. Statutes must comply with applicable federal law. The State Nurse Practice Acts are examples of statutory law. Statutes frequently require written rules and regulations for enforcement. Administrative agencies write administrative law, the rules and regulations that enforce the statute. The State Boards of Nursing are administrative agencies that promulgate administrative law.[4] Case law, or judicial law, varies from state to state. Legal issues brought before the courts are interpreted based on the facts of a particular case.

Criminal law permits legal action to be filed by the state for behavior that is offensive or harmful to society. Flight nurses may be charged with a criminal offense if there is violation of either the State Nurse Practice Act or safe nursing practices. Civil law, in contrast to criminal law, permits an action to be filed by an individual for monetary compensation. Tort law is used most commonly in civil cases related to medical and nursing care. Compensation is requested for the person(s) wrongfully injured by the actions of another.[3,4]

Negligence and malpractice are often incorrectly used as interchangeable terms. *Negligence* is a deviation from accepted standards of performance.[3,4,8,9] *Malpractice* is based on a professional standard of care, as well as the professional statutes of the care giver.[9] The same types of acts form the basis for negligence and malpractice.

Elements of Malpractice

The elements of malpractice that must be present are presented in order of priority in the box. First, a *duty* must be present. The duty may be a contract, statute, or when a flight nurse voluntarily assumes care of a patient.[1,3,4,9] A duty is created by the development of a nurse-patient relationship and not merely employment status.[4]

Once it is established that a duty exists, the second element is a *breach of duty*. Breach of duty may occur as a result of malfeasance (act of commission) or nonfeasance (act of omission).[3,4] Administering the wrong medication would be malfeasance, whereas failure to follow a procedure would be nonfeasance.

The third element is *foreseeability;* that is, one could reasonably expect certain events to cause specific results.[1,4]

ELEMENTS OF A MALPRACTICE CASE

Presence of duty
Breach of duty
Foreseeability
Causation
Injury
Damages

The fourth element in malpractice is *causation*. There must be a reasonable cause-and-effect relationship between the breach of duty and injury.[1,3,4,9,10] There are two types of causation: (1) in fact and (2) proximate. Proximate cause occurs when the result is directly related to the act. Cause in fact occurs when the breach of duty owed causes the injury.

The fifth element is *injury*. The patient must be harmed either physically, financially, or emotionally in a discernible way.[1,3,4,9,10]

The sixth element is *damages*. Damages are compensatory in nature and may be of different types. General damages are inherent to the injury itself. Special damages are losses and expenses incurred as a result of stress and emotional pain produced by the injury. Punitive damages are requested when there was alleged malicious intent, or willful or wanton misconduct.[4]

In certain circumstances the doctrine of *res ipsa loquitor*, "let the thing speak for itself," is used. The elements that must be proved are causation, injury, and damages. Commonly, *res ipsa loquitor* is used in situations where the patient was unconscious or in surgery at the time the injury occurred.[1,3,4,9]

Statute of Limitations

Filing a lawsuit is under a statute of time limitations. Generally, if malpractice is alleged after a traumatic injury, the statute of limitations is 2 years, whereas in cases of disease it is at the time discovered.[3,4] The exception is in pediatric cases. The statute of limitations is extended until the minor is emancipated or reaches the age of majority (established by state law).[3]

Types of Liability

Intentional Torts or Criminal Acts

Assault or battery, or both, may be either criminal or tort (civil). *Assault* is placing an individual without consent in a situation in which he or she fears immediate bodily harm. *Battery* is the touching of a person without his or her consent. Battery can also occur with the touching of anything connected with a person (clothing, purse, jewelry) without consent.[3,4] Damages for battery may be punitive or nominal as well as compensatory.[3]

Other types of intentional torts are, briefly, false imprisonment, the unjustifiable detention of a person without his or her consent, and invasion of privacy, a key concept in issues related to confidentiality. The patient has the right to privacy of medical information. Photographs cannot be taken without consent as well as information. There are some situations that are newsworthy, and the public's right to know can exceed the patient's right to privacy.[4] Obviously, knowledge of statutes related to consent is vital. Defenses used against intentional torts are consent (discussed later in this chapter), self-defense, defense of others, and necessity.[4]

Vicarious Liability

Vicarious liability is defined as one party being responsible for the actions of another. The doctrine of *respondeat superior,* "let the master respond," has been used frequently when nurses are accused of malpractice. As a result of this doctrine, the employer has an obligation to ensure that employees perform duties in a competent, safe manner. Two elements must be demonstrated: (1) the injured party must prove that the employer had control over the employee, and (2) the negligent act occurred within the scope and course of the employment.[4] Vicarious liability can occur for malfeasance or nonfeasance.

Recently courts have attached judgments directly against institutions for corporate negligence. Hospitals have found themselves accountable as an entity when the duty is owed directly to the patient and not through employees. Types of corporate duties attached directly to the institution are outlined in the box.[8]

Product Liability

There has been an increase in product liability cases, which are mixtures of tort and contract law. The sale of a product places the manufacturer, processor, or nonmanufacturing seller at risk for a product liability case should injury to a person or person's property occur. Delivery of a service without the sale of the product is generally not substantial enough for a successful product liability suit. However, court decisions have been inconsistent in separating the sale of product from delivery of a service.[4] Collective liability may occur when several manufacturers have participated in a cooperative activity. Alternative liability occurs when two or more manufacturers commit separate acts.

Abandonment

The principles related to abandonment are important to flight nurse practice. Abandonment occurs with unilateral termination of the nurse-patient relationship without consent from the patient.[3] Abandonment can also occur if the care of the patient is transferred to someone less qualified.[5,6] Questions may arise regarding abandonment any time there is a

EXAMPLES OF CORPORATE DUTIES OWED DIRECTLY TO PATIENT

- Duty of reasonable care in maintenance and use of equipment
- Availability of equipment and services
- Duty of reasonable care in selecting and retaining employees
- Adoption and assurance of compliance with rules related to administrative responsibility for patient care
- Selection and retention of medical staff

demonstration of disregard for the patient's welfare, or unreasonable practices, or both.[1] The various types of air medical transports should be reviewed by each program and evaluated to ensure that potential abandonment issues are addressed. George suggested that the act of dispatching an ambulance was presumptive of voluntary assumption of a duty to a patient.[3] This should be considered when developing Communication Center protocols.

Consent Issues

Most medical tort claims are related to consent issues.[4] Informed consent requires more than a patient's signature on a consent form. The suggested treatment must be presented to the patient with a discussion of risks, consequences, and available alternatives.[1-4,6] If the first treatment option is refused by the patient, other treatment options should be explained. Informed consent requires *understanding* on the part of the patient.

Consent can be written or oral. Nurses are frequently asked to obtain signatures on consent forms. Before having the patient sign, one should determine that he or she understands the purpose of the consent. *Expressed consent* occurs with written or oral acknowledgement. *Implied consent* occurs when a patient is compliant with a request (extending arm for phlebotomy, allowing placement of nasal prongs, and so on). Implied consent is frequently operational in emergency situations. Most consent statutes allow for treatment of life-threatening emergencies if the patient is unable to consent because it is the reasonable thing to do.[1,2] One should be cautious, however, not to exceed the limits of implied consent. If the patient is physically or mentally incapable of consenting, implied consent is operative in the case of a true emergency. Absent a true emergency, consent should be obtained before treatment from a person whose relationship is such that he or she is authorized to consent.[2]

Consent for treatment of minors is reserved for a parent or legal guardian. Implied consent is used for minors with life-threatening, emergency conditions. The parent(s) or legal guardian should be contacted as soon as possible for notification and consent. Most states have laws related to emancipated minors who can consent before the age of majority. In addition, minors may be allowed to consent for treatment of certain conditions such as sexually transmitted diseases, pregnancy, and substance abuse.[1,4]

Refusal to consent or withdrawal of consent is sometimes a murky question. A common issue is the refusal of a blood transfusion because of religious beliefs. If it is the opinion of the treating physician that a blood transfusion is necessary and the patient refuses, an attempt can be made to obtain a court order. The court uses a balancing test to weigh one right against the other. The court leans to the right of the patient to make a knowing choice in refusing consent. The exception is in the case of minors. If the court is convinced a child requires lifesaving measures, compelling state's interest in the child usually overrides the parent's interest.

Documentation

The medical record of a patient is owned by the hospital, although the patient has a right to the information contained therein.[1,4] The medical record is the documentation of the patient's course of treatment. It serves as a means of communication between various providers of service. It protects the legal interests of the patient, the hospital, and the health care practitioner.[4] The medical record may also be used for research and continuing education. The contents of the medical record should be factual and based on objective data.

Standard abbreviations should also be used. The entries should be readable, concise, and complete.[4] The patient should be described objectively. The patient's appearance, signs and symptoms, interventions, and responses to them should be documented in a timely fashion. If an untoward incident occurs, an incident report should be completed and appropriate hospital personnel notified.

The COBRA Law

The Consolidated Omnibus Budget Reconciliation Act was passed in 1986. This contained the Emergency Medical Treatment and Active Labor Act of 1986.[7,10] The initial components of this act directed hospitals to do the following[7]:

1. Examine all patients who come to the emergency department and provide them with necessary medical care
2. Patients are not to be transferred until their condition is stable
3. It must be documented that the patient will receive better care at the receiving facility
4. Ambulances, fixed winged aircrafts, and helicopters must have appropriate personnel and equipment to make the transfer

In 1990 the COBRA law underwent further revisions that broadened who is subject to the law. The law now includes all participating physicians and any other physician responsible for the examination, treatment, or the transfer of the participating hospital.[10] Violations of COBRA legislation include financial penalties and potential loss of government funding.

The COBRA law itself does not directly affect the practice of flight nursing. However, flight nurses need to be aware when a potential violation is occurring, for example, recognizing when a transfer may be based on financial reasons instead of patient need.[10]

SCOPE OF PRACTICE

The scope of practice is defined by statutes, rules, or a combination of the two. The initial statutes that govern flight nursing scope of practice are State Nurse Practice Acts. The Nurse Practice Acts establish licensure requirements for nurses. Most states require mandatory licensure before either the title or actions are permitted. Exceptions are generally related to students, new graduates, and transport through a state's jurisdiction.[4] The box illustrates the common elements of nurse practice acts.[4]

ELEMENTS OF NURSE PRACTICE ACTS

- Definition of professional nursing
- Requirements for licensure
- Exemptions
- Licensure across jurisdictions
- Disciplinary action and due process requirements
- Creation of Board of Nursing
- Penalties for practicing without a license

Flight nursing, in most situations, is an expanded role. Before practicing in an expanded role, flight nurses should review the pertinent nurse, medical, and pharmacy practice acts, attorney general's opinions, and recent judicial decisions.[4] The institution's policies and procedures should be investigated and followed to ensure that the scope of practice for the flight nurse is clearly defined. In addition to scope of practice, the standard of care must be reviewed. Internal standards are set by the role of the nurse, job descriptions, and policies and procedures. External standards are established by state boards of nursing, professional and specialty nursing organizations, and federal guidelines.[4] In cases of purported deviation from the standard of care, the external standards may be submitted as evidence, or expert witnesses used, or both. Professional publications may be submitted to assist the jury in understanding the expected standard of care.[1]

The National Flight Nurses Association revised "Practice Standards for Flight Nursing" in 1995. A summary of these standards is presented in the box. The flight nurse practice standards are external standards.

SUMMARY

Risk management in the air medical environment requires a thorough understanding of all applicable legal issues. Specific questions are best addressed by a legal authority. The risk management and CQI program go hand in hand to reduce potential liability. The flight nurse can reduce the liability risks by maintaining open and honest communications with patients and family members. A knowledge of the law and legal doctrine is also necessary, as is staying within the defined scope of practice and individual competence.

STANDARDS OF PROFESSIONAL PERFORMANCE

Standard I. Quality of Care

The flight nurse systematically and continuously evaluates the quality, appropriateness, and effectiveness of client care and nursing practice in the air medical transport environment.

Measurement Criteria:

1. The flight nurse participates in quality management activities to evaluate care in the transport environment. Such activities may include but are not limited to:
   a. Delineation of scope of care
   b. Development of standards of care
   c. Identification of aspects of care important for quality monitoring
   d. Identification of indicators used to monitor quality and effectiveness of care delivered by flight nurses
   e. Data collection to monitor quality and effectiveness of client care
   f. Data assessment to identify opportunities for improving flight nursing practice and client care
   g. Formulation of recommendations to improve flight nursing practice and client outcomes
   h. Action to improve care and service
   i. Evaluation
   j. Report of findings
2. The flight nurse utilizes the results of the quality management activities to initiate appropriate changes in client care procedures and flight nursing practice.
3. The flight nurse utilizes the results of the quality management activities to initiate appropriate changes in air medical services.
4. The flight nurse uses the results of the quality management activities to initiate appropriate changes throughout the health care delivery system.
5. The flight nurse identifies safety concerns.
6. The flight nurse ensures that appropriate infection control measures are implemented according to: (a) Centers for Disease Control and Prevention (CDCP) guidelines; (b) Occupational Safety Health Administration (OSHA) standards; (c) individual program and institution procedures.
7. The flight nurse advises appropriate personnel if actual or potential risk exists from exposure to infectious organisms.
8. The flight nurse participates in ongoing infection control educational activities.

Standard II. Performance Appraisal

Flight nurse evaluates his/her own nursing practice.

Measurement Criteria:

1. The flight nurse engages in performance appraisal on a regular basis, identifying areas of strength as well as areas for professional/practice development.
2. The nurse seeks constructive feedback regarding his/her own practice.
3. The flight nurse takes steps to achieve goals identified during performance appraisal.
4. The flight nurse participates in peer review as appropriate.

Standard III. Education

The flight nurse acquires and maintains knowledge necessary for competent flight nursing practice.

Measurement Criteria:

1. The flight nurse successfully completes an initial training/orientation program, which includes didactic and clinical topics pertinent to flight nursing practice and specialty area(s) of practice.
2. The flight nurse participates in ongoing educational activities pertinent to flight nursing practice and specialty area(s).
3. The flight nurse seeks learning experiences to maintain a knowledge base and clinical skills necessary for flight nursing practice.
4. The flight nurse maintains documentation of educational activities

Excellence Criteria:

1. The flight nurse independently seeks advanced learning experiences to expand knowledge base and clinical skills to enhance flight nursing practice.
2. The flight nurse attains advanced educational degrees.

Standard IV. Collegiality

The flight nurse contributes to the knowledge base of peers, colleagues, and health care providers.

Measurement Criteria:

1. The flight nurse shares knowledge and skills with colleagues and other health care providers.

From National Flight Nurses Association: *Standards of flight nursing practice,* St Louis, 1995, Mosby.

Continued.

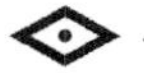

2. The flight nurse provides peers with constructive feedback regarding their flight nurse practice.
3. The flight nurse contributes to an environment that is conducive to clinical education of other health care providers.

Excellence Criteria:

1. The flight nurse organizes educational presentations for other health care providers to promote optimal health care for the community.

Standard V. Ethics

The flight nurse's decisions and actions on behalf of clients are determined in an ethical manner.

Measurement Criteria:

1. Flight nurse practice is guided by the American Nurses Association's Code of Ethics.
2. Flight nursing practice is guided by the Nurse Practice Act as defined by each state.
3. The flight nurse delivers care in a nonjudgmental and nondiscriminatory manner that is sensitive to client diversities.
4. The flight nurse provides information to assist the client or significant other in making an informed decision for transfer.
5. The flight nurse will be a client advocate.
6. The flight nurse maintains client confidentiality at all times.
7. The flight nurse delivers care in a manner that preserves/protects client autonomy, dignity, and rights.
8. The flight nurse uses available resources to help formulate ethical decisions.
9. The flight nurse uses available mechanisms to identify and resolve ethical issues related to client care.

Standard VI. Collaboration

The flight nurse collaborates with the client, significant others, and other health care providers in providing client care.

Measurement Criteria:

1. The flight nurse communicates with the client, significant others, and health care professionals regarding client care and nursing's role in the provision of care.
2. The flight nurse consults with health care providers for client care, as needed.
3. The flight nurse makes referrals, including provisions for continuity of care, as needed.

Standard VII. Research

The flight nurse enhances and supports practice through the use of research findings.

Measurement Criteria:

1. The flight nurse incorporates into practice validated research outcomes.
2. The flight nurse disseminates validated research findings to others.
3. The flight nurse complies with ethical research principles.
4. The flight nurse utilizes the results of validated research to initiate changes in air medical services.

Excellence Criteria:

1. The flight nurse initiates and actively participates in formal research through participation in one or more of the following areas: (a) research design; (b) grant application; (c) research analysis; (d) abstract presentation; (e) research contribution to literature.

Standard VIII. Resource Utilization

The flight nurse considers factors related to safety, effectiveness, and cost in planning and delivering care.

Measurement Criteria:

1. The flight nurse practices safety measures through applied knowledge of:
   a. General aviation safety procedures
   b. FAA rules and regulations pertaining to safety
   c. Emergency aircraft equipment and procedures
   d. Ground operations
   e. Safe use of client care procedures and equipment used in the aircraft environment
   f. Scene hazards
2. The flight nurse evaluates factors related to safety, effectiveness, and cost when two or more practice options would result in the same expected client outcomes.
3. The flight nurse assigns or delegates care based on the needs of the client and the knowledge and skill of the provider.
4. The flight nurse assists the client and significant others to identify and secure appropriate services.

From National Flight Nurses Association: *Standards of flight nursing practice,* St Louis, 1995, Mosby.

REFERENCES

1. Cushing M: *Nursing jurisprudence,* East Norwalk, Conn, 1988, Appleton & Lange.
2. Cisar NS: Informed consent: an ethical dilemma, *Nurs Forum* 30(303):20, 1995.
3. George JE: *Law and emergency care,* St Louis, 1980, Mosby.
4. Guido GW: *Legal issues in nursing: source book for practice,* East Norwalk, Conn, 1988, Appleton & Lange.
5. Hepp R: *Standards of flight nursing practice,* St Louis, 1995, Mosby.
6. Lazar RA: *EMS law: a guide for EMS professionals,* Rockville, Md, 1989, Aspen.
7. Southard P: COBRA legislation: complying with ED provisions, *J Emerg Nurs* 15:23-25, 1989.
8. Southwick AF: *The law of hospital and health administration,* ed 2, Ann Arbor, Mich, 1988, Health Administration Press.
9. Youngberg BJ: Medical-legal considerations involved in the transport of critically ill patients, *Crit Care Clin* 8(3): 501-514, 1992.
10. Youngberg BJ: Legal issues related to transport. In Mc-Closkey K, Orr RA, editors: *Pediatric transport medicine,* St Louis, 1995, Mosby.

CHAPTER 36

Quality Management

COMPETENCIES

1. Identify the differences between quality management and continuous quality improvement.
2. Identify two indicators that could be used in a specific flight program to monitor quality management.
3. Design a remedy for a specific problem related to a transport program.

Air medical services have become a familiar part of the American health care system. As health care faces dwindling financial resources, ongoing financial justification and proof of its positive effect on patient outcomes are imperative for air medical services.

Flight nurses, as an indispensable part of the air medical system, have the professional responsibility to provide sound documentation that quality nursing care is being provided to patients in a timely and cost-effective manner. It is crucial to the flight nursing profession that flight nurses prove their contribution to patient outcomes through their autonomous approach to patient care. With the advent of the accrediting body CAAMS (Commission on the Accreditation of Air Medical Services), there is now a method of external review to ensure programs are homogenous in their approach to quality care.

For many air medical programs, quality management (QM) is often viewed as a time-consuming activity with little measurable impact on actual patient care and outcomes. This chapter provides an overview of the QM process for air medical transport and flight nursing and provides several practical methods for evaluating air medical clinical practice and improving systems of care. The external quality review process, as administered by CAAMS, will also be discussed.

DEFINITION OF TERMS: QUALITY ASSURANCE VERSUS CONTINUOUS QUALITY IMPROVEMENT

A veritable alphabet soup of quality terms has glutted the health care market. For the sake of clarity, it is important to define the terminology that will be used in this text. *Quality assurance* (QA) implies a traditional approach to evaluation. It includes such activities as monitoring of indicators and comparison of results to a predetermined threshold or standards. Unfortunately, traditional QA is sometimes perceived negatively by health care providers because it is associated with the perception that people are doing a bad job or not complying with certain standards. As an alternative to traditional QA, continuous quality improvement (CQI), total quality management (TQM), and many derivations of these terms have deluged the health care arena over the past decade. These terms are often used interchangeably and essentially embrace the same concepts. They are radically different from traditional QA, but not all individuals who use these terms appreciate the differences.

CQI and QA differ in four major categories: motivation, leadership, methodologic differences, and organization. The motivations for pursuing QA and CQI are radically different. Traditionally, health care providers have been motivated to perform QA activities mainly to meet externally mandated requirements (regulatory, Joint Commission for the Accreditation of Healthcare Organizations, etc.). In the CQI environment, health care providers pursue CQI activities as a way to please their customers. This is the era of choice in health care, and patients are informed consumers with discriminating taste in health care facilities. Although patient choice may not be much of an issue in the emergency setting of air medical transport, patients and their families have certain expectations of health care providers, regardless of the setting.

The leadership component of CQI versus QA also differs dramatically. In the QA environment, quality initiatives are typically the responsibility of a middle manager or "QA coordinator." The entire responsibility for quality is relegated to this individual. In the CQI environment, primary accountability for quality rests with lead tier management. The lead tier must be committed to the CQI initiative in both word and deed.

Perhaps the greatest difference between CQI and QA is the methodology used. QA has often depended on retrospective audits, indicators, and less rigorous QA studies. Decisions are often based on unfounded or spurious data and opinions. In the CQI environment, there is much greater reliance on statistics and hard facts, not feelings and assumptions. Additionally, CQI uses a standardized problem-solving formula that, if followed carefully, yields a more predictable result than traditional problem-solving techniques.

Finally, the organizational culture of a CQI environment is fundamentally different. In the CQI environment, all processes and plans are centered around the customer (patients and families). Good customer service is a core value of the individuals who work in a CQI environment. Also, employees, to meet the needs of the customer, are empowered to implement changes and decisions, not encumbered by bureaucratic rules and regulations.

QUALITY MANAGEMENT MODEL FOR AIR MEDICAL TRANSPORT

Despite their inherent limitations, some traditional QA activities still have merit in air medical transport. Programs might be inclined to discard QA methods completely and adopt CQI exclusively. This approach is not recommended. An integration of the two methods is the most effective way to evaluate and improve care. This model suggests the integration of QA and CQI in an overall QM strategy in which select QA activities serve as a stimulus for multidisciplinary CQI teams. With the significant differences between traditional QA and CQI now elucidated, this chapter will use the term "quality management," or QM, to imply a blending of the best aspects of traditional QA and CQI/TQM.

ASSIGNING ACCOUNTABILITY: THE STAFF-BASED APPROACH TO QUALITY MANAGEMENT

Ultimate accountability for the results of quality activities is held by managers of the air medical program. However, air medical personnel (AMP) involvement in the QM program from its inception through the process of monitoring, data collection, and change is the only way to achieve "buy-in" at the provider level. Managers can delegate much of the monitoring, evaluation, and multidisciplinary team activities to a committee of AMP or to one individual such as a QM coordinator, but top-down support and involvement are hallmarks of effective QM. Top-down support is demonstrated by financial support for individuals assigned QM responsibilities to receive specialized training and by allowing paid time away from flight duty to complete QM activities and projects. Some air medical services have elected to hire QM coordinators who are assigned most of this workload. Whether the QM coordinator is a full-time staff nurse or an individual who flies part time, it is important that one individual be accountable for overseeing the process. Failure to assign accountability will result in disorganization and lack of direction for the QM program.

The success or failure of an air medical QM program is also related to the degree to which the AMP have been involved in its development, implementation, and ongoing maintenance. If a QM program is conceived and implemented with little or no involvement on the part of those who deliver care, the program may be perceived negatively by the staff. If, on the other hand, the AMP are given the opportunity to contribute to the development of the QM program, the personal investment on the part of the staff will improve the chance for greater success of the program.

THE QUALITY MANAGEMENT COMMITTEE

Development of a QM committee is one way to ensure staff involvement in the air medical QM process. The QM committee approach promotes "ownership" of the QM program on the part of the flight nurses. Also, participation on the multidisciplinary air medical QM committee may be used as a part of the program's clinical advancement system. Committee membership may be made by application, appointment, or election. Whatever the approach, the flight nurse member must be committed to the goals of the committee. Establishment of bylaws for the QM committee that address its structure, reporting mechanisms, voting privileges, attendance requirements, and so on will aid in making the committee more "official" and will serve to heighten the members' sense of commitment to the aims of the committee.

QUALITY MANAGEMENT PROGRAM ORGANIZATIONAL STRATEGIES

The most effective QM program is well organized and multifaceted. Programs that depend too heavily on one monitoring method risk missing opportunities for improvement. However, managing multiple simultaneous studies of indicators and multidisciplinary teams can be overwhelming.

The written QA plan is an effective organizational tool to manage the air medical QM effort. The written plan serves as an infrastructure for all quality efforts and assures that monitoring and evaluation are systematic and organized.

Table 36-1 displays a generic air medical written QM plan. The development of such a plan is straightforward; however, some essential components must be included.

First and foremost, the content of the monitoring plan is based on the air medical service's scope of service. The scope of service delineates the types of patients transported and how they are transported. For instance, a flight program that transports 80% scene patients will have a different scope of care than a neonatal transport program. A statement that clearly summarizes the essence of the care provided by the particular air medical service and by its flight nurses could read something like this: "LifeFlight provides for the rapid assessment, diagnosis, and treatment of critically or injured patients of all ages from the scene of an accident or from intraagency transports." With this statement as the framework, QM personnel can begin to develop standards; identify high-risk, high-volume aspects of care; and develop ways to monitor them.

TABLE 36-1

Generic air medical QA and improvement plan (1996)

Indicator(s)*	Rate based (RB) or sentinel event (SE)	Goal benchmark threshold	Collection schedule/method	Collection responsibility	Date of next review
ASPECT: TIMELY AND APPROPRIATE CARE OF THE PEDIATRIC PATIENT					
Pediatric IV fluid rates Maintenance flow rates based on patient weight	RB	95%	Quarterly review of sample (5% or 30 cases) of pediatric patients transported	Pediatric representative	Quarter 2, 1996
Fluid boluses appropriate for patient age/weight	RB	95%	Same	QM committee	Quarter 2, 1996
Fluid bolus effect documented	RB	95%	Same	QM committee	Quarter 2, 1996
ASPECT: APPROPRIATE AND TIMELY AIRWAY MANAGEMENT					
Intubation of pediatric patient Airway size appropriate for weight/age	RB	95%	Quarterly review of all pediatric intubations	Pediatric representative, QM committee	Quarter 3, 1996
Documentation of placement confirmed in nursing notes	RB	95%	Semi-annual review of documentation of all intubations	QM committee	Quarter 3, 1996
Intubation (all patients) Tube confirmed in trachea on arrival at receiving facility	SE	100%	All intubation reported to be esophageal reviewed by medical director/team member involved	QM coordinator/ medical director	Quarter 3, 1996
Documentation of all intubation attempts and reasons attempts not successful	RB	95%	Retrospective quarterly review N = all intubations or attempted intubations	QM committee	Quarter 3, 1996

*From Samaritan Air Evac, Phoenix, Ariz, 1996.

IDENTIFYING IMPORTANT ASPECTS

Important aspects of care are high-risk, problem-prone, high-volume areas of air medical transport with the greatest impact on patient outcome, cost, and efficient functioning of the program. Nursing responsibilities such as physical assessment, documentation, medication administration, timely response for requests for service, and invasive procedures are examples of important aspects of flight nursing care. Several examples are shown in Table 36-1.

INDICATOR DEVELOPMENT

Indicators are well-delineated, objective measures of compliance with a particular standard. Two indicators dealing with patient physical assessments after intubation might be:

1. Bilateral breath sounds will be documented on all patients postintubation.
2. Esophageal intubations will be recognized and corrected.

THRESHOLDS AND BENCHMARKS

The final step in developing a written QM plan is to establish the level at which lack of compliance with the given standard or indicator of quality will be unacceptable and will require intervention. This level, usually expressed as a percentage, is known as the threshold. Some experts prefer the use of the term *benchmark* to imply an externally determined level of performance. Several nationally determined thresholds or benchmarks have been published for air medical quality indicators.[1,4,5] Several of these thresholds or benchmarks have been validated through research and evaluation of large data sets.[5]

When no national data are available with which to validate a certain level of performance, how does one realistically assign thresholds? First, thresholds must be attainable and pragmatic. There is no sense in establishing thresholds so high they can never be met. Likewise, in high-risk areas in which failure to meet the threshold 100% of the time could result in a deleterious outcome for a patient—for example, esophageal intubations—the threshold should be set at 100%.

Although some national benchmark data are available for air medical transport, a great opportunity exists for flight nurses to take an active role in collecting data and establishing thresholds based on realistic clinical settings.

ESTABLISHING PRIORITIES FOR MONITORING, EVALUATION, AND MULTIDISCIPLINARY TEAMS

The written plan outlines all general categories of care to be monitored in a given year, how often these aspects of care are to be monitored, and the method to be used. The actual implementation of these activities can be a daunting task. A prioritization tool is needed to determine which activities should be undertaken first.

The decision matrix is a simple but valuable way to prioritize the QM efforts. It is usually most effective if completed in a group by the QM committee or similar planning structure. The following case study describes the use of the decision matrix.

The Life Flight XYZ QM committee meets the first week of January to determine "quality initiatives" for the coming year. During this meeting, they hold a brainstorming session to identify all possible clinical and operational nursing, paramedic, respiratory, administration, pilots, and communications. As a result of brainstorming, they target 10 potential opportunities for improvement. These include interfacility AMP bedside time, intubation success rate, documentation of contact with medical control, team composition for maternal transports, improved documentation of chest pain management during cardiac transport, fetal monitor interpretation, and refueling turnaround time, flight following compliance, referring hospital satisfaction, and fluid management in the pediatric patient. To decide which of these issues they will address first during the coming year, the QM committee uses a decision matrix (Table 36-2). After completion of the decision matrix, the five highest ranking issues were (1) team composition for maternal transports, (2) AMP bedside time for interfacility transports, (3) intubation success rate, (4) flight-following compliance, and (5) documentation of contact with medical control. This exercise determines where the QA committee should focus the greatest efforts.

UTILIZATION APPROPRIATENESS

The comprehensive QM plan for air medical transport monitors indicators as appropriate and uses this monitoring activity as a stimulus for multidisciplinary team development. Another facet of the comprehensive QM program is the evaluation of *appropriateness* of the transport. Appropriate use of expensive air medical transportation is as important to the greater quality picture as indicator monitoring and multidisciplinary teams. Yet this important component is often overlooked by the air medical service.

What constitutes a medically appropriate transport remains controversial and has not yet been scientifically proven. Several professional organizations have proposed utilization appropriateness criteria.[2,3] It is incumbent on the air medical program to develop a mechanism to screen medical appropriateness both prospectively and retrospectively. In the development of a method to evaluate the appropriateness of the air transport, several general considerations should be kept in mind. First, does the patient's condition dictate an optimal scene or interhospital transport time? Second, what are the distances covered, the local geography, and traffic conditions that might

TABLE 36-2

Sample decision matrix

Process chosen for improvement	Patient outcomes	Patient satisfaction	Personnel satisfaction	Safety	Cost savings	Customer satisfaction	Total
Interfacility AMP bedside times	3	3	2	1	3	4	14
Team composition—maternal transports	4	2	4	2	4	4	20
Chest pain management	4	3	1	1	1	3	13
Fetal monitor interpretation	4	2	1	1	1	3	12
Refueling turnaround time	2	2	3	4	4	4	12
Flight-following compliance	2	2	4	4	2	2	16
Referring hospital satisfaction	1	3	4	1	1	4	14
Pediatric fluid management	4	3	2	1	1	3	14
Contact with medical control	4	3	4	2	1	4	18
Intubation success rate	4	4	3	2	1	4	14

Rating: 4 = High/significant improvements will occur if changes made to the process, 3 = moderate improvements will occur if changes made to the process, 2 = low/minimal improvements will occur if changes made to the process, 1 = changes in the process will not affect this area.

preclude ground transportation alternatives. Third, what is the availability of ground transportation and personnel? Next, what are the prevailing weather conditions that might warrant air transport? Finally, what is the cost of air transport as opposed to ground transportation?[3]

With these factors as a framework, the air medical program can develop criteria for an appropriate versus inappropriate air medical transport.

EXTERNAL ACCREDITATION

Several professional organizations with a stake in air medical transport collaborated in the formation of CAAMS in the early 1990s. The first CAAMS accreditation standards were published in 1991. By participating in the voluntary accreditation process of CAAMS, air medical programs can verify their compliance with quality accreditation standards to themselves, their peers, medical professionals, and the general public. Participation in the CAAMS accreditation process is important because it demonstrates an air medical program's philosophical and financial commitment to the provision of quality care that is based on national standards.

The process of accreditation is straightforward. To become accredited, the air medical program must submit a proposal to CAAMS before an on-site visit by a team of air medical experts. At the time of site visit, two to three specially trained site surveyors measure compliance with standards relating to all aspects of air transport including medical care, aviation safety, management, and administration. Although the QM program is a large component of the site visit, the entire operation of the air medical program is carefully evaluated and scrutinized.

The CAAMS accreditation process is an important step for the air medical profession. It demonstrates self-regulation, responsibility, and accountability on the part of air medical professionals.

LEGAL CONSIDERATIONS FOR QUALITY MANAGEMENT

One of the most underacknowledged considerations in the development of an air medical QM program are the legal issues that surround the quality evaluation process. Laws protecting QM activities and personnel involved in data collection from the threat of subpoena and liability vary significantly from state to state. This section examines the importance of state discoverability, immunity, and admissibility laws to the air medical QM program and the protection of the QM program and its employees from litigation issues. The legal terminology of QM activities must be defined for the ramifications of state legislation on the QM process to be understood.

Discovery is a term used to describe the acquisition of information and evidence before a trial by oral or written deposition, or other means. Admissible evidence is that which is allowed as evidence in court. State laws governing rules of procedure and evidence vary significantly. Information that is not discoverable, however, does not automatically preclude its admissibility by means other than discovery. For example, if a plaintiff's attorney stumbles upon undiscoverable QM data stored in sloppy personnel files or carelessly placed in patient records, certain states will allow this information to be admitted.

A *subpoena* is a directive of the court requiring a witness to appear before the court. A subpoena can also force a witness to produce any written evidence that may be pertinent to the case. The difference between subpoena and discoverability becomes problematic because there are two separate legal processes. State laws that prevent discoverability may not necessarily prevent subpoenability. These issues are further confused by the often unclear and ambiguous language used in these laws, which often leave interpretation to the courts.

State laws defining the protection of QM data and QM activities from discoverability, subpoena, and admissibility have a considerable impact on the planning, design, and implementation of the QM plan in the air medical services. These laws have bearing on the protection of the flight nurses and other health care providers being monitored and the protection of data obtained from QM monitoring activities from being used against the air medical service in court. Without protective legislation, persons in air medical programs whose activity initiates QM activities are placing themselves and their employees at risk. Air medical programs that implement QM plans with inadequate knowledge of the peer-review statutes in their state are placing the air medical service at risk. The scope and nature of the protection for QM activities vary dramatically from state to state. The air medical program should request help from an attorney to determine the rules within their state.

Once the air medical program has adequate knowledge of the state's discoverability and peer-review statutes, several additional precautions may be taken to ensure protection under the laws:

1. Written memoranda regarding adverse patient outcomes, medication errors, and reasons for delay of flights (whether valid or otherwise) should not be circulated through the flight service for review.
2. Written documentation of such incidents should never be kept in the employee's personnel file, which may be discoverable and admissible in court.
3. Data derived from all QM studies should be kept in the QM system. It is also helpful to title all QM data, reports, and summaries with "LifeFlight XYZ Quality Management Program: Confidential." If the actual number of the peer-review protective statute and its wording are known, the air medical program can stamp it on all documents relating to QM. Explicit discussion of sensitive patient care information should not occur in the open forum of the air medical service's weekly or monthly chart review. This practice, though it does have certain educational merit, is essentially placing all of the crew members who attend the forum and hear about the incident at risk for subpoena; these crew members, on hearing the details of the incident, can theoretically be subpoenaed to testify in court about the details of the incident.
4. Any memoranda or other written materials such as incident reports or other sensitive appropriateness-of-care issues should not make references to the source of the data.

Laws affecting QM activities are diverse and often ambiguous. Statutes in many states have gone unchallenged. Because of the laws' complexities, it is imperative that program administrators obtain legal assistance in tackling these issues.

SUMMARY

The evaluation and documentation of quality care in the air medical environment remain one of the greatest challenges a program must face. This chapter has proposed a framework for this evaluation process that is practical and comprehensive. The CAAMS accreditation process adds another dimension to the quality picture for air medical transport. As health care moves into the twenty-first century, these tools will be invaluable for sustaining the viability of air medical transport.

USE OF A MULTIDISCIPLINARY TEAM CASE STUDY

In addition to the activity of indicator monitoring and evaluation, multidisciplinary problem-solving teams are a powerful component of the air medical QM model. The process of identifying issues that might be appropriate for development of a multidisciplinary team was described previously. The following case study will demonstrate the use of this QM problem solving tool.

Life Flight XYZ was facing increasing budget restraints as the health care market in the area became more heavily penetrated by managed care. After a great deal of fiscal analysis, Life Flight XYZ identified the need to change the manner in which maternal transport services were being provided to the community. Two maternal flight nurses were on duty 24 hours a day, which equated 14 full time equivalents (FTEs) to cover the fixed-wing, rotor-wing, and ground transports. These 14 FTEs transported approximately 1000 maternal patients per year. Life Flight XYZ determined that all but five maternal flight nurses would have to be laid off. Maternal transports would be handled by the adult/pediatric flight nurses after they had received sufficient cross-training. The QM committee sponsored a multidisciplinary team with the goal of improving the maternal transport process using the cross-trained flight nurses.

The multidisciplinary team comprised the Life Flight XYZ program director, perinatal medical director, adult/pediatric medical director, QM coordinator, perinatal flight nurse manager, a maternal flight nurse, neonatal flight nurse, adult/pediatric flight nurse, and a trained team facilitator. Over the next 9 months, this team worked through a carefully prescribed problem-solving process to remedy the problem and develop a sound solution (box).

SYMPTOM DIAGNOSIS

The first step of the team was to diagnose the symptoms of the problem. To accomplish this goal, the team used a flow diagram (Fig. 36-1) to outline the current maternal transport process. Next, data were collected to determine historical statistics on the annual volume of maternal transports, average length of each transport (by mode of transportation), severity of the patient's conditions, accuracy of initial reports from the referring facility, number of concurrent transports, response times, cost by mode of transport, and reimbursement rate by payor.

THEORY FORMULATION

After months of data collection and analysis, the team was then left to formulate theories of the root causes of the problem. The original assumption of the team was that all maternal patients required spe-

Text continued on p. 681.

STEPS THAT CAN BE USED BY A MULTIDISCIPLINARY TEAM TO SOLVE A QUALITY MANAGEMENT PROBLEM

Symptom diagnosis
Theory formulation
Designing a remedy
Holding the gains

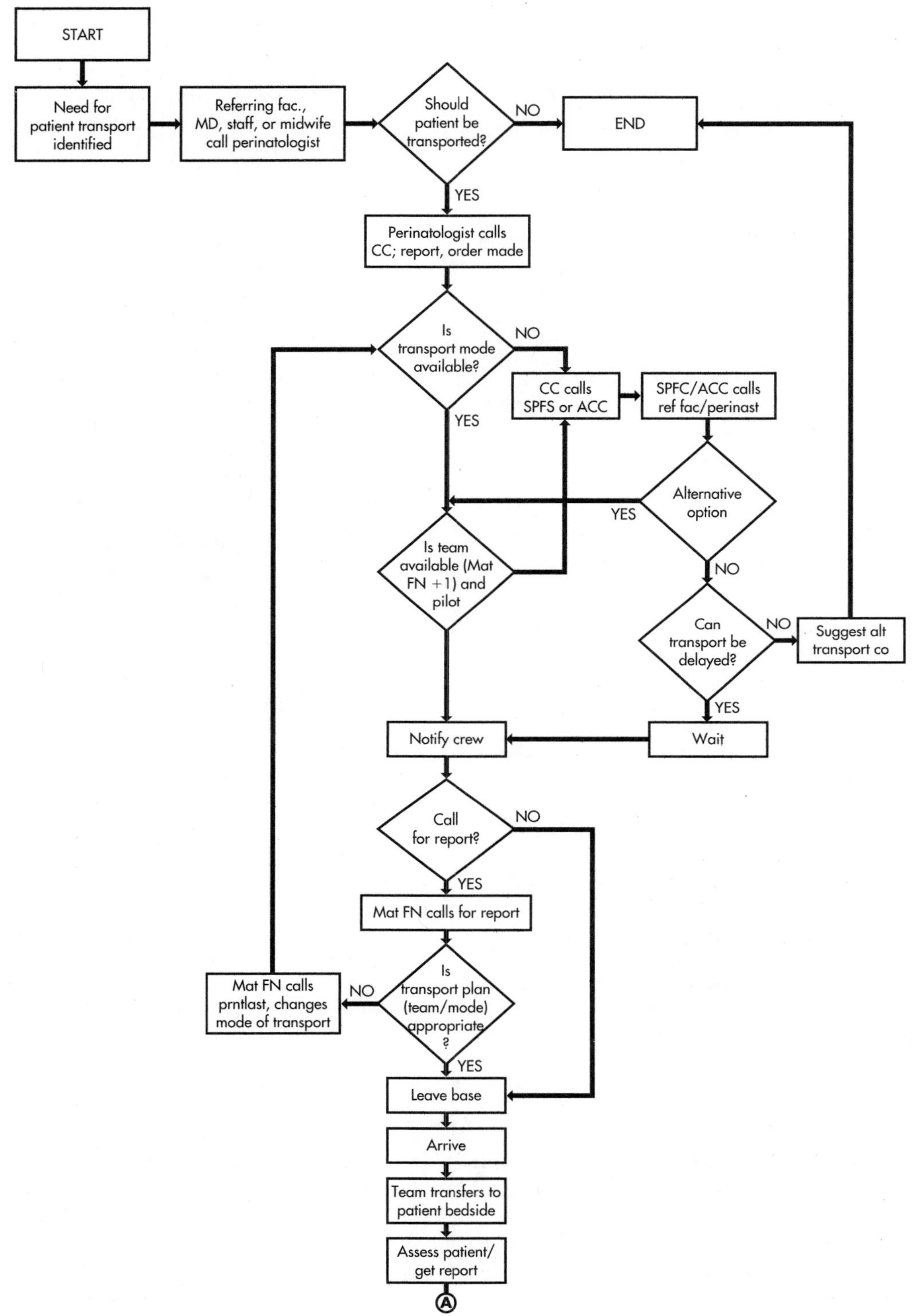

Fig. 36-1. Maternal transport process. (Courtesy Samaritan AirEvac, Phoenix, Ariz.)

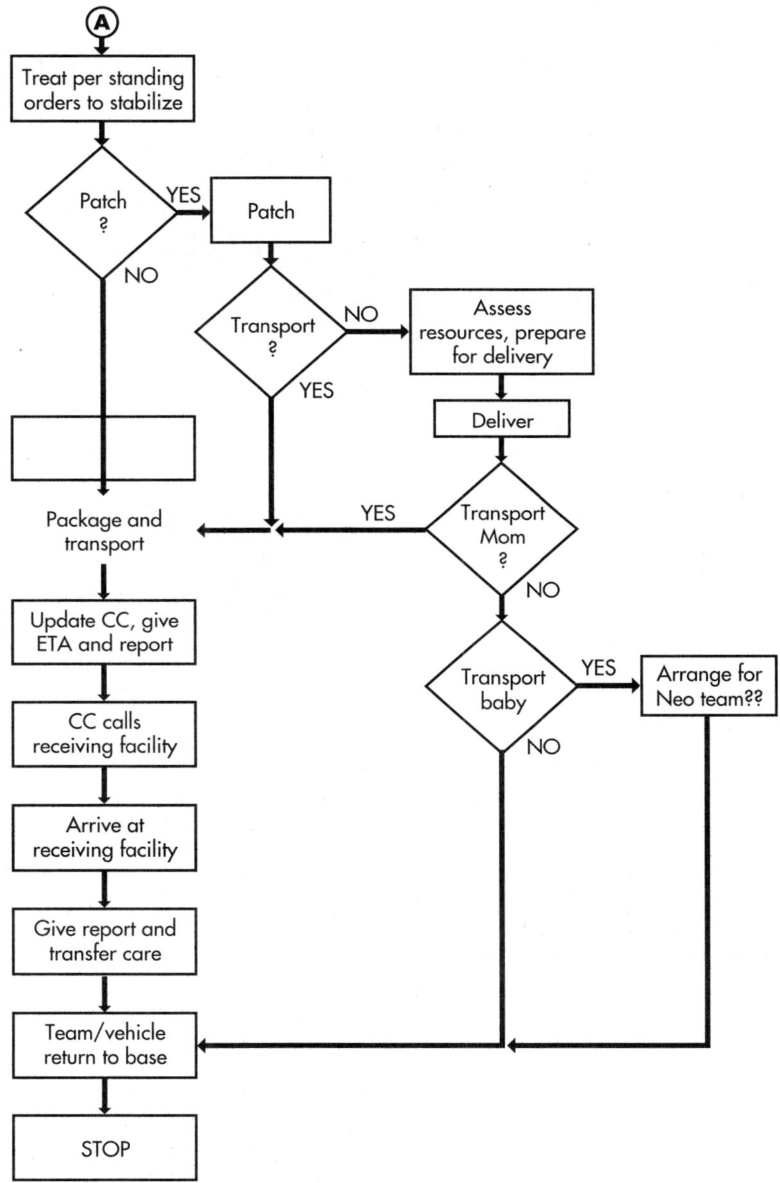

Fig. 36-1, cont'd. Maternal transport process. (Courtesy Samaritan AirEvac, Phoenix, Ariz.)

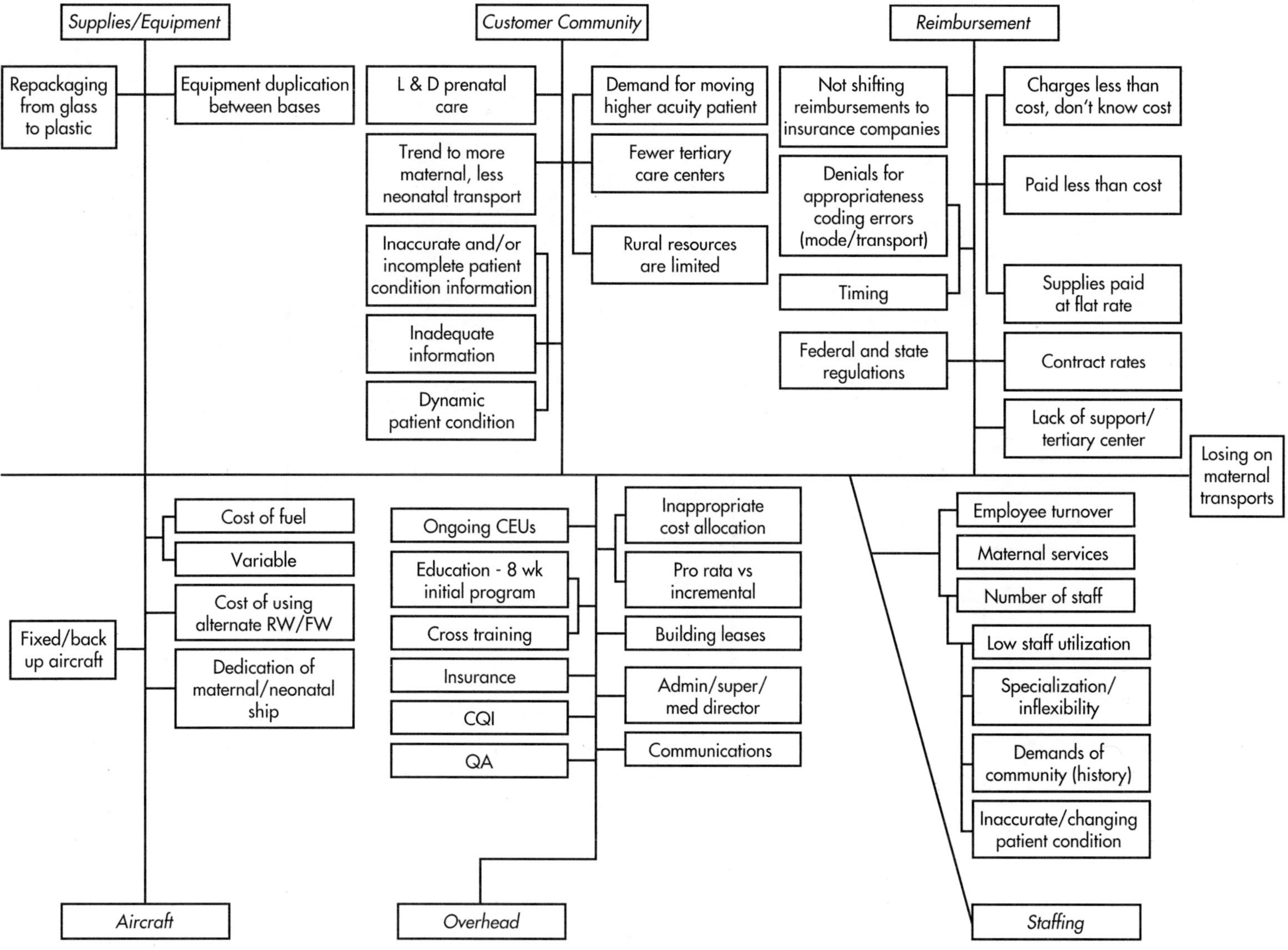

Fig. 36-2. Cause-and-effect diagram. (Courtesy Samaritan AirEvac, Phoenix, Ariz.)

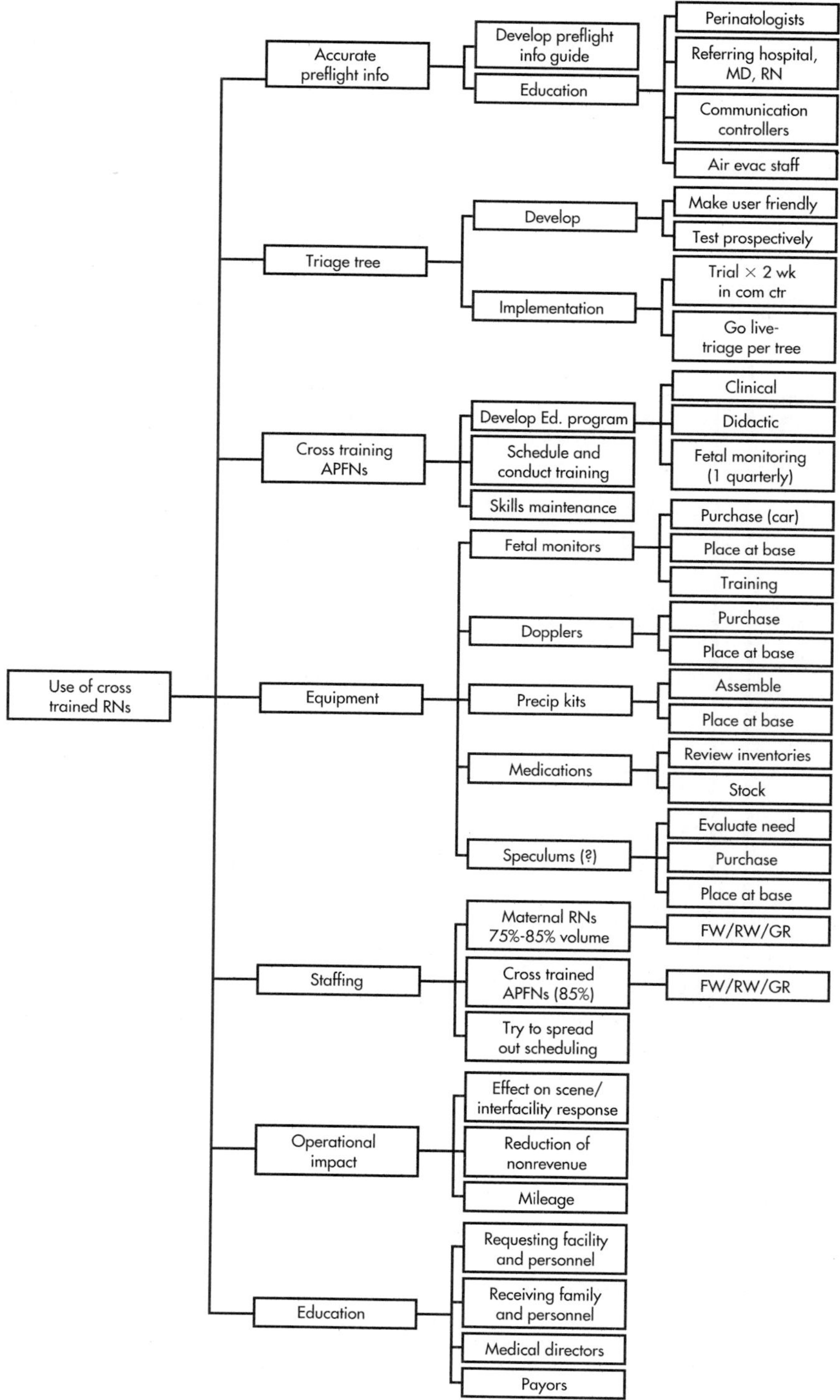

Fig. 36-3. Planning tree for use of cross-trained adult/pediatric flight nurses. (Courtesy Samaritan AirEvac, Phoenix, Ariz.)

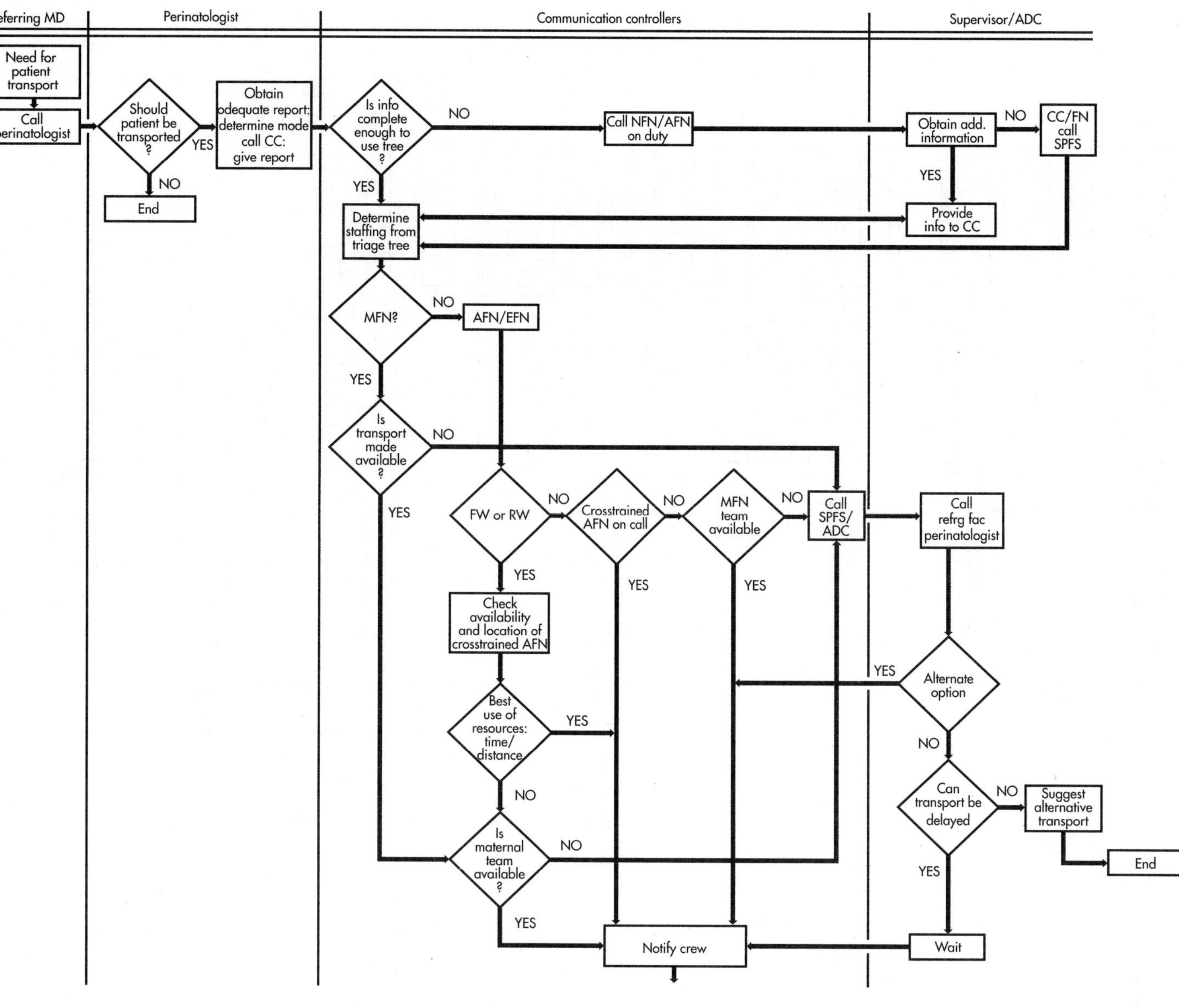

Fig. 36-4. Maternal transport process. (Courtesy Samaritan AirEvac, Phoenix, Ariz.)

cialized care. The team tested this hypothesis by defining major diagnoses requiring the need for the maternal flight nurse. These definitions were based on the possibility of delivery or fetal distress. Ten primary diagnosis categories were identified that might cause major maternal patient complications. Retrospective data were collected to show what percentage of maternal transports could have been cared for by a maternal flight nurse, a cross-trained adult/pediatric flight nurse, or either of the two teams. The data showed that as many as 30% of the maternal patients did not require specialized care.

A cause-and-effect diagram was created to identify the root causes of monetary losses on maternal transports (Fig. 36-2). This diagram helped the team recognize the major root cause of the problem: that Life Flight XYZ had created a system whereby all maternal transports had to be completed by maternal flight nurses and options for triaging any maternal calls to the nonspecialized team were limited.

DESIGNING THE REMEDY

The most rigorous challenge the team faced was to remedy the cause and design a solution for this complex and emotional issue. The team used the following solutions:

1. Maternal transports were triaged through the communication center with the aid of a maternal decision tree developed by the multidisciplinary team.
2. Communications specialists, referring physicians, referring labor-and-delivery departments, and perinatologists began using preflight information notepads. The purpose of these pads was to assist the AMP in obtaining complete, accurate information.
3. The team prospectively collected data on all maternal transports to determine whether the decision tree was functioning appropriately.
4. Life Flight XYZ implemented cross-training of all adult/pediatric flight nurses in maternal transport. Competency was verified by written and oral examinations. A planning tree (Fig. 36-3) was developed to assign accountability for carrying out the steps required to make the new process successful.
5. The team developed a new flow diagram (Fig. 36-4) to show the new transport process.

HOLDING THE GAINS

The final challenge the multidisciplinary team faced was holding the gains made by this successful project. To accomplish this objective, the team implemented an ongoing review of all maternal transports to assess the appropriateness of the triage decision and patient management. Life Flight XYZ also provided continuing education regarding the new process for AMP, communications specialists, and referring facilities and physicians.

LESSONS LEARNED

This multidisciplinary project was a combination of clinical and administrative budgetary dilemmas. The team faced an enormous problem that was emotionally charged. The team met weekly for 2 hours over a period of 9 months. They found it important to continue to meet intermittently to review the new process and identify additional modifications that might be required. Although not everyone was happy with the radical changes brought on by this process, AMP had the sense that an appropriate cross-section of personnel were given the opportunity to scientifically develop a new process to meet the budget constraints of Life Flight XYZ while maintaining high-quality patient care.

REFERENCES

1. AAMS Quality Assurance Committee: AAMS resource document for air medical quality assurance, *J Air Med Transport* 9:23-26, 1990.
2. American Academy of Pediatric Committee on Hospital Care: Guidelines for air and ground transportation of pediatric patients, *Pediatrics* 78(5):943-949, 1986.
3. Falcone RE: Indication for air medical transport: practical applications. In Rodenberg H, Blumen IJ, editors: *Air medical physician handbook,* Salt Lake City, Utah, 1994, Air Medical Physicians Association.
4. Rodenberg H, Blumen IJ, editors: *Air medical physician handbook,* Salt Lake City, Utah, 1994, Air Medical Physicians Association.
5. Thompson CB, et al: Intubation quality assurance thresholds, *Air Med J* 13:10, 416, 1994.

CHAPTER 37

Marketing the Air Medical Program

This chapter presents an overview of the components of the marketing process and how marketing relates to the air medical program and offers direct applications for flight nurses and program directors to consider for their specific air medical programs.

Marketing is a planned, multistep, strategic process and not a single or isolated event. Each component is one carefully interwoven building block in the overall marketing plan. The main components are the mission statement of the program, market research, market planning, and public relations. Two critical elements of the marketing process are quality of service and customer relations.

Marketing activities should be designed so that the end results are measurable. This is important for the nurse manager in evaluating current and past marketing activities and setting strategy for future market potentials. Marketing is not the distribution of program paraphernalia such as calendars, pens, and buttons. The expenditure of resources for such materials must be carefully planned, budgeted, and evaluated in terms of other marketing activities that are significantly more important. Marketing is not primarily a sales activity. Rather, it is the preparation and delivery of information and support to those on whom the program depends. Through marketing, the program attempts to influence the decision-making and buying practices of the users. The air medical program has no control over these external agencies. However, through the informational value of the marketing program, the public relations function, the nurse manager can influence user selection.

A marketing plan is a written document that identifies the more promising growth opportunities for the program. It describes the strategies necessary to successfully penetrate, capture, and retain "market share" of the patient catchment area. Essentially, it is the foundation on which the air medical program's other operating plans are built.

Unfortunately, air medical programs have a history of initiating operations with a limited scope of market planning. From inception, marketing may be viewed administratively as a luxury to be addressed later. Quick program start-ups as a response to competition have often left strategic planning processes on the back burner.

It is not unusual to find the budget line item for marketing, advertising and public relations, and program promotion to be the lowest allocation in the overall air medical program. In addition, nurse managers are often neutralized by the sponsor hospital's marketing resources and marketing departments, which are assigned responsibility for promoting the air medical service along with an array of other hospital services and programs. Thus the involvement of the nurse manager is limited and often quite latent. At a minimum, the air medical program leader must strive to influence the informational environment in which the "marketing department" makes decisions that can affect the program's success.

MISSION OF THE AIR MEDICAL PROGRAM

A program's mission is generally expressed as a broad statement that defines the roles and purpose of the organization and the environment in which it will operate. The mission reflects the primary reasons for the organization's existence.

Mission and scope may refer to the nature of the program's product and activities in terms of its ability to serve its market area. The mission statement should address the basic questions "What business are we in?" and "What markets should we serve?"

In defining the air medical program's mission, the nurse manager should consider the following key questions:

1. What groups will our organization initially serve and need to serve in the future?
2. What are the requirements and characteristics of these groups?
3. Are these groups satisfied with the services they are receiving?
4. Are there any individuals, groups, organizations, or agencies that our program is not servicing but should be?
5. What should the program's posture be toward competition?
6. Is the present mission of our sponsor organization (hospital) patient service mix adequate to meet the needs of the air medical program's market?
7. What is our program's responsibility for controlling prehospital care costs and services?

The nurse manager must also be able to see the mission of the air medical program through the eyes of the chief executive officers, board of directors, and administrators of the sponsor organization(s). By understanding their expectations for the air medical service and operations, the nurse manager can then begin to plan marketing strategies and activities that will support that mission or help to reshape administrative thinking.

For example, administration's priorities and expectations may be to bring 90% of the patients transported by helicopter back to the home base. The nurse manager may need to balance administration's expectations, the institution's clinical resources and expertise, and the projected helicopter patient market. If in the patient catchment area there is a high incidence of coronary artery disease, and the institution has very limited specialties in cardiology, the market and the resources may not match to yield the expected transport share for the institution. Integrating the institution's strengths into the air medical program's mission will enhance the success of both.

Another common area of confusion in addressing the mission of the air medical program is found in the expectations regarding service scene versus interhospital transports. The nurse manager might see the mission of the program as being primarily a second responder to scene requests. Thus energies can be focused on this market segment, whereas administration's priorities have been placed exclusively on the interhospital transport market.

The mission statement will give clarity to the air medical program with regard to what it does and whom it serves. Through the mission, the program can communicate its identity to its members and the outside community. In essence, the mission statement is the foundation for the behavior of the organization.

Goals of the air medical program are driven by the mission statement. They are an ideal condition or end result. Goals state the overall long-term intent of the program's management. They define areas of concentration for the organization's financial and human resources.

The goals, or the specific desired results of the program's operating plan, should be driven by what the program sees itself doing in the future, as well as whom it will serve in the future. Clarity of the mission enables the nurse manager to set goals that will be supported by the administration.

The goals specified for the accomplishment of the mission of the program should include projected results from each of the defined market segments.

MARKET SEGMENTATION: IDENTIFY THE CLIENT BASE

Market segmentation is concerned with finding, identifying, and serving consumer and user groups in the organization's service area. An air medical program's service area can be divided into groups of people with similar needs and characteristics to which the program can provide specific services. For example, a program goal may be to provide rapid transport services to a group of people aged 40 to 65 years with a high incidence of coronary artery disease. Thus the market segment, defined in this case by age, is targeted for education regarding heart disease and the role of helicopter transport.

A primary mode for success in marketing is to segment the multiple macromarkets into homogeneous micromarket segments. This subclassification allows implementation by the management of an affordable, focused plan of action. Market segmentation reveals who the customers are and prioritizes the provision of information addressed to their specific needs.

Air medical programs have two groups of clients: patients who receive direct care and program activators who initiate the air medical response. The challenge is to serve the patients clinically and provide the education and training, followed with timely, appropriate, and supportive feedback to the system activators.

Program activators are the main target of the marketing plan. Because air medical programs are generally not accessed directly by patients, an activator network must be created or focused on. The following section discusses the development of an effective network for activators to access the service and patient systems provided by the air medical program.

CREATING THE "WEB" OF AN EFFECTIVE MARKETING PLAN

The nurse manager must first identify the potential activators of the service. The identification process evaluates the external and internal environments in which the program will operate. The most objective means to gather data to service these environments is through market research.

Market Research

Market research is a systematic analysis of the market to obtain objective data relevant to the goals or objectives of the air medical program. Market research facilitates informed management decision making. Data from market research will help identify and solve marketing problems, but these data are not a substitute for management decision making.

With respect to the air medical program, market research is focused on people from agencies that would activate an air medical response. Having projected the largest potential group of activators, a survey instrument such as a questionnaire can be developed to obtain information from each specific market segment (physicians, law enforcement agencies, and so on) about the perceived servicing needs of the air medical program. From this information, marketing strategies can be formulated.

In addition to the questionnaire, the nurse manager can use air medical staff personnel to interact with activators in a community. For example, brief discussions at local hospital medical staff meetings, or in groups as small as a specific physician practice group, may elicit information from the physician activators. Whether the interview method or survey instrument is used, questions should be constructed in such a manner that an objective analysis can be made on the data gathered. Reliability of the instrument must be carefully considered before management decisions on the basis of the information derived are weighted.

In the case of competing programs, market research can objectively identify the perceived strengths and weakness of each of the air medical services. It can also identify the parameters by which activators decide that an air medical response is most appropriate, which helps the nurse manager plan how to sway those not firmly convinced of the efficiency of air medical transport.

Internal Environmental Support

Although the external environment is the main user of the air medical service, the internal environment—the hospital organization(s) sponsoring the service—must also be addressed. This internal environment allocates the resources that support the air medical service, as well as what areas are lacking in resources.

The influence of physicians of the sponsor institution is often overlooked. This component of the internal environment needs as much care, support, and organizational framework to function in as possible. Key physician leaders should be brought on board to help develop marketing strategies for the air medical service, as well as be encouraged and reimbursed by the sponsor organizations for their time in developing physician outreach, networking, or physician speaker bureaus. Other institutional resources such as the marketing department or training and development can be used in planning to develop marketing strategies for establishing collaborative relationships with neighboring and system hospitals. The sponsor institutions' resources or strengths in marketing or staff development may well be a supportive asset to the smaller community hospitals' development and/or participation in a health care network/ system.

External Market Strategies

External groups are generally hospitals, physicians, and public safety agencies such as ambulance services, fire departments, county sheriff departments, and special rescue teams. A major force supporting or obstructing interhospital transports is the hospital networking and physician-to-physician bridge building that takes place. Experience demonstrates that patients have strong preference for their personal physician and generally prefer to remain in the local community for health care services. Both of these factors can work as significant obstacles if ignored by the air medical program. The role of the nurse manager is to develop the appropriate policies that support these natural patient linkages and keep patients in their defined health care system as is appropriate.

The nurse manager must identify and overcome a hospital's resistance to referral. A key resistance may arise from economic issues—specifically, the perceived loss of patient revenue. Intense economic pressure and a patient's strong desire to remain close to home at a time of illness may hamper air medical intervention even when it is most appropriate. Also to be considered is the difficulty for many smaller community and rural hospital employees to have "a patient taken away because we couldn't do the job," and their personal financial effect in realizing the institution's need to keep patients and the revenues that they generate. This may be perceived as an equivalent to the admission of failure.

Given these obstacles, the nurse manager can develop several strategies for smaller community and/ or rural hospital team participation on the air medical service. First is the emphasis on the health care team. Referring hospital staff must have a participatory role in the patient's road to recovery, rather than that of an inadequate health care provider. The air medical program can implement several different types of strategies to include and enhance rural hospital team participation. Several of the strategies are:

1. *Patient returns home for recovery.* In this program, patients are returned to their local community hospitals for the rehabilitative or final recovery stage of their illness or injury. Strategy must be carefully planned to ensure that reimbursements by payers are not compromised by the program. However, such a program encourages the continuum of health

care and appropriate use of tertiary health care services and supports the linkage between the patient, the private physician, and the community. It also supports a critical objective of health care systems and managed care organizations: matching the intensity of the health care resources with the intensity of the patient's health care needs.

2. *Enhancing the lines of communication.* Each outlying hospital brought on board as a participant in the air medical program should be given "preferred status" reception each time they request support. The conveyance of this attitude begins with the initial interaction with the air medical communications center. Responding to the hospital that has the preferred status begins with a service-oriented attitude reflected by the communications staff on the radio and on the telephone with the hospital team. A request for the services of the air medical program should be a two-sided, participatory event. Special phone lines can be an asset in conveying the preferred status to the rural hospital network. The nurse manager should streamline the information required to ensure a simple, easy way for the outlying hospitals to access the medical helicopter and/or airplane. A "no-questions-asked" approach is afforded if the time is taken proactively to compile the referring institution's information and have it quickly available in the communications center.
3. *Proactive involvement.* Proactively involving the air medical program with the health care team at the outlying hospital can be accomplished through a physicians' speakers bureau, continued education courses or seminars, and visible support of the hospital's marketing efforts. The air medical program can gain positive goodwill exposure by assisting the rural hospitals in marketing and promoting *their* services.
4. *Promote aviation service and training.* This program involves ongoing continuing safety training and education for the hospital personnel and focuses on making the air medical transport vehicle part of their hospital services. Helipad and landing site selection reviews can all be provided through the resources of the air medical program. In addition, emergency procedures and on-line radio communications should be preestablished in light of the outlying hospital's ability to facilitate them. For example, if the hospital radio is not in a convenient location, then the air medical team should limit this type of communication.

Patients and Their Families

Patients being transported by an air medical service have a unique set of needs. The first is the need for clinical intervention; the second, often overlooked, is for emotional support. Often, patients have not made or even been involved in the decision to be flown to another institution for care. This factor can be a major obstacle during the transfer of the patient to the air medical team. The nurse manager must prepare the air medical staff for dealing with this on a proactive, rather than reactive, basis. The team should take time to meet the needs of the patients and their families before transporting. In the crisis of the moment, this will tend to be a very hurried and rushed encounter. Using the resources at the referring institution, such as other health team members, can facilitate the air medical staff's explanations to patients and families if they are informed and encouraged to assist. Taking a few extra minutes to discuss with the family their fears or concerns and provide written directions to the destination hospital can be most helpful. The air medical team should explain the nature of the transport, the length of time of the flight, and most important, the clinical care to be delivered during the flight. It is often helpful to have maps already prepared to direct the family to the destination hospital. The family should know how to reconnect with the flight team after the transport, and the team members should schedule a follow-up visit as soon as they return. This may be more difficult if the destination hospital is not a participating hospital, and the follow-up visit may be limited to telephone contact.

Patients and their families, as well as the utilizers or activators of the service, need feedback about the air medical mission. The nurse manager must adequately prepare the staff to handle and facilitate these follow-up, feedback calls, including physician-to-physician contacts.

Prehospital Personnel

Prehospital personnel use of the air medical service is usually less than that of the hospital and physician network. Marketing activities and resources should be proportionately focused on this group.

Prehospital decision-making algorithms should be collaboratively established with each public service and EMS service entity in the catchment area. These should outline a mutual set of expectations for when the helicopter will be called directly to the scene or when interception at the closest hospital is more appropriate.

In meeting with the prehospital personnel, it is highly advantageous to involve local hospital personnel and local physicians as well. Thus, the hospital staff and physician community will be less likely to perceive the air medical program as a threat, again emphasizing the strategy for team participation with the air medical service as one of the members. The development of objective scoring systems for prehospital use when triaging or decision-making for air medical transport is also highly encouraged. Application of guidelines published by national associations representing air medical transport is encouraged. It is important to emphasize the involvement and input of the hospital and local physicians.

Seminars are often efficient marketing tools. Generally, they work because they offer the personal contact needed to present the program's expertise and services in a low-key, nonthreatening environment. The training and education of prehospital personnel, if considered part of an overall marketing plan, may create unfounded expectations for increased numbers of calls. These expectations may color and consequently defeat the goals of the educational programs. It may also leave prehospital personnel feeling used or propositioned: "They are only doing this so we'll call them."

Training and education can be separate activities of the air medical program yet complement marketing strategies. By identifying the needs of prehospital personnel through surveys or personal communication, the nurse manager may discover a market demand for specific programs to improve the level of prehospital care. Many of these programs should be conducted in conjunction with local training, physicians, or community hospitals. Specifically in the rural communities, hospitals may appreciate and need the additional support of the air medical team and its sponsor hospital resources to provide continuing education opportunities for prehospital and hospital staff. Networking programs such as these have a subtle but positive public relations effect. They can have a dramatic impact on creating the desired team approach and collaboration with the air medical service through recognition of the valued role of each primary care giver.

The team approach must also be emphasized on any scene response. Before the initiation of the request for service, the air medical program personnel and prehospital personnel should have decided who is in charge. Coordination on the scene will directly reflect collaboration that has already taken place.

Many air medical services have follow-up and callback programs for user agencies. These programs should be constructed in such a way that they focus on quality improvement (QI) activities for both organizations. A comprehensive QI program will review the clinical, operational, and aviation components of each mission. The services should each independently evaluate performance against mutually developed standards and share their discoveries about the positive areas, as well as areas for future improvement. The nurse manager should develop the comprehensive, collaborative quality improvement program with a progressive and positive tone. Focusing feedback on predetermined standards, rather than on emotionally charged assumptions, creates clarity for communicating and avoids a negative, policing attitude that might otherwise be conveyed.

Many of the marketing strategies involve the external environment of the air medical service. In brief, it looks at opportunities for expansion of services, as well as carefully critiquing areas in which services may be threatened. The air medical program depends on external sources over which it has little control. Without control, the focus turns to providing information, influence, and support to achieve the desired outcomes. The external environment is the main user of the air medical service, but the internal environment, the hospital organization sponsoring the service, must also be addressed.

PUBLIC RELATIONS: CREATING THE PROGRAM'S IMAGE

Marketing activities and public relations efforts are often confused. They are not one and the same. The nurse manager should consider public relations a part of the overall marketing plan. The public relations activities of the air medical program involve those tasks that foster positive regard for the program. It is the building of goodwill and the enhancement of relations with patients and users of the service. It is, in effect, the "image-building" aspect of the overall marketing plan.

Public relations policy should be consistent with and driven by the organization's mission and goals. The policy objectives should ensure two-way communication between the program and the internal and external communities. Image-building results of a good public relations program may be difficult to measure. This is the biggest obstacle for the nurse manager to overcome in justifying the budget needs for the public relations aspect of the marketing plan.

The benefits of public relations are important not only to sales but also to cooperation and two-way communication with the community. There are two basic elements of the public relations program to be explored. They are community involvement and publicity.

Community Involvement

Obtaining successful community support uses the same techniques employed in networking with hospitals. Enlisting local resources such as government representatives by making them part of the team essentially makes or breaks the service's welcome to their jurisdiction. The nurse manager should be knowledgeable about local government activities and recognize opportunities for the flight program or air medical personnel to support these activities.

The goal of the community-involvement aspect of the public relations program is to have the flight team and management contribute to the community's social and economic development. In an effective program, program representatives become active in the community and community members are invited to participate in the air medical program.

The range of community activities for involvement of the flight team is limited only by management's imagination. Possible areas include:

1. *Medical programs.* The program can cosponsor CPR or wellness training with local emergency medical services (EMS), fire department, and hospital personnel. Opportunities to support primary health care activities such as immunization clinics in remote areas should also be considered.
2. *Educational assistance.* An effective method for promoting goodwill is to provide scholarships, speakers, equipment, and other assistance to local high schools, colleges, and universities.
3. *Recreation and sports.* Sponsoring sporting events such as golf outings or long-distance runs to raise money for charity can enhance the organization's image in the communities it serves.
4. *Fund-raising drives.* Participation by the organization in fund-raising activities to support local charities is good PR.
5. *Leadership activities.* Air medical personnel can become active in the Chamber of Commerce, professional associations, and political advisory groups.
6. *Cultural activities.* The organization can demonstrate goodwill through sponsoring cultural activities such as concerts, plays, or excursions and field trips for the disadvantaged or disabled.

Publicity

Through publicity, the program can develop good relations with media audiences by informing them about the organization, its services, and its contributions to the communities. In order to be effective, publicity must be newsworthy and have special interest for the media's audiences.

Publicity begins with the development of appropriate topics that will enable the organization to translate corporate mission and goals into publicity goals. Such goals may include gaining the competitive edge over other services, influencing the decisions of service users, and improving relations in specific communities.

Through a strategic use of publicity, the organization can maintain a continuous flow of program information to the community. Publicity is a proven technique for achieving specific corporate objectives with a smaller financial investment than other marketing methods. "Free" publicity that is used in conjunction with paid advertising and other marketing methods is especially effective. It is important to remember, however, that the success of a publicity program is reflective of its role in the overall marketing plan.

Working with the press and media has often been outside the responsibilities of the nurse manager. However, inadequate or inappropriate press relations will directly reflect the air medical program. Thus the nurse manager must become involved with the press and media either directly or indirectly through the hospital's normal network. Proactively, it is important that the nurse manager form a positive relationship between the media and the program.

Methods of Publicity

The nurse manager has several options for effectively communicating the objectives and performance of the program through the use of the media. Several methods for obtaining publicity are as follows.

Press Releases. The press release is the foundation of the publicity program. It is an inexpensive method for the dissemination of program news through the media. Releases contain a brief description of the subject, often accompanied by a diagram.

The media generally welcomes press releases, and releases can be an especially successful means of stimulating positive coverage and increasing the visibility of the program. One can significantly increase the chances of generating coverage of events that are of marginal news value by minimizing the effort needed by reporters. The release should be well written in a style appropriate for the media. The nurse manager should meet the media contacts personally and, after sending releases, make follow-up courtesy calls. Releases should be sent as far in advance of the event as possible to facilitate scheduling. Including photographs of the program in action may increase the likelihood of media coverage, especially in smaller newspapers.

Feature Articles. Generally longer than press releases, feature articles include materials such as a case history of the program (or product news item), an explanation of how the product is properly used, or a description of how the product helped solve a specific problem. Photographs provided are an asset to your article.

The chances of having an article accepted are dramatically increased by developing strong working relationships within the media. A major part of publicity work is in establishing and maintaining rapport with the media representatives.

Press Conferences. Through effective press conferences, program management has the opportunity to disseminate news about the program and its services. These events can be somewhat complex and intimidating, and therefore require extensive planning and preparation to successfully execute. Nurse managers should look to their sponsor hospital resources for involvement in planning and executing a press conference.

Trade Shows. The opportunity to disseminate information about the program to a specific audience can be enhanced by participation at trade shows. The types of shows to consider including in the public relations budget should be reflective of the primary users of the program, such as hospital associations, physicians' conferences, EMS conferences, and public safety agency trade shows.

Public Speaking Engagements. Participation as a public speaker is important to both community involvement and publicity aspects of the public relations program. This public relations tool can keep the air medical program's name visible in the community while enabling the program to publicize its objectives. Steps involved in the process of using speakers from the sponsor and/or participating hospital effectively include identifying speaker opportunities accessing the primary program users, constructing presentations to ensure consistency in the message delivered, and developing the list of probable questions that will be asked.

Press Relations Day. Representatives of the media can be invited for a formal luncheon to encourage open dialogue and conversation. The agenda should include expectations of both air medical program and media in terms of information that is needed for a successful news release and explanation of why some information cannot be made available (i.e., patient confidentiality). The nurse manager can create the appropriate environment in which the media learns that the program will provide the information needed within the constraints of patient privacy. The media can provide feedback on how best to supply information, including the framework and content for news releases, as well as how to hold a press conference. Establishing a collaborative relationship between the press and the program will aid in future coverage, but should not carry expectation that the program will be shown favoritism by the news media.

Evaluating Results in a Public Relations Program

The means by which to monitor and evaluate the public relations program are recording activities and measuring success. The record of activities should include the number of press releases mailed versus the number used and by whom; press conferences and speaking engagements, including numbers and lists of participants for future follow-up; and newsletters and brochures produced with documentation of follow-up activities, including solicitation of feedback regarding material content.

Measuring the success of the public relations program is somewhat difficult in that the results are generally seen in changes of attitudes of the program activators. A successful program may result in increased service utilization, but this is not a reliable indicator because it is dependent upon an event triggered external to the targeted audience. Success may be measured through appropriate air medical use, tracking the numbers of times one service is used versus that of a competitor, and monitoring ground transports that potentially were appropriate to be flown. Other program outputs can be measured on the basis of projections of the response expected through marketing the physicians' speakers bureau versus actual numbers of programs delivered.

THE MARKETING PROCESS

The marketing plan begins with an analysis of the results of market research, public relations activities, strengths identified in the internal and external environment, identification of the market segments, program goals, and ultimately the program mission. Specific objectives are derived from this information that focus program management and staff on the development of a plan that will have specific, measurable outcomes.

Writing a marketing plan is similar to developing a nursing care plan. It involves assessment, identification of objectives, development of a plan of action, monitoring, and reevaluation. Tools for measuring results must also be established. There is no secret ingredient to a marketing plan outside of commitment to documenting and following it. The marketing plan should be simple, clear, and open to accommodating new strategies. The effectiveness of the plan should be evaluated on a regularly scheduled basis.

Major pitfalls in strategic marketing or planning generally derive from incomplete market information and failure to follow through. Poor communication of the marketing plan also add to the demise of successful marketing strategies. A collaborative goal-setting and strategic-planning process involving internal and external organizational players is critical to the success of the plan.

Advertising must be carefully integrated and should support the objectives of the marketing plan. For example, the advertising budget should reflect both indirect and direct costs of advertising and marketing. Creative methods to maximize the budget dollar involve use of existing overhead (personnel salaries) to accomplish the marketing plan. Advertising and publicity can be a perfect union for a low-dollar high-impact marketing strategy. Detailed programs should be formulated and evaluated in terms of the following factors:

1. Profitability
2. Market share
3. Continued program use
4. The overall marketing objectives

THE NURSE MANAGER AND PROGRAM MARKETING

Approaching marketing as a process, with each of the components developed to support program goals and mission, is important. Integrated into the marketing process components are strategies specific to air medical program activity. The air medical industry involves a great deal of one-on-one contact with clients and hospital personnel. Technical skills are less important to the clients than are how they perceive they are received and treated. An important theme the flight team can convey is captured in one sentence: "How might I help you?" This attitude is one of the strongest marketing approaches to introduce.

The nurse manager is responsible for weaving service management into the overall marketing process. Service management attitudes of, "Keep it simple, add a personal touch, and treat everyone like a VIP," are all important approaches for the program, beginning at the grass roots level. A service-oriented attitude supports marketing strategies and processes that are focused on influencing decision-makers.

CHAPTER 38

Stress and Stress Management

Seyle was one of the first scientists to report the physical and psychological effects of stress and the stress response. He defined stress as the "rate of wear and tear in the body as it adapts to change or threat."[10,15] The concept of stress has been further described as an adverse state during which tension, fatigue, unpleasant emotions, and, occasionally, a sense of hopelessness and futility may be experienced.[15] Stress has also been characterized as a dynamic, progressive relationship between a person and the environment.[10]

Stress is an integral part of flight nursing practice. There are numerous sources of stress that the flight nurse must learn to cope with to maintain physical and mental health. Some of the major sources of stress encountered in flight nursing include the types of patient situations, the work environment, and social responsibilities such as a family.

Multiple studies have documented the effect of stress on nurses.[7,10] Excessive exposure to stress may result in physical and psychological reactions. Some of these reactions may lead to long-term physical effects such as migraine headaches or psychological harm such as burnout or posttraumatic stress disorder (PTSD).[2,7]

This chapter will discuss the sources of stress, the factors that contribute to reactions to stress, the physical and psychological reactions to stress, and coping mechanisms that can be used to contend with stress.

Factors Influencing Reaction to Stress

The ability to cope with stress depends on several factors, including the intensity of the stress (physical and psychological components); the number of times one encounters the same stress; the amount of time one is exposed to the stress; the perceived or real threat that the stress may cause; the individual's previous experience with the stress or similar stressors; and the presence of support systems. It is important to keep in mind that the *individual's perception* of the stress is a major contributor to one's reactions to stress. Each of us has a particular world view that influences how the source of stress is perceived. In other words, what one person may find stressful another may not. Lachman notes, "The difference is not in the quantity as it is in the quality of the stress."[10]

Sources of Stress

The sources of stress in flight nursing are many and varied. They come from both physical and psychological origins and sometimes may be a combination of the two. The work environment, the organization in which one is employed, and one's social environments are additional factors that may contribute to stress.

Physical stressors include limited work space, malfunctioning equipment, noise, odors, and vibration. The physical condition of the flight nurse also contributes to stress. The long shifts, changes in weather, and illness or injury influence physical well-being and work response. The box contains a summary of physical stressors.

One of the most cited sources of stress is patient illness or injury (Fig. 38-1). The patient with a difficult-to-maintain airway that tries the flight nurse's skills or a patient who dies despite aggressive care may produce a stress reaction. There are other psychological sources of stress that are summarized in the box on the top of p. 694.

PHYSICAL SOURCES OF STRESS

- Limited space in which to provide patient care
- Lack of appropriate patient care equipment
- Malfunctioning equipment
- Malfunctioning transport equipment
- Changes in the outside environment
- Noise, odors, and vibration
- Work hours
- Lack of sleep
- Illness or injury
- Significant exposure to infectious diseases

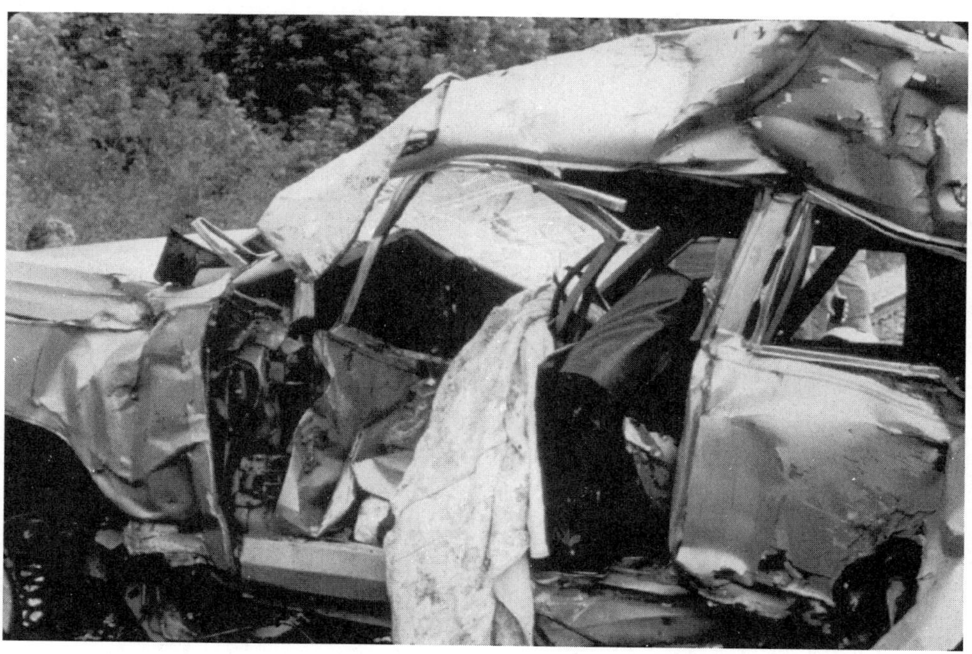

Fig. 38-1. A patient's illness or injury may be a source of stress for the flight nurse, particularly the patient who has been severely injured like the victim of this motor vehicle crash.

PSYCHOLOGICAL SOURCES OF STRESS

Age of the patient (particularly pediatric patients)
Death of the patient
Patient's illness or injury (particularly as the result of violence)
Grief and anxiety of the patient's family or friends
Team member interactions
Lack of organizational support
Lack of autonomy in making decisions
Lack of a support group

EXAMPLES OF ACUTE REACTIONS TO STRESS

Physical

Exhaustion
Headaches
Nausea and vomiting
Diarrhea
Sweating
Increased heart rate
Difficulty breathing

Emotional

Nightmares
Inability to sleep
Fear
Guilt
Feelings of helplessness
Anger
Irritability

Cognitive

Confusion
Inability to prioritize tasks
Loss of attention
Calculation problems
Loss of concentration
Easy distraction

Reactions to Stress

As previously stated, many studies have described and documented nurses and other prehospital care providers' reactions to stress.[1,4,6,7,10] Stress reactions can be physical, psychological, social, or a blend of both physical and psychological. They can have serious physical and psychological aftermaths. The boxes below each contain a summary of the physical and psychological reactions to acute and long-term stressors.

There may be an initial acute reaction to stress such as sweating, tachycardia, and shortness of breath. If the stressors continue, long-term effects may occur. Some of the long-term consequences of stress include deficits in relationship skills, less sensitivity to patients, less tolerance of patients, and aggressive behavior.[6]

Burnout

Burnout has been attributed to long-term exposure to stress. Burnout generally manifests itself as a psychological, physical, and behavioral reaction to stress.[7] Signs and symptoms of burnout include emo-

EXAMPLES OF LONG-TERM EFFECTS OF STRESS

Physical

Headache
Nausea and vomiting
Chronic illness

Emotional

Setting inflexible rules
Alterations in personal finances
Depression
Burnout

Cognitive

Anomia
Inability to make decisions
Memory loss
Hyperexcitability

tional exhaustion, fatigue, irritability, anxiety, helplessness, and hopelessness. Physical symptoms of burnout include headaches, backaches, and gastrointestinal disturbances.[7]

Posttraumatic Stress Disorder

One of the most serious reactions to stress is PTSD. It arises from the exposure to a traumatic event that involves real or threatened death or injury to an individual or a group of individuals. The person experiencing PTSD may have nightmares or flashbacks; avoids people, places, or things that bring back the event, and may experience such things as hypervigilance or an increased startle response.[2]

STRESS MANAGEMENT

Learning to manage stress should be one of the most important self-interventions practiced by the flight nurse. Individuals learn to manage stress through coping, and these coping mechanisms may be adaptive or maladaptive. Adaptive coping mechanisms reduce the physical and psychological consequences of stress. Maladaptive coping mechanisms increase the negative effects of stress.[10] Flight nurses must recognize what coping mechanisms work for them and which ones do not. As a member of a team, the flight nurse must be able to recognize when other team members are not coping with stress.

Adaptive Coping Mechanisms

Many coping mechanisms have been identified to decrease the aftermath of stress. These include a sense of competence or pleasure in one's work, autonomy, planned problem-solving, assertiveness exercises, lifestyle management, personal philosophy, hobbies, continuing education, interpersonal support, and a sense of humor.[2,6,7,8,10,11]

A study by McAbee[11] revealed that both personal and organization coping strategies were needed to decrease nursing stress. More than 600 employed women including oncology, nononcology, and female university employees completed a self-administered questionnaire that included questions about such things as work stress, coping mechanisms, and work-setting ways to decrease stress.

Personal coping mechanisms used by the oncology nurses to manage stress involved exercise, talking with coworkers, taking breaks, humor, music, and praying. Work-setting methods to decrease stress encompassed formal support such as critical incident stress (CIS) debriefing, informal support in the form of an atmosphere that allowed open discussion among employees, formal counseling, continuing education—particularly related to stress management—and massage.[11] It would appear that adaptive coping mechanisms have both a personal and organizational component.

Two important things detected in this study were not only the need for personal coping mechanisms, but also a supportive work environment. The combination of these factors contributed to decreasing stress both from a personal and organizational point of view. Duquette et al[7] note that ". . . support from superiors and colleagues plays an important role in protecting nursing personnel from burnout."

Maladaptive Coping Mechanisms

Maladaptive coping mechanisms to stress include inability to sleep, nightmares, desensitization to patient needs, aggressive behavior, excessive use of caffeine, smoking, overeating, use of drugs (legal and illegal), and increased alcohol consumption.[6,10] When people have difficulty adapting to stress or develop maladaptive behavior, the effects go beyond the individual to their coworkers, families, and friends.

Buffering Factors Related to Stress

Duquette et al.[7] described "buffering factors" that help nurses deal with and manage the stress such as hardiness, social support, and coping. Social support and coping were previously discussed.

Hardiness has been described as a psychological concept. Hardy individuals are open to change, are committed to their work, and feel in control of their lives no matter what challenge is directed at them.[7] "To be committed requires the action to proceed ahead and avoid passivity and situations seen as distasteful or disagreeable."[7]

Flight nursing requires commitment. There are always challenges, and one needs the ability to at least "feel" in control in onerous situations. It is essential that flight nurses recognize the signs and symptoms of stress and develop methods of coping.

Methods of Stress Management

Multiple methods to manage stress have been proposed over the years. Research has demonstrated that physical and emotional care, diversions, and interpersonal care are some of the most effective techniques that can be employed to manage stress.[3,4,5,7,9,10] In addition, organizations that promote autonomy, staff participation, and recognition have employees with decreased levels of stress.[10,11]

Exercise has long been recognized as one of the best methods of managing stress.[10,11] Flight nursing requires physical exertion, as well as the ability to physically adapt to a variety of environments. If one does not feel physically well, it is difficult to cope with stress.

Use of relaxation techniques in stressful situations may also reduce the effects of stress. Imagery, deep breathing, meditation, and praying are some useful approaches that can be used no matter where the flight nurse is.

Emotional and interpersonal care is probably most often neglected by flight nurses. Commitment to the job can be both a good and a bad thing. If commitment excludes social support, the nurse may feel isolated and emotionally drained in a continuously stressful situation. Learning time-management skills, taking a break, and spending time with people who do different work are examples of ways to provide emotional care for ourselves.

Diversions such as hobbies, keeping a journal, listening to music, and caring for a pet not only decrease stress but also expand the view of the world. Photography (Fig. 38-2) can capture feelings that are difficult to express and also provide a method of

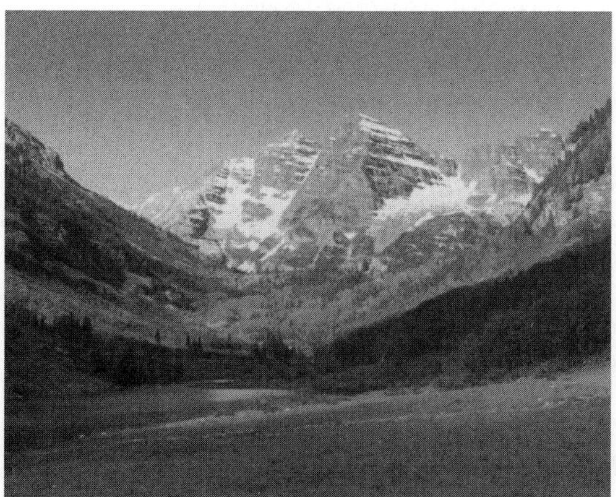

Fig. 38-2. Photography can provide a method of stress management. Looking at pictures of past pleasant experiences can decrease stress.

STRESS MANAGEMENT

Physical Care

Participating in an exercise program
Using relaxation techniques
- Imagery
- Deep breathing
- Meditation

Appropriate diet
Limiting or eliminating the use of tobacco and alcohol

Emotional care

Learning and using time management techniques
Acquiring problem-solving skills
Using humor
Spending time with people who do not do the same work

Diversions

Setting aside some private time each day
Keeping a journal
Volunteering for work different from current work
Finding a hobby
Listening to music
Caring for a pet
Planning group activities away from work

Interpersonal care

Spending time with one's family
Sharing one's feelings with others
Attending assertiveness training

relaxation when the photographer looks at pleasant images. The box (on opposite page) contains a summary of some selected methods of stress management.

Humor

Humor has been suggested as a useful antidote to stress.[5] It has been described as a "quality of perception that enables us to experience joy even when faced with adversity."[15] Humor also has been found to positively affect both physical and spiritual well-being. It has been determined that laughter decreases serum cholesterol, and it increases the number of T-cells and the number and activity of natural killer cells, boosting the immune system. Laughter can increase the energy of the spirit.

There are many sources of humor that can be used by the flight nurse to decrease stress. One of these is cartoons. "The Far Side," "Herman," and other favorite comics routinely picture common occurrences in nursing and medicine. A great series, *I Am Not an Ambulance Driver I-III,*[5] contains some hilarious cartoons about rotor-wing transport.

It is important that humor is used in the appropriate context. Laughing at the expense of others' feelings or in the potential presence of some who may not understand could produce very serious consequences.

Wooten[15] notes, "Humor and laughter can be effective self-care tools to cope with stress. They can improve the function of the body, the mind, and the spirit."

CRITICAL INCIDENT STRESS

In the early 1980s, CIS was recognized as a potential source of stress in emergency practice. Nurses, paramedics, physicians, and emergency medical technicians were being exposed to incidents involving serious illness and injury rarely experienced by others. Some individuals exhibited signs and symptoms of stress similar to those who had returned from Vietnam and described as PTSD. Interest was generated in why this was occurring and exactly what it was.[1,4,9,12]

As a part of our practice, we experience first-hand both individual and community disasters. The stress response that can occur from such experiences has been characterized as CIS. CIS has been described as a heightened state of physical, cognitive, behavioral, and emotional arousal.[14] Examples of CIS are outlined in the box below and shown in Fig. 38-3.

The effects of CIS include a tendency to reexperience the trauma when confronted with similar patients or situations; avoiding similar care situations; flashbacks; nightmares; and excessive startle reaction.[9,12] The care provider may find it increasingly difficult to function and may attempt to cope with maladaptive mechanisms or actually leave work.

To prevent and help people cope with CIS, CIS management (CISM) was developed. The components of CISM include the formation of CIS teams, education about stress and stress management, significant other and family support, management support, peer support, and mutual aid to community stress management programs. CISM teams are located around the world. Most of these teams are composed of multiple disciplines and include EMS providers, nurses, physicians, and mental health workers.

One function of the CISM team is to provide defusings and debriefings. A defusing is a short ver-

SOURCES OF CRITICAL INCIDENT STRESS

- A fellow worker who has been taken hostage
- Serious injury, illness, or death of a co-worker
- Violent, threatening patients
- Suicide or unexpected death of a co-worker
- Loss of life of a patient after prolonged extrication or resuscitation
- Caring for a patient who is a friend, relative, or co-worker
- Incidents attracting extensive media attention
- Any incident in which the sights, sounds, odors are so distressing as to produce a high level of immediate or delayed emotional response

Modified from Mitchell J: Comprehensive traumatic stress management in the emergency department, *Leadership Manage* 1(8):3-14, 1992; O'Rear, JA: Post-traumatic stress disorder: when the rescuer becomes the victim, *JEMS* 17(1):30-35, 1992; Bell NA: Critical incident stress debriefing, *Emergency* 23(9):30-35, 58, 1991.

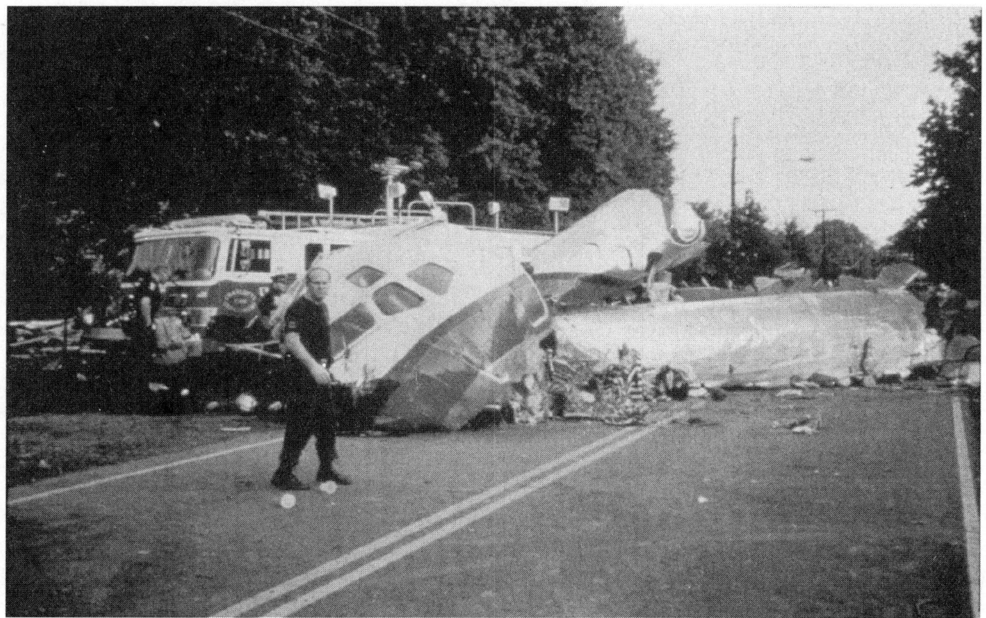

Fig. 38-3. The USAir 1016 crash, which had multiple victims, is an example of critical incident stress. Of the 57 passengers on board, only 20 survived. (Courtesy Bob Weir, Charlotte, NC.)

PHASES OF DEBRIEFING

Phase I

Introduction of group members, encouragement of active participation if members feel comfortable with it.

Phase II

Each person is asked to discuss and describe his or her role in the incident. It is easy to initiate this phase by reconstructing the entire incident.

Phase III

In this phase, participants are encouraged to discuss and describe their initial feelings after the incident.

Phase IV

A discussion of which parts of the incident elicited the most physical or emotional response.

Phase V

CISM asks the group what signs and symptoms of stress they have experienced since the incident.

Phase VI

The reentry phase, in which the team elicits any questions or comments about the process.

Phase VII

Wrap-up of the session. Some groups provide refreshments and additional time to socialize.

Modified from Mitchell J: Comprehensive traumatic stress management in the emergency department, *Leadership Manage* 1(8):3-14, 1992.

sion of a debriefing that is held within a few hours of the critical incident. A defusing comprises an introduction, discussion of the incident, and a description of some of the reactions those involved in the incident may experience.[12]

A debriefing is a formal process that generally occurs within 72 hours of the incident. Debriefings are conducted by the CISM team, composed of peer counselors and a mental health professional. The debriefing generally transpires over seven steps summarized in the box.

SUMMARY

Flight nursing practice requires that the nurse be physically and spiritually ready to care for patients in diverse situations. Stress and exposure to critical incident stress are tangible realities in flight nursing practice. Learning how to recognize, avert, and manage stress should decrease the potential devastating effects stress may have. Flight nursing requires commitment not only to our patients and colleagues, but also to ourselves.

REFERENCES

1. Armstrong KR et al: Multiple stressor debriefing and the American Red Cross: the East Bay fire experience, *Social Work* 40(1):83-90, 1995.
2. Baldwin D: Personal communication, 1995.
3. Bell N: Critical incident stress debriefing, *Emergency* 23(9): 30-35, 58, 1991.
4. Bell N: Exorcizing stress, *Emergency* 23(9):36-39, 57, 1991.
5. Berry S: *I am not an ambulance driver.*, Woodland Park, Colorado.
6. Cydulka R et al: Stress levels in EMS personnel: a longitudinal study with work-schedule modification, *Acad Emerg Med* 1(3):240-246, 1994.
7. Duquette A et al: Factors related to nursing burnout: a review of empirical knowledge, *Issu Mental Health Nurs* 15: 337-358, 1994.
8. Hardin S: Chronic occupational distress in nursing. In McClosky J, Grace H, editors: *Current issues in nursing*, St Louis, 1985, Mosby.
9. Hopkins M: Caring for our own, *Air Med* 1(2):33-37, 1995.
10. Lachman V: Stress and self-care revisited: a literature review, *Holistic Nurs Pract* 10(2):1-12, 1996.
11. McAbee R: Job stress and coping strategies among nurses, *AAOHN* 42(10):483-487, 1994.
12. Mitchell J: Comprehensive traumatic stress management in the emergency department, *Leadership Manage* 1(8):3-14, 1992.
13. O'Rear J: Post traumatic stress disorder: when the rescuer becomes the victim, *JEMS* 17(1):30-35, 1992.
14. Porter B: Learning how to cope with tragedy, *Nursing* 96: 32, 1996.
15. Wooten P: Humor: an antidote for stress, *Holistic Nurs Pract* 10(2);49-56, 1996.

Index

Tables are indicated by *t.*

G

J

K

L

O

ISBN 0-8151-7471-3